The American Psychiatric Press

Textbook of Geriatric Neuropsychiatry

The American Psychiatric Press

Textbook of Geriatric Neuropsychiatry

Editors

C. Edward Coffey, M.D.

Allegheny Neuropsychiatric Institute, Pittsburgh, Pennsylvania

Jeffrey L. Cummings, M.D.

UCLA School of Medicine, Los Angeles, California

Associate Editors

Mark R. Lovell, Ph.D.

Medical College of Pennsylvania, Allegheny Campus, Pittsburgh, Pennsylvania

Godfrey D. Pearlson, M.D.

Johns Hopkins University School of Medicine, Baltimore, Maryland

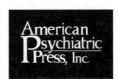

Washington, DC   London, England

Note: The editors and contributors have worked to ensure that all information in this book concerning drug dosages, schedules, and routes of administration is accurate as of the time of publication and consistent with standards set by the U.S. Food and Drug Administration and the general medical community. As medical research and practice advance, however, therapeutic standards may change. For this reason and because human and mechanical errors sometimes occur, we recommend that readers follow the advice of a physician who is directly involved in their care or the care of a member of their family.

Books published by the American Psychiatric Press, Inc., represent the views and opinions of the individual authors and do not necessarily represent the policies and opinions of the Press or the American Psychiatric Association.

American Psychiatric Press, Inc.
1400 K Street, N.W., Washington, DC   20005

Library of Congress Cataloging-in-Publication Data

The American Psychiatric Press textbook of geriatric neuropsychiatry /
    edited by C. Edward Coffey, Jeffrey L. Cummings. — 1st ed.
        p.   cm.
    Includes bibliographical references and index.
    ISBN 0-88048-391-1 (alk. paper)
    1. Geriatric neuropsychiatry.   I. Coffey, C. Edward., 1952–   .
II. Cummings, Jeffrey L., 1948–   .   III. Title: Textbook of
    geriatric neuropsychiatry.
    [DNLM: 1. Geriatric Psychiatry.   2. Mental Disorders—in old age.
3. Neuropsychology—in old age.   WT 150 A5123 1994]
RC451.4.A5A52   1994
618.97′68—dc20
DNLM/DLC
for Library of Congress   93-46298
                                                                      CIP

British Library Cataloguing in Publication Data

A CIP record is available from the British Library.

Contents

Contributors ix

Foreword xiii
     Gene D. Cohen, M.D., Ph.D.

Preface xv

Section I
Introduction to Geriatric Neuropsychiatry
Jeffrey L. Cummings, M.D., and C. Edward Coffey, M.D., Section Editors

1. Geriatric Neuropsychiatry 3
    Jeffrey L. Cummings, M.D.
    C. Edward Coffey, M.D.

2. Epidemiology of Aging 17
    Roberta Malmgren, Ph.D.

3. Neurobiology of Aging 35
    Richard E. Powers, M.D.

4. Neurobiological Basis of Behavior 71
    Jeffrey L. Cummings, M.D.
    C. Edward Coffey, M.D.

Section II
Neuropsychiatric Assessment of the Elderly
Mark R. Lovell, Ph.D., Section Editor

5. Neuropsychiatric Assessment 99
    Raymond Faber, M.D.

6. Mental Status Examination 111
    David L. Sultzer, M.D.

7. Neuropsychological Assessment 129
    Mark R. Lovell, Ph.D.
    Paul D. Nussbaum, Ph.D.

8. Age-Associated Memory Impairment 145
    Graham Ratcliff, D.Phil.
    Judith Saxton, Ph.D.

9. Anatomic Imaging of the Aging Human Brain: Computed Tomography and
    Magnetic Resonance Imaging 159
        C. Edward Coffey, M.D.

10. Functional Neuroimaging: Positron-Emission Tomography in the Study of
    Cerebral Blood Flow and Glucose Utilization in Human Subjects at Different Ages 195
    Pietro Pietrini, M.D.
    Stanley I. Rapoport, M.D.

11. Quantitative Electroencephalography: Neurophysiological Alterations in
    Normal Aging and Geriatric Neuropsychiatric Disorders 215
        Andrew Leuchter, M.D.
        Daniel Holschneider, M.D.

Section III
Neuropsychiatric Aspects of Psychiatric Disorders in the Elderly
Godfrey D. Pearlson, M.D., Section Editor

12. Mood Disorders 243
        Marsden H. McGuire, M.D.
        Peter V. Rabins, M.D., M.P.H.

13. Late-Life–Onset Psychoses 261
        Godfrey D. Pearlson, M.D.
        Richard G. Petty, M.D.

14. Anxiety Disorders 279
        Javaid I. Sheikh, M.D.

15. Substance Abuse 297
        Roland M. Atkinson, M.D.
        Linda Ganzini, M.D.

16. Sleep Disorders in Late Life: A Biopsychosocial Model for Understanding
    Pathogenesis and Intervention 323
        Charles F. Reynolds III, M.D.
        Mary Amanda Dew, Ph.D.
        Timothy H. Monk, Ph.D.
        Carolyn C. Hoch, Ph.D.

17. Pain 333
        James M. Schuster, M.D., M.B.A.
        Kenneth L. Goetz, M.D.

18. Delirium 351
        Larry Tune, M.D.
        Christopher Ross, M.D., Ph.D.

Section IV
Neuropsychiatric Aspects of Neurological Disease in the Elderly
Jeffrey L. Cummings, M.D., Section Editor

19. Nondegenerative Dementing Disorders 369
    William E. Reichman, M.D.

20. Alzheimer's Disease and Frontal Lobe Dementias 389
    Bruce L. Miller, M.D.
    Linda Chang, M.D.
    Grace Oropilla, M.D.
    Ismael Mena, M.D.

21. Hyperkinetic Movement Disorders 405
    Joanne M. Wojcieszek, M.D.
    Anthony E. Lang, M.D, F.R.C.P.

22. Parkinson's Disease and Parkinsonism 433
    William C. Koller, M.D., Ph.D.
    Bernard B. Megaffin, M.D.

23. Neuropsychiatric Aspects of Stroke 457
    Sergio E. Starkstein, M.D., Ph.D.
    Robert G. Robinson, M.D.

24. Traumatic Brain Injury 479
    Robert B. Fields, Ph.D.
    C. Edward Coffey, M.D.

25. Neuropsychiatric Aspects of Epilepsy 509
    Mario F. Mendez, M.D., Ph.D.

26. Neuropsychiatric Aspects of Neoplastic, Demyelinating, Infectious, and
    Inflammatory Brain Disorders 523
    Douglas W. Scharre, M.D.

27. Neuropsychiatric Aspects of Medical Therapies 549
    Harry McConnell, M.D., F.R.C.P.C.
    James Duffy, M.D.

Section V
Principles of Neuropsychiatric Treatment of the Elderly
C. Edward Coffey, M.D., Section Editor

28. Pharmacological and Neuroendocrine Probes in Neuropsychiatric Illness 577
    Marc Cantillon, M.D.
    Susan E. Molchan, M.D.
    John Little, M.D.
    Trey Sunderland, M.D.

29. Geriatric Neuropsychopharmacology 595
    Steven L. Dubovsky, M.D.

30. Electroconvulsive Therapy in Geriatric Neuropsychiatry 633
    John T. Pritchett, M.D.
    Charles H. Kellner, M.D.
    C. Edward Coffey, M.D.

31. Psychosocial Therapies 661
    Linda Teri, Ph.D.
    Susan M. McCurry, Ph.D.

32. Neuropsychiatry in Nursing Homes 683
    Barry W. Rovner, M.D.
    Ira R. Katz, M.D.

Index 695

Contributors

Roland M. Atkinson, M.D.
Professor of Psychiatry, School of Medicine, Oregon Health Sciences University, and Chief, Psychiatry Service, Portland Veterans Affairs Medical Center, Portland, Oregon

Marc Cantillon, M.D.
Assistant Professor of Psychiatry, Georgetown University; Senior Clinical Investigator, National Institute of Mental Health, Bethesda, Maryland

Linda Chang, M.D.
Assistant Professor of Neurology, Department of Neurology, Harbor-UCLA Medical Center, Torrance, California

C. Edward Coffey, M.D.
Professor of Psychiatry (Neuropsychiatry) and Medicine (Neurology), Director, Division of Neuropsychiatry, Medical College of Pennsylvania, Allegheny Campus, and Clinical Director, Allegheny Neuropsychiatric Institute, Oakdale, Pennsylvania

Gene D. Cohen, M.D., Ph.D.
Deputy Director, National Institute on Aging, Washington, DC

Jeffrey L. Cummings, M.D.
Professor of Neurology and Psychiatry & Biobehavioral Sciences and Director, UCLA Alzheimer's Disease Center, University of California, Los Angeles, School of Medicine, and Chief, Behavioral Neuroscience Section, Psychiatry Service, West Los Angeles Veterans Affairs Medical Center, Los Angeles, California

Mary Amanda. Dew, Ph.D.
Associate Professor of Psychiatry, Psychology, and Epidemiology, Department of Psychiatry, University of Pittsburgh, School of Medicine, Western Psychiatric Institute and Clinic, Pittsburgh, Pennsylvania

Steven L. Dubovsky, M.D.
Professor of Psychiatry and Medicine, University of Colorado, and Vice Chairman, Department of Psychiatry, University of Colorado, Denver, Colorado

James Duffy, M.D.
Assistant Professor of Psychiatry (Neuropsychiatry), Medical College of Pennsylvania, Allegheny Campus, and Associate Clinical Director, Allegheny Neuropsychiatric Institute, Oakdale, Pennsylvania

Raymond Faber, M.D.
Associate Professor of Psychiatry and Medicine, University of Texas Health Sciences at San Antonio, and Chief, Neuropsychiatry Program, Audie L. Murphy Memorial Veterans Affairs Hospital, San Antonio, Texas

Robert B. Fields, Ph.D.
Assistant Professor of Psychiatry (Psychology), Division of Neuropsychiatry, Medical College of Pennsylvania, Allegheny Campus, Oakdale Pennsylvania

Linda Ganzini, M.D.
Assistant Professor of Psychiatry, School of Medicine, Oregon Health Sciences University, and Director, Geriatric Psychiatry, Portland Veterans Affairs Medical Center, Portland, Oregon

Kenneth L. Goetz, M.D.

Assistant Professor of Psychiatry, Medical College
of Pennsylvania, Allegheny Campus, and
Associate Director, Inpatient Psychiatry,
Allegheny General Hospital, Pittsburgh,
Pennsylvania

Carolyn C. Hoch, Ph.D.

Assistant Professor of Psychiatry, Department of
Psychiatry, University of Pittsburgh, School of
Medicine, Western Psychiatric Institute and
Clinic, Pittsburgh, Pennsylvania

Daniel Holschneider, M.D.

Fellow, UCLA/VAMC Multicampus Geriatric
Psychiatry, Training Program, UCLA School of
Medicine, Los Angeles, California

Ira R. Katz, M.D.

Professor of Psychiatry, University of
Pennsylvania, and Director, Psychiatric Research,
Philadelphia Geriatric Center, Philadelphia,
Pennsylvania

Charles H. Kellner, M.D.

Professor of Psychiatry and Neurology, Director,
ECT Program, Medical University of South
Carolina, Charleston, South Carolina

William C. Koller, M.D., Ph.D.

Professor and Chairman, Department of
Neurology, University of Kansas Medical Center,
Kansas City, Kansas

Anthony E. Lang, M.D., F.R.C.P.

Associate Professor of Neurology, Department of
Neurology, University of Toronto, and Director,
Movement Disorders Clinic, The Toronto
Hospital, Toronto, Ontario, Canada

Andrew Leuchter, M.D.

Assistant Professor of Psychiatry and
Biobehavioral Sciences, UCLA School of
Medicine, and Director, Quantitative
Electroencephalography (QEEG) Laboratory,
UCLA Neuropsychiatric Institute and Hospital,
Los Angeles, California

John Little, M.D.

Senior Staff Fellow, National Institute of Mental
Health; Bethesda, Maryland

Mark R. Lovell, Ph.D.

Assistant Professor of Psychiatry (Psychology),
Medical College of Pennsylvania, Allegheny
Campus, and Director, Section of Psychology and
Neuropsychology, Allegheny General Hospital
and Allegheny Neuropsychiatric Institute,
Pittsburgh, Pennsylvania

Roberta Malmgren, Ph.D.

Adjunct Assistant Professor, Department of
Epidemiology, School of Public Health,
University of California, Los Angeles, California

Harry McConnell, M.D., F.R.C.P.C.

Director, Behavioral Epilepsy Program, and Staff
Neuropsychiatrist, Allegheny Neuropsychiatric
Institute, Oakdale, Pennsylvania

Susan M. McCurry, Ph.D.

Acting Assistant Professor, Department of
Psychiatry and Behavioral Sciences, University of
Washington, Seattle, Washington

Marsden H. McGuire, M.D.

Assistant Professor of Psychiatry, Johns Hopkins
University School of Medicine, Francis Scott Key
Medical Center, Baltimore, Maryland

Bernard B. Megaffin, M.D.

Assistant Professor of Neurology, University of
Kansas Medical Center, Kansas City, Kansas

Ismael Mena, M.D.

Professor of Radiological Science and Director,
Nuclear Medicine, Harbor-UCLA Medical
Center, Torrance, California

Mario F. Mendez, M.D., Ph.D.

Associate Professor of Neurology, University of
California, Los Angeles, School of Medicine, and
Chief, Neurobehavior Unit, Psychiatry Service,
West Los Angeles Veterans Affairs Medical
Center, Los Angeles, California

Bruce L.Miller, M.D.

Associate Professor of Neurology, Department of Neurology, Harbor-UCLA Medical Center, Torrance, California

Susan E. Molchan, M.D.

Senior Clinical Investigator, National Institute of Mental Health, Bethesda, Maryland

Timothy H. Monk, Ph.D.

Associate Professor of Psychiatry, Department of Psychiatry, University of Pittsburgh, School of Medicine, Western Psychiatric Institute and Clinic, Pittsburgh, Pennsylvania

Paul D. Nussbaum, Ph.D.

Assistant Professor of Psychiatry (Psychology), Medical College of Pennsylvania, Allegheny Campus, and Neuropsychologist, Allegheny Neuropsychiatric Institute, Oakdale, Pennsylvania

Grace Oropilla, M.D.

Research Associate, Department of Neurology, Harbor-UCLA Medical Center, Torrance, California

Godfrey D. Pearlson, M.D.

Professor of Psychiatry and Behavioral Science and Director, Division of Psychiatric Neuro-Imaging, Johns Hopkins University School of Medicine, Baltimore, Maryland

Richard G. Petty, M.D.

Senior Registrar, Institute of Psychiatry, De Crespigny Park, London, United Kingdom

Pietro Pietrini, M.D.

Senior Staff Fellow, Laboratory of Neurosciences, National Institute on Aging, National Institutes of Health, Bethesda, Maryland

Richard E. Powers, M.D.

Associate Professor of Pathology, University of Alabama (Birmingham), and Director, Bureau of Geriatric Psychiatry, Alabama Department of Mental Health and Mental Retardation, Birmingham, Alabama

John T. Pritchett, M.D.

Fellow in ECT, Medical University of South Carolina, Charleston, South Carolina

Peter V. Rabins, M.D., M.P.H.

Professor of Psychiatry and Behavioral Science, Johns Hopkins University School of Medicine, Baltimore, Maryland

Stanley I. Rapoport, M.D.

Chief of Laboratory of Neurosciences, National Institute on Aging, National Institutes of Health, Bethesda, Maryland

Graham Ratcliff, D. Phil.

Adjunct Assistant Professor of Psychiatry and Neurology, University of Pittsburgh, and Director of Neurobehavioral Services, Harmarville Rehabilitation Hospital, Pittsburgh, Pennsylvania

William E. Reichman, M.D.

Assistant Professor of Psychiatry, University of Medicine and Dentistry of New Jersey, Community Mental Health Center of Piscataway, Piscataway, New Jersey

Charles F. Reynolds III, M.D.

Professor of Psychiatry and Neurology and Director, Sleep and Chronobiology Center, Western Psychiatric Institute and Clinics, University of Pittsburgh, Pittsburgh, Pennsylvania

Robert G. Robinson, M.D.

Professor and Chairman, Department of Psychiatry, University of Iowa College of Medicine, Iowa City, Iowa

Christopher Ross, M.D., Ph.D.

Associate Professor, Division of Genetics, Departments of Psychiatry and Neuroscience, and Program in Molecular and Cellular Medicine, Johns Hopkins University School of Medicine, Baltimore, Maryland

Barry W. Rovner, M.D.
Associate Professor of Psychiatry and Human Behavior and Director, Division of Geriatric Psychatiry, Jefferson Medical College, and Medical Director, Wills/Jefferson Geriatric Psychiatry Inpatient Unit, Wills Eye Hospital, Philadelphia, Pennsylvania

Judith Saxton, Ph.D.
Assistant Professor of Psychiatry, Univeristy of Pittsburgh, Pittsburgh, Pennsylvania

Douglas W. Scharre, M.D.
Assistant Professor of Neurology, Ohio State University, Columbus, Ohio

James M. Schuster, M.D., M.B.A.
Assistant Professor of Psychiatry, Medical College of Pennsylvania, Allegheny Campus, and Director of Emergency Psychiatry, Allegheny General Hospital, Pittsburgh, Pennsylvania

Javaid I. Sheikh, M.D.
Assistant Professor, Department of Psychiatry and Behavioral Sciences, and Director, Geriatric Psychiatry Program, Stanford University School of Medicine, Stanford, California

Sergio E. Starkstein, M.D., Ph.D.
Director, Department of Behavioral Neurology, Raúl Carrea Institute of Neurological Research, Buenos Aires, Argentina

David L. Sultzer, M.D.
Assistant Clinical Professor, Department of Psychiatry and Biobehavioral Sciences, UCLA School of Medicine, and Psychiatrist, Behavioral Neuroscience Section, West Los Angeles Veterans Administration Medical Center, Los Angeles, California

Trey Sunderland, M.D.
Chief, Section on Geriatric Psychiatry, National Institute of Mental Health, Bethesda, Maryland

Linda Teri, Ph.D.
Professor, Department of Psychiatry and Behavioral Sciences, University of Washington, and Director, Geriatric Family Service Clinic, Seattle, Washington

Larry Tune, M.D.
Professor, Department of Psychiatry and Behavioral Sciences, and Chief, Division of Geriatric Psychiatry, Wesley Woods Geriatric Center, Emory University, Atlanta, Georgia

Joanne M. Wojcieszek, M.D.
Instructor in Neurology, Department of Neurology, University of Rochester Medical Center, Rochester, New York

Foreword

The American Psychiatric Press Textbook of Geriatric Neuropsychiatry, edited by Coffey and Cummings, represents another important contribution to the scientific literature in the field of aging and reflects the increasingly dynamic and rich interplay between geriatrics and related fields. It also illustrates the increasing magnification under which age-related problems are being placed and the concomitant growth in understanding about these problems.

As Coffey and Cummings point out in the Chapter 1, "Geriatric neuropsychiatry has a wide interface with geriatric psychiatry, and geriatric neuropsychiatry can be regarded as a subdiscipline of geriatric psychiatry, as well as of neuropsychiatry." Whenever questions can be raised or looked at from a different vantage point, chances increase that new insights will be gained about them. Such are the contributions of many subdisciplines: in this case, a neuropsychiatric perspective on aging with its emphasis on brain-behavior relationships. The perspectives and information in this book add to our road map for raising research questions and defining clinical approaches to improve health care for older adults.

Twenty years ago, our clinical road map in geriatrics was analogous to having a map of the United States that provided only the outlines of the states. With the growth of geriatrics in the realms of research, training, services, and public policy, that road map began to become more sophisticated. Interstate highways were added that started to connect related areas of the field as a whole. Then, gradually, other roads were added within the given states (disciplines), followed by other roads connecting towns (subdisciplines) within the states. Today we have a rich network of increasingly well-constructed roadways with increasingly well-defined junctions speeding the course to new discoveries and applications.

It is the mind that most defines our species. And the fate of the mind in later life has emerged as the greatest health concern among older adults. This concern is completely consistent with the fact that the greatest risk factors driving the need for long-term care involve problems that cause cognitive impairment and result in the loss of ability to function independently. Alzheimer's disease (which affects approximately two-thirds of nursing home residents) highlights this situation, bringing about the triple hardship of high personal suffering, family burden, and societal costs. Hence, our best chance of reducing risk factors that influence the need for long-term care is through maximizing the application of present knowledge and generating new research breakthroughs in the field of aging. The questions and answers offered by a neuropsychiatric approach to these problems are many and important and are well developed in the chapters that follow.

Gene D. Cohen, M.D., Ph.D.

Preface

Geriatric psychiatry is an emerging clinical discipline devoted to the diagnosis and treatment of psychiatric or behavior disorders in aging patients with disturbances of brain structure or function. Such disturbances are particularly common in older individuals, and the continued expansion of the elderly segment of our population has recently resulted in considerable interest in the study of neuropsychiatric illness associated with normal and "abnormal" brain aging. *The American Psychiatric Press Textbook of Geriatric Neuropsychiatry* bridges the fields of geriatric neurology and geriatric psychiatry and emphasizes the relationships that exist between neuropsychiatric illness and aging of the nervous system. The book is intended for health care professionals—psychiatrists, neurologists, psychologists, geriatricians, and other clinicians—who desire to understand and manage disturbed behavior in elderly patients through a comprehensive approach based on a thorough knowledge of contemporary neuroscience. *The American Psychiatric Press Textbook of Geriatric Neuropsychiatry* endeavors to establish a link between the neurobiology of major psychiatric illness and the neurobiology of brain disorders that cause disturbed behavior in elderly individuals, and in so doing stimulate consideration of fundamental brain-behavior relationships.

The *Textbook* is organized into five sections, each edited by one or more of the book's editors or associate editors. The section editors have assembled an outstanding collection of respected neuropsychiatrists and neuroscientists, who in turn have endeavored to produce chapters that impart clinically relevant information within the context of the very latest in neuroscience research.

Section I begins with an overview of the emerging clinical specialty of geriatric neuropsychiatry, followed by the demography of aging and the neurobiology of brain aging. The final chapter in this section provides an integrative model linking neurobiology with behavior and thus sets the stage for the subsequent sections in the book.

Section II, Neuropsychiatric Assessment of the Elderly, comprises three practical chapters on clinical and neuropsychological examination of the elderly, a chapter on memory changes in senescence, and three chapters on the role of advanced brain imaging technologies (magnetic resonance imaging, positron-emission tomography, and computerized topographic electroencephalography) in the evaluation of the aging patient. This section accomplishes the essential and fundamental task of defining the acceptable limits of "normal aging" as assessed at the bedside and in the neuroscience laboratory.

Sections III and IV provide the clinical core of the book and focus on the neuropsychiatric aspects of psychiatric and neurological disorders, respectively, in the elderly. The comprehensive chapters in these sections highlight the influence of the aging nervous system on the pathophysiology, neuropsychiatric manifestations, clinical course, and prognosis of psychiatric and neurological illness in elderly patients.

Section V emphasizes the special considerations that are essential for safe and effective treatment of neuropsychiatric disorders in the elderly. This final section features up-to-date chapters on neurobiological probes of treatment response, pharmacotherapy, electroconvulsive therapy, psychosocial and family therapies, and extended care for the elderly population. The discussions and recommendations for treatment are anchored as much as possible in a firm foundation of clinical science research.

We would like to acknowledge the associate editors, Mark R. Lovell, Ph.D., and Godfrey Pearlson, M.D., for the incredible effort they devoted to this volume. We would also like to thank each of the authors for their contribution. Writing a chapter takes thought, time, and energy, all of which must be redirected from other pressing projects. We are grateful that the associate editors and chapter authors shared our vision and made this textbook a priority. Carol Nadelson, M.D., Claire Reinburg, Edward Winkleman, and Joanie Lefkowitz of American Psychiatric Press, Inc., provided much valuable guidance and were always available to answer questions.

We also acknowledge Trevor R. P. Price, M.D., Chairman of Psychiatry, Medical College of Pennsylvania, Allegheny Campus, and the Board of Directors of Allegheny Neuropsychiatric Institute, who understand and value the role of research in the provision of quality medical care to patients with neuropsychiatric illness. Further, we acknowledge Robert Collins, M.D., Chair of Neurology, and Gary Tischler, M.D., Chair of Psychiatry and Biobehavioral Sciences at UCLA, for creating an environment that encourages the growth of neuropsychiatry. The consistent support of D. Frank Benson, M.D., a pioneer in exploring the psychiatric manifestations of neurological disease, is also gratefully acknowledged. We thank Barbara Amadio and Regina Klein for the administrative assistance they provided. Finally, this project could not have come to fruition without the tremendous support offered by our wives and children.

C. Edward Coffey, M.D.
Jeffrey L. Cummings, M.D.

SECTION

I

Introduction to Geriatric Neuropsychiatry

Section Editors
Jeffrey L. Cummings, M.D., and C. Edward Coffey, M.D.

chapter 1
Geriatric Neuropsychiatry

chapter 2
Epidemiology of Aging

chapter 3
Neurobiology of Aging

chapter 4
Neurobiological Basis of Behavior

1

Geriatric Neuropsychiatry

Jeffrey L. Cummings, M.D.
C. Edward Coffey, M.D.

Grow old along with me!
The best is yet to be,
The last of life, for which the first was made.

Robert Browning
Rabbi Ben Ezra

Introduction

Neuropsychiatry is the discipline devoted to understanding the neurobiological basis of human behavior. Neuropsychiatry has patient care, research, and educational dimensions emphasizing, respectively, the application, expansion, and dissemination of neuropsychiatric information. The growth of neuropsychiatry has been enhanced by advances in neuroscience, neuroimaging, neuropsychopharmacology, geriatrics, and psychiatry. *Geriatric neuropsychiatry* represents the application of neuropsychiatry to older individuals. Geriatric neuropsychiatry is an integrative discipline bridging the fields of psychiatry, neurology, neuroscience, and geriatrics. The emergence of geriatric neuropsychiatry is a response to the increasing size of the elderly population and the high prevalence of brain diseases and behavioral disorders among them. Geriatric neuropsychiatry is committed to the principle that improved understanding of brain-behavior relationships can lead to a higher quality of life for older individuals through minimization of excess disability, early recognition of diseases, and improved therapeutic interventions in behavioral disturbances.

The *Textbook of Geriatric Neuropsychiatry* is the first volume devoted exclusively to the discipline of geriatric neuropsychiatry. It is intended to serve as a guide to the practice and further development of this field. In this introductory chapter, we review the major issues in geriatric neuropsychiatry. Our purpose is to provide a neurobiological perspective on behavioral disturbances in elderly individuals, to create a context for the remaining chapters of this book, and to define and describe geriatric neuropsychiatry. In this chapter, we

also review important aspects of training and research in geriatric neuropsychiatry.

Geriatric Neuropsychiatry as a Discipline

Geriatric Neuropsychiatry

Most subspecialization results from concentration on a small part of the parent discipline. With the explosion of information relevant to behavioral alterations in the elderly, however, geriatric neuropsychiatry arises from a different imperative. Geriatric neuropsychiatry is an integrative specialty that draws from a diversity of fields (psychiatry, neuropsychiatry, neurology, neuroscience, neuroimaging, neuropsychopharmacology, neuropsychology, gerontology, molecular biology, genetics, epidemiology, and psychodynamics) to improve the care of behaviorally impaired elderly individuals and to stimulate research in this critical area (Figure 1–1).

The practice of geriatric neuropsychiatry depends on distinguishing normal age-related changes from those of disease and disordered brain function. Slowing of cognition, diminished access to specific bits of memory (e.g., names), and reduced cognitive flexibility may occur in the course of normal aging (Van Gorp and Mahler 1990). These changes must be differentiated from the effects of dementia, depression, and systemic illness. Geriatric neuropsychiatry provides expertise in this area.

Geriatric Neuropsychiatry and Neuropsychiatry

Neuropsychiatry is an old discipline that has been resurrected recently to assume a prominent place in con-

Supported by Department of Veterans Affairs and a National Institute on Aging Alzheimer's Disease Core Center Grant AG 10123 (to JLC), and by Allegheny Singer Research Institute (to CEC).

temporary psychiatry. There is no consensus definition of *neuropsychiatry*. Lishman (1992) suggested that it is that aspect of psychiatry that seeks to advance understanding of clinical problems through increased knowledge of brain structure and function. Yudofsky and Hales (1989a, 1989b) defined *neuropsychiatry* as the discipline concerned with the assessment and treatment of patients with psychiatric illnesses or symptoms associated with brain abnormalities. Trimble (1993) emphasized that neuropsychiatry attempts to understand the effects of central nervous system structural or functional change on behavior, recognizing the essentially dynamic and individualistic nature of behavioral dispositions.

Neuropsychiatry is an umbrella discipline under which geriatric neuropsychiatry is subsumed. Geriatric neuropsychiatry, however, integrates information from geriatrics, gerontology, and aging research not specifically relevant to all areas of the broader discipline of neuropsychiatry.

Geriatric Neuropsychiatry and Geriatric Psychiatry

Geriatric neuropsychiatry has a wide interface with geriatric psychiatry and can be regarded as a subdiscipline of geriatric psychiatry, as well as of neuropsychiatry. Both geriatric psychiatry and geriatric

Psychiatry ——→	Geriatric psychiatry	**N**
Psychiatry ——→	Neuropsychiatry	**e**
Neurology ——→	Geriatric neurology	**u**
Neurology ——→	Behavioral neurology	**G r**
Medicine ——→	Geriatrics	**e o**
Psychology ——→	Neuropsychology	**r p**
Psychology ——→	Geriatric psychology	**i s**
Pharmacology ——→	Neuropsycho- pharmacology	**a y t c**
Radiolgy ——→	Neuroimaging	**r h**
Basic science ——→	Neuroscience	**i a**
Sociology ——→	Gerontology	**c t r y**

Figure 1–1. Geriatric neuropsychiatry is an integrative discipline importing information from a number of specialties relevant to behavioral alterations in elderly individuals.

neuropsychiatry are concerned with care, education, and research related to behavioral changes in elderly individuals. The principle difference between the two is one of emphasis. Geriatric neuropsychiatry emphasizes its relationship to the neurosciences, the application of pharmacological treatments, and the assessment and management of psychiatric aspects of neurological diseases in elderly patients. Geriatric neuropsychiatry is committed to the proposition that the cure of neuropsychiatric disorders of elderly patients, improved management of behavioral disturbances, and amelioration of adverse age-related changes in brain function are linked to advances in neuroscience, as well as to progress in psychology, sociology, and related disciplines. While accepting the incontestable importance of social, cultural, and psychological aspects of aging and diseases of the elderly population, geriatric neuropsychiatry emphasizes importing and developing neuroscience information with the goal of better understanding and treatment.

Geriatric Neuropsychiatry and Behavioral Neurology

There are no definitional boundaries between neuropsychiatry and behavioral neurology or between geriatric neuropsychiatry and behavioral neurology. Traditionally, behavioral neurology has been devoted to the study of "deficit disorders" such as aphasia, amnesia, agnosia, and apraxia, whereas neuropsychiatry has been concerned with the diagnosis and management of syndromes with "productive symptoms" such as hallucinations, delusions, and mood changes. In addition, behavioral neurologists have usually been trained in neurology, whereas neuropsychiatrists have usually had a background in psychiatry. Neither discipline, however, completely prepares a clinician for the broad range of behavioral disorders associated with acquired and idiopathic brain dysfunction. Both disciplines produce behavioral neuroscientists who use similar concepts to relate abnormal behavior to brain dysfunction. Furthermore, individual patients often manifest both deficit and productive disorders, making it imperative that clinicians have knowledge of both neuropsychiatry and behavioral neurology. This is particularly important in geriatric neuropsychiatry where the prevalence of acquired brain disease as a cause of altered behavior is high.

A corollary of the absence of boundaries between behavioral neurology and neuropsychiatry is the transcendence of traditional restrictive definitions of individual diseases as "neurological" or "psychiatric." Alzheimer's disease and Parkinson's disease are examples of disorders traditionally considered as "neurological," whereas depression and obsessive-compulsive disorder have been thought of as "psychiatric." Neither of these assumptions proves to be true from the perspective of geriatric neuropsychiatry. Alzheimer's disease and Parkinson's disease both have major behavioral manifestations, whereas depression and obsessive-compulsive disorder are increasingly well understood as brain disorders. It is ever more evident that designating disorders as "neurological" or "psychiatric"—although convenient for some purposes—is arbitrary and may be misleading. These designations are clinically unhelpful and may hinder the evolution of a behavioral neuroscience commensurate with optimum patient care.

Geriatric Neuropsychiatry: Clinical Training

There is a gross lack of availability of individuals with expertise in geriatric neuropsychiatry and a dearth of training programs to provide experience in this area. This reflects the widespread lack of training in clinical care and research regarding both behavioral neuroscience and the care of elderly patients. Investigators have found that only 16 of 122 United States neurology residencies provide formal research training (Griggs et al. 1987), and only 12% of psychiatric faculty members have postgraduate research training (Burke et al. 1986). Geriatric psychiatry and geriatric

medicine are decidedly undermanned (Rowe 1987; Small et al. 1988). Development of a cadre of individuals with expertise in the assessment and management of geriatric neuropsychiatric abnormalities is an essential response to the expanding elderly population.

Converging Information in Geriatric Neuropsychiatry

There are two principal dimensions in geriatric neuropsychiatry: the psychiatric manifestations of neurological disorders and the neurobiological basis of psychiatric illnesses. One exciting aspect of contemporary neuropsychiatry is the convergence of conclusions emanating from these two avenues of research (Table 1–1). For example, Robinson and Starkstein (1990) have demonstrated that depression is most common among stroke patients when the lesion involves the anterior structures of the left hemisphere, whereas studies of idiopathic depression have found evidence of reduced frontal lobe volume (Coffey et al. 1993) and metabolism (Baxter et al. 1985, 1989). Recent neuropathological investigations in schizophrenia have revealed abnormalities in the cellular architectonics in the temporal lobe (Altshuler et al. 1987), and studies of neurological disease with psychosis demonstrated that the temporal lobe is a common site of pathological changes (Cummings 1992b).

Similarly, in studies of idiopathic obsessive-compulsive disorders, Baxter et al. 1987 found increased metabolism in the orbitofrontal cortex, and Cummings (1993) observed that obsessions and com-

Table 1–1. Convergent results of investigations of the psychiatric complications of neurological disorders and the neurobiological basis of psychiatric illness

Neuropsychiatric abnormality	Neurological disorder	Psychiatric illness
Depression	Poststroke depression after left frontal stroke	Reduced metabolism in the frontal lobes in idiopathic depression with PET; reduced frontal lobe volume in depression with MRI
Psychosis	Increased prevalence in temporal lobe disorders	Histologic changes in the temporal lobes in schizophrenia
Obsessive-compulsive disorder (OCD)	Increased prevalence of OCD in diseases affecting frontal-subcortical circuits originating in orbitofrontal cortex	Increased glucose metabolism in orbitofrontal cortex in idiopathic OCD
Anxiety	Occurs with lesions of the temporal cortex	Increased blood flow in the temporal lobes during episodes of anxiety

Note. PET = positron-emission tomography; MRI = magnetic resonance imaging.

pulsions occur in neurological disease when there is involvement of structures participating in the frontal-subcortical circuit originating in orbitofrontal cortical regions. Preliminary studies with positron-emission tomography (PET) have suggested altered regional metabolic activity in anxiety disorders (Reiman et al. 1989; Wu et al. 1991), and anxiety symptoms have been associated with structural lesions of related cortical areas in neurological diseases (Drubach and Kelly 1989). The convergence of information from these two approaches to neuropsychiatry has many implications. It suggests that when clinical neuropsychiatric symptoms are similar, even in seemingly different disorders, there may be involvement of the same underlying neuroanatomic structures and common pathobiological mechanisms may be present. These observations also support the use of the same therapeutic agents in patients with diverse underlying diseases, but similar neuropsychiatric symptoms. In addition, many idiopathic psychiatric illnesses appear to be inherited, and the observations relating symptoms to regional brain dysfunction suggest which brain areas may be most affected by the abnormal gene products.

The emergence of these convergent data in neuropsychiatric research justifies the working assumption of geriatric neuropsychiatry that the relationship between brain dysfunction and behavioral disturbances is rule governed, that the axioms relating structure and function are discoverable, and that the rules will apply regardless of the etiology of the underlying disorder.

Aging, the Brain, and Geriatric Neuropsychiatry

The brain undergoes various neurochemical, structural, and neurophysiological alterations in the course of normal aging (Creasey and Rapoport 1985; see also Chapter 3). Grossly, there is a small decrease in brain weight in the course of normal aging with widening of cerebral cortical sulci and enlargement of the lateral ventricles.

Microscopically, there is neuronal loss in specific cortical and subcortical structures (Brody 1982; Terry et al. 1987). In addition, lipofuscin, granulovacuolar changes, neuritic plaques, and neurofibrillary tangles also accumulate in the course of aging, and there is a progressive shrinkage of the dendritic domain of some cortical and subcortical neurons (Brody 1982).

Neurochemical changes also accompany aging. Decreased activity of catecholamine synthesis enzymes and increased activity of monoamine oxidase (an enzyme involved in catecholamine catabolism) have been documented (Bowen and Davison 1982; Van Gorp and Mahler 1990). These biochemical changes may underlie the psychomotor retardation of elderly individuals, as well as the mild parkinsonian habitus associated with aging, and they may contribute to the occurrence of depression in elderly people (Veith and Raskind 1988). Neurochemical alterations may also have a role in the age-associated memory impairment observed in elderly individuals.

The underlying mechanisms of aging remain mysterious, but strides are being made in understanding some of the processes that contribute to age-related changes in function. Oxidative metabolism catalyzed by oxygen-free radicals damages enzymes, and this in turn leads to a reduced synthetic ability and compromise of the aged organism's ability to respond to changing biological contingencies (Stadtman 1992). Trophic factors may be responsible for maintaining cellular connectivity, and changes in tropism with aging may contribute to some age-related brain alterations (Creasey and Rapoport 1985). Finally, some cells have genetically determined lifespans, whereas other cell populations manifest few, if any, changes in the course of aging (Finch 1990). Deciphering these molecular mechanisms responsible for programmed aging is critical to a comprehensive understanding of the neurobiology of aging.

The brain is continuously changing from its fetal developmental period through senescence. The changes associated with aging are not global, and they affect specific cellular populations, structures, and transmitters more than they do others. The neurobiological changes of aging, as well as the differential involvement of functional systems, may influence the types of neuropsychiatric disorders to which elderly people are vulnerable.

Aging, Brain Diseases, and Geriatric Neuropsychiatry

The emergence and growth of geriatric neuropsychiatry are driven by four circumstances: 1) the growth of the size of the elderly population, 2) the increased prevalence of brain diseases among the elderly, 3) the recognition that behavioral disturbances are often manifestations of brain dysfunction, and 4) a high frequency of psychiatric disorders among elderly people.

Demography of Aging

People over age 65 comprised only 4% of the United States population in 1900; this population will increase to 13% by the year 2000 and to 22% by 2030 (Department of Health and Human Services 1990; see also Chapter 2). The growth of the old-old population is proceeding at a disproportionately rapid pace. Those over age 80 numbered 6 million in 1985 and comprised 22% of the elderly population; by 2005, 31% of elderly Americans will be over age 80 (Torrey et al. 1987). In 1980, there were approximately 15,000 centenarians (people 100 years old or older) in the United States; this number increased to 25,000 by 1986 and is projected to reach 100,000 by the year 2000 (Spencer et al. 1987).

Aging and the diseases of elderly people present a global challenge (Torrey et al. 1987). The world's elderly population is growing at a rate of 2.4% per year, faster than the rest of the population. In 1985, there were 290 million individuals over age 65 in the world; this number will rise to 410 million by the year 2000. Twenty-three countries had two million or more elderly individuals in 1985; 50 countries will have this number by 2025. The growth of the world's elderly population will occur disproportionately in the countries least able to provide services; by the year 2025, 69% of the world's elderly people will live in developing countries (Torrey et al. 1987).

Neurological Diseases With Behavioral Manifestations Among the Elderly

The three neurological conditions most responsible for neuropsychiatric morbidity in elderly individuals are 1) Alzheimer's disease and other dementing disorders, 2) Parkinson's disease, and 3) stroke. The prevalence of dementia increases dramatically with age. A recent demographic study of dementia in Stockholm, Sweden (Fratiglioni et al. 1991), found that 5.7% of individuals 75–79 years old had mental status changes indicative of dementia and 9.6% of those 80–84 had dementia; the proportion rose to 20.4% in those 85–89 and to 32% in those over age 90. Evans et al. (1989) found the rate of Alzheimer's disease among the elderly in a United States community to be 3% in those 65–74 years old, 18.7% in those 75–84, and 47.2% in those over age 84. Parkinson's disease also exhibits an age-related prevalence. The reported frequency varies among studies, but a representative investigation

(D'Alessandro et al. 1987) revealed a prevalence of 0.8% among people 55–59 years old, 3.8% in those 60–64, 5.7% in those 65–69, 12.4% in those 70–74, 19.5% in those 75–79, and 9.5% in those 80–84 years old. The prevalence of stroke and vascular dementia also increases with age. The prevalence of cerebrovascular disease rises from 2.3% in those 55–64 to 4.2% in those 65–74, 8.1% in those 75–84, and 10% of those over age 85 (National Center for Health Statistics 1986). The cumulative prevalence of neurological disease among the elderly and the chronic nature of many neurological illnesses make brain diseases a major source of morbidity and mortality among elderly individuals.

Neurological diseases of elderly people are often manifested by alterations in behavior. The dementia syndromes are defined by loss of cognitive abilities, and many dementia patients also exhibit delusions, depression, anxiety, agitation, and aggressiveness (Cummings and Benson 1992; Cummings et al. 1987; Merriam et al. 1988; Reisberg et al. 1987; Teri et al. 1988). Dementia occurs in 41% of patients with Parkinson's disease (Mayeux et al. 1992), and 40%–60% of Parkinson's disease patients have depressive disorders (Cummings 1992a). Eighty percent of strokes involve the cerebral hemispheres where they produce neurobehavioral and neuropsychiatric syndromes such as aphasia, amnesia, visuospatial disturbances, depression, or psychosis (Beckson and Cummings 1991; Robinson and Benson 1981). One-fourth of all patients hospitalized with stroke meet criteria for vascular dementia (Hershey et al. 1987). Thus behavioral disturbances are the principal clinical manifestations of many brain diseases of elderly people. Recognition and management of geriatric neuropsychiatric disorders is critical in an aging society.

Psychiatric Illness in the Elderly Population

Psychiatric illness is present in 12.3% of the elderly population (Regier et al. 1988; see also Chapter 2 and Section III). Approximately 5.5% of elderly individuals have anxiety disorders (4.8% phobia, 0.1% panic), 4.9% have severe cognitive impairment, 2.5% have a mood disorder (0.7% major depressive episode; 1.8% dysthymia), 1% manifest alcohol abuse or dependence, 0.8% have obsessive-compulsive disorder, and 0.1% have schizophrenia or a schizophreniform disorder. These figures were derived from a household study (Regier et al. 1988) of individuals in five United States cities using the DSM-III criteria (American Psychiatric Association 1980). In a similar community survey (Myers et al. 1984), the four most common psychiatric disorders in men over age 65 were severe cognitive impairment, phobia, alcohol abuse and dependence, and dysthymia; in women of the same age, the four most frequent diagnoses were phobia, severe cognitive impairment, dysthymia, and major depressive episode.

Thus dementia, alcoholism, anxiety, and mood disorders are the most common psychiatric conditions among elderly people. Each of these diseases has an important neurobiological dimension. Dementia is an overt brain disorder produced by Alzheimer's disease, cerebrovascular disease, or other encephalopathic process (Cummings and Benson 1992). In alcoholic individuals, PET reveals diminished brain glucose metabolism (Volkow et al. 1992), and dysfunction of basal ganglia–limbic circuits is implicated in alcohol craving (Modell et al. 1990). Patients with anxiety disorders have an increased frequency of structural alterations of the right temporal lobe (Fontaine et al. 1990), exhibit regional alterations in metabolism (Reiman et al. 1989; Wu et al. 1991), and evidence functional disturbances involving a variety of neurotransmitter systems (Hoehn-Saric 1982).

Depression occupies a particularly important place in geriatric neuropsychiatry. It is disabling and treatable and may occur for the first time in elderly individuals. If not detected and treated, depression may be fatal; men 65–74 years old have the highest suicide rate of any age group in the United States (Department of Health and Human Services 1990). Imaging studies suggest that depression is associated with alterations in brain structure and function, particularly in elderly people (see Chapters 12 and 23). Reported structural abnormalities include cortical atrophy (especially of the frontal lobes), ventricular enlargement, and subcortical encephalomalacia (Coffey 1991; Coffey et al. 1990, 1993; Nasrallah et al. 1989). These findings may be related to the onset of the mental disorder in late life (Coffey 1991), and they are associated with a poor long-term prognosis (Jacoby et al. 1981). Functional imaging studies reveal evidence of altered regional cerebral blood flow and metabolism in depressive disorders. The frontal lobes are most prominently affected (Baxter et al. 1985, 1989; Sackeim et al. 1990; see also Chapter 12). Although relatively few studies have examined elderly subjects, data suggest that functional brain imaging may be useful in distinguishing the neurodegenerative dementias from the dementia of de-

pression. Together, these observations indicate that alterations of brain structure and function may interact with the aging process to facilitate the emergence of affective disorders in late life.

Late-onset psychoses, although considerably more rare than late-occurring depression or anxiety, may occur. Investigations of patients with late-onset delusional disorders reveal that about half have an identifiable underlying brain disease (Leuchter and Spar 1985; Miller et al. 1992). Thus delusions may be the heralding feature of a neurological disease.

Together these studies indicate that mental disorders are an important aspect of geriatric care, that there is an emerging understanding of the neurobiology of these psychiatric conditions, and that brain abnormalities are associated with many late-onset psychiatric disturbances. Geriatric neuropsychiatry addresses both the neurobiology of idiopathic psychiatric disorders and the psychiatric disturbances associated with neurological condition.

The Cost of Brain Disorders

The annual cost of brain disease has recently been calculated and the yearly expense is staggering (National Foundation for Brain Research 1992). The annual cost (direct and indirect total) in billions of dollars for psychiatric illnesses is $136.1, for neurological disease $103.7, for alcohol abuse $90.1, and for drug abuse $71.2. Together, these diseases cost United States society $401.1 billion annually. Fifteen percent of the average annual income of American workers is devoted to brain diseases. Although the costs of diseases of the elderly were not separately calculated, dementia accounted for the largest share (45%) of the costs of all neurological illnesses, and it is obvious that a substantial share of the funds expended on brain disorders concerns diseases of elderly patients.

Aging, Medical Illness, Drugs, and Geriatric Neuropsychiatry

The rise of geriatric neuropsychiatry is fueled in part by the marked rise in medical illness in the elderly population and the increased frequency of associated behavioral disturbances. Medical disorders become increasingly common among elderly people, medications are more frequently administered, and there are changes in drug metabolism with aging. These alterations create a neurophysiological setting that is conducive to brain dysfunction and behavioral abnormalities (Figure 1–2).

Medical illnesses are common in elderly people, and many of these affect brain function and produce behavioral alterations. Among the 10 most common nonneurological diseases of elderly people are hypertension, ischemic heart disease, diabetes, and arteriosclerosis (Cassel and Brody 1990). These may involve the brain through direct mechanisms such as stroke or through indirect mechanisms including hypoxia and renal failure. Epidemiological studies (Cohen-Cole 1989; Derogatis and Wise 1989) have revealed that approximately 20% of medically ill patients have significant depressive symptoms and 5%–20% experience major depressive episodes; 10%–15% of medically ill patients manifest anxiety disorders. The coexistence of medical and psychiatric illness increases the length of stay of hospitalized patients and is associated with a poorer postdischarge prognosis (Mayou et al. 1991; Saravay et al. 1991). Conversely, about 50% of elderly psychiatric patients have significant medical illnesses. Nearly 60% of these conditions are undiagnosed before psychiatric admission, and in 10%–20% the behavioral changes are directly attributable to the physical pathology (Koranyi 1982).

The high prevalence of medical illness among elderly people results in an increase in the number of medications ingested (see Chapter 29). Elderly people take more prescribed and over-the-counter medications than any other age group. They comprise 12% of the population and take 25%–30% of all prescribed drugs. The average older United States citizen receives 4.5 prescribed medications, and two-thirds also take at least one over-the-counter agent (Beers 1992; Lamy 1985). Forty percent of the elderly individuals who take medications receive prescriptions from more than one physician, and 12% take drugs prescribed for someone else (Lamy 1985). These practices are further complicated by intentional or accidental noncompliance with prescribing instructions. Up to 30% of elderly patients make serious errors in the way they take their medications, and up to 50% default on one or more prescribed agent (Lamy 1985).

Drug metabolism is altered in elderly patients, and the changes may have marked consequences for brain function and the treatment of behavioral abnormalities. There is an increased sensitivity of receptors for most classes of drugs in the course of aging, making lower levels more effective and more likely to induce toxicity (Avorn and Gurwitz 1990). Changes also occur in drug distribution with aging. There is a relative increase in body fat and decrease in muscle; this produces a greater volume of distribution for fat-soluble drugs (e.g., benzodiazepines) and smaller volume of distribution for drugs absorbed primarily in lean body mass (e.g., lithium). There is reduced liver blood flow and impaired oxidative metabolism by hepatic enzymes in the course of normal aging, leading to reduced hepatic clearance of many pharmacological

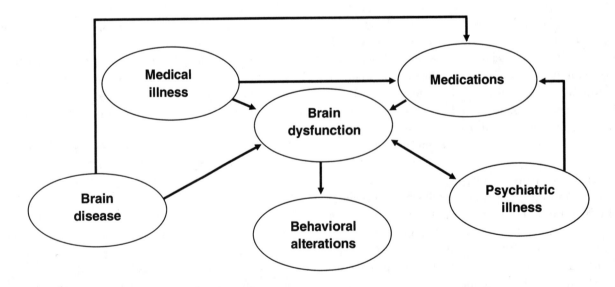

Figure 1–2. Interactions of medical illness, medications, brain disease, and psychiatric disorders to produce brain dysfunction and behavioral changes.

agents. Renal function also declines with age; glomerular filtration rate is reduced by approximately one-third in elderly individuals (Avorn and Gurwitz 1990). These changes all tend to increase the risk of toxicity when medications are administered to elderly patients. Adverse drug reactions account for 12%–17% of all hospital admissions of elderly patients, and 21% of all elderly patients experience adverse side effects while in the hospital (Davison 1985; Lamy 1985).

The higher frequency of medical illness in the elderly population and concomitant need for more drug administration place elderly patients at a substantially increased risk of toxic-metabolic neuropsychiatric disturbances. Delirium, dementia, depression, mania, psychosis, and anxiety have all been observed in patients with brain dysfunction secondary to systemic illnesses and drug toxicity (Cummings 1985; Estroff and Gold 1986).

New Diagnostic Technologies and Advances in Treatment

Neuroimaging

The emergence of new diagnostic technologies has accelerated the development of geriatric neuropsychiatry. Among these, neuroimaging has had the greatest impact. Neuroimaging plays an increasingly large role in the diagnosis, differential diagnosis, and treatment monitoring of behavioral disturbances in the elderly. Structural and functional imaging has provided new insights into brain function, the pathophysiology of brain disorders, and the neurobiology of normal aging.

Imaging brain structure, metabolism, and chemical composition are now possible (Mazziotta and Gilman 1992). In addition, specialized techniques allow visualization of arterial and venous blood flow. Images of brain structure are generated by computed tomography (CT) and magnetic resonance imaging (MRI). These techniques allow visualization of the brain structure and the ventricular system. Tumors, large strokes, subdural hematomas, large demyelinating lesions, arteriovenous malformations, and hydrocephalus are revealed by both techniques. MRI is more sensitive to changes in white matter of the central nervous system and is superior to CT in revealing evidence of ischemic and inflammatory disease.

MRI has been shown recently to have a potential role in predicting adverse responses to therapy. Depressed patients with basal ganglia lesions and increased white matter abnormalities are more likely to exhibit prolonged interictal confusion during electroconvulsive therapy and a higher frequency of antidepressant-induced delirium than are depressed elderly patients with normal MRI results (Coffey 1991; Figiel et al. 1990). Depressed elderly patients with enlarged ventricles and cortical atrophy may have a poorer prognosis for recovery than elderly depressed patients without these structural changes (Jacoby et al. 1981).

Magnetic resonance spectroscopy is a specialized application of magnetic resonance technology that allows the determination of the concentration of specific chemicals in the brain, and new fast imaging techniques using MRI can be used to determine cerebral blood flow. The rapid advances in MRI technology suggest that this tool will be of increasing importance in neuropsychiatry.

Except for the marked caudate nucleus atrophy associated with Huntington's disease, degenerative brain diseases (e.g., Alzheimer's disease and Parkinson's disease) produce no pathognomonic changes that are detectable on conventional structural imaging. In these disorders, structural imaging techniques such as CT and MRI provide little diagnostic information. Moreover, idiopathic neuropsychiatric disorders such as depression, mania, psychosis, and anxiety are not associated with diagnostic structural brain alterations.

Functional brain imaging such as PET and single photon emission computed tomography (SPECT) provide a new approach to these neuropsychiatric disorders. PET may be used to study cerebral glucose metabolism (with radiolabeled glucose), cerebral blood flow (with radiolabeled oxygen), or neurotransmitter function (with radiolabeled receptor ligands) (see Chapter 10). SPECT is typically used to measure cerebral blood flow, but may also be applied to assessment of neurotransmitters. Degenerative diseases and idiopathic neuropsychiatric illnesses may have distinctive alterations on metabolic imaging studies. For example, Alzheimer's disease typically causes reduced metabolism or perfusion in the temporo-parieto-occipital junction region, frontal lobe degenerations cause decreased metabolism or perfusion of the frontal lobes, depression may be associated with diminished frontal lobe metabolism, and obsessive-compulsive disorder has been shown to be associated with increased metabolism of the orbitofrontal cortex (Holcomb et al. 1989).

These investigations demonstrate that there are reliable relationships between behavioral changes and brain metabolism or perfusion. Imaging research is beginning to provide important insights into the pathophysiology of neuropsychiatric disorders.

Advances in Treatment

The value of accurate diagnosis is enhanced when it proceeds in concert with advances in treatment. In this regard, the past decade has seen an unparalleled increase in the availability of medications to treat behavioral disturbances. Antidepressant agents have proliferated and become highly differentiated, with relative selectivity for inhibition of reuptake of norepinephrine or serotonin. A variety of anxiolytics have been discovered, and the clinician can now choose an agent that best fits the patient's needs according to the rapidity of onset, duration of action, and side effects. Conventional neuroleptic agents are gradually giving way to a new generation of antipsychotic drugs that have little affinity for dopamine, subtype 2 (D_2), receptors and therefore produce few acute or chronic extrapyramidal side effects (Baldessarini and Frankenburg 1991). With the evolution of these agents, patients should no longer have to weigh risk of dystonia, parkinsonism, or tardive dyskinesia against control of their psychiatric disorders. The discovery that anticonvulsants such as carbamazepine and sodium valproate have antimanic benefits has improved the treatment of mania, while emphasizing that common neurophysiological processes are shared by some neurological and psychiatric illnesses (Post et al. 1984).

Relevant advances have also been made in the pharmacological treatment of neurological disorders. Most remarkably, selegiline (a monoamine oxidase–B inhibitor) appears to have neuroprotective effects, slowing the progress of Parkinson's disease (Tetrud and Langston 1989). If confirmed, this will represent a revolutionary treatment advance and will be the first success in intervening in a degenerative disease. The action of this agent in neuronal rescue implies that the behavioral aspects of Parkinson's disease such as depression and dementia may also be delayed or ameliorated. Alzheimer's disease has many treatable behavioral complications, but the underlying degenerative process has proven to be more resistant to pharmacological intervention. Nevertheless, modest symptomatic improvement is observed in some patients treated with tacrine, an anticholinesterase inhib-

itor that facilitates central cholinergic function (Farlow et al. 1992), and intensive investigation at the molecular biological level has revealed a systematic cascade of events with individual steps that might be amenable to pharmacological manipulation. Finally, ticlopidine (a potent platelet antiaggregant) has been shown to be more powerful than aspirin in preventing stroke and improving the prognosis for patients with cerebrovascular disease (Gent et al. 1989).

The rapid advances in neuropsychopharmacology provide the clinician with a varied and powerful armamentarium with which to meet the challenges of neuropsychiatric disease in the elderly patient. They also require that the clinician be familiar with the pharmacokinetics, side effects, and drug interactions of each of these new agents. Geriatric neuropsychiatry is the clinical discipline committed to implementation of these advances for the benefit of elderly individuals with behavioral disorders.

Geriatric Neuropsychiatry and Ethical Issues

Ethical issues arise often in geriatric neuropsychiatry. The main challenges concern the ability of individuals to take responsibility for their own actions and the responsibility of society to preserve the rights of elderly citizens. With regard to driving, for example, at what point are the wishes of the patient to maintain independence and mobility in conflict with the safety of other drivers and pedestrians who might be endangered by the patient? At what point do patients relinquish their right to make decisions regarding disposition of property and money; when do they lose their right to decide when they can no longer live at home; when do they need a surrogate decision maker for questions of life support, treatment of infections, and postmortem autopsy? Who should make decisions for the patients when the patients themselves cannot? Should such decisions be based on family beliefs about what the patient would want, advanced directives from the patient, or an assessment of the apparent daily life satisfaction of the individual with dementia (Dresser 1992; Moody 1992; see also Chapter 32)? Is euthanasia a viable societal response to severe dementia? These questions do not have categorical answers; they must be answered individually for each patient, taking into account the needs and abilities of the patient, the family context, and other patient-specific contingencies.

Geriatric neuropsychiatric illnesses strike at the

self and alter the individual's personal identity; whereas a patient may *have* pneumonia, he or she *is* "demented." How does and how should this change in identity affect decision making for the patient? How can the dignity of the patient be preserved when institutional caregivers know only the postdisease person and are unacquainted with the unique biography of the individual under their care? For the individual with dementia, how can extended care become an extended meaningful life?

The great majority of elderly people and many of those in institutions are competent, if physically infirm. How can we best preserve their autonomy, dignity, and quality of life? These ethical dilemmas must be given careful consideration as the elderly population grows, more and more elderly individuals require institutional care, and the resources available to care for them come steadily under more pressure.

An Agenda for Geriatric Neuropsychiatry

Patient Care

The growth of geriatric neuropsychiatry can improve the quality of patient care. Appropriate treatment depends on accurate diagnosis, and diagnosis in elderly patients depends on a comprehensive understanding of brain-behavior relationships. In addition, diagnosis increasingly demands familiarity with neuroimaging, electrophysiology, and a variety of laboratory tests, and geriatric neuropsychiatry incorporates data from these techniques into diagnostic formulations. New medications have been developed and are able to effectively ameliorate many behavioral disturbances and improve the quality of life of elderly patients with brain disorders. Many of these agents have potentially serious side effects and practitioners in this area must be familiar with the effects, as well as the adverse consequences, of these new agents.

Education

The growth of the elderly population demands greater availability of practitioners of geriatric neuropsychiatry. This field incorporates information from psychiatry, neurology, geriatrics, and neuroscience. Training opportunities must be developed and expanded. These may arise in conjunction with existing programs providing training in psychiatry or neurology.

Research

Geriatric neuropsychiatry is a nascent field. The research agenda of geriatric neuropsychiatry must include the application of advanced technologies to diagnosis in the elderly population: the utility of PET, SPECT, and magnetic resonance spectroscopy has yet to be defined in detail. Their sensitivity in early disease, specificity in differential diagnosis, and predictive ability for determining prognosis and treatment response have not been established. The correlations between behavior and metabolic and structural brain imaging changes, as well as between behavior and pathological alterations, must be described. Complex behavioral changes such as delusions and mood disorders are unlikely to correspond to single specific lesions, and the shared characteristics of lesions and conditions producing similar syndromes demand investigation. New treatments are continuously emerging and must be integrated into clinical practice to provide the most benefit for elderly patients. The effects, side effects, and drug interactions of these new agents must be discovered. Effective nonpharmacological interventions must also be identified and perfected. Molecular underpinnings of aging must be identified and explored. The appropriate ethical responses of society to severe illness in elderly individuals must be carefully considered. Finally, a means of bridging the gap between neuroscience and human experience must be found. Geriatric neuropsychiatry will succeed to the extent that advances in the neurosciences can be related to the suffering of elderly people and its relief. We hold the conviction that research advances will translate directly into improved care and a higher quality of life for elderly individuals.

References

Altshuler LL, Conrad A, Kovelman JA, et al: Hippocampal pyramidal cell orientation in schizophrenia. Arch Gen Psychiatry 44:1094–1098, 1987

American Psychiatric Association: Diagnostic and Statistical Manual of Mental Disorders, 3rd Edition. American Psychiatric Association, Washington, DC, 1980

Avorn J, Gurwitz J: Demography, epidemiology, and aging, in Geriatric Medicine, 2nd Edition. Edited by Cassel CK, Riesenberg DE, Sorensen LB, et al. New York, Springer-Verlag, 1990, pp 66–77

Baldessarini RJ, Frankenburg FR: Clozapine: a novel antipsychotic agent. N Engl J Med 324:746–754,1991

Baxter LR Jr, Phelps ME, Mazziotta JC, et al: Cerebral metabolic rates for glucose in mood disorders. Arch Gen Psychiatry 42:441–447, 1985

Baxter LR Jr, Phelps ME, Mazziotta JC, et al: Local cerebral glucose metabolic rates in obsessive-compulsive disorder. Arch Gen Psychiatry 44:211–218, 1987

Baxter LR Jr, Schwartz JM, Phelps ME, et al: Reduction of prefrontal cortex glucose metabolism common to three types of depression. Arch Gen Psychiatry 46:243–250, 1989

Beckson M, Cummings JL: Neuropsychiatric aspects of stroke. Int J Psychiatry Med 21:1–15, 1991

Beers MH: Medication use in the elderly, in Practice of Geriatrics, 2nd Edition. Edited by Calkins E, Ford AB, Katz PR. Philadelphia, PA, WB Saunders, 1992, pp 33–49

Bowen DM, Davison AN: The biochemistry of the ageing brain, in Neurological Disorders in the Elderly. Edited by Caird FI. London, Wright PSG, 1982, pp 33–43

Brody H: Age changes in the nervous system, in Neurological Disorders in the Elderly. Edited by Caird FI. London, Wright PSG, 1982, pp 17–24

Burke JD Jr, Pincus HA, Pardes H: The clinician-researcher in psychiatry. Am J Psychiatry 143:968–975, 1986

Cassel CK, Brody JA: Demography, epidemiology, and aging, in Geriatric Medicine, 2nd Edition. Edited by Cassel CK, Riesenberg DE, Sorensen LB, et al. New York, Springer-Verlag, 1990, pp 16–27

Coffey CE: Structural brain abnormalities in the depressed elderly, in Brain Imaging in Affective Disorders. Edited by Hauser P. Washington, DC, American Psychiatric Press, 1991, pp 89–111

Coffey CE, Figiel GS, Djang WT, et al: Subcortical hyperintensity on magnetic resonance imaging: a comparison of normal and depressed elderly. Am J Psychiatry 147:187–189, 1990

Coffey CE, Wilkinson WE, Weiner RD, et al: Quantitative cerebral anatomy in depression: a controlled magnetic resonance imaging study. Arch Gen Psychiatry 50:7–16, 1993

Cohen-Cole SA: Depression and heart disease, in Depression and Co-Existing Disease. Edited by Robinson RG, Rabins PV. New York, Igaku-Shoin, 1989, pp 27–39

Creasey H, Rapoport SI: The aging human brain. Ann Neurol 17:2–10, 1985

Cummings JL: Clinical Neuropsychiatry. New York, Grune & Stratton, 1985

Cummings JL: Depression and Parkinson's disease: a review. Am J Psychiatry 149:443–454, 1992a

Cummings JL: Psychosis in neurologic disease: neurobiology and pathogenesis. Neuropsychiatry, Neuropsychology, and Behavioral Neurology 5:144–150, 1992b

Cummings JL: Frontal-subcortical circuits and human behavior. Arch Neurol 50:873–880, 1993

Cummings JL, Benson DF: Dementia: A Clinical Approach, 2nd Edition. Boston, MA, Butterworths, 1992

Cummings JL, Miller B, Hill MA, et al: Neuropsychiatric aspects of multi-infarct dementia and dementia of the Alzheimer type. Arch Neurol 44:389–393, 1987

D'Alessandro R, Gamberini G, Granieri E, et al: Prevalence of Parkinson's disease in the Republic of San Marino. Neurology 37:1679–1682, 1987

Davison W: Adverse drug reactions in the elderly: general considerations, in The Aging Process: Therapeutic Implications. Edited by Butler RN, Bearn AD. New York, Raven, 1985, pp 101–113

Department of Health and Human Services: Healthy People 2000. Washington, DC, Department of Health and Human Services, US Government Printing Office, 1990

Derogatis LR, Wise TN: Anxiety and Depressive Disorders in the Medical Patient. Washington, DC, American Psychiatric Press, 1989

Dresser RS: Autonomy revisited: the limits of anticipatory choices, in Dementia and Aging: Ethics, Values, and Policy Choices. Edited by Binstock RH, Post SG, Whitehouse PJ. Baltimore, MD, Johns Hopkins University Press, 1992, pp 71–85

Drubach DA, Kelly MP: Panic disorder associated with a right paralimbic lesion. Neuropsychiatry, Neuropsychology, and Behavioral Neurology 2:282–289, 1989

Estroff TW, Gold MS: Medication-induced and toxin-induced psychiatric disorders, in Medical Mimics of Psychiatric Disorders. Edited by Extein I, Gold MS. Washington, DC, American Psychiatric Press, 1986, pp 163–198

Evans DA, Funkenstein H, Albert MS, et al: Prevalence of Alzheimer's disease in a community of older persons: higher than previously reported. JAMA 262:2552–2556, 1989

Farlow M, Gracon SI, Hershey LA, et al: A controlled trial of tacrine in Alzheimer's disease. JAMA 268:2523–2529, 1992

Figiel GS, Coffey CE, Djang WT, et al: Brain magnetic resonance imaging findings in ECT-induced delirium. J Neuropsychiatry Clin Neurosci 2:53–58, 1990

Finch CE: Longevity, Senescence, and the Genome. Chicago, IL, University of Chicago Press, 1990

Fontaine R, Breton G, Dery R, et al: Temporal lobe abnormalities in panic disorder: an MRI study. Biol Psychiatry 27:304–310, 1990

Fratiglioni L, Grut M, Forsell Y, et al: Prevalence of Alzheimer's disease and other dementias in an elderly urban population: relationship with age, sex, and education. Neurology 41:1886–1892, 1991

Gent M, Easton JD, Hachinski VC, et al: The Canadian American Ticlopidine Study (CATS) in thromboembolic stroke. Lancet 2:1215–1220, 1989

Griggs RC, Martin TB, Penn AS, et al: Training clinical neuroscientists. Ann Neurol 21:197–201, 1987

Hershey LA, Modic MT, Greenough PG, et al: Magnetic resonance imaging in vascular dementia. Neurology 37:29–36, 1987

Hoehn-Saric R: Neurotransmitters in anxiety. Arch Gen Psychiatry 39:735–742, 1982

Holcomb HH, Links J, Smith C, et al: Positron emission tomography: measuring the metabolic and neurochemical characteristics of the living human nervous system, in Brain Imaging: Applications in Psychiatry. Edited by Andreasen NC. Washington, DC, American Psychiatric Press, 1989, pp 235–370

Jacoby RJ, Levy R, Bird JM: Computed tomography and the outcome of affective disorder: a follow-up study of elderly patients. Br J Psychiatry 139:288–292, 1981

Koranyi EK: Undiagnosed physical illness in psychiatric patients. Annual Review of Medicine 33:309–316, 1982

Lamy PP: Patterns of prescribing and drug use, in The Aging Process: Therapeutic Implications. Edited by Butler RN, Bearn AD. New York, Raven, 1985, pp 53–82

Leuchter AF, Spar JE: The late-onset psychoses. J Nerv Ment Dis 173:488–494, 1985

Lishman WA: What is neuropsychiatry? J Neurol Neurosurg Psychiatry 55:983–985, 1992

Mayeux R, Denaro J, Hemenegildo N, et al: A population-based investigation of Parkinson's disease with and without dementia: relationship to age and gender. Arch Neurol 49:492–497, 1992

Mayou R, Hawton K, Feldman E, et al: Psychiatric problems among medical admissions. Int J Psychiatry Med 21:71–84, 1991

Mazziotta JC, Gilman S (eds): Clinical Brain Imaging: Principles and Application. Philadelphia, PA, FA Davis, 1992

Merriam AE, Aronson MK, Gaston P, et al: The psychiatric symptoms of Alzheimer's disease. J Am Geriatr Soc 36:7–12, 1988

Miller BL, Lesser IM, Mena I, et al: Regional cerebral blood flow in late-life-onset psychosis. Neuropsychiatry, Neuropsychology, and Behavioral Neurology 5:132–137, 1992

Modell JG, Mountz JM, Beresford TP: Basal ganglia/limbic striatal and thalamocortical involvement in craving and loss of control in alcoholism. J Neuropsychiatry Clin Neurosci 2:123–144, 1990

Moody HR: A critical view of ethical dilemmas in dementia, in Dementia and Aging: Ethics, Values, and Policy Choices. Edited by Binsstock RH, Post SG, Whitehouse PJ. Baltimore, MD, Johns Hopkins University Press, 1992, pp 86–100

Myers JK, Weissman MM, Tischler GL, et al: Six-month prevalence of psychiatric disorders in three communities. Arch Gen Psychiatry 41:959–967, 1984

Nasrallah HA, Coffman JA, Olson SC: Structural brain-imaging findings in affective disorders: an overview. J Neuropsychiatry Clin Neurosci 1:21–26, 1989

National Center for Health Statistics: Statistics on older persons: United States, 1986 (Vital and Health Statistics). Washington, DC, Department of Health and Human Services, 1986

National Foundation for Brain Research: The Cost of Disorders of the Brain. Washington, DC, National Foundation for Brain Research, 1992

Post RM, Uhde TW, Ballenger JC: Efficacy of carbamazepine in affective disorders: implications for underlying physiological and biochemical substrates, in Anticonvulsants in Affective Disorders. Edited by Emrich HM, Okuma T, Muller AA. New York, Elsevier, 1984, pp 93–115

Regier DA, Boyd JH, Burke JD Jr, et al: One-month prevalence of mental disorders in the United States. Arch Gen Psychiatry 45:977–986, 1988

Reiman EM, Fusselman MJ, Tox PT, et al: Neuroanatomical correlates of anticipatory anxiety. Science 243:1071–1074, 1989

Reisberg B, Borenstein J, Salob SP, et al: Behavioral symptoms in Alzheimer's disease: phenomenology and treatment. J Clin Psychiatry 48 (suppl):9–15, 1987

Robinson RG, Benson DF: Depression in aphasic patients: frequency, severity, and clinicopathologic correlations. Brain Lang 14:282–291, 1981

Robinson RG, Starkstein SE: Current research in affective disorders following stroke. J Neuropsychiatry Clin Neurosci 2:1–14, 1990

Rowe J: Report of the Institute of Medicine: academic geriatrics in the year 2000. N Engl J Med 316:1425–1428, 1987

Sackeim HA, Prohovnik II, Moeller JR, et al: Regional cerebral blood flow in mood disorders. Arch Gen Psychiatry 47:60–70, 1990

Saravay SM, Steinberg MD, Weinschel B, et al: Psychological comorbidity and length of stay in the general hospital. Am J Psychiatry 148:324–329, 1991

Small GW, Fong K, Beck JC: Training in geriatric psychiatry: will supply meet the demand? Am J Psychiatry 145:476–478, 1988

Spencer G, Goldstein AA, Taeuber CM: America's Centenarians. Washington, DC, US Department of Commerce, Bureau of Statistics, US Government Printing Office, 1987

Stadtman ER: Protein oxidation and aging. Science 257:1220–1224, 1992

Teri L, Larson EB, Reifler BV: Behavioral disturbances in dementia of the Alzheimer's type. J Am Geriatr Soc 36:1–6, 1988

Terry RD, DeTeresa R, Hansen LA: Neocortical cell counts in normal human adult aging. Ann Neurol 21:530–539, 1987

Tetrud JW, Langston JW: The effect of deprenyl (selegiline) on the natural history of Parkinson's disease. Science 245:519–522, 1989

Torrey BB, Kinsella K, Taeuber CM: An Aging World. Washington, DC, US Department of Commerce, Bureau of the Census, US Government Printing Office, 1987

Trimble MR: Neuropsychiatry or behavioral neurology. Neuropsychiatry, Neuropsychology, and Behavioral Neurology 6:60–69, 1993

Van Gorp W, Mahler M: Subcortical features of normal aging, in Subcortical Dementia. Edited by Cummings JL. New York, Oxford University Press, 1990, pp 231–250

Veith RC, Raskind MA: The neurobiology of aging: does it predispose to depression? Neurobiol Aging 9:101–117, 1988

Volkow ND, Hitzemann R, Wang G-J, et al: Decreased brain metabolism in neurologically intact healthy alcoholics. Am J Psychiatry 149:1016–1022, 1992

Wu JC, Buchsbaum MS, Hershey TG, et al: PET in generalized anxiety disorder. Biol Psychiatry 29:1181–1199, 1991

Yudofsky SC, Hales RE: The reemergence of neuropsychiatry: definition and direction. J Neuropsychiatry Clin Neurosci 1:1–6, 1989a

Yudofsky SC, Hales RE: When patients ask ...What is neuropsychiatry? J Neuropsychiatry Clin Neurosci 1:362–365, 1989b

2

Epidemiology of Aging

Roberta Malmgren, Ph.D.

Introduction

Aging populations present one of the world's major health care challenges. Industrialized countries currently face this challenge; but developing nations, with anticipated increases in the numbers and proportion of their elderly populations, will also soon need to deal with problems of growing geriatric populations. Concerns about the elderly population arise from two characteristics of that group: 1) the recent and continuing increases in the population aged 65 and older ("65+") and 2) the increasing number and severity of health problems associated with aging. (Unless otherwise noted, "elderly" and "older people" refer to people 65 years old and older.)

Epidemiology characterizes groups rather than individuals. As cultural background and gender play an important role in an individual's health, so, too, do characteristics of an age group, such as "the elderly," affect and reflect the well-being of its members. Although the subject of this book is neuropsychiatric disorders, it is important to understand how a range of other factors may impact the neuropsychiatric realm. Therefore, in this chapter, I first define the population at risk, the elderly population, and describe some of the most salient epidemiological characteristics of this population, particularly its physical health. Through most of this chapter, I focus on the elderly population in the United States. However, many of the concepts and problems apply to other industrialized countries now and presage issues that will affect developing nations in the near future. What, then, are some of the major epidemiological characteristics of the elderly?

Graying of the Population

One of the most remarkable and far-reaching demographic developments of the 20th century has been the "graying" of populations. The phrase, the "graying of the population," often evokes the image of a horrendous set of problems resulting from an increasingly elderly population. The specific problems—medical, social, financial, and psychological—are not all necessarily new. But what is unique are the great increases in the numbers and proportions of older people.

The graying of the population has three components (Table 2–1). First are the increases in the absolute numbers of people 65 and older. Between 1900 and 1990, the number of elderly people in the United States increased tenfold, from 3 million to 31 million. Second are the increases in the proportion of the population that is elderly. In 1900, the elderly represented only 4% of the total United States population, whereas currently they represent over 12%. Third are the increases in the oldest old, those who are 85 or older ("85+"), as a proportion of the 65+ group. The 1990 census counted 3 million people who were 85+. This was 25 times their number in 1900 and more than double their proportion in the total elderly population (Taueber 1992).

Table 2–1 shows that the graying of our population will continue well into the next century. In the year 2030, there will be 70 million elderly people, more than twice as many as there are now. As a proportion of the total population, today one out of eight Americans is 65 or older; in 2030, one out of five will be. In the next century, the 85+ group will be one of the fastest growing age groups, increasing from 3 million in 1990 to almost 18 million in 2050. Currently only 10% of the elderly population are 85+. In 2050, 22% of the 65+ group will be 85 or older.

The major reason for future increases in the 65+ population is past increases in birth rates: the Baby Boomers, a large cohort born between 1946 and 1964, will start to turn 65 in 2011 and will continue to inflate the numbers of 65+ until 2030 (Taueber 1992). Past birth rates strongly affect the proportion of the total population that is 65+. Improvements in mortality rates

Table 2–1. Population 65 and older (65+)—United States 1900–2050

Population	1900	1920	1940	1960	1980	1990	2010[a]	2030[a]	2050[a]
65+ population (in millions)	3.1	4.9	9.0	16.6	25.6	31.1	39.7	69.8	78.9
(As % of total population)	(4.1)	(4.7)	(6.8)	(9.2)	(11.3)	(12.5)	(13.3)	(20.2)	(20.6)
85+ population (in millions)	0.1	0.2	0.4	0.9	2.2	3.0	5.7	8.4	17.6
(As % of total 65+ population)	(4.0)	(4.3)	(4.0)	(5.6)	(8.8)	(9.7)	(14.4)	(12.0)	(22.4)

[a]Middle series projections.
Sources.   1900–1990: Taueber 1992; 2010–2050: Day 1992.

among the elderly population have only a small effect on this proportion, but do affect the absolute numbers of elderly people and the age composition within the 65+ group (Olshansky 1988).

Changing Racial Composition

In the coming century, the racial composition of the elderly population will also change (Table 2–2). In 1990, 10% of the United States elderly population was non-white. In 2050, 21% will be non-white. By 2050, the black[1] elderly population is projected to increase from 8% to 12% of the 65+ group, whereas Hispanic elderly people (who may be of any race) will have more than quadrupled as a percentage of the United States elderly population. In that year, there will be 16 times the number of elderly people of Asian and Pacific Islander ancestry, an increase from 1.4% to 8.2% of the total 65+ group.

Sex Ratio

Because of increased mortality rates among men, the ratio of men to women decreases strikingly from ages 65–69 (when there are 81 men to every 100 women) to ages 90+ (when the ratio is 31 to 100) (Figure 2–1). Many social and medical consequences of aging in developed countries are associated with the sex ratio imbalance. With increasing age, women are more likely to be unmarried and living alone (Saluter 1992). Both of these characteristics are linked to poverty (Social Security Administration 1992; US Bureau of the Census 1990) and other disadvantages, such as increased likelihood of admission to nursing homes (Cohen et al. 1986; Hing and Bloom 1990).

Marital Status[*]

Elderly men are most likely to be married, and elderly women are more likely to be widowed. According to the U.S. Bureau of the Census (Saluter 1992), in 1991 15% of all men 65+ were widowers, whereas 48% of all women 65+ were widows. As a corollary of this, 74% of elderly men lived with spouses compared to 40% of elderly women.

Living Arrangements[*]

The percentage of elderly people living alone increases with age and is greater for women than for men. In 1991, 13% of men 65–74 years old lived alone, whereas 34% of women these ages did so; 21% of men 75+ lived alone compared to 53% of women 75+ (Saluter 1992).

Income[*]

The median income of the elderly population decreases with age, is lower for nonmarried people, and is lowest for nonmarried women (Social Security Administration 1992). In terms of median income and total assets, today's elderly people are financially better off than in the past (Chen 1991; Social Security Administration 1992). However, in 1991, 20% lived either below the federally established poverty level or had incomes that were only 25% above that level (US Bureau of the Census 1992). The risk of poverty rises with age (Social Security Administration 1992) and is associated with race and sex: in 1991, 34% of black elderly peo-

Table 2–2. Racial and ethnic changes in population of people 65 and older (65+)—United States 1990–2050

	1990	2010[a]	2030[a]	2050[a]
All non-white				
Population (in millions)	3.1	5.3	11.6	16.5
As % of total 65+ population	(9.8)	(13.4)	(16.7)	(20.9)
Black				
Population (in millions)	2.5	3.6	7.4	9.4
As % of total 65+ population	(8.0)	(8.9)	(10.6)	(12.0)
Asian and Pacific Islander				
Population (in millions)	0.4	1.5	3.8	6.5
As % of total 65+ population	(1.4)	(3.9)	(5.5)	(8.2)
American Indian, Eskimo, and Aleut				
Population (in millions)	0.1	0.2	0.4	0.6
As % of total 65+ population	(0.4)	(0.6)	(0.6)	(0.7)
Hispanic origin[b]				
Population (in millions)	1.1	2.8	7.4	12.0
As % of total 65+ population	(3.7)	(7.1)	(10.6)	(15.3)

[a]Middle series projections.
[b]May be of any race.
Sources. 1990: Taueber 1992; 2010–2050: Day 1992.

---

[1] Although the term *African American* is preferred by many people, "black" is the race category used in the Census and other cited research in this chapter.

[*]Statistics for marital status, living arrangements, and income are all based on surveys of noninstitutionalized elderly.

ple, compared to 10% of white elderly people and 21% of elderly Hispanic people, had incomes below the poverty level (US Bureau of the Census 1992). Older women are twice as likely as older men to be poor: in 1991, 15.5% of women 65+ were below the poverty level, whereas only 7.9% of men 65+ were (US Bureau of the Census 1992).

Worldwide Aging

The aging of populations is a worldwide phenomenon. As Table 2–3 shows, in 1990, 323 million people, 6% of the world's population, were 65+. Their numbers will more than double in 2020, when 9% of the world will be 65+. In that year, two-thirds of the world's elderly people will live in developing countries. The greatest numerical gain will be in Asia, which will have nearly 400 million elderly people. Within industrialized countries, there are wide variations in the projected increases of elderly people: by 2025, when the United States elderly population will have increased by 100%, Japan's elderly population will have increased by 136%, Canada's by 200%, France's by 60%, but the United Kingdom's by only 25% (Dean 1990).

Life Expectancy

The single statistic that best summarizes a population's health is life expectancy—the average number of years a person or group can be expected to live from a given age. Although life expectancy from birth is the most commonly quoted, life tables generate life expectancy values for all ages of a population (Palmore and Gardner 1983). Thus we can compare the longevity of elderly people in different groups or at different times using life expectancy at, for example, age 65 or age 85.

Older Americans have many years of life yet to live. In 1991, a 65-year-old person had a life expectancy of 17.4 years—over 20% of his or her life still remained (National Center for Health Statistics 1993a). In the same year, a 75-year-old person had an expected 11.1 more years of life, and an 85-year-old person could expect to live, on average, 6.2 more years. Life expectancy for elderly people has, in general, been improving since 1900. At the turn of the century, the life expectancy of a 65-year-old person was 11.9 years, and that of an 85-year-old person was 4.0 years ("Trends in Longevity" 1987). Thus in less than 100 years, life expectancy has increased 46% for 65-year-old people and 55% for those 85+.

As is true of virtually all health measures, life expectancy for elderly people varies by race and sex, with

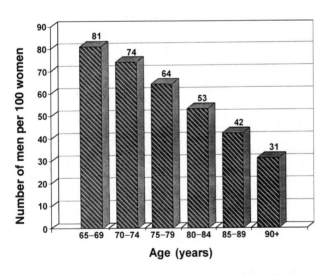

Figure 2–1. Ratio of men to women, by age group—United States 1990.
Source. From Taueber 1992.

Table 2–3. World population (in millions) of people 65 and older, by region—1990–2020

Region	1990 Number	1990 % of total region population	2020 Number	2020 % of total region population
World	322.7	6.0	742.0	9.0
Developing	175.7	4.3	491.6	7.2
Developed	147.1	12.1	250.4	18.4
Sub-Saharan Africa	14.5	2.7	41.7	3.3
Near East and North Africa	9.7	3.8	30.1	6.0
Asia	145.1	4.8	395.9	8.8
Developing	130.4	4.5	362.5	8.3
China only	65.9	5.8	179.6	11.7
Developed	14.6	11.8	33.4	26.2
Latin American/ Caribbean	20.9	4.7	56.9	8.1
North America	34.6	12.5	58.5	17.9
Europe	68.1	13.6	107.3	20.6
Soviet Union	27.5	9.4	46.6	13.1
Oceania	2.4	9.3	5.1	13.6
Developing	0.2	2.7	0.4	4.3
Developed	2.3	11.2	4.6	17.1

Source. From Jamison 1991.

elderly women having a definite, but declining, survival advantage over men. Table 2–4 lists expectancies for elderly subgroups in 1989, the year of the most recent official data for race and sex subgroups.[2] In that year, a 65-year-old man had a life expectancy of 15.2 years, compared to a woman's 18.8 years. For ages 85+, men-women differences in life expectancy shrank to 1.3 years (5.3 for men versus 6.6 for women). For blacks and whites as well, the gap in life expectancy narrows with age: in 1989 life expectancy for 65-year-old white men was 1.6 years more than that for black men that age, whereas 65-year-old white women that age could expect to live 2 years longer than black women that age. However, at age 85, life expectancy of black people was longer than that of white people: black men and women had life expectancies that were, respectively, 0.3 and 0.2 years longer than those of their white counterparts. This reversal of racial survival has been reported for many years and reflects a phenomenon known as the "black-white mortality crossover," in which at very old ages mortality rates for whites exceed those of blacks (Wing et al. 1985).

Mortality Rates

Life expectancy, though a succinct summary of a population's health, tells nothing of the specific components of survival: who dies, what people die from, and how these causes change over time. Mortality data, from which life expectancies are calculated, are needed to provide this information.

In the United States, 5 of every 100 elderly people die each year (Table 2–5). Mortality rises dramatically with age: in 1991, the death rates were 2.6% for those 65–74 years old; 5.9% for those 75–84 years old; and 15.1% for those 85+. Men are at higher risk of dying than are women; and, up to very old ages, blacks have higher mortality rates than do whites (National Center for Health Statistics 1993a). However, after 65, with increasing age, differences in mortality rates lessen between the sexes and between the races; and, as noted in the previous section, at very old ages, mortality rates for whites of both sexes exceed those of blacks.

High mortality rates in the elderly result in a large turnover of this population in a short time and may result in considerable changes in the characteristics of the 65+ population in a short period. Myers (1990) estimated that 50% of those who were 65+ in 1970 had died by 1980. Thus the elderly population in one decade may be quite different from that in the next in terms of health, lifestyles, and attitudes.

The three leading causes of death in elderly people are heart disease, cancer, and stroke (Table 2–5). In 1991, these accounted for almost 70% of all elderly deaths (National Center for Health Statistics 1993a). The major fatal cancers in elderly men are lung, colon, prostate, and bladder; in elderly women, the major sites are colon, lung, breast, and uterus (Brock et al. 1990).

Chronic obstructive pulmonary disease is the fourth leading cause of death, and the combination category of pneumonia and influenza is the fifth. This last cause particularly affects the oldest old: in 1991, the pneumonia/influenza death rate among those 85+ was almost 20 times that occurring in 65–74 year olds.

In developed countries, virtually all deaths are recorded, so that, of all health status measures, mortality data are the most complete. Cause-specific mortality, however, has a number of limitations, especially for older persons (Havlik and Rosenberg 1992). Diagnos-

Table 2–4. Life expectancy (in years) at ages 65, 75, and 85, by sex and race—United States 1989

	All races	White	Black
At age 65			
Men	15.2	15.2	13.6
Women	18.8	19.0	17.0
At age 75			
Men	9.4	9.4	8.8
Women	11.9	11.9	11.0
At age 85			
Men	5.3	5.3	5.6
Women	6.6	6.5	6.7

Source. From National Center for Health Statistics 1992.

---

[2] The National Center for Health Statistics, which provides official life expectancy figures for the United States population, publishes life expectancy data by age group alone before it publishes values further broken down by race and sex. At this writing, the most recent life expectancies by age group alone were for 1991 (National Center for Health Statistics 1993a), whereas the most recent published data for age groups, by race and sex, shown in Table 2–4, were for 1989 (National Center for Health Statistics 1992).

tic accuracy of cause of death partly reflects much lower autopsy rates in the elderly (Ahronheim et al. 1983), as well as attending physicians' perceptions of what is normal aging and what is disease. But even with thorough and accurate medical assessment of an elderly decedent, determining the underlying cause of death can be very difficult because of the presence of multiple, chronic disorders.

Alzheimer's disease exemplifies the limitations of mortality data. In a seminal article on the senile type of Alzheimer's disease, Katzman (1976) estimated that it was the fourth or fifth leading cause of death in the United States, despite the fact that it was not among the 263 leading causes of death listed in United States vital statistics. (In fact, at that time, there was no specific cause-of-death code for Alzheimer's disease.) Katzman's article greatly increased awareness of Alzheimer's disease as a major health problem of the elderly population. However, even with both improved recognition of Alzheimer's disease and assignment of a code for it, it is unlikely that current mortality rates precisely describe the severity of this disease.

The International Classification of Diseases, used to code conditions on death certificates, now includes Alzheimer's disease (Department of Health and Human Services 1991). Also multiple cause-of-death coding allows assessment of all conditions listed on a death certificate, both underlying and associated. Havlik and Rosenberg (1992) analyzed all 1987 United States deaths using multiple cause-of-death codes: 11,311 people died with Alzheimer's disease coded as the underlying cause of death, but an additional 14,639 had

Alzheimer's disease listed as a contributing, but not underlying, cause of death. Thus 1987 mortality rates, based on underlying cause-of-death codes, identified less than half of the death certificates on which Alzheimer's disease was listed. Although there is much evidence that people with dementia, and Alzheimer's disease in particular, have a much lower survival rate than expected (Barclay et al. 1985; Breteler et al. 1992; Molsa et al. 1986), many patients diagnosed in life as having dementia may not have it mentioned anywhere on their death certificates (Martyn and Pippard 1988). It is important to remember, however, that determining whether a chronic disorder is truly the underlying cause of death or only contributes to mortality is difficult and applies to many conditions other than the dementing disorders. Therefore, we cannot use all mentions of Alzheimer's disease on death certificates to rank its importance in mortality without doing the same for many other chronic diseases, such as diabetes and osteoporosis.

With increasing physician awareness of Alzheimer's disease and its effects, more deaths will be appropriately attributed to this cause. Though this means that mortality data will thus be a better measure of the frequency of Alzheimer's disease, it also means that we must be cautious when interpreting reports of secular increases in Alzheimer's disease mortality (Centers for Disease Control 1990).

In the United States, mortality has been declining for all three older age groups for many years (Figure 2–2). Between 1950 and 1990, mortality rates for people 65–84 years old decreased by more than one-third;

Table 2–5. Leading causes of death in the population 65 and older (65+)—United States 1991

Cause	Death rates per 100,000 people			
	65+	65–74	75–84	85+
All Causes	4,924	2,618	5,890	15,108
Diseases of the heart	1,881	872	2,219	6,613
Malignant neoplasms	1,117	872	1,352	1,774
Cerebrovascular diseases	394	140	479	1,588
Chronic obstructive pulmonary diseases	241	156	327	447
Pneumonia and influenza	217	56	238	1,080
Diabetes mellitus	115	76	142	254
Accidents and adverse effects	83	44	98	258
Nephritis/necrosis	57	24	70	202
Atherosclerosis	52	12	51	292
Septicemia	50	21	61	183

Source. From National Center for Health Statistics 1993a.

for those 85+, the rates declined by one-quarter (National Center for Health Statistics 1993b). Much of this remarkable decline in mortality is due to improvements in cardiovascular disease mortality (Beaglehole 1990; Cooper et al. 1990). Between 1950 and 1990, there was a 50% decline in the age-adjusted rates for heart disease mortality and a 69% decrease in age-adjusted mortality rates for stroke in the total United States population (National Center for Health Statistics 1993b). These improvements occurred in the elderly population as well: in the past 40 years, death rates from both heart disease and stroke have decreased in all three of the elderly age groups; however, death rates for cancer have increased in the elderly (National Center for Health Statistics 1993b). These increases in cancer mortality have not been enough to offset the effects of improvements in cardiovascular disease mortality.

Risk of Severe Medical Disease

The risk of developing a disease is not the same as the risk of dying from it. Even diseases that are the leading causes of death do not always result in death and so do not give a complete picture of the occurrence of those diseases in a population. The two epidemiological measures most often used to describe the occurrence of disease are incidence and prevalence. *Incidence* is the number of new cases of a disease or condition arising in a population within a certain period (usually a year). *Prevalence* is the number of existing cases in a

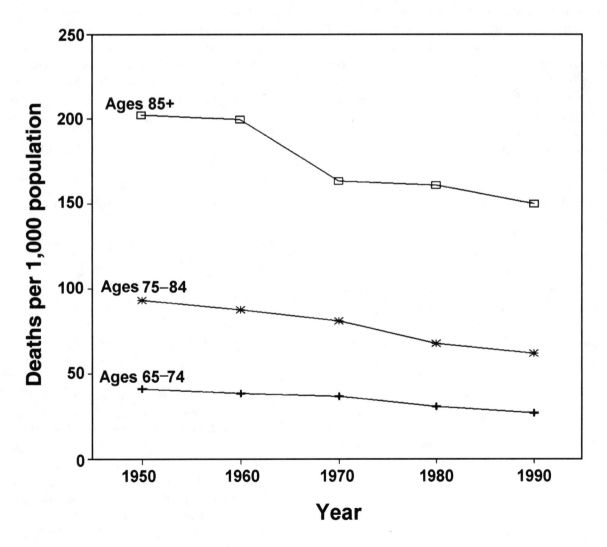

Figure 2–2.   Death rates in the elderly population, all causes—United States 1950–1990.
Source.   From National Center for Health Statistics 1993b.

population at a certain point in time (or in a short period). Though incidence is the only valid way to measure risk of developing disease, incidence studies are usually expensive and time-consuming to conduct. Because of this, relatively few community-based incidence studies have been conducted on even the three leading causes of death: heart disease, cancer, and stroke. Fewer still have collected information on any but the youngest of the elderly. Where adequate data exist, they show that the prevalence and incidence of severe diseases increase greatly in elderly people.

Heart Disease

Considering that four-fifths of all heart disease deaths in the United States occur in people 65+ (National Center for Health Statistics 1993a), there is remarkably little information on their risk of developing heart disease. Rochester, Minnesota, has an excellent medical record linkage system that covers virtually all residents (Leibson et al. 1992). In Rochester, between 1979 and 1982, the average annual incidence of coronary heart disease for people 70+ was 1.7/100 for men and 1.4/100 for women (Elveback et al. 1986). The coronary heart disease rate in men 70+ was almost eight times greater than that observed in 30- to 49-year-old men; whereas the rate in women 70+ was 24 times that of women who were 30–49. As has been shown in other studies (Burke et al. 1989; Centers for Disease Control 1992b), though, older men continue to have a higher risk of heart disease than do women; the gender difference narrows with age.

Unlike the clear decline in heart disease mortality observed, evidence for decreases in heart disease incidence is mixed. Both the Framingham Heart Study (D'Agostino et al. 1989) and the Minnesota Heart Survey (Burke et al. 1989) could detect no statistically significant changes in coronary heart disease incidence over 15- to 20-year periods. In Rochester, between 1965–1969 and 1979–1982, the risk of myocardial infarction and sudden unexpected death declined for 50- to 69-year-old men but increased for women (Elveback et al. 1986). For those 70+, rates of these manifestations of heart disease declined only slightly over time for men (9%) and not at all for women.

Cancer

The Surveillance and Epidemiology End Results program is the major source of data on cancer incidence in this country and has population-based cancer registries in nine areas of the United States (Frey et al. 1992). The leading cancer incidence sites in elderly people are lung, colon, breast, and prostate (Brock et al. 1990). As with cancer mortality, cancer incidence in the elderly has been increasing with time for a number of sites (Hoel et al. 1992).

Stroke

More than heart disease or cancer, stroke is a disease of elderly people. In 1991, 87% of all stroke deaths occurred in the elderly population (National Center for Health Statistics 1993a). Stroke is also one of the most disabling conditions to affect elderly people (Verbrugge et al. 1989), and the risk of it increases with age (Bonita 1992). In well-designed studies of stroke incidence, 2%–4% of the 85+ age group have a first-ever stroke each year; and men have a somewhat greater risk of stroke than do women (Malmgren et al. 1987).

Detailed evidence for secular changes in stroke incidence with time comes from Rochester, Minnesota, where average annual stroke rates were calculated for five-year periods starting in 1945 (Broderick et al. 1989). Between 1945–1949 and 1975–1979, total age-adjusted stroke rates dropped by 45% in this city but then increased by 17% between 1975–1979 and 1980–1984. Changes occurred in all age groups, but were most pronounced in the 85+ group (Figure 2–3).

Neuropsychiatric Disorders

Dementia

Progressive loss of cognition and eventual total incapacitation make dementia one of the most dreaded consequences of aging. It is a major cause of functional disability (Manton 1989); need for long-term care, including admission to nursing homes (Hing et al. 1989); and enormous burden to family caregivers (Office of Technology Assessment Task Force 1988).

If there is an "epidemic" among the elderly population, it is Alzheimer's disease and related dementias. The Office of Technology Assessment Task Force (1988) conducted an extensive research review on dementia and estimated the prevalence of severe dementia in the United States. The prevalence of severe dementia in all elderly Americans was estimated to be 6%. By age group, estimated prevalence rates were 1%

in those 65–74 years old, 7% in those 75–84 years old, and 25% in those 85+. When these rates are applied to 1990 census data (Taueber 1992), the results indicate that 1.6 million elderly people had severe dementia in that year. Forecasts of these same rates combined with population projections (Day 1992) indicate that, in the year 2050, more than 6 million elderly Americans will have severe dementia.

Studies have been done in many parts of the world and have produced wildly differing estimates of dementia prevalence (Hafner 1990). However, for no other disorder of the elderly population are methodological issues of doing community-based studies so complex or variation in study design so great (Colsher and Wallace 1991; Jorm 1990). These methodological variations, rather than true differences in frequency of dementia, are a major reason why estimates of prevalence rates of dementia are so disparate.

Another cause of differences in rates of overall prevalence of dementia is the type of dementia identi-

fied. The Office of Technology Task Force (1988) lists more than 80 conditions that cause or simulate dementia. In the United States, Alzheimer's disease is the most frequent cause and vascular dementias the next most frequent (Gorelick and Mangone 1991). The exact proportion of dementia attributable to each cause depends in part on the stroke risk in the population of interest: where stroke risk is higher, for example among blacks (Centers for Disease Control 1992a) or in Japan (Jorm 1991), the proportion of dementia attributable to vascular causes will be higher. Similarly, secular declines in stroke risk should have an effect on the total risk of dementia, as well as on the type of dementia seen.

Few population-based studies of dementia incidence have been conducted. In Rochester, Minnesota, data were collected on all new cases occurring between 1970 and 1974 (Kokmen et al. 1988). The average annual incidence rates of all dementias there were 1.4/1,000 for those 60–69 years old, 6.4/1,000 for

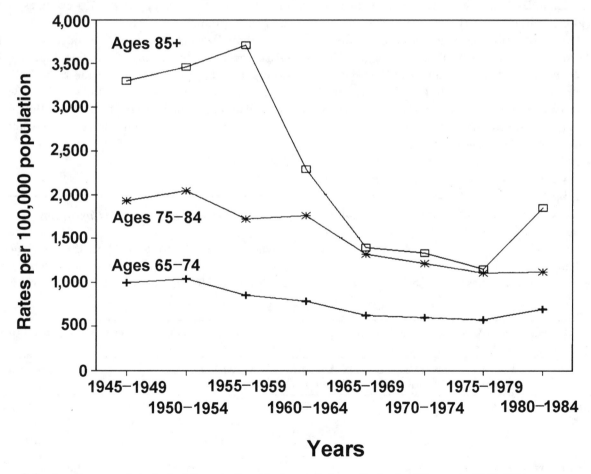

Figure 2–3. Average annual stroke incidence in the elderly population—Rochester, Minnesota, 1945–1984.
Source. From Broderick et al. 1989.

those 70–79 years old, and 20.5/1,000 for those 80+. Alzheimer's disease was the diagnosis in 38% of new dementia cases in people who were 60–69, 71% of those 70–79, and 82% in those 80+. Most, but not all, studies suggest a somewhat greater frequency (incidence and prevalence) of Alzheimer's disease in women and of vascular dementia in men (Jorm 1990).

A few studies have looked at changes over time in the incidence of dementia. In Lundby, Sweden, residents were followed from 1947 until 1972 (Rorsman et al. 1986). No change in the incidence of "age psychosis" was detected. Similarly, in Rochester, Minnesota, no statistically significant differences were found in the incidence of either dementia or Alzheimer's disease between 1960 and 1975 (Kokmen et al. 1988).

Other Mental Disorders

Except for dementia, the frequency of most mental disorders does not increase in the elderly population. The Epidemiologic Catchment Area Program provides the largest sample of population-based data on mental illness in the United States (Eaton et al. 1989). In the early 1980s, staff from this research program interviewed residents in five cities (Baltimore, Maryland; St. Louis, Missouri; Los Angeles, California; New Haven, Connecticut; and Durham, North Carolina), identifying major types of mental disorders using a questionnaire based on DSM-III criteria (American Psychiatric Association 1980). The prevalence of all types of mental disorder combined in elderly people was 12.3%, lower than that for any other age group (Regier et al. 1988) (Table 2–6). By type of disorder, the prevalence was also lower in all categories except severe cognitive impairment: as measured by the Mini-Mental State Exam (Folstein et al. 1975), 5% of the elderly in this sample had severe cognitive impairment. There were differences by sex for some of the disorders: the preva-

lence of alcohol abuse was 6 times greater in elderly men than in elderly women, whereas the prevalence of affective disorders in women was more than double that in men. Elderly men had a higher prevalence of severe cognitive impairment than did women at ages 65–74 and a similar rate at ages 75–84, but for those 85+, the prevalence in men was less than half that observed in women (8.2% compared to 19.5%).

The Epidemiologic Catchment Area Program reinterviewed subjects 1 year after the baseline interview to determine the incidence (rate of new cases) in their population (Eaton et al. 1989). The authors found that the onset of major depressive disorder was rare in elderly subjects (except in St. Louis), as was the onset of panic disorders. Not surprisingly, the risk of developing severe cognitive impairment increased with age: approximately 5 of every 100 subjects 65+ developed severe cognitive impairment each year. Unlike the prevalence data, the incidence of alcohol abuse increased after age 60: in men 75+ older, the rate was six times as high as that for men 65–74. For women, the incidence was twice as high in the 75+ group as in the 65–74 age group.

Although elderly people do not appear to be at increased risk for most forms of functional mental disorders, they have the highest suicide rate of all age groups, due primarily to the high rates in elderly white men (National Center for Health Statistics 1993b). In 1989, the rates for white men were 35/100,000 for those 65–74, 55/100,000 for those 75–84, and 72/100,000 for those 85+.

Prevalence of Chronic Conditions

A major source of information about the prevalence of chronic conditions in the United States comes from the National Health Interview Survey, a continuing

Table 2–6. Epidemiologic Catchment Area Program 1-month prevalence of mental disorders in persons 65 and older (per 100 subjects)

	Anxiety disorders[a]	Severe cognitive impairment	Affective disorders[b]	Alcohol abuse	Schizophrenia	Antisocial personality
Both sexes	5.5	4.9	2.5	0.9	0.1	0.0
Men	3.6	5.1	1.4	1.8	0.1	0.1
Women	6.8	4.7	3.3	0.3	0.1	0.0

[a]Phobia, panic, and obsessive-compulsive disorders.
[b]Manic episode, major depressive episode, and dysthymia.
Source. From Regier et al. 1988.

survey of the noninstitutionalized United States population (Havlik et al. 1987). Table 2–7 lists the 10 most prevalent chronic conditions reported by the 65+ population in 1982–1984. Almost 50% of elderly Americans reported that they had arthritis, 31% reported hearing impairments, and 10% had visual impairments (not corrected by glasses). Surprisingly, the prevalence of many of these conditions did not increase with age. However, the National Health Interview Survey excludes nursing home residents. In very old subjects, some of the listed conditions are likely to result in institutionalization or death, removing subjects with these conditions from the target population.

Many of the most prevalent conditions in the elderly population are not necessarily acute nor fatal, but have a major impact on the quality of life. Both visual and hearing problems often lead to significant physical, social, and emotional problems (Branch et al. 1989; Lichtenstein 1992; Mulrow et al. 1990). Stroke, reported by 6% of the subjects in Table 2–7, is one of the most disabling of all chronic conditions (Verbrugge et al. 1989); but arthritis, too, is associated with considerable dysfunction in elderly people (Manton 1989; Verbrugge et al. 1989).

Comorbidity

Comorbidity, the coexistence of multiple conditions—physical and psychiatric—is common in elderly individuals. The Supplement on Aging, a supplement to the 1984 National Health Interview Survey, focused on the elderly population (Fitti and Kovar 1987). Half of the Supplement's subjects 60+ reported two or more of nine medical conditions, the most frequent combination being arthritis and high blood pressure (Guralnik et al. 1989). Comorbidity complicates diagnosis and management of health problems in elderly patients and is associated with a number of health problems, including functional limitations (Guralnik et al. 1989; Verbrugge et al. 1991) and mortality (Dunn et al. 1992).

Psychiatric disorders also often coexist with organic illnesses of the elderly (see Section IV, this volume). For example, depression is frequently reported in Alzheimer's disease (Alexopoulos and Abrams 1991), stroke (Finch et al. 1992), and Parkinson's disease (Cummings 1992). Exactly how frequently depression occurs in these diseases is an unresolved issue. Methodological problems beset the accurate estimation of comorbidity and complicate the determination of whether depression is primarily reactive or pathobiological in origin. Authors reviewing the literature have noted a wide range of reported depression in patients with one of these three diseases: none to 87% of Alzheimer's patients (Alexopoulos and Abrams 1991), 25%–65% of stroke patients (Finch et al. 1992), and 4%–70% of Parkinson's patients (Cummings 1992). Moreover, all three of these organic disorders have clinical features that overlap with those of depression (Alexopoulos and Abrams 1991; Kramer and Reifler 1992; Ring 1993). Whatever the precise risk of depression in Alzheimer's disease, stroke, or Parkinson's disease, any such comorbidity in these devastating disorders will add to an already heavy burden of dysfunction. Because depression can often be alleviated in such patients, it is extremely important that they be evaluated for depression (Alexopoulos and Abrams 1991; Cummings 1992; Kramer and Reifler 1992).

Table 2–7. Percentage of self-reported conditions of noninstitutionalized elderly individuals—United States 1982–1984

Condition	Age			
	65+	65–74	75–84	85+
Arthritis	49	48	50	52
Hypertension	39	39	40	39
Hearing impairment	31	26	36	50
Deformity or orthopedic impairment	17	17	16	21
Cataract	15	9	22	33
Ischemic heart disease	14	14	14	12
Visual impairment	10	7	12	22
Diabetes	9	9	9	8
Cerebrovascular disease	6	4	8	10
Chronic bronchitis	6	6	5	4

Source. From Havlik et al. 1987.

Functional Limitations

The well-being of the elderly population, more than any other age group, is measured in terms of functional abilities. Kane (1990) wrote, "Function is the common language of gerontology" (p. 15). Impairment of physical and psychological function is associated with an enormous number of health problems, including greater risk of specific diseases and conditions, such as fractures (Grisso et al. 1991), increased probability of institutionalization (Cohen et al. 1986), and higher mortality (Harris et al. 1989).

If, however, function is the lingua franca of geriatric research and practice, it is a language with many dialects: functional ability has many components, and for each there is a multitude of assessment instruments (Applegate et al. 1990; Guralnik and LaCroix 1992). In population-based surveys, the most common assessments are of activities of daily living (ADLs) and instrumental activities of daily living (IADLs). ADLs reflect basic personal care activities: eating, bathing, dressing, getting in and out of bed or a chair ("transferring"), using the toilet, and mobility. IADLs measure more complex (and also more culture- and gender-specific) functions of daily living: shopping, preparing meals, using the telephone, managing money, and doing light and heavy housework.

The Supplement on Aging provided estimates of functional limitations for the noninstitutionalized United States population. Figure 2–4 shows the percentage of all elderly people, as well as those 85+, who reported difficulties with ADLs. Walking was the most prevalent ADL limitation: 19% of the 65+ group and 40% of those 85+ had problems walking. However, only 2% of all elderly in the community and 4% of those 85+ had difficulties with eating activities. The most frequent IADL difficulty was with heavy housework (Figure 2–5). Among those 85+, one-fifth or more reported that they had problems with all IADLs except using the telephone.

Most studies indicate that the prevalence of ADL and IADL limitations is greater for women than for men (Taueber 1992). This may be due to the increased survival of women with the same disabilities rather than to differences in risks (i.e., incidence) of developing functional limitations (Harris et al. 1989; Manton 1988; Strawbridge et al. 1992).

Figures 2–4 and 2–5 indicate only whether the elderly have problems performing the various ADLs. Receipt of help from others defines dependency in performing these activities. Figure 2–6 shows the percentage of Supplement on Aging respondents who reported receiving help with IADLs and ADLs. Three-quarters did not get help with any of these activities, and only 4.2% received help with three or more ADLs.

Institutionalization

For the elderly population, ultimate dependency is symbolized by admission to nursing homes (see Chapter 32, this volume). Kemper and Murtaugh (1991) estimated that 43% of all people reaching age 65 will enter a nursing home at some time in their lives. Nevertheless, at any one time, the proportion of the el-

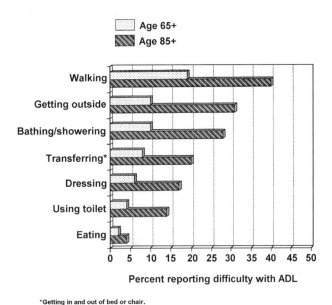

Figure 2–4. Activity of daily living (ADL) difficulties in the elderly population (ages 65 and older [65+] and 85 and older [85+])—United States 1984.
Source. From Taueber 1992.

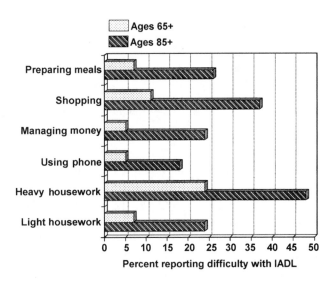

Figure 2–5. Instrumental activity of daily living (IADL) difficulties in the elderly population (ages 65 and older [65+] and 85 and older [85+])—United States 1984.
Source. From Taueber 1992.

derly population in nursing homes is not high. According to the National Nursing Home Survey (Hing et al. 1989), in 1985 the percentage of elderly in nursing homes was approximately 5%. The percentage increased from 1% for those 65–74 years old to 6% for those 75–84 years old and to 22% for those 85+. A greater proportion of women are in nursing homes, a difference that becomes especially pronounced at very old ages (Figure 2–7). This disparity is due to the fact that women, with their greater longevity, are less likely to have spouses available as caretakers.

Conclusions

Aging is associated with increased vulnerability to a number of interacting disadvantages: physical, functional, social, psychological, and economic. Assessment of each of these dimensions is needed to give a complete picture of the health of the elderly individual (Fillenbaum 1990). Beyond the specific impact that each dimension has on the well-being of elderly people, together they create a complex matrix of cause-and-effect (Fried and Wallace 1992). Furthermore, the health of an elderly person often greatly affects others. In the United States in 1984, an estimated 4.2 million spouses and children provided help with ADLs and IADLs for elderly people living in the community (Stone and Kemper 1989). More than one-third of these caregivers were themselves over 65 years old. Informal caregivers, often female relatives of the elderly person, are at increased risk for health problems, both physical and psychological (Office of Technology Task Force 1988). In many instances, the caregiver is as appropriate an intervention target as the patient (Brown et al. 1990).

Characterizing and treating health problems of

the elderly population is much more complex than doing so in younger groups. The traditional medical model of diseased versus not diseased is not adequate for older people, and health professionals need to expand and refocus expectations regarding health and prevention. As an example, elderly patients may have several impairments, with no obvious link to a specific disease. Halting or slowing progression of any one of these impairments may make a critical difference in their quality of life and ability to remain independent.

Although many dimensions of well-being worsen with age, the 65+ population is an extraordinarily diverse group. This open-ended classification includes people whose ages range from 65 to more than 100. With increasing age, there are increases in the percentage of people who are female, who are poor, and who live alone. The elderly population is also racially diverse, and this racial and ethnic diversity will increase in the next century.

One of the most overlooked characteristics of the elderly population is its diversity in health (Berkman 1988). For every morbidity statistic presented in this chapter, there is a complementary one of health. For example, 75% of the noninstitutionalized elderly population receive no help with ADLs and IADLs (Hing and Bloom 1990); and almost four-fifths of the 85+ population live in the community, not in nursing homes (Hing et al. 1989).

The demographic heterogeneity of elderly Americans explains, in part, the diversity of health. The wide

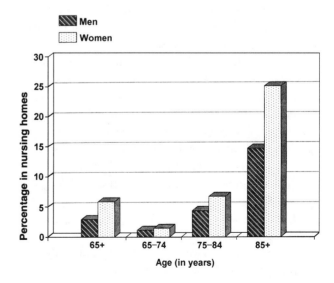

Figure 2–7. Percentage of elderly residents in nursing homes, by age and sex—United States 1985.
Source. From Hing et al. 1989.

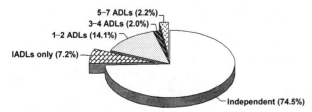

Figure 2–6. Percentage of noninstitutionalized elderly individuals who are dependent in activities of daily living (ADLs) and instrumental activities of daily living (IADLs)—United States 1984.
Source. From Hing and Bloom 1990.

age range is itself a major contributing factor. With each successive 10 years of age, health worsens. Functional limitations, incidence and prevalence of specific conditions, and mortality all increase enormously. Sex and race are also associated with different health risks. As has been described, women live longer than men, but risks for specific types of morbidity vary between the sexes. Further, each of the minority elderly groups in the United States has a different health profile (Miles and Bernard 1992; Mutchler and Burr 1991; "Older Americans' Health" 1988), and with future changing racial and ethnic proportions the health needs of American elderly will change accordingly.

As the 65+ population in the United States is diverse, so are the elderly in other countries, both within those countries and compared with the data presented in this chapter. Although many of the general concepts outlined here will apply to the elderly in other nations, measures of specific morbidity, functional limitations, and institutionalization are not always comparable (Feinleib 1993; B. E. Fries et al. 1991). Even when standardized methods are used to study the elderly populations of other countries, cultural, social, and economic differences may affect clinical presentation, as well as use of health services.

Much has been written about the compression of morbidity, that is, delaying or preventing the onset of illness and disability so that the amount of active, self-sufficient life in the elderly person increases as a proportion of total life expectancy (J. Fries 1980; Katz et al. 1983). Although there is debate regarding whether many measures of health, such as functional ability, are improving (Kane et al. 1990), there is no doubt that, according to mortality and some morbidity measures, the health of the elderly population is improving (J. Fries 1989; Leibson et al. 1992). Increasingly there are calls to focus on the vigorous, or successful, elderly (Rowe and Kahn 1987) and to enhance life, as well as to extend it (Lonergan 1991). More than for any other age group, the health of the elderly population is a continuum, and this heterogeneity strongly suggests that much ill-health in the elderly is preventable (Berg and Cassells 1990).

Besides health, other factors are changing that will have a positive effect on the well-being of older people. For example, women today are better educated than in the past: today 11% of women 55 and older have completed at least four years of college education, compared to only 4% in 1960 (Kominski and Adams 1992). Because of such changes, women have been able, more than in the past, to make lives outside their immediate families. When they reach advanced age, these women are likely to be more socially and financially independent than their past cohorts.

Thus in the future, older people are likely to be healthier than the elderly of today, and a number of concerns regarding the future needs of the elderly population may prove to be unfounded. For geriatric health professionals, a commitment to understanding the unique characteristics of elderly people and the complexity of their health will help ensure that, in the coming century, these improvements will take place.

References

Ahronheim S, Bernholc A, Clark W: Age trends in autopsy rates. JAMA 250:1182–86, 1983

Alexopoulos GS, Abrams RC: Depression in Alzheimer's disease. Psychiatr Clin North Am 14:327–340, 1991

American Psychiatric Association: Diagnostic and Statistical Manual of Mental Disorders, 3rd Edition. Washington, DC, American Psychiatric Association, 1980

Applegate WB, Blass JD, Williams TF: Instruments for the functional assessment of older patients. N Engl J Med 322:1207–1214, 1990

Barclay LL, Zemcov A, Blass JP, et al: Survival in Alzheimer's disease and vascular dementias. Neurology 35:834–840, 1985

Beaglehole R: International trends in coronary heart disease mortality, morbidity, and risk factors. Epidemiol Rev 12:1–15, 1990

Berg R, Cassells J (eds): The Second 50 Years: Promoting Health and Preventing Disability. Washington, DC, National Academy Press, 1990

Berkman L: The changing and heterogenous nature of aging and longevity: a social and medical perspective. Annual Review of Gerontology and Geriatrics 8:37–68, 1988

Bonita R: Epidemiology of stroke. Lancet 339:342–344, 1992

Branch LG, Horowitz A, Carr C: The implications for everyday life of incident self-reported visual decline among people over age 65 living in the community. Gerontologist 29:359–365, 1989

Breteler MB, Claus JJ, van Duijn CM, et al: Epidemiology of Alzheimer's disease. Epidemiol Rev 14:59–82, 1992

Brock D, Guralnik J, Brody J: Demography and epidemiology of aging in the United States, in Handbook of the Biology of Aging, 3rd Edition. Edited by Schneider E, Rowe J. San Diego, CA, Academic Press, 1990, pp 3–23

Broderick JP, Phillips SJ, Whisnant JP, et al: Incidence rates of stroke in the eighties: the end of the decline in stroke? Stroke 20:577–582, 1989

Brown LJ, Potter JF, Foster BG: Caregiver burden should be evaluated during geriatric assessment. J Am Geriatr Soc 38:455–460, 1990

Burke GL, Sprafka JM, Folsom AR, et al: Trends in CHD mortality, morbidity, and risk factor levels from 1960 to 1986: the Minnesota Heart Survey. Int J Epidemiol 18 (suppl 1):S73–S81, 1989

Centers for Disease Control: Mortality from Alzheimer's disease—United States, 1979–1987. MMWR 39:785–786, 1990

Centers for Disease Control: Cerebrovascular disease mortality and Medicare hospitalization: United States, 1980–1990. MMWR 41:477–480, 1992a

Centers for Disease Control: Coronary heart disease incidence, by sex: United States, 1971–1987. MMWR 41:526–529, 1992b

Chen Y: Improving the economic security of minority persons as they enter old age, in Minority Elders: Longevity, Economics and Health. Edited by Gerontological Society of America. Washington, DC, Gerontological Society of America, 1991, pp 14–23

Cohen MA, Tell EJ, Walleck SS: Client-related risk factors of nursing home entry among elderly adults. J Gerontol 41:785–792, 1986

Colsher PL, Wallace RB: Epidemiologic considerations in studies of cognitive function in the elderly: methodology and nondementing acquired dysfunction. Epidemiol Rev 13:1–27, 1991

Cooper R, Sempos C, Hsieh S, et al: Slowdown in the decline of stroke mortality in the United States, 1978–1986. Stroke 21:1274–1279, 1990

Cummings JL: Depression and Parkinson's disease: a review. Am J Psychiatry 149:443–454, 1992

D'Agostino RB, Kannel WB, Belanger AJ, et al: Trends in CHD and risk factors at age 55–64 in the Framingham Study. Int J Epidemiol 18 (suppl 1):S67–S72, 1989

Day JC: Population Projections of the United States by Age, Sex, Race, and Hispanic Origin: 1992 to 2050 (US Bureau of the Census, Current Population Reports, Series P-25, No 1092). Washington, DC, US Government Printing Office, 1992

Dean M: Grey growth. Lancet 335:1330–1331, 1990

Department of Health and Human Services: International Classification of Diseases, 9th Revision. Clinical Modification, 4th Edition, Vol I. Washington, DC, Public Health Service, 1991

Dunn JE, Rudberg MA, Furner SE, et al: Mortality, disability, and falls in older persons: the role of underlying disease and disability. Am J Public Health 82:395–400, 1992

Eaton WW, Kramer M, Anthony JC, et al: The incidence of specific DIS/DSM-III mental disorders: data from the NIMH Epidemiologic Catchment Area Program. Acta Psychiatr Scand 79:163–178, 1989

Elveback LR, Connolly DC, Melton LJ: Coronary heart disease in residents of Rochester, Minnesota, VII: incidence, 1950 through 1982. Mayo Clin Proc 61:896–900, 1986

Feinleib M (ed): Proceedings of the 1991 International Symposium on Data on Aging (National Center for Health Statistics). Vital Health Stat [5] 7:1–69, 1993

Fillenbaum GG: Assessment of health and functional status: an international comparison, in Improving the Health of Older People: A World View. Edited by Kane R, Evans J, MacFayden D. Oxford, England, Oxford University Press, 1990, pp 69–90

Finch EJ, Ramsay R, Katona CL: Depression and physical illness in the elderly. Clin Geriatr Med 8:275–287, 1992

Fitti JE, Kovar MG: The Supplement on Aging to the 1984 National Health Interview Survey. Vital Health Stat [1] 21:1–115, 1987

Folstein MF, Folstein SE, McHugh PR: Mini-Mental State: a practical method for grading the cognitive state of patients for the clinician. J Psychiatr Res 12:189–198, 1975

Frey CM, McMillen, MM, Cowan CD, et al: Representativeness of the Surveillance, Epidemiology, and End Results program data: recent trends in cancer mortality rates. J Natl Cancer Inst 84:872–877, 1992

Fried L, Wallace R: The complexity of chronic illness in the elderly: from clinic to community, in The Epidemiologic Study of the Elderly. Edited by Wallace R, Woolson R. New York, Oxford University Press, 1992, pp 10–19

Fries BE, Ljunggren C, Winblad B: International comparison of long-term care: the need for resident level classification. J Am Geriatr Soc 39:10–16, 1991

Fries J: Aging, natural death, and the compression of morbidity. N Engl J Med 303:130–135, 1980

Fries J: The compression of morbidity: near or far? Milbank Q 67:208–230, 1989

Gorelick PB, Mangone CA: Vascular dementias in the elderly. Clin Geriatr Med 7:599–615, 1991

Grisso JA, Kelsey JL, Strom BL, et al: Risk factors for falls as a cause of hip fracture in women. N Engl J Med 324:1326–1331, 1991

Guralnik JM, LaCroix AZ: Assessing physical function in older populations, in The Epidemiologic Study of the Elderly. Edited by Wallace R, Woolson R. New York, Oxford University Press, 1992, pp 159–181

Guralnik JM, LaCroix AZ, Everett DF, et al: Aging in the eighties: the prevalence of co-morbidity and its association with disability (Advance Data). Vital Health Stat 170:1–8, 1989

Hafner H: Epidemiology of Alzheimer's disease, in Alzheimer's Disease: Epidemiology, Neuropathology, Neurochemistry, and Clinics. Edited by Maurer K, Riederer P, Beckmann H. New York, Springer-Verlag, 1990, pp 23–39

Harris T, Kovar MG, Suzman R, et al: Longitudinal study of physical ability in the oldest old. Am J Public Health 79:698–702, 1989

Havlik R, Rosenberg H: The quality and application of death records of older persons, in The Epidemiologic Study of the Elderly. Edited by Wallace R, Woolson R. New York, Oxford University Press, 1992, pp 262–280

Havlik R, Liu B, Kovar M, et al: Health statistics on older persons: United States, 1986. Vital Health Stat [3] 25:1–157, 1987

Hing E, Bloom B: Long-term care for the functionally dependent elderly. Vital Health Stat [13] 104:1–50, 1990

Hing E, Sekscenski E, Strahan G: The National Nursing Home Survey: 1985 summary for the United States. Vital Health Stat [13] 97:1–249, 1989

Hoel DG, Davis DL, Miller AB, et al: Trends in cancer mortality in 15 industrialized countries, 1969–1986. J Natl Cancer Inst 84:313–320, 1992

Jamison E: World Population Profile: 1991 (US Bureau of the Census, Report WP/91). Washington, DC, US Government Printing Office, 1991

Jorm AF: The Epidemiology of Alzheimer's Disease and Related Disorders. London, Chapman & Hall, 1990

Jorm AF: Cross-national comparisons of the occurrence of Alzheimer's and vascular dementias. Eur Arch Psychiatry Clin Neurosci 240:218–222, 1991

Kane RL: Introduction, in Improving the Health of Older People: A World View. Edited by Kane R, Evans J, MacFayden D. Oxford, England, Oxford University Press, 1990, pp 15–18

Kane RL, Radosevich DM, Vaupel JW: Compression of morbidity: issues and irrelevancies, in Improving the Health of Older People: A World View. Edited by Kane R, Evans J, MacFayden D. Oxford, England, Oxford University Press, 1990, pp 30–49

Katz S, Branch LG, Branson MH, et al: Active life expectancy. N Engl J Med 309:1218–1224, 1983

Katzman R: The prevalence and malignancy of Alzheimer Disease. Arch Neurol 33:217–218, 1976

Kemper P, Murtaugh C: Lifetime use of nursing home care. N Engl J Med 324:595–600, 1991

Kokmen E, Chandra V, Schoenberg B: Trends in incidence of dementing illness in Rochester, Minnesota, in three quinquennial periods, 1960–1974. Neurology 38:975–980, 1988

Kominski R, Adams A: Educational attainment in the United States: March 1991 and 1990 (U.S. Bureau of the Census, Current Population Reports, Series P-20, No 462). Washington, DC, US Government Printing Office, 1992

Kramer SI, Reifler BV: Depression, dementia, and reversible dementia. Clin Geriatr Med 8:289–297, 1992

Leibson CL, Ballard DJ, Whisnant JP, et al: The compression of morbidity hypothesis: promise and pitfalls of using record-linked data bases to assess secular trends in morbidity and mortality. Milbank Q 70:127–154, 1992

Lichtenstein MJ: Hearing and visual impairments. Clin Geriatr Med 8:173–182, 1992

Lonergan E (ed): Extending Life, Enhancing Life: A National Research Agenda on Aging. Washington, DC, National Academy Press, 1991

Malmgren R, Warlow C, Bamford J, et al: Geographical and secular trends in stroke incidence. Lancet 2:1196–1200, 1987

Manton KG: A longitudinal study of functional change and mortality in the United States. J Gerontol 43:S153–S161, 1988

Manton KG: Epidemiological, demographic, and social correlates of disability among the elderly. Milbank Q 67 (suppl 2, pt 1):13–58, 1989

Martyn CN, Pippard EC: Usefulness of mortality data in determining the geography and time trends of dementia. J Epidemiol Community Health 42:134–137, 1988

Miles TP, Bernard MA: Morbidity, disability, and health status of black American elderly: a new look at the oldest old. J Am Geriatr Soc 40:1047–1054, 1992

Molsa PK, Marttila RJ, Rinne UK: Survival and cause of death in Alzheimer's disease and multi-infarct dementia. Acta Neurol Scand 74:103–107, 1986

Mulrow C, Aguilar C, Velez R, et al: Association between hearing impairment and the quality of life of elderly individuals. J Am Geriatr Soc 38:45–50, 1990

Mutchler JE, Burr JA: Racial differences in health and health care service utilization in later life: the effect of socioeconomic status. J Health Soc Behav 32:342–356, 1991

Myers G: Demography of aging, in Handbook of Aging and the Social Sciences, 3rd Edition. Edited by Binstock R, George L. San Diego, CA, Academic Press, 1990, pp 19–44

National Center for Health Statistics: Vital Statistics of the United States, 1989, Vol II, Sec 6: Life Tables. Washington, DC, Public Health Service, 1992

National Center for Health Statistics: Advance report of final mortality statistics, 1991. Monthly Vital Stat Report. Vol 42, No 2, suppl. Hyattsville, MD, Public Health Service, 1993a

National Center for Health Statistics: Health, United States, 1992. Hyattsville, MD, Public Health Service, 1993b

Office of Technology Assessment Task Force: Confronting Alzheimer's Disease and Other Dementias. Washington, DC, Science Information Resource Center, 1988

Older Americans' health. Stat Bull Metrop Life Insur Co 69:10–17, 1988

Olshansky SJ: On forecasting mortality. Milbank Q 66:482–530, 1988

Palmore JA, Gardner RW: Measuring mortality, fertility and natural increase. Honolulu, HI, East-West Center, 1983

Regier DA, Boyd JH, Burke JD, et al: One-month prevalence of mental disorders in the United States. Arch Gen Psychiatry 45:977–986, 1988

Ring H: Psychological and social problems of Parkinson's disease. Br J Hosp Med 49:111–116, 1993

Rorsman B, Hagnell O, Lanke J: Prevalence and incidence of senile and multi-infarct dementia in the Lundby study: a comparison between the time periods 1947–1957 and 1957–1972. Neuropsychobiology 15:122–129, 1986

Rowe JW, Kahn RL: Human aging: usual and successful. Science 237:143–149, 1987

Saluter AF: Marital status and living arrangements: March, 1991 (US Bureau of the Census, Current Population Reports, Series P-20, No 461). Washington, DC, US Government Printing Office, 1992

Social Security Administration: Income of the aged chartbook, 1990. Washington, DC, US Government Printing Office, 1992

Stone RI, Kemper P: Spouses and children of disabled elders: how large a constituency for long-term care reform? Milbank Q 67:485–506, 1989

Strawbridge WJ, Kaplan GA, Camacho T, et al: The dynamics of disability and functional change in an elderly cohort: results from the Alameda County Study. J Am Geriatr Soc 40:799–806, 1992

Taueber C: Sixty-Five Plus in America (US Bureau of the Census, Current Population Reports, Special Studies, P23-178). Washington, DC, US Government Printing Office, 1992

Trends in longevity after age 65. Stat Bull Metrop Insur Co 68:10–17, 1987

US Bureau of the Census: Housing arrangements of the elderly (US Bureau of the Census Statistical Brief, SB-2-90). Washington, DC, US Government Printing Office, 1990

US Bureau of the Census: Poverty in the United States: 1991 (Current Population Reports, Series P-60, No 181). Washington, DC, US Government Printing Office, 1992

Verbrugge LM, Lepkowski JM, Imanaka Y: Comorbidity and its impact on disability. Milbank Q 67:450–484, 1989

Verbrugge LM, Lepkowski JM, Konkol LL: Levels of disability among US adults with arthritis. J Gerontol 46:S71–S83, 1991

Wing S, Manton KG, Stallard E, et al: The black/white mortality crossover: investigation in a community-based study. J Gerontol 40:78–84, 1985

3

Neurobiology of Aging

Richard E. Powers, M.D.

Introduction

Overview

The brain, like most other organs in the human body, undergoes senescent changes. The boundary between normal aging and age-related disease can be difficult to mark. Most causes of age-related neurological degeneration and death are unclear.

Senescent alterations of the brain usually become apparent to the neuropathologist in the fourth or fifth decade and evolve at a variable pace. The rate of progression ranges from linear to parabolic; however, the aging process is progressive in most instances.

It is unknown whether human brain aging follows Gompertz Law stating mortality rates increase exponentially with age. Theories attributed to the gerontologist James Fries indicate that the body naturally wears out around age 85 (Comfort 1979). Newer theories suggest that death rates may level off for the oldest old (Barinaga 1992).

Many species undergo neurological aging identifiable with gross, microscopic, molecular biological, and chemical techniques. These alterations may be affected by genetic (Hayflick 1985) and environmental variables (Van Gool et al. 1987), as well as by systemic disease outside the central nervous system (CNS).

Theories of Aging

Many theories attempt to explain the age-related degeneration that occurs across mammalian species. The theories of aging can be divided into the organ-based, physiological, and genomic theories (Hayflick 1985). Organ-based theories hypothesize that human aging results from incremental loss of organ function driven by the immune system or alterations in neuroendocrine function of the CNS. Physiological theories include damage from free radicals, cross-linkage of vital molecules (e.g., collagen, deoxyribonucleic acid [DNA], or vital proteins), and the concept that toxic levels of cellular waste products accumulate over time. The genomic theories hypothesize the effect of aging as the consequence of somatic mutations and multiple genetic errors and include the concept that there may be programmed cell death.

A conceptual disagreement exists in human aging research between proponents of theories that human neurological degeneration results from disuse versus overuse (i.e., the "use it or lose it" theory) and those who attribute aging to cumulative damage (i.e., the "wearing it out" theory) (Davies 1991; Greenamyre 1991; McEwen 1991; Scheff 1991; Swaab 1991). Most experimental aging data come from nonhuman models and provide the basis for this conceptual disagreement. Mammalian aging is best described in the rodent, in which metabolic rates may influence the rate of aging (Hofman 1983, 1991). Rodent studies have shown that diminished feeding will slow aging and prolong reproductive life span (Swaab 1991) and consistent exercise will enhance brain vascularity (Black et al. 1987). The effect of environmental factors on human aging is unknown, although rodent studies demonstrate a positive relationship between environmental stimulation and brain size (Anthony and Zerweck 1979; Van Gool et al. 1987). The effect of chronic physical and emotional stress on aging is unclear, but elevated glucocorticoids are toxic to rodent hippocampal neurons (Sapolsky 1987a, 1987b). Free radical production may damage senescent neurons and is presently considered a pathogenetic mechanism in Alzheimer's disease and parkinsonism (Volicer and Crino 1990).

Linkages may exist between senescent brain changes and non-CNS organ damage. Studies like those linking numbers of senile plaques in brain to severity of coronary artery disease are few (Sparks et al. 1990), but may provide helpful information about the effect of extracranial systemic disease on the CNS.

Normal Versus Abnormal Brain Aging

The neuropathological distinctions between "normal" aging and disease are frequently obscure and confused by conflicting literature. For example, senile plaques, amyloid deposits, and cholinergic deficits were considered disease markers until studies demonstrated similar alterations in brains of some cognitively intact elderly humans (Crystal et al. 1988; Katzman et al. 1988). Subtle anoxic neuronal injury can be extremely difficult to identify, and considerable damage may escape detection by standard histopathological methods (Garcia 1992). Clinicopathological correlations can be confused by the lack of diagnostic sophistication and understanding of neurodegenerative disorders by pathologists (Powers et al. 1989). Some neuropathologists propose a continuum from normal aging through abnormal aging to disease states. These unresolved clinical and pathological distinctions between aging and disease will continue until more sophisticated markers of disease are available.

Neurons, astrocytes, oligodendrocytes, microglia, and blood vessels are the major cellular constituents of human CNS (Figure 3–1). The neuropil is the woven fabric of the cortex that includes neuronal and astrocytic processes. A normal neuron has a large nucleus, prominent nucleolus, conspicuous dendrites, and axons that are straight and thin (Figure 3–1). Neuronal atrophy is defined by a decrease in size of the cell body (perikaryon), nucleus, nucleolus, or extent of dendritic arborization. Although dysfunction atrophy or death of neurons is central to age-related changes and neurodegenerative disorders, senescent changes of glia and vascular tissue may also cause dysfunction. Neurons do not replicate in the mature brain; however, plasticity allows them to reorganize synapses and dendritic arborizations (Coleman and Flood 1987; Geddes and Cotman 1991). The number and affinity of receptors for transmitters depleted by senescent changes can either increase or decrease (Gottfries 1990). The mo-

lecular promoters of neuronal plasticity and reinnervation are probably altered in aging (Hefti and Mash 1989; Hefti et al. 1989). Trophic factors, such as nerve growth factor, may play important roles in preventing or slowing the aging process. Each of these brain components changes with senescence; however, none will discriminate normal brain aging from disease. No scientific consensus exists for the definition, causes, or consequences of normal brain aging. Few studies examine these issues in the very old (i.e., those who are over age 85).

In this chapter, I describe important gross, microscopic, neurochemical, and molecular biological alterations of aging human brain. Aging human neurons may enter a complicated cascade of atrophy, hypertrophy, synaptic reorganization, or death. The presence of changes such as cortical atrophy, senile plaques, amyloid deposits, or cholinergic deficits does not always predict neuropsychiatric sequelae (Crystal et al. 1988;

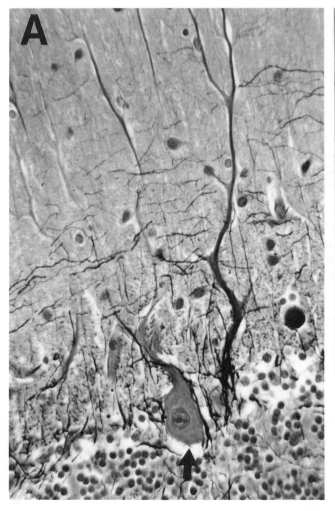

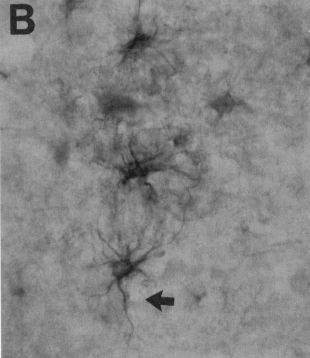

Figure 3–1. Normal neurons and reactive astrocytes. *Panel A:* A silver preparation of cerebellum demonstrating a Purkinje cell (*arrow*) with a prominent nucleus and nucleolus. Many straight, thin axons are seen. *Panel B:* An immunocytochemical stain of reactive astrocytes using antibodies to glial fibrillary acidic protein (GFAP). These astrocytes have many long, thin processes and variable amounts of cytoplasm (*arrow*).

Katzman et al. 1988). The severity of histopathological alterations, lesion location, and other cumulative brain damage is also important.

Neuronal Alteration in Aging: The Hippocampus as a Model

Normal Intrinsic Hippocampal Connections

The structural and functional homology of hippocampus across mammalian species makes it an excellent model (Rosene and Van Hoesen 1986) to study age-related damage occurring with senescence in humans. This allocortical structure (i.e., three-layered cortex) and adjacent parahippocampal cortices are consistently damaged in aging and disease (Figure 3–2, *panel A*) (Braak and Braak 1991; Hyman et al. 1984).

The hippocampus and associated parahippocampal cortices span 3–5 cm of the mesial temporal lobe (Figure 3–2, *panels A and B*). The hippocampal formation is important for short-term memory, and transmission through this allocortical structure proceeds in an orderly fashion (Figure 3–2, *panel C*). Afferent inputs, originating from the superficial entorhinal cortex, synapse on dendrites of granule cells in the molecular layer of the dentate gyrus (Figures 3–2 and 3–3). Transmission proceeds to the CA$_4$-CA$_3$ region via mossy fibers (Figure 3–2) and then to the CA$_1$-subiculum via axons termed the *Schaffer collaterals*. Information is relayed out to the deeper layers of the entorhinal cortex and to neocortical regions such as the temporal lobe (Figure 3–3). Important basal forebrain cholinergic inputs project to the dentate gyrus (Decker 1987) and synapse on the dendrites of granule cells in the molecular layer (Rosene and Van Hoesen 1986). Noradrenergic and serotonergic fibers project onto neurons in the CA$_4$ through CA$_1$ (Powers et al. 1988; Rosene and Van Hoesen 1986). Adrenergic and serotonergic receptors are present in hippocampus, and rodent studies show these catecholamines will facilitate or synchronize hippocampal transmission (Rosene and Von Hoesen 1986). GABAergic[1] and peptidergic neurons are present in CA$_4$ and provide inhibitory transmission. Proper hippocampal function depends on a balance of these excitatory, inhibitory, and neuromodulatory transmitters (Figure 3–2, *panel C*).

Cellular Hippocampal Alterations With Normal Aging

A range of neuronal alterations occurs in hippocampus of aged human brains. For example, the number of granule cell neurons in the dentate gyrus (Figure

---

[1] GABA = γ-aminobutyric acid.

Figure 3–2. *(at right)* The gross and microscopic appearance of hippocampus from elderly control subjects and an individual with Alzheimer's disease. A schematic drawing depicts hippocampal neuronal pathways. (See Figure 3–3 for the cytoarchitectonics discussed here.) *Panel A:* Comparison of temporal lobes and hippocampi (*arrows*) from an elderly control subject (*upper*) and a subject with Alzheimer's disease (*lower*). A normal hippocampus and inferior horn of lateral ventricle are seen in the control subject. The Alzheimer's disease subject has atrophy of the hippocampus, widening of the collateral sulcus, and ventriculomegaly. *Panel B:* A low-magnification photomicrograph of a normal hippocampus stained with cresyl violet. Important anatomical regions include dentate gyrus (d), the Cornu Ammonis (Ammons horn [CA$_4$ through CA$_1$]), the subiculum (SUB), entorhinal cortex (ERC), parahippocampal cortex (P) aside the collateral sulcus (CS), and fimbria (f). This hippocampus is depicted in *panel C.* The granule cell layer is part of the dentate gyrus. Boundaries between the four fields CA$_4$ through CA$_1$ are determined by microscopic examination. *Panel C:* Schematic drawing of hippocampus depicting the complicated neuronal interactions in a typical 65-year-old human. Inputs from ERC neurons synapse on granule cell dendrites in the molecular layer (ML) of the dentate (intact afferents). Axons (mossy fibers) from the granule cells (GCL) synapse on CA$_4$–CA$_3$ neurons that project to CA$_1$-subiculum neurons via Schaffer collateral axons. Neurons in CA$_1$-subiculum complete the loop with axons that synapse on neurons in ERC or temporal cortex. Each granule cell neuron is receiving many types of inputs from intact (IA) and damaged afferents (DA), from temporal cortices (e.g., from neurons in ERC), aminergic inputs from noradrenaline- or serotonin-producing neurons in brain stem (AI), cholinergic inputs from basal forebrain neurons, trophic factors (TF) such as nerve growth factor, and inhibitory inputs (II) such as γ-aminobutyric acid (GABA). Age-related decrease or loss of each type of input can affect granule cell firing and synaptic density. The vacant dendritic fields of some damaged granule cells may be partially occupied by dendritic sprouting (S) from adjacent healthy granule cells. Age-related loss of neurons in CA$_1$ region or subiculum (Sub) will eliminate targets for axons from CA$_3$ neurons. Loss of neurons in deep layers of ERC will disrupt outflow from CA$_1$-subicular neurons. Hippocampal neurons and astrocytes (A) also respond to alterations of blood-brain barrier resulting from vascular damage (BV) such as arteriolar sclerosis. F = fimbria.

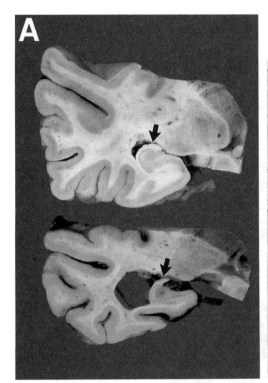

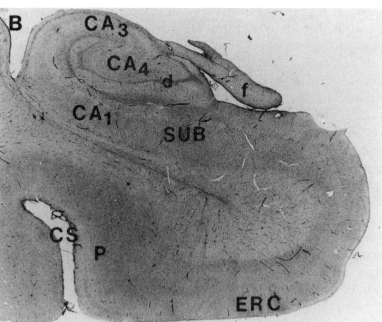

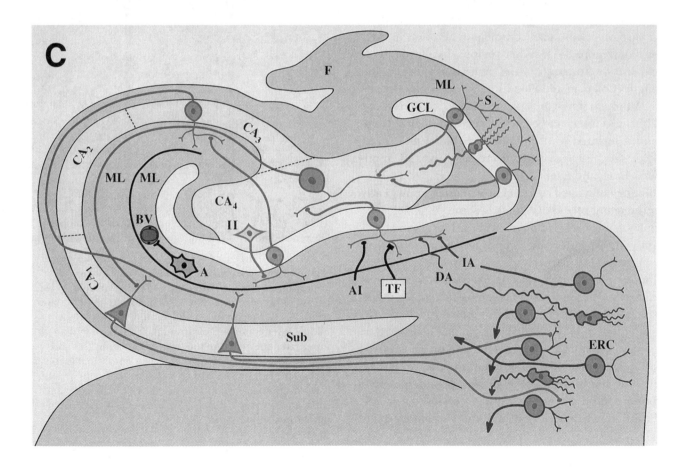

3–2) is reduced by 15% when counts from young subjects (21–56 years) are compared to those of older subjects (69–91 years) (Dam 1979), and these small neurons provide a useful model for age-related changes (Figure 3–2). The dendritic tree of granule cells increases in 50- to 70-year-old humans and declines in the very old (those over 90) or those with Alzheimer's disease (Flood and Coleman 1988). This proliferation may reflect attempts by intact granule cell neurons to compensate for the senescent loss of neighboring neurons (Flood et al. 1985). Loss of inputs from neurons in entorhinal cortex results in sprouting by axons from other afferent neurons to fill the vacant synapses. Collateral axons develop from cholinergic neurons, intrinsic hippocampal neurons, and neurons of other temporal lobe areas (Geddes and Cotman 1991). Dendritic extent in the neighboring CA3-CA2 region shows no change with aging (Figure 3–3), although neuronal loss occurs at 5.4% per decade from age 50 through 90 years (Ball 1977). Dendritic length of CA1 neurons may also remain constant in normal aging but is significantly shortened in Alzheimer's disease (Hanks and Flood 1991). Loss of neurons may provoke gliosis (i.e., increased numbers of astrocytes with more conspicuous amounts of cytoplasm) (Figure 3–1). Other regions, like frontal cortex, will demonstrate a net reduction of dendritic length (Coleman and Flood 1987) in subjects over age 65. Although senescent changes in synaptic density are difficult to interpret because of methodological problems associated with quantitation (Ball 1986), most reports suggest age-related decreases in synaptic numbers (Haug and Eggers 1991).

The entorhinal cortex neurons sustain injury early in the aging process (Figures 3–2 and 3–3). Selective injury to one group of neurons in the hippocampal circuit can disconnect the hippocampus, a mechanism proposed in Alzheimer's disease (Hyman et al. 1984). Cholinergic, serotonergic, and noradrenergic inputs can be lost early as a result of damage to neurons in the basal forebrain (Decker 1987), raphe, or locus coeruleus (Table 3–1). Intrinsic hippocampal neurons that employ excitatory amino acids can be damaged by neurofibrillary tangles, ischemic injury, or other processes. Intrinsic inhibitory GABAergic and peptidergic neurons are also damaged by these processes, disturbing the inherent balance of excitatory and inhibitory trans-

mission. While this process of neuronal injury and death proceeds, undamaged hippocampal neurons attempt reinnervation and reorganization (Figure 3–2, *panel C*).

Age-related alterations in hippocampus demonstrate the complicated cellular events associated with aging. Hippocampal circuits are important because they are severely damaged in a range of neurodegenerative disorders (e.g., Alzheimer's and Pick's diseases) (Hyman et al. 1984). Subtle anoxic brain injury causes hippocampal neuronal ischemic damage or loss.[2] The resulting damage provides a simple model for aging of more complex circuits in neocortical regions.

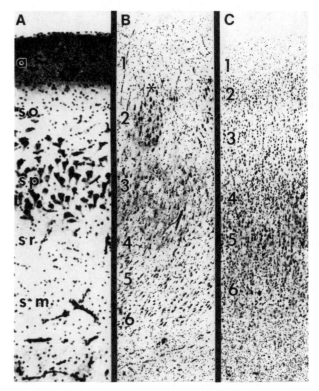

Figure 3–3. Three types of cortex seen in human mesial temporal lobe. (See Figure 3–2 for the macroscopic appearance.) *Panel A:* Three-layered cortex from the CA3 region of hippocampus. This allocortex has an outer layer consisting of the alveus (a) and stratum oriens (so), a middle layer composed of pyramidal cells (sp), and an inner layer composed of the stratum radiatum (sr) and stratum moleculare (sm). *Panel B:* The entorhinal cortex, a transition region from 3-layered to 6-layered cortex. Neurons in layer 2 (*star*) are damaged early in aging and Alzheimer's disease. *Panel C:* Six-layered isocortex in the parahippocampal gyrus.

---

[2] See Figure 3–10, *panel H.*

Structural Brain Alterations in Aging

Changes in Gross Anatomy

Normal adult human brain volume varies by approximately 15% (Haug 1987) for given age groups. The average brain weight of a healthy man at age 65 is 1,360 grams and at age 90 1,290 grams (Dekaban and Sadowsky 1978). Although the female brain is typically 150 grams lighter than the male brain, both sexes have equal numbers of neurons (Haug 1987; Haug and Eggers 1991). Rates of atrophy are similar among the sexes (Kemper 1984), although men have larger lateral ventricles than do women (Table 3–2) (Kaye et al. 1992).

Visible atrophy of the human brain typically is apparent (to the neuropathologist) between ages 60 and 65, although brain weight begins to decline after age 30 and cellular changes occur between ages 40 and 50 (Figure 3–4). Dura mater, the fibrous covering of the brain that contains the venous system and the arachnoid granulations, thickens and ossifies with age.

The volume of the frontal lobes decreases approximately 10% with aging, and white matter is reduced 11% when brain volumes from younger subjects (20–40 years) are compared with those of elderly subjects (75–85 years) (Haug and Eggers 1991). This atrophy expands the subarachnoid space, increases the length of bridging veins spanning from the cerebral hemisphere to the sagittal sinus, and may account for the higher rate of subdural hematomas in elderly people

(Adams and Duchen 1992). Little is known about the senescent changes in the production, circulation, and resorption of cerebrospinal fluid (CSF) despite the occurrence of normal pressure hydrocephalus in older subjects (Katzman 1978) (Figure 3–5).

Cerebral cortical volume is reduced in aging based on premortem image analysis estimates (see Chapter 9) and postmortem studies. Brain volume peaks in the second or third decade and begins a gradual decline that is readily apparent after age 60 (Haug and Eggers

Table 3–2. Comparisons of age- and disease-related alterations usually present in brains of elderly (65 years or older) people

Pathology	Cortical alterations in elderly, cognitively intact subjects	Cortical alterations in Alzheimer's disease subjects
Atrophy and/or ventriculomegaly	0–2+	0–3+
Senile plaques	0–2+	3+
Neurofibrillary tangles	0–1+	0–3+
Presence of A68 (Alz-50) epitope[a]	0–3+	2+ –3+
Presence of amyloid	0–2+	1+ –3+
Cholinergic deficit	0–1+	2+ –3+

Note. 0 = none; 1+ = mild or few; 2+ = moderate; 3+ = severe or many.
[a]Epitope as determined by immunocytochemical staining of neurons, neuropil, neurites, and senile plaques.
Sources. From Blessed et al. 1968; Katzman et al. 1988; Matsuyama and Nakamura 1978; J. L. Price et al. 1991; Ulrich 1982.

Table 3–1. Alterations in the number of neurons in selected brain regions of individuals over age 65

Location of neuronal count	Brain region	Change in neuronal count	Studies
Cortex	Middle frontal gyrus	28%–40% decrease in large neurons	Terry et al. 1987
		None to 28% increase in small neurons	Coleman and Flood 1987
	Calcarine (area 17)	None	Haug and Eggers 1991
Hippocampus	Ammon's horn	19%–43% decrease	Dam 1979
Subcortical	Nucleus basalis of Meynert	None to 50% decrease	Whitehouse et al. 1981; Coleman and Flood 1987; de Lacalle et al. 1991
Cerebellum	Purkinje cell layer	10%–40% decrease	Hall et al. 1975
Brain stem	Substantia nigra	35% decrease	McGeer et al. 1977
	Locus coeruleus	40% decrease	Mann et al. 1983; Vijayashankar and Brody 1977
	Inferior olivary complex	None to 20% decrease	Moatamed 1966; Coleman and Flood 1987

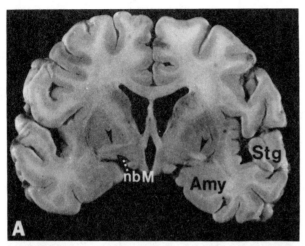

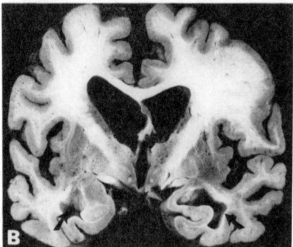

1991). *Atrophy* is defined as widening of sulci and narrowing of gyri (Figures 3–6, 3–7, and 3–8). Frontal (Figure 3–6), parasagittal, and temporal lobe atrophy are present in both aging and Alzheimer's disease (Figure 3–9) (Blessed et al. 1968; Kemper 1984; Tomlinson et al. 1970). Severe cortical atrophy is quite rare in cognitively intact individuals (Table 3–2); however, mild to moderate ventriculomegaly is sometimes present (Figure 3–4) (Blessed et al. 1968; Kemper 1984; Tomlinson et al. 1970). The volumes of basal ganglia and thalamus are reduced by approximately 20% in aging (Haug et al. 1983); however, the volume of parieto-occipital region remains constant (Eggers et al. 1984) when comparing brains from young individuals (20–40 years) with those from people over age 75.

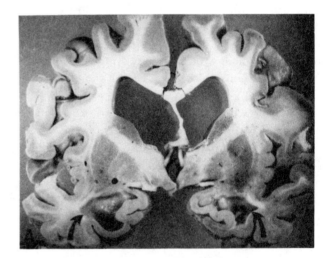

Figure 3–4. The coronal sections of normal (*panel A*) and atrophic (*panel B*) brain. *Panel A:* The brain from a 67-year-old control subject with minimal atrophy and normal ventricle size. The anterior commissure is highlighted by *arrow heads,* and the nucleus basalis of Meynert (nbM) is seen immediately beneath the anterior commissure (*arrow*). Normal appearing amygdala (Amy) and superior temporal gyrus (Stg) are present. The third ventricle is normal in size, and hypothalamic nuclei are located immediately adjacent to the third ventricle. Histological examination of this brain showed occasional senile plaques. *Panel B:* A coronal brain section from a 70-year-old subject with Alzheimer's disease demonstrating atrophy, ventriculomegaly, and dilation of the lateral sulci. The inferior horns of the lateral ventricles (*arrows*) and lateral ventricles are dilated. The hippocampus and amygdala are reduced in volume. The third ventricle is moderately dilated. Histological examination of this brain showed numerous senile plaques, neurofibrillary tangles, and neuronal loss.

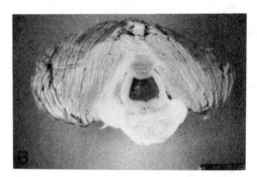

Figure 3–5. A coronal section of brain (*panel A*) and horizontal sections of brain stem (*panel B*) from a 72-year-old man with normal pressure hydrocephalus. This man had ataxia, dementia, and incontinence. All ventricles, including inferior horn of lateral ventricles (*arrows*), lateral, third, and fourth, are markedly dilated. This brain had a normal histological appearance. Normal lateral and third ventricles are seen in Figure 3–4, *panel A.*

Cellular Changes in Aging

The cellular substrate of brain volume reduction is obscure. Atrophy may result from a net loss of neurons and fibers, but quantitative data are inconclusive. The human brain contains approximately 13.9 billion neurons (Haug and Eggers 1991). Although early studies described generalized senescent neuronal loss (Brody 1955), recent reports have shown relatively stable numbers of cortical neurons in many brain regions as compared with younger subjects (Haug and Eggers 1991). Hippocampal and subcortical neurons are depleted in subjects over age 65 (Table 3–2) (Coleman and Flood 1987; Katzman et al. 1988). These discrepancies may result from methodological problems, such as variations of sampling, and shrinkage artifact. Several authors (Haug 1987; Haug and Eggers 1991; Haug et al. 1984) have demonstrated reduction of neuronal perikaryal diameter and diminished cortical thickness, but stable numbers of neurons (Tables 3–2 and 3–3). This neuronal atrophy is reported to begin around age 60 by most investigators and may be layer specific. For example, neurons in layer 3 of gyrus rectus (Figure 3–8) are shrunken, but those in layer 5 remain constant in subjects over age 65 (Haug et al. 1984). Neuronal atrophy is reported after age 40 in a few cortical regions, such as area 6 (Haug and Eggers 1991). Neuronal shrinkage may explain the net increase in the numbers of small neurons with aging (i.e., shrunken large neurons are counted with small neurons) (Finch 1993). There is variable reduction in the number of synapses in aging. Haug and Eggers (1991) cited stable numbers of synapses in area 6 but diminished (10%) numbers in area 11 (gyrus rectus) of subjects over 65.

Reduction in the volume of neurons may be offset by a net increase in the number or volume of astrocytes (Table 3–3). Studies in rodent and human have demonstrated increased glial fibrillary acidic protein (Figure 3–1), an intermediate filament specific for astrocytes, and increased glial markers (e.g., glutamate synthetase) (Finch and Morgan 1990; Frederickson 1992). However, some authors have described a mini-

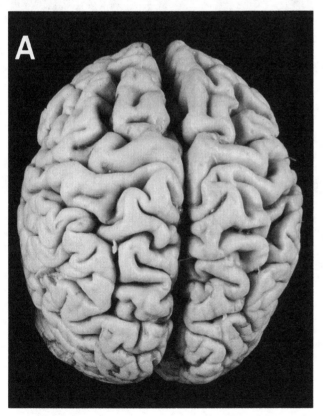
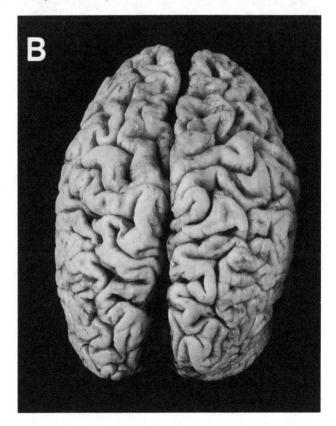

Figure 3–6. Mild atrophy seen in the brain of an 82-year-old control subject compared with severe atrophy in the brain of an 81-year-old Alzheimer's disease subject (see also Figures 3–7 and 3–8). The superior surfaces of both brains are shown with frontal poles facing inferiorly. The control brain (*panel A*) weighs 1,150 grams and has mild atrophy in the frontal lobes (e.g., widening of bilateral superior frontal sulci) and normal occipital lobes. The Alzheimer's disease brain (*panel B*) weighs 960 grams and has diffuse reduction in the gyral volume, as well as widening of the sulci.

mal increase in astrocytic numbers in aging (Haug and Eggers 1991; Haug et al. 1984). Oligodendrocytes have not been studied in aging. Blood vessels do not change in number or diameter with aging, although senescent changes in the blood-brain barrier occur with alterations of tight junctions (Haug and Eggers 1991). Detailed counts are not available for microglia in the brains of elderly human subjects.

Molecular Neuropathology of Aging

Aging neurons undergo a series of histological and molecular biological changes (Figure 3–10). Lipofuscin, a brown, wear-and-tear pigment, begins to accum-

ulate within neuronal bodies. Neuromelanin, a brown pigment common to catecholamine-producing neurons, becomes visible in the brains of adolescent humans and progressively accumulates over years (Graham 1979). Neuronal inclusions, such as Hirano bodies, and granulovacular degeneration begin to appear in hippocampal pyramidal neurons (Figure 3–10). Lewy bodies are seen usually in catecholamine-producing neurons and occasionally in cortical neurons (Figure 3–10). Corpora amylacea, dense spherical inclusions, appear around the ventricles and in the neuropil, where they are numerous in aging and neurodegenerative disorders (Adams and Duchen 1992).

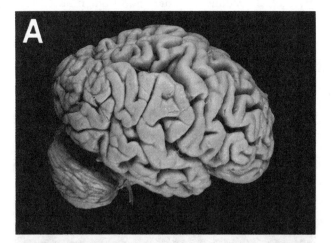

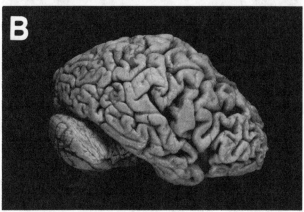

Figure 3–7. Mild atrophy seen in the brain of an 82-year-old control subject compared with severe atrophy in the brain of an 81-year-old Alzheimer's disease subject (see also Figures 3–6 and 3–8). The right lateral views of the control brain (*panel A*) and the Alzheimer's disease (*panel B*) brain are shown. The frontal gyri are mildly atrophic in the control brain and markedly atrophic in the Alzheimer's disease brain. The lateral sulcus is dilated in the Alzheimer's disease brain.

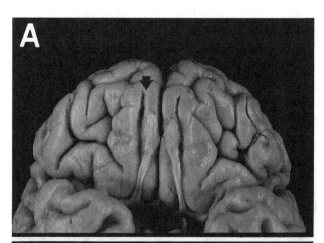

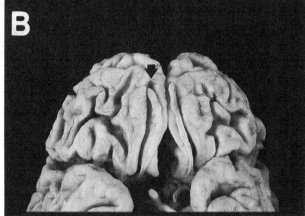

Figure 3–8. Mild atrophy seen in brain of an 82-year-old control subject compared with severe atrophy in brain of an 81-year-old Alzheimer's disease subject (see also Figures 3–6 and 3–7). The orbitofrontal regions of the control brain (*panel A*) and the Alzheimer's disease brain (*panel B*) are shown. The orbitofrontal gyri and olfactory nerves (immediately adjacent the gyrus rectus) are markedly shrunken in the Alzheimer's disease brain, but mildly reduced in the control brain (*arrows*).

The neuronal cytoskeleton undergoes important, age-related alterations. The cytoskeleton is the delicate meshwork of microtubules, neurofilaments, and other proteins (e.g., microtubule-associated proteins). This matrix, barely visualized with the electron microscope, provides structure to neurons and participates in transport. The cytoskeleton is a dynamic system constantly cycling through production, transport, and degradation (Peng et al. 1986). Age-related alteration of axonal transport in human neurons is unknown, but slow transport is decreased by 30% in aged rodent brain (Finch and Morgan 1990). The production of antibodies to specific cytoskeletal antigenic sites (i.e., epitopes) allows the identification of molecular constituents within neurons. Immunocytochemical methods show collection of abnormal cytoskeletal constituents in neurons of human neocortex and allocortex in the fifth or sixth decade (Figure 3–11) prior to developing neurofibrillary tangles (Figure 3–12).

For example, phosphorylated neurofilament epitope is normally present in the axon but not in the neuronal perikarya (Goldman and Yen 1986). Immunocytochemical methods demonstrate accumulation of phosphorylated neurofilament epitope in the body of aging neurons. Cytoskeleton is the major constituent of most age- and disease-related histopathology. Hirano bodies contain actin (Goldman 1983), granulovacuolar degenerations contain tubulin (Maurer et al.

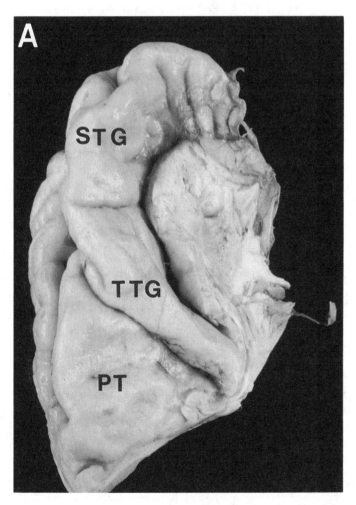
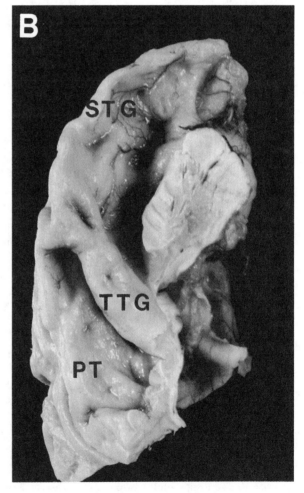

Figure 3–9. Comparison of the supratemporal plane (STP) of an 82-year-old control subject (*panel A*) with that of a patient with Alzheimer's disease (*panel B*). The temporal poles are oriented upward, and the superior surface of dissected temporal lobes are shown. The three main components of the supratemporal plane include the superior temporal gyrus (STG), the transverse temporal gyrus (TTG), and the planum temporale (PT); and these appear normal in *panel A*. The supratemporal plane from the Alzheimer's disease subject demonstrates severe atrophy of superior temporal gyrus (auditory association cortex); however, transverse temporal gyrus (primary receptive cortex) is less severely shrunken. Association cortex is preferentially damaged in Alzheimer's disease over primary sensory cortex.

1990), Lewy bodies contain filaments (Goldman et al. 1983), dystrophic neurites contain paired helical filament and tau, and neurofibrillary tangles contain many cytoskeletal constituents (Figures 3–11 and 3–12) (Goldman and Yen 1986; Maurer et al. 1990). Tau, a low molecular weight, microtubule-associated protein, is present in most forms of age- and disease-related microscopic pathology (Figure 3–11) (Kowall and Kosik 1987). Selected abnormal proteins also begin to appear in the aged brains. Epitopes of the A68 protein, recognized by the Alz-50 antibody, are not present in young control subjects (Hyman et al. 1988; Nukina et al. 1988). This epitope begins to appear in neurons of elderly, non-dementia subjects and is abundant in the brains of Alzheimer's disease subjects (Carlsson 1990; Giaquinto 1988). Amyloid protein precursor appears in neurons and blood vessels of cognitively intact elderly subjects (Coria et al. 1992). Amyloid deposits are frequently present in brains of elderly control subjects (Braak and Braak 1991).

Aging and Genomic Function

Alteration of the human genome plays an undefined role in the natural history of aging; however, genetics is involved in selected neurodegenerative disorders. The genetic locus for the β-amyloid precursor protein is on chromosome 21 (Kosik 1992; Mattson and Rydel 1992), as is the marker for familial Alzheimer's disease and Down's syndrome. Patients with Down's syndrome frequently develop accelerated Alzheimer's disease, and familial Alzheimer's disease is an autosomal dominant disorder that maps to chromosome 14 or 21. These observations demonstrate the role of genetics in age-related disease.

The role of genetic regulation on human brain aging is unclear, as is the effect of aging on genetic function. Most research is conducted in rodents because methodological obstacles limit the study of DNA and RNA from human brain tissues. Messenger RNAs for many proteins are present in low abundance and are difficult to study in all species (Finch et al. 1990). Integrity of genomic function depends on accuracy of base pair sequences, as well as on histone content, three-dimensional conformation, methylation states, and multiple other biochemical variables that affect the accuracy and speed of genetic transcription. Nongenomic DNA (i.e., mitochondrial) has no repair

Table 3–3. Neuronal and astrocytic alterations usually present in neocortex of aged human brain as compared with young brain

Measurement	Neuron	Astrocyte
Cell number	NC or decrease	NC or increase
Cytoplasmic volume	Increase or decrease	Increase
Nucleus size	Decrease	Increase
RNA content	Decrease	?

Note. NC = no significant change; ? = definitive data unavailable.
Sources. From Coleman and Flood 1987; Finch 1993; Finch and Morgan 1990; Haug 1987; Haug and Eggers 1991; Haug et al. 1983.

Figure 3–10. *(on following 2 pages)* Eight hematoxylin and eosin preparations showing microscopic alterations frequently observed in the brains of elderly humans, including lipofuscin (*panel A*), ischemic neuronal injury (*panel B*), Hirano bodies (*panel C*), granulovacular degenerations (*panel D*), Lewy bodies (*panel E*), loss of neuromelanin-containing neurons (*panel F*), atherosclerosis (*panel G*), and arteriosclerosis (*panel H*). *Panel A:* Several neurons are shown. Two (*straight arrows*) contain abundant lipofuscin, a light-brown pigment. A normal neuron with abundant Nissl substance is present (*curved arrow*). *Panel B:* Photomicrograph of human hippocampus from a 68-year-old cognitively intact individual who had brief hypoxia. Normal neurons surround a single shrunken pyramidal neuron in the center of the field with ischemic, eosinophilic degeneration (*arrow*). *Panel C:* Hirano bodies in hippocampal neurons from CA1 region. A Hirano body, the cigar-shaped, eosinophilic rod immediately adjacent to the nucleus, is seen in the center of the field (*arrow*). *Panel D:* Granulovacuolar degenerations in the pyramidal neurons of CA3 region. In the cytoplasm of the neuron in the center of the field, there are multiple round, clear spaces with a central, slightly basophilic core (*arrow*). *Panel E:* Lewy bodies, circular eosinophilic masses with a thin, peripheral clear space (*arrow*) that displaces the neuromelanin, in the cytoplasm of substantia nigra neurons. Neurons that contain neuromelanin are also present. *Panel F:* Age-related damage of substantia nigra. Two normal-appearing pigmented neurons are shown (*arrows*); however, most neuromelanin is present in macrophages or in the neuropil (*arrowheads*). *Panel G:* Atherosclerotic damage in a branch of the posterior cerebral artery. The intima is detached and badly damaged with cholesterol deposition (CD), but the media is intact. *Panel H:* Arteriosclerosis in basal ganglia from a 74-year-old hypertensive individual. A small penetrating blood vessel in the center of the field contains pink, hyalinized material in the media and adventitia.

Richard C. Josiassen, Ph.D.
MCP / EPPI
Department of Psychiatry
3200 Henry Avenue
Philadelphia, PA 19129

mechanisms and may also undergo senescent changes. Studies in rodent and primate suggest that aging may alter DNA base pair sequence, genetic repair mechanisms, mRNA metabolism, posttranslational modifica-

tion, protein biochemistry, and axonal transport.

Some theories suggest that aging results from multiple genomic errors accumulated over time. Experimental models involving irradiated animals or others

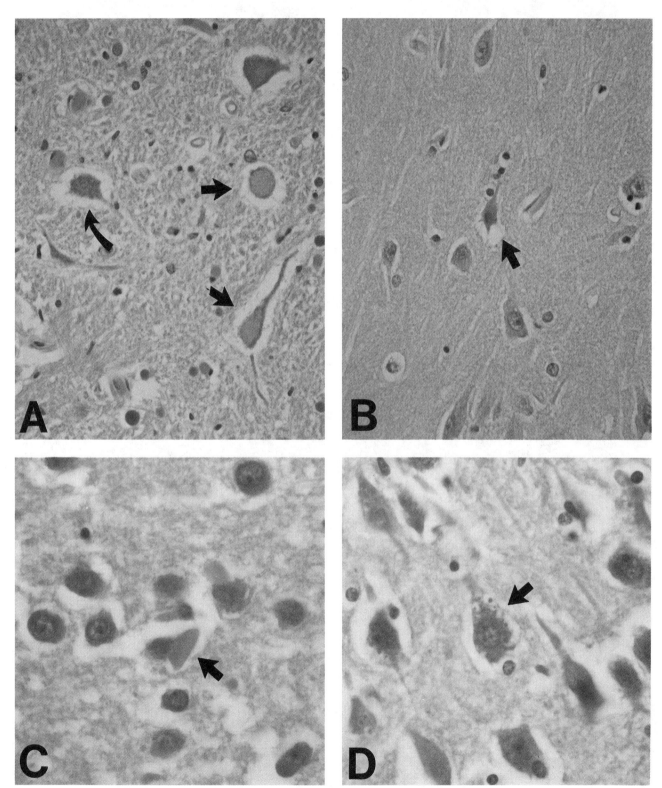

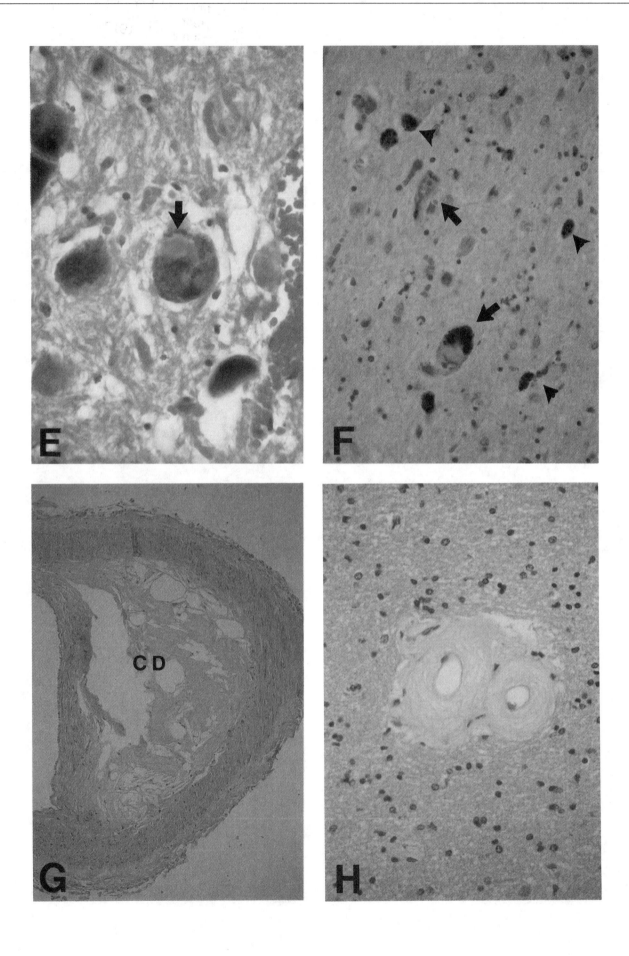

exposed to mutagens fail to show accelerated aging (Hayflick 1985). Age-related reactivation of X-linked genes may increase the expression in females of steroid sulfatase and monoamine oxidase–A (MOA-A) (Wareham et al. 1987). Age-related demethylation of 5-methyldeoxycitidine may also occur in aging. Studies in aged rodent DNA show age-dependent change of excision repair and reduction of single strand break repair (Niedermüller et al. 1985).

Brain RNA content changes with age. The RNA repertoire is not drastically altered with aging; however, selected RNAs are increased or decreased (Finch and Morgan 1990). For instance, the abundance of pro-opiomelanocortin mRNA decreases by 30% in aged rodents, whereas luteinizing hormone-releasing hormone production remains constant (Finch and Morgan 1990). Total RNA content and poly(A)-RNA do not significantly change in aged rodent or primate brain, but selected human RNA is increased, such as tachykinin message in hypothalamus (Rance and Young 1991). Reductions of nuclear or nucleolar size in neurons of elderly humans suggest diminished gene or RNA activity. Selected human neuronal populations have reductions in nuclear and nucleolar volumes that reflect perikaryal atrophy (Tables 3–2 and 3–3). Nucleolar shrinkage may result from decreased transcription of ribosomal RNA cistrons and diminished assembly of ribosomes. Neuron populations damaged by neurofibrillary tangles have reduced RNA metabolism as well (Doebler et al. 1987).

Studies in aged rodents show slowing of protein synthesis and axonal transport. Increased amounts of conformationally altered, inactive enzymes accumulate in aged rodents; however, similar data in human neurons are unavailable (Finch and Morgan 1990; Ingvar et al. 1985). Some proteins are produced by both astrocytes and neurons. The interpretation of neuronal protein content is complicated by age- and disease-related increases in the numbers of astrocytes (Frederickson 1992). For example, stability in the number of β-adrenergic receptors in aged rodents may reflect diminished numbers of neuronal receptors counterbalanced by increased numbers of astrocytes with this molecule. The increased number of astrocytes in aged human brain may obscure similar alterations (Finch and Morgan 1990).

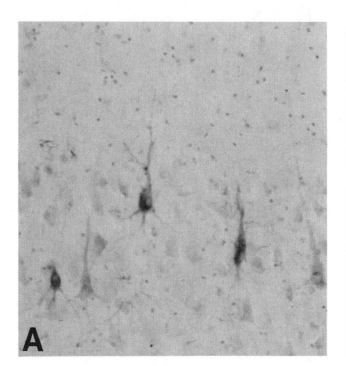
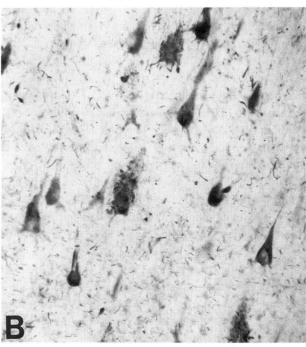

Figure 3–11.   Immunocytochemical preparations of hippocampal cortex with anti-tau antibodies. *Panel A:* This preparation is counterstained with cresyl violet and shows normal-appearing, immunostained (brown-colored) neurons that are accumulating tau epitope. Normal neurons are not stained. *Panel B:* A similar preparation of the same area from an Alzheimer's disease subject. Numerous neuronal cell bodies, neurofibrillary tangles, and dystrophic neurites (i.e., thick, swollen processes) are immunostained with anti-tau antibodies.

Information about senescent changes in human genome and protein synthesis is limited. Morphological assessments and molecular biological techniques suggest age-related reductions of DNA and RNA function in some neuronal populations or increased expression of selected genes in others. Further research is necessary to clarify this complicated scientific picture. However, molecular biological probes demonstrate great promise in distinguishing normal aging from senescent disease.

Pathological Overlap of Aging and Alzheimer's Disease

The pathological hallmarks of Alzheimer's disease include senile plaques, neurofibrillary tangles, and amyloid deposits (McKhann et al. 1984). Senile plaques are abnormal collections of neurites, microglia, and astrocytes that disrupt the normal woven appearance of the neuropil (Figure 3–12). Senile plaques have a range of features and may contain amyloid deposits or cores (Figure 3–12). The appearance of senile plaques ranges from "immature" (i.e., amorphous amyloid deposits) to "burned-out" with few remaining neurites (Probst et al. 1987) and amyloid cores. Neuritic plaques contain many dystrophic neurites and glia. Neurofibrillary tangles are masses of abnormal straight and paired helical filaments (Figure 3–12). Neurofibrillary tangles are usually located within neuronal perikarya, although "ghost" tangles are seen in the neuropil. Amyloid deposits include beta pleated sheets of fibrillar material composed partially of beta protein (A4), the cleavage product of beta amyloid precursor protein, a large transmembrane protein (Mattson and Rydel 1992). Amyloid deposition occurs in aging or Alzheimer's disease (Braak and Braak 1991; Ikeda et al. 1989) and is present around blood vessels, in senile plaques and in the neuropil. The role of amyloid in aging and disease is controversial and is the focus of considerable research.

Dystrophic neurites are swollen, tortuous neuronal processes that contain multiple cytoskeletal constituents including tau and paired helical filaments (Figure 3–11). It is unknown whether neurites are axons or dendrites, nor whether they are degenerative or regenerative. Neurites contain many types of neurotransmitters (Powers et al. 1988; Struble et al. 1987)

and are seen in aging and Alzheimer's disease (Braak and Braak 1991; Braak et al. 1986).

Lewy bodies, spherical neuronal inclusions with an eosinophilic core and clear halo, are composed of neurofilaments (Figure 3–10, *panel E*) (Goldman et al. 1983). Lewy bodies are present in catecholamine-producing neurons in normal aging (Giaquinto 1988), as well as in diseases such as idiopathic parkinsonism and Lewy body dementia.[3]

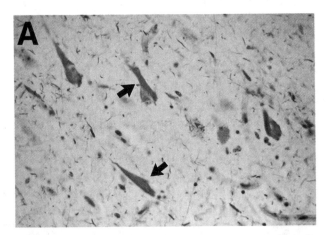

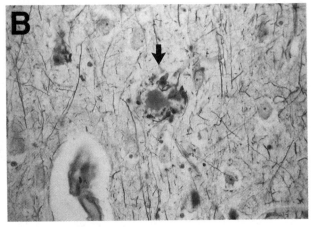

Figure 3–12. Photomicrographs showing the appearance of neurofibrillary tangles (*panel A*) and senile plaques (*panel B*) in a 100-year-old subject. *Panel A:* Four hippocampal pyramidal neurons with neurofibrillary tangles (i.e., flame-shaped masses of filamentous material [*arrows*]). Tangles were not present in neocortex. *Panel B:* A silver preparation of neocortex. A senile plaque (*arrow*) contains swollen neurites, an amyloid core, glia, and microglia. Insufficient numbers were present in neocortex to warrant Alzheimer's disease diagnosis.

_____

[3]See Figure 3–14.

National Institute for Neurological and Communicative Disorders and Stroke (NINCDS) criteria for Alzheimer's disease are consensus values that are based on age-adjusted numbers of senile plaques per square millimeter in the neocortex (McKhann et al. 1984). Senile plaque counts in the hippocampus are not used because the hippocampus is frequently damaged in normal aging. In fact, mesial temporal cortex is damaged in the early stages of Alzheimer's disease (Braak and Braak 1991) and is a brain region in which the morphological features of aging and disease frequently overlap (Figure 3–2).

An important exception to the NINCDS criteria for Alzheimer's disease is a group of cognitively intact elderly individuals with large numbers of senile plaques in neocortex (Katzman et al. 1988). Further, the small group of elderly dementia subjects with morphologically normal brains also demonstrates the limitations of histopathological assessments (Heilig et al. 1985).

Several studies have shown that cognitively intact elderly patients can have numerous senile plaques, occasional neurofibrillary tangles (Figure 3–12), amyloid deposits, and many neurons immunoreactive with Alz-50 antisera (Crystal et al. 1988; Katzman et al. 1988; J. L. Price et al. 1991). Matsuyama (see Matsuyama and Nakamura 1978) demonstrated an age-dependent increase in the intensity of Alzheimer's disease pathology in brains from a large retrospective study of 897 Japanese subjects who had no history of neurological disease. In a retrospective study of neurologically intact patients ages 55 to 64, Ulrich (1982) demonstrated Alzheimer's disease-type pathology in 25% of brains. Katzman et al. (1988) described a small percentage (10%) of cognitively intact elderly individuals who met NINCDS histopathological criteria for Alzheimer's disease and had cholinergic deficits.

Neurofibrillary tangles may be a more reliable indicator of brain damage despite a subpopulation of Alzheimer subjects without neurofibrillary degeneration (Terry et al. 1987). No single histopathological, neurochemical, or molecular biological marker always distinguishes normal aging from Alzheimer's disease (Table 3–1); however, some researchers contend that cognitively intact individuals with Alzheimer's disease pathology would have developed clinical symptoms in time. Other scientists contend that some elderly individuals develop nonprogressive injury (i.e., senile plaques) to selected brain regions. This overlap of pathology between aging and Alzheimer's disease explains the difficulty in creating a premortem marker for Alzheimer's disease.

Alterations of White Matter With Aging

The integrity of myelin and oligodendrocytes is important to neural transmission, and alterations of white matter occur in aging. White matter damage occurs in Alzheimer's disease (Brun and Englund 1986), and neuroradiological studies have demonstrated white matter hyperintensities in deep white matter and pons (Coffey et al. 1992).

Autopsy data show an 11% reduction in white matter volume of elderly subjects (Haug and Eggers 1991) that may reflect decreased numbers of axons or reduced volume of myelin. The subtle boundary between cortex and white matter obscures small reductions in the volume of white matter.

Studies in human occipital cortex from ages 30 through 90 reveal a linear, age-dependent myelin loss in the stripe of Gennari (Lintl and Braak 1983). The optic nerve loses more than 5,600 axons per year (Lintl and Braak 1983) from childhood through senescence. Morphological data on white matter are limited by methodological problems with measuring the volume of myelin or packing densities of axis cylinders in postmortem material. Magnetic resonance imaging (MRI) may be more sensitive for identifying alterations in the density of white matter than are standard postmortem histological methodologies.

The terminology for white matter alterations depends on imaging methods, is sometimes inconsistent, and includes subcortical hyperintensities, leukoaraiosis (Hachinski et al. 1987), subcortical encephalomalacia, and Binswanger's disease (Figure 3–13) (Coffey and Figiel 1991; Giaquinto 1988). White matter lucencies are reported in 4% to 35% of computed tomography evaluations of elderly individuals and up to 92% of MRI examinations of elderly control subjects (Awad et al. 1986; Coffey et al. 1992). White matter alterations are also present in Alzheimer's disease (Bennett et al. 1992) and in depression (Coffey et al. 1993).

Neuropathological correlates for these radiological white matter lesions range from normal myelin to Binswanger's disease (Figure 3–13) (Coffey and Figiel 1991; Gupta et al. 1988; Kirkpatrick and Hayman 1987; Sze et al. 1986). Hypertensive vascular changes (i.e., arteriosclerosis) is frequently noted (Inzitari et al. 1987) in areas of abnormal white matter. *Arteriosclerosis* is damage to the media of small blood vessels, in contrast to *atherosclerosis,* which is damage to the intima of larger caliber vessels (Figure 3–10). Significant atherosclerosis is uncommon beyond secondary divisions of the cerebral arteries. Arteriosclerosis is hyalinized degeneration of small caliber arteries or arterioles in white matter and basal ganglia and is present in aged human, monkey, and dog. Arteriosclerotic vascular injury may precede lacunar infarctions, which are common in elderly hypertensive patients (Giaquinto 1988). Arteriosclerosis is usually detected by microscopic examination showing loss of brain parenchyma sur-

rounding damaged blood vessels. Brains of patients with Binswanger's disease (Figure 3–13) can be distinguished from other white matter lesions by plaque-like areas of demyelination (Caplan and Schoene 1978). Microscopic examination reveals concentric, obliterative, hyalinized thickening of medium and small caliber blood vessels.

Although the number of brain astrocytes increases with age (Figure 3–1), alterations in the number of oligodendrocytes are not reported. Few studies have examined the composition of myelin and the biological activity of oligodendrocytes in aging human brain.

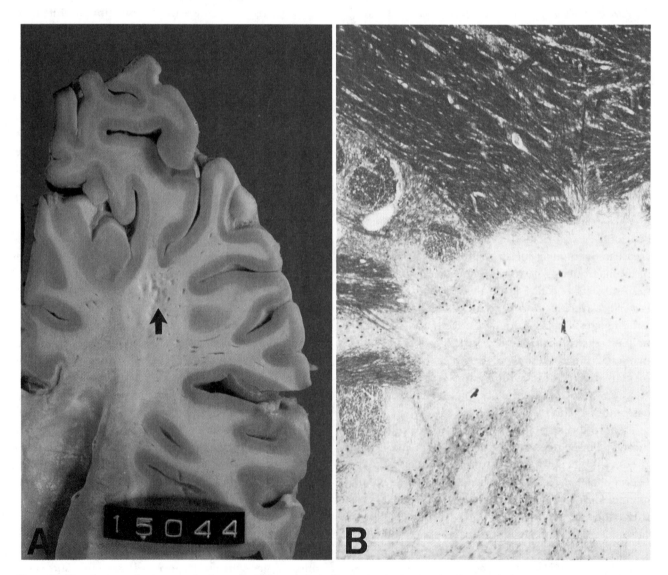

Figure 3–13.   Gross and microscopic damage of Binswanger's disease in the brain of a 62-year-old hypertensive woman. *Panel A:* A horizontal section of brain with multiple punched-out lesions in white matter of the frontal lobe (*arrow*). The cortex appears normal. *Panel B:* A myelin (Luxol fast blue) stain through a periventricular area with a similar lesion. There is discrete loss of blue-staining myelin in areas with severe vascular damage. A brain with leuko-araiosis would show only slight pallor of blue staining.

There is no evidence that aging oligodendrocytes develop degenerative changes (like neurons) or hypertrophy (like astrocytes).

Age-Related Changes of the Blood-Brain Barrier

The blood-brain barrier has two major functions: transport of essential materials and protection of brain homeostasis. The blood-brain barrier is located in the brain's small vessels and consists of tight junctions and fenestration of brain capillary endothelium that use selective pinocytosis. It is the locus of transport for critical nutrients, hormones, and drugs, as well as export of metabolic waste products. The blood-brain barrier's second function is protection against influx of toxins and osmotically damaging agents (Mooradian 1988). Unlike capillaries of non-CNS organs, brain capillary pores do not allow free movement of substances. Carrier-mediated transport in the brain capillaries selects only appropriate substances for entrance into the CNS. This barrier function is mediated by tight junctions between endothelial cells (Giaquinto 1988).

Histochemical studies of brains from human subjects over age 45 show alterations in the biochemical composition of arterioles, capillaries, and venules (Sobin et al. 1992). Aging of brain microvasculature may result in minor leakage through the blood-brain barrier. Human serum proteins, such as IgG, IgA, IgM, and α_2-macroglobulin are leaked into the cortical tissue of elderly subjects and are found in some neurons (Mooradian 1988). Systemic diseases common in the elderly such as hypertension and diabetes mellitus damage the blood-brain barrier. Transport of high molecular weight proteins increases with hypertension and mild ischemia. Blood-brain barrier permeability is increased by brief periods of ischemia through acceleration of transendothelial transport and transcytosis. More severe ischemia worsens this leakage and loosens the tight junctions of endothelium. The significance of blood-brain barrier alterations is unclear, although this damage may contribute to the cumulative injury seen in aging brain.

Alterations of Transmitter Systems in Aging

The impact of aging on transmitter systems can be measured at the presynaptic or postsynaptic level. Presynaptic levels of chemical transmitters can be reduced by death or dysfunction of neurons that produce the transmitter, diminished release, and alterations of reuptake. Postsynaptic effects include alteration of postsynaptic receptor density, alterations of the receptor, and changes in signal transduction mechanisms that translate the receptor activation into cellular or membrane events. It is likely that signal transmission is altered at several levels, confusing the interpretation of human data. Although many human brain transmitter markers are altered in aging, in this chapter, I focus on systems of most importance to the geriatric neuropsychiatrist (Table 3–4).

Cholinergic Systems

Acetylcholine innervation is widely present throughout the mammalian CNS. Most cortical cholinergic fibers originate from neurons in the nucleus basalis of Meynert, a band of large neurons in the basal forebrain that is most conspicuous beneath the anterior commissure (Figure 3–4) (Hedreen et al. 1984; Mesulam and Geula 1988). This band begins anteriorly in the medial septal region and is present posteriorly beneath the basal ganglia. This nucleus has an organized projection to cortex with medial septal neurons projecting to hippocampus.

A plexus of cholinergic fibers is seen in cortex (Divac 1975; Mesulam et al. 1983), and immunocytochemical methodologies with antisera directed against nicotinic receptors demonstrate postsynaptic densities over neurons in layers 2, 3, and 5 (Schröder et al. 1991) of neocortex. Cholinergic fibers are altered in aged humans and primates (Decker 1987), and cholinergic deficits in rodents, primates, and humans are correlated to cognitive impairment (Olton et al. 1991).

It is unclear whether acetylcholine content is significantly reduced in the brains of cognitively intact elderly humans. Although acetylcholinetransferase, the synthetic enzyme for acetylcholine, is reduced in Alzheimer's disease, the data in normal aging are conflicting (Giaquinto 1988; Müller et al. 1991) and demonstrate minimal reductions or no change. This minor senescent cholinergic loss may reflect complex alterations in the number and size of neurons in nucleus basalis of Meynert with aging (Figure 3–4). The diameters of some human forebrain cholinergic neurons increase until age 60. Nucleus basalis of Meynert neurons in elderly humans (over age 60) begin to atrophy, and neuronal loss varies according to region sampled (i.e., 0% in the anterior portion and 65% in posterior subdivisions) (de Lacalle et al. 1991; Finch 1993). A similar sequence of changes is seen in rodent and monkey. The large cholinergic neurons of the nucleus basalis of Meynert are frequently referred to as *magnocellular* and may contain occasional neurofibrillary tangles or Lewy bodies in older human subjects. Aging has a minimal effect on high-affinity choline uptake, the rate-limiting step in the production of acetylcholine (ACh). Levels of acetylcholinesterase are increased in CSF of elderly subjects (Table 3–5) (Hartikainen et al. 1991; Müller et al. 1991).

Cholinergic receptors change with aging (Table 3–4). Release of ACh may be reduced in aging brains because of diminished autoreceptor sensitivity. Many alterations of both muscarinic and nicotinic receptors occur in senescent human brain. There is a 10%–30% reduction of muscarinic receptors in samples of cortex, hippocampus, and striatum and diminished nicotinic receptors in hippocampus. However, in thalamus, there is decreased density of nicotinic receptors, but increased density of muscarinic receptors (Giacobini 1990, 1991). Nicotinic receptors are also reduced in Alzheimer's disease (Nordberg and Winblad 1986).

It is unknown whether the structure of cholinergic receptors is altered in aging and Alzheimer's disease. Genetic messages code for multiple subtypes of muscarinic and nicotinic receptors. The effect of aging on the ratios of receptors and encoding messages is unknown. Studies in rodents demonstrate age-related decrease in receptor plasticity and diminished neural response to ACh stimulation (Giacobini 1990; Müller et al. 1991). Similar studies are not available in human subjects.

Although our knowledge of senescent alterations of cholinergic systems is incomplete, there is a clear relationship between cholinergic deficits and cognitive impairment (Fields et al. 1986). Cholinergic systems

Table 3–5. Age-related alterations of transmitter metabolites reported in human cerebrospinal fluid

Transmitter system	Marker	Effect with age
Cholinergic	Acetylcholinesterase	Increase
Noradrenergic	MHPG	Increase
Serotonergic	5-HIAA	No change
Dopaminergic	Homovanillic acid	No change
Peptidergic	Somatostatin	No change
	β-Endorphin	No change

Note. MHPG = 3-methoxy-4-hydroxyphenylglycol; 5-HIAA = 5-hydroxyindoleacetic acid.
Sources. From Giaquinto 1988; Gottfries 1990; Hartikainen et al. 1991.

Table 3–4. Senescent changes of selected cholinergic and catecholaminergic markers usually present in aged human brain

Transmitter	Location of neurons	Senescent change in neuronal numbers	Receptor location	Alternations of receptor densities with aging
Serotonin	Raphe	?	Neocortex	Decrease in 5-HT$_1$ Decrease in 5-HT$_2$
Noradrenaline	Locus coeruleus	Decrease	Neocortex	Decrease in α-adrenergic Decrease in β-adrenergic
Dopamine	Substantia nigra	Decrease	Basal ganglia	Increase in postsynaptic D$_1$ Decrease in postsynaptic D$_2$ Decrease in presynaptic D$_1$ Decrease in presynaptic D$_2$
	Ventral tegmental area	?	Neocortex	Unknown —
Acetylcholine	Nucleus basalis of Meynert	No change or decrease	Neocortex	Decrease in M$_1$ Decrease in M$_2$ Decrease in N
	Medial septal region	?	Hippocampus	Decrease in M$_1$ M$_2$ unknown Decrease in N (^{3}H tubocurarine)

Note. ? = definitive data unavailable; 5-HT$_1$ = serotonin (5-hydroxytryptamine), subtype 1; 5-HT$_2$ = serotonin, subtype 2; D$_1$ = dopamine, subtype 1; D$_2$ = dopamine, subtype 2; M$_1$ = muscarinic, subtype 1; M$_2$ = muscarinic, subtype 2; N = nicotinic.
Sources. From Coleman and Flood 1987; Giacobini 1990; Gottfries 1990; Mendelsohn and Paxinos 1991; Müller et al. 1991.

are damaged in many neurodegenerative disorders including Alzheimer's disease, progressive supranuclear palsy, parkinsonism with dementia, and other disorders. Improving cholinergic function is presently the focus of pharmacological interventions for Alzheimer's disease.

Noradrenergic Systems

A relationship may exist between the aging of the human catecholaminergic system and neuropsychiatric diseases such as depression (Mann 1991; Procter and Bowen 1987; Veith and Rasking 1988). Poststroke depression may be linked to catecholaminergic function (Robinson et al. 1984, 1987), and depression in Alzheimer's disease may correlate with loss of neurons in the locus coeruleus (Zubenko and Moossy 1988).

Noradrenergic systems in human brain include an extensive network of fibers and receptors in neocortex, allocortex, selected diencephalic structures, and brain stem (Fallon and Loughlin 1987). Noradrenaline in the human forebrain is produced by the locus coeruleus, a band of neurons located immediately beneath the fourth ventricle in the pons (Figure 3–14). A variable mixture of α- and β-adrenergic receptors are present throughout the cerebral cortices (Mendelsohn and Paxinos 1991; Reznikoff et al. 1986). There is a progressive loss of noradrenergic neurons throughout the aging human brain stem, commencing between ages 30 and 40 and progressing with a linear relationship to age (Tables 3–2 and 3–4) (Mann et al. 1983, 1984). In the locus coeruleus, 40% of pigmented neurons are lost by age 90, and similar losses are sustained by the A-2 cell groups in the medulla (i.e., the dorsal motor nucleus of the vagus) (Figure 3–14). Occasional neurofibrillary tangles or Lewy bodies are present in these neurons after age 60. Noradrenergic neurites (i.e., abnormal, swollen processes that contain dopamine β-hydroxylase) are present in the neuropil and within senile plaques of elderly subjects (Powers et al. 1988), as well as within the pineal gland (Jengeleski et al. 1989). Enzymatic activities are reduced for tyrosine hydroxylase, the rate-limiting enzyme in the production of both dopamine and noradrenaline, as well as dopamine β-hydroxylase, the committed enzyme for the production of noradrenaline. Brain concentrations of 3-methoxy-4-hydroxylphenylglycol (MHPG) may remain constant in aging (Gottfries 1990), but CSF levels are increased (Table 3–5).

Age-related loss of β-adrenergic receptors is region dependent (Table 3–4). Receptor numbers remain constant in the frontal cortex (Kalaria et al. 1989); however, cingulate, precentral, temporal, and occipito-temporal regions demonstrate a linear age-dependent loss (Mendelsohn and Paxinos 1991). α_2-Adrenergic receptors demonstrate a substantial decline in aging human brain (Pascual et al. 1992). Rodent studies also demonstrate age-related loss of β-adrenergic receptors in all regions except cortex, a phenomenon possibly due to diminished receptor synthesis (Miller and Zahniser 1988; Scarpace and Abrass 1988). Other studies in rodent show a progressive age-dependent loss of postsynaptic response to noradrenaline and serotonin (Bickford-Wimer et al. 1988). Similar human studies are not available. This cumulative evidence suggests a gradual senescent loss of noradrenergic production and region-dependent loss of adrenergic receptors in human brain.

Serotonergic Systems

Serotonin is produced by raphe nuclei, clusters of neurons in the midline of the midbrain and pons (Figure 3–14) (Fallon and Loughlin 1987). Quantitation of serotonergic neurons in human brain stem is limited by methodological problems with serotonin markers. There is extensive serotonergic innervation of human neocortex, allocortex, and some diencephalic structures. Serotonin content is reduced in selected neocortical and allocortical regions of aged human brain (Gottfries 1990; Morgan and Finch 1987). Concentrations of 5-hydroxyindoleacetic acid, the primary metabolite of serotonin, are not reduced in brain or CSF (Table 3–5). However, imipramine binding, a putative marker for serotonin re-uptake, is reduced in aging. Activity of tryptophan hydroxylase, the synthetic enzyme for the production of serotonin, is reduced in the brains of aged rodents.

Two major types of serotonin receptor are described: the S_1 (5-hydroxytryptamine, subtype 1 [5-HT$_1$]) and the S_2 (5-HT$_2$), and the densities of both are reduced in brains of aged humans (Table 3–4) (Mendelsohn and Paxinos 1991). The density of S_2 is reduced 20% to 50%, and S_1 declines up to 70%. Depletion of neurons in the raphe nuclei would explain the decreased serotonin content, but not the decreased serotonin receptor density. These limited data on serotonergic systems in human aging suggest a gradual loss of serotonin production and receptors with aging.

Dopaminergic Systems

Dopaminergic systems are altered in aging and in many neurodegenerative disorders, including Alzheimer's disease, idiopathic parkinsonism, and progressive supranuclear palsy (Gibb et al. 1989; Morgan and Finch 1987; Morgan et al. 1987). The brain stem neurons of the mesocortical and nigrostriatal dopaminergic pathways are well defined in human brain (Figure 3–14). Although dopaminergic neurons are present in the human septal and hypothalamic regions (Gaspar et al. 1985), the tuberoinfundibular system is poorly defined in humans. There is a progressive loss of neurons in the substantia nigra (Uchihara et al. 1992) in aging and disease. The number of pigmented neurons in the substantia nigra may begin to drop between ages 30 and 50, and substantial loss (35%) is reported after age 65 (Table 3–2) (Mann et al. 1984; McGeer et al. 1977). Nucleolar volume of substantia nigra neurons is reduced after age 65 and neurofibrillary tangles or Lewy bodies begin to appear in small numbers (Mann et al. 1984) (Figure 3–10, *panels E and F*). The loss of neurons in the ventral tegmental area has not been determined (Hirai 1968; Jellinger 1987).

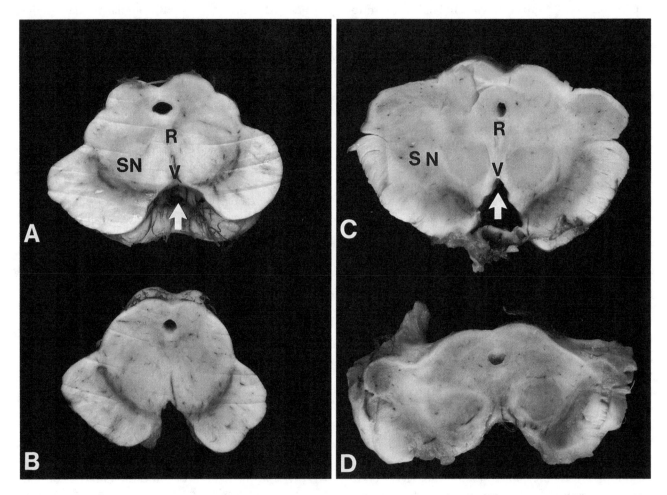

Figure 3–14.   Comparisons of midbrain and pons from elderly control subjects and individuals with depigmentation. Regions that produce dopamine and noradrenaline can be distinguished by the brown-black neuromelanin pigment. Serotonin-producing neurons are located in the midline of the brain stem (i.e., raphe [R]) but cannot be distinguished from adjacent structures with either gross or microscopic examination. The ventral tegmental area (V) is present in the midline between the substantia nigrae (SN) and above the interpeduncular fossa (*arrow*). *Panel A:* A substantia nigra from an 85-year-old subject with some mild loss of pigment. *Panel B:* A subject with Alzheimer's disease who has moderate depigmentation. *Panels C and D:* A patient with idiopathic parkinsonism with more severe depigmentation on the left than on the right. *Panel E: (at right)* The appearance of locus coeruleus in an elderly control subject: a discrete area of brown-black pigment beneath the fourth ventricle (*arrow*). *Panel F: (at right)* Depigmentation in an aged subject with diffusion of neuromelanin into adjacent neuropil (*arrow*).

Surviving catecholaminergic neurons progressively accumulate neuromelanin (Graham 1979), which displaces perikaryal RNA and reduces nucleolar volume (McGeer et al. 1977). The ventral tegmental area is damaged by Alzheimer's disease (Torack and Morris 1988). Senescent alterations of dopamine-producing neurons in hypothalamus are unknown. Concentrations of dopamine are reduced in the striatum of individuals over age 65; however, homovanillic acid content, the primary dopamine metabolite, remains constant in tissue and CSF (Table 3–5) (Gottfries 1990; Hartikainen et al. 1991).

The cortical anatomy of the mesocortical and mesolimbic dopaminergic innervation is poorly defined in humans and few studies examine alterations of these systems in aging. The number of presynaptic striatal dopamine, subtype 1 (D1), receptors decreases (Table 3–4) and the number of postsynaptic receptors increases with aging (Morgan and Finch 1987). The density of both pre- and postsynaptic dopamine, subtype 2 (D2), striatal receptors is decreased, according to multiple investigators (Morgan et al. 1987). The senescent loss of neurons in the basal ganglia may par-

tially explain the loss of receptors. The relationship is unclear between these neurochemical alterations and movement disorders such as spontaneous dyskinesia in the elderly.

Alterations of Monoamine Oxidase and Aging

Monoamine oxidase (MAO) activity is significantly altered in the aged human brain. MAO-A, which facilitates the oxidative deamination of noradrenaline, serotonin, and partially dopamine, is not drastically altered in aging. MAO-B, which catalyzes the oxidative deamination of several amines and partially dopamine, increases with age (Gottfries 1990). The importance of these age-related alterations is unclear, although increased quantities of this catabolic enzyme may result in depletion of dopamine and other catecholamines. MAO activity is also significantly altered in neurodegenerative disorders such as Alzheimer's disease (Morgan and Finch 1987; Perry et al. 1991; Procter and Bowen 1987).

Alterations of Peptidergic Transmission in Aging

A wide array of neuropeptides function as neuromodulators and colocalize with other classical transmitters such as noradrenaline and serotonin. Corticotropin-releasing factor is diminished in aging; however, other more abundant peptides such as somatostatin and neuropeptide Y are not (Giaquinto 1988; Gottfries 1990). A variety of neuropeptides are present in dystrophic neurites and senile plaques of aged subjects, including somatostatin, neuropeptide Y, and corticotropin-releasing factor (Struble et al. 1987). CSF contents (Table 3–5) of somatostatin and β-endorphin are not changed in elderly humans (Hartikainen et al. 1991). Peptide receptors are not adequately characterized in human cortex to assess age-related alterations (Mendelsohn and Paxinos 1991). Studies in aging rodents show no loss of enkephalinergic receptors or diminished receptor affinity (Ueno et al. 1988).

Alteration of Other Transmitter Systems in Aging

Excitatory amino acids are common transmitters in the human brain. Quantitative methodologies are not sufficient to precisely define subtle age-related neurochemical or histochemical changes; however, glutamate receptors are reduced in Alzheimer's disease (Cotman et al. 1987b). Inhibitory transmitter systems

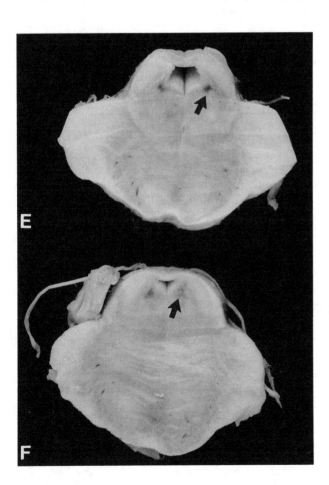

are probably altered in aging. For example, GABA-ergic systems in human hippocampus are altered in disease and possibly in aging (Giaquinto 1988). Patients with Alzheimer's disease have reductions of hippocampal GABAergic receptors (Shimohama et al. 1988), suggesting a loss of GABAergic input or target neurons.

Signal Transduction and Aging

Signal transduction is transmitter dependent and mediated through a variety of mechanisms. Senescent alterations of second messenger systems are unclear. Phosphoinositide-derived second messengers, calbindin, and protein kinase C–derived systems are altered in several neurodegenerative disorders; however, similar data are not available for normal human aging. It is likely that subtle alterations of signal transduction systems occur in the brains of elderly subjects (Fowler et al. 1992; Mattson 1991).

Aging of the Autonomic Nervous System

Autonomic regulation involves a balance between sympathetic and parasympathetic innervation. These two systems include neurons in hypothalamus, brain stem, spinal cord, and peripheral ganglia. Small-diameter myelinated and unmyelinated axons conduct impulses to target organs (McLeod and Tuck 1987). There is a reduction in number or density of peripheral or autonomic myelinated fibers in aging rodents and humans (Knox et al. 1989).

Aging of the human sympathetic nervous system results in a mixed clinical picture. Essential hypertension is an age-related disorder that has both central and peripheral causes (Evans and Williams 1992), and orthostatic hypotension is a common problem in the elderly. Postural hypotension occurs in 20% of selected geriatric patients and complicates the prescription of psychotropic medications (Mader 1989; see also Chapter 29). Antihypertensive agents can cause depression in elderly patients. Individuals over age 65 are sensitive to the orthostatic effects of the tricyclic antidepressants. Although senescent changes occur in brain stem and spinal cord (Clark et al. 1984), the age-related alterations of central nuclei that control autonomic function are unknown. There is a progressive, age-related loss of sympathetic neurons in the intermediolateral column of the spinal cord. These neurons span from

T1 to L2 and are involved with vasomotor tone.

Sympathetic blood pressure is maintained through a complicated interaction of central, peripheral, and neuroendocrine interactions. The sympathetic nervous system is inhibited in the medullary brain stem and spinal cord through centrally located α_2-adrenergic mechanisms. Obesity is associated with increasing plasma norepinephrine levels, and older subjects have higher total body fat. Plasma norepinephrine is elevated in aging; however, the net effect of aging on the peripheral sympathetic tone is unknown (Rowe 1987). Age-related pathologies (e.g., neurofibrillary tangles, senile plaques, and dystrophic neurites) occur rarely in the human spinal cord and peripheral nervous system, although neurofibrillary tangles are reported in the human superior cervical ganglion (Kawasaki et al. 1987). Lewy bodies are present in Auerbach's and Meissner's plexuses in elderly subjects, as well as in those with Parkinson's disease (Wakabayashi et al. 1988).

The aging of the human parasympathetic nervous system is poorly understood. There is a senescent loss of small-diameter peripheral nerve fibers that may contribute to parasympathetic dysfunction. Sacral parasympathetic neurons are damaged in parkinsonism (Oyanagi et al. 1990). Many drugs with anticholinergic side effects alter parasympathetic function (Peters 1989).

Trophic Factors and Aging

Trophic factors are substances that maintain or promote the growth and integrity of cell populations. Neuronal trophic factors are best characterized; however, similar substances exist for glia. Receptors for trophic factors are present on neurons (Hefti and Mash 1989), and synthesis of these substances is regulated by specific transmitter systems (Thoenen et al. 1991).

A variety of neuronal trophic factors are the focus of future therapeutic interventions for neurodegenerative disorders. The presently known family of neurotrophins includes nerve growth factor, brain-derived neurotrophic factor, neurotrophin-3, and neurotrophin-4 (Fuxe and Agnati 1992).

Nerve growth factor is best characterized and is composed of three subunits: α, β, and γ. All biological activity appears to be present in the β subunit. Nerve growth factor receptors are present in the human nucleus basalis of Meynert (Figure 3–4) and in sympathetic neurons (Hefti and Mash 1989; Hefti et al. 1989). This peptide promotes neurite extension and stimulates the activity of tyrosine hydroxylase and dopamine beta hydroxylase (Fuxe and Agnati 1992). Nerve growth factor is essential to the normal development and maintenance of cholinergic neurons. Administration of nerve growth factor to aging rodents will reverse the age-related dendritic spine loss of cortical pyramidal neurons (Mervis et al. 1991).

At the cellular level, nerve growth factor may increase the degradation of superoxide radicals and hydrogen peroxides. Preliminary data in humans suggest an age-related reduction in the synthesis of nerve growth factor (Hefti et al. 1989). Nerve growth factor will protect damaged cholinergic forebrain neurons in monkeys, and a similar protective role is postulated for human neurons.

Other peptides such as insulin-like growth factor, platelet-derived growth factor, and fibroblast growth factor affect the production of neurites, development of glia, and regulation of nigrostriatal neurons in nonhuman models (Fuxe and Agnati 1992; Otto and Unsicker 1992). Many of these also are present in human CNS. Growth factors may arrest or reverse some of the atrophic changes in aging and are the focus of pharmacological research (Fuxe and Agnati 1992).

Aging and the Hypothalamus

The human hypothalamus consists of multiple nuclei adjacent to the third ventricle (Figure 3–4). These neurons control a range of neuroendocrine functions such as regulation of gonadotropins and releasing factors for adrenal, thyroid, or growth hormones.

Humans undergo a series of senescent sexual and neuroendocrinological alterations (Rance et al. 1993). Sexual drive, circulating gonadotropins, and hypothalamic nuclei change with age and are gender dependent. Senescent hypothalamic neuronal alterations may include either atrophy or hypertrophy.

The sexually dimorphic nucleus and the preoptic area of the human hypothalamus contain neurons whose density and size are gender specific (Hofman and Swaab 1989). These neurons undergo a series of orderly, predictable changes with age. Sexually dimorphic structures have a sex-dependent pattern of growth and decay (Hofman and Swaab 1989). There is a 43% reduction in males and a 62% reduction in females of the volume of the sexually dimorphic nucleus-preoptic

area of young (20–30 years) versus old (70–90 years) control subjects. This contrasts to 6% reductions of net brain volume and 20%–25% reductions of basal forebrain structures (Hofman and Swaab 1989). Alterations of these nuclei may reflect the gender-dependent patterns of human sexual aging.

Menopause occurs in most women around age 50 and includes many physiological and psychological alterations. Menopause is caused by disruption of the gonadal-hypothalamic-pituitary cycle through loss of ovarian estrogen production (Rance 1992). The number of human ova peaks in utero at mid-gestation (seven million), is one million at birth, and is four hundred thousand at menarche. This gradual ovarian attrition from ages 20 to 50 that ends in ovarian follicles unresponsive to gonadotropins results in subsequent increases of serum follicle-stimulating hormone (FSH) and luteinizing hormone (LH) and falling levels of serum estrogens (Evans and Williams 1992; Hazzard et al. 1990).

The cyclical nature of the menstrual cycle may be partially driven by neurons in the anterior hypothalamus, which receive a variety of catecholaminergic inputs (Wise et al. 1987). Rodent studies have indicated that the release of LH is influenced by noradrenergic, serotonergic, dopaminergic, and peptidergic inputs. The loss of steroid negative feedback results in elevated serum gonadotropins. In postmenopausal senescent women, some hypothalamic nuclei hypertrophy to include marked increase in the diameter of infundibular neurons expressing estrogen receptors (Rance et al. 1990) and increased tachykinin message in selected hypothalamic nuclei (Rance and Young 1991).

The senescent changes of gonadotropic nuclei that provoke the decline of sexual function in elderly men are undefined. The male sexually dimorphic nucleus also is reduced in size with aging, and there is a decline of circulating testosterone in individuals 40–60 years old. Although the relationship between senescent changes of hypothalamic nuclei and circulating gonadotropins is unclear, significant physiological and neuropsychiatric sequelae may result from these changes.

Other functions of the hypothalamic-pituitary axis are altered in aging and selected neuropsychiatric disorders. The hypothalamus receives noradrenergic, serotonergic, and cholinergic innervation (Mendelsohn and Paxinos 1991) affecting control of many pituitary-releasing factors. The control of three important releasing factors, corticotropin-releasing factor, thyrotropin-releasing hormone, and growth hormone is well characterized in humans. The function of the hypothalamic-pituitary-adrenal axis has been extensively described in "normal" (Evans and Williams 1992) and depressed elderly patients (Veith and Raskind 1988). Basal levels of plasma cortisol increase with age, but the reactivity of the axis as determined by suppression with oral dexamethasone is unchanged (Hazzard et al. 1990; Veith and Raskind 1988). The age-related loss of noradrenergic neurons in the locus coeruleus may partially explain the increased levels of plasma cortisol. The dexamethasone suppression test is altered in depression and is discussed elsewhere (see Chapter 28).

Noradrenaline affects the release of growth hormone via control of growth hormone–releasing factor and somatostatin. Growth hormone secretion is increased by α-adrenergic and dopaminergic receptor activation and inhibited by β-adrenergic stimulation. Somatostatin release is increased in aging (Hazzard et al. 1990). The peak of growth hormone secretion occurs in adolescence followed by a progressive decline over years and diminished number of growth hormone immunoreactive pituicytes in the glands of elderly ssubjects (Veith and Raskind 1988). Recent studies have shown that growth hormone injection in older humans will increase lean body mass (8.8%), skin thickness (7.1%), and bone density, while lowering adipose tissue mass (14.4%) (Rudman et al. 1990). The expense of growth hormone—$10,000–$20,000 per year—and its potential side effects limit the usefulness of this therapeutic modality (Schoen 1991).

Abnormalities of thyroid function are common in elderly patients. Between 4% and 12% of subjects over age 60 may have chemical hypothyroidism. Individuals over age 60 have a sevenfold increase in the prevalence of hyperthyroidism (Evans and Williams 1992). Fifteen percent of patients over age 60 will have elevated blood levels of thyroid-stimulating hormone (TSH), and one-third will develop thyroid failure when followed for 4 years (Hazzard et al. 1990). Some elderly individuals have diminished pituitary responsiveness to thyrotropin-releasing hormone (TRH) (Evans and Williams 1992), although blunting of TSH response is present with depression (Veith and Raskind 1988).

The mechanism for central control of TRH is unclear, and adrenergic, dopaminergic, histaminergic, or serotonergic mechanisms are postulated (Veith and Raskind 1988). Age-related alterations of TRH secretion remain controversial.

Age-Related Alterations of the Special Senses

Aging may affect all five of the special senses. Increased thresholds for touch-pressure, vibration, and cooling are present in aging; however, deficits of olfaction, sight, and hearing are most significant and best characterized. Alterations of these senses will have significant impact on psychological testing and clinical management of patients.

Sensory association cortices are heavily damaged by Alzheimer's disease, but adjacent primary receptive cortices (Figure 3–1) are usually spared (Morrison et al. 1991; J. L. Price et al. 1991). Sensory association cortices have reciprocal connections with hippocampus and parahippocampal cortices (Hyman et al. 1984), structures involved with memory. These mesial temporal cortices are frequently damaged in aging (Braak and Braak 1991; Morrison et al. 1991), and this may add to dysfunction of sensory information processing.

Olfactory Senses

Aging humans lose multiple olfactory abilities (Kesslak et al. 1988) including the ability to perceive odors, odor discrimination, odor recognition, and olfactory memory (Figure 3–8) (Giaquinto 1988; Hazzard et al. 1990). The rate and age at onset for olfactory deficits are unclear. Multiple factors contribute to olfactory loss including alteration of mucosa, cribriform plate stenosis, airway pathology, and others (Doty 1991). The role of environmental and other factors (e.g., smoking) on olfactory function is unclear. Age-related histopathology, such as neurofibrillary tangles, begins to occur in individuals over age 50 (Doty 1991). Olfactory association areas such as amygdala and uncal cortices are frequently damaged in aging (Figure 3–4) (Braak and Braak 1991; Kemper 1984). Most studies of olfactory systems in Alzheimer's disease patients demonstrate olfaction deficits and neuropathology (Figure 3–7) in all components of the olfactory pathway (Hyman et al. 1991; Kesslak et al. 1988; Talamo et al. 1989).

Visual Impairment

Senescent visual loss results from environmental, genetic, metabolic, and vascular etiologies (Evans and Williams 1992). Visual impairment is common in elderly individuals, and frequent causes include opacification of the cornea (cataracts), retinal damage (diabetic retinopathy), deterioration of the macula (macular degeneration), or disturbance of ocular optics (presbyopia) (Hazzard et al. 1990). Visual thresholds begin to decline between ages 30 and 40. Approximately 36% of individuals over age 80 have opacification of the lens (Giaquinto 1988). Low vision and blindness are common in those over age 85; however, one-half may never seek specialty care, and many can be assisted with simple interventions such as improved home lighting (Evans and Williams 1992). Diabetic retinopathy accounts for 10%–20% of blindness in subjects 65–74 years old and macular degeneration for 50% of those over age 85 (Evans and Williams 1992; Hazzard et al. 1990).

Primate studies show that visual information is processed along two pathways involving temporal and parietal cortices. A striate–inferior temporal circuit processes information about form and color distinction (Morrison et al. 1991). A striate-parietal pathway processes visuospatial and motor data. The effect of aging on these interconnected, high-level association cortices is not known; however, these brain regions are damaged in Alzheimer's disease (Hof and Morrison 1990).

Low vision can worsen neuropsychiatric symptoms and complicate management. Recognition of low vision, correction of refractive error, and maximal use of environmental light are important in management of the geriatric population.

Auditory Functions

Auditory impairment progresses with age and involves approximately 60% of individuals ages 71–80 (Davis et al. 1990). High-frequency hearing loss increases with aging and is usually caused by mechanical failure. Causes of hearing loss in elderly people include disorders of the outer, middle, and inner ear. Cerumen impaction is a common problem of the outer ear (Gulya 1992). Hearing loss from damage to the inner ear has four primary causes: 1) sensory presbycusis, 2) neural presbycusis, 3) strial presbycusis, and 4) cochlear conductive presbycusis. Precise epidemiological data are limited because correlative histopathological studies of the auditory apparatuses are few and many conditions have mixed pathology. Most age-related hearing loss is mechanical, and age-related histopathology (i.e., senile plaques or neurofibrillary tangles) is not reported in the peripheral auditory system. Conduc-

tive or sensorineural hearing loss can be improved with appropriate hearing aids. Auditory cortex can be severely damaged in Alzheimer's disease (Esiri et al. 1986) in which a specific pattern of atrophy shows shrinkage of the association cortex (i.e., the superior temporal gyrus [Brodmann areas 22 and 52]), with sparing of the primary auditory cortex (i.e., the transverse temporal gyrus [Brodmann areas 41 and 42]) (Figure 3–9).

Subtle auditory impairment may be difficult to detect in the elderly patient who has developed accessory methods such as lip and face reading. Even mild (10 dB) hearing loss can significantly lower quality of life. Hearing loss can remain undetected by caregivers, and this communication problem can be misinterpreted by caregivers as patient obstinacy. Unrecognized hearing loss can complicate the management of neuropsychiatric problems.

Aging and the Immune System

The interaction of brain aging and the immune system can be viewed two ways: the effect of aging brain on immune function or the effect of an aging immune system on the brain. Components of the immune system, such as spleen and thymus, receive direct innervation and respond to substances produced by the neuroendocrine system (e.g., cortisol). Selected products of the immune system are CNS-active (Cotman et al. 1987a) and may complete the feedback loop to the CNS.

The brain does not have a system of lymphatics or lymphoid tissue like other organs (e.g., lung or gastrointestinal tract) (Adams and Duchen 1992). Microglia, the immune cells of the brain, are of hematogenous origin. Senescent alterations in the function of brain microglia are not described (Thomas 1992).

Immunologically active substances are present in the brain. Interleukin-1, a cytokine that mediates acute phase reaction, innervates key endocrine and autonomic neurons in human hypothalamus that affect many components of the acute phase immune reaction (Breder et al. 1988). Interleukin-2 is centrally active and affects firing of locus coeruleus neurons (Nisticò and De Sarro 1991). Some neuronal populations involved in neuroimmunological circuits are altered in aging, such as depopulation of the locus coeruleus and selected hypothalamic nuclei. Immunological consequences of catecholaminergic neuron loss are unknown.

Many systemic diseases of the elderly population, such as arthritis, are immune mediated. There is little evidence to suggest that age-related brain changes result from autoimmunity. The intact blood-brain barrier provides some protection against autoimmunity; however, age- and disease-related changes increase its permeability for selected immunoglobulins. Brain-directed autoantibodies are absent in young subjects, but some older humans produce antibodies that recognize neurons and astrocytes (Gaskin et al. 1987). Some antibodies recognize cholinergic neurons, although the significance of this is unclear (Lopez et al. 1991). Astrocytes and microglial cells participate in the immune response of the brain by presenting antigen to T cells (Cotman et al. 1987a). Microglia are the intrinsic brain immune cells (Thomas 1992), and their numbers have not been calculated in elderly subjects. Microglia are associated with senile plaques (Figure 3–12), as well as with intracellular and extracellular neurofibrillary tangles (Cras et al. 1991). The fragmentary understanding of interactions between the brain and the immune system limits the identification of neuroimmunological alterations in senescence and neurodegenerative disorders.

Neurobiology of Aging in Chronically Mentally Ill Patients

Brains of patients with chronic mental illnesses may age differently than those of mentally healthy individuals. Assessment of age-related alterations in chronically mentally ill patients is complicated by the effect of chronic neuroleptic usage, nutrition, environment, and health status. Current hypotheses suggest schizophrenia results from neuronal migrational abnormalities, genetic factors, and environmental influences (Barta et al. 1990; Weinberger 1987). Neuropathological correlates do not exist for neuroradiological studies that show individuals from lower socioeconomic strata have smaller brains. Some disorders such as mental retardation, autism (Bauman and Kemper 1985), and dyslexia (Hier et al. 1978; Galaburda et al. 1985) may involve abnormalities of neuronal migration in brain regions such as hippocampus and planum temporale (Figure 3–9). The neurobiology of aging in migrationally disordered brain is unknown.

Aging of organ systems such as cardiovascular and renal is not accelerated in seriously mentally ill populations. Postmortem studies do not suggest accelerated death rates caused by atherosclerosis, arteriosclerosis, or other age-dependent pathological processes in patients with schizophrenia or affective disorder. Excessive rates of natural death may result from psychosocial complications of physical disorders (Black et al. 1987; Kuperman et al. 1988), such as noncompliance and unavailability of health services.

Brain image analysis studies of elderly individuals with depression show a 7% reduction in the volume of frontal lobes and subcortical encephalomalacia (Coffey et al. 1993). Correlative neuropathological studies on aging and depression are not available. Studies of brains from elderly schizophrenic subjects have demonstrated senile plaques, neurofibrillary tangles, and vascular alterations similar to those of age-matched control subjects (Brown et al. 1986; Bruton et al. 1990). Recent immunocytochemical studies of hippocampus from schizophrenic subjects have demonstrated abnormal expression of the cytoskeletal epitopes, microtubule-associated protein 2, and microtubule-associated protein 5 in subicular neurons (Arnold et al. 1991). These findings are distinct from those of other pathological studies (Bogerts et al. 1990) showing cytoarchitectonic abnormalities of hippocampus in young schizophrenic subjects. Little information is available about histopathological or neurochemical alterations of brains from elderly patients with affective disorders or individuals with other major psychiatric disorders (Procter and Bowen 1987).

Animal Models for the Neurobiology of Aging

Several animal aging models have been described including ones for monkey, bear, and dog (Brizzee et al. 1978; Cork et al. 1988; Maurer et al. 1990). Dystrophic neurites and senile plaques are described in all models, and substantial numbers of neurofibrillary tangles are described in the brains of aged bears (Cork et al. 1988). Other age-related changes such as granulovacuolar degeneration, Hirano bodies, and Lewy bodies are not described (Figure 3–10). Chronic hypertension injures rodent neocortex; however, animal models do not exist for idiopathic parkinsonism, progressive supranuclear palsy, or other neurodegenerative disorders (Wyss and Van Groen 1992; Wyss et al. 1992). Monkeys with surgically induced hypertension will manifest cognitive deficits and multiple cortical infarctions.

Older primates demonstrate subtle cognitive decline similar to that of elderly humans (D. L. Price et al. 1991). Aged monkey brain develops senile plaques, dystrophic neurites, and congophilic angiopathy closely resembling that in aged human brain. Neurofibrillary tangles are seen in bears and very old primates with advanced disease. Individual bear and monkey neurons atrophy, accumulate abnormal cytoskeletal proteins, and express amyloid precursor protein. Markers for cholinergic, noradrenergic, serotonergic, and peptidergic systems are decreased in brains of aged primates suggesting that age-related pathology is not species specific, but rather reflects the longevity of the animal (D. L. Price et al. 1991).

Systemic Effects of Aging of Importance to Geriatric Neuropsychiatry

Most organ systems in the human body are altered by the aging process; however, age-related loss of function is frequently overestimated in disease-free organ systems of elderly patients. Cardiovascular alterations, resulting from common diseases in the elderly such as hypertension and atherosclerosis, are immensely important to the geriatric neuropsychiatrist. Age-related loss of cardiovascular function is not as dramatic as anticipated in healthy elderly patients (Evans and Williams 1992; Hazzard et al. 1990). Loss of exercise

tolerance is partially explained by disuse (Evans and Williams 1992), rather than by atrophy. Age-related effects on systemic organ systems are displayed in Table 3–6, and alterations of renal function and pharmacodynamics are discussed elsewhere (see Chapter 29).

Conclusions

The secret of successful aging is unknown. The distinction between "normal" senescent phenomena and age-related disease remains unclear. Human neuronal aging includes a complex mixture of atrophy, hypertrophy, synaptic reorganization, or cell death. Genetic, environmental, systemic, and immunological factors may influence human brain aging. The neurobiology of aging in the very old (i.e., those over age 85) remains to be studied.

References

Adams JH, Duchen LW (eds): Greenfield's Neuropathology, 5th Edition. New York, Oxford University Press, 1992

Anthony A, Zerweck C: Scanning-integrating microdensitometric analysis of age-related changes in RNA content of cerebrocortical neurons in mice subjected to auditory stimulation. Exp Neurol 65:542–551, 1979

Arnold SE, Lee VM-Y, Gur RE, et al: Abnormal expression of two microtubule-associated proteins (MAP2 and MAP5) in specific subfields of the hippocampal formation in schizophrenia. Proc Natl Acad Sci U S A 88:10850–10854, 1991

Awad IA, Johnson PC, Spetzler RF, et al: Incidental subcortical lesions identified on magnetic resonance imaging in the elderly, II: postmortem pathological correlations. Stroke 17:1090–1097, 1986

Ball MJ: Neuronal loss, neurofibrillary tangles and granulovacuolar degeneration in the hippocampus with ageing and dementia: a quantitative study. Acta Neuropathol (Berl) 37:111–118, 1977

Ball MJ: Challenges and opportunities of clinicopathological investigation in longitudinal studies of Alzheimer's disease. Can J Neurol Sci 13 (suppl 4):452–455, 1986

Barinaga M: Mortality: overturning received wisdom. Science 258:398–399, 1992

Barta PE, Pearlson GD, Powers RE, et al: Auditory hallucinations and smaller superior temporal gyral volume in schizophrenia. Am J Psychiatry 147:1457–1462, 1990

Bauman M, Kemper TL: Histoanatomic observations of the brain in early infantile autism. Neurology 35:866–874, 1985

Bennett DA, Gilley DW, Wilson RS, et al: Clinical correlates of high signal lesions on magnetic resonance imaging in Alzheimer's disease. J Neurol 239:186–190, 1992

Table 3–6. Age-related alterations of cardiovascular, renal, and pulmonary function in the absence of intrinsic diseases

Function	Alteration
Cardiac	
Heart rate	No significant change
Ejection fraction	No significant change
Physical exercise capacity	Slight decrease
Pulmonary	
Total lung capacity (TLC)	No significant change
Forced vital capacity (FVC)	Decrease
Diffusion capacity (CDco)	Decrease
Physical work capacity $VO_{2\,max}$	Decrease
Partial pressure of arterial oxygen (PaO_2)	Decrease
Renal	
Renal mass	Decrease
Renal blood flow	Decrease
Glomerular filtration rate (GFR)	Decrease

Sources. From Evans and Williams 1992; Hazzard et al. 1990.

Bickford-Wimer PC, Granholm A-CH, Gerhardt GA: Cerebellar noradrenergic systems in aging: studies in situ and in oculo grafts. Neurobiol Aging 9:591–599, 1988

Black DW, Winokur G, Nasrallah A: Is death from natural causes still excessive in psychiatric patients? a follow-up of 1593 patients with major affective disorder. J Nerv Ment Dis 175:674–680, 1987

Blessed G, Tomlinson BE, Roth M: The association between quantitative measures of dementia and of senile change in the cerebral grey matter of elderly subjects. Br J Psychiatry 114:797–811, 1968

Bogerts B, Falkai P, Haupts M, et al: Post-mortem volume measurements of limbic system and basal ganglia structures in chronic schizophrenics: initial results from a new brain collection. Schrizophr Res 3:295–301, 1990

Braak H, Braak E: Neuropathological staging of Alzheimer's-related changes. Acta Neuropathol (Berl) 82:239–259, 1991

Braak H, Braak E, Grundke-Iqbal I, et al: Occurrence of neuropil threads in the senile human brain and in Alzheimer's disease: a third location of paired helical filaments outside of neurofibrillary tangles and neuritic plaques. Neurosci Lett 65:351–355, 1986

Breder CD, Dinarello CA, Saper CB: Interleukin-1 immunoreactive innervation of the human hypothalamus. Science 240:321–324, 1988

Brizzee KR, Ordy JM, Hofer H, et al: Animal models for the study of senile brain disease and aging changes in the brain, in Alzheimer's Disease: Senile Dementia and Related Disorders. Edited by Katzman R, Terry RD, Bick KL. New York, Raven, 1978, pp 515–553

Brody H: Organization of the cerebral cortex, III: a study of ageing in the cerebral cortex. J Comp Neurol 102:511–556, 1955

Brown R, Colter N, Corsellis JAN, et al: Postmortem evidence of structural brain changes in schizophrenia: differences in brain weight, temporal horn area, and parahippocampal gyrus compared with affective disorder. Arch Gen Psychiatry 43:36–42, 1986

Brun A, Englund E: A white matter disorder in dementia of the Alzheimer type: a pathoanatomical study. Ann Neurol 19:253–262, 1986

Bruton CJ, Crow TJ, Frith CD, et al: Schizophrenia and the brain: a prospective cliniconeuropathological study. Psychol Med 20:285–304, 1990

Caplan LR, Schoene WC: Clinical features of subcortical arteriosclerotic encephalopathy (Binswanger disease). Neurology 12:1206–1215, 1978

Carlsson A: The aging brain and its disorders, in Alzheimer's Disease: Epidemiology, Neuropathology, Neurochemistry, and Clinics. Edited by Maurer K, Riederer P, Beckmann H. New York, Springer-Verlag, 1990, pp 7–20

Clark AW, Parhad IM, Griffin JW, et al: Neurofilamentous axonal swellings as a normal finding in the spinal anterior horn of man and other primates. J Neuropathol Exp Neurol 43:253–262, 1984

Coffey CE, Figiel GS: Neuropsychiatric significance of subcortical encephalomalacia, in Psychopathology and the Brain. Edited by Carroll BJ, Barrett JE. New York, Raven, 1991, pp 243–264

Coffey CE, Wilkinson WE, Parashos IA, et al: Quantitative cerebral anatomy of the aging human brain: a cross-sectional study using magnetic resonance imaging. Neurology 42:527–536, 1992

Coffey CE, Wilkinson WE, Weiner RD, et al: Quantitative cerebral anatomy in depression: a controlled magnetic resonance imaging study. Arch Gen Psychiatry 50:7–16, 1993

Coleman PD, Flood DG: Neuron numbers and dendritic extent in normal aging and Alzheimer's disease. Neurobiol Aging 8:521–545, 1987

Comfort A: The Biology of Senescence, 3rd Edition. New York, Elsevier, 1979

Coria F, Moreno A, Torres A, et al: Distribution of Alzheimer's disease amyloid protein precursor in normal human and rat nervous system. Neuropathol Appl Neurobiol 18:27–35, 1992

Cork LC, Powers RE, Selkoe DJ, et al: Neurofibrillary tangles and senile plaques in aged bears. J Neuropathol Exp Neurol 47:629–641, 1988

Cotman CW, Brinton RE, Galaburda A, et al (eds): The Neuro-Immune-Endocrine Connection. New York, Raven, 1987a

Cotman CW, Geddes JW, Monaghan DT, et al: Excitatory amino acid receptors in Alzheimer's disease, in Molecular Neuropathology of Aging. Edited by Davies P, Finch CE. Cold Spring Harbor, NY, Cold Spring Harbor Laboratory, 1987b, pp 67–83

Cras P, Kawai M, Siedlak S, et al: Microglia are associated with the extracellular neurofibrillary tangles of Alzheimer disease. Brain Res 558:312–314, 1991

Crystal H, Dickson D, Fuld P, et al: Clinico-pathologic studies in dementia: nondemented subjects with pathologically confirmed Alzheimer's disease. Neurology 38:1682–1687, 1988

Dam AM: The density of neurons in the human hippocampus. Neuropathol Appl Neurobiol 5:249–264, 1979

Davies I: Comments on review by Swaab: brain aging and Alzheimer's disease: "wear and tear" versus "use it or lose it." Neurobiol Aging 12:328–330, 1991

Davis AC, Ostri B, Parving A: Longitudinal study of hearing. Acta Otolaryngol (Stockh) 476 (suppl):12–22, 1990

Decker MW: The effects of aging on hippocampal and cortical projections of the forebrain cholinergic system. Brain Research Reviews 12:423–438, 1987

Dekaban AS, Sadowsky BS: Changes in brain weights during the span of human life: relation of brain weights to body height and weight. Ann Neurol 4:345–357, 1978

de Lacalle S, Iraizoz I, Ma Gonzalo L: Differential changes in cell size and number in topographic subdivisions of human basal nucleus in normal aging. Neuroscience 43:445–456, 1991

Divac I: Magnocellular nuclei of the basal forebrain project to neocortex, brain stem, and olfactory bulb: review of some functional correlates. Brain Res 93:385–398, 1975

Doebler JA, Markesbery WR, Anthony A, et al: Neuronal RNA in relation to neuronal loss and neurofibrillary pathology in the hippocampus in Alzheimer's disease. J Neuropathol Exp Neurol 46:28–39, 1987

Doty RL: Olfactory capacities in aging and Alzheimer's disease: psychophysical and anatomic considerations. Ann N Y Acad Sci 640:20–27, 1991

Eggers R, Haug H, Fischer D: Preliminary report on macroscopic age changes in the human prosencephalon: a stereologic investigation. J Hirnforsch 25:129–139, 1984

Esiri MM, Pearson RCA, Powell TPS: The cortex of the primary auditory area in Alzheimer's disease. Brain Res 366:385–387, 1986

Evans JG, Williams TF (eds): Oxford Textbook of Geriatric Medicine. New York, Oxford University Press, 1992

Fallon JH, Loughlin SE: Monoamine innervation of cerebral cortex and a theory of the role of monoamines in cerebral cortex and basal ganglia, in Cortex, Vol 1. Edited by Jones EG, Peters A. New York, Plenum, 1987, pp 41–127

Fields SD, MacKenzie CR, Charlson ME, et al: Reversibility of cognitive impairment in medical inpatients. Arch Intern Med 146:1593–1596, 1986

Finch CE: Neuron atrophy during aging: programmed or sporadic? Trends Neurosci 16:104–110, 1993

Finch CE, Morgan DG: RNA and protein metabolism in the aging brain. Annu Rev Neurosci 13:75–88, 1990

Flood DG, Coleman PD: Neuron numbers and sizes in aging brain: comparisons of human, monkey, and rodent data. Neurobiol Aging 9:453–463, 1988

Flood DG, Buell SJ, Defiore CH, et al: Age-related dendritic growth in dentate gyrus of human brain is followed by regression in the "oldest old." Brain Res 345:366–368, 1985

Fowler CJ, Cowburn RF, O'Neill CO: Brain signal transduction disturbances in neurodegenerative disorders. Cell Signal 4:1–9, 1992

Frederickson RCA: Astroglia in Alzheimer's disease. Neurobiol Aging 13:239–253, 1992

Fuxe K, Agnati LF: Neurotrophic factors and central dopamine neurons. Neuroscience Facts 3:81, 1992

Galaburda AM, Sherman GF, Rosen GD, et al: Developmental dyslexia: four consecutive patients with cortical anomalies. Ann Neurol 18:222–233, 1985

Garcia JH: The evolution of brain infarcts: a review. J Neuropathol Exp Neurol 51:387–393, 1992

Gaskin F, Kingsley BS, Fu SM: Autoantibodies to neurofibrillary tangles and brain tissue in Alzheimer's disease and aging, in Molecular Neuropathology of Aging. Edited by Davies P, Finch CE. Cold Spring Harbor, NY, Cold Spring Harbor Laboratory, 1987, pp 321–336

Gaspar P, Berger B, Alvarez C, et al: Catecholaminergic innervation of the septal area in man: immunocytochemical study using TH and DBH antibodies. J Comp Neurol 241:12–33, 1985

Geddes JW, Cotman CW: Plasticity in Alzheimer's disease: too much or not enough? Neurobiol Aging 12:330–333, 1991

Giacobini E: Cholinergic receptors in human brain: effects of aging and Alzheimer disease. J Neurosci Res 27:548–560, 1990

Giacobini E: Nicotinic cholinergic receptors in human brain: effects of aging and Alzheimer, in Plasticity and Regeneration of the Nervous System: Advances in Experimental Medicine and Biology, Vol 296. Edited by Timiras PS, Privat A, Giacobini E, et al. New York, Plenum, 1991, pp 303–315

Giaquinto S: Aging and the Nervous System. New York, Wiley, 1988

Gibb WRG, Mountjoy CQ, Mann DMA, et al: The substantia nigra and ventral tegmental area in Alzheimer's disease and Down's syndrome. J Neurol Neurosurg Psychiatry 52:193–200, 1989

Goldman JE: The association of actin with hirano bodies. J Neuropathol Exp Neurol 42:146–152, 1983

Goldman JE, Yen S-H: Cytoskeletal protein abnormalities in neurodegenerative diseases. Ann Neurol 19:209–223, 1986

Goldman JE, Yen S-H, Chiu F-C, et al: Lewy bodies of Parkinson's disease contain neurofilament antigens. Science 221:1082–1084, 1983

Gottfries CG: Neurochemical aspects on aging and diseases with cognitive impairment. J Neurosci Res 27:541–547, 1990

Graham DG: On the origin and significance of neuromelanin. Arch Pathol Lab Med 103:359–362, 1979

Greenamyre JT: Neuronal bioenergetic defects, excitotoxicity and Alzheimer's disease: "use it or lose it." Neurobiol Aging 12:334–336, 1991

Gulya AJ: Disorders of hearing, in Oxford Textbook of Geriatric Medicine. Edited by Evans JG, Williams TF. New York, Oxford University Press, 1992, pp 580–585

Gupta SR, Naheedy MH, Young JC, et al: Periventricular white matter changes and dementia: clinical, neuropsychological, radiological, and pathological correlation. Arch Neurol 45:637–641, 1988

Hachinski VC, Potter P, Merskey H: Leuko-araiosis. Arch Neurol 44:21–23, 1987

Hall TC, Miller AKH, Corsellis JAN: Variations in human Purkinje cell population according to age and sex. Neuropathol Appl Neurobiol 1:267–292, 1975

Hanks SD, Flood DG: Region-specific stability of dendritic extent in normal human aging and regression in Alzheimer's disease, I: CA1 of hippocampus. Brain Res 540:63–82, 1991

Hartikainen P, Soininen H, Reinikainen KJ, et al: Neurotransmitter markers in the cerebrospinal fluid of normal subjects: effects of aging and other confounding factors. J Neural Transm Gen Sect 84:103–117, 1991

Haug H: Brain sizes, surfaces, and neuronal sizes of the cortex cerebri: a stereological investigation of man and his variability and a comparison with some mammals (primates, whales, marsupials, insectivores, and one elephant). American Journal of Anatomy 180:126–142, 1987

Haug H, Eggers R: Morphometry of the human cortex cerebri and corpus striatum during aging. Neurobiol Aging 12:336–338, 1991

Haug H, Barmwater U, Eggers R, et al: Anatomical changes in aging brain: morphometric analysis of the human prosencephalon, in Brain Aging: Neuropathology and Neuropharmacology. Edited by Cervós-Navarro J, Sarkander HI. New York, Raven, 1983, pp 1–11

Haug H, Kühl S, Mecke E, et al: The significance of morphometric procedures in the investigation of age changes in cytoarchitectonic structures of human brain. J Hirnforsch 25:353–374, 1984

Hayflick L: Theories of biological aging. Exp Gerontol 20:145–159, 1985

Hazzard WR, Andres R, Bierman EL, et al (eds): Principles of Geriatric Medicine and Gerontology, 2nd Edition. New York, McGraw-Hill, 1990

Hedreen JC, Struble RG, Whitehouse PJ, et al: Topography of the magnocellular basal forebrain system in human brain. J Neuropathol Exp Neurol 43:1–21, 1984

Hefti F, Mash DC: Localization of nerve growth factor receptors in the normal human brain and in Alzheimer's disease. Neurobiol Aging 10:75–87, 1989

Hefti F, Hartikka J, Knusel B: Function of neurotropic factors in the adult and aging brain and their possible use in the treatment of neurodegenerative diseases. Neurobiol Aging 10:515–533, 1989

Heilig CW, Knopman DS, Mastri AR, et al: Dementia without Alzheimer pathology. Neurology 35:762–765, 1985

Hier DB, LeMay M, Rosenberg PB, et al: Developmental dyslexia: evidence for a subgroup with a reversal of cerebral asymmetry. Arch Neurol 35:90–92, 1978

Hirai S: [Histochemical study on the regressive degeneration of the senile brain, with special reference to the aging of the substantia nigra.] Advances in Neurological Science (Tokyo) 12:845–849, 1968

Hof PR, Morrison JH: Quantitative analysis of a vulnerable subset of pyramidal neurons in Alzheimer's disease, II: primary and secondary visual cortex. J Comp Neurol 301:55–64, 1990

Hofman MA: Energy metabolism, brain size and longevity in mammals. Q Rev Biol 58:495–512, 1983

Hofman MA: From here to eternity: brain aging in an evolutionary perspective. Neurobiol Aging 12:338–340, 1991

Hofman MA, Swaab DF: The sexually dimorphic nucleus of the preoptic area in the human brain: a comparative morphometric study. J Anat 164:55–72, 1989

Hyman BT, Van Hoesen GW, Damasio AR, et al: Alzheimer's disease: cell-specific pathology isolates the hippocampal formation. Science 225:1168–1170, 1984

Hyman BT, Van Hoesen GW, Wolozin BL, et al: Alz-50 antibody recognizes Alzheimer-related neuronal changes. Ann Neurol 23:371–378, 1988

Hyman BT, Arriagada PV, Van Hoesen GW: Pathologic changes in the olfactory system in aging and Alzheimer's disease. Ann N Y Acad Sci 640:14–19, 1991

Ikeda SI, Allsop D, Glenner GG: Morphology and distribution of plaque and related deposits in the brains of Alzheimer's disease and control cases: an immunohistochemical study using amyloid β-protein antibody. Lab Invest 60:113–122, 1989

Ingvar MC, Maeder P, Sokoloff L, et al: Effects of ageing on local rates of cerebral protein synthesis in Sprague-Dawley rats. Brain 108:155–170, 1985

Inzitari D, Diaz F, Fox A, et al: Vascular risk factors and leukoaraiosis. Arch Neurol 44:42–47, 1987

Jellinger K: Quantitative changes in some subcortical nuclei in aging, Alzheimer's disease and Parkinson's disease. Neurobiol Aging 8:556–561, 1987

Jengeleski CA, Powers RE, O'Connor DT, et al: Noradrenergic innervation of human pineal gland: abnormalities in aging and Alzheimer's disease. Brain Res 481:378–382, 1989

Kalaria RN, Andorn AC, Tabaton M, et al: Adrenergic receptors in aging and Alzheimer's disease: increased β2-receptors in prefrontal cortex and hippocampus. J Neurochem 53:1772–1781, 1989

Katzman R: Normal pressure hydrocephalus, in Alzheimer's Disease: Senile Dementia and Related Disorders, Vol 7. Edited by Datzman R, Terry RD, Bick KL. New York, Raven, 1978, pp 115–124

Katzman R, Terry R, DeTeresa R, et al: Clinical, pathological, and neurochemical changes in dementia: a subgroup with preserved mental status and numerous neocortical plaques. Ann Neurol 23:138–144, 1988

Kawasaki H, Murayama SA, Tomonaga M, et al: Neurofibrillary tangles in human upper cervical ganglia: morphological study with immunohistochemistry and electron microscopy. Acta Neuropathol 75:156–159, 1987

Kaye JA, DeCarli C, Luxenberg JS, et al: The significance of age-related enlargement of the cerebral ventricles in healthy men and women measured by quantitative computed x-ray tomography. J Am Geriatr Soc 40:225–231, 1992

Kemper T: Neuroanatomical and neuropathological changes in normal aging and dementia, in Clinical Neurology of Aging. Edited by Albert ML. New York, Oxford University Press, 1984, pp 9–52

Kesslak JP, Cotman CW, Chui HC, et al: Olfactory tests as possible probes for detecting and monitoring Alzheimer's disease. Neurobiol Aging 9:399–403, 1988

Kirkpatrick JB, Hayman LA: White-matter lesions in MR imaging of clinically healthy brains of elderly subjects: possible pathologic basis. Radiology 162:509–511, 1987

Knox CA, Kokmen E, Dyck PJ: Morphometric alteration of rat myelinated fibers with aging. J Neuropathol Exp Neurol 48:119–139, 1989

Kosik KS: Alzheimer's disease: a cell biological perspective. Science 256:780–783, 1992

Kowall NW, Kosik KS: Axonal disruption and aberrant localization of tau protein characterize the neuropil pathology of Alzheimer's disease. Ann Neurol 22:639–643, 1987

Kuperman S, Black DW, Burns TL: Excess mortality among formerly hospitalized child psychiatric patients. Arch Gen Psychiatry 45:277–282, 1988

Lintl P, Braak H: Loss of intracortical myelinated fibers: a distinctive age-related alteration in the human striate area. Acta Neuropathol (Berl) 61:178–182, 1983

Lopez OL, Rabin BS, Huff FJ: Serum auto-antibodies in Alzheimer's disease. Acta Neurol Scand 84:441–444, 1991

Mader SL: Aging and postural hypotension: an update. J Am Geriatr Soc 37:129–137, 1989

Mann DMA: Is the pattern of nerve cell loss in aging and Alzheimer's disease a real, or only an apparent, selectivity? Neurobiol Aging 12:340–343, 1991

Mann DMA, Yates PO, Hawkes J: The pathology of the human locus ceruleus. Clin Neuropathol 2:1–7, 1983

Mann DMA, Yates PO, Marcyniuk B: Monoaminergic neurotransmitter systems in presenile Alzheimer's disease and in senile dementia of Alzheimer type. Clin Neuropathol 3:199–205, 1984

Matsuyama H, Nakamura S: Senile changes in the brain in the Japanese: incidence of Alzheimer's neurofibrillary change and senile plaques, in Alzheimer's Disease: Senile Dementia and Related Disorders. Edited by Katzman R, Terry RD, Bick KL. New York, Raven, 1978, pp 287–297

Mattson MP: Activities in cellular signalling pathways: a two-edged sword? Neurobiol Aging 12:343–346, 1991

Mattson MP, Rydel RE: β-Amyloid precursor protein and Alzheimer's disease: the peptide plot thickens. Neurobiol Aging 13:617–621, 1992

Maurer K, Riederer P, Beckmann (eds): Alzheimer's Disease: Epidemiology, Neuropathology, Neurochemistry, and Clinics. New York, Springer-Verlag, 1990

McEwen BS: When is stimulation too much of a good thing? Neurobiol Aging 12:346–348, 1991

McGeer PL, McGeer EG, Suzuki JS: Aging and extrapyramidal function. Arch Neurol 34:33–35, 1977

McKhann G, Drachman D, Folstein M, et al: Clinical diagnosis of Alzheimer's disease: report of the NINCDS-ADRDA work group under the auspices of department of health and human services task force on Alzheimer's disease. Neurology (NY) 34:939–944, 1984

McLeod JG, Tuck RR: Disorders of the autonomic nervous system, I: pathophysiology and clinical features. Ann Neurol 21:419–430, 1987

Mendelsohn FAO, Paxinos G (eds): Receptors in the Human Nervous System. San Diego, CA, Academic Press, 1991

Mervis RF, Pope D, Lewis R, et al: Exogenous nerve growth factor reverses age-related structural changes in neocortical neurons in the aging rat: a quantitative Golgi study. Ann N Y Acad Sci 640:95–103, 1991

Mesulam M-M, Geula C: Nucleus basalis (ch 4) and cortical cholinergic innervation in the human brain: observations based on the distribution of acetylcholinesterase and choline acetyltransferase. J Comp Neurol 275:216–240, 1988

Mesulam M-M, Mufson EJ, Levey AI, et al: Cholinergic innervation of cortex by the basal forebrain: cytochemistry and cortical connections of the septal area, diagonal band nuclei, nucleus basalis (substantia innominata), and hypothalamus in the Rhesus monkey. J Comp Neurol 214:170–197, 1983

Miller JA, Zahniser NR: Quantitative autoradiographic analysis of ^{125}I-pindolol binding in Fischer 344 rat brain: changes in β-adrenergic receptor density with aging. Neurobiol Aging 9:267–272, 1988

Moatamed F: Cell frequencies in human inferior olivary nuclear complex. J Comp Neurol 128:109–115, 1966

Mooradian AD: Effect of aging on the blood-brain barrier. Neurobiol Aging 9:31–39, 1988

Morgan DG, Finch CE: Neurotransmitter receptors in Alzheimer's disease and nonpathological aging, in Molecular Neuropathology of Aging. Edited by Davies P, Finch CE. Cold Spring Harbor, NY, Cold Spring Harbor Laboratory, 1987, pp 21–35

Morgan DG, Marcusson JO, Nyberg P, et al: Divergent changes in D-1 and D-2 dopamine binding sites in human brain during aging. Neurobiol Aging 8:195–201, 1987

Morrison JH, Hof PR, Bouras C: An anatomic substrate for visual disconnection in Alzheimer's disease. Ann N Y Acad Sci 640:36–43, 1991

Müller WE, Stoll L, Schubert T, et al: Central cholinergic functioning and aging. Acta Psychiatr Scand 366 (suppl): 34–39, 1991

Niedermüller H, Hofecker G, Skalicky M: Changes of DNA repair mechanisms during the aging of the rat. Mech Ageing Dev 29:221–238, 1985

Nisticò G, De Sarro G: Is interleukin 2 a neuromodulator in the brain? Trends Neurosci 14:146–150, 1991

Nordberg A, Winblad B: Reduced number of [3H]nicotine and [3H]acetylcholine binding sites in the frontal cortex of Alzheimer brains. Neurosci Lett 72:115–119, 1986

Nukina N, Kosik KS, Selkoe DJ: The monoclonal antibody, Alz 50, recognizes tau proteins in Alzheimer's disease brain. Neurosci Lett 87:240–246, 1988

Olton D, Markowska A, Voytko ML, et al: Basal forebrain cholinergic system: a functional analysis, in The Basal Forebrain Anatomy to Function, Advances in Experimental Medicine and Biology, Vol 295. Edited by Napier TC, Kalivas PW, Hanin I. New York, Plenum, 1991, pp 353–371

Otto D, Unsicker K: Effects of FGF-2 on dopamine neurons. Neuroscience Facts 3:82–83, 1992

Oyanagi K, Wakabayashi K, Ohama E, et al: Lewy bodies in the lower sacral parasympathetic neurons of a patient with Parkinson's disease. Acta Neuropathol 80:558–559, 1990

Pascual J, del Arco C, Gonzàlez AM, et al: Quantitative light microscopic autoradiographic localization of α2-adrenoceptors in the human brain. Brain Res 585:116–127, 1992

Peng I, Binder LI, Black MM: Biochemical and immunological analyses of cytoskeletal domains of neurons. J Cell Biol 102:252–262, 1986

Perry EK, McKeith I, Thompson P, et al: Topography, extent, and clinical relevance of neurochemical deficits in dementia of Lewy body type, Parkinson's disease, and Alzheimer's disease. Ann N Y Acad Sci 640:197–202, 1991

Peters NL: Snipping the thread of life: antimuscarinic side effects of medications in the elderly. Arch Intern Med 149:2414–2420, 1989

Powers RE, Struble RG, Casanova MF, et al: Innervation of human hippocampus by noradrenergic systems: normal anatomy and structural abnormalities in aging and in Alzheimer's disease. Neuroscience 25:401–417, 1988

Powers RE, Powell SK, Schlough CN, et al: Autopsy services for dementia patients. Gerontologist 29:120–123, 1989

Price DL, Martin LJ, Sisodia SS, et al: Aged non-human primates: an animal model of age-associated neurodegenerative disease. Brain Pathology 1:287–296, 1991

Price JL, Davis PB, Morris JC, et al: The distribution of tangles, plaques and related immunohistochemical markers in healthy aging and Alzheimer's disease. Neurobiol Aging 12:295–312, 1991

Probst A, Brunnschweiler H, Lautenschlager C, et al: A special type of senile plaque, possibly an initial stage. Acta Neuropathol (Berl) 74:133–141, 1987

Procter AW, Bowen DM: Aging, the cerebral neocortex, and psychiatric disorder, in Molecular Neuropathology of Aging. Edited by Davies P, Finch CE. Cold Spring Harbor, NY, Cold Spring Harbor Laboratory, 1987, pp 3–21

Rance NE: Hormonal influences on morphology and neuropeptide gene expression in the infundibular nucleus of post-menopausal women. Prog Brain Res 93:221–236, 1992

Rance NE, Young WS III: Hypertrophy and increased gene expression of neurons containing neurokinin-B and substance-P messenger ribonucleic acids in the hypothalami of postmenopausal women. Endocrinology 128:2239–2247, 1991

Rance NE, McMullen NT, Smialek JE, et al: Postmenopausal hypertrophy of neurons expressing the estrogen receptor gene in the human hypothalamus. J Clin Endocrinol Metab 71:79–85, 1990

Rance NE, Uswandi SV, McMullen NT: Neuronal hypertrophy in the hypothalamus of older men. Neurobiol Aging 14:337–342, 1993

Reznikoff GA, Manaker S, Rhodes CH, et al: Localization and quantification of beta-adrenergic receptors in human brain. Neurology 36:1067–1073, 1986

Robinson RG, Kubos KL, Starr LBN, et al: Mood disorders in stroke patients. Importance of location of lesion. Brain 107 (pt 1):81–93, 1984

Robinson RG, Bolduc PL, Price TR: Two-year longitudinal study of poststroke disorders: diagnosis and outcome at one and two years. Stroke 18:837–843, 1987

Rosene DL, Van Hoesen GW: The hippocampal formation of the primate brain: a review of some comparative aspects of cytoarchitecture and connections, in Cerebral Cortex, Vol 6. Edited by Jones EG, Peters A. New York, Plenum, 1986, pp 345–456

Rowe JW: Plasma norepinephrine as an index of sympathetic activity in aging man, in Molecular Neuropathology of Aging. Edited by Davies P, Finch CE. Cold Spring Harbor, NY, Cold Spring Harbor Laboratory, 1987, pp 137–143

Rudman D, Feller AG, Nagraj HS, et al: Effects of human growth hormone in men over 60 years old. N Engl J Med 323:1–6, 1990

Sapolsky RM: Glucocorticoids and hippocampal damage. Trends Neurosci 10:346–349, 1987a

Sapolsky RM: Protecting the injured hippocampus by attenuating glucocorticoid secretion, in Molecular Neuropathology of Aging. Edited by Davies P, Finch CE. Cold Spring Harbor, NY, Cold Spring Harbor Laboratory, 1987b, pp 191–201

Scarpace PJ, Abrass IB: Alpha- and beta-adrenergic receptor function in the brain during senescence. Neurobiol Aging 9:53–58, 1988

Scheff SW: Use or abuse. Neurobiol Aging 12:349–351, 1991

Schoen EJ: Growth hormone in youth and old age (the old and new déjà vu) (letter). J Am Geriatr Soc 39:839, 1991

Schröder H, Giacobini E, Struble RG, et al: Cellular distribution and expression of cortical acetylcholine receptors in aging and Alzheimer's disease. Ann N Y Acad Sci 640:189–192, 1991

Shimohama S, Taniguchi T, Fujiwara M, et al: Changes in benzodiazepine receptors in Alzheimer's type-dementia. Ann Neurol 23:404–406, 1988

Sobin SS, Bernick S, Ballard KW: Histochemical characterization of the aging microvasculature in the human and other mammalian and non-mammalian vertebrates by the periodic acid-Schiff reaction. Mech Ageing Dev 63:183–192, 1992

Sparks DL, Hunsaker JC III, Scheff SW, et al: Cortical senile plaques in coronary artery disease, aging and Alzheimer's disease. Neurobiol Aging 11:601–607, 1990

Struble RG, Powers RE, Casanova MF, et al: Neuropeptidergic systems in plaques of Alzheimer's disease. J Neuropathol Exp Neurol 46:567–584, 1987

Swaab DF: Brain aging and Alzheimer's disease, "wear and tear" versus "use it or lose it." Neurobiol Aging 12:317–324, 1991

Sze G, De Armond SJ, Brant-Zawadzki M, et al: Foci of MRI signal (pseudo lesions) anterior to the frontal horns: histologic correlations of a normal finding. American Journal of Neuroradiology 7:381–387, 1986

Talamo BR, Rudel RA, Kosik KS, et al: Pathological changes in olfactory neurons in patients with Alzheimer's disease. Nature 337:736–739, 1989

Terry RD, Hansen LA, DeTeresa R, et al: Senile dementia of the Alzheimer type without neocortical neurofibrillary tangles. J Neuropathol Exp Neurol 46:262–268, 1987

Thoenen H, Zafra F, Hengerer B, et al: The synthesis of nerve growth factor and brain-derived neurotrophic factor in hippocampal and cortical neurons is regulated by specific transmitter systems. Ann N Y Acad Sci 640:86–90, 1991

Thomas WE: Brain macrophages: evaluation of microglia and their functions. Brain Research Reviews 17:61–74, 1992

Tomlinson BE, Blessed G, Roth M: Observations on the brains of demented old people. J Neurol Sci 11:205–242, 1970

Torack RM, Morris JC: The association of ventral tegmental area histopathology with adult dementia. Arch Neurol 45:497–501, 1988

Uchihara T, Kondo H, Kosaka K, et al: Selective loss of nigral neurons in Alzheimer's disease: a morphometric study. Acta Neuropathol (Berl) 83:271–276, 1992

Ueno E, Liu DD, Ho IK, et al: Opiate receptor characteristics in brains from young, mature and aged mice. Neurobiol Aging 9:279–283, 1988

Ulrich J: Senile plaques and neurofibrillary tangles of the Alzheimer type in nondemented individuals at presenile age. Gerontology 28:86–90, 1982

Van Gool WA, Pronker HF, Mirmiran M, et al: Effect of housing in an enriched environment on the size of the cerebral cortex in young and old rats. Exp Neurol 96:225–232, 1987

Veith RC, Raskind MA: The neurobiology of aging: does it predispose to depression? Neurobiol Aging 9:101–117, 1988

Volicer L, Crino PB: Involvement of free radicals in dementia of the Alzheimer type: a hypothesis. Neurobiol Aging 11:567–571, 1990

Wakabayashi K, Takahashi H, Takeda S, et al: Parkinson's disease: the presence of Lewy bodies in Auerbach's and Meissner's plexuses. Acta Neuropathol 76:217–221, 1988

Wareham KA, Lyon MF, Glenister PH, et al: Age-related reactivation of an X-linked gene. Nature 327:725–727, 1987

Weinberger DR: Implications of normal brain development for the pathogenesis of schizophrenia. Arch Gen Psychiatry 44:660–669, 1987

Whitehouse PJ, Price DL, Clark AW, et al: Alzheimer disease: evidence for selective loss of cholinergic neurons in the nucleus basalis. Ann Neurol 10:122–126, 1981

Wise PM, Cohen IR, Weiland NG: Hypothalamic monoamine function during aging: its role in the onset of reproductive infertility, in Molecular Neuropathology of Aging. Edited by Davies P, Finch CE. Cold Spring Harbor, NY, Cold Spring Harbor Laboratory, pp 159–164, 1987

Wyss JM, Van Groen T: Early breakdown of dendritic bundles in the retrosplenial granular cortex of hypertensive rats: prevention by antihypertensive therapy. Cerebral Cortex 2:468–476, 1992

Wyss JM, Fisk G, Van Groen T: Impaired learning and memory in mature spontaneously hypertensive rats. Brain Res 592:135–140, 1992

Zubenko GS, Moossy J: Major depression in primary dementia: clinical and neuropathologic correlates. Arch Neurol 45:1182–1186, 1988

4

Neurobiological Basis of Behavior

Jeffrey L. Cummings, M.D.
C. Edward Coffey, M.D.

Introduction

All behavior and experience are mediated by the brain. No behavior, thought, or emotion lacks a corresponding cerebral event, and abnormalities of human behavior are frequently a reflection of abnormal brain structure and are accompanied by aberrant brain function. This premise does not deny the influence of learning, life events, education, or the sociocultural dimension of human existence; these factors create the context of human behavior and exert powerful developmental and situational influences. In all cases, however, sociocultural effects are mediated through brain function. Thus, a comprehensive approach to human behavior demands an understanding of the neurological basis of human cognition, emotion, and psychopathology.

A life-span perspective adds another dimension to understanding behavior: brain function alters dramatically from uterine life, through infancy, childhood, adolescence, adulthood, and old age. Physiological functions vary more widely in elderly people than in young people, tolerance of injury and potential for recovery are diminished in elderly patients, and the types of behaviors associated with brain dysfunction may differ depending on the age of the patient.

In this chapter, we provide a review of the neuroanatomical and neurochemical basis of human behavior. First we present a synoptic model of behavioral neuroanatomy as a framework for the remaining discussion. The model divides the nervous system into three behaviorally relevant zones: an inner zone surrounding the ventricular system, a middle zone encompassing the basal ganglia and limbic system, and an outer zone comprised primarily of the neocortex. We present the anatomy of each zone and describe the behavioral consequences of injury to each. Next we describe two distributed systems; these cross the three zones to allow information to enter the brain (thalamocortical system) and allow impulses mediating action to exit the brain (frontal-subcortical circuits). We also present neuropsychiatric syndromes associated with abnormalities of these systems. Finally, we integrate the biochemical basis of behavior with this anatomical approach.

A Model of Behavioral Neuroanatomy

Yakovlev provided a comprehensive model of the nervous system in terms relevant to behavior (Yakovlev 1948, 1968; Yakovlev and Lecours 1967). He adopted an evolutionary perspective and noted that the brain consists of three general regions: a median zone surrounding the ventricular system; a paramedian-limbic zone consisting primarily of limbic system structures, basal ganglia, and parts of the thalamus; and a supralimbic zone containing the neocortex.

In this chapter, we present the Yakovlev approach—updated with information from more recent anatomical studies (Mesulam 1985)—as a foundation for understanding brain-behavior relationships (Figure 4–1). The *median zone* is immediately adjacent to the central canal, is poorly myelinated, and has neurons with short axons that synapse on nearby cells, as well as on cells with longer axons that project to more distant nuclei. The median zone contains the hypothalamus, medial thalamus, and periventricular gray matter of the brain stem. The system mediates energy metabolism, homeostasis, peristalsis, respiration, and circulation. The median zone contains the reticular activating system and the nonspecific thalamocortical projections that maintain consciousness and arousal in the awake state and participate in sleep mechanisms. No lateral specialization is evident in the median zone. This system is fully functional at birth and is responsible for the early survival of the infant.

The *paramedian-limbic zone* has more myelin than the median zone, and neurons here are grouped in nuclear structures that are connected in series. Many of the thalamic nuclei, the basal ganglia, cingulate gyrus, insula, orbitofrontal region, hippocampus, and parahippocampal gyri are included in this zone. The paramedian-limbic zone includes the structures comprising the limbic system (Papez 1937). Structures of this zone mediate the experiential aspects of emotional states. They also mediate posture and the outward expression of emotion in vocalization, gestures, and facial affective display. There is little lateral specialization of the paramedian structures. Phylogenetically, this level of brain development is present in reptiles (MacLean 1990). The paramedian-limbic zone is partially func-

This project was supported by the Department of Veterans Affairs and by a National Institute on Aging Alzheimer's Disease Core Center grant (AG010123) (to CEC) and by the Allegheny Singer Research Institute (to CEC).

tional at birth, and its emerging integrity becomes evident in smiling and crawling. Disorders of motivation, mood, and emotion are associated with paramedian-limbic dysfunction, and this zone is the anatomic site of structures involved in many neuropsychiatric disorders. Parkinson's disease with its depression, apathy, akinesia, masked face, hypophonic voice, and marked postural changes is an example of a common disease of elderly people affecting the paramedian-limbic zone.

The *supralimbic zone* is outermost in the brain and includes the neocortex and the lateral thalamic nuclei. The neurons of this zone have long, well-myelinated axons that project via white matter tracts to more distant targets. The supralimbic neocortex contains the neurons mediating higher cortical (association) functions, as well as the pyramidal neurons projecting to limbs, lips, and tongue. It mediates highly skilled fine motor movements evident in human speech and hand control. Ontogenetically, this zone first finds expres-

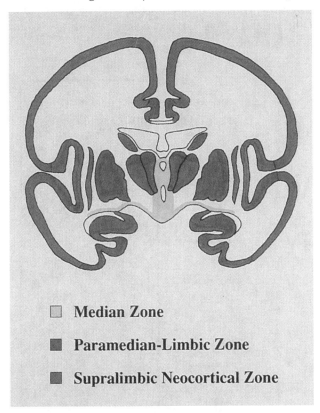

□ **Median Zone**

■ **Paramedian-Limbic Zone**

■ **Supralimbic Neocortical Zone**

Figure 4–1. Updated version of Yakovlev's model of the nervous system demonstrating the median zone (*yellow*), paramedian-limbic zone (*green*), and supralimbic zone (*red*) *Source.* Modified from Yakovlev PI, Lecours A-R: "The Myelogenetic Cycles of Regional Maturation of the Brain," in *Regional Development of the Brain in Early Life.* Edited by Minkowski A. Oxford, England, Blackwell Scientific, 1967, pp. 3–65. Used with permission.

sion in the pincer grasp and articulate speech. Phylogenetically, the supralimbic zone first appears in mammals and is most well-developed in humans (MacLean 1990). The supralimbic zone is expressed in human cultural achievements including art, manufacture, speech, and writing. The supralimbic zone exhibits lateral specialization with marked differences between the functions of the neocortex within the two hemispheres. This zone is vulnerable to some of the most common neurological disorders associated with aging, including stroke and Alzheimer's disease. For example, the expansion of the neocortex has been at the expense of a secure vasculature. The enlarged association areas have created border zone areas between the territories of the major intracranial blood vessels that are at risk of stroke because of limited interconnections and poor collateral flow; reduced cerebral perfusion with carotid artery disease or cardiopulmonary arrest regularly results in border zone infarctions at the margins between these vascular territories. In addition, penetrating branches form arterial end zones that have no collateral supply as they project through the white matter to the borders of the ventricles. This creates an area of vulnerability to ischemia at the margins of the lateral ventricles. Periventricular brain injury has been associated with depression (Coffey et al. 1988) and vascular dementia. Along with the hippocampus, the supralimbic zone is the major site of pathological changes in Alzheimer's disease. Focal lesions of the neocortex result in restricted neurobehavioral deficits such as aphasia, apraxia, and agnosia.

This model of behavioral neuroanatomy provides an ontogenetic life-span perspective showing the emerging function of these structures in early life and their disease-related vulnerability in later life. The model reflects an evolutionary perspective of the brain emphasizing its development through time and its increasing complexity in response to evolutionary pressures. From a clinical point of view, most neuropsychological deficit syndromes such as disorders of language and praxis are associated with dysfunction of the supralimbic neocortex, whereas disorders of mood, psychosis, and personality alterations are more likely to occur with abnormalities in the paramedian-limbic system. The median zone is responsible for more primitive life-sustaining functions, and disturbances there are reflected in disorders of consciousness and abnormalities of metabolism, respiration, and circulation. Thus the patterns of neuropsychiatric disturbance occurring with brain disorders are highly organized events that reflect the history, structure, and function of the nervous system.

Neocortex (Supralimbic Zone)

Histological Organization of the Cortex and Behavior

Brodmann originally described 46 cortical areas with distinctive histological characteristics, and Brodmann's maps have remained the classical guide to the histological organization of the cerebral mantle. Within Brodmann's areas, three types of cortex relevant to understanding behavior have been identified: a three-layered allocortex, six-layered neocortex, and an intermediate paralimbic cortex. The limbic system cortex such as the hippocampus has a three-layered allocortical structure, whereas the sensory, motor, and association cortices of the hemispheres have a six-layered organization (Kelly 1991). Layer I is outermost and consists primarily of axons connecting local cortical areas; layers II and III have a predominance of small pyramidal cells and serve to connect one region of cortex with another; layer IV has mostly nonpyramidal cells, receives most of the cortical input from the thalamus, and is greatly expanded in primary sensory cortex; layer V is most prominent in motor cortex and has large pyramidal cells that have long axons descending to subcortical structures, brain stem, and spinal cord; and layer VI is adjacent to the hemispheric white matter and contains pyramidal cells, many of which project to thalamus (Figure 4–2) (Kelly 1991). Layers II and IV have the greatest cell density and the smallest cells; conversely, layers III and V have the lowest density and the largest cells. Cell size correlates with the extent of dendritic ramification, implying that cells of the layers III and V projecting to other cortical regions have the largest dendritic domains (Schade and Groeningen 1961).

Functional Organization of the Neocortex

The *neocortex* is highly differentiated into primary motor and sensory areas and unimodal and heteromodal association regions (Table 4–1) (Mesulam 1985). Figure 4–3 shows the anatomical distribution of the different cortical types in the cerebral hemispheres (Mesulam 1985). Association cortex occupies 84% of the human neocortex, whereas primary motor

and sensory areas account for only 16%; this indicates the marked importance of association cortex in human brain function (Rapoport 1990). The neocortex is organized in a mosaic of cortical columns, and local circuit neurons (confined to the cortex) comprise approximately 25% of the cellular population (Rapoport 1990). Cortical regions receive and send information via white matter tracts.

Primary motor cortex occupies the motor strip in the posterior frontal lobe and serves as the origin of the pyramidal motor system (Figure 4–4). Lesions of the motor cortex produce contralateral weakness, particularly of the leg flexors and arm extensors, hyperreflexia, and an extensor plantar response. *Primary somatosensory cortex* is located in the postcentral gyrus in the anterior parietal lobe, *primary auditory cortex* occupies Heschl's gyrus in the superior temporal lobe anterior to Wernicke's area, and *primary visual cortex* is situated in the calcarine region of the occipital lobe (Figure 4–4). Lesions of these regions typically result in contralateral hemisensory deficits (the auditory system is an exception).

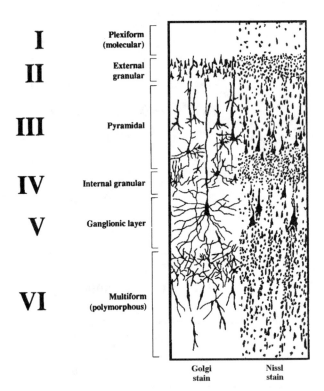

Figure 4–2.   Histological structure of six-layered neocortex.
Source.   Reprinted from Carpenter MB: *Core Text of Neuroanatomy,* 4th Edition. Philadelphia, PA, Williams & Wilkins, 1991, p. 391. Copyright 1991 Williams & Wilkins. Used with permission.

Unimodal association areas mediate the second level of information processing in the cerebral cortex after the primary sensory cortex. Unimodal somatosensory cortex is located in the superior parietal lobule, unimodal auditory cortex is situated in Wernicke's region in the left hemisphere and the equivalent area of the posterior superior temporal cortex of the right hemisphere, and unimodal visual cortex occupies peristriate, midtemporal, and inferotemporal cortical regions (Figure 4–5). Lesions of these regions produce deficits confined to a single sensory modality; the syndromes associated with dysfunction of these regions reflect the higher level of information processing. Wernicke's area lesions produce fluent aphasia; lesions of right-sided auditory unimodal cortex produce sensory aprosodia (i.e., the inability to comprehend speech inflection and melody); and lesions of the unimodal visual association cortex produces visual agnosias (e.g., visual object agnosia, prosopagnosia, and environmental agnosia) (Kirshner 1986).

The highest level of information processing in the cerebral hemispheres occurs in the *heteromodal association cortices*. It is also in these regions that sensory information from primary sensory and unimodal association cortex is integrated with limbic and paralimbic input (Mesulam 1985). Two heteromodal association regions are recognized in the human brain: the inferior parietal lobule and the prefrontal cortex (Figure 4–6). Dysfunction of these areas produces complex behavioral deficits that transcend single modalities. Lesions of the left inferior parietal lobule produce the angular gyrus syndrome with alexia, agraphia, acalculia, right-left disorientation, finger agnosia, anomia, and constructional disturbances (Benson et al. 1982).

Right-sided inferior parietal lesions produce visuospatial deficits affecting constructions, spatial attention, and body-environment orientation. Prefrontal cortical dysfunction produces deficits in motor programing, memory retrieval, abstraction, and judgment (Stuss and Benson 1986). Posterior heteromodal association cortex dysfunction observed with inferior parietal lobe

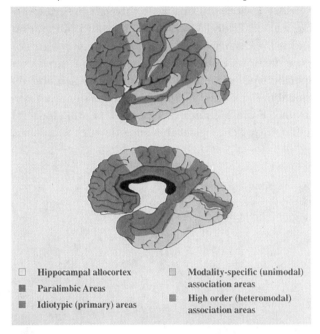

☐ Hippocampal allocortex	☐ Modality-specific (unimodal) association areas
■ Paralimbic Areas	
■ Idiotypic (primary) areas	■ High order (heteromodal) association areas

Figure 4–3. Distribution of different histological types of cortex in the human cerebrum. The hippocampal allocortex is shown in *white,* paralimbic cortex in *green,* unimodal association cortex in *yellow,* multimodal association cortex in *red,* and primary motor and sensory cortex in *blue.*
Source. Modified from Mesulam M-M (ed): *Principles of Behavioral Neurology.* Philadelphia, PA, F. A. Davis, 1985. Used with permission.

Table 4–1. Structure and function of different types of cerebral cortex

Cortex	Layer number	Brain regions	Relevant behaviors
Neocortex			
Primary cortex			
Koniocortex	6	Primary sensory cortex (parietal)	Vision, hearing, somatic sensation
Macropyramidal	6	Primary motor cortex (motor cortex)	Movement
Unimodal association cortex	6	Secondary association (parietal, temporal, occipital cortex)	Modality-specific processing of vision, hearing, and somatic sensation
Heteromodal association cortex	6	Multimodal association (inferior parietal lobule, prefrontal cortex)	Higher-order association
Allocortex			
Archicortex	3	Hippocampus	Memory
Paleocortex	3	Piriform cortex	Olfaction
Paralimbic (mesocortex)	4, 5	Orbitofrontal cortex, insula, temporal pole, parahippocampal gyrus, cingulate gyrus	Emotional behavior

lesions reflects abnormalities of the highest level of processing of incoming sensory information; anterior heteromodal association cortex dysfunction in conjunction with prefrontal disturbances produces deficits in active organizational or "executive" behaviors.

Thus a behavioral neuroanatomy can be discerned in the histological organization of the cerebral cortex. Sensory processing proceeds through progressively more complicated levels of analysis and integration and is then translated into action through a series of executive processes. Each cortical region carries on specific types of neurophysiological activities, and regional injury or dysfunction produces a signature syndrome. From a clinical perspective, neurobehavioral and neuropsychological abnormalities such as aphasia,

aprosodia, and agnosia are associated with neocortical lesions. Although each region has unique functions, each also contributes to more complex integrative processes required for human experience and behavior.

White Matter Connections

White matter of the brain consists of myelinated axons of neurons and contains three types of fibers: 1) projection fibers that connect the cortex with the basal ganglia, thalamus, brain stem, and spinal cord; 2) association fibers that interconnect cortical regions of the same hemisphere; and 3) commissural fibers that connect the two hemispheres with each other (Carpenter and Sutin 1983). The principal *projection tracts* include the efferent corticostriatal projections, corticothalamic connections, corticobulbar, corticopontine, and corticospinal fibers and the afferent thalamocortical radiations. There are also short and long *association fibers*. The short association or "U" fibers connect adja-

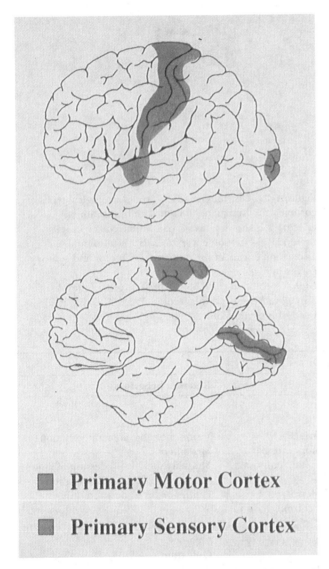

Figure 4–4. Primary motor (*red*) and sensory (*blue*) cortex.

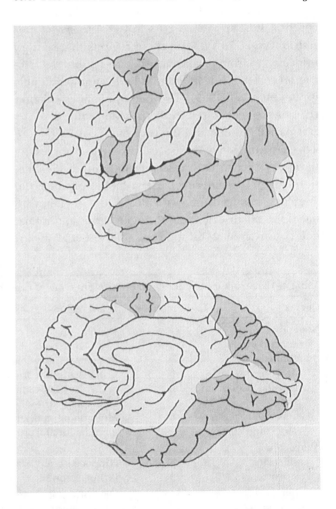

Figure 4–5. Unimodal association cortex (*yellow*).

■ **Primary Motor Cortex**

■ **Primary Sensory Cortex**

cent sulci; the long association fibers form robust tracts connecting more distant regions within each hemisphere. The main long association tracts are the uncinate gyrus connecting the orbitofrontal region with the anterior temporal cortex, the arcuate fasciculus projecting between the temporal lobe and the superior and middle frontal gyri, the superior longitudinal fasciculus reaching between parieto-occipital and frontal cortices, the inferior longitudinal fasciculus connecting the parieto-occipital region with the temporal lobe, and the cingulum containing fibers connecting frontal and parietal regions with the hippocampus (Figure 4–7). The commissural fibers are situated in the massive corpus callosum interconnecting all lobes of one hemisphere with corresponding areas of the contralateral hemisphere and in the more diminutive anterior commissure interconnecting the olfactory regions and the middle and inferior temporal gyri of the hemispheres (Figure 4–8).

Intact cerebral function depends on the integrity of the axons of the white matter, as well as on the activ-

ity of the neurons of the gray matter. White matter diseases with diffuse or multifocal demyelination produce memory abnormalities, dementia, depression, mania, delusions, and personality alterations. Focal lesions of white matter tracts produce a number of *disconnection syndromes* that arise when critical neuronal areas are uncoupled by an intervening lesion (Geschwind 1965; Kirshner 1986). Table 4–2 summarizes the principal disconnection syndromes.

Disruption of *commissural fibers* by stroke, surgery, or trauma disconnects the left and right hemispheres,

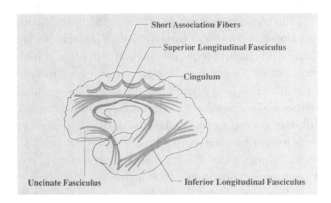

Figure 4–7. Major association fiber tracts of the hemispheres.

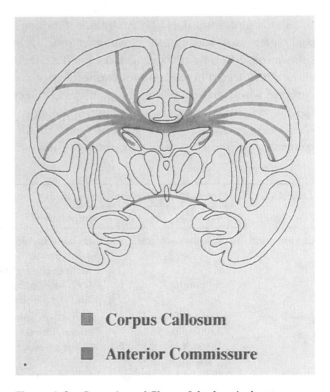

Figure 4–8. Commissural fibers of the hemispheres including the corpus callosum (*blue*) and the anterior commissure (*red*).

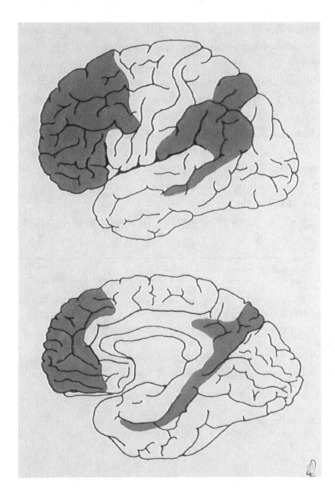

Figure 4–6. Heteromodal association cortex (*red*).

and several commissural or callosal syndromes are recognized clinically. With an anterior callosal lesion, the right hemisphere controlling the left hand becomes disconnected from the left hemisphere; thus the left hand no longer has access to the verbal and motor skills of the left hemisphere, and apraxia results. When the splenium of the corpus callosum is damaged in association with injury to the left occipital cortex (usually from a left posterior cerebral artery occlusion), the visual information available to the right hemisphere cannot be transferred to the left for semantic decoding, and alexia without agraphia results.

Disconnection syndromes also occur with lesions of *association fiber tracts.* Interruption of the arcuate fasciculus is responsible for conduction aphasia and parietal apraxia. Lesions of the right inferior longitudinal fasciculus produce prosopagnosia and environmental agnosia, whereas bilateral inferior longitudinal fasciculus damage causes visual object agnosia. Hemisensory deficits and homonymous hemianopsia result from lesions affecting the thalamocortical projections, and hemimotor syndromes occur with lesions of the descending corticospinal projections. The locked-in syndrome occurs with bilateral lesions of descending corticobulbar and corticospinal projection tracts at the pontine level.

The complex histological organization of the cerebral cortex, with its different cytoarchitectonic areas subsuming different processing tasks (as described above), is reflected in the complex connectivity of the cerebral white matter. White matter tracts connect specialized cortical regions, and neuropsychological syndromes may reflect focal cortical injury or disconnection of the cortical regions through injury to the associated white matter connections. Disconnection syndromes occur with lesions of commissural, long association, or projection fibers. Discrete neurobehavioral syndromes have been identified only when lesions of callosal or association fibers disconnect unimodal association areas (e.g., interruption of visual processing in the agnosias or motor activities in the apraxias); no multimodal disconnection syndromes have been described.

Hemispheric Specialization, Laterality, and Dominance

Anatomic asymmetries. The two cerebral hemispheres, although grossly symmetrical, differ in some aspects of development, structure, and biochemical constitution. Differences between the right and left hemispheres have been shown in both the upper surface of the temporal lobes and the inferolateral surface of the frontal lobe (Figure 4–9). The temporal lobe area corresponding to Wernicke's area (in 65% of cases) and the frontal region corresponding to Broca's area (in 83% of cases) are both larger than the corresponding right-brain regions (Falzi et al. 1982; Galaburda et al. 1978). The superior temporal surface is longer and the total area is approximately one-third larger in the left hemisphere. The Sylvian fissure is longer and more horizontal on the left, whereas it is curved upward on the right (Galaburda et al. 1978). Cytoarchitectonic differences correspond to these morphological asymmetries: there is a larger region corresponding to Wernicke's area on the left compared to on the right.

Other gross asymmetries of the human brain in-

Table 4–2. Fiber tracts and related disconnection syndromes of the cerebral hemispheres

Fiber type	Tract	Symptoms
Commissural	Corpus callosum	Left hand tactile anomia, left hand agraphia, left hand apraxia, inability to match hand postures or tactile stimuli of the two hands, reduced constructional skills in the right hand
	Splenium	Alexia without agraphia (this syndrome occurs when there is a left occipital injury and right homonymous hemianopsia in addition to the splenial lesion)
Association	Arcuate fasciculus	Conduction aphasia
	Arcuate fasciculus	Parietal apraxia
	Inferior longitudinal fasciculus (right)	Prosopagnosia, environmental agnosia
	Inferior longitudinal fasciculus (bilateral)	Visual object agnosia
Projection	Corticospinal tract	Locked-in syndrome

clude a wider and longer left occipital lobe, wider right frontal lobe, larger left occipital horn of the lateral ventricular system, and a tendency for the left descending pyramidal tract to decussate before the right in the medulla (Galaburda et al. 1978). Asymmetries of neurotransmitter concentrations have also been identified. Cortical choline acetyltransferase activity is greater in the left than in the right temporal lobe (Amaducci et al. 1981).

Cerebral asymmetries do not occur in the brains of nonprimates but are present in gorillas, chimpanzees, and orangutans, as well as in humans (LeMay 1976). Studies of endocasts of fossil skulls reveal that brain asymmetries similar to those of modern humans were evident in the brains of Neanderthal people 40,000 years ago and may have been present as early as 400,000 years ago in Peking Man (Galaburda et al. 1978).

Investigations of asymmetries between the two hemispheres have identified differences at the gross morphological level, in the cytoarchitectonic structure of the hemispheres, in the shape of the brain, in the shape of specific aspects of the ventricular system, and

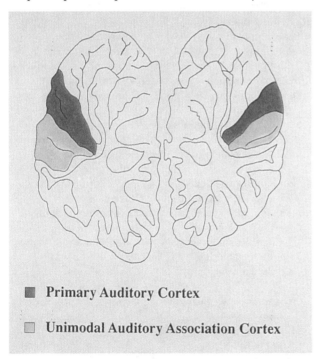

■ Primary Auditory Cortex

☐ Unimodal Auditory Association Cortex

Figure 4–9. Asymmetries of the temporal cortex. Note the larger planum temporale (*yellow*) corresponding to Wernicke's area in the left hemisphere.
Source. Reprinted from Galaburda AM, LeMay M, Kemper TL, et al: "Right-Left Asymmetries in the Brain." *Science* 199:852–856, 1978. Copyright 1978 by the AAAS. Used with permission.

in the concentrations of neurotransmitters. The magnitude of these differences is relatively small and does not correspond to the marked differences in hemispheric function. The means by which the dramatic differences in function of the two hemispheres are achieved remain enigmatic. The advantage of hemispheric specialization and lateralized development of functional capacities is that the capacity of the human brain is nearly doubled (Levy 1977). The principal disadvantage is that reduced redundancy exaggerates the effects of lateralized cerebral injury; in humans, a unilateral lesion often has devastating behavioral consequences because of the limited compensatory capability of the contralateral hemisphere.

Asymmetric cognitive function of the hemispheres. Hemispheric specialization refers to the differential functions of the two hemispheres. Nearly all human behavior has contributions from both hemispheres, and complex behavior requires the integrated action of both halves of the brain. Almost no skills are completely unique to one hemisphere. Nevertheless, the two hemispheres differ substantially in their potential for many skills and are differentially engaged in most tasks. There have been numerous attempts to identify antinomies of function that characterize the right and left hemispheres (i.e., verbal versus nonverbal, propositional versus appositional, and holistic versus analytic); none of these have been entirely successful, and it is unlikely that the brain is organized along such polar dimensions. A more accurate approach is to acknowledge that the two hemispheres perform different but not necessarily correlated or complementary roles. Table 4–3 lists capacities mediated to a significantly different extent by the two hemispheres.

Language is the best known example of a lateralized function. The left hemisphere is specialized for symbol usage including words (spoken, written, heard, and read), mathematical symbols, symbolic gesture, and verbal memory. The left brain is language dominant in nearly all right-handed individuals and in most left-handed people. The lateralization of language functions is not complete, and rudimentary language skills are present in the right brain.

Praxis refers to the ability to execute learned movements on command. This ability is mediated by the left hemisphere, and most instances of apraxia occur in patients with left-sided brain injury.

The right hemisphere is dominant for visuospatial functions, but the left hemisphere has considerable visuospatial ability and left-hemishpere injuries frequently produce at least minor visuospatial deficits. The most marked and enduring visuospatial abnormalities occur with lesions of the posterior right hemisphere. Elementary visuoperceptual skills (e.g., judging line orientation and depth perception), complex visual discrimination and recognition abilities (e.g., discriminating between two unfamiliar faces or recognizing familiar faces), and visuomotor skills (e.g., drawing, copying, and dressing) are mediated primarily by the right hemisphere (Kimura and Durford 1974).

Components of music appear to be differentially processed in the hemispheres. At least in nonprofessionals, the left hemisphere appears to be involved primarily in the mediation of rhythm, whereas the right brain mediates the perception and execution of melody (Gordon 1983).

Cortically mediated processes are well lateralized, and neurobehavioral phenomena such as aphasia, alexia, agraphia, amusia, abnormalities of visual discrimination and recognition, and altered affective expression occur with local damage to the left or right hemisphere. The cortex is composed of regionally specialized modules that can be rendered dysfunctional by local cortical injury or by disconnection from other regions by white matter lesions.

Limbic System (Paramedian Zone)

Limbic system structures comprise a critical neuroanatomic substrate for the mediation of mood and motivation. Limbic dysfunction contributes to a variety of neuropsychiatric syndromes including psychosis, depression, mania, personality alterations, and obsessive-compulsive disorder.

"Limbic" means "border" or "hem" and was first used in its anatomical sense by Broca, the French anatomist, to describe the structures that lie beneath the neocortex and that surround the brain stem (Isaacson 1974). In 1937, Papez authored an important article titled "A Proposed Mechanism of Emotion" in which he hypothesized that the structures surrounding the upper brain stem formed a functional system mediating human emotion. Since then, research and clinical observations have largely confirmed the idea that limbic structures are involved in the mediation of behaviors and experiences that share the common feature of having an emotional component.

As currently conceived, the limbic system includes the hippocampus, olfactory cortex, caudal orbitofrontal cortex, insula, temporal pole, parahippocampal

Table 4–3. Abilities mediated primarily by the right or left hemisphere and corresponding clinical deficits resulting from lateralized lesions

Hemispheric function	Correlated clinical deficit
Left hemisphere	
Language	Aphasia
Execution	Nonfluent aphasia
Comprehension	Comprehension defect
Reading	Alexia
Writing	Agraphia
Verbal memory	Verbal amnesia
Verbal fluency (word list generation)	Reduced verbal fluency
Mathematical abilities	Anarithmetia
Praxis	Apraxia
Musical rhythm (execution)	Impaired rhythm in singing
Contralateral spatial attention	Right-sided neglect
Contralateral motor function	Right hemiparesis
Contralateral sensory function	Right hemisensory loss
Contralateral visual field perception	Right homonymous hemianopia
Right hemisphere	
Speech prosody	Aprosodia
Executive	Executive aprosodia
Receptive	Receptive aprosodia
Nonverbal memory	Nonverbal amnesia
Design fluency (novel figure generation)	Reduced design fluency
Elementary visuospatial skills	
Depth perception	Reduced depth perception
Angle discrimination	Reduced angle discrimination
Complex visuospatial skills	
Familiar face recognition	Prosopagnosia
Familiar place recognition	Environmental agnosia
Unfamiliar face discrimination	Impaired facial discrimination
Visuomotor abilities	
Constructional ability	Constructional disturbance
Dressing (body-garment orientation)	Dressing disturbance
Musical melody (perception and execution)	Amusia
Contralateral spatial attention	Left-sided neglect
Contralateral motor function	Left hemiparesis
Contralateral sensory function	Left hemisensory loss
Contralateral visual field perception	Left homonymous hemianopia
Miscellaneous	
Familiar voice recognition	Phonagnosia

gyrus, cingulate cortex, amygdala, septal nuclei, hypothalamus, and selected thalamic nuclei (see Figure 4–10) (Carpenter 1991; Mesulam 1985). The limbic system is poised between the hypothalamus with its neuroendocrine control systems of the internal milieu and the neocortex mediating action on the external environment.

The principal known function of the hippocampus is the mediation of new learning and recent memory. Localized injury of hippocampus produces an amnestic disorder with deficient storage of new information. This syndrome has been described with hippocampal injury secondary to stroke, anoxia, trauma, early Alzheimer's disease, and herpes encephalitis.

Paralimbic cortex includes the orbitofrontal area, insula, temporal pole, parahippocampal gyrus, and cingulate gyrus. Paralimbic cortex is represented in brain regions critical to emotional control, social judgment, civility, and motivated behavior. Lesions of the orbitofrontal cortex produce marked personality changes with disinhibition, impulsiveness, loss of tact, and coarsened behavior. Cingulate dysfunction results in marked apathy with disinterest and loss of motivation (Cummings 1993).

Portions of the basal ganglia are included in the limbic system. The head of the caudate nucleus consists of ventromedial and dorsolateral portions. The ventromedial section has major limbic system connections and receives projections from the hippocampus, amygdala, cingulate cortex, and the orbitofrontal cortex. The dorsolateral portion, in contrast, receives projections from the lateral prefrontal cortex and has little limbic input (Nauta 1986). The globus pallidus is divided similarly into dorsal-nonlimbic portions and ventral-limbic portions. As predicted by these anatomic observations, basal ganglia diseases are commonly accompanied by emotional dysfunction and psychopathology.

Various clinical neuropsychiatric disorders are associated with limbic system dysfunction (Table 4–4) (Cummings 1985; Doane 1986). There is no single unifying function served by the limbic system, and the only common feature shared by limbic system disorders is that they have an emotional dimension. Limbic system lesions produce emotional disturbances and rarely cause intellectual deficits (an exception is the amnesia produced by hippocampal system lesions).

Psychosis, mood disorders, obsessive-compulsive behavior, personality alterations, and disturbances of sexual behavior have all been linked to limbic system dysfunction. *Psychosis* occurs with lesions of the temporal lobes and subcorticolimbic system structures. The schizophrenia-like disorder of epilepsy occurs almost exclusively in patients with seizure foci in the temporolimbic cortex (Perez et al. 1985). Stroke, tumors, herpes encephalitis, and Alzheimer's disease are other disorders that affect the temporal cortex and produce psychotic features in the elderly. At the subcorticolimbic level, Huntington's disease, idiopathic basal ganglia calcification, and lacunar state are examples of conditions with pathology of the limbic system and increased frequencies of psychosis.

Mood disorders have also been related to limbic system dysfunction. Depression occurs with basal ganglia dysfunction in stroke, movement disorders, and idiopathic depressive disorders (Baxter et al. 1985; Cummings 1992; Starkstein et al. 1987, 1988a). Manic behavior has been associated with disorders affecting the caudate nuclei, thalamus, and basotemporal areas

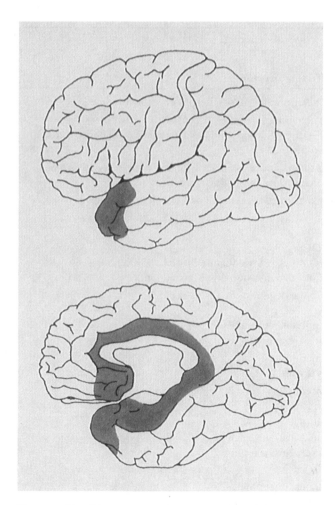

Figure 4–10. The cortical components of the limbic system (*green*).

(Bogousslavsky et al. 1988; Cummings and Mendez 1984; Folstein 1989; Starkstein et al. 1988b).

Investigation of idiopathic *obsessive-compulsive behavior* has revealed increased metabolism in the obitofrontal cortex (Baxter et al. 1987). Focal lesions and neurological disorders producing obsessive-compulsive behavior frequently involve the caudate nucleus or globus pallidus (Cummings and Cunningham 1992).

A variety of *personality alterations* have been correlated with limbic system lesions. Orbitofrontal or orbitofrontal-subcortical circuit lesions produce disinhibited, impulsive, and tactless behavior; temporolimbic epilepsy has been associated with a rigid, viscous demeanor with hypergraphia, circumstantiality, and hyperreligiosity (Brandt et al. 1985); and bilateral amygdala lesions produce behavioral placidity as part of the Klüver-Bucy syndrome (Lilly et al. 1983).

Idiopathic *anxiety* is associated with increased tem-poral and decreased basal ganglia glucose metabolism (Wu et al. 1991). Anxiety has been associated with temporal lobe and basal ganglia disorders including Parkinson's disease and Alzheimer's disease (Reisberg et al. 1989; Stein et al. 1990).

Disorders of sexual function may also reflect limbic system disturbances. Diminished libido has been associated with hypothalamic injury and with the interictal state of patients with temporal lobe seizure foci. Hypersexuality has been observed in patients with orbitofrontal injury or trauma to the septal region and as an ictal manifestation in the course of temporal lobe seizures (Gorman and Cummings 1992). Paraphiliac behavior including pedophilia, transvestism, sadomasochistic behavior, and exhibitionism has been observed in patients with temporal lobe injury and epilepsy, basal ganglia disorders, and brain tumors involving limbic structures (Cummings 1985; Miller et al. 1986). Opiate and cocaine *addictions* appear to be me-

Table 4–4.   Neuropsychiatric disorders with evidence of limbic system dysfunction

Neuropsychiatric disorder	Anatomical structure implicated	Diseases affecting structure
Amnesia	Hippocampus, hypothalamus	Stroke, anoxia, trauma, tumors, herpes encephalitis
Psychosis	Temporal cortex	Epilepsy, stroke, tumors, herpes encephalitis, Alzheimer's disease
	Striatum	Huntington's disease, idiopathic basal ganglia calcification, lacunar state, schizophrenia
Depression	Striatum	Stroke, Huntington's disease, Parkinson's disease, idiopathic basal ganglia calcification, idiopathic depression
Mania	Striatum	Huntington's disease, idiopathic basal ganglia calcification
	Thalamus	Stroke
	Temporal cortex	Stroke, trauma
OCD	Orbitofrontal cortex	Idiopathic OCD
	Striatum	Huntington's disease, Sydenham's chorea, PEPD, manganese intoxication, carbon monoxide intoxication
Personality alterations	Orbitofrontal cortex	Trauma, tumors, degenerative disorders
	Temporal cortex	Epilepsy
	Amygdala	Herpes encephalitis, trauma
	Striatum	Huntington's disease
Anxiety	Temporal cortex	Idiopathic anxiety
	Striatum	Parkinson's disease
Hyposexuality	Temporal cortex	Epilepsy (interictal)
	Hypothalamus	Trauma (surgical)
Hypersexuality	Orbitofrontal cortex	Tumors, trauma
	Temporal cortex	Epilepsy (ictal)
	Amygdala	Herpes encephalitis, trauma
	Septal nuclei	Trauma
Paraphilias	Hypothalamus	Tumors, trauma, encephalitis
Addictions	Septal nuclei, hypothalamus	Idiopathic addictive behavior

Note.   OCD = obsessive-compulsive disorder; PEPD = postencephalitic Parkinson's disease.

diated in part by receptors located in limbic brain regions (Gawin 1991).

Thus neocortical disorders and white matter lesions tend to produce deficit disorders of language, praxis, and gnosis. Limbic system disorders have little associated intellectual impairment and produce diverse disorders of emotional function.

Limbic System Asymmetries and Lateralized Neuropsychiatric Syndromes

Anatomic and biochemical asymmetries of the limbic system. Asymmetries of subcortical structures are less marked than are asymmetries of cortical regions, but the left globus pallidus, right medial geniculate nucleus of the thalamus, and left lateral posterior nucleus of the thalamus have been found to be larger than the corresponding nuclei of the contralateral hemisphere (Eidelberg and Galaburda 1982; Kooistra and Heilman 1988). Asymmetries of neurotransmitter concentrations in limbic system structures have been identified. The content of dopamine and choline acetyltransferase (a marker of cholinergic function) are increased in the left globus pallidus compared with in the right (Glick et al. 1982), norepinephrine concentrations are greater in the left pulvinar and in the right somatosensory nuclei of the thalamus (Oke et al. 1978), and choline acetyltransferase activity is greater in the left than in the right temporal lobe (Amaducci et al. 1981). Transmitter asymmetries may underlie the differential occurrence of mood disorders and anxiety with lesions of the left and right hemispheres.

Lateralized neuropsychiatric syndromes. Some aspects of emotional function are lateralized, with greater representation in one hemisphere than in the other (Coffey 1987). Emotional functions include the perception of emotional stimuli in the environment (e.g., apprehending facial expression, comprehending voice inflection, and interpreting postural adjustments), the expression of emotion (e.g., facial affective display and inflection of voice), and the subjective experience of emotion. Emotional perception and expression appear to be mediated primarily by the right hemisphere. For example, the right hemisphere is superior to the left in discriminating among unfamiliar faces, recognizing familiar faces, and interpreting facial emotional expression (Borod et al. 1986). The right brain is also better able to recognize familiar voices than is the left (Van Lancker et al. 1989) and to

comprehend the emotional inflection of spoken language (Tucker et al. 1977). Emotion is more intensely expressed on the left side of the face, suggesting that the right brain has more efficient access to cerebral mechanisms required for affective expression (Moscovitch and Olds 1982). Finally, the right hemisphere also shows evidence of electroencephalographic (EEG) "activation" when processing emotional stimuli (Davidson 1992), and emotional information may serve to activate the right hemisphere (Bryden and Ley 1984).

Experiential aspects of emotion are more difficult to study, and the underlying neurobiology is less securely established. Information has been derived from depth electrode investigations, from emotional changes reported in association with epileptic seizures, from temporary hemispheric inactivation with intracarotid amobarbital injections (Wada test), and from lesion studies. Stimulating depth electrodes located in and around the amygdala produce the sense of déjà vu, anxiety, visceral sensations, hallucinations (Halgren et al. 1978), and occasionally intense fear of anger (Girgis 1981), irrespective of which hemisphere is stimulated. Fear is the most common affect experienced in the course of spontaneous epileptic seizures. Some studies have found a predominance of right-sided lesions (Hermann et al. 1992), but fear is also observed in patients with left-sided lesions, suggesting that this experience is not consistently lateralized (Strauss et al. 1982). Depression is the second most common ictal affect and occurs with both left- and right-sided foci (Williams 1956). A small number of patients have positive emotional experiences as ictal manifestations, and laughter as an ictal behavior may be more common with left- than with right-sided seizure foci (Sackeim et al. 1982), although a consensus is lacking regarding interpretation of this observation (Coffey 1987). Taken together, these data suggest that many experiential aspects of emotion are mediated by non-lateralized limbic system structures.

Another source of information regarding the laterality of emotional processing is the Wada test. In this technique, amobarbital is injected into the carotid artery of patients with epilepsy before temporal lobectomy to establish which side of the brain is dominant for language function. The carotid is the principal arterial supply for the ipsilateral hemisphere, and transient hemispheric inactivation follows the injection. About 50% of patients undergoing this procedure evidence a marked change in emotion soon after the amobarbital perfusion. When the left hemisphere is inactivated, a depressive or catastrophic reaction occurs; when the right hemisphere is involved, patients manifest euphoria or an indifference reaction (Loring et al. 1992). Thus in most studies, the mood effects of transient hemispheric inactivation differ markedly according to which hemisphere is affected.

Studies of emotional changes in patients with unilateral lesions lead to conclusions similar to those suggested by the Wada test. Patients with left-hemisphere lesions have more catastrophic reactions and are more anxious and depressed; patients with right-hemisphere lesions evidence more indifference and tend to joke about, minimize, or deny their disability (Gainotti 1972). Recent investigation of stroke patients have found a higher prevalence of severe depression among those with left frontal lobe lesions, whereas patients with right-brain lesions exhibited more undue cheerfulness or, occasionally, frank mania (Robinson and Starkstein 1990; see also Chapter 23). Van Lancker (1991) observed that many functions of the right hemisphere subserve determination of the personal relevance of environmental stimuli, and Weintraub and Mesulam (1983) reported that children who had sustained right-brain injury characteristically had interpersonal difficulties, shyness, and impaired prosody and gesture. An impaired ability to comprehend personally relevant information or to execute interpersonal cues appropriately may lead to difficulties in establishing interpersonal relationships and subsequent social isolation. In elderly individuals, right-hemisphere dysfunction may contribute to the disengagement and interpersonal abnormalities evident in many patients with right-brain strokes and dementia syndromes.

Another avenue for investigating the hemisphericity of emotion is to search for evidence of lateral brain dysfunction in idiopathic psychiatric disorders. A number of neuropsychological studies have suggested preferential right-hemisphere dysfunction during depressed mood states that normalizes during euthymia, and a few patients have been reported to exhibit frank neurological deficits referable to the right hemisphere that were present only during the depressed period (for a review, see Coffey 1987). Electrophysiological studies have demonstrated EEG changes referable to the right hemisphere during depressed mood states (Davidson 1992), but studies of regional cerebral blood flow and metabolism have produced conflicting findings, with dysfunction in either or both hemispheres accompanying depression (Baxter et al. 1985;

Delvenne et al. 1990; Dolan et al. 1992; Drevets et al. 1992; Sackeim et al. 1990).

As for other psychiatric disorders, several lines of evidence point toward dysfunction of left temporal lobe structures in schizophrenia, but this hypothesis is controversial (Gruzelier 1983; Sedvall 1992; Suddath et al. 1989). Even more tentative are data suggesting greater left-hemisphere dysfunction in violent individuals and obsessive-compulsive disorder, as well as more right-brain involvement in patients with conversion hysteria and alexithymia (Flor-Henry 1983; Nachson 1983; Stern 1983; TenHouten et al. 1986). Most idiopathic disorders have not been found to be strongly linked to a single hemisphere. Table 4–5 summarizes the neuropsychiatric syndromes associated with lateralized brain dysfunction.

Reticular Formation (Median Zone)

The median zone contains the reticular formation including the ascending reticular activating system, vasopressor and respiratory mechanisms, and the central

Table 4–5. Neuropsychiatric disorders associated with lateralized brain dysfunction

Neuropsychiatric disorder	Predominant laterality of an associated lesion
Disorders of personal relevance	
Prosopagnosia (inability to recognize familiar faces)	Right
Environmental agnosia (inability to recognize familiar places)	Right
Phonagnosia (inability to recognize familiar voices)	Right
Affective dysprosody (inability to inflect one's voice or to comprehend emotional inflection)	Right
Mood disorders	
Depression (major)	Left
Catastrophic reaction	Left
Mania	Right
Euphoria, undue cheerfulness	Right
Indifference	Right
Possible hemispheric relationships to other psychiatric disorders	
Schizophrenia	Left
Violent behavior	Left
Obsessive-compulsive behavior	Left
Conversion hysteria	Right
Alexithymia	Right

components of the sympathetic and parasympathetic nervous systems (Carpenter 1991). The reticular formation is a dense network of neurons with short and long axons that form nuclei in the periventricular gray areas surrounding the cerebral aqueduct in the brain stem, is adjacent to the floor of the fourth ventricle in the pons, and extends into the medulla. The ascending reticular activating system projects to the intralaminar nuclei of the thalamus, and these in turn project to the cerebral cortex. The intralaminar nuclei project primarily to layer I of the cortex, the layer composed of parallel fibers whose stimulation results in local cortical activation (Figure 4–11).

The thalamic reticular nucleus is a unique structure that forms a thin shell around the anterior aspects of the thalamus and governs cortical arousal. It receives projections from the cerebral cortex, dorsal intralaminar nucleus, and dorsal specific sensory nuclei. It has no projections to the cerebral cortex but projects back to the dorsal thalamic nuclei. It is positioned to serve as a "gate," modifying and censoring information projected from thalamus to cortex, and its principal effect is to inhibit cortical activity (Carpenter and Sutin 1983; Plum and Posner 1980).

Increased input from the brain stem reticular activating system reduces the tonic inhibition of the reticular nucleus and activates the cortex by disinhibiting the cortical projections of other thalamic nuclei (Plum and Posner 1980). The ascending reticular activating system is responsible for the maintenance of consciousness, and disturbances of the system result in impaired

arousal varying from drowsiness, to obtundation, stupor, and finally coma.

Nuclei of the reticular formation are also involved in control of heart rate, blood pressure, and respiratory rhythms (Carpenter 1991). Dysfunction of these nuclei results in alterations in blood pressure, cardiac arrhythmias, and respiratory irregularities. The hypothalamus is contained in the median zone, and abnormalities of basic life functions (e.g., appetite, libido, and sleep) may occur in individuals who sustain hypothalamic injury. The hypothalamus influences endocrine function via its connections with the pituitary gland, and endocrine abnormalities are produced by hypothalamic lesions.

Connections Between the Cerebral Cortex and Subcortical Structures

There is one principal way for information to enter the nervous system and one principal exit pathway by which humans act on their environment. The entry pathway is via thalamocortical afferents that receive sensory information from peripheral sensory receptors and convey the data to the cortex. The principal exit pathway is via the descending corticospinal tracts, particularly the pyramidal system. Thus the flow of information is from the thalamus to the primary sensory cortex, unimodal association cortex, and then heteromodal association cortex. From there the long association fibers connect the posterior heteromodal cortex to the anterior (frontal lobe) heteromodal cortex that in turn connects to the subcortical nuclei. After processing through frontal-subcortical circuits, executive commands flow to the primary motor cortex and then to bulbar and spinal effector mechanisms. The thalamocortical afferents and frontal-subcortical efferents are distributed systems that include portions of both the paramedian (limbic) and supralimbic (neocortical) zones. Activation of brain structures is not limited to the sequence described above; there is simultaneous activation of many brain regions, as well as feedback mechanisms from on-going activity.

Thalamic-Cortical Relationships

The thalamus plays several crucial roles in human brain function (Figure 4–12). Specific thalamic nuclei receive input from a relatively restricted number of sources and project to layers 3 and 4 of the cortex.

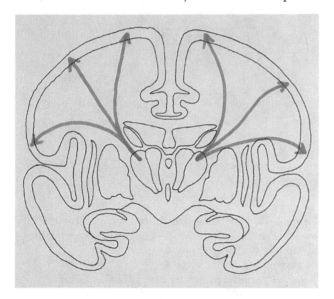

Figure 4–11. The thalamocortical components of the reticular activating system.

The specific nuclei include sensory nuclei that process all incoming sensory information except olfaction (ventral posterior, medial geniculate, and lateral geniculate); nuclei that participate in the motor pathways (ventral anterior and ventral lateral); association nuclei that have major connections with frontal (dorsomedial nuclei) or temporoparietal (lateral nuclei) association cortex; and nuclei that are included in the limbic circuits (anterior and medial nuclei) (Carpenter and Sutin 1983; Nauta and Feirtag 1986). Table 4–6 presents a functional classification of thalamic nuclei with their principal afferents and efferents.

A number of distinctive behavioral disorders have been associated with dysfunction of the associative and sensory thalamic nuclei. Disorders of the associative dorsal medial nuclei produce amnesia and a frontal lobe–type syndrome (Cummings 1993; Stuss et al. 1988). Lesions of the specific thalamic sensory nuclei cause deficits in primary sensation. Ventral posterior nuclear lesions disrupt all sensory abilities of the contralateral limbs, trunk, and face. In some cases, spontaneous disabling pain of the affected side occurs (Dejerine-Roussy syndrome) (Adams and Victor 1981). Lesions of the lateral geniculate bodies produce a contralateral visual field defect. Mania has been observed in several patients with right-sided thalamic lesions involving the paramedian thalamic nuclei (Bogousslavsky et al. 1988; Cummings and Mendez 1984; Starkstein et al. 1998b).

Frontal Subcortical Circuits

The frontal lobe is the origin of executive processes that guide action. The output from the frontal lobe is through subcortical circuits that eventually reach motor pathways. Five circuits connecting the frontal lobes and subcortical structures are currently recognized: a motor circuit originating in the supplementary motor area, an oculomotor circuit with origins in the frontal eye fields, and three circuits originating in prefrontal cortex (dorsolateral prefrontal cortex, lateral orbital cortex, and anterior cingulate cortex) (Alexander and Crutcher 1990; Alexander et al. 1986, 1990). The prototypic structure of all circuits is an origin in the frontal lobes, projection to striatal structures (caudate, putamen, and ventral striatum), connections from striatum to globus pallidus and substantia nigra, projections from these two structures to specific thalamic nuclei, and a final link back to the frontal lobe (Figure 4–13).

The *motor circuit* originates from neurons in the supplementary motor area, premotor cortex, motor cortex, and somatosensory cortex (Alexander and Crutcher 1990; Alexander et al. 1986). Throughout the circuit, the discrete somatotopic organization of move-

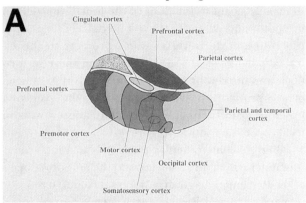

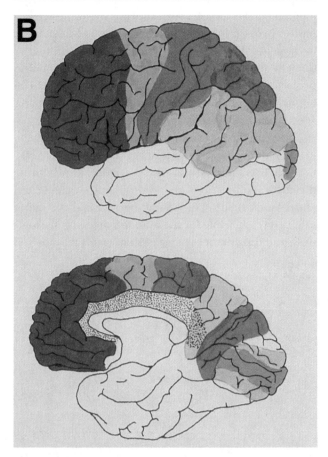

Figure 4–12. Thalamocortical relationships. Thalamic nuclei (*Panel A*) and the areas of the cortex receiving the thalamocortical projections are shown in the corresponding colors (*Panel B*).
Source. Reprinted from Carpenter MB: *Core Text of Neuroanatomy,* 4th Edition. Philadelphia, PA, Williams & Wilkins, 1991, pp. 262–263. Copyright 1991 Williams & Wilkins. Used with permission.

ment-related neurons is maintained. Distinct types of motor disturbances are associated with lesions at different sites in the motor circuit. Motor initiation abnormalities (akinesia) are associated with supplementary motor area lesions; parkinsonism and dystonia are observed with putamenal dysfunction; and choreiform movements occur with caudate and subthalamic nucleus damage.

The *oculomotor circuit* originates in the frontal eye fields, as well as in the prefrontal and posterior parietal cortex. Acute lesions of the cortical eye fields produce ipsilateral eye deviation, whereas more chronic lesions produce ipsilateral gaze impersistence; lesions in other areas of the circuit produce supranuclear gaze palsies such as those seen in Parkinson's disease, progressive supranuclear palsy, and Huntington's disease.

Three distinct frontal lobe neurobehavioral syndromes are recognized, and each corresponds to a region of origin of one of the three prefrontal-subcortical circuits. Dysfunction of any of the member structures of the circuits results in similar circuit-specific behavioral complexes, and these frontal-subcortical circuits comprise major anatomic axes governing behavior (Cummings 1993). The *dorsolateral prefrontal circuit* originates in the convexity of the frontal lobe and pro-

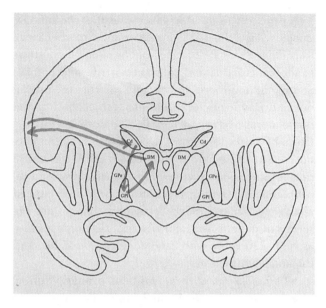

Figure 4–13. Organization of the prefrontal-subcortical circuits. The prefrontal cortical regions (dorsolateral prefrontal, orbitofrontal, and anterior cingulate) project to specific striatal regions, that in turn project to globus pallidus and substantia nigra. These structures project to thalamic nuclei that connect to frontal lobe, completing the circuit. GPe = globus pallidus externa; GPi = globus pallidus interna; Cd = caudate; DM = dorsomedial nucleus of the thalamus.

Table 4–6. Function and anatomic relationships of the thalamic nuclei

Nuclei	Input	Output	Function
Limbic nuclei			
Anterior	Mammillary body	Cingulate	Emotional function
Motor nuclei			
Ventroanterior	Globus pallidus	Frontal cortex	Motor function
Ventrolateral	Cerebellum	Frontal cortex	Motor function
Sensory nuclei			
Ventral posterolateral	Sensory tracts from body	Parietal sensory cortex	Touch, temperature vibration, position
Ventral posteromedial	Sensory tracts from face	Parietal sensory cortex	Touch, temperature vibration, position
Lateral geniculate	Optic tracts	Occipital cortex	Vision
Medial geniculate	Inferior colliculi	Temporal cortex	Hearing
Association nuclei			
Dorsomedial	Globus pallidus, amygdala, temporal and frontal cortex	Prefrontal cortex	Intellectual and emotional function
Lateral[a]	Sensory thalamic nucleus, parietal and temporal cortex	Temporo-parietal cortex	Intellectual function
Nonspecific nuclei			
Midline	Hypothalamus	Amygdala, cingulate hypothalamus	Visceral function
Intralaminar	Reticular formation, precentral and premotor cortex	Striatum, cortex	Activation
Reticular	Thalamic nucleus and cortex	Dorsal thalamic nuclei	Samples, gates, and focuses thalamo-cortical output

[a]Includes lateral dorsal nucleus, lateral posterior nucleus, and the pulvinar.

jects primarily to the dorsolateral head of the caudate nucleus (Figure 4–14) (Alexander and Crutcher 1990; Alexander et al. 1986). This caudate region connects to globus pallidus and substantia nigra, and pallidal and nigral neurons of the circuit project to the medial dorsal thalamic nuclei that in turn project back to the dorsolateral prefrontal region. The dorsolateral prefrontal syndrome is characterized primarily by "executive function" deficits. Abnormalities include developing poor strategies for solving visuospatial problems or learning new information and reduced ability to shift sets. Such behavioral changes are observed in patients with dorsolateral prefrontal lesions, as well as in those with caudate, globus pallidus, and thalamic dysfunction.

The *orbitofrontal circuit* contains primarily limbic system structures. It begins in the inferolateral prefrontal cortex and projects to ventromedial caudate nucleus (Figure 4–14) (Alexander and Crutcher 1990; Alexander et al. 1986). This caudate region projects to the pallidum and substantia nigra. Pallidum and nigra connect to medial portions of the ventral anterior and medial dorsal thalamic nuclei that project back to the orbitofrontal cortex. Disorders involving cortical or subcortical structures of the orbitofrontal circuit feature marked changes in personality, including a tendency to be more outspoken, more irritable, and more tactless and to worry less and have an elevated mood.

The anterior cingulate circuit begins in the cortex of the anterior cingulate gyrus (Brodmann area 24) and projects to the ventral striatum (also known as the *limbic striatum*), which includes nucleus accumbens and the ventromedial portions of the caudate and putamen (Figure 4–14) (Alexander and Crutcher 1990; Alexander et al. 1986). The most dramatic cases of anterior cingulate injury exhibit akinetic mutism. The patients are profoundly apathetic: they typically have their eyes open, do not speak spontaneously, answer questions in monosyllables if at all, and are profoundly indifferent. Apathy has been associated with lesions of nucleus accumbens, globus pallidus, and thalamus, the principal subcortical members of the anterior cingulate circuit. Table 4–7 summarizes the behaviorally relevant frontal-subcortical circuits including the anatomical structures involved, the behavioral disturbances observed with circuit dysfunction, and the common diseases affecting each circuit.

Frontal-subcortical circuits are involved in several neuropsychiatric disorders. In addition to personality alterations (e.g., apathy and disinhibition), mood changes and obsessive-compulsive behaviors are associated with focal brain lesions affecting these circuits. Depression occurs with lesions of the dorsolateral prefrontal cortex and the head of the caudate nucleus, particularly when the left hemisphere is affected (Robinson et al. 1984; Starkstein et al. 1987, 1988a; see also Chapter 23). Positron-emission tomography in patients with idiopathic unipolar depression reveals diminished glucose metabolism in the prefrontal cortex and the caudate nuclei, suggesting that dysfunction of frontal-subcortical circuits may be a shared substrate for both idiopathic and acquired mood disorders (Baxter et al. 1985). Lesions producing secondary mania also involve nuclei and connections of frontal-subcortical circuits. Mania has been observed with lesions of the medial orbitofrontal cortex, diseases of the caudate nuclei such as Huntington's disease, and injury to the right thalamus (Bogousslavsky et al. 1988; Cummings and Mendez 1984; Folstein 1989; Starkstein et al. 1988b).

Both acquired and idiopathic obsessive-compulsive disorders have been related to dysfunction of fron-

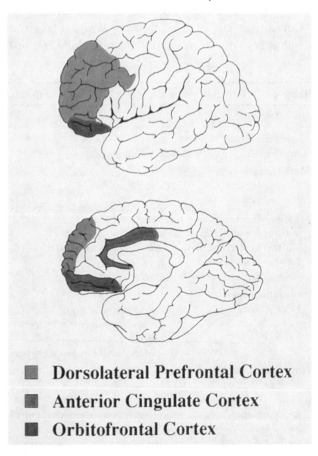

Dorsolateral Prefrontal Cortex

Anterior Cingulate Cortex

Orbitofrontal Cortex

Figure 4–14. Prefrontal cortical origins of the dorsolateral, anterior cingulate, and orbital circuits.

tal-subcortical circuits. Obsessive-compulsive behavior has been observed in patients with caudate dysfunction in Huntington's disease and following Sydenham's chorea (Cummings and Cunningham 1992; Swedo et al. 1989), as well as with globus pallidus lesions in postencephalitic Parkinson's disease, progressive supranuclear palsy, manganese-induced parkinsonism, and following anoxic injury (Laplane et al. 1989; Mena et al. 1967; Schilder 1938). Idiopathic obsessive-compulsive disorder has been associated with increased glucose metabolism in the left orbitofrontal frontal gyrus and caudate nuclei (Baxter et al. 1987) and with increased blood flow in the medial frontal area (Machlin et al. 1991).

Frontal-subcortical circuits are affected in patients who have diseases of the basal ganglia. The high frequency of neuropsychological alterations, the increased prevalence of personality and mood disturbances, the occurrence of obsessive-compulsive disorder, and the similarity between behaviors of patients with basal ganglia diseases and patients with frontal lobe injury are attributable to dysfunction of multiple frontal-subcortical circuits in basal ganglia disorders.

Neurochemistry and Behavior

The anatomical organization of the brain is complemented by an equally complex neurochemical organization. Many behavioral disorders reflect biochemical dysfunction, and the most effective interventions available are neurochemical in nature. Neurobehavioral deficits stemming from focal cortical lesions (e.g., aphasia and apraxia) have no available neurochemical treatments; neuropsychiatric disorders associated with limbic system dysfunction are frequently modifiable through neurochemical interventions.

There are two types of cerebral transmitters: 1) projection or extrinsic transmitters that originate in subcortical and brain stem nuclei and project to brain targets and 2) local or intrinsic transmitters that originate in neurons of the brain and project locally to adjacent or nearby cells. Projection transmitters or their synthetic enzymes must be transported within neurons for long distances from subcortical nuclei to distant regions and are vulnerable to disruption by stroke, tumors, and other processes. Transmitters are highly conserved from an evolutionary point of view, and

Table 4–7. Behavioral abnormalities associated with frontal-subcortical circuit disorders

Disease	Personality change	Mania	Depression	Obsessive-compulsive disorder	Neuropsychological impairment
Prefrontal cortical disorders					
Lateral prefrontal syndrome	No	No	Yes	No	Yes
Orbitofrontal syndrome	Yes	Yes	No	Yes	No
Medial frontal syndrome	Yes	No	No	No	No
Caudate disorders					
Parkinson's disease	Yes	No	Yes	No	Yes
Progressive supranuclear palsy	UD	No	Yes	Yes	Yes
Huntington's disease	Yes	Yes	Yes	Yes	Yes
Sydenham's chorea	Yes	No	No	Yes	No
Wilson's disease	Yes	Yes	Yes	No	Yes
Neuroacanthocytosis	Yes	Yes	Yes	Yes	Yes
Fahr's disease	UD	Yes	Yes	No	Yes
Infarction	Yes	No	Yes	Yes	Yes
Globus pallidus disorders					
Postencephalitic Parkinson's disease	Yes	Yes	Yes	Yes	Yes
Manganese toxicity	Yes	UD	UD	Yes	Yes
Carbon monoxide toxicity	Yes	No	No	Yes	Yes
Infarction	Yes	UD	UD	No	Yes
Thalamic disorders					
Infarction	Yes	Yes	No	No	Yes
Degeneration	Yes	UD	UD	UD	Yes

Note. UD = undetermined.

many function locally in some neuronal systems and function as projection transmitters in others. The classic neurotransmitters have served neuronal communication for some 600 million years of evolution (Rapoport 1990). Table 4–8 summarizes the origins and destinations of the extrinsic transmitters. Behavioral effects can rarely be assigned to alterations in a single transmitter, but some aberrant behaviors are associated with changes that affect predominantly one type of transmitter; Table 4–9 presents the principal transmitter-behavior relationships currently identified.

There are two main *cholinergic* projections from subcortical sites to the brain (Figure 4–15). The first originates in the reticular formation and projects via the dorsal tegmental pathway to the thalamus. This pathway is the essential component of the ascending reticular activating system (Nieuwenhuys 1985). The second cholinergic projection begins in the cells of the nucleus basalis in the basal forebrain and projects to the hippocampus, hypothalamus, amygdala, and diffusely to the neocortex. The afferents to nucleus basalis are primarily from cortical and subcortical limbic

Table 4–8. Origins and destinations of the major extrinsic transmitter projections

Neurotransmitter	Origin	Destination
Acetylcholine		
Reticular system	Reticular formation	Thalamus
Basal forebrain system	Nucleus basalis and nucleus of diagonal band of Broca	Neocortex, hippocampus, hypothalamus, and amygdala
Dopamine		
Nigrostriatal system	Substantia nigra	Putamen and caudate nucleus
Mesolimbic system	Ventral tegmental area	Nucleus accumbens, septal nucleus, and amygdala
Mesocortical system	Ventral tegmental area	Medial temporal and frontal lobes and anterior cingulate cortex
Noradrenaline		
Dorsal pathway	Locus ceruleus	Thalamus, amygdala, basal forebrain, hippocampus, and neocortex
Ventral pathway	Locus ceruleus	Hypothalamus and midbrain reticular formation
Serotonin	Raphe nuclei	Entire nervous system
Histamine	Posterior hypothalamus	Entire nervous system
GABA	Zona incerta	Neocortex, basal ganglia, and brain stem
	Caudate and putamen	Globus pallidus and substantia nigra
	Globus pallidus and substantia nigra	Thalamus
Glutamate	Neocortex	Caudate, putamen, thalamus, and nucleus accumbens
	Subthalamic nucleus	Globus pallidus
	Thalamus	Neocortex
	Hippocampus, subiculum	Septal region
	Entorhinal cortex	Hippocampus

Note. GABA = γ-aminobutyric acid.

Table 4–9. Behavioral alterations associated with transmitter disturbances

Neurotransmitter	Reduced function	Increased function
Acetylcholine	Memory impairment, delirium, and delusions	Depression, aggression
Dopamine		
Motor function	Parkinsonism	Chorea, tics
Behavior	Dementia and depression	Psychosis, anxiety, confusion, elation, obsessive-compulsive behavior, and paraphilias
Noradrenaline	Depression, dementia, and reduced attention	Anxiety
Serotonin	Depression	Anxiety and obsessive-compulsive behavior

system structures establishing the nucleus basalis as a relay between the limbic system afferents and efferents to the neocortex (Mesulam and Mufson 1984).

Cholinergic systems mediate a wide range of behaviors. Disruption of cholinergic function (e.g., through the administration of cholinergic receptor–blocking agents like scopolamine) produces amnesia (Bartus et al. 1982), and intoxication with anticholinergic compounds produces delirium and delusions. Alzheimer's disease is one major disorder associated with cholinergic deficiency. This disease produces atrophy of the nucleus basalis with consequent reduction in the synthesis of choline acetyltransferase, the enzyme that synthesizes acetylcholine; loss of synthetic activity leads to interruption of cortical cholinergic function (Katzman and Thal 1989). Cholinergic hyperactivity has been posited to play a role in the genesis of depression (Dilsaver and Coffman 1989), and in some species cholinergic stimulation of limbic system structures produces aggression (Valzelli 1981).

There are three main dopaminergic projections from the brain stem to the cerebral hemispheres: 1) a nigrostriatal projection arising from the compact portion of the substantia nigra and projecting to the putamen and caudate, 2) a mesolimbic projection originating in the ventral tegmental area and projecting to limbic system structures, and 3) a mesocortical system beginning in the ventral tegmental area and projecting to frontal and temporal areas (Figure 4–16) (Nieuwenhuys 1985). Targets of the mesolimbic dopaminergic projection include the nucleus accumbens, septal nucleus, and amygdala. The mesocortical projections terminate primarily in the medial frontal lobe, medial temporal lobe, and the anterior cingulate region.

Dopamine plays a key role in motoric functions and behavior. Dopamine deficiency or blockade leads to parkinsonism: dopamine excess produces chorea, dyskinesia, or tics. Behaviorally, dopamine deficiency causes at least mild cognitive impairment and may contribute to the depression that commonly accompanies Parkinson's disease and other parkinsonian syndromes. Dopamine excess leads to psychosis, elation or hypomania, and confusion. Dopamine hyperactivity may contribute to the pathophysiology of schizophrenia, obsessive-compulsive behavior, anxiety, and some paraphiliac behaviors (Cummings 1985, 1991).

The locus ceruleus and adjacent nuclei comprise the origin of the *noradrenergic* projection system. A dorsal noradrenergic bundle courses in the dorsal brain

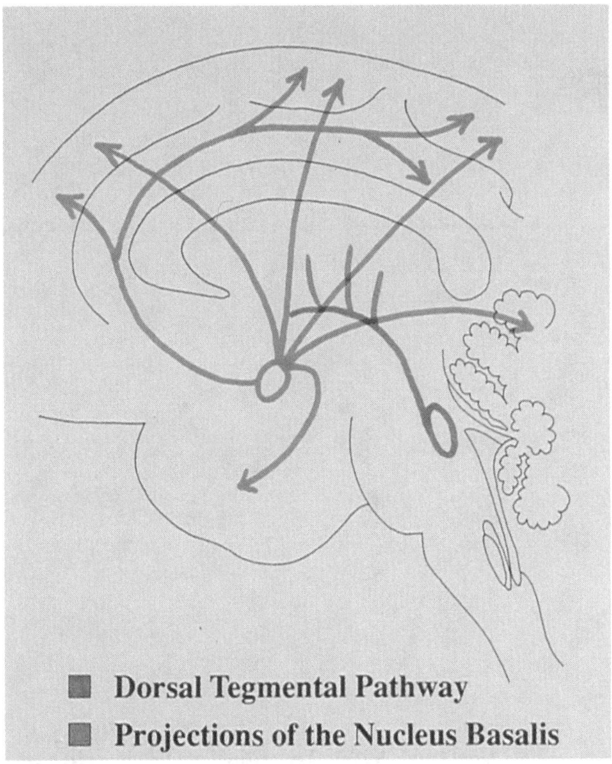

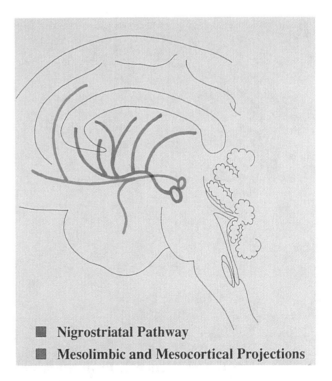

■ Dorsal Tegmental Pathway
■ Projections of the Nucleus Basalis

■ Nigrostriatal Pathway
■ Mesolimbic and Mesocortical Projections

Figure 4–15. Dorsal (*blue*) and ventral (*red*) cholinergic pathways.

Figure 4–16. Nigrostriatal (*blue*) and mesolimbic and mesocortical (*red*) dopaminergic pathways.

stem to the septum, thalamus, amygdala, basal forebrain, hippocampus, and neocortex (Figure 4–17; *panel A*) (Nieuwenhuys 1985). A ventral noradrenergic bundle projects to the hypothalamus and midbrain reticular formation (Figure 4–17; *panel B*). Noradrenergic hypofunction has been linked to depression, dementia, and diminished alertness and concentration (Agid et al. 1987). Increased noradrenergic activity has been linked to anxiety (Lechin et al. 1989).

Serotonergic neurons are located almost exclusively in the median and paramedian raphe nuclei of the medulla, pons, and midbrain (Figure 4–18). The projection system of these serotonergic neurons is a complex highly branched fiber system that embraces virtually the entire central nervous system (Nieuwenhuys 1985). Serotonin deficiency has been hypothesized to play a major role in suicide and depression (Agid et al. 1987), and serotonin hyperactivity may play a role in obsessive-compulsive behavior and anxiety (Lechin et al. 1989; Zohar et al. 1987).

γ-Aminobutyric acid (GABA) is an inhibitory neurotransmitter present in both projection systems and local neuronal circuits. The principal GABA projection system begins in the zona incerta and projects bilaterally to the entire neocortex, basal ganglia, and brainstem (Lin et al. 1990). In subcortical regions, one projection system originates in the caudate and putamen and projects to the globus pallidus and substantia nigra, another begins in the globus pallidus and substantia nigra with projections to the thalamus (Alexander and Crutcher 1990; Nieuwenhuys 1985). Local circuit neurons using GABA are found in the raphe nuclei, reticular nucleus of the thalamus, and basal ganglia. Local circuit neurons of the cerebral cortex also use GABA as their principal neurotransmitter (Rapoport 1990). GABA concentrations are decreased in the basal ganglia of Huntington's disease patients and the GABA deficiency may contribute to the dementia, mood disorders, obsessive-compulsive disorder, and psychoses occurring with increased frequency in this condition (Morris 1991).

Glutamate is an excitatory neurotransmitter that is used in the massive projection from the neocortex to the ipsilateral caudate, putamen, and nucleus accumbens. Glutamate is the principal neurotransmitter of projections from cortex to thalamus, from thalamus to cortex, and from one region of cortex to another. Glutamatergic neurons also project from subthalamic nucleus to globus pallidus. Glutamate functions in several hippocampus-related projections, including the per-

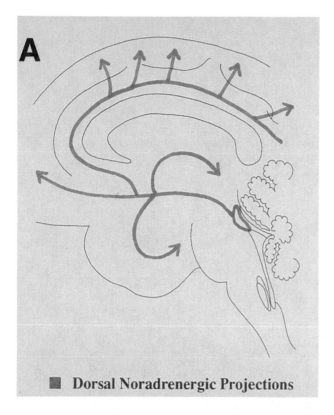

■ **Dorsal Noradrenergic Projections**

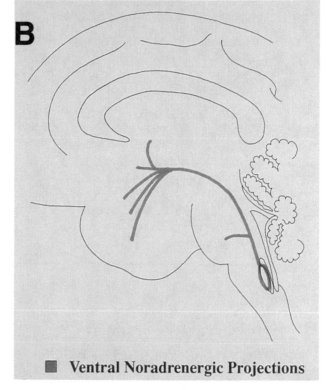

■ **Ventral Noradrenergic Projections**

Figure 4–17.   Dorsal (*blue; panel A*) and ventral (*red; panel B*) noradrenergic pathways.

forant pathway projecting from entorhinal cortex to hippocampus and the pathways originating in hippocampus and adjacent subiculum and projecting to the septal region (Alexander and Crutcher 1990; Nieuwenhuys 1985). The behavioral consequences of alterations in glutamate function are unknown.

Several other transmitters occur in behaviorally relevant areas, but their role in human behavior remains to be determined. *Histaminergic* neurons are

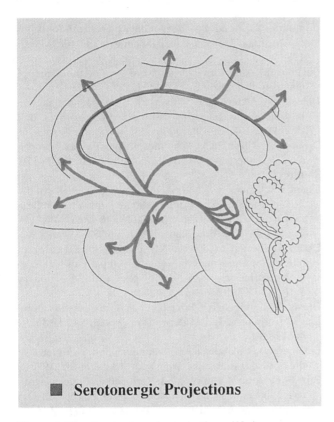

■ **Serotonergic Projections**

Figure 4–18. Serotoninergic projections (*blue*).

situated in the posterior hypothalamus and project diffusely to most brain structures including the neocortex, amygdala, septum, caudate, and putamen (Nieuwenhuys 1985). *Glycine* is an inhibitory transmitter that may function in local circuit neurons in the substantia nigra, caudate, and putamen. *Substance P* is present in the projection from caudate and putamen to the substantia nigra, and *enkephalin*-containing neurons project from caudate and putamen to the globus pallidus (Alexander and Crutcher 1990; Nieuwenhuys 1985). *Vasoactive intestinal peptide* neurons are intrinsic to the cortex and participate in local neuronal circuits (Nieuwenhuys 1985).

Summary

The brain consists of a median zone mediating arousal and basic life-sustaining functions such as respiration, digestion, circulation, and neuroendocrine function; a paramedian-limbic zone mediating extrapyramidal function and many aspects of emotional experience; and a supralimbic-neocortical zone mediating instrumental cognitive functions such as language and praxis (see Table 4–10). Injury of the supralimbic-neocortical zone is associated with neurobehavioral deficit syndromes such as aphasia and apraxia; dysfunction of the paramedian-limbic zone correlates with neuropsychiatric syndromes including mood disorders, psychoses, anxiety, and obsessive-compulsive disorder. Within each zone, behavioral deficits can be related to dysfunction of specific neurotransmitters. This approach provides a comprehensive framework for understanding brain-behavior relationships.

Table 4–10. Summary of the anatomy, functions, and syndromes of the median, paramedian-limbic, and supralimbic-neocortical zones of the brain

Zone	Myelination	Neuronal connectivity/ anatomy	Ontogeny	Function	Behavioral syndromes
Median	Poor	Feltwork; reticular	Functional at birth	Arousal	Disturbances of arousal, neuroendocrine control, respiration, and circulation
Paramedian-limbic	Substantial	Series; limbic system and basal ganglia	Functional within first few months	Emotion and extra-pyramidal function	Neuropsychiatric disorders; movement disorders
Supralimbic-neocortical	Well	Parallel; neocortex	Functional in adulthood	Sensory cortex, motor cortex, and association cortex	Neurobehavioral disorders

References

Adams RD, Victor M: Principles of Neurology, 2nd Edition. New York, McGraw-Hill, New York, 1981

Agid Y, Ruberg M, Dubois B, et al: Anatomoclinical and biochemical concepts of subcortical dementia, in Cognitive Neurochemistry. Edited by Stahl SM, Iversen SD, Goodman EC. New York, Oxford University Press, 1987, pp 248–271

Alexander GE, Crutcher MD: Functional architecture of basal ganglia circuits: neural substrates of parallel processing. Trends Neurosci 13:266–271, 1990

Alexander GE, DeLong MR, Strick PL: Parallel organization of functionally segregated circuits linking basal ganglia and cortex. Annu Rev Neurosci 9:357–381, 1986

Alexander GE, Crutcher MD, DeLong MR: Basal ganglia-thalamocortical circuits: parallel substrates for motor, oculomotor, "prefrontal" and "limbic" functions. Prog Brain Res 85:119–146, 1990

Amaducci L, Sorbi S, Albanese A, et al: Choline acetyltransferase (ChAT) activity differs in right and left human temporal lobes. Neurology 31:799–805, 1981

Bartus RT, Dean RL III, Beer B, et al: The cholinergic hypothesis of geriatric memory dysfunction. Science 217:408–417, 1982

Baxter LR Jr, Phelps ME, Mazziotta JC, et al: Cerebral metabolic rates for glucose in mood disorders. Arch Gen Psychiatry 42:441–447, 1985

Baxter LR Jr, Phelps ME, Mazziotta JC, et al: Local cerebral glucose metabolic rates in obsessive-compulsive disorder. Arch Gen Psychiatry 44:211–218, 1987

Benson DF, Cummings JL, Tsai SY: Angular gyrus syndrome simulating Alzheimer disease. Arch Neurol 39:616–620, 1982

Bogousslavsky J, Ferrazzini M, Regli F, et al: Manic delirium and frontal-like syndrome with paramedian infarction of the right thalamus. J Neurol Neurosurg Psychiatry 51:116–119, 1988

Borod JC, Koff E, Lorch MP, et al: The expression and perception of facial emotion in brain-damaged patients. Neuropsychologia 24:169–180, 1986

Brandt J, Seidman LJ, Kohl D: Personality characteristics of epileptic patients: a controlled study of generalized and temporal lobe cases. J Clin Exp Neuropsychol 7:25–38, 1985

Bryden MP, Ley RC: Right-left hemispheric involvement in the perception and expression of emotion in normal humans, in Neuropsychology of Human Emotion. Edited by Heilman KM, Satz P. New York, Guilford, 1984, pp 6–44

Carpenter MB: Core Text of Neuroanatomy, 4th Edition. Baltimore, MD, Williams & Wilkins, 1991

Carpenter MB, Sutin J: Human Neuroanatomy, 8th Edition. Baltimore, MD, Williams & Wilkins, 1983

Coffey CE: Cerebral laterality and emotion: the neurology of depression. Compr Psychiatry 28:197–219, 1987

Coffey CE, Figiel GS, Djang WT, et al: Leukoencephalopathy in elderly depressed patients referred for ECT. Biol Psychiatry 24:143–161, 1988

Cummings JL: Clinical Neuropsychiatry. New York, Grune & Stratton, 1985

Cummings JL: Behavioral complications of drug treatment of Parkinson's disease. J Am Geriatr Soc 39:708–716, 1991

Cummings JL: Depression and Parkinson's disease: a review. Am J Psychiatry 149:443–454, 1992

Cummings JL: Frontal-subcortical circuits and human behavior. Arch Neurol 50:873–880, 1993

Cummings JL, Cunningham K: Obsessive-compulsive disorder in Huntington's disease. Biol Psychiatry 31:263–270, 1992

Cummings JL, Mendez MF: Secondary mania with focal cerebrovascular lesions. Am J Psychiatry 141:1084–1087, 1984

Davidson RJ: Anterior cerebral asymmetry and the nature of emotion. Brain Cogn 20:125–151, 1992

Delvenne V, Delecluse F, Hubain Ph P, et al: Regional cerebral blood flow in patients with affective disorders. Br J Psychiatry 157:359–365, 1990

Dilsaver SC, Coffman JA: Cholinergic hypothesis of depression: a reappraisal. J Clin Psychopharmacol 9:173–179, 1989

Doane BK: Clinical psychiatry and the physiodynamics of the limbic system, in The Limbic System: Functional Organization and Clinical Disorders. Edited by Doane BK, Livingston KE. New York, Raven, 1986, pp 285–315

Dolan RJ, Bench CJ, Brown RG, et al: Regional cerebral blood flow abnormalities in depressed patients with cognitive impairment. J Neurol Neurosurg Psychiatry 55:768–773, 1992

Drevets WC, Videen TO, Price JL, et al: A functional anatomical study of unipolar depression. J Neurosci 12:3628–3641, 1992

Eidelberg D, Galaburda AM: Symmetry and asymmetry in the posterior thalamus. Arch Neurol 39:325–332, 1982

Falzi G, Perrone P, Vignolog LA: Right-left asymmetry in anterior speech region. Arch Neurol 39:239–240, 1982

Flor-Henry P: Cerebral Basis of Psychopathology. Boston, MA, John Wright-PSG, 1983

Folstein SE: Huntington's Disease. A Disorder of Families. Baltimore, MD, Johns Hopkins University Press, 1989

Gainotti G: Emotional behavior and hemispheric side of lesion. Cortex 8:41–55, 1972

Galaburda AM, LeMay M, Kemper TL, et al: Right-left asymmetries in the brain. Science 199:852–856, 1978

Gawin FH: Cocaine addiction: psychology and neurophysiology. Science 251:1580–1586, 1991

Geschwind N: Disconnection syndromes in animals and man. Brain 88:237–294, 585–644, 1965

Girgis M: Neural Substrates of Limbic Epilepsy. St. Louis, MO, Warren H. Green, 1981

Glick SD, Ross DA, Hough LB: Lateral asymmetry of neurotransmitters in human brain. Brain Res 234:53–63, 1982

Gordan HW: Music and the Right Hemisphere, in Functions of the Right Cerebral Hemisphere. Edited by Young AW. New York, Academic Press, 1983, pp 65–87

Gorman DG, Cummings JL: Hypersexuality following septal injury. Arch Neurol 49:308–310, 1992

Gruzelier JH: A critical assessment and integration of lateral asymmetries in schizophrenia, in Hemisyndromes: Psychobiology, Neurology, and Psychiatry. Edited by Myslobodsky MS. New York, Academic Press, 1983, pp 265–326

Halgren E, Walter RD, Cherlow DG, et al: Mental phenomena evoked by electrical stimulation of the human hippocampal formation and amygdala. Brain 101:83–117, 1978

Hermann BP, Wyler AR, Blumer D, et al: Ictal fear: lateralizing significance and implications for understanding the neurobiology of pathological fear states. Neuropsychiatry, Neuropsychology, and Behavioral Neurology 5:205–210, 1992

Isaacson RL: The Limbic System. New York, Plenum, 1974

Katzman R, Thal L: Neurochemistry of Alzheimer's disease, in Basic Neurochemistry, 4th Edition. Edited by Siegel GJ, Agranoff BW, Albers RW, et al. New York, Raven, 1989, pp 827–838

Kelly JP: The neural basis of perception and movement, in Principles of Neural Science, 3rd Edition. Edited by Kandel ER, Schwartz JH, Jessell TM. New York, Elsevier, 1991, pp 283–295

Kimura D, Durnford M: Normal studies on the function of the right hemisphere in vision, in Hemisphere Function in the Human Brain. Edited by Dimond SJ, Beaumont JG. London, Elek Science, 1974, pp 25–47

Kirshner HS: Behavioral Neurology. A Practical Approach. New York, Churchill Livingstone, 1986

Kooistra CA, Heilman KM: Motor dominance and lateral asymmetry of the globus pallidus. Neurology 38:388–390, 1988

Laplane D, Levasseur M, Pillon B, et al: Obsessive-compulsive and other behavioral changes with bilateral basal ganglia lesions. Brain 112:699–725, 1989

Lechin F, van der Dijs B, Amat J, et al: Central neuronal pathways involved in anxiety behavior: experimental findings, in Neurochemistry and Clinical Disorders: Circuitry of Some Psychiatric and Psychosomatic Syndromes. Edited by Lechin F, van der Dijs B. Boca Raton, FL, CRC Press, 1989, pp 49–64

LeMay M: Morphological cerebral asymmetries of modern man, fossil man, and nonhuman primate. Ann N Y Acad Sci 280:349–366, 1976

Levy J: The mammalian brain and the adaptive advantage of cerebral asymmetry. Ann N Y Acad Sci 299:264–272, 1977

Lilly R, Cummings JL, Benson DF, et al: The human Kluver-Bucy syndrome. Neurology 33:1141–1145, 1983

Lin C-S, Nicolelis MAL, Schneider JS, et al: A major direct GABAergic pathway from zona incerta to neocortex. Science 248:1553–1556, 1990

Loring DW, Meador KJ, Lee GP, et al: Amobarbital effects and lateralized brain function. New York, Springer-Verlag, 1992

Machlin SR, Harris GJ, Pearlson GD, et al: Elevated medial-frontal cerebral blood flow in obsessive-compulsive patients: a SPECT study. Am J Psychiatry 148:1240–1242, 1991

MacLean PD: The Triune Brain in Evolution. New York, Plenum, 1990

Mena I, Marin O, Fuenzalida S, et al: Chronic manganese poisoning. Neurology 17:128–136, 1967

Mesulam M-M: Patterns of behavioral neuroanatomy: association areas, the limbic system, and hemispheric specialization, in Principles of Behavioral Neurology. Edited by Mesulam M-M. Philadelphia, PA, FA Davis, 1985, pp 1–70

Mesulam M-M, Mufson EJ: Neural inputs into the nucleus basalis of the substantia innominata (Ch4) in the rhesus monkey. Brain 107:253–274, 1984

Miller BL, Cummings JL, McIntyre H, et al: Hypersexuality or altered sexual preference following brain injury. J Neurol Neurosurg Psychiatry 49:867–873, 1986

Morris M: Psychiatric aspects of Huntington's disease, in Huntington's Disease. Edited by Harper PS. Philadelphia, PA, WB Saunders, 1991, pp 81–126

Moscovitch M, Olds J: Asymmetries in spontaneous facial expressions and their possible relation to hemispheric specialization. Neuropsychologia 20:71–81, 1982

Nachson I: Hemisphere dysfunction in psychopathy and behavior disorders, in Hemisyndromes: Psychobiology, Neurology, and Psychiatry. Edited by Myslobodsky MS. New York, Academic Press, 1983, pp 389–414

Nauta WJH: Circuitous connections linking cerebral cortex, limbic system, and corpus striatum, in The Limbic System: Functional Organization and Clinical Disorders. Edited by Doane BK, Livingston KE. New York, Raven, 1986, pp 43–54

Nauta WJH, Feirtag M: Fundamental Neuroanatomy. New York, WH Freeman, 1986

Nieuwenhuys R: Chemoarchitecture of the Brain. New York, Springer-Verlag, 1985

Oke A, Keller R, Mefford I, et al: Lateralization of norepinephrine in human thalamus. Science 200:1411–1413, 1978

Papez JW: A proposed mechanism of emotion. Arch Neurol Psychiatry 38:725–743, 1937

Perez MM, Trimble MR, Murray NMF, et al: Epileptic psychosis: an evaluation of PSE profiles. Br J Psychiatry 146:155–163, 1985

Plum F, Posner JB: The Diagnosis of Stupor and Coma. Philadelphia, PA, FA Davis, 1980

Rapoport SI: Integrated phylogeny of the primate brain, with special reference to humans and their diseases. Brain Res Brain Res Rev 15:267–294, 1990

Reisberg B, Franssen E, Sclan SG, et al: Stage specific incidence of potentially remediable behavioral symptoms in aging and Alzheimer's disease. Bulletin of Clinical Neurosciences 54:95–112, 1989

Robinson RG, Starkstein SE: Current research in affective disorders following stroke. J Neuropsychiatry Clin Neurosci 2:1–14, 1990

Robinson RG, Kubos KL, Starr LB, et al: Mood disorders in stroke patients: importance of location of lesion. Brain 107:81–93, 1984

Sackeim HA, Greenburg MS, Weiman AL, et al: Hemispheric asymmetry in the expression of positive and negative emotions. Arch Neurol 39:210–218, 1982

Sackeim HA, Prohovnik I, Moeller JR, et al: Regional cerebral blood flow in mood disorders. Arch Gen Psychiatry 47:60–70, 1990

Schade JP, Groeningen VV: Structural organization of the human cerebral cortex. Acta Anat 47:79–111, 1961

Schilder P: The organic background of obsessions and compulsions. Am J Psychiatry 94:1397–1416, 1938

Sedvall G: The current status of PET scanning with respect to schizophrenia. Neuropsychopharm 7:41–54, 1992

Starkstein SE, Robinson RG, Price TR: Comparison of cortical and subcortical lesions in the production of post-stroke mood disorders. Brain 110:1045–1059, 1987

Starkstein SE, Robinson RG, Berthier ML, et al: Differential mood changes following basal ganglia vs thalamic lesions. Arch Neurol 45:725–730, 1988a

Starkstein SE, Boston JD, Robinson RG: Mechanisms of mania after brain injury: twelve case reports and review of the literature. J Nerv Ment Dis 176:87–100, 1988b

Stein MB, Heuser IJ, Juncos JL, et al: Anxiety disorders in patients with Parkinson's disease. Am J Psychiatry 147:217–220, 1990

Stern DB: Psychogenic somatic symptoms on the left side: review and interpretation, in Hemisyndromes: Psychobiology, Neurology, and Psychiatry. Edited by Myslobodsky MS. New York, Academic Press, 1983, pp 415–445

Strauss E, Risser A, Jones MW: Fear responses in patients with epilepsy. Arch Neurol 39:626–630, 1982

Stuss DT, Benson DF: The Frontal Lobes. New York, Raven, 1986

Stuss DT, Guberman A, Nelson R, et al: The neuropsychology of paramedian thalamic infarction. Brain Cogn 8:348–378, 1988

Suddath RC, Casanova MF, Goldberg TE, et al: Temporal lobe pathology in schizophrenia: a quantitative magnetic resonance imaging study. Am J Psychiatry 146:464–472, 1989

Swedo SE, Rapoport JL, Cheslow DL, et al: High prevalence of obsessive-compulsive symptoms in patients with Sydenham's chorea. Am J Psychiatry 146:246–249, 1989

TenHouten WD, Hoppe KD, Bogen JE, et al: Alexithymia: an experimental study of cerebral commissurotomy patients and normal control subjects. Am J Psychiatry 143:312–316, 1986

Tucker DM, Watson RT, Heilman KM: Discrimination and evocation of affectively intoned speech in patients with right parietal disease. Neurology 27:947–950, 1977

Valzelli L: Psychobiology of Aggression and Violence. New York, Raven, 1981

Van Lancker D: Personal relevance and the human right hemisphere. Brain Cogn 17:64–92, 1991

Van Lancker D, Kreiman J, Cummings JL: Voice perception deficits: neuroanatomical correlates of phonagnosia. J Clin Exp Neuropsychol 11:665–674, 1989

Weintraub S, Mesulam M-M: Developmental learning disabilities of the right hemisphere. Arch Neurol 40:463–468, 1983

Williams D: The structure of emotions reflected in epileptic experiences. Brain 79:29–67, 1956

Wu JC, Buchsbaum MS, Hershey TG, et al: PET in generalized anxiety disorder. Biol Psychiatry 29:1181–1199, 1991

Yakovlev PI: Motility, behavior and the brain. J Nerv Ment Dis 107:313–335, 1948

Yakovlev PI: Telencephalon "impar," "semipar," and "totopar." Int J Neurol 6:245–265, 1968

Yakovlev PI, Lecours A-R: The myelogenetic cycles of regional maturation of the brain, in Regional Development of the Brain in Early Life. Edited by Minkowski A. Oxford, England, Blackwell Scientific, 1967, pp 3–65

Zohar J, Mueller EA, Insel TR, et al: Serotonergic responsivity in obsessive-compulsive disorder. Arch Gen Psychiatry 44:946–951, 1987

SECTION

II

Neuropsychiatric Assessment of the Elderly

Section Editor
Mark R. Lovell, Ph.D.

chapter 5
Neuropsychiatric Assessment

chapter 6
Mental Status Examination

chapter 7
Neuropsychological Assessment

chapter 8
Age-Associated Memory Impairment

chapter 9
Anatomic Imaging of the Aging Human Brain:
Computed Tomography and Magnetic
Resonance Imaging

chapter 10
Functional Neuroimaging: Positron-Emission
Tomography in the Study of Cerebral Blood
Flow and Glucose Utilization in Human
Subjects at Different Ages

chapter 11
Quantitative Electroencephalography:
Neurophysiological Alterations in Normal Aging and
Geriatric Neuropsychiatric Disorders

5

Neuropsychiatric Assessment

Raymond Faber, M.D.

Time waits for no one.

Mick Jagger
Keith Richards

Introduction

The clinical assessment of behavior remains the bedrock of psychiatric practice. Although the management of neuropsychiatric disorders has progressed impressively with advances in brain imaging technology and somatic therapies, it is in the observation, elicitation, and elucidation of relevant patient behaviors that the successful neuropsychiatrist makes his or her mark. In this chapter, after reviewing fundamental principals of the neuropsychiatric evaluation of the geriatric patient, I concentrate on neuropsychiatric assessment as epitomized in the mental status examination.

Purpose of the Clinical Encounter

As clinicians, our depth of inquiry is always limited by time. Similarly, the setting in which we see a patient will also greatly influence the scope of an examination. We must proceed at different paces in the emergency room, critical care unit, general psychiatry inpatient unit, or outpatient office where an appointment was set up several weeks previously. A comprehensive neuropsychiatric assessment can take several hours, and, as examiners, we must prioritize a hierarchy of interwoven management and diagnostic issues. Our main effort is to increase the probability of a "correct" diagnosis, while being cognizant of the impossibility of absolute certitude without a tissue diagnosis.

Interview Style

No two interviewers are identical in how they examine a patient, and the same interviewer will not examine different patients in exactly the same way. An exception would be a computer driven interview or an interview done by a robot. The effective interviewer allows

his or her personality to enter into, but not intrude on, the line of inquiry. Likewise, every patient has a unique personality that should be appreciated if at all possible. The rationale for these beliefs is that the interview is enhanced by being conversational in style, albeit unidirectionally focused. Such an approach will generally put the patient at ease and facilitate a full elaboration of affect and cognition. At best, this is a "pseudoconversation"; the interviewer's goal, however, is not simply to befriend a patient, but to gain an understanding of certain specific capabilities and experiences and ultimately to design and implement a treatment program that addresses psychiatric issues.

Although conversational in style, the interview should be far from being unstructured or nondirected. To the extent possible, a patient's leads should be followed as long as the information generated is relevant. A patient certainly should be allowed to repeat or reiterate a point about which he or she feels strongly. This conveys to the examiner the strength of the patient's feelings on a matter. Sometimes the repetition can reach the point of perseveration, for a very germane observation. On the other hand, a passive, unstructured, nondirected interview, which simply lets the patient talk, wastes valuable time. For the reasonably astute patient, this can result in the conclusion that "the doctor doesn't know what he's [she's] doing, he [she] just let me talk." A patient's confidence is not gained by naively listening to whatever he or she might say but by maintaining a professional attitude while gaining a thorough understanding of the patient. Likewise, an overly structured interview can be disastrous. Perfunctory questions concerning orientation, serial subtractions, and abstracting ability can be highly inappropriate and even insulting if the preceding portion of the interview made it clear the patient was obviously oriented, well able to sustain attention, and able to spontaneously use abstract concepts and relevant analogies. Embarrassment and hostility can be avoided in such instances with a simple explanation as to the purpose of such inquiries.

The interview should begin with introductions and a clarification of the goals and objectives of the examiner. This should be followed by customary social questions including age, handedness, marital status, family composition, employment, and living situation. These should generally precede questions regarding the "chief complaint." The rationale for this strategy is to convey an interest in the patient as a person rather than the repository of a (hopefully) interesting neuropsychiatric condition. In addition, the patient's initial responses usually dictate some direction to subsequent questions, such as consideration of confusion, attentional deficits, aphasias, cognitive dysfunction, depression, or psychosis (Leon et al. 1989).

Patients benefit greatly by being given some immediate feedback at the conclusion of an interview. Clear and concise communication of diagnostic impressions often provides great relief for the patient in providing some kind of label for what may have been a morass of emotional and cognitive distress. Alleviating uncertainty and instilling hope should be high priorities. Unless both of these occur, an interview cannot be considered successful (except in unusual circumstances such as a profound dementia or severe delirium). Another priority is to remain genuine and realistic; one of the worst possible outcomes of an interview is for the patient to conclude that the examiner lacks credibility.

Phenomenology of Behavior

Descriptive psychopathology and *descriptive phenomenology* are two terms inextricably involved in psychiatric assessment. The former term refers to the signs of aberrant behavior that include patients' verbalizations enumerated from an atheoretical point of view. The latter term, best discussed by Jaspers (1963), is the attempt to depict as clearly as possible the psychological experiences of the patient. In this vein, it is important to distinguish between the form of psychopathology and the content of symptoms. *Form* refers to the structure of psychopathology and is a reflection of the illness process. For example, manic hyperactivity, social intrusiveness, colorful attire, and rapid and pressured speech represent the form of manic symptoms. These are readily apparent, even in individuals from different cultures who speak a foreign language. The form

of delusions include their fixity and imperviousness to logical challenge. The form of auditory hallucinations includes speech versus nonspeech sounds, loudness, clarity, perceived source of sound, and hearing complex sentences versus the simple repetition of a few words. *Content* refers to the subject matter of symptoms. The statements a patient makes, what auditory hallucinations may "say" to a patient, and the theme of delusions are examples of content. Understanding content helps in appreciating the patient as a unique person; understanding the form of symptoms tends to have more diagnostic import (Slater and Roth 1969). The form of behavior can be assessed most systematically through the mental status examination.

Mental Status Examination

The mental status examination is sometimes referred to as the *physical examination of psychiatry*. This is odd as it suggests the physical examination has no place in psychiatry. Nothing could be further from the truth in neuropsychiatry. Although a detailed discussion is outside the scope of this chapter, a physical exam, even if "normal," is a vital component of a complete assessment. Naturally, a sufficiently detailed longitudinal history must be obtained from the patient or a knowledgeable collateral historian, because an isolated, cross-sectional view such as the mental status examination can lead to erroneous conclusions. Patients may present with long-standing developmental problems or behavioral alterations with acute, subacute, or insidious onset. The rapidity and progression of symptom evolution must be determined in the context of premorbid functioning and achievement. For example, highly intelligent individuals and those with marginal premorbid intellect can demonstrate widely disparate abilities, even if both are identically afflicted with Alzheimer's disease for 2 years. Table 5–1 outlines the components of the mental status examination.

Appearance

A patient's appearance is an extremely germane aspect of the overall assessment. Apparent age is particularly important in geriatric neuropsychiatry. Generally, people appear as they feel. Typically, patients in the early to middle stages of Alzheimer's disease look young and healthy for their age. Also it is important to note obvious physical stigmata, general state of physical health ranging from cachectic to robust, overt emotional displays, manner of relating, and level of cooperation.

Early on in an interview the clinician should try to assess the reliability and accuracy of a patient's statements. Facial expressions may convey elated, sad, anxious, disgruntled, or perplexed states of mind. Melancholic patients classically exhibit both an omega sign (a furrowed brow wrinkling the glabellar area into the shape of the Greek letter *omega,* caused by sustained contraction of the corrugator muscle) and Veraguth's folds (an upward, inward peaking of the upper eyelids).

Grooming and hygiene tend to be poor among most patients with schizophrenia, and these and other social niceties deteriorate among patients with progressive dementia. Patients with mania often appear in colorful and bizarre clothing, including head decorations with scraps of debris, excessive jewelry, and layering of mismatched clothing. Patients with antisocial personality disorders and substance use disorders tend to adopt slick, au courant garb (Leon et al. 1989).

Patients with right parietal lobe lesions can display signs of both unilateral neglect and dressing apraxia. They may not properly shave, comb their hair, or secure buttons on their left side. Patients with dressing apraxia can wind up with garments that are upside-down or inside-out; likewise they may wear their trousers backward. Such patients may be completely unaware of these seemingly obvious difficulties, and friends and relatives may be the first to notice.

Activity

Motor activity may be appropriate, increased, decreased, or catatonic in character. With normal aging

Table 5–1. Mental status examination

Appearance
Activity (including catatonic features)
Emotional state (including affect and mood)
Speech and language (including formal thought disorder)
Thought content (including Schneiderian first-rank symptoms)
Perceptual disturbances
Personality
Insight and judgment

there is a generalized slowing of psychomotor activity. The average octogenarian is much less active than the average young adult. Classic movement disorders including tremors, dystonias, and choreiform movements including tardive dyskinesia should be noted. Repetitive, unvarying movements, if goal directed, are termed *mannerisms,* whereas repetitive purposeless movements are *stereotypes.* Likewise, increased motor activity, if purposeful and goal directed, is *hyperactivity,* whereas an increase of purposeless activity is called *agitation.* The latter often includes pacing, handwringing, foot tapping, scalp rubbing, and carphologic movements such as picking at clothing and bed linens. Agitation is commonly seen in delirium, is frequent in dementias, and tends to reflect intense emotions accompanying anxiety states, mood disorders, and psychoses. Antipsychotic medication–induced akathisia mimics agitation.

Decreased activity as manifested by a diminution of movement, speech, and thinking is known as *psychomotor retardation.* It typically includes prolonged speech latency before answering a question. Such slowing of activity can be prominent in depressions, schizophrenias, dorsolateral frontal lobe syndromes, medial frontal lobe damage, and dementias, especially subcortical dementias. In subcortical dementias due to Parkinson's disease, the term *bradyphrenia* has been used to characterize slowed thinking (Rodgers 1992). Stupor is extreme psychomotor retardation and includes mutism, immobility, and unresponsiveness to vigorous, even painful, stimuli. Mute patients will usually become verbally responsive under the influence of sodium amobarbital or other sedatives. In performing an "Amytal interview," the examiner injects amobarbital at a rate between 25 and 50 mg iv per minute until the patient begins to speak or becomes grossly sedated. The information gained by this procedure can have substantial diagnostic importance.

Catatonic behaviors tend to be overlooked if they are subtle and may require skillful examination (Taylor 1981). Components of catatonic behaviors include mannerisms and stereotypes. Catalepsy is the maintenance of an awkward posture or position. Psychological pillow involves keeping one's head several inches from a bed surface as if a pillow were present. Automatic obedience is a category of catatonic behavior wherein seemingly understood verbal instructions are overridden by more recent tactile or visual stimuli (e.g., the patient tries to shake hands with the examiner contrary to firm verbal instructions whenever the examiner extends his or her right hand). In *Mitmachen* the patient allows a body part to be put into any position without resistance in response to light pressure, despite instructions to the contrary. In ambitendency the patient makes a series of back-and-forth movements that approach but never reach a goal, such as shaking hands or walking to a particular location. Echolalia is the automatic repetition of the examiner's utterances. This is easily tested by asking the patient to say "1, 2, 3" after the examiner says "A, B, C." Echopraxia is the automatic copying of the examiner's posture or position; it may be found on asking the patient to "touch your nose, when I touch my chest." Negativism, the opposite of obedience, may also be part of catatonia. This may include refusal to speak, eat, or move (stupor) and paratonia (or *Gegenhalten*) wherein the patient resists attempts to move his or her limbs by a force equal to that being applied by an examiner.

Emotional State

Mood refers to sustained emotional state and can include feelings such as joy, sadness, anxiety, shame, anger, and indifference. *Affect* refers to more transitory and immediate emotional expressions. Other aspects of affect include 1) range, which is constricted if a spectrum of moods is not elicitable or expanded if excesses of joyfulness or sadness are seen; 2) intensity, which can be increased as in vituperative, invective speech laced with dogmatic insistence regarding convictions or diminished when patients appear shallow and vacuous with little conviction in their statements; 3) stability versus lability (rapid, often unpredictable changeability); 4) appropriateness of affective display to the content of speech and thought; and 5) relatedness, which is the ability to establish rapport and interpersonal connectedness.

To assess mood and affect fully, the interview must cover a variety of topics in sufficient depth and breadth. If the interview is limited to an enumeration of symptoms, a comprehensive analysis of affect is impossible. Patients' unique, individually experienced joys and disappointments must be brought out. Asking about personal losses and the ensuing reactions are invaluable, as are questions concerning loved ones and career achievements. By inquiring about hobbies and interests, different aspects of affect will be elicited, as well as information about drive and motivation and whether anhedonia is present (Klein 1974). It is im-

portant to distinguish apathy without sadness from the sad and lowered mood present in depressions and grief states.

The fixity of a depressed mood can have diagnostic and therapeutic implications. This can be gauged by observers' reports of persistent glumness and by observing patients' reactions to the punch line of jokes (as, for example, drawn from Magliozzi and Magliozzi [1991]). Autonomous, nonreactive sadness suggests an endogenous, biological process that typically responds well to somatic therapy. Reactive depressions are adjustment disorders that may respond as equally well to placebo as to medication, and psychotherapy may be their treatment of choice.

The expression "emotional [or affective] blunting" can best be applied to apathetic, indifferent patients in whom affects are diminished in intensity and constricted to a narrow neutral range. Such patients do not display happiness or sadness, have no depth to their convictions, lack relatedness to the examiner, and lack concern for other people. If manifested to an extreme degree, such as just shrugging their shoulders when asked what they would do if they won the lottery, the term *flattened affect* is appropriate. This limitation in affective expression is a core negative symptom of schizophrenia. Interestingly, it also often accompanies damage to the dorsolateral frontal cortex, and this brain region has been implicated as dysfunctional in many schizophrenic patients.

Sometimes confused with *affective blunting* is the term *motor dysprosody*, which is a typical sequelae of right anterior cerebral and subcortical lesions (Ross and Mesulam 1979). Motor dysprosody consists of monotonous, sparse speech without inflection or affective coloring; however, patients with motor dysprosody can experience strong and painful emotions. Although such patients may complain of severe dysphoria, examiners may be misled into minimizing its importance, much to the patient's disadvantage.

Inappropriate affect with lability is characteristic of pseudobulbar palsy, wherein patients laugh while describing depression or cry while claiming to be happy. Increased mood intensity is allegedly a characteristic of limbic epilepsy, as is humorlessness. Frontal lobe lesions can cause a plethora of affective disturbances including depression, mania, shallow jocularity (*Witzelsucht*), irritability, lability, impulsivity, apathy, and indifference.

Suicide potential is assessed by asking a graded series of questions beginning with feelings of hopelessness, feeling life is not worth living, thoughts about death, wishing to die in one's sleep, thoughts of taking one's life, and having a means and plan to commit suicide. If the latter is the case, the next inquiry should be to establish how long that patient is willing to live before acting on his or her plan. This is a very practical means of determining the urgency of the situation.

Determining a particular patient's potential to harm others is even more problematic. Patients should be asked whether they have any intention of deliberately hurting another person. If a specific victim is identified, psychiatrists have a legal duty to warn that third party. Command hallucinations to inflict harm must be taken seriously, although in most instances they do not lead to overt violence.

Speech and Language

Speech or language disturbances can reflect brain pathology, psychiatric disturbance, or both. The form of language disturbance can be of diagnostic importance and must be considered separately from the content of speech. Aphasic language may reflect previously unrecognized coarse (identifiable) brain disease, such as a stroke, tumor, migraine, or infection. Misidentifying aphasic language as "functional" can lead to dire consequences.

Speech fluency, comprehension, naming, repetition, reading, writing, and prosody should all be assessed (see Chapter 6, this volume). Mutism, excessive latency of response, paucity of speech, dysarthria, anomia, agrammatism, and paraphasic errors are all pathological. Loud, insistent (pressured) speech is characteristic of mania.

When the accompanying content of speech is colorful or unusual, it may be difficult to focus on the form of language and possible disturbance. This can be overcome by the deliberate, separate characterization of speech form irrespective of content. Circumstantiality is overly detailed, often tedious speech that eventually reaches its intended goal. Tangential speech initially seems relevant but continuously veers from its intended goal, never getting back to it. Blocking is the stopping of speech prematurely; if it begins again on an unrelated topic, this is termed *derailment*. In loosening of associations there is a continuing shifting of topics. If this becomes nearly incomprehensible, it is called *word salad*, an apropos descriptive denoting jumbled and often incomprehensible speech. Psychotic pa-

tients will use words idiosyncratically (stock words), abruptly change the subject, defy logic in their conclusions, and yet often use a rich vocabulary with complex grammar. The latter symptoms would be highly atypical of patients with an organic aphasia and are useful points for differentiation (Faber and Reichstein 1981; Faber et al. 1983). Lack of formal education and local dialects can complicate language evaluations. Manic flight of ideas typically includes understandable linkages often by sound (clanging) in a kind of speech romp. Manic speech is also rapid and pressured and vulnerable to distraction by irrelevant, external stimuli. Non sequiturs are responses totally irrelevant to the question. Inappropriately, often incessantly, repeated words (palilalia), phrases (verbigeration), or themes are types of verbal perseveration. In logoclonia, the last syllable of the last word is repeated.

Thought Content

Disorders of thought content range from transient preoccupations to intractable delusions. Ruminations are recurring mood-congruent concerns that typically reflect the presence of anxiety or depression. Obsessions are unwanted and unwarranted ideas, images, memories, or impulses that incessantly intrude into consciousness. They are intensely unpleasant and can cause great distress. Obsessions are frequently accompanied by compulsions—stereotyped actions or action sequences, which typically include checking, counting, cleaning, rearranging, or other rituals. If not performed expediently and precisely, compulsions become a source of intense dysphoria. Obsessions and compulsions are common in Gilles de la Tourette's syndrome. Phobias are unrealistic fears of objects, locations, or situations that the individual tries to avoid at almost any cost.

Delusional ideas represent a particular form of cognitive intransigence. These unshakable beliefs are not in keeping with a particular patient's social, cultural, or religious background. They may by chance be true, as is occasionally the case with delusions of infidelity, but almost always delusions are false and often outlandish. Table 5–2 lists common delusional themes.

A primary delusional idea is one that cannot be understood as arising from preexisting psychopathology, such as hallucinations or an aberrant mood. It is therefore important to ask how patients became aware of any delusional ideas. The examiner should not challenge a patient's delusional ideas. Sometimes, on hearing a delusional idea, it may be useful to react with mild surprise or disbelief at the ideas expressed to assess the fixity of these beliefs. If examiners have no noticeable reaction to a blatantly bizarre statement, patients with partial insight regarding their delusions may conclude the examiner is patronizing and insincere.

Overvalued idea is a very useful term for quasi-delusional beliefs that are plausible, although generally unlikely. They are not bizarre, but patients realize their concerns are relatively unique. They will not concede, however, that the inordinate amount of time and energy expended on overvalued ideas is pathological. Overvalued ideas are found in a broad spectrum of psychiatric conditions.

Delusions of persecution, often known somewhat imprecisely as *paranoid delusions,* are the most common delusions found in neuropsychiatric disorders. They may concern being influenced or harmed by outside forces or being the object of strangers' notice and conversation (ideas of reference). Patients with such delusions are usually guarded and mistrustful of the examiner. To elicit delusions in this situation, patients should be asked if they feel they have been singled out from the populace at large for some type of mistreatment. Delusional patients emphasize their uniqueness in being harassed.

Table 5–2. Common delusional themes

Delusion	Content
Persecution	Feeling threatened or mistreated
Grandeur	Possessing special abilities, talents, or powers
Somatic, hypochondriacal	Having physical ailments
Guilt	Feeling unduly responsible for misdeeds or misfortune
Poverty	Being without financial resources
Nihilism (Cotard's syndrome)	Conviction of nonexistence of self
Jealousy	Feeling spouse or lover is engaged in illicit relationship
Capgras syndrome	Claiming an impostor is posing as spouse or familiar person
Fregoli syndrome	Claiming a known persecutor has assumed the guise of a stranger
Erotomania; de Clerambault syndrome	Believing an uninvolved party, often a celebrity, is in love with the patient

Less common delusions include grandiose delusions of wealth, power, healing ability, and friendships with famous personages, as typify manic states. Somatic or hypochondriacal delusions of ill-health include false convictions of having fatal diseases, infestations, or degeneration of internal organs. Related delusions of guilt and poverty can occur in psychotic depressions as can, in the extreme, nihilistic delusions (Cotard's syndrome), wherein patients say they no longer exist or have a body. (Such patients are often overly agreeable to electroconvulsive therapy, the treatment of choice in such situations, based on their hope that complications, however unlikely, will result in their permanent demise.) Delusions of jealousy are not rare, and delusions involving misidentification are common. One subtype of the latter is the Capgras syndrome—the delusion that a significant person (often the spouse) has been replaced by a nearly identical impostor. The Capgras syndrome is prevalent in Alzheimer's disease and other dementias. This can be a cruel experience for a devoted spouse who has made self-sacrificing efforts to be supportive and loving.

A related, though rarer, condition is the Fregoli syndrome—the belief that a known persecutor has taken on the appearance of a stranger. Erotomania, or de Clerambault syndrome, is the delusion that a stranger, usually a celebrity, is in love with the patient. Other types of delusions are somewhat rare and esoteric, though fascinating.

It should be appreciated that the term *delusion* can also refer to delusional mood and delusional perception. In a delusional mood, patients are convinced that something in their environment has changed for the worse. They become preoccupied with fears of impending doom, though they cannot identify specifics. A delusional perception is a Schneiderian first-rank symptom of schizophrenia (see below). This phenomenon has two components: a normal perception, immediately followed by a delusional conclusion. An example would be an American concluding he belonged to the British monarchy after receiving a letter from England posted by the Royal Mail.

Of substantial historic interest and current importance are "symptoms of the first rank" described by Schneider, who asserted their specificity (in the absence of identifiable brain disease) in schizophrenia (see Hamilton 1984). It is now known that these symptoms can also occur in affective psychoses, but they, nonetheless, provide the phenomenological pillars for all modern diagnostic schemes for schizophrenia. In addition to delusional perception, other first-rank symptoms mainly involve thought content.

In experiences of influence, patients believe that their thoughts, speech or actions are controlled by some outside agency that cannot be resisted or overcome by the patient. In experiences of alienation, patients perceive thoughts, feelings, speech, and body parts as not belonging to them. They will describe, for instance, that some thoughts that come into their minds are qualitatively distinct from their own usual thoughts and have been placed there by some external source. This phenomenon is called *thought insertion.* Thought withdrawal is the converse and involves the patient's mind going blank as if his or her thoughts had been sucked away into a psychic vacuum cleaner. In thought broadcasting, patients are convinced that their thoughts are audible to anyone in their vicinity. This is typically accompanied by secondary delusional explanations involving radar or mental telepathy. Finally, complete auditory hallucinations are loud, clear, well-formed, sustained voices perceived as coming from an external source. Subtypes include hearing two or more voices converse about the patient in the third person, voices continually commenting on the patient's actions, and thought echo, in which a patient's thoughts are repeated audibly. Linguaphiles refer to the latter as *echo de pensees* or *Gedankenlautwerden* (Hamilton 1984).

Perceptual Disturbances

Any sensory modality can be disturbed to a greater or lesser extent. Illusions are misinterpreted perceptions (e.g., shadows mistaken for threatening figures). Stimulus intensity or quality may be distorted as in hyperacusis. Distorted visual perceptions are termed *dysmegaiopsia;* if objects appear in miniature this is micropsia, if enlarged, macropsia. Such visual disturbances may occur in all varieties of temporal lobe lesions (Hamilton 1985). Occurrences of this nature are common on falling asleep (hypnagogic) or arising (hypnopompic) and then are not pathological.

Hallucinations are sensory experiences occurring without external stimulation. Pseudohallucinations have been variously defined and consist of hallucinations accompanied by the insight that they are unreal. Elementary hallucinations consist of flashes of light, noises, or sounds that are not formed into a coherent organization. Functional hallucinations occur only when there is a concurrent real perception in the same sensory modality (e.g., hearing voices only when a water tap is running). Autoscopic hallucinations occur when patients have a visual hallucination of themselves. Extracampine hallucinations occur outside of a known sensory field (e.g., seeing objects through a solid wall—Superman hallucinations). Hallucinations of voices may range from one or two muffled or softly spoken words emanating from inside the patient's head (incomplete auditory hallucinations) to loud, clear sentences from space external to the patient (complete auditory hallucinations). The former may be nearly innocuous; the latter is grossly pathological. Studies of epileptic patients with psychoses have found complete auditory hallucinations to be associated with left temporal lobe abnormalities (Trimble 1990).

The apperception of self can be disturbed in many neuropsychiatric conditions. Body image is distorted in patients with eating disorders, borderline personality, and schizophrenia. In depersonalization, patients feel that their sense of identity has been altered, and they, therefore, feel strange and unreal concerning their personhood. In derealization, patients feel the environment has changed and is unreal. They may feel as if life were a play on a stage—one step removed from reality.

Though visual hallucinations may be predominant in states of delirium, no hallucinations, in and of themselves, are pathognomonic for any specific psychiatric or neurological condition. Visual hallucinations are, however, especially relevant in geriatric neuropsychiatry. Approximately 50% of patients in delirium or acute confusion states experience visual hallucinations. These are also highly prevalent in states of alcohol withdrawal and drug toxicity. Although numerous drugs may be responsible, anticholinergics and antiparkinsonian medication are leading offenders. A variety of nervous system lesions cause visual hallucinations (Cummings 1985). Ocular pathology can result in hallucinations ranging from unformed, brief streaks to clear, fully formed complex images. Cerebral lesions, especially of the posterior right hemisphere, can cause release hallucinations of novel formed images lasting from minutes to hours. Epilepsy, migraine, and narcolepsy are common neuropsychiatric disorders also associated with visual hallucinations.

It is important to inquire about disturbances of touch, taste, and smell as they may reflect an epileptic aura. Furthermore, multiple concurrent types of hallucinations are more the rule then the exception in psychiatric disorders. Tactile hallucinations of insects crawling under the skin, termed *formication,* often accompany drug-induced psychotic states.

In initial inquiries about major forms of psychopathology, such as hallucinations or delusions, it is best to start asking rather general questions, such as "Have you noticed anything unusual happening around you?" or "Are you concerned about matters that other people are probably unaware of?" This allows the patient to elaborate on concerns without suggestions as to what the examiner is looking for. However, negative responses by the patient obviously require more focused inquiries.

Personality

Appraising a patient's personality is an important part of any assessment. Contemporary diagnostic schemes propose three clusters of personality disorders. Cluster A includes paranoid, schizoid, and schizotypal personality disorders; cluster B contains antisocial, borderline, histrionic, and narcissistic types; and cluster C contains avoidant, dependent, obsessive-compulsive, and passive-aggressive types. Many of these have dubious validity generally, and their application in geriatric populations is unknown. What is relevant in any assessment are personality traits that, taken together, constitute the unique personal attributes and idiosyncrasies that define a person. No patient can be fully understood without understanding his or her personality. Traits including neuroticism, extraversion, novelty seeking, and agreeableness have been validated in research studies and have practical utility.

Any alteration in a patient's personality may be secondary to a neuropsychiatric condition. This would constitute an organic personality disorder. Typical characteristics include 1) mood lability with depression, irritability, or anxiety; 2) inappropriate aggression; 3) impaired, typically disinhibited, social judgment; 4) apathy and indifference; and 5) severe suspiciousness.

A specific, though controversial, constellation of behavioral changes has been suggested to result from chronic complex partial seizures. These are the tetrad of hypergraphia, hyposexuality, severe circumstantiality, and hyperreligiosity. Although of unknown sensitivity and specificity, when present these behavioral changes should lead the clinician to a consideration of heretofore undiagnosed epilepsy.

Insight and Judgment

Insight refers to subjective awareness of the pathological nature of neuropsychiatric disturbances. Lack of insight or denial of illness is termed *anosognosia* and is classically associated with right parietal lobe lesions. It is also characteristic of many dementias with widespread brain pathology. The phenomenon spans a spectrum that includes denial of hemiparesis or blindness to a minimization of problems, indifference to the disability (*anosodiaphoria*), and a calm attitude toward any disability (*la belle indifference*). The extent of insight is a strong predictor of compliance with treatment plans, be they pharmacological or psychosocial.

Insight correlates strongly, but not absolutely, with judgment, as lack of insight indicates poor judgment, but the presence of insight does not insure sound judgment. Hypothetical questions about mailing letters are of much less value than inquiries and observations about real-life issues such as financial management. Traditionally, the ability to interpret proverbs has served to assess cognitive skills and thought process and reflect ultimately on judgment. The same has held for class similarities of objects. Both tend to correlate with current intelligence and educational level but, because of problems of reliability and validity, should serve only as minor adjuncts in an evaluation.

If insight and judgment are impaired so that harm to self or others is deemed likely, the difficult issues of competence and forced intervention must be addressed. Early Alzheimer's disease is the classic setting in which neuropsychiatrists confront such thorny problems as privileges to drive a car, management of finances, and even the ability to live freely outside an institution. Common sense strategies, (e.g., safety first and treating others as one would hope to be treated) represent the most prudent approach. Because of potential legal ramifications, thorough documentation of assessments, explanations, and attempted interventions is especially important. The psychiatrist is not necessarily responsible for a patient's misadventures, unless he or she has failed to document assessment efforts and treatment recommendations adequately.

Rating Scales

There are a number of rating scales that can serve as useful adjuncts in a neuropsychiatric evaluation. The Mini-Mental State Exam (MMSE; Folstein et al. 1975) is used widely and is well established as an instrument to screen for cognitive dysfunction. It is somewhat insensitive for picking up non–dominant-hemisphere lesions and dementias with predominant frontal lobe features. In my experience, the Neurobehavioral Cognitive Status Examination (NCSE; Kiernan et al. 1987; Schwamm et al. 1987) serves better as a screening instrument for cognitive dysfunction than does the MMSE. The Executive Interview (Exit; Royall et al. 1992) is a recently developed screen for frontal executive cognitive functions that correlates highly with level of care requirements and problem behaviors.

A range of behavioral disturbances can be rated on a number of instruments. The best established is the Brief Psychiatric Rating Scale (BPRS; Overall and Gorham 1988), which uses 18 items to cover a broad range of psychopathology. The Neurobehavioral Rating Scale (NRS; Levin et al. 1987; Sultzer et al. 1992) incorporates BPRS items and adds measures of behavioral disturbances and cognitive impairment. Severity of depression is usually determined using the Hamilton Rating Scale for Depression (HRSD [or Ham-D]; Hamilton 1967). Screening for depression in geriatric populations is usually determined using the Geriatric Depression Scale (Yesavage et al. 1983). The Hamilton Anxiety Scale (Hamilton 1959) is helpful in measuring anxiety symptoms. The BEHAVE-AD (Reisberg et al. 1987) is useful in assessing psychosis and behavioral disturbances in Alzheimer's disease.

Conclusions

In the final analysis, the goal of neuropsychiatric assessment is to understand the patient and explain his or her predicament, leading to maximally effective treatment. Mainly through empathy and pertinent observation, clinicians can understand psychologically the patient's pain, distress, and dysphoria. Knowledge of brain functioning and dysfunctioning can allow a biological explanation of symptomatology. The intent of this chapter was to foster both of these ends. Topics discussed were the context of the clinical encounter and interview style. Both require an integration of structure and flexibility. Details concerning appearance, activity (including underappreciated signs of catatonia), emotional state, speech and language, thought content, perceptual disturbances, and insight and judgment were discussed. The latter included suggestions for appraising competence and potential for

harm to the patient or others. Chapter 6 focuses on the assessment of sensorium attention and concentration, language, visuospatial skills, memory, and higher executive functions.

References

Cummings JL: Clinical Neuropsychiatry. Orlando, FL, Grune & Stratton, 1985

Faber R, Reichstein MB: Language dysfunction in schizophrenia. Br J Psychiatry 139:519–522, 1981

Faber R, Abrams R, Taylor MA, et al: Comparison of schizophrenic patients with formal thought disorder and neurologically impaired patients with aphasia. Am J Psychiatry 140:1348–1351, 1983

Folstein M, Folstein S, McHugh P: Mini-Mental State: a practical method for grading the cognitive state of patients for the clinician. J Psychiatry Res 12:189–198, 1975

Hamilton M: The assessment of anxiety stated by rating. Br J Med Psychol 32:50–55, 1959

Hamilton M: Development of a rating scale for primary depressive illness. British Journal of Social and Clinical Psychology 6:278–296, 1967

Hamilton M (ed): Fish's Schizophrenia, 3rd Edition. Bristol, England, Wright-PSG, 1984

Hamilton M (ed): Fish's Clinical Psychopathology, 2nd Editon. Bristol, England, Wright, 1985

Jaspers K: General Psychopathology. Translated by Hoenig J, Hamilton MW. Manchester, England, Manchester University Press, 1963

Kiernan RJ, Mueller J, Langston W, et al: The Neurobehavioral Cognitive Status Examination: a brief but quantitative approach to cognitive assessment. Ann Intern Med 107:481–485, 1987

Klein DF: Endogenomorphic depression: a conceptual and terminological revision. Arch Gen Psychiatry 31:447–454, 1974

Leon RL, Bowden CL, Faber RA: The psychiatric interview, history and mental status examination, in Comprehensive Textbook of Psychiatry, 5th Edition. Edited by Kaplan HI, Sadock BJ. Baltimore, MD, Williams & Wilkins, 1989, pp 449–462

Levin HS, High WM, Goethe KE, et al: The neurobehavioral rating scale: assessment of the behavioral sequelae of head injury by the clinician. J Neurol Neurosurg Psychiatry 50:183–193, 1987

Magliozzi T, Magliozzi R: Car Talk. New York, Dell, 1991

Overall JE, Gorham DR: Introduction: the Brief Psychiatric Rating Scale (BPRS): recent developments in ascertainment and scaling. Psychopharmacol Bull 24:97–99, 1988

Reisberg B, Borenstein J, Salob SP: Behavioral symptoms in Alzheimer's disease: phenomenology and treatment. J Clin Psychiatry 48 (suppl):9–15, 1987

Rodgers D: Bradyphrenia in Parkinson's disease, in Parkinson's Disease: Neurobehavioral Aspects. Edited by Huber SJ, Cummings JL. New York, Oxford University Press, 1992

Ross ED, Mesulam MM: Dominant language functions of the right hemisphere: prosody and emotional gesturing. Arch Neurology 36:144–148, 1979

Royall DR, Mahurin RK, Gray KF: Bedside assessment of executive cognitive impariment: the executive interview. J Am Geriatr Soc 40:1221–1226, 1992

Schwamm LH, Van Dyke C, Kiernan RJ, et al: The Neurobehavioral Cognitive Status Examination: comparison with the Cognitive Capacity Screening Examination and the Mini-Mental State Examination in a neurological population. Ann Intern Med 107:486–491, 1987

Slater E, Roth M: Clinical Psychiatry, 3rd Edition. Baltimore, MD, Williams & Wilkins, 1969

Sultzer DL, Levin HS, Mahler ME, et al: Assessment of cognitive, psychiatric, and behavioral disturbances in patients with dementia: the neurobehavioral rating scale. J Am Geriatr Soc 40:549–555, 1992

Taylor MA: The Neuropsychiatric Mental Status Examination. New York, SP Medical and Scientific Books, 1981

Trimble MR: First-rank symptoms of Schneider: a new perspective. Br J Psychiatry 156:195–200, 1990

Yesage JA, Brink TL, Rose TL, et al: Development and validation of a geriatric depression screening scale: a preliminary report. J Psychiatr Res 17:37–49, 1983

6

Mental Status Examination

David L. Sultzer, M.D.

Introduction

Mental status examination is a fundamental part of the neuropsychiatric assessment of older patients. The examination explores the integrity of cognitive skills, which include intellectual abilities such as thinking, perception, and problem solving. Performance in several cognitive domains is assessed, including attention, memory, language, visuospatial skills, calculation, and executive skills.

Cognitive evaluation adds an important dimension to neuropsychiatric assessment. The psychiatric examination reveals abnormal experiences, thoughts, interpersonal skills, and behavior; the neurological evaluation primarily examines motor skills and sensory integrity, thus exploring the function of a limited part of the brain. The cognitive mental status examination expands the assessment of regional brain function and can reveal the presence of cerebral pathology that contributes to the expression of psychiatric symptoms or intellectual deficits. Although a trichotomy is implied, the psychiatric, cognitive, and neurological examinations overlap considerably. Together they identify a pattern of neuropsychiatric signs that the clinician uses to formulate the differential diagnosis and to select additional diagnostic tests.

Assessment of cognitive skills is particularly important in older patients because the prevalence of delirium, dementia, and neurological insults increases with age. In addition, the care of older patients is affected by cognitive impairment: medication compliance may be low and self-reported medical symptoms may be unreliable. Other goals of mental status assessment in elderly patients include

1. Distinguishing the subtle cognitive changes of normal aging from the deficits of a dementing illness.
2. Distinguishing cognitive changes of dementia from those associated with depression or delirium.
3. Promoting early recognition of dementia, as even moderate cognitive decline may not be detected by family members or the primary physician (Kallman and May 1989). Cognitive impairment in patients with reversible dementia is often less severe and of shorter duration than in those with irreversible dementia (Larson et al. 1984).

4. Distinguishing dementia, or multidimensional cognitive impairment, from the neuropsychiatric syndromes characterized by impairment in only one cognitive domain, such as aphasia or amnesia.
5. Identifying and localizing cerebral pathology that is neurologically silent.
6. Monitoring changes in cognition over time to assess illness progression or the effect of therapeutic interventions.
7. Identifying cognitive strengths in patients with mild dementia. Use of preserved cognitive skills can maximize a patient's functional skills.

In this chapter, I review the clinical mental status examination of elderly patients. I first discuss history taking and examination technique and then describe evaluation of each cognitive domain. I identify regional neuroanatomic pathology associated with impairment in specific cognitive domains and the clinical features of four neuropsychiatric syndromes of cognitive impairment: disorders of attention, memory disorders, aphasia, and frontal lobe disorders. Finally, I review the assessment of functional skills and the use of screening instruments to detect and measure cognitive impairment in elderly patients. (The neurobiology of specific neuropsychiatric syndromes are described in detail in Sections III and IV of this volume, and an overview of the neuroanatomical and neurochemical underpinnings of human cognition and emotion is provided in Chapter 4.)

Clinical History

The mental status examination begins with a thorough historical review of cognitive symptoms. The patient should be invited to describe current or past difficulties with memory or thinking, such as problems concentrating, forgetting what was learned recently, forgetting where things are located, difficulty finding the right word to say, difficulty understanding what others are saying, getting lost in previously familiar places, or difficulty with calculations. Specific features and the time course of the difficulties are diagnostically relevant and indicate which cognitive domains should be explored in detail in the examination. A history of head trauma, meningitis, encephalitis, seizure

Supported in part by the National Institute of Mental Health (No. MH00910) and the Department of Veterans Affairs.

disorder, psychiatric symptoms, neurological symptoms, or substance abuse should be identified.

Because memory or language impairment may interfere with the patient's ability to provide an accurate history, collateral information from a family member or close friend is useful. Family members may feel uncomfortable discussing difficulties with the patient present; if so, a separate interview should be conducted. The patient's age, educational background, cultural background, occupation, and handedness should be noted, as these factors affect the interpretation of cognitive performance.

Examination Technique

The scope of mental status evaluation depends on the clinical circumstances. All patients with suspected neuropsychiatric illness require at least a screen for competence in each cognitive domain. In some cases, the history of symptoms or results of a screening evaluation point toward a cognitive area that needs to be investigated in detail and may warrant formal neuropsychological assessment. The clinical mental status examination offers the opportunity to vary the length or focus of the examination depending on clinical circumstances. The examiner develops and tests hypotheses during the course of the examination, beginning with observations of behavior and language during the history. Throughout the examination, the *kind* of errors that occur are as important as the *presence* of errors.

A patient may become anxious or defensive during the evaluation. Briefly describing the purpose and content of the examination at the beginning usually helps reduce anxiety. The patient should be reminded that "some of these questions may seem relatively easy and others may be very difficult." The evaluation is not an interrogation; an empathic approach improves the interpersonal quality of the interview and increases the reliability of the assessment.

The principal cognitive domains to be assessed are listed in Table 6–1. These are not hierarchical, but competence in some domains is required for adequate performance in others. Adequate attention (arousal and concentration) is required for optimal performance of all other cognitive tasks. A patient who is stuporous or markedly distractible will have difficulty in other areas. Some executive skills require reasonable competence in other cognitive areas because integration of several cognitive abilities (memory, language,

and visuospatial skills) is necessary. As a result of these two principles, attention is usually assessed at the beginning of the evaluation, and executive skills are often assessed at the end. The order in which other domains are assessed is less important.

Clinical Mental Status Examination

Attention

Attention is the ability to focus, sustain, and appropriately shift mental activity. Arousal and concentration both contribute to attention. *Arousal, alertness,* and *level of consciousness* are terms that describe the patient's awareness of stimuli. Level of arousal is evident during the interview and falls along a continuum from fully alert to comatose. Intermediate levels of arousal include lethargy, obtundation, and stupor (Plum and Posner 1982); these levels are defined by the amount of stimulus required to maintain an awake state. A patient with mild impairment of arousal appears drowsy or may fall asleep during the interview. Marked impairment of arousal can be monitored using the Glasgow Coma Scale (Teasdale and Jennett 1974).

Poor concentration is evident in a patient who has difficulty focusing on a conversation or task. The patient may be easily distracted by extraneous events in the room, the television, or a sound outdoors. Ability to concentrate is further assessed by asking the patient to perform tasks that require focused mental activity:

1. *Digit span.* The patient is asked to repeat a string of digits that is presented by the examiner at a rate of one digit per second. A string of 3 digits is initially

Table 6–1. The principal cognitive domains of the mental status examination

Attention	Visuospatial skills
Arousal	Calculation
Concentration	Praxis
Memory	Executive skills
Learning	Drive
Recall	Programming
Recognition	Response Control
Language	Synthesis
Spontaneous speech; fluency	
Comprehension	
Repetition	
Naming	

presented, followed by a string of 4 digits, then 5 digits, and so on. Normal performance is correctly repeating a string of at least 5 digits.

2. *Reverse digit span.* The examiner presents a string of digits, and the patient is asked to repeat the string in reverse order. Normal aging is associated with a decline in the ability to perform reverse digit span, but forward digit span is usually relatively unaffected by age (Lezak 1983). Older patients can normally reverse a string of at least 3 digits.

3. *Reverse sequences.* The patient is asked to state the days of the week, or months of the year, in reverse order (e.g., "December, November, October, . . .").

4. *Serial 7s.* The patient is asked to subtract 7 from 100, and to continue subtracting 7 from the result. Arithmetic skills are a prerequisite for accurate performance, and the patient's educational background and lifelong occupation often provide clues to the expected level of performance.

5. *Continuous performance.* The patient is asked to tap the table "each time you hear the letter *A*." The examiner then presents a string of random letters that contains embedded *A*'s. Letters are presented one per second and the task continues for at least 30 seconds. Errors of omission (not tapping for an *A*) and errors of commission (tapping for a letter other than *A*) are noted. Normally no errors occur.

Arousal is normally maintained by the reticular activating system. This system originates with cells of the pons and midbrain and projects diffusely to cortical and subcortical regions of the brain via the thalamic projection system. Concentration requires an intact reticular activating system, as well as intact cortical (particularly frontal) and limbic structures that focus and modulate attention. (Specific disorders of attention are discussed below.) Patients with impaired arousal or concentration have difficulty with other cognitive tasks because attention is required to stay awake, understand directions, and maintain the mental control required for optimal cognitive performance. Thus all cognitive deficits must be interpreted cautiously when attention is impaired. Diagnoses of dementia or amnesia cannot be reliably made when marked disturbance of arousal or concentration is present.

Memory

Although there has been increased understanding of the synaptic changes and neuroanatomic systems that

are associated with different aspects of memory function (Kupfermann 1991), specific strategies to clinically assess these neurobiological systems have remained elusive. In addition, theoretical constructs of memory function and terms used to describe the features of memory often differ among physicians and psychologists (Loring et al. 1989). For the purpose of clinical assessment, memory can be divided into the abilities to learn, retain, and recall information.

Learning and *recall* can be assessed using a word list test. In this test, a list of words is presented to the patient who is asked to immediately recall as many words as possible from the list. The process is repeated, using the same list, 3 or 4 times. This technique assesses the patient's immediate or "working" memory, which requires intact attention. Immediate recall of more words on each trial indicates that learning has occurred. Later in the mental status examination, the patient is asked to recall the word list. Patients with normal memory will recall the majority of the words. The examiner should give the patient clues for those words that are not recalled spontaneously. Clues can be either a category that contains the missed word (e.g., "an article of clothing") or a multiple choice list (e.g., "Was the word *hat, belt,* or *shoes?*"). Poor free recall of the word list and inability to recognize the words with clues indicate that the information has not been stored and retained. Poor free recall, but accurate recognition of many of the words with clues, suggests dysfunction of the memory retrieval process and indicates that some learning has occurred. Although a word list containing 3 words may suffice for cognitive screening, a list of 8–10 words can demonstrate the learning curve and provides a more sensitive and specific test of learning and recall. *Orientation* questions also assess memory function. Accurately stating the current date and location indicates that new information is being learned and recalled.

Learning requires the integrity of limbic structures: the medial temporal lobes, the fornix, the dorsomedial thalamic nuclei, and the mammillary bodies (Squire 1987). Severe memory impairment is usually a result of bilateral or midline brain dysfunction; unilateral brain dysfunction (usually a medial temporal lobe lesion) may cause mild memory impairment. Preferential impairment of verbal memory occurs with left-hemisphere dysfunction, whereas impairment in visuospatial memory often occurs with right-hemisphere dysfunction (Signoret 1985). Verbal memory is assessed with the word list test. Visuospatial memory can be assessed by asking the patient to reproduce drawings, either immediately after a brief presentation ("working" memory) or later in the examination (retention and recall). Alternatively, visuospatial memory can be assessed by asking the patient to locate objects that were hidden in the room while the patient observed. Ability to *retrieve* previously learned information may be mildly reduced in association with normal aging or more dramatically reduced in patients with frontal-subcortical systems dysfunction.

Tests of *remote memory* assess the ability to recall information that was learned in the distant past. Accurate remote memory requires the integrity of diffuse cortical systems that are required for storage and recall of data. Patients with limbic dysfunction who are unable to learn new information (as in Korsakoff's syndrome or after head trauma or herpes encephalitis) may be able to recall information that was learned prior to limbic disturbance. Remote memory is assessed by asking the patient to recall historical data: birthplace, family birth dates, work history, past presidents, or details of important historic events. For reliable assessment, the correct information must be known by the examiner and must have clearly been learned in the past by the patient. Therefore, it is helpful to validate remote memory loss with collateral sources.

Language

Language skills are essential for human communication. In the mental status examination, language competence also contributes to accurate performance in other cognitive domains, as the majority of information required for normal cognitive functioning is verbally mediated. Right- or left-handedness must be noted in the examination because handedness predicts the hemisphere that is dominant for language. Knowledge of hemispheric dominance allows neuroanatomic localization of lesions that cause language disturbance. Nearly all right-handed individuals and the majority of left-handed people are left-hemisphere dominant for language. Some left-handed individuals, particularly those with a strong family history of left-handedness, have language function distributed across both hemispheres.

Language assessment explores four principal areas: spontaneous speech, comprehension, repetition, and naming. *Spontaneous speech* is evaluated during the clinical interview by listening to the linguistic

features of the patient's discourse. Dysarthria, a motor disorder of speech, is distinguished from aphasia, a disorder of language. Two categories of aphasia are considered. In fluent aphasia, spontaneous output is generally effortless, with normal or increased word output, normal melody and inflection (prosody), and normal phrase length. Paraphasias, or intrusions of incorrect words or phonemes, may occur (e.g., "I was *leading* the newspaper"). The information content, or "efficiency" of language, is often reduced: long sentences may contain many grammatical connecting words, nonspecific nouns ("thing," "the other one"), and limited meaning. Nonfluent aphasia, in contrast, is characterized by effortful but reduced word output, short phrase length, and dysprosody. Dysarthria is often present, and sentences efficiently convey meaning with few words; grammar and syntax are usually abnormal. Fluent aphasia occurs with lesions of the posterior left hemisphere; nonfluent aphasia occurs with lesions of the left frontal cortex or underlying white matter.

Comprehension is assessed by asking the patient to

1. *Follow simple commands.* Single-step or multiple-step commands are given, such as "Point to your nose" or "Point to the window, then to the floor, and then to the chair."
2. *Follow commands, using objects.* Several items are placed on the table (e.g., a pen, a key, a paper clip, and a nickel). The patient is asked to follow instructions, such as "Touch the pen, then pick up the paper clip" or "With the key, touch the nickel, then point to the floor."
3. *Answer yes-or-no questions.* These might include "Does a rock float on water?" or "Do you put your shoes on before your socks?"

Reading comprehension can be assessed by presenting similar commands and questions to the patient in writing. Reduced hearing in elderly patients can contribute to impaired performance of spoken commands. Language comprehension is impaired with dysfunction of the left posterior temporal or parieto-temporal cortex.

Repetition is assessed by asking the patient to repeat sentences of increasing length and linguistic complexity. Abnormal repetition occurs with disruption of peri-Sylvian structures of the left hemisphere.

Naming ability can be assessed in the course of spontaneous speech; word-finding difficulty may be evidence of a naming disturbance. Naming is further assessed by asking the patient to name objects or parts of the body. Both high-frequency names (elbow, nose, shoe, watch, and pen) and low-frequency names (eyebrow, earlobe, sole of the shoe, and watch crystal) are tested. Poor naming may result from focal brain lesions (usually the left inferior parietal lobule) or with diffuse hemispheric dysfunction. Other tasks, such as verbal fluency (asking the patient to name as many animals as possible in 1 minute), reading skills, or writing ability can help identify specific aphasic disorders and can provide additional information on regional brain function (Strub and Black 1985). The syndromes of aphasia are discussed later in this chapter.

Visuospatial Skills

Visuospatial impairment is one of the most sensitive indicators of brain dysfunction. Patients with mild delirium or with posterior brain lesions that are otherwise neurologically silent may have marked visuospatial deficits. In contrast, patients with primary psychiatric illness usually have minimal difficulty with visuospatial tasks.

Visuospatial skills include visually guided attention, perception, use of internal visual images, visuospatial memory, and constructional abilities. The history can reveal important indications of visuospatial impairment: getting lost in previously familiar environments, difficulty estimating distance, or difficulty orienting objects to perform a task. Visuospatial skills can be clinically assessed by asking the patient to copy drawings provided by the examiner and by asking the patient to spontaneously draw a clock face, a house, or a person. Drawings to be copied should include a simple geometric shape, a design that is not easily verbally described, and a more complex drawing that has three-dimensional perspective (Figure 6–1). The patient's drawings may reveal a variety of visuospatial errors: poor use of the space available to draw, hemineglect, unusual drawing strategy (focusing on detail while missing overall layout), overlapping or "closing in" on the stimulus drawing, loss of details, loss of three-dimensionality, scattering parts of the drawing, or poor spatial relationships among elements of the drawing (reversals, rotations, and inaccurate angles). Figure 6–2 provides examples of inaccurate reproduction drawings. Visual acuity and motor skills are obviously required for accurate drawing. Complete understanding of visuospatial deficits may require formal neuropsychological assessment using standardized tests of

block design, object assembly, and line orientation.

Visuospatial impairment is more common and usually more severe among patients with a focal brain lesion in the posterior hemisphere (Black and Strub 1976). Patients with right-hemisphere lesions more often have visuospatial deficits than do those with left-hemisphere lesions. Characteristic visuoconstructive deficits that depend on the laterality of brain injury have been identified, although the specificity of these findings is limited (Benson and Barton 1970). Characteristic features of the deficits associated with lateralized lesions are shown in Table 6–2.

Among elderly patients, visuospatial disturbance is a sensitive indicator of delirium and may occur in any dementia syndrome. Patients with Alzheimer's disease typically have visuospatial impairment early in the course of illness. Visuospatial impairment may also occur with a focal brain lesion due to cortical infarction or tumor.

Calculation

Calculation skill is assessed by asking the patient to perform simple addition and multiplication (e.g., 7 + 6, 5 × 7, or 8 × 9), then more difficult arithmetic (e.g., 18 + 29, or 15 × 7) without using paper and pencil. Calculation is further assessed by asking the patient to answer arithmetic questions with paper and pencil

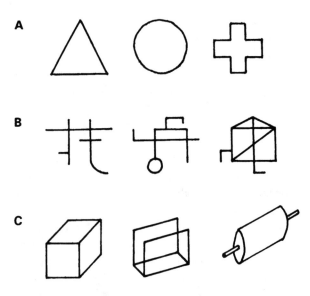

Figure 6–1. Examples of designs to be reproduced to assess visuospatial skill. *Panel A:* Simple geometric shapes. *Panel B:* Designs that are not easily verbally described. *Panel C:* Three-dimensional designs.

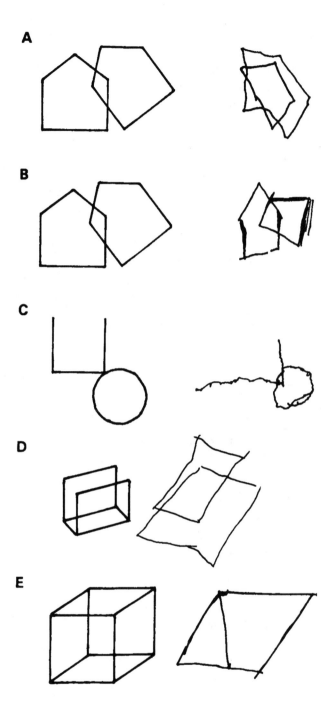

(e.g., 129 + 87 or 423 × 18). The ability to perform calculations requires attention, an understanding of mathematical operations (namely, addition, subtraction, multiplication, and division), memorized knowledge of simple sums and the "times table," and the visuospatial ability to maintain number alignment. The patient's premorbid arithmetic skills must be considered in assessing current performance.

Dyscalculia may result from a variety of neurological conditions. Patients with impaired concentration caused by metabolic or toxic disturbance usually perform poorly, as do patients with diffuse degenerative brain conditions such as Alzheimer's disease. Dyscalculia has been demonstrated in patients with focal involvement of a wide range of brain regions, although it often occurs in association with aphasia and is most common with lesions of the dominant parietal lobe (Luria 1980). Acalculia, dysgraphia, right-left disorientation, and finger agnosia may co-occur with a discrete lesion of the left angular gyrus (Gerstmann's syndrome) (Strub and Geschwind 1983).

Executive Skills

Executive skills are the mental abilities that facilitate performance of complex cognitive tasks or behaviors. Several intellectual abilities are included: recognizing patterns, developing strategies to accomplish complex tasks, adjusting strategies as needed, monitoring cognitive performance, and developing abstract formula-

Figure 6–2. Examples of inaccurate reproduction drawings. The design to be reproduced is shown on the left; the patient's reproduction is to the right. *Panel A:* Inaccurate angles and rotation of one of the pentagons; patient with delirium. *Panel B:* Inaccurate angles; patient with Alzheimer's disease. *Panel C:* Missing parts of the design and evidence of tremor; patient with Alzheimer's disease. *Panel D:* Missing parts of the design and loss of three-dimensionality; patient with vascular dementia. *Panel E:* Simplified drawing with loss of three-dimensionality; patient after resection of a left occipital astrocytoma.

Table 6–2. Visuoconstructive deficits that are characteristic of left-hemisphere versus right-hemisphere brain lesions

Left-hemisphere lesions
 Few lines in drawings
 "Simplified" drawings; lacking details
 Preserved symmetry of drawings
 Drawing is done slowly
 Drawing skill improves with practice

Right-hemisphere lesions
 Complicated structure and elaborate details
 Fragmented, disorganized drawings
 Extra lines in drawings; extraneous scribbling
 Larger drawings with poor symmetry
 Particular impairment of 3-dimensional drawings
 Left hemineglect
 "Piecemeal" approach to construction of drawings
 Drawing is done rapidly
 Drawing skill does not improve with visual cues or
  practice

tions. Executive skills are required for routine daily activities and extend beyond the elementary cognitive skills of memory, language, calculation, andvisuospatial skills.

Executive skills can be divided into 4 categories: drive, programming, response control, and synthesis (Table 6–3). These categories provide a useful framework for clinical assessment of executive function and for interpretation of executive deficits, although there is overlap among the categories, and skills within one category may facilitate performance of skills in other categories.

Drive includes the patient's initiation of cognitive activity and motivation to perform tasks. Drive is subjectively assessed during the mental status examination. Reduced drive may have a marked impact on performance in other cognitive domains.

Programming is the ability to recognize patterns and to generate motor programs to perform motor sequences. There are several strategies to assess programming skill:

1. *Rhythm tapping.* The patient is asked to reproduce a simple rhythm that the examiner taps out on the table.

Table 6–3.   Categories of executive skills

Category	Executive skills
Drive	Initiation of activity Motivation
Programming	Recognizing patterns Recognizing timing sequence Fluid output of alternating or rhythmic patterns

Response control	Divided attention
	Inhibition of incorrect responses
	Nonperseverative responses
	Cognitive speed and fluency
	Ordering the steps to accomplish a task;
	   planning
	Mental flexibility: changing strategies, as
	   required
	Freedom from environmental dependence:
	   ability to resist imitation, utilization, or
	   stimulus-bound behavior

Synthesis	Abstraction:
	   Similarities
	   Proverb interpretation
	Monitoring cognitive performance; use of
	   feedback
	Anticipation

2. *Alternating programs.* The examiner provides the patient with an alternating pattern. The patient is asked to copy the pattern and continue the pattern across the page. Examples of inability to generate or maintain a pattern are shown in Figure 6–3.

3. *Hand sequences.* The patient is asked to perform a three-step hand sequence: "slap" (palm down on the table), "fist" (hand in a fist on the table), and "cut" (side of the hand on the table) (Christensen 1975). The examiner demonstrates the sequence, then the patient makes serial attempts to produce the sequence. Normally, a subject will learn to perform the pattern smoothly after about 5 trials. If there is difficulty, the patient is encouraged to "say the words out loud as you do each step" ("slap"-"fist"-"cut"). Inability to produce smooth three-step sequences and verbal-manual dissociation (saying "fist," while doing "slap") are noted.

Response control is the ability to plan and efficiently execute a strategy to complete a complex cognitive

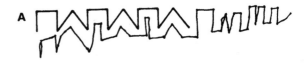

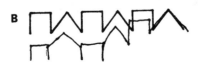

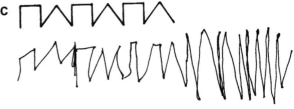

Figure 6–3.   Alternating patterns. The patient is asked to copy the pattern (shown at the top of each example) and to continue the pattern across the page. *Panel A:* The patient's drawing initially moves toward the stimulus, and the alternating pattern deteriorates as it progresses across the page. *Panel B:* The patient's drawing "closes in" on the stimulus and is not continued after the stimulus ends. The patient, with mild dementia and severe bifrontal hypoperfusion on single photon emission computed tomography (SPECT) scan, was able to understand and repeat the instructions. *Panel C:* Marked inability to maintain the alternating pattern.

task. Mental flexibility, divided attention, and a balance between autonomous thought and use of environmental cues are required for response control. Tasks that assess response control at the bedside include

1. *Flexible attention.* The patient is asked to continue the sequence, "1-A, 2-B, 3-C, . . ."
2. *Verbal fluency.* The patient is asked to name as many animals as possible in 1 minute. Alternatively, the patient is asked to name as many words as possible that begin with the letter *F.* Normal performance is at least 12 animals or 10 "F" words in 1 minute.
3. *Design fluency.* The patient is asked to create as many free-form designs as possible in 1 minute, with the constraint that each design must be novel and contain exactly four lines (Jones-Gotman and Milner 1977). Normally, at least eight unique designs are drawn. Perseveration is noted.
4. *Reciprocal programs and "go–no go."* The patient is asked to tap the table twice if the examiner taps the table once and to tap once if the examiner taps twice (reciprocal programs). The examiner then randomly taps once or twice and notes the patient's response. When this task is mastered (usually after a few presentations), the patient is told, "Now I would like to change the rule. If I tap once, you tap twice, but if I tap twice, you should not tap at all" (go–no go). The patient's ability to perform the tasks and to resist the impulse to tap is noted.
5. *Multiple loops.* The patient is asked to draw a set of loop figures with the same number of loops in each figure as drawn by the examiner. Perseveration of loop drawing is noted, as shown in Figure 6–4.
6. *Planning.* Planning ability is revealed by the patient's strategy for drawing complex figures and ability to place the numbers correctly on a clock face. Poor spacing of clock face numbers or perseveration may occur (Figure 6–5).
7. *Stimulus boundedness.* The patient is asked to draw the hands on a clock face as they would appear when the time is 11:10. The patient may be unable to resist placing the hands on the "11" and the "10" (Figure 6–6). In another task, the examiner writes the word *brown* in large black letters. The patient is asked to name the color that the word is written in. The patient may be unable to ignore the word *brown.* Stimulus boundedness may also appear in a patient's reproduction drawings with overdrawing of the stimulus figure (Figure 6–7).
8. *Imitation behavior.* The examiner rapidly flexes and

extends his or her thumb, while pointing to it with the other hand. The patient is asked, "What is this finger called?" Spontaneous movement of the patient's thumb is noted.

Synthesis is the ability to appreciate meaning, form an intellectual gestalt, and monitor cognitive performance. These skills are influenced by educational background. Clinical assessment includes evaluation of

1. *Similarities.* The patient is asked to describe how a pair of words are alike. Examples are *hat-coat, rabbit-elephant, bicycle-train,* and *watch-ruler.*
2. *Proverbs.* The patient is asked to describe the meaning of a proverb, such as "Don't change horses in the middle of a stream." The patient's appreciation of the abstract meaning is noted.
3. *Monitoring.* The patient's ability to learn from errors and to self-correct during performance of cognitive tasks is subjectively assessed during the examination.

Executive skills require the integrity of diffuse or multifocal neuronal systems. Drive, programming, and response control depend on intact function of discrete

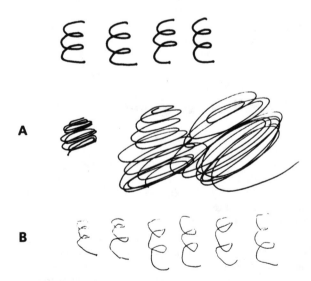

Figure 6–4. Multiple loops. The patient is asked to draw a set of loop figures that contain the same number of loops as the examples provided by the examiner (*top*). The patient, who had recently undergone resection of a left frontal astrocytoma, had great difficulty terminating each loop figure drawn with her right hand, which felt "out of control" (*panel A*). She was able to draw the correct number of loops with her left (nondominant) hand (*panel B*).

circuits that include the frontal cortex, basal ganglia, thalamus, and connecting white matter tracts (Cummings 1993). These executive skills are often impaired in patients with frontal lobe damage (Mesulam 1986;

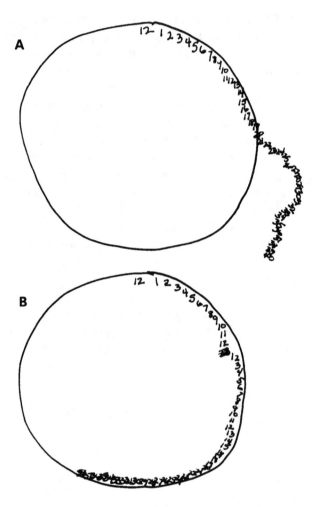

Figure 6–5. Poor planning and perseveration on the clock face drawing. The patient, with moderate subcortical dementia and parkinsonism, was asked to put all the numbers on the clock face in their appropriate places. The patient produced the drawing shown in *panel A.* The spacing between numbers is not correct for 12 evenly spaced numbers and there is perseveration of micrographic number-writing up to 40. The patient was able to correctly state that a clock has 12 numbers on it and that the *12* is at the top. When asked to redraw the 12 numbers on a clock face, he produced the drawing shown in *panel B.* Poor planning for the space between numbers and micrographia are again evident. When he reached the number *12,* he hesitated, added a *13,* crossed it out, restarted the sequence at *1,* and continued up to *38.* He was again able to state that a clock has 12 numbers on it. He was able to put all 12 numbers in correct position on a clock face (*not shown*), when the examiner dictated the numbers to him one-by-one in random order.

Shallice and Burgess 1991; Stuss and Benson 1986).

Among elderly patients, impairment of executive skills can result from a variety of conditions: toxic and/or metabolic disturbance, cerebral or systemic infection, head trauma, cerebral neoplasm, infarctions, and degenerative brain diseases such as Alzheimer's disease. Patients with schizophrenia also may exhibit deficits in executive skills (Figure 6–6). Drive, programming, and response control may be particularly impaired in older patients with dysfunction of frontal cortex, as in Pick's disease, frontal lobe degeneration, and some cases of Alzheimer's disease, or with disruption of frontal-subcortical circuits that often occurs in vascular dementia (Ishii et al. 1986). Executive deficits are associated with problem behaviors and reduced ability for self-care among elderly individuals (Royall et al. 1992).

Other Cognitive Skills

Apraxia. The term *apraxia* is used with variable meaning. Generally, it refers to the inability of a patient

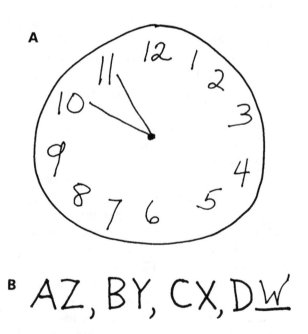

Figure 6–6. Stimulus boundedness. The patient is asked to put the hands on the clock as they would appear when the time is 11:10. *Panel A:* The hands are placed on the *11* and the *10,* as the patient is unable to resist the stimulus numbers. This example was drawn by a 73-year-old man with schizophrenia, who showed no evidence of memory, language, calculation, or visuospatial deficits. Other executive skills were intact; he was able to correctly identify the letter that follows the *D* in the sequence of letters shown in *panel B.*

with normal elementary motor function to execute the required sequence of skilled movements to complete a complex motor task (Luria 1980). In "dressing apraxia," for example, the coordinated sequence of movements required to put on clothes is disrupted: the steps are out of order, or coordinated simultaneous movements do not occur. This type of apraxia usually reflects right parietal or bilateral diffuse brain dysfunction.

In ideomotor apraxia, the patient is unable to pantomime a motor task on command that can be performed spontaneously (Geschwind 1975). Ideomotor apraxia is identified by asking the patient to briefly pantomime a motor skill that involves muscle groups of the face, trunk, or limbs. Examples include, "Show me how you blow out a match, . . . suck through a straw, . . . hold a baseball bat, . . . wave goodbye, . . . [or] brush your teeth." Ideomotor apraxia is an inability to smoothly perform the movement altogether or the substitution of a part of the body for the imitated object (e.g., substituting a finger for the toothbrush). Ideomotor apraxia reflects left-hemisphere dysfunction or lesion of the anterior corpus callosum.

Agnosia. Patients with agnosia have intact primary sensory skills and normal perception, but lack the ability to recognize or associate meaning to the sensory perception. In visual agnosia, the patient can "see" the outline, color, and lighting of an object, but is unable to recognize what the object is or what it is used for (Benson and Greenberg 1969). Visual agnosia occurs with bilateral lesions of visual association cortex. Patients with prosopagnosia have normal visual percep-

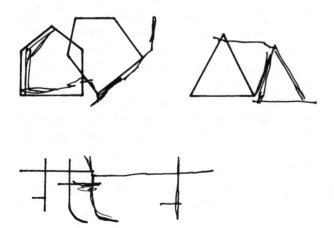

Figure 6–7. Stimulus boundedness in reproduction drawings. In each example, the patient correctly begins the drawing in the space next to the stimulus, but the drawing then "closes in" and overlaps the stimulus.

tion and do not have visual agnosia, except for impaired recognition of familiar faces. In environmental agnosia, the patient can describe details of a familiar environment, but the scene lacks any sense of familiarity (Landis et al. 1986). In astereognosis, the patient with normal somatosensory perception is unable to recognize an object by tactile exploration with eyes closed (Adams and Victor 1985). Agnosia in an elderly patient is usually caused by a discrete cortical infarction.

Right-left disorientation. Ability to distinguish right from left is tested by asking the patient to identify body parts on the left and right side of the examiner's body (e.g., "Point to my right thumb" or "Point to my left wrist"). This is performed with the examiner's arms in the usual position and with the examiner's arms crossed. Acquired right-left disorientation occurs as a result of aphasia, diffuse brain dysfunction, or a focal lesion of the dominant angular gyrus.

Syndromes of Cognitive Impairment

Disorders of Attention

Abnormal attention is the hallmark of delirium, or acute confusional state, which is one of the most common causes of behavioral disturbance among hospitalized elderly patients (see Chapter 19). Poor attention is also an important clinical feature that distinguishes delirium from dementia (see Chapters 20 and 21).

Reduced *arousal* occurs on a spectrum: drowsiness, obtundation, stupor, or coma. These states occur with impairment of the reticular activating system or widespread cortical dysfunction. Conditions that cause reduced arousal in older patients include brain stem infarction or compression, metabolic disturbances, drug intoxication, bilateral cortical infarction, brain infection, and head trauma. Increased arousal with anxiety, hypervigilance, and signs of autonomic activation can occur with drug intoxication (stimulants), drug withdrawal (alcohol, benzodiazepine, opioid, or barbiturate), or metabolic disturbances.

Akinetic mutism and *catatonia* resemble the syndrome of reduced arousal. Patients with akinetic mutism appear alert and may follow stimuli with their eyes. However, spontaneous movement and speech are rare and tend to occur in brief episodes in response to vigorous stimulation (Benson 1990; Plum and Posner 1982). Akinetic mutism is caused by lesions of the midbrain, bilateral cingulate gyri, or septal area. Patients with catatonia can present with a variety of motor signs and alterations of attention, including reduced response to stimuli, mutism, posturing, waxy flexibility, and repetitive stereotypic movements (Taylor 1990). Catatonia may occur in patients with schizophrenia, mood disorders, diffuse neurological illness, or metabolic disorders. Focal brain dysfunction can also result in catatonia; lesions of the frontal lobes or subcortical structures are most often implicated.

Unilateral *neglect* is a syndrome of inattention to half the body or half the external space. In sensory neglect, sensory input from one hemispace is neglected or extinguished. Sensory neglect may occur in a single sensory modality (e.g., somatosensory or visual) or may be multimodal. In motor neglect, movement in or toward one hemispace is reduced. Neglect of the left hemispace occurs more frequently than does neglect of the right hemispace, and the extent of neglect does not depend on the extent of primary sensory or motor impairment. With either sensory or motor neglect, the patient is strikingly unaware of the neglected halfspace. Sensory neglect usually occurs with right parietal dysfunction, and motor neglect may occur with frontal lesions, although the neuroanatomic specificity of the sensory versus motor components of neglect syndromes is limited (Mesulam 1985).

Patients with normal arousal, but poor *concentration,* appear awake and alert but are easily distracted and have difficulty focusing on cognitive tasks. Poor concentration can result from dysfunction of the brain stem, midbrain, limbic system, or diffuse cortical systems that modulate and focus mental activity. Poor concentration can occur with metabolic, toxic, or infectious conditions that affect brain function diffusely or with bilateral cortical lesions as in head trauma or bilateral infarction. Prefrontal cortex appears to play an important role in modulating concentration (Knight 1991). Older patients with primary psychiatric disorders such as schizophrenia, mania, major depression, and dissociative states may also have reduced ability to concentrate.

Memory Disorders

Amnesia is the inability to learn new information. Patients with amnesia are often able to recall information that was learned before the onset of the memory disorder. Anterograde amnesia is the lack of ability to learn during a period that begins at the time of cerebral insult and extends forward in time. Retrograde amnesia is the lack of recall for events that occurred during the recent period before the cerebral insult. Amnesia occurs with bilateral damage to the medial temporal lobes or midline limbic structures. Conditions that cause amnesia in elderly people include dementia, head trauma, posterior cerebral artery occlusion, anoxia, neoplasms involving midline limbic structures, herpes encephalitis, and Korsakoff's syndrome. Anterograde amnesia may improve over time, and there may be concomitant shrinkage of the period of retrograde amnesia.

Age-associated memory impairment is the term applied to subtle alterations in recent memory that occur with normal aging (see Chapter 8). Elderly people often describe a subjective sense of reduced memory, may require more trials to learn a list of words, and may be less efficient in memory retrieval.

Memory impairment occurs in concert with other cognitive deficits in patients with dementia. Patients with Alzheimer's disease have difficulty learning new information (anterograde amnesia), as well as difficulty recalling information that was learned before onset of the dementia. The recall deficit is due to widespread impairment of diffuse cortical systems that are required for continued storage and recall of memory and may be mild in the early stage of illness. In Pick's disease, memory impairment often occurs after the onset of behavioral changes, whereas in Alzheimer's disease memory impairment is often the first indication of illness. In subcortical dementias, such as those associated with Parkinson's disease or Huntington's disease, memory impairment usually occurs early in the course of dementia, as in Alzheimer's disease. However, the memory impairment of subcortical dementia is characterized by improvement in recall when clues are given, spared recognition memory, and relatively spared declarative memory (facts or knowledge) compared with procedural memory (acquisition of motor skills or cognitive strategies) (Huber and Shuttleworth 1990). The memory impairment of patients with Alzheimer's disease does not robustly improve when clues are given, and deficits in declarative memory are greater than deficits in procedural memory (Cummings and Benson 1992).

Aphasia

Syndromes of aphasia are distinguished by the pattern of specific language skills that are impaired: fluency, comprehension, repetition, or naming (Cummings 1985; Goodglass and Kaplan 1983). The principal aphasia syndromes, the specific language skills that are impaired in each syndrome, and the region of the brain involved are shown in Table 6–4. Disorders of language provide relatively sensitive and specific indications of regional brain dysfunction.

Among elderly patients with language impairment and no other cognitive deficits, the aphasia syndromes usually occur as a result of infarction, hemorrhage, or tumor that affects the brain regions identified in Table 6–4. Occlusion of the left-middle cerebral artery causes global aphasia and right hemiparesis, if the occlusion disrupts perfusion of a wide area of the left hemisphere. If the occlusion is more distal, Broca's aphasia, conduction aphasia, or Wernicke's aphasia may occur, depending on the vascular territory that is compromised. Border zone infarctions, caused by anoxia, hypotension, or carotid stenosis, affect the watershed regions between the vascular territories served by the anterior, middle, and posterior cerebral arteries and produce transcortical motor or transcortical sensory aphasia.

Elderly patients with dementia often have aphasia along with other cognitive deficits. The involvement of specific language skills depends on the regional distribution of brain lesions that cause the dementia. In Alzheimer's disease, a characteristic pattern of language disturbance occurs. Very early in the illness, word-finding difficulty and "empty speech" (language output that contains little information) are common.

Subsequently, naming difficulty, mild comprehension deficit, and reduced fluency (e.g., animals per minute) occur. Paraphasias may be apparent in spontaneous speech. Elements of transcortical sensory aphasia are present during the course of Alzheimer's disease, reflecting the prominence of the neuropathological changes of Alzheimer's disease in the inferior parietal lobe.

In vascular dementia, speech abnormalities are more common than in Alzheimer's disease (Sultzer et al. 1993). Language disturbance also occurs; the characteristics of language impairment depend on the brain regions affected by cerebrovascular disease. In general, patients with vascular dementia are more likely than Alzheimer patients to have nonfluent aphasia and are less likely to have naming impairments (Cummings and Mahler 1991). Marked impairment of language does not occur in patients with dementia associated with subcortical extrapyramidal disorders (Huber and Shuttleworth 1990).

Frontal Lobe Disorders

The frontal lobe disorders are particularly important in neuropsychiatric evaluation because the brain lesions that are responsible are often not detected by the traditional neurological examination and the psychiatric symptoms that occur do not usually fit the characteristic pattern of common psychiatric disorders. The neuropsychiatric symptoms that occur in each of the three principal syndromes of frontal lobe impairment

Table 6–4. The principal syndromes of aphasia

| Aphasia syndrome | Language skills | | | | Regional brain dysfunction[a] |
	Fluency	Comprehension	Repetition	Naming	
Broca's	Nonfluent	Intact	Impaired	Impaired	Left frontal operculum, left insular cortex, and adjacent white matter
Transcortical motor	Nonfluent	Intact	Intact	Impaired	Left supplementary motor area
Global	Nonfluent	Impaired	Impaired	Impaired	Wide area of left-hemisphere convexity
Wernicke's	Fluent	Impaired	Impaired	Impaired	Posterior, superior left temporal lobe; left inferior parietal lobe may also be involved
Transcortical sensory	Fluent	Impaired	Intact	Impaired	Left inferior parietal lobule
Conduction	Fluent	Intact	Impaired	Impaired	Left arcuate fasciculus (usually in the the left parietal operculum) or left insula and adjacent white matter
Anomic	Fluent	Intact	Intact	Impaired	Left angular gyrus or left posterior middle temporal gyrus

[a]In patients with left-hemisphere dominance for language.

are shown in Table 6–5. Each syndrome is associated with dysfunction of a particular region of the frontal lobe, its connections with other cortical centers, or connections with subcortical nuclei. The relationship between anatomy and symptomatology is incomplete: patients with extensive frontal dysfunction may not manifest the full spectrum of "frontal" symptoms, and these symptoms may occur following lesions outside the frontal circuits.

The *medial frontal syndrome* is primarily a disturbance of drive and motivation and includes a spectrum of symptoms from mild disinterest to akinetic mutism (Stuss and Benson 1986). Apathy, aspontaneity, reduced verbal output, and reduced spontaneous movement may occur. The syndrome occurs with lesions of the anterior cingulate gyrus, white matter tracts that connect this region to the ventral striatum, or medial dorsal thalamus. More severe symptoms usually occur with bilateral lesions. Conditions that cause the medial frontal syndrome in the elderly include anterior cerebral artery occlusion, thalamic infarction, hydrocephalus, or tumors of the diencephalon or third ventricle.

Lesions of the *dorsolateral frontal convexity* produce a syndrome of impaired motor programing and reduced cognitive flexibility. Deficits that appear on the mental status examination include perseveration (e.g., extra loops on the multiple loops and intrusion of a prior response in a new task), difficulty with alternating programs or changing mental set, or reduced verbal or design fluency. Dorsolateral frontal convexity insults include head trauma, frontal infarction, frontal lobe tumor, and degenerative dementias. Lesion of the dorsolateral caudate nucleus may produce a similar pattern of executive deficits.

The *orbitofrontal syndrome* occurs with lesions of the inferior aspect of the frontal lobe. This region of the frontal lobe is intimately associated with the limbic system, and dysfunction often appears as a striking change of personality (Fuster 1989). Disinhibition is common and patients may show a marked inability to conform behavior to social customs. Mood is often expansive or irritable, affect is labile, and there may be impulsive outbursts of jocularity. When lesions are confined to the orbitofrontal cortex, there may be no formal neurological deficits and no other cognitive deficits. Orbitofrontal damage occurs with head trauma, inferior frontal meningiomas, rupture of anterior cerebral artery aneurysms, and frontal dementias such as frontal lobe degeneration and Pick's disease.

Rating Scales for Cognitive Assessment

Rating scales can be used to screen for cognitive impairment or to quantify the results of a thorough mental status examination. Measurement of cognitive deficits permits the clinician to identify changes over time or to determine the response to therapeutic intervention. In addition, structured assessment facilitates reliable communication of cognitive skills among clinicians.

Many different rating scales are available and reviews of their use have been published (Kluger and Ferris 1991; Raskin and Niederehe 1988; Schmitt et al. 1989; Siu 1991). Rating scales differ in the time required for administration and the spectrum of symptoms assessed (cognition, cognition and functional skills, or cognition and psychiatric symptoms). Some scales are screening instruments, whereas others are more comprehensive. Further, some scales provide subscores for individual cognitive domains, whereas others generate only an overall score. Each rating scale accomplishes a different clinical goal:

1. The Mini-Mental State Exam (Folstein et al. 1975), a 30-item instrument that is widely used to screen for cognitive impairment and to assess the severity

Table 6–5. Neuropsychiatric symptoms that occur with lesions of the frontal lobe or related subcortical structure

Lesion site	Symptoms
Medial frontal	Apathy
	Aspontaneity
	Low motivation
	Motor retardation
	Reduced verbal output
	Akinetic mutism
Dorsolateral frontal convexity	Perseveration
	Motor impersistence
	Reduced verbal or design fluency
	Impaired motor programming
	Inability to change rules
Orbitofrontal	Disinhibition
	Failure to appreciate social customs
	Childlike jocularity
	Labile affect
	Expansive mood
	Irritability
	Lack of empathy

of impairment. The examination takes about 10 minutes and provides a reliable overall cognitive score. Sensitivity for mild impairment is limited (Tombaugh and McIntyre 1992).

2. The Short Portable Mental Status Questionnaire (Pfeiffer 1975), a very brief screening instrument. The 10 items assess orientation, concentration, and remote memory. Reliability and validity have been shown to be acceptable, although mild impairment may not be detected.

3. The Mattis Dementia Rating Scale (Mattis 1976), which assesses a wider range of cognitive skills: attention, memory, visuospatial skills, and executive abilities. The instrument requires about 30–45 minutes to complete with an impaired patient. It provides an overall cognitive score, with a maximum of 144 points.

4. The Neurobehavioral Cognitive Status Examination (Kiernan et al. 1987), which assesses attention, memory, calculation, visuoconstructive skills, language, and abstraction. A subscore for each of these cognitive domains is generated. The examination requires specific testing materials and takes about 20 minutes to complete with an impaired patient.

5. The Neurobehavioral Rating Scale (Levin et al. 1987), a 27-item instrument that measures psychiatric and behavioral disturbances, in addition to cognitive impairment. The evaluation takes about 40 minutes to complete. The instrument provides six factor scores that measure the cognitive and noncognitive symptoms in patients with dementia (Sultzer et al. 1992).

6. The Global Deterioration Scale (Reisberg et al. 1988), a 7-point scale that measures the overall severity of dementia. Cognitive deficits, psychiatric symptoms, and functional impairment are all considered by the clinician to determine the global severity score.

Functional Assessment

The ability to accomplish functional activities at home is important information that complements the assessment of cognitive skills in the mental status examination. Reduced functional skills can be a sensitive indicator of dementia (Barberger-Gateau et al. 1992). Functional assessment also reveals the impact of medical problems and cognitive deficits on living skills and indicates the need for assistance with activities, which are both of importance to the patient and family.

At least a brief review of functional skills should be included in the assessment of each geriatric patient, and whether the patient currently drives a car should be noted. Two groups of activities are considered in functional assessment: physical activities of daily living (ADLs) and instrumental activities of daily living (IADLs) (Lawton and Brody 1969). Physical ADLs include the basic skills required for self-maintenance: dressing, bathing, toileting, transferring, and feeding. IADLs include more complex skills required for independent living: shopping, cooking, housekeeping, laundry, using the telephone, using transportation, managing money, and managing medications. An observer determines whether the patient is independently able to perform each of these activities. Rating scales can be used to improve the reliability of functional assessment (Lawton 1988).

Summary

Mental status examination is a fundamental part of the neuropsychiatric assessment of elderly patients. The examination focuses on cognitive abilities, which include perception, "thinking," intellect, and problem-solving skills. Several cognitive domains are explored: attention, memory, language, visuospatial skills, calculation, praxis, and executive skills. Deficits in these domains reveal dysfunction of specific neuroanatomic structures or dysfunction of neural systems that integrate functionally related brain regions. In addition, the pattern of particular deficits is used to identify syndromes of cognitive impairment, such as delirium, other disorders of attention, dementia, aphasia, amnesia, and frontal lobe disorders. The results of the mental status examination can also reveal the contribution of regional brain dysfunction to the expression of psychiatric symptoms in elderly patients.

The scope of cognitive assessment depends on the particular clinical circumstances and the goals of the evaluation; at least a screening evaluation is recommended for all geriatric patients. Rating scales can be used to help screen for cognitive impairment or to quantify the extent of impairment in patients with known deficits. Assessment of functional skills provides additional evidence of cognitive ability and helps identify those clinical features that deserve particular attention in the treatment plan.

References

Adams RD, Victor M: Principles of Neurology, 3rd Edition. New York, McGraw-Hill, 1985

Barberger-Gateau P, Commenges D, Gagnon M, et al: Instrumental activities of daily living as a screening tool for cognitive impairment and dementia in elderly community dwellers. J Am Geriatr Soc 40:1129–1134, 1992

Benson DF: Psychomotor retardation. Neuropsychiatry, Neuropsychology, and Behavioral Neurology 3:36–47, 1990

Benson DF, Barton MI: Disturbances in constructional ability. Cortex 6:19–46, 1970

Benson DF, Greenberg JP: Visual form agnosia. Arch Neurol 20:82–89, 1969

Black FW, Strub RL: Constructional apraxia in patients with discrete missile wounds of the brain. Cortex 12:212–220, 1976

Christensen A-L: Luria's Neuropsychological Investigation: Text. New York, Spectrum, 1975

Cummings JL: Clinical Neuropsychiatry. New York, Grune & Stratton, 1985

Cummings JL: Frontal-subcortical circuits and human behavior. Arch Neurol 50:873–880, 1993

Cummings JL, Benson DF: Dementia: A Clinical Approach, 2nd Edition. Boston, MA, Butterworth-Heinemann, 1992

Cummings JL, Mahler ME: Cerebrovascular dementia, in Neurobehavioral Aspects of Cerebrovascular Disease. Edited by Bornstein RA, Brown GG. New York, Oxford University Press, 1991, pp 131–149

Folstein M, Folstein S, McHugh P: "Mini-Mental State": a practical method for grading the cognitive state of patients for the clinician. J Psychiatr Res 12:189–198, 1975

Fuster JM: The Prefrontal Cortex: Anatomy, Physiology, and Neuropsychology of the Frontal Lobe, 2nd Edition. New York, Raven, 1989

Geschwind N: The apraxias: neural mechanisms of disorders of learned movement. American Scientist 63:188–195, 1975

Goodglass H, Kaplan E: The Assessment of Aphasia and Related Disorders, 2nd Edition. Philadelphia, PA, Lea & Febiger, 1983

Huber SJ, Shuttleworth EC: Neuropsychological assessment of subcortical dementia, in Subcortical Dementia. Edited by Cummings JL. New York, Oxford University Press, 1990, pp 71–86

Ishii N, Nishihara Y, Imamura T: Why do frontal lobe symptoms predominate in vascular dementia with lacunes? Neurology 36:340–345, 1986

Jones-Gotman M, Milner B: Design fluency: the invention of nonsense drawings after focal cortical lesions. Neuropsychologia 15:653–674, 1977

Kallman H, May HJ: Mental status assessment in the elderly. Prim Care 16:329–347, 1989

Kiernan RJ, Mueller J, Langston JW, et al: The Neurobehavioral Cognitive Status Examination: a brief but differentiated approach to cognitive assessment. Ann Intern Med 107:481–485, 1987

Kluger A, Ferris SH: Scales for the assessment of Alzheimer's disease. Psychiatr Clin North Am 14:309–326, 1991

Knight RT: Evoked potential studies of attention capacity in human frontal lobe lesions, in Frontal Lobe Function and Dysfunction. Edited by Levin HS, Eisenberg HM, Benton AL. New York, Oxford University Press, 1991, pp 139–153

Kupfermann I: Learning and memory, in Principles of Neural Science, 3rd Edition. Edited by Kandel ER, Schwartz JH, Jessell TM. New York, Elsevier, 1991, pp 997–1008

Landis T, Cummings JL, Benson DF, et al: Loss of topographic familiarity: an environmental agnosia. Arch Neurol 43:132–136, 1986

Larson EB, Reifler BV, Featherstone HJ, et al: Dementia in elderly outpatients: a prospective study. Ann Intern Med 100:417–423, 1984

Lawton MP: Scales to measure competence in everyday activities. Psychopharmacol Bull 24:609–614, 1988

Lawton MP, Brody EM: Assessment of older people: self-maintaining and instrumental activities of daily living. Gerontologist 9:179–186, 1969

Levin HS, High WM, Goethe KE, et al: The Neurobehavioral Rating Scale: assessment of the behavioral sequelae of head injury by the clinician. J Neurol Neurosurg Psychiatry 50:183–193, 1987

Lezak MD: Intellectual ability tests, I: the Wechsler Intelligence Scales, in Neuropsychological Assessment, 2nd Edition. New York, Oxford University Press, 1983, pp 239–286

Loring DW, Lee GP, Meador KJ: Issues in memory assessment of the elderly. Clin Geriatr Med 5:565–581, 1989

Luria AR: Higher Cortical Functions in Man, 2nd Edition. New York, Basic Books, 1980

Mattis S: Mental status examination for organic mental syndrome in the elderly patient, in Geriatric Psychiatry. Edited by Bellak R, Karasu TE. New York, Grune & Stratton, 1976, pp 77–121

Mesulam M-M: Attention, confusional states, and neglect, in Principles of Behavioral Neurology. Edited by Mesulam M-M. Philadelphia, PA, FA Davis, 1985, pp 125–168

Mesulam M-M: Frontal cortex and behavior (editorial). Ann Neurol 19:320–325, 1986

Pfeiffer E: A short portable mental status questionnaire for the assessment of organic brain deficit in elderly patients. J Am Geriatr Soc 23:433–441, 1975

Plum F, Posner JB: The Diagnosis of Stupor and Coma, 3rd Edition. Philadelphia, PA, FA Davis, 1982

Raskin A, Niederehe G (eds): Assessment in diagnosis and treatment of geropsychiatric patients. Psychopharmacol Bull 24:501–510, 1988

Reisberg B, Ferris SH, de Leon MJ, et al: Global deterioration scale. Psychopharmacol Bull 24:661–663, 1988

Royall DR, Mahurin RK, Gray KF: Bedside assessment of executive cognitive impairment: the executive interview. J Am Geriatr Soc 40:1221–1226, 1992

Schmitt FA, Ranseen JD, DeKosky ST: Cognitive mental status examinations. Clin Geriatr Med 5:545–564, 1989

Shallice T, Burgess P: Higher-order cognitive impairments and frontal lobe lesions in man, in Frontal Lobe Function and Dysfunction. Edited by Levin HS, Eisenberg HM, Benton AL. New York, Oxford University Press, 1991, pp 125–138

Signoret J-L: Memory and amnesias, in Principles of Behavioral Neurology. Edited by Mesulam M-M. Philadelphia, PA, FA Davis, 1985, pp 169–192

Siu AL: Screening for dementia and investigating its causes. Ann Intern Med 115:122–132, 1991

Squire LR: Memory and Brain. New York, Oxford University Press, 1987

Strub RL, Black FW: The Mental Status Examination in Neurology, 2nd Edition. Philadelphia, PA, FA Davis, 1985

Strub RL, Geschwind N: Localization in Gerstmann syndrome, in Localization in Neuropsychology. Edited by Kertesz A. New York, Academic Press, 1983, pp 295–321

Stuss DT, Benson DF: The Frontal Lobes. New York, Raven, 1986

Sultzer DL, Levin HS, Mahler ME, et al: Assessment of cognitive, psychiatric, and behavioral disturbances in patients with dementia: the Neurobehavioral Rating Scale. J Am Geriatr Soc 40:549–555, 1992

Sultzer DL, Levin HS, Mahler ME, et al: A comparison of psychiatric symptoms in vascular dementia and Alzheimer's disease. Am J Psychiatry 150:1806–1812, 1993

Taylor MA: Catatonia: a review of a behavioral neurologic syndrome. Neuropsychiatry, Neuropsychology, and Behavioral Neurology 3:48–72, 1990

Teasdale G, Jennett B: Assessment of coma and impaired consciousness: a practical scale. Lancet 2:81–84, 1974

Tombaugh TN, McIntyre NJ: The Mini-Mental State Examination: a comprehensive review. J Am Geriatr Soc 40:922–935, 1992

7

Neuropsychological Assessment

Mark R. Lovell, Ph.D.
Paul D. Nussbaum, Ph.D.

Introduction

The neuropsychological evaluation of older adults has become increasingly important over the past decade and is often a standard component of the neuropsychiatric evaluation. Neuropsychological assessment can be considered an extension and quantification of the mental status examination (see Chapter 6) and as such is focused on the psychometric assessment of cognitive processes. A thorough neuropsychological evaluation can add much to the clinical diagnostic process and can complement information gathered through physiological and anatomical imaging technologies (see Chapters 9 and 10).

In this chapter, we review the applications of neuropsychological assessment to geriatric patients and discuss relevant issues regarding the establishment of appropriate normative data bases for this population, the selection and use of neuropsychological tests, the interpretation of test results, and the use of these results in the treatment planning process. We also discuss the use of fixed neuropsychological test batteries and contrast them with more flexible approaches to assessment of elderly patients.

Goals of the Neuropsychological Evaluation

Neuropsychological test results are used in various ways depending on the training of the neuropsychologist, the setting, the referral question, and the treatment program. However, despite differing approaches to assessment, the three primary goals of neuropsychological assessment are the same: 1) to establish an individual's cognitive and behavioral strengths and weaknesses, 2) to interpret findings from a diagnostic viewpoint, and 3) to extrapolate treatment and rehabilitation recommendations from the neuropsychological assessment findings (La Rue 1992). In addition to providing specific information that may be useful in differential diagnosis and the localization of brain dysfunction, the neuropsychological evaluation is relatively unique among neurodiagnostic techniques in its ability to provide information regarding the functional capabilities of geriatric patients. This aspect of neuropsychological assessment has become increasingly important as a greater number of individuals are living well into their eighth decade and clinicians are routinely faced with decisions regarding their patients' ability to live alone, operate an automobile, and manage their financial affairs.

Methodological Issues in Geriatric Neuropsychology

The aging process is accompanied by subtle declines in specific domains of cognitive functioning (Albert 1981; Kaszniak 1987; Nussbaum, in press) with motor speed, speed of cognitive processing, and mental flexibility most affected (La Rue 1992). This decline is a function of the synergistic effects of the "normal aging process" in combination with the multitude of medical and psychosocial variables that impact elderly individuals. The concept of "normal aging," particularly as it pertains to memory decline in older adults, is an extremely important issue and is discussed more thoroughly in Chapter 8. However, a brief discussion of how this issue has affected the clinical neuropsychological evaluation of the geriatric patient is germane to the current chapter.

The clinical neuropsychological evaluation is highly dependent on appropriate comparison groups that allow the cognitive dysfunction related to pathological processes to be separated from the decline secondary to the normal aging process. The normative sample provides the basis for this comparison of individual patient performance to established standards for a given age group and is an important prerequisite to the assessment process. However, to date, the usefulness of neuropsychological testing with older adults has been limited by a relative dearth of normative data. The development of valid normative data for geriatric patients continues to be a major challenge for geriatric neuropsychology, particularly with regard to the psychometric assessment of patients over the age of 75 years. Indeed, as La Rue (1992) recently pointed out, there still are substantial limitations in age-based normative data, with limited heterogeneity of education and health variables among normative samples. Along similar lines, Kaszniak (1989) noted a lack of reliability, validity, and normative data relevant to "old-old" patient groups (i.e., those 75 or older) and stressed the importance of continued development in this area. This lack of an adequate normative base has at times fostered a reliance on norms obtained on younger subject groups—a practice that can lead to an overdiagnosis of pathological cognitive impairment in geriatric patients.

In the absence of age-appropriate and current normative data, there has also been a tendency by some clinicians to rely on data that were collected many years earlier, from samples of geriatric subjects who may have differed significantly from the individual patient whose performance is being evaluated. Given generational differences in the availability of medical treatment, education, nutrition, and a host of other factors that can influence performance on neuropsychological tests, it is indeed risky to compare the test performance of an elderly patient in the 1990s to normative data gathered during the 1970s or before. This cohort effect (Schaie and Schaie 1977) limits the usefulness of previously established normative data to current samples of patients.

Yet another methodological issue that has affected the neuropsychological evaluation of elderly patients has been differing definitions of what constitutes the expected cognitive pattern of "normal aging." For example, some researchers have distinguished between *usual aging*, in which the effects of the aging process are influenced by extrinsic factors such as nutrition and psychosocial factors, and *successful aging*, in which these factors play a neutral or positive role (Rowe and Kahn 1987). Still others have studied unusually healthy groups of geriatric subjects, documenting cognitive functioning in patients who are uncharacteristically free of the medical problems that often afflict the elderly (MacInnes et al. 1983). Obviously, the comparison of a patient's performance to norms gathered from these disparate samples could lead to markedly different conclusions regarding pathological cognitive decline in a given patient. Comparison of the typical elderly patient with norms derived from a sample of unusually healthy individuals may result in an overdiagnosis of pathological cognitive dysfunction (Albert 1981).

Despite past limitations in the development of normative data on cognitive functioning in geriatric patients, there has recently been a significant increase in the development of neuropsychological tests that provide geriatric norms. For example, the Wechsler Memory Scale–Revised (WMS-R; Wechsler 1987), and the Wechsler Adult Intelligence Scale–Revised (WAIS-R; Wechsler 1981), two of the most popular tests used by neuropsychologists, have supporting normative data through age 74. Even more recently, these norms have been augmented by data specific to the old-old population that provide information on normal subjects well into their 90s (Ivnik et al. 1992). Along similar lines, demographic corrections have been developed for the Halstead-Reitan Neuropsychological Battery (HRNB; Heaton et al. 1991). Relatively new cognitive screening instruments have also included older age normative data that permit appropriate global mental status examinations in the elderly (Osato et al. 1989).

Neuropsychological Evaluation Process

Neuropsychological assessment of older patients requires attention to at least four basic elements: 1) understanding of the neurobiology, clinical neurology, pharmacology, clinical medicine, and psychology of aging; 2) understanding of the methodological and conceptual framework unique to the experimental and clinical neuropsychology of aging; 3) knowledge of when neuropsychological assessment of an older adult is indicated; and 4) familiarity with neuropsychological assessment procedures, psychometric properties of specific tests, and age-relevant normative data (Kaszniak 1989). The evaluation typically consists of a clinical interview, selection of tests to be used in the evaluation, interpretation of test results, and specification of treatment and rehabilitation recommendations based on these results.

The primary goal of the clinical interview should be to develop hypotheses regarding the patient's overall cognitive status and his or her capacity to engage in further neuropsychological evaluation. In addition, the clinical interview provides an opportunity for the examiner to develop rapport with the patient and explain the nature of the evaluation; it permits the patient time to express his or her concerns. A thorough interview should yield relevant demographic background information (e.g., age, education, occupational history, and handedness), medical and psychiatric history (including past and present medication use), substance use or abuse, familial and developmental information, current living situation and support network, any recent losses (i.e., death of a spouse or loss of driving license), information pertaining to activity level and hobbies, motivation, and the patient's understanding of why he or she was referred for neuropsychological evaluation.

Through the clinical interview, the neuropsychologist gathers important qualitative information regarding cognitive functioning through direct interaction with the patient. This includes a general sense of the patient's orientation, level of arousal, motivation, awareness of impairment, engagement in the testing process, social appropriateness, integrity of gross language and motor function, memory capacity, and stamina. The older patient may have limitations that affect his or her performance during the neuropsychological evaluation, including reduced vision and hearing and the effects of overmedication (Goreczny and Nussbaum, in press; Russell 1984). As a result of these factors, the questions may need to repeated and presented louder and slower. In addition, the patient should be encouraged to continue working on tasks even after specified time limits have been reached. This testing-the-limits approach can help to establish the patient's capacity to perform a cognitive task when motor abnormalities (e.g., as in Parkinson's disease) and sensory deficits are taken into account.

The administration of neuropsychological tests usually begins directly after the clinical interview. Selection of tests should be based on the following four factors: 1) the referral question, 2) level of functioning of the patient as ascertained during the clinical interview, 3) hypotheses regarding the differential diagnosis, and 4) the need to document cognitive deficiencies and relative strengths. The latter point has relevance to the patient's ability to function in everyday life.

The selection of tests may differ based on individual patient needs. For example, older patients with severe cognitive or medical disturbances may lack the stamina or attentional capacity to undergo an intensive neuropsychological evaluation. For these patients, the selection of tests that tap specific domains of cognitive functioning in combination with the use of a more broad-based screening instrument may be the most useful approach. In contrast, a patient with relatively preserved cognitive abilities and without serious medical complications may be engaged in a more thorough cognitive assessment involving the in-depth assessment of multiple domains of neuropsychological functioning (Russell 1984). Regardless of the estimated level of cognitive functioning or the hypothesized nature of the cognitive impairment, we recommend the use of a brief cognitive screen as part of the interview process with the older patient. This permits not only an initial assessment of the patient's general cognitive capacity but also provides direction for the selection of instruments to be used in the neuropsychological evaluation. The use of cognitive screening instruments within the more general context of the neuropsychological evaluation also promotes the comparison of test results across different testing sessions, even when the patient

has deteriorated to a degree that precludes more comprehensive evaluation (for a discussion of representative screening instruments and rating scales, see Chapter 6).

Approaches to the Neuropsychological Evaluation of Geriatric Patients

As a discipline, clinical neuropsychology is generally concerned with the study of brain-behavior relationships. However, clinical approaches to the assessment of these relationships vary widely (Kane 1991). Currently well-accepted strategies for neuropsychological assessment include the use of fixed batteries of neuropsychological tests, flexible evaluation strategies, and use of a combination of both of these approaches. In this section, we review the application of these different approaches with adults 65 years old or older.

Fixed Test Battery Approaches

A fixed neuropsychological battery approach assumes that the same test instruments are administered to every patient in a standard manner regardless of the patient's presenting illness or referral question (Kane 1991; Kaszniak 1989). The two most popular neuropsychological batteries are currently the HRNB and the Luria-Nebraska Neuropsychological Battery (see Incagnoli et al. 1986). Advantages of the fixed battery approach to neuropsychological assessment include the fact that it provides a comprehensive assessment of multiple cognitive domains and, because of its standardized format, the test data can be incorporated into data bases for clinical and scientific analysis. Disadvantages of the fixed battery approach include time and labor intensiveness and a lack of flexibility in different clinical situations.

Use of fixed test batteries with geriatric patients.   A large literature exists on the psychometric properties of fixed batteries such as the HRNB (Anthony et al. 1980; Heaton and Pendleton 1981; Kane 1991; Parsons 1986; Reitan 1976; Reitan and Davison 1974; Reitan and Wolfson 1985) and the Luria-Nebraska Neuropsychological Battery (Golden and Maruish 1986; Golden et al. 1980; Kane 1991; Purisch and Sbordone 1986). However, there is relatively little empirical research on the psychometric properties of flexible and fixed battery approaches with the elderly population (Kaszniak 1989).

HRNB. The HRNB represents one of the most popular battery approaches to neuropsychological assessment (Table 7–1). This battery measures cognitive functioning across a number of cognitive domains, but is often too difficult for individuals with more than mild cognitive impairment. Despite its widespread use in nongeriatric patients, the use of this battery with the elderly has been criticized, and several recent studies have established age as an important moderator variable for several of the battery's subtests (Heaton et al. 1986, 1991). Indeed, in a comparison of the HRNB Impairment Index (a summary score based on seven different measures) with non-neurologically impaired young, middle-aged, and old subgroups stratified on age and education, older subjects were misclassified as having brain damage more often than the other two groups. Additionally, older patients with lower educational levels were disproportionately classified more often as having brain damage using the impairment index (Heaton et al. 1991).

The principle concerns with reliance on the HRNB in assessment of older adults are 1) the HRNB may overestimate brain damage in otherwise non-neurologically impaired older adults; 2) the HRNB is time consuming and effort demanding and may be inappropriate for elderly patients who are prone to fatigue easily; and 3) the HRNB uses subtests that measure primarily fluid abilities (i.e., novel problem-solving, reasoning, and spatial processes) known to decline with normal aging. For these reasons, some have argued against the use of the HRNB with the elderly (La Rue 1992). Despite these concerns, some subtests from the HRNB can be included with screening procedures in the initial overall assessment of the older patient's cognitive capacity. Subtests that can provide useful clinical information during an initial assessment include trail making test (parts A and B) as a measure of cognitive flexibility and attention, aphasia screening test as a gross measure of language, finger oscillation test as a measure of bilateral fine motor speed, and seashore rhythm test and speech sounds perception test as measures of verbal and nonverbal auditory attentional capacity. Additionally, efforts have been made to develop HRNB age and education corrections for older adults (see Heaton et al. 1991) and a brief form of the HRNB has been developed (Storrie and Doerr 1980). Finally, the HRNB has been found to be useful for treatment and rehabilitation planning because some of the subtests from the battery correlate with occupational, social, and independent living criteria (Heaton and Pendleton 1981).

Luria-Nebraska Neuropsychological Battery. The Luria-Nebraska Neuropsychological Battery yields a number of empirically derived summary scores (Table 7–2). This battery requires less time to administer than the HRNB (which takes 2 to 3 hours), making it more appealing for use with the geriatric population. The

Table 7–1. The Halstead-Reitan Neuropsychological Battery (HRNB) with measures of general intellect and memory

Halstead-Reitan Battery
Tactual performance test
  Total time[a]
  Localization[a]
  Memory[a]
Finger oscillation test (dominant hand)[a]
Category test[a]
Seashore rhythm test[a]
Speech sounds perception test[a]
Aphasia screening test
Sensory-perceptual examination
Strength of grip test
Tactile form recognition test

General Intelligence
Wechsler Adult Intelligence Scale–Revised

Memory
Wechsler Memory Scale–Revised

[a]These scores make up the Impairment Index.
Source. See Heaton et al. 1991.

Table 7–2. The Luria-Nebraska Neuropsychological Battery

Clinical scales	Summary scales
Scale 1 (Motor functions)	S1 (Pathognomonic)
Scale 2 (Rhythm)	S2 (Left hemisphere)
Scale 3 (Tactile functions)	S3 (Right hemisphere)
Scale 4 (Visual functions)	S4 (Profile elevation)
Scale 5 (Receptive speech)	S5 (Impairment)
Scale 6 (Expressive speech)	**Localization scales**
Scale 7 (Writing)	L1 (Left frontal)
Scale 8 (Reading)	L2 (Left sensorimotor)
Scale 9 (Arithmetic)	L3 (Left parietal-occipital)
Scale 10 (Memory)	L4 (Left temporal)
Scale 11 (Intellectual functions)	L5 (Right frontal)
Scale 12 (Intermediate memory)	L6 (Right sensorimotor)
	L7 (right parietal-occipital)
	L8 (right temporal)

Source. See Incagnoli et al. 1986.

battery also promotes an analysis of both quantitative and qualitative aspects of performance (Franzen and Lovell 1987). However, although the Luria-Nebraska yields standardized summary scores that correct for age and education, relatively little research has been specifically conducted with geriatric subjects. One study (MacInnes et al. 1983) demonstrated good dissociation between healthy elderly patients and older adults with brain injury on all scales of the Luria-Nebraska, but to date additional studies have not been completed. Additionally, a short form of the Luria-Nebraska has been developed, reducing the number of total items from 269 to 141, which might address older adults' tendency to fatigue during administration of the full battery. The short form of the Luria-Nebraska was found to correlate significantly (r = .8 to .9) with the long form of the battery, suggesting relatively good equivalence of the two forms (McCue et al. 1989). Although the Luria-Nebraska and, in particular, the short form has the advantage of a relatively brief administration time (1 to 2 hours), its diagnostic accuracy has been questioned (for a complete discussion, see Lezak 1983). Overall, additional research is needed prior to the widespread use of this battery with older adults.

The Flexible Approach To Neuropsychological Assessment

A flexible strategy to neuropsychological evaluation is a more tailored approach that enables the examiner to select specific individual tests based on the patient's presenting illness or referral question (Goodglass 1986; Kane 1991; Kaszniak 1989; Lezak 1983; Schear 1984). Primary advantages of the flexible approach to neuropsychological evaluation include a potentially shorter administration time, economical favorability, and adaptability to differing patient situations and needs. Some (Goodglass 1986; Russell 1984) have argued that the flexible approach permits better specification of the nature of the brain impairment rather than simply documenting the presence or absence of brain damage. Others use the flexible approach because it permits easy evaluation of qualitative features such as the patient's use of problem-solving strategies (Kaplan 1983). Finally, the flexible approach can be modified easily and therefore is adaptable to a wide variety of clinical situations (Kane 1991).

Disadvantages of the flexible approach include a lack of standardization of administration rules for some tests, a potential lack of comprehensiveness, and limitations in establishing systematic data bases (Kane 1991; Tarter and Edwards 1986). Also, examiners who use the flexible battery approach require extensive clinical training and experience as the interpretation of test results is qualitative rather than solely quantitative in nature.

The flexible approach does not lend itself well to empirical investigation because of the individualized nature of the tasks and the difficulty comparing results across institutions or centers. However, this individualized approach to neuropsychological assessment remains popular with many neuropsychologists because of its adaptability, efficiency with severely impaired patients, and applicability with patients who are vulnerable to fatigue, distress, or sensory limitations (Kane 1991; La Rue 1992). For these reasons, the flexible neuropsychological evaluation appears to be a useful approach for the clinical assessment of older adults. An understanding of developmental normal aging, age-related cognitive decline, neuropathological conditions in the elderly, and other issues pertinent to differential diagnosis are particularly important when using the flexible neuropsychological assessment approach with elderly patients.

Individual Tests of Cognitive Functioning

Even when a flexible approach to neuropsychological assessment is adopted, a broad range of cognitive processes should be evaluated. The major domains of cognitive functioning that should be assessed include attention and concentration, general intelligence, conceptual processes and executive functioning, memory and learning, visuospatial skills, language, and fine motor speed, coordination, and strength (see Albert and Moss 1988; Russell 1984). Table 7–3 lists individual neuropsychological tests that are commonly used in evaluating the major domains of cognitive functioning in older adults. (A complete review of these cognitive domains and the instruments that measure them is beyond the scope of this chapter; for excellent reviews on this topic, see Albert and Moss 1988; La Rue 1992.)

Assessment of Attentional Processes

After the informal assessment of the patient's basic level of arousal, alertness, and level of orientation, the patient's attentional capacity should be evaluated. Assessment of attention is necessary because attention is

Table 7–3. Cognitive domains and representative
neuropsychological tests

Attention
Digit Span (Wechsler Adult Intelligence Scale–Revised
[WAIS-R; Wechsler 1981], Wechsler Memory Scale–
Revised [WMS-R; Wechsler 1987])
Visual Memory Span (WMS-R)
Cancellation tests (number, letter, or figure)
Continuous Performance Test (Rosvold and Mirsky
1956; Loong 1988)
Stroop Test (Golden 1978)
Trail Making Test (see Reitan and Wolfson 1985)

Memory
WMS-R
California Verbal Learning Test (Delis et al. 1987)
Rey-Osterrieth Complex Figure Test (memory)
(Osterrieth 1944)
Hopkins Verbal Learning Test (Brandt 1991)
Rey Auditory-Verbal Learning Test (1964)

Intelligence
WAIS-R

Executive functions
Category Test (see Reitan and Wolfson 1985)
Wisconsin Card Sorting Test (Berg 1948; Heaton 1981)
Tower of London (Shallice 1982)
Trail Making Test
Tinkertoy Test (Lezak 1983)
Porteus Maze Test (Porteus 1965)
Stroop Test

Language
Boston Diagnostic Aphasia Examination (Goodglass and
Kaplan 1972)
Multilingual Aphasia Examination (Benton and
Hamsher 1978)
Reitan-Indiana Aphasia Screening Test (see Reitan and
Wolfson 1985)
Wepman Auditory Discrimination Test (Wepman and
Jones 1961)

Visuospatial and visuomotor processes
Facial Recognition Test (see Benton et al. 1983)
Judgment of Line Orientation (see Benton et al. 1983)
Visual Form Discrimination Test (see Benton et al.
1983)
Benton Visual Retention Test (Benton 1974)
Rey-Osterrieth Complex Figure (copy) (Osterrieth
1944)

Motor Processes
Finger Oscillation Test (see Reitan and Wolfson 1985)
Grooved Pegboard Test (Matthews and Kløve 1964)
Purdue Pegboard Test (Purdue Research Foundation
1948)
Strength of Grip Test (see Reitan and Wolfson 1985)

a prerequisite for successful performance in other cognitive domains (Albert 1981). If the patient appears to fatigue in the course of testing, it may be necessary to reassess attention to determine the effect of exhaustion on test performance.

Attention is not a unitary phenomenon; it is a multifactorial and complex cognitive activity. Attentional processes can be impaired in patients with delirium and with dementing disorders, but may also be significantly impaired in the depressed geriatric patient and patients with focal brain lesions. For the purposes of the clinical evaluation of the geriatric patient, it is useful to evaluate both verbal and nonverbal aspects of attention, as these components of attention can be variably impaired depending on the etiology of the cognitive dysfunction.

Auditory attentional processes are most readily assessed by the use of span procedures such as the Digit Span from the WMS-R. In this procedure, strings of numbers are read to the patient in increasing length in both forward and backward order. Visual attention span can be evaluated through the use of the Visual Memory Span subtest of the WMS-R and requires the patient to tap progressively longer sequences of colored boxes printed on a card, after watching the test administrator do so in a specific order. The patient's ability to perform this task in both forward and backward order is evaluated. Letter and number cancellation tasks (Talland and Schwab 1964) can be used to assess visual attentional processes and require the patient to cross off designated stimuli on a sheet of paper within a short period of time. Visual cancellation tests are particularly useful in patients with hearing loss but are contraindicated in patients with decreased visual acuity.

The Continuous Performance Test (Rosvold and Mirsky 1956) measures sustained attention or vigilance and is currently available in a computer-based format (Loong 1988). This group of procedures involves the presentation of stimuli (letters or numbers) via a computer monitor. The subject is instructed to depress a key when a specific number or letter appears on the screen. The test sequence can be varied to assess the patient's ability to sustain attention over variable time spans.

Divided attention (i.e., the ability to ignore extraneous information, while focusing on specific stimuli) can be assessed by the Stroop Test (Golden 1978; Stroop 1935). This test first involves the presentation of a 100-item list of words, which the patient reads aloud. Next, the patient is required to name the colors of a series of *X*'s. Finally, the patient is presented with a list of words that are printed in a different color ink than the word implies and is asked to name the color of the ink, ignoring the word. For example, the word *Red* is presented in green ink and the patient must suppress the tendency to read the word rather than name the color. This test is considered to be a measure of executive functioning, as well as being sensitive to divided attention, and is particularly sensitive to frontal lobe lesions. Once the patient's ability to focus and sustain attention has been evaluated, the patient's level of cognitive functioning in other domains can be evaluated. If the patient's ability to attend is judged to be severely impaired, further neuropsychological assessment beyond a brief cognitive screen may not be useful.

Assessment of Intellectual Processes

Intellectual processes are differentially affected by the aging process and by dementing disorders. Overlearned crystallized intellectual functions (Cattell 1963) such as fund of general information and vocabulary development are often preserved, whereas the ability to use abstract reasoning and cognitive flexibility (fluid intelligence) usually declines both with normal aging and with disease-associated processes. The WAIS-R is the most commonly used test of general intelligence but may take more than 2 hours to administer to an elderly patient, making it impractical in many cases. When the complete administration of the

WAIS-R is not possible because of limitations in the patient's stamina or severity of cognitive impairment, the administration of selected subtests can be useful. In particular, the Vocabulary and Information subtests are relatively good indicators of the patient's premorbid level of functioning, although the best estimate of the patient's life-long level of functioning may be educational level and occupational history (Albert 1981). The ability to think abstractly is most commonly assessed through the use of the Similarities subtest of the WAIS-R, and the Comprehension subtest provides a sample of the patient's judgment when placed in hypothetical situations.

Executive Functioning

Executive functioning involves drive, programming, control of behavior, and synthesis (see Chapter 6), and different components of executive processes can be assessed psychometrically. Performance on tasks that require mental flexibility, set shifting, and learning in novel situations such as the Wisconsin Card Sorting Test (Berg 1948; Heaton 1981) or the Category Test (Halstead 1947) from the HRNB is often impaired in patients with neuropsychiatric illnesses, particularly when there is involvement of frontal-subcortical circuits. Planning can be assessed through an analysis of how the patient approaches tasks such as the Block Design subtest of the WAIS-R or the Rey-Osterrieth Complex Figure (Osterrieth 1944) (Figure 7–1), or it can be evaluated using the Tinkertoy Test (Lezak 1983),

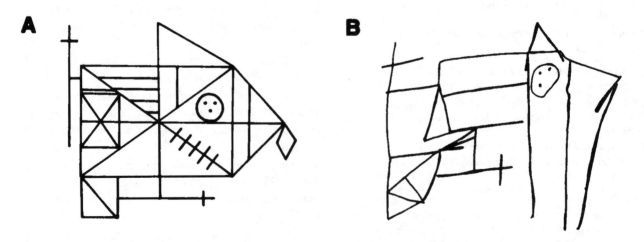

Figure 7–1. Rey-Osterrieth Complex Figure Test (*panel A*) and reproduction of this figure by a 77-year-old man with suspected Alzheimer's disease (*panel B*). His copy of the figure demonstrates severe impairment of visuoconstructional processes often associated with parietal lobe damage.
Source. See Osterrieth 1944.

the Tower of London Test (Shallice 1982), or the Porteus Maze Test (Porteus 1965). As its name implies, the Tinkertoy Test requires the patient to build a design using a 50-piece Tinkertoy set. The resulting construction is then scored on eight dimensions, which include the number of pieces used in building the design, the symmetry of the design, and whether or not the construction has moving parts. The Tower of London Test requires the patient to fit colored beads onto pegs based on a model, in the fewest number of moves possible. The Porteus Maze Test requires the patient to solve a series of mazes of increasing complexity that are presented on paper.

Memory

The evaluation of memory represents an extremely important component of the neuropsychological assessment of the geriatric patient and can yield important diagnostic information. The patient's performance can help discriminate the effects of brain impairment from normal aging and can also help differentiate dementias of different etiologies. For example, one dissociation of memory performance includes the difference between impaired free recall and recognition of recent information versus impaired free recall but relatively preserved recognition of recent information. Impaired free recall and recognition performance may be classified as a "pure amnesia" with concomitant dysfunction of encoding, storage, and retrieval mechanisms. This type of memory loss is typically associated with medial-temporal lobe damage, particularly the hippocampus, and is characteristic of Alzheimer's disease. Impaired free recall with relatively preserved recognition performance suggests a retrieval deficit consistent with dysfunction of the frontal-subcortical circuitry and characteristic of basal ganglia diseases and frontal lobe disorders (Cummings 1992).

Both verbal and visuospatial memory should be assessed and may have relevance for the localization of brain dysfunction to either the left or right hemisphere. Verbal memory processes are most often assessed through the use of word lists that are presented a specified number of times or through the presentation of "stories" that the patient is asked to memorize and recall at some later time. The Rey Auditory-Verbal Learning Test (Rey 1964) and the California Verbal Learning Test (Delis et al. 1987) are commonly used list-learning tasks, although these tests are challenging

because of the length of the lists (15 and 16 words, respectively) and the five required repetitions of the lists. These tests may be too difficult for geriatric patients who have more than a mild level of dementia or who have reduced stamina. The Hopkins Verbal Learning Test (Brandt 1991) may be preferable because it is shorter (12 words) and involves only three repetitions of the material. However, the usefulness of this test is currently limited by the unavailability of normative data for delayed recall, making an accurate evaluation of memory retention and retrieval more qualitative than quantitative. The most commonly used story recall tasks used to evaluate verbal memory are taken from the Wechsler Memory Scale (Wechsler 1945), and the revision of this test (i.e., the WMS-R).

Evaluation of the patient's ability to learn and remember abstract, spatial information is also an important component of the neuropsychological assessment process, and disruption of spatial memory relative to other test results may suggest right-hemisphere dysfunction. Testing most often involves the reproduction and subsequent recall of abstract designs such as are provided by the Visual Reproduction subtest of the WMS-R or the Rey-Osterrieth Complex Figure Test. In the evaluation of spatial memory, it is particularly important to dissociate the patient's ability to reproduce the designs (constructional disturbance) from memory, per se. One way of conveniently accomplishing this is by asking the patient to copy the design before the memory component of the evaluation is completed. Figure 7–1 provides an example of severe constructional disturbance in a 77-year-old patient with suspected Alzheimer's disease. In addition, other assessment procedures such as the Benton Visual Retention Test (Benton 1974) allow separation of constructional disturbance from impairment of spatial memory by providing normative data for both the reproduction and retention of figural information.

Remote memory, also referred to as *tertiary memory*, refers to the recall of events that occurred during the early years of one's life (La Rue 1992). Interestingly, older adults typically report the ability to recall events from remote memory (i.e., names of grade school teachers), while complaining of memory loss for recent events (what they had for lunch 2 days ago). Traditional measures of remote memory include the Famous Faces Test or Famous Events Test (see Lezak 1983), which assess the individual's ability to recall famous faces or events during different decades of the 20th century.

The assessment of remote memory is difficult because the examiner is usually uncertain about the amount of initial exposure to the stimuli or the subsequent rehearsal of this information over time (Craik 1977). In other words, what may appear as remote memory failure in a given patient may actually be a lack of exposure to the event in question. Research documents significant age differences in a comparison of remote memory (public events) between young, middle-aged, and older adults (Howes and Katz 1988). Specifically, the elderly group demonstrated significantly poorer performance in recall of remote events during the time periods when both groups had lived. However, the elderly demonstrated consistent recall across all decades that covered 50 years. The issue of whether older subjects demonstrate consistent recall across decades remains a controversial issue (Squire 1974; Warrington and Sanders 1971). Overall, remote memory appears to be affected by age, but this finding should continue to be interpreted with caution as there remain methodological differences across studies (La Rue 1992).

Visuospatial and Visuoconstructive Processes

Just as it is important to separate disorders of memory from difficulties secondary to impairment of constructional processes, it is also necessary to separate disorders of visuospatial analysis from those of visuoconstructive processes, because this can have localizing value and may aid in differential diagnosis. The separation of these different, but related, neuropsychological processes can be most effectively accomplished by comparing the results of constructional tasks such as Block Design from the WAIS-R to performance on motor-free spatial tasks such as the Visual Form Discrimination Test, Judgment of Line Orientation, and Facial Recognition tests developed by Benton and his colleagues (see Benton et al. 1983). The Rey-Osterrieth Complex Figure Test, used in combination with these motor-free tasks, can be quite useful in separating visuospatial from visuoconstructive deficits. Poor performance in copying the figure with better performance on motor-free tests suggests a constructional rather than visuospatial disorder.

Speech and Language

The clinical evaluation of speech and language processes is also a necessary component in the neuropsychological evaluation of geriatric patients. Language processes in the elderly can be affected by the normal aging process (Albert et al. 1988), depression (Speedie et al. 1990), and dementia (Hill et al. 1989), and a thorough evaluation of language can help differentiate these disorders clinically. In particular, disorders of object naming (tested by presenting the patients with pictures of common objects) have been found to be associated with dementing illness (Albert 1981; Hill et al. 1989) and to a lesser degree with cognitive impairment secondary to depression (Speedie et al. 1990).

Other aspects of language should also be assessed during the neuropsychological evaluation, including comprehension, repetition, and verbal fluency, as well as reading and writing. Fluency can be easily assessed via the Animal Naming subtest of the Boston Diagnostic Aphasia Examination (Goodglass and Kaplan 1972) or the Controlled Oral Word Association Test (Benton and Hamsher 1978). Both types of verbal fluency tests provide the patient with 1 minute to produce as many words that fall under the category of "animals" or that begin with a specific letter. The total number of words generated by the patient in 1 minute represents a total verbal fluency score and is compared to age-appropriate normative data. The Aphasia Screening Test (Halstead and Wepman 1959) from the HRNB is also useful and provides a brief assessment of multiple aspects of language, as well as allowing an evaluation of basic reading, writing, and calculational abilities. Other tests that measure more specific problems of cognitive processing including arithmetic, orientation, object recognition, color recognition, and facial recognition are available (see Lezak 1983).

Motor Processes and Psychomotor Speed

Although motor speed and coordination decrease with normal aging, impairment of motor processes can also signal underlying neuropathological process. Decreased motor strength or speed can suggest a lateralized brain lesion such as a stroke, tumor, or metastases or may occur with other neurological disorders such as Parkinson's disease. In addition, a disruption in the ability to produce complex motor acts (e.g., dressing and eating) may represent an apraxia and may point to a specific lesion in the parietal lobes.

Motor speed is most commonly evaluated through the use of the Finger Oscillation Test from the HRNB or through the use of the Grooved Pegboard Test (Matthews and Kløve 1964) or Purdue Pegboard Test (Purdue Research Foundation 1948). In general, better performance is expected of the dominant (usually right) hand relative to the nondominant hand and the absence of this pattern may help to localize a brain lesion to the contralateral hemisphere. Similarly, a relative difference is expected in motor strength between the dominant and nondominant hands, and the absence of this pattern may suggest a contralateral brain lesion. The evaluation of upper-extremity motor strength is most often measured formally via a dynamometer as is used in the HRNB (Reitan 1955). The cautions concerning the use of age-appropriate norms are particularly germane to a discussion of the evaluation of motor processes. Comparison of an elderly patient's performance on a motor task to a younger normative group can result in spurious and misleading information.

Use of Neuropsychological Testing in Differential Diagnosis

As highlighted throughout this chapter, geriatric patients are at risk for a number of neuropathological disorders that affect cognitive functioning, and these disorders are often difficult to distinguish clinically. Although the neuropsychological evaluation can often be helpful in the differential diagnosis of neurological disorders, it must be emphasized that the results of neuropsychological testing should not be interpreted "in a vacuum," but should be integrated with other diagnostic information gathered within the broader con-

text of the neuropsychiatric evaluation. This should involve a thorough medical, social, and psychiatric history; mental status examination; the application of appropriate neuroimaging technologies; and appropriate laboratory studies. With these guidelines in mind, in the following section we review the use of neuropsychological testing in the differential diagnostic process.

Dementia

Dementing disorders are not a homogeneous group of conditions; they vary greatly with regard to etiology, neurological substrate, disease course, and treatment. Therefore, it is not surprising that different types of dementia are associated with different neuropsychological profiles (Table 7–4).

The neuropsychological profile of Alzheimer's disease is most often characterized by impairment of memory, visuospatial processes, intellectual processes, and language, although impairment in all of these areas may not be present in every patient, particularly early in the disease. Memory impairment is usually the first sign of the disorder, although detailed neuropsychological evaluation may reveal subtle deficits in other areas (e.g., executive functioning). Dysnomia and decreased verbal fluency are also common, even very early in the disease process, and can be documented through the use of tests such as the Boston Naming Test and Animal Naming Test of the Boston Diagnostic Aphasia Examination. Memory impair-

Table 7–4.   Profiles of neuropsychological dysfunction in elderly patients

Syndrome	Neuropsychological profile
Alzheimer's disease	Impaired recent memory, intrusive errors on list learning tasks, poor performance on memory recognition and retention measures, impaired naming and other signs of aphasia, visuospatial processing deficits, general intellectual decline, apraxia, and agnosia (in advanced illness)
Frontal lobe dementias	Executive functioning deficits (perseveration, impaired planning, stimulus boundedness, impaired synthesis, impaired mental flexibility), reduced fluency (verbal and nonverbal), impaired insight, marked personality change early in illness characterized by apathy and inertia, impaired selective attention, and relatively preserved memory
Vascular dementia	"Patchy" pattern of deficits depending on location of infarcts, general intellectual decline over time, step-wise decline in cognitive functioning over time, and lateralized cognitive deficits depending on site of infarct or infarcts
Subcortical dementias	Psychomotor slowing, prominent memory impairment, speech or motor-system difficulties, impaired concept formation and mental flexibility, impaired insight, and depression
Dementia syndrome of depression	Mildly impaired naming, impaired attentional processes and immediate memory but intact retention of new material, normal primacy effects on memory tasks, normal learning curve on list learning tasks, normal retrieval and recognition of material, and intact visuospatial processing

ment is characterized by relatively spared immediate memory (as measured by the Digit Span procedure) but marked impairment in the retention of newly learned material. Intrusive errors (i.e., the inclusion of extraneous items) are common, both on list learning and story recall tasks.

Early in Alzheimer's disease, there is often subtle impairment of mental flexibility and executive functioning that may be viewed by the patient (and by his or her family) as being part and parcel of the normal aging process. Visuospatial impairment may be evident in the patient's drawings and range from mild distortions of designs to a complete inability to reproduce even simple, two-dimensional copies. At later stages in the disease, more severe impairment of intellectual processes is observed, and agnosia and apraxia are often seen. Severe visuospatial impairment may take the form of an inability to tell time on an analog clock or by spatial disorientation. This problem may become so severe that the patient is unable to find his or her room consistently.

The label *frontal lobe dementia* is used to describe a number of disorders that primarily affect the frontal lobes of the brain. Pick's disease, the dementia accompanying motor neuron disease, and syphilis represent disorders that have primary frontal lobe involvement. Frontal lobe dementia is most often characterized by marked personality change and impairment of executive functioning (Cummings 1992). Unlike dementia of the Alzheimer type, the first signs of the disease are usually neuropsychiatric rather than cognitive in nature. Personality change is characterized by apathy and by behavioral inertia. Executive functioning impairment takes the form of perseveration, stimulus boundedness, impaired synthesis, and impaired ability to plan. In contrast to those with the dementia of Alzheimer's disease, patients with frontal lobe dementia often have preserved visuospatial abilities and relatively preserved memory functions (Neary and Snowden 1991). Although basic motor processes are usually intact, executive processes that involve a significant motor component may be impaired. Language comprehension and expression are often preserved, but echolalia may be present. The neuropsychiatric and cognitive difficulties seen in frontal lobe dementia may become so severe as to limit the patient's ability to complete a comprehensive evaluation. Short bedside procedures are often useful and should be part of the mental status examination (see Chapter 6).

Vascular dementia is characterized by "patchy"

performance on neuropsychological measures with islands of preserved and impaired performance, depending on the site of the infarct or infarcts. As the disease progresses, a "stepwise" decline in cognitive functioning is typically observed and can be documented through serial neuropsychological evaluations. Left-hemisphere lesions often result in language and verbal memory impairment, whereas right-hemisphere lesions result in greater impairment of visuospatial processes and visual memory. Small infarcts that do not affect motor or speech areas may go unnoticed by the patient or family, but can be documented through neuropsychological evaluation.

The subcortical dementias are a group of disorders that are characterized by primary dysfunction in subcortical brain areas. Unlike dementing conditions that primarily affect cortical areas, leading to aphasia, apraxia, agnosia, and anomia, subcortical dementia features motor dysfunction, speech impairment, memory dysfunction, executive disorders, and disturbances in mood and personality (Cummings 1985). Subcortical dementia occurs with extrapyramidal syndromes such as Parkinson's disease, Wilson's disease, progressive supranuclear palsy, and Huntington's disease. Although there is often a general decline in intellectual processes over time, this decline is usually much less severe than in other dementing disorders. Parkinson's disease is relatively common in elderly individuals. Performance on neuropsychological testing varies across patients, but deficits are often found on tests that require psychomotor speed, visuospatial processing, executive functioning, and memory (Pirozzolo et al. 1982). In addition, performance may be impaired on tests that measure concept formation and problem solving in new situations (Matthews and Haaland 1979), category fluency, and mental flexibility (Beatty et al. 1989).

Patients with Huntington's disease often exhibit executive functioning impairment that involves difficulty with mental flexibility and abstraction with relatively preserved "overlearned" verbal skills (i.e., on the Information and Vocabulary subtests on the WAIS-R). Memory impairment also commonly occurs with Huntington's disease and is characterized by impairment in the acquisition and retrieval of new information, as well as by impaired remote memory later in the disease process (Albert et al. 1981). In contrast to the dysnomia that characterizes Alzheimer's disease, the Huntington's patient may perform normally on confrontation naming tests (Butters et al. 1978).

Depression-Related Cognitive Dysfunction

It is estimated that from 10% to 20% of depressed patients have significant cognitive impairment (Reynolds and Hoch 1988). In addition, depression frequently accompanies neurological disorders such as Alzheimer's disease (Kaszniak 1987), stroke (Robinson and Price 1982), and extrapyramidal diseases such as Parkinson's and Huntington's (Cummings 1985). The labels *pseudodementia* (Kiloh 1961), *dementia syndrome of depression* (Folstein and McHugh 1978), *depression-induced organic mental disorder* (McAllister 1983), and, more recently, *depression-related cognitive dysfunction* (Stoudemire et al. 1989) have been used to describe the reversible cognitive impairment in elderly depressed patients. Since Kiloh's initial characterization of pseudodementia (1961), there have been numerous articles describing the clinical features of cognitive impairment secondary to depression and its differentiation from progressive and irreversible conditions such as Alzheimer's disease (Bulbena and Berrios 1986; Cummings 1989; Jeste et al. 1990; Kaszniak 1987). Although the concept of depression-related cognitive impairment is well accepted and has had value in identifying potentially treatable forms of dementia, the term *pseudodementia* has come under criticism (Arie 1983; Lamberty and Bieliuskas 1993; Reifler 1982; Shraberg 1978, 1980). These criticisms have stemmed primarily from the implication that cognitive dysfunction secondary to depression does not represent a "real" or "organic" phenomenon. Additional criticisms have been based on the lack of diagnostic specificity of the term and from the lack of utility of the concept in predicting response to treatment.

Understanding of the complexity of cognitive dysfunction in depressed elderly patients has increased substantially over the last decade, and there has been an increasing number of systematic studies designed to assist in the separation of the potentially reversible (and treatable) dementia of depression from irreversible and often progressive conditions such as Alzheimer's disease and vascular dementia. Although there is currently no universally accepted neuropsychological template for the differentiation of depression-related cognitive dysfunction from cognitive impairment secondary to specific brain disease, recent research has suggested that neuropsychological test results may be useful in this regard. For example, several studies have pointed to the usefulness of confrontation naming tests such as the Boston Naming Test (Kaplan et al.

1983) in the differential diagnostic process (Caine 1981; Hill et al. 1989; Petrick and Mittenberg 1992), although this finding has not been found by all researchers (Speedie et al. 1990). Further complicating the issue is relatively recent research suggesting that depression might represent an early marker for later developing progressive dementia (Kral and Emery 1989; Nussbaum et al. 1991; Reding et al. 1985). The issue of cognitive dysfunction in depressed elderly patients is a complicated one that deserves further study.

Ecological Validity of Neuropsychological Tests

Generalization and predictive validity of neuropsychological test performance to the patient's functional capacity is emerging as an important issue for clinical neuropsychology and is particularly relevant to the assessment of older adults. Indeed, the utility of neuropsychological assessment lies not only in its ability to aid in the diagnostic process, but also in its ability to provide information regarding the patient's ability to function in his or her natural environment. Most of the available research suggests a moderate relationship between neuropsychological test performance and outcome measures (Acker 1990; Chelune and Moehle 1986), with the predictive accuracy of neuropsychological test performance being greater for functional skills demanding complex information processing such as writing a check than for basic functional capacity such as performance of a personal hygiene skill (McCue et al. 1990). Other research has suggested that specific neuropsychological tests correlate best with specific functional skills in specific older populations (Goldstein et al. 1992). In addition, initial neuropsychological test performance has been found to successfully predict longitudinal functional capacity of geropsychiatric inpatients (Rogers et al., in press).

The clinical neuropsychologist is often asked to recommend optimal residential placement and determine if driving should be continued for older patients (see Blaustein et al. 1988; Kaszniak and Nussbaum 1990). Unfortunately, relatively few empirical data exist to support the predictive validity of neuropsychological test performance on these functional domains in older patients. The development of new neuropsychological tasks that more closely parallel activities in daily life is much needed (Zappala et al. 1989). Currently, decisions are more often based on estimates of the patient's performance on more traditional neuropsychological measures that have no direct corollary "in real life." In particular, decisions regarding the patient's ability to drive are often based on performance on visuospatial, attentional, memory, and executive functioning tasks, as these processes are generally thought to be requisite to the safe operation of an automobile. The development of ecologically valid neuropsychological tests to more directly assess the patient's ability to perform real-life activities requires continued attention and represents one of the biggest challenges for the field of geriatric neuropsychology.

Conclusions and Future Directions

In this chapter, we have reviewed several important issues related to the neuropsychological assessment of older patients. First, the use of a flexible, individualized approach to neuropsychological assessment with older patients is advocated because it typically requires less time than standard fixed batteries, is cost effective, and is patient driven, thus providing the opportunity to address specific cognitive deficits. Second, despite recent developments in geriatric neuropsychology, there is a continued need for empirical-clinical investigation of the utility of different evaluation approaches to the assessment of older adults. Third, age-appropriate normative data for individuals over the age of 74 are currently lacking, and although progress has been made in this area, there remains a need for normative data for individuals in this age group. Fourth, the use of neuropsychological testing in the differential diagnosis of dementing illnesses, particularly subcortical versus cortical dementia, remains an important area deserving of continued attention. Fifth, the ecological validity of neuropsychological assessment is a relatively new area of concern that deserves sophisticated empirical investigation. Cognitive tests that predict the functional capacity of older patients are needed and will enhance the usefulness of the neuropsychological evaluation. Finally, continued specialized training of the clinical neuropsychologist in the assessment and treatment of older patients is needed.

References

Acker MB: A review of the ecological validity of neuropsychological tests, in The Neuropsychology of Everyday Life. Edited by Tupper DE, Cicerone KD. Boston, MA, Kluwer Academic Press, 1990, pp 19–55

Albert MS: Geriatric neuropsychology. J Consult Clin Psychol 49:835–850, 1981

Albert MS, Moss MB: Geriatric Neuropsychology. New York, Guilford, 1988

Albert MS, Butters N, Brandt J: Development of remote memory loss in patients with Huntington's disease. J Clin Neuropsychology 3:1–12, 1981

Anthony WZ, Heaton RK, Lehman RAW: An attempt to cross-validate two actuarial systems for neuropsychological test interpretation. J Consult Clin Psychol 48:317–326, 1980

Arie T: Pseudodementia. BMJ 286:1301–1302, 1983

Beatty W, Staton RD, Weir WS, et al: Cognitive disturbances in Parkinson's disease. J Geriatr Psychiatry Neurol 2:22–23, 1989

Benton AL: The Revised Visual Retention Test, 4th Edition. New York, Psychological Corporation, 1974

Benton AL, Hamsher K: Multilingual Aphasia Examination. Iowa City, IA, University of Iowa Press, 1978

Benton AL, Hamsher K, Varney N, et al: Contributions to Neuropsychological Assessment: A Clinical Manual. New York, Oxford University Press, 1983

Berg GE: A simple objective test for measuring flexibility in thinking. J Gen Psychol 39:15–22, 1948

Blaustein MJL, Filipp CL, Dungan C, et al: Driving in patients with dementia. J Am Geriatr Soc 36:1087–1091, 1988

Brandt J: The Hopkins verbal learning test: development of a new memory test with six equivalent forms. Clinical Neuropsychologist 5:125–142, 1991

Bulbena A, Berrios GE: Pseudodementia: facts and figures. Br J Psychiatry 148:87–94, 1986

Butters N, Sax D, Montgomery K, et al: Comparison of the neuropsychological deficits associated with early and advanced Huntington's disease. Arch Neurol 35:585–589, 1978

Caine ED: Pseudodementia: current concepts and future directions. Arch Gen Psychiatry 38:1359–1364, 1981

Catell RB: Theory of fluid and crystallized intelligence: a critical experiment. Journal of Educational Psychology 54:1–22, 1963

Chelune GJ, Moehle KA: Neuropsychological assessment and everyday functioning, in The Neuropsychology Handbook: Behavioral and Clinical Perspectives. Edited by Wedding AM, Horton J, Webster J. New York, Springer, 1986, pp 489–525

Craik FIM: Age differences in human memory, in Handbook of the Psychology of Aging. Edited by Birren JE, Schaie KW. New York, Van Nostrand Reinhold, 1977, pp 384–420

Cummings JL: Clinical Neuropsychiatry. Orlando, FL, Grune & Stratton, 1985

Cummings JL: Dementia and depression: an evolving enigma. J Neuropsychiatry Clin Neurosci 1:236–242, 1989

Cummings JL: Neuropsychiatric aspects of Alzheimer's disease and other dementing illnesses, in The American Psychiatric Press Textbook of Neuropsychiatry, 2nd Edition. Edited by Yudofsky SC, Hales RE. Washington, DC, American Psychiatric Press, 1992, pp 605–620

Delis D, Kramer JH, Kaplan E, et al: The California Verbal Learning Test—Adult Version. San Antonio, TX, Psychological Corporation, 1987

Folstein MF, McHugh PR: Dementia syndrome of depression, in Alzheimer's Disease: Senile Dementia and Related Disorders. Edited by Katzman R, Terry RD, Bick KL. New York, Raven, 1978, pp 281–289

Franzen MD, Lovell MR: Neuropsychological assessment, in The American Psychiatric Press Textbook of Neuropsychiatry. Edited by Hales RE and Yudofsky SC. Washington, American Psychiatric Press, 1987, pp 41–53

Golden CJ: The Stroop Color and Word Test: A Manual for Clinical and Experimental Use. Chicago, IL, Stoelting, 1978

Golden CJ, Maruish M: The Luria-Nebraska Neuropsychological Battery, in Neuropsychological Test Batteries. Edited by Incagnoli T, Goldstein G, Golden CJ. New York, Plenum, 1986, pp 193–227

Golden CJ, Hammeke TA, Purisch AD: The Luria-Nebraska Neuropsychological Battery Manual. Los Angeles, Western Psychological Services, 1980

Goldstein G, McCue M, Roger J, et al: Diagnostic differences in memory test based predictions of functional capacity in the elderly. Neuropsychological Rehabilitation 2:307–317, 1992

Goodglass H: The flexible battery, in Neuropsychological Assessment. Edited by Incagnoli T, Goldstein G, Golden CJ. New York, Plenum, pp 121–131, 1986

Goodglass H, Kaplan E: Assessment of Aphasia and Related Disorders. Phliadelphia, PA, Lea & Febiger, 1972

Goreczny AJ, Nussbaum PD: Behavioral medicine with military veterans, in Progress in Behavior Modification. Edited by Hersen M, Eisler RM, Miller PM. Sycamore, IL, Sycamore Publishing Company (in press)

Halstead WC: Brain and Intelligence. Chicago, IL, University of Chicago Press, 1947

Halstead WC, Wepman JM: The Halstead-Wepman aphasia screening test. Journal of Speech and Hearing Disorders 14:9–15, 1959

Heaton RK: The Wisconsin Card Sorting Test Manual. Odessa, FL, Psychological Assessment Resources, 1981

Heaton RK, Pendleton MG: Use of neuropsychological tests to predict adult patient's everyday functioning. J Consult Clin Psychol 49:807–821, 1981

Heaton RK, Grant I, Matthews CG: Differences in neuropsychological test performance associated with age, education, and sex, in Neuropsychological Assessment of Neuropsychiatric Disorders. Edited by Grant I, Adams KM. New York, Oxford, 1986 pp 100–120

Heaton RK, Grant I, Matthews CG: Comprehensive Norms for an Expanded Halstead-Reitan Battery. Odessa, FL, Psychological Assessment Resources, 1991

Hill C, Stoudemire A, Morris R, et al: Dysnomia in the differential diagnosis of major depression, depression-related cognitive dysfunction, and dementia. J Neuropsychiatry Clin Neurosci 4:64–69, 1989

Howes JL, Katz AN: Assessing remote memory with an improved public events questionnaire. Psychol Aging 3:142–150, 1988

Incagnoli T, Goldstein G, Golden CJ: Neuropsychological Test Batteries. New York, Plenum, 1986

Ivnik RV, Malec JF, Smith GE, et al: Mayo's older American study. Clinical Neuropsychologist 6:1–30, 1992

Jeste DV, Gierz M, Harris MJ: Pseudodementia: myths and realities. Psychiatric Annals 20:71–79, 1990

Kane R: Standardized and flexible batteries in neuropsychology: an assessment update. Neuropsychology Review 2:281–339, 1991

Kaplan E: Process and achievement revisited, in Towards a Holistic Developmental Psychology. Edited by Wapner S, Kaplan B. Hillsdale, NJ, Lawrence Erlbaum Associates, 1983, pp 143–156

Kaplan EF, Goodglass H, Weintraube S: The Boston Naming Test. Philadelphia, PA, Lea & Febiger, 1983

Kaszniak AW: Neuropsychological consultation to geriatricians: issues in the assessment of memory complaints. Clinical Neuropsychologist 1:35–46, 1987

Kaszniak AW: Psychological assessment of the aging individual, in Handbook of the Psychology of Aging. Edited by Birren JE, Schaie KW. San Diego, CA, Academic Press, 1989, pp 427–445

Kaszniak AW, Nussbaum PD: Driving in older patients with dementia and depression. Paper presented at the annual meeting of the American Psychological Association, Boston, MA, August 1990

Kiloh LG: Pseudo-dementia. Acta Psychiatrica Scandinavica 37:336–351, 1961

Kral VA, Emery OB: Long-term follow-up of depressive pseudo-dementia of the aged. Can J Psychiatry 34:445–446, 1989

Lamberty CJ, Bieliuskas LA: Distinguishing between depression and dementia in the elderly: a review of neuropsychological findings. Archives of Clinical Neuropsychology 8:149–170, 1993

La Rue A: Aging and Neuropsychological Assessment. New York, Plenum, 1992

Lezak M: Neuropsychological Assessment, 2nd Edition. New York, Oxford University Press, 1983

Loong WK: The Continuing Performance Test. San Luis Obispo, CA, Wang Neuropsychological Laboratory, 1988

MacInnes WD, Gillen RW, Golden CJ, et al: Aging and performance on the Luria-Nebraska Neuropsychological Battery. Int J Neurosci 19:179–190, 1983

Matthews CG, Haaland KY: The effect of symptom duration on cognitive and motor performance in Parkinson's. Neurology 29:951–956, 1979

Matthews CG, Kløve H: Instruction Manual for the Adult Neuropsychological Text Battery. Madison, WI, University of Wisconsin Medical School Press, 1964

McAllister TW: Overview: pseudodementia. Am J Psychiatry 140:528–533, 1983

McCue M, Goldstein G, Shelly C: The application of a short form of the Luria-Nebraska Neuropsychological Battery to discrimination between dementia and depression in the elderly. Int J Clin Neuropsychol 11:21–29, 1989

McCue M, Rogers J, Goldstein G: Relationships between neuropsychological and functional assessment in elderly neuropsychiatric patients. Rehabilitation Psychology 35:91–,95, 1990

Neary D, Snowden JS: Dementia of the frontal lobe type, in Frontal Lobe Function and Dysfunction. Edited by Levin HS, Eisenberg HM, Benton AL. New York, Oxford University Press, 1991, pp 304–317

Nussbaum PD: Aging: issues in health and neuropsychological functioning, in Handbook of Recent Advances in Behavioral Medicine. Edited by Goreczny AJ. New York, Plenum (in press)

Nussbaum PD, Kaszniak AW, Allender J, et al: Cognitive deterioration in elderly depressed: a follow-up study. Paper presented at the annual meeting of the International Neuropsychological Society, San Antonio, TX, February 1991

Osato S, La Rue A, Yang J: Screening for cognitive deficits in older psychiatric patients. Paper presented at the annual meeting of the Gerontological Society of America, Minneapolis, MN, November 1989

Osterrieth PA: Le test de copie d' une figure complexe. Archives de Psychologie 30:306–356, 1944

Parsons OA: Overview of the Halstead-Reitan Battery, in Clinical Applications of Neuropsychological Test Batteries. Edited by Incagnoli T, Goldstein G, Golden C. New York, Plenum, 1986, pp 155–189

Petrick JD, Mittenberg W: The course of naming dysfunction in dementia and depressive pseudodementia. Paper presented at annual meeting of the National Academy of Neuropsychology, Pittsburgh, PA, November 1992

Pirozzolo FJ, Hansch EC, Mortimer JA: Dementia in Parkinson's disease: a neuropsychological analysis. Brain Cogn 1:71–83, 1982

Porteus SD: Porteus Maze Test: Fifty Year's Application. Palo Alto, CA, Pacific Books, 1965

Purdue Research Foundation: Examiners Manual for the Purdue Pegboard. Chicago, IL, Science Research Associates, 1948

Purisch AD, Sbordone RJ: The Luria-Nebraska Neuropsychological Battery, in Advances in Clinical Neuropsychology. Edited by Goldstein G, Tarter RE. New York, Plenum, 1986, pp 291–316

Reding M, Haycox J, Blass J: Depression in patients referred to a dementia clinic. Arch Neurol 42:894–896, 1985

Reifler BV: Arguments for abandoning the term pseudodementia. J Am Geriatr Soc 30:665–668, 1982

Reitan RM: An investigation of the validity of Halstead's measures of biological intelligence. Archives of Neurology and Psychiatry 73:28–35, 1955

Reitan RM: Neurological and physiological bases of psychopathology. Ann Rev Psychol 27:189–216, 1976

Reitan RM, Davison LA: Clinical Neuropsychology: Current Status and Applications. New York, Winston-Wiley, 1974

Reitan RM, Wolfson D: The Halstead-Reitan Neuropsychological Test Battery. Tempe, AZ, Neuropsychology Press, 1985

Rey A: L'Examen Clinique En Psychologie. Paris, Press Universitaires de France, 1964

Reynolds CF, Hoch CC: Differential diagnosis of depressive pseudodementia and primary degenerative dementia. Psychiatric Annals 17:743–749, 1988

Robinson RG, Price TR: Poststroke depressive disorders: a follow-up study of 103 patients. Stroke 13:635–641, 1982

Rogers JC, Holm M, Goldstein G, et al: Stability and change in functional assessment of geropsychiatric inpatients. Journal of Occupational Therapy (special issue) (in press)

Rosvold HE, Mirsky AF: A continuous performance test of brain damage. Journal of Consulting Psychology 20:343–350, 1956

Rowe JW, Kahn RL: Human aging: usual and unusual. Science 237:143–149, 1987

Russell EW: Theory and development of pattern analysis methods related to the Halstead-Reitan battery, in Clinical Neuropsychology: A Multidisciplinary Approach. Edited by Logue PE, Schear JM. Springfield, IL, Charles C Thomas, 1984, pp 50–62

Shallice T: Specific impairment of planning. Philos Trans R Soc Lond Biol 298:199–209, 1982

Schaie KW, Schaie J: Clinical assessment in aging, in Handbook of the Psychology of Aging. Edited by Birren J, Schaie KW. New York, Van Nostrand Reinhold, 1977, pp 692–723

Schear JM: Neuropsychological assessment of the elderly in clinical practice, in Clinical Neuropsychology: A Multidisciplinary Approach. Edited by Logue PE, Schear JM. Springfield, IL, Charles C Thomas, 1984, pp 199–236

Shraberg D: The myth of pseudodementia: depression and the aging brain. Am J Psychiatry 135:601–603, 1978

Shraberg D: Questioning the concept of pseudodementia. Am J Psychiatry 137:260–261, 1980

Speedie L, Rabins P, Pearlson G, et al: Confrontation naming deficit in dementia and depression. J Neuropsychiatry Clin Neurosci 2:59–63, 1990

Squire LR: Remote memory as affected by aging. Neuropsychologia 12:429–435, 1974

Storrie MC, Doerr HO: Characterization of Alzheimer's type dementia utilizing an abbreviated Halstead-Reitan Battery. Clinical Neuropsychology 2:78–82, 1980

Stoudemire A, Hill C, Gulley LR, et al: Neuropsychological and biomedical assessment of depression-dementia syndromes. J Neuropsychiatry Clin Neurosci 1:347–361, 1989

Stroop JR: Studies of interference in serial verbal reactions. Journal of Experimental Psychology 18:643–662, 1935

Talland GA, Schwab RS: Performance with multiple sets in Parkinson's disease. Neuropsychologia 2:45–53, 1964

Tarter RE, Edwards KL: Neuropsychological batteries, in Clinical Application of Neuropsychological Test Batteries. Edited by Incagnoli T, Goldstein G, Golden CJ. New York, Plenum, 1986, pp 135–152

Warrington EK, Sanders HI: The fate of old memories. Q J Exp Psychol 23:432–442, 1971

Wechsler D: A standardized memory scale for clinical use. Journal of Psychology 19:87–95, 1945

Wechsler D: Wechsler Adult Intelligence Scale–Revised Manual. New York, Psychological Corporation, 1981

Wechsler D: Wechsler Memory Scale–Revised Manual. New York, Psychological Corporation, 1987

Wepman JM, Jones LV: Studies in Aphasia: An Approach to Testing. Chicago, IL, Education Industry Service, 1961

Zappala G, Martini E, Crook T, et al: Ecological memory assessment in normal aging: a preliminary report on an Italian population. Clin Geriatr Med 5:583–594, 1989

8

Age-Associated Memory Impairment

Graham Ratcliff, D.Phil.
Judith Saxton, Ph.D.

Introduction

In this chapter, we review the memory changes associated with aging, paying particular attention to the phenomenon of age-associated memory impairment (AAMI). We begin the chapter with a brief overview of what is known about memory loss in older adults and a discussion of some current theoretical interpretations of these data. We then turn to the specific, well-defined phenomenon of AAMI, reviewing and critiquing proposed diagnostic criteria for this condition, exploring its clinical significance, and considering alternate constructs. We make the points that age-related memory changes can be conceptualized in a number of different ways and that different constructs, associated with different sets of diagnostic criteria, are appropriate for different purposes. We consider the prime distinguishing feature of currently available constructs to be the comparison group (young adults or the elderly individual's age peers) with reference to which memory is compared, approaches which we see as relevant to the study of normal aging, and pathological aging, respectively.

We then undertake a brief review of the characteristics of individuals who exhibit age-related memory changes and explore some possible biological bases for these conditions. Finally, we discuss some principles and practical considerations relating to clinical memory assessment in elderly individuals and describe some of the tests available for this purpose.

Background

There is solid, converging evidence from a variety of sources that some otherwise healthy, normally aging individuals experience a deterioration in memory as they grow older (Kaszniak et al. 1986; Poon 1985). The literature of experimental psychology suggests that this decline typically affects secondary memory, also known as *long-term* or *recent memory*, more than primary (*short-term* or *immediate*) memory or tertiary (*remote*) memory (Schacter et al. 1991). Age effects also sometimes appear in working memory (Baddeley 1986), tasks that require the individual not only to hold information in mind for a short time, but also to perform some mental operation on that information or perform another task simultaneously (Bromley 1958; Craik 1977; Dobbs and Rule 1989; Salthouse et al. 1989).

The net main effect of these changes is to reduce the ability to encode new information into memory, hold it over time, and recall it after an interval. Although the processes involved in remembering, particularly encoding and retrieval, become less effective as we grow older, the content of our memories—our knowledge base—can continue to increase (Perlmutter et al. 1987). Older people may, therefore, perform nearly as well as young people on tests such as digit span (in which information need only be held temporarily in a short-term memory store) or on tests assessing general knowledge or vocabulary (which assess well-learned factual or semantic knowledge rather than memory for specific events). They are likely to perform less well on tests such as backward digit span or delayed recall of recently presented material exceeding their immediate memory spans. The balance of opinion seems to be that the reported memory impairments cannot be entirely explained by other age-related changes in cognition or behavior or any of the other cohort effects that complicate aging research. They can thus be regarded as true *memory impairments* by most ordinary definitions of the term.

Psychometric evidence confirms that the decline of memory with increasing age is of substantial proportions. Performance on standard tests of secondary memory declines with age such that the norms for people 70 to 74 years old on the Wechsler Memory Scale–Revised (WMS-R; Wechsler 1987) call for scores up to 50% lower than those expected of 25- to 34-year-old individuals, and further declines are seen in individuals age 75 and older (Ivnik et al. 1992b). Age seems to have a more deleterious effect on the subtests involving memory for nonverbal material than on memory for verbal material, and recall is more affected than recognition memory.

In the clinical literature, the phenomenon of "benign senescent forgetfulness" (Kral 1958) has been recognized for more than 30 years. The disorder was described as being the forgetting of details of events without loss of awareness of the events themselves. Remote memories were more affected than recent memories and sufferers were aware of their problem, attempting to compensate for it. Kral et al. (1964) thought that this relatively mild and inconsistent memory impairment was nonprogressive and originally attributed it to normal aging (Kral 1962). They distinguished it in these respects from the "malignant" forgetfulness of the organic amnestic syndrome and dementia.

However, although this general picture is easily discerned and consistent from several viewpoints, the details are less clear and more controversial. Craik (1990, 1991) has argued that the degree of age-related impairment on memory tasks depends on the degree to which the task demands more active, less routine, and more internally organized processing on the part of the subject rather than on the type of memory involved. Older subjects have more difficulty with, or are less inclined to use, this kind of processing and perform less well on tasks that require it. Certainly, some of the factors that affect the degree of age-related decline on memory test performance affect performance on other cognitive tasks in a similar way. For example, the differential difficulty of verbal and visuospatial memory tests for elderly patients is mirrored in differential rates of decline on the verbal and performance subtests of the Wechsler Adult Intelligence Scale–Revised (WAIS-R; Wechsler 1981), and it may be that the decline in visuospatial memory can be more usefully regarded as a facet of impaired visuospatial ability rather than as a problem primarily of memory (Koss et al. 1991). Similarly, the changes in working memory may be regarded primarily as information-processing deficits rather than memory impairments, per se, and the age effect seems to appear only when certain kinds of processing are required (Salthouse et al. 1991).

In this view, memory can be regarded as just one aspect of cognition, an emergent property of the human information processing system, which, like other aspects of cognition, is affected by changes in the efficiency of that system. This analysis is similar to those that emphasize the difference between "fluid" and "crystallized" abilities (Cattell 1963), linking age-related changes in cognitive test performance to a decline in the fluid aspects of intelligence. The implication is that we may learn more about age-related changes in cognition if we do not think of them as changes in memory, perception, attention, and so on, but instead attempt to analyze the memory, perceptual, and attentional tests we use to identify the information-processing requirements involved.

Just as the magnitude of the age-related decline in memory and the nature of the underlying cognitive processes affected are less well established than the fact of a decline in memory performance, so the defining characteristics, epidemiology, and clinical significance of benign senescent forgetfulness have not been well delineated although the existence of the disorder is recognized. Kral (1958) described some of the characteristics of his subjects' forgetfulness, but he did not define operational criteria for diagnosing the disorder and he did not objectively quantify the impairment. Although he initially regarded the disorder as a part of normal aging (Kral 1962), his subjects were nursing home residents and patients in a psychiatric hospital. More than half of them exhibited neurological signs suggesting lesions in the brain, as did nearly half of his unimpaired subjects. They were thus certainly not drawn from a "normal" population, and Kral himself subsequently speculated (Kral et al. 1964) that benign and malignant forgetfulness might differ only in degree and might both be reflections of a single underlying pathological process. Of course, this would not necessarily make them "abnormal" if the "usually aging" individual who exhibits the range of physiological and even pathological changes typically associated with aging (Caine et al. 1991), rather than the optimally healthy "successfully aging" individual (Rowe and Kahn 1987), is accepted as the norm.

Constructs of Age-Related Memory Decline

Definitions

Before discussing the specific construct of AAMI (Crook et al. 1986a) in detail, we need to define some of the terms used in this chapter. Our purpose in doing so is emphatically not to introduce yet more terms into the literature; we simply wish to simplify communication for the purposes of this review. To this end, *age-associated memory impairment* (AAMI) is used strictly as defined by Crook et al. (1986a) and only designates phenomena meeting all the National Institute of Mental Health (NIMH) work group's diagnostic criteria. We also at times refer separately to the NIMH "psychometric criteria for AAMI." By these we mean the conditions set out in criteria c, d, and e, which define memory impairment but not the population eligible for diagnosis (see below). We also make a general distinction between "age-appropriate forgetfulness," implying a decline in memory from young adult levels (of which AAMI is a specific example), and "age-inappropriate forgetfulness," implying memory impairment in comparison with age peers. The distinction between age-appropriate and age-inappropriate forgetfulness was recently recognized by Blackford and La Rue (1989) in their definitions of *age-consistent memory impairment* (ACMI) and *late-life forgetfulness*

(LLF), the terms apparently being chosen for their similarity to those designating the similar constructs of AAMI and benign senescent forgetfulness, respectively, but we use their terms only to refer to phenomena meeting their specific diagnostic criteria. Finally, we use the general phrase *age-related memory decline* as an all embracing, vaguely defined term to refer to any and all changes in memory allegedly associated with aging.

Diagnostic Criteria for AAMI

The construct of AAMI was introduced by an NIMH work group (Crook et al. 1986a). It was the group's declared intention to facilitate communication and stimulate research into late-life memory loss, particularly its treatment, by introducing research diagnostic criteria, with the expectation that the criteria would be modified as research in the area developed. Modifications have indeed been suggested (Blackford and La Rue 1989; Rosen 1990; Smith et al. 1991), but have not yet been universally agreed on. The NIMH work group made a great contribution by providing a focus for discussion and emphasizing the importance of a detailed operational definition of the construct with which they were dealing. Their original criteria for AAMI are summarized as follows:

a. Age 50 years or over
b. Complaint of memory loss affecting everyday functioning with gradual onset
c. Memory test performance at least one standard deviation below the mean established for young adults on a standardized test of secondary memory with adequate normative data
d. Adequate intellectual function as determined by a scaled score of at least 9 on the Vocabulary subtest of the Wechsler Adult Intelligence Scale (WAIS; Wechsler 1955)
e. Absence of dementia as determined by a score of 24 or higher on the Mini-Mental State Exam (MMSE; Folstein et al. 1975)
f. Exclusion criteria including absence of a number of medical conditions, depression, risk factors for stroke, history of repeated minor or single major head injury, drug or alcohol abuse, or recent use of psychotropic medications that might affect cognitive function together with, in many cases, guidelines for determining whether these conditions were present

Also it should be noted that this definition of *age-associated memory impairment* differs from Kral's concept of *benign senescent forgetfulness* (Kral 1958) in several important respects. First, these criteria are attempting to capture a different phenomenon than that described by Kral, and the comparison group is different in the two cases. The AAMI criteria define *impairment* with respect to healthy young adult levels, not to those of the older individual's age peers as was implied in the description of benign senescent forgetfulness. Thus it would logically be possible for all older individuals to meet criteria for AAMI, by exhibiting poorer memory than young adults, without exhibiting benign senescent forgetfulness in the sense of poorer memory than would be expected of a healthy older individual. Conversely, except for those who failed the AAMI exclusion criteria (including at least 53% of Kral's original group), cases of benign senescent forgetfulness would generally meet criteria for AAMI unless the clinical evidence of forgetfulness was not substantiated by poor performance on standardized memory tests. In practice this is probably relatively infrequent if the judgment is based on a reasonably thorough clinical evaluation and not just subjective report of memory impairment. With these provisos, *benign senescent forgetfulness* can be regarded as a subset of *age-associated memory impairment,* but the terms are not equivalent.

Second, the term *age-associated memory impairment* is "non-specific with regard to etiology and does not necessarily imply that the disorder is non-progressive" (Crook et al. 1986a, pp. 269–170). Thus patients whose memory impairment is subsequently shown to be the earliest stage of a dementing illness are not necessarily excluded from the category of AAMI and it is sensible to ask how often AAMI is, in fact, a dementia prodrome. This also implies that AAMI is not necessarily to be regarded as nonpathological, although the lengthy and detailed exclusion criteria clearly indicate that Crook and his colleagues had an optimally healthy cohort in mind when they defined it.

Utility of the Construct of AAMI

The construct of AAMI can be criticized on several grounds. First, is the phenomenon it attempts to define—decline from presumed young adult levels rather than an age-inappropriate impairment of memory relative to older individuals' age peers—the appropriate one to define? Second, if so, do the proposed criteria actually capture it clearly? Third, is the term *age-associated memory impairment* appropriate, and should it be regarded as a diagnosis? Finally, although the specification of diagnostic criteria has undoubtedly helped clarify some issues, is a focus on classification and diagnosis the best way of investigating and describing the changes in memory associated with aging?

When we rate the memory of elderly people, should we compare it with the presumably better memory of young adults as Crook et al. (1986a) suggested, or should we compare older adults with each other to identify a subgroup with poorer memory more in the spirit of Kral's benign senescent forgetfulness? Both approaches are feasible and have their merits, but both have practical and theoretical disadvantages. Only the former approach can tell us whether the memories of older people are, in fact, worse than the memories of younger people. However, it is very difficult to be sure that the memory of a given older individual has changed over time without reference to test scores obtained from that individual in youth. Cross-sectional studies comparing older individuals' data with normative data collected from young people suffer from the obvious risk of cohort effects, as well as the more general problems involved in referencing performance to published norms based on populations whose demographics are incompletely specified or frankly different. Conversely, only the latter approach can tell us whether an individual has an abnormally poor memory given his or her age, but normative data on cognitive test performance in the old-old has, until recently, been virtually nonexistent, although some progress is being made in this regard. A number of studies from the Mayo Clinic, for example, promise to be very useful in the psychometric assessment of the elderly (Ivnik et al. 1992a, 1992b, 1992c).

As is often the case, the answer depends on what question one is interested in. Arguing for the "decline from young adult" model, Crook and Ferris (1992) pointed out that elderly people typically complain that their memories are worse than they used to be, not that their memories are worse than those of their age peers, and that the decline is sufficiently common and sufficiently severe to justify therapeutic trials, whether it is normal or not. They compared the situation to other conditions, such as presbyopia, which are "defined by reference to normative standards for young adults and . . . so common among the elderly as to be considered 'normal.' Nevertheless, few clinicians would compare the vision of an 80-year-old with norms established for other people of the same age and prescribe corrective lenses only to those whose visual performance falls outside those norms" (Crook and Ferris 1992, p. 714). If the primary purpose is to select subjects for trials of treatments for a potentially normal age-related decline in memory, the NIMH concept of AAMI is appropriate and the strict exclusion of other possible causes of memory impairment is necessary.

Alternative Approaches to Age-Related Memory Decline

On the other hand, if one is interested in defining a disease state, identifying a dementia prodrome, or performing clinical evaluation of the mass of elderly individuals who are referred for neuropsychological assessment, the "impaired relative to age peers" approach may be more appropriate or, at least, provide a useful additional conceptual framework. Several different ways of defining an age-inappropriate memory impairment have been proposed, and, where the evidence is available, these do seem to identify abnormal memory functioning, although whether the condition is benign has not been conclusively established. In this vein, Larrabee et al. (1986) identified individuals with "senescent forgetfulness" on the basis of memory test performance significantly worse than performance in other cognitive domains and significantly below an age-residualized mean (i.e., they conceptualized it as an age-atypical deficit specific to memory without necessarily implying change from a higher level earlier in life). Senescent forgetfulness defined in this way did not seem simply to be one end of a continuum of memory function because memory test performance in their sample was bimodally distributed, raising the possibility of some causative disease process. Larrabee and Crook (1989) also identified a subgroup of AAMI subjects whose performance on more ecologically valid, everyday memory tests was impaired relative to an age-residualized mean. In both studies, the prevalence of age-inappropriate memory impairment actually increased with increasing age suggesting that the pathological process involved, if any, is age related. Larrabee and Crook (1989) also pointed out that their age-residualized, cross-sectional data suggest that this form of memory impairment is not evenly distributed across the adult age range (i.e., those individuals who are shown to be abnormally forgetful after age 65 are not all likely to have been abnormally forgetful earlier in life).

Clinical Significance of Age-Inappropriate Forgetfulness

The value of the construct of an age-inappropriate, selective impairment of memory lies chiefly in its clinical significance, particularly whether it is a correlate of disease and whether it is truly benign or heralds an impending dementia. The evidence on this point is, as yet, inconclusive, although the topic clearly deserves further investigation. Larrabee et al. (1986), for example, failed to find any progression of memory deficit in their subjects with age-inappropriate "senescent forgetfulness" at 1-year follow-up, whereas Katzman et al. (1989) reported that 37% of the "functioning individuals with memory impairment (who) might well have been considered to have benign senescent forgetfulness" in their sample of elderly volunteers had dementia at 5-year follow-up. Further, O'Brien et al. (1992) reported an intermediate rate of progression to dementia of 8.8% in a group of 68 patients with benign senescent forgetfulness followed for an average of 3 years. However, they based the diagnosis of forgetfulness entirely on subjective report, specifically excluding subjects who showed objective evidence of memory impairment on psychological tests. This is a different construct from the senescent forgetfulness of Larrabee et al. (1986), which was objectively demonstrable, and highlights the importance of the use of comparable terms in diagnostic criteria.

Another important aspect of the concept of age-inappropriate forgetfulness advanced here and by Larrabee et al. (1986) is that memory should be selectively impaired, or at least disproportionately affected, in comparison with other cognitive functions. This is another difference from the NIMH concept of AAMI in which the memory impairment could be associated with age-related decline in other cognitive functionsm, provided that these were not sufficient to justify the diagnosis of dementia and did not substantially affect vocabulary test performance. The disproportionately severe impairment of memory in comparison with other cognitive functions may also distinguish the concept of age-inappropriate forgetfulness advanced here in principle, although possibly not in practice, from other concepts of "mild cognitive impairment not amounting to dementia" (World Health Organization 1978) or "questionable dementia" as used in the Clinical Dementia Rating Scale (Hughes et al. 1982) in which the preservation of nonmnemonic cognitive functions is either not required or only implied. On the whole, studies using these kinds of classifications seem to find rather higher rates of progression to dementia than those attempting to isolate senescent forgetfulness, although the line of demarcation is not well defined (Dawe et al. 1992). It is not certain for example, to what extent the baseline impairment in Katzman et al.'s subjects (1989) was specific to memory. Although Reisburg et al. (1986) found that the extent to which subjects deteriorated was dependent on initial degree of impairment (i.e., the more impaired subjects tending to show more deterioration), this was based on a global assignment of "magnitude of cognitive decline" rather than on an assessment of memory performance in comparison to other cognitive functions.

The essential difference between the two principal concepts of age-related memory decline discussed so far has been the standard against which memory is compared—the young or the healthy elderly. A third approach is to look for qualitative rather than quantitative differences between the memory of healthy older individuals and the other groups of interest. Generally, the memory of individuals with dementia is much worse than that of healthy elderly people, but not qualitatively different (Huppert, in press). However, Grober and colleagues (Grober and Buschke 1986; Grober et al. 1988) have suggested that a failure to benefit to the normal extent from semantic cuing may distinguish the memory impairment of dementia and this, rather than absolute score, may also be a way of identifying age-inappropriate memory impairment in individuals without dementia.

The significance of abnormal rates of forgetting (Cullum et al. 1990) and slow rates of learning (Petersen et al. 1992) have also been emphasized. Although such studies of qualitative aspects of memory in aging are important, we do not believe that they should be incorporated into the diagnostic criteria. The memory of individuals with AAMI may be qualitatively different from the memory of young adults, as well as quantitatively worse; however, the construct of AAMI is not defined by that difference.

To summarize, there are two distinct concepts of age-related memory decline and both are useful. The concept of a potentially normal age-related decline from young adult levels envisaged by the NIMH criteria for AAMI is appropriate for studies of normal aging and memory. On the other hand, the phenomenon of selective, age-inappropriate forgetfulness in elderly people does appear to exist (Larrabee et al. 1986), and this concept is likely to be more useful in clinical evaluations and research looking for the antecedents of dementia (Blackford and La Rue 1989; Smith et al. 1991).

Applicability of Current Diagnostic Criteria

There have been several criticisms of the NIMH criteria for AAMI (Bamford and Caine 1988; Blackford and La Rue 1989; Rosen 1990; Smith et al. 1991). Some of these criticisms are somewhat technical and may be overly strident, but the issue of precise diagnosis is so important that we review these criticisms here.

First, the criterion of memory test performance one standard deviation below the mean for young adults does not make adequate provision for individuals whose memory functioning as a young adult was substantially above or below average. Assuming a normal distribution of scores, about 16% of young adults will always have had memory test scores more than one standard deviation below the mean and will thus become eligible for the diagnosis of AAMI on attaining the age of 50 without having experienced any decline in their memory as they grew older. Conversely, individuals who initially enjoyed superior levels of memory functioning (e.g., more than one standard deviation above the mean) could experience a substantial decline in memory with aging (up to two standard deviation units) without meeting criteria for AAMI.

There is a similar problem with respect to the inclusion criterion of a Vocabulary subtest scaled score of at least 9 on the WAIS. A scaled score of 9 or above represents performance at or above a level corresponding to the 37th percentile of the reference group. If we consider the normative data for the updated WAIS-R rather than for the older WAIS, this corresponds to a raw score of at least 43, which, in turn, was almost exactly the median score of adults 70–74 years old in the normative sample. Thus about half of the elderly population are ineligible for the diagnosis of AAMI on the grounds that their general intellectual functioning may not be adequate. There seems to be no a priori reason for supposing that individuals whose general intellectual functioning is in the lower half of the average range should not experience age-related declines in memory. Although it may be prudent to ensure some minimal level of general intellectual functioning when selecting subjects for research studies, the current criterion seems overstrict, and results obtained with it may not be generalizable to individuals with even slightly below-average intelligence.

Blackford and La Rue (1989) have criticized the

Vocabulary subtest requirement as a way of estimating level of intellectual function on the grounds that it is an imperfect correlate of intelligence and have recommended full-scale IQ scores instead. These investigators also pointed out that preservation of vocabulary does not imply that deterioration has not taken place in other cognitive domains. However, as discussed above, the AAMI construct does not require that decline be specific to memory, provided that other cognitive changes are not sufficient to warrant a diagnosis of dementia. It is not, therefore, required that such changes be excluded.

A possible way of overcoming the problems inherent in the use of fixed cutoff scores to ensure adequacy of intellectual function and impairment of memory was suggested by Rosen (1990) and is in use in our laboratory. Vocabulary is moderately well correlated with memory test performance in young adults and relatively resistant to decline with age. To the extent that this is true, one can calculate expected memory test scores for young adults with different levels of intellectual functioning. Following the spirit, but not the letter, of the NIMH criteria one can then classify as "impaired" those older individuals whose observed memory test performance is at least one standard deviation below that expected for young adults of an equivalent intellectual level as reflected in their WAIS-R Vocabulary scores. This allows one to identify memory impairment in high-functioning individuals whose memories have declined below their presumably superior premorbid levels, but are not yet below average.

When we applied this modified criterion to define memory impairment in a sample of more than 600 community-resident elderly individuals in Pittsburgh, Pennsylvania, we found that twice as many people were classified as "impaired" as when the NIMH criteria were applied to the same sample (52% versus 26%). The difference was almost entirely attributable to the fact that we were able to identify impairment in individuals in the lower part of the range of intellectual functioning (who would have been ineligible by virtue of low Vocabulary subtest scores under the NIMH criteria) and in a higher proportion of individuals functioning at superior levels (who would have been classified as "unimpaired" by those criteria). Like other authors, we found that the prevalence of impairment increased with increasing age, consistent with an age-related change. Although this method of classification is associated with its own error, we believe that the error is less than that inherent in the use of uncorrected mean scores of young adults as a benchmark for impairment and that the group classified as "impaired" by the modified criterion is more representative of the population of memory-impaired elderly individuals. Note that the figures mentioned above are simply the proportions of elderly adults classified as "impaired" by the two sets of psychometric criteria without applying any exclusion criteria and without requiring subjective report of memory decline. They thus simply reflect the prevalence of age-related memory decline in our sample, not the prevalence of AAMI.

The third main criticism of the original NIMH criteria involves the requirement for complaints of memory loss affecting everyday life with gradual onset and without sudden worsening in recent months. Subjective report of memory impairment has been associated with depressed mood (Kahn et al. 1975; Popkin et al. 1982), neuroticism (Poitrenaud et al. 1989), age stereotypes of failing memory to which the complainant subscribes (Scogin et al. 1985; Zarit et al. 1981), and self-reported health status and number of functional limitations (Cutler and Grams 1988), as well as to actual memory impairment (Zelinski et al. 1980).

The frequency with which older individuals "complain" of memory problems is probably also crucially dependent on how the question is asked. Only about half of Cutler and Grams's 14,564 subjects (1988) reported trouble remembering things "frequently" or "sometimes" as opposed to "rarely" or "never," whereas Sunderland et al. (1986) reported a "universal belief" among their elderly subjects that their memories failed them more frequently "now" than "when age 30." Sunderland and colleagues did find evidence of age-related memory impairment on objective tests in their group, but the frequency of reported memory failures was related to performance on only a few of the memory tests and very few subjects regarded memory failures in everyday life as "even a minor handicap." Sunderland et al. (1986) also reported only moderate agreement between different subjective methods of memory assessment, and their questionnaire (although carefully designed and based on one that had been used effectively with younger individuals with memory impairment resulting from head injury and their families [Sunderland et al. 1983]) showed low test-retest reliability. Even though studies involving clinical samples show more relationship between complaint and performance than community-based studies and progress is being made in the design and selection of appropriate instruments (Zelinski and Gilewski

1988), these observations cast serious doubt on the validity of current methods of subjective memory assessment and suggest that subjective complaints should not be a necessary condition for the diagnosis of AAMI.

A counter argument is that individuals' subjective assessments of their own memories are important in themselves because perceived memory loss, rather than poor memory test performance, brings patients to a clinic. Further, laboratory memory tests may not themselves be good predictors of real-life memory function. Thus the failure to find correlations between subjective report of memory impairment and poor performance on standard memory tests may be attributable to the fact that laboratory memory test performance does not reflect the everyday memory abilities that are accurately reported by the subjects. In at least one study (Larrabee et al. 1991), good correlations were obtained between performance on a battery of computerized memory tests ingeniously designed to simulate everyday memory functions (Crook et al. 1986b) and responses to a subjective memory questionnaire with good psychometric properties (Crook and Larrabee 1990). Unlike many previous authors, Crook and Larrabee did not find that subjective memory complaint was related to depressed mood. Nevertheless, in spite of this result, subjective reports of memory impairment are currently so difficult to interpret that their place in the diagnostic criteria for AAMI should be questioned.

Differential Sensitivity of Memory Tests

Even if general diagnostic criteria are agreed, the differential sensitivity of different memory tests to aging indicates that the particular test used will determine the size of the population defined. Smith et al. (1991) found at least twice as many of their two groups of elderly subjects met NIMH psychometric criteria for AAMI when a less verbal memory test—Visual Reproduction from the Wechsler Memory Scale (Wechsler 1945) or WMS-R, rather than Logical Memory from the same tests—was used as the index of memory impairment. Even when two verbal tests with a different format (Logical Memory and the Rey Auditory Verbal Learning Test [RAVLT; Rey 1964]) were compared (Lezak 1983), the proportion of cases identified varied by a factor of more than 4 (20% to 96% in one group and 11% to 58% in the other). Similar results were reported by Raffaele et al. (1992) with classification rates varying from 22.7% for immediate Logical Memory to

53% for delayed Visual Reproduction. The general tendency is for more subjects to be classified as "impaired" by visuospatial tests than by verbal tests, by delayed recall than by immediate recall, and, at least within the verbal domain, by list learning tasks than by narrative recall. The difference in sensitivity appears to be attributable partly to the modality involved, but also to the psychometric properties (e.g., ceiling effects) of the tests themselves (Raffaele et al. 1992).

Blackford and La Rue (1989) addressed the issue of differential sensitivity of memory tests by requiring that the test battery include at least four memory tests and recommended a number of instruments from which the clinician may select. They defined three levels of impairment on the basis of such a battery: AAMI (performance at least 1 SD below the mean established for young adults on one or more tests); ACMI (performance within + 1 SD of the mean established for age on 75% or more of the tests administered); or LLF (performance between 1 and 2 SD below the mean established for age on 50% or more of the tests administered). Although this reduces the problem of differential sensitivity, it does not eliminate it, as studies using, for example, the four secondary memory tests from the WMS-R would still be expected to yield different rates of LLF than would those including a list learning task like the RAVLT.

A possible compromise is to use a composite score based on the weighted averages of scores on a group of individual tests (rather than looking at the percentage of tests on which performance falls below a certain level). The General Memory Index and Delayed Recall Index derived from the WMS-R are based on such weighted averages of four tests including both verbal and nonverbal material, and a composite score based on these tests is considerably more sensitive than each of the component tests individually (Smith et al. 1991). Though it may be premature to specify the particular tests that should be used in assessing age-related memory decline as Smith et al. (1991) suggested, the WMS-R meets some of the requirements and has the advantages that it is widely used and that normative data for the older old are becoming available.

Blackford and La Rue (1989) also suggested minor modifications to the AAMI exclusion criteria, tightening some, loosening some, and elaborating others. The medical exclusion criteria eliminate from consideration at least one-third to one-half of the community-resident elderly (Smith et al. 1991), and although this may be appropriate for some research purposes in which the exclusion of other possible causes of memory impairment is regarded as being of paramount importance, the criteria are likely to be overly restrictive for other purposes, excluding persons whose memories are unaffected by their medical conditions. An MMSE score of 24 is, at best, an approximate criterion by which to judge whether older individuals have dementia and can be expected to yield both false negatives and false positives. The standard will be harder to meet for older and less educated individuals who typically obtain lower MMSE scores (Holzer et al. 1984). If individuals over age 65 who may have MMSE scores below 24 (approximately 20% [Folstein et al. 1985]) are added to those whose Vocabulary subtest scores are below the specified level and the substantial proportion of older individuals who fail medical exclusion criteria, well under half of the community-resident elderly without dementia would be left. We agree with Blackford and La Rue that these exclusion criteria may be overstrict.

AAMI as a Diagnostic Entity

It was not the stated intention of the NIMH work group to imply that AAMI was a disease or that it was necessarily abnormal or that it had a known and defined pathological basis for which a diagnostic laboratory test might, in principle, be developed. Instead, as stated above, they proposed to introduce a "diagnostic term" (Crook et al. 1986a) and associated diagnostic criteria to facilitate communication and promote research, particularly into pharmacological treatment for the condition they defined. Nevertheless, a number of subsequent authors have objected to the term on the grounds that it does imply a clinical diagnosis, which in turn implies a disease although the phenomenon it demotes does not merit such a status (Bamford and Caine 1988; O'Brien and Levy 1992; Rosen 1990). Perhaps because of these kinds of criticism, future diagnostic systems such as DSM-IV (American Psychiatric Association 1994) are likely to modify the construct (Caine 1992), distinguishing between age-appropriate and age-inappropriate impairments on the one hand and between those associated with and independent of other systemic or central nervous system disease on the other.

Even if AAMI (or LLF or any other form of age-related memory decline) does constitute a diagnostic entity, one can ask whether the construct is appropriately named and whether it is likely to be useful. Just as the term *benign senescent forgetfulness* can be criticized because it is not clear that the implication of non-progression is necessarily justified, so the term *age-associated memory impairment* has been criticized because *impairment* connotes abnormality, which is not a necessary part of the AAMI construct (Smith et al. 1991). *Decline* or *loss*, which connote deterioration from a previously higher level but not abnormality, might be better. Ironically, the more descriptive and less evaluative term *forgetfulness* has been used in two contexts (*benign senescent forgetfulness* and *late-life forgetfulness*) in which abnormality is implicitly or explicitly involved.

Possible Biological Bases of Age-Related Memory Decline

A number of neuroanatomical and neurochemical changes are known or suspected to occur with aging, and some of these might plausibly be related to deterioration in memory. Modest age-related decreases are known to occur in the size of the mammillary bodies (Raz et al. 1992) and temporal lobe structures (Coffey et al. 1992). Both these brain areas are known to be involved in memory, and reduced hippocampal volume has been reported in amnesic patients (Press et al. 1989) and in patients with Alzheimer's disease (Kesslak et al. 1991; Seab et al. 1988), although Seab and colleagues did not find that the degree of atrophy was related to severity of memory impairment. White matter changes documented by computed tomography or magnetic resonance imaging are a frequent incidental finding in the elderly (Coffey et al. 1992). Whereas some authors have found that these are both more severe and related to severity of cognitive impairment in individuals with dementia, this is certainly not universally agreed to be the case (Kozachuk et al. 1990). Similarly, changes in cholinergic neurotransmitter systems are well documented in Alzheimer's disease and may also be found in normal aging (Morgan 1992). These changes have been suggested as a possible basis for AAMI (Bartus et al. 1982). Crook and Larrabee (1988) have reviewed other potential underpinnings of AAMI and recommended trials of pharmacotherapy on this basis.

These and other potential causes of AAMI deserve further study, but, to date, we are not aware of any empirical evidence that conclusively links age-related memory decline to specific neurochemical or anatomical changes. In the search for such evidence, it will be necessary to bear in mind the distinctions between age-appropriate and age-inappropriate forgetfulness and, consequently, to look for correlates in both successfully and unsuccessfully aging individuals.

Future Research Strategies

The availability of diagnostic criteria for AAMI should not thwart the pursuit of other goals for aging research or other approaches to the study of age-related memory decline. As discussed above, memory can be regarded as an emergent property of the human information-processing system, as well as a cognitive domain in which an individual may or may not exhibit impaired functioning. The information-processing system could be affected in a number of different ways, any or all of which could cause the individual to meet criteria for AAMI but have different theoretical, prognostic, and, possibly, therapeutic implications. A different kind of research focused on the processes involved in remembering is required to determine what age-related memory decline is, rather than simply whether it is present in a given individual.

We also need to supplement AAMI-oriented research with studies of aging individuals in which some form of psychometrically defined age-related memory decline is the independent variable and medical conditions, demographics, and subjective report are treated as dependent variables, rather than as exclusion criteria. Certainly, it is important to know what proportion of the community-resident elderly exhibit a decline in memory and, for those that do, what the typical causes or, at least, correlates of that decline are. As we have seen, the NIMH exclusion criteria render a large proportion of the population ineligible for the diagnosis of AAMI, and many of these individuals do not exhibit memory impairment in spite of the "threats to memory" (Smith et al. 1991) represented by the condition causing their ineligibility. Conversely, it is likely that some of the ineligible individuals who do exhibit memory impairment do so because of age-related changes, rather than because of their medical conditions. It is our impression that, in community samples, rather than patient groups, the adverse effect of medical and psychiatric illness on cognition is minimal. In our sample of community-resident elderly individuals (described above), we evaluated self-reported depressive symptomatology in the previous week using the Center for Epidemiological Studies Depression Scale (CES-D; Radloff 1977) and assessed memory using the WMS-R. Although there was a significant correlation between depression score and Delayed Recall weighted raw score, this accounted for less than 3% of the variance. Furthermore, individuals with CES-D scores exceeding a conventional cutoff score of 17, raising the possibility of clinically significant depression, were found only slightly more frequently among individuals meeting psychometric criteria for AAMI (11% compared to 7% of individuals not meeting these criteria).

Clinical Memory Assessment in the Elderly

The way in which the clinician investigates the memory of the elderly patient and the thoroughness of the assessment will depend on the purposes and circumstances of the evaluation. It is clear that the assessment must involve some form of objective memory test, rather than relying on subjective report. The minimum requirement for such a test is that it involve the delayed recall of recently presented information and be sufficiently difficult that it is not subject to a marked ceiling effect. The word list learning test used by the Consortium to Establish a Registry of Alzheimer's Disease (CERAD; Morris et al. 1989) meets these minimal requirements, but the three words from the MMSE (Folstein et al. 1975) do not, as the test is too easy to be sensitive to mild or even moderate memory impairment. Preferably, the test should also involve multitrial learning, as well as memory, providing a way of comparing the ability to encode, retain, and recall information (e.g., immediate and delayed recall trials); use both verbal and nonverbal material; and have norms for elderly individuals. A combination of measures is probably required if all these requirements are to be met adequately, and some suggestions were made by Blackford and La Rue (1989). A selection of memory tests was also reviewed by Lezak (1983) and by Spreen and Strauss (1991), and the subject was discussed more extensively in *Clinical Memory Assessment of Older Adults* by Poon (1986).

Although it is not ideal, our usual practice in routine memory assessments is to use the WMS-R. As noted above, the WMS-R goes some way to overcoming the problem of differential sensitivity of different tests by providing summary scores based on the weighted averages of four subtests involving immediate and delayed recall of verbal and nonverbal material. It is true that the more age-sensitive list-learning type of task is underrepresented in these weighted averages, but this is partially compensated by fact that the Logical Mem-

ory subtest (recall of short passages of prose, similar to news items) weighs heavily and is one of the more ecologically valid memory tests in common clinical use (Sunderland et al. 1983). If prediction of everyday memory function is crucial, however, it would be more appropriate to use the Rivermead Behavioral Memory Test (Wilson et al. 1985) or a research instrument of the kind described by Crook et al. (1986b). The WMS-R also allows one to compare verbal and nonverbal memory, although the tests are not terribly well matched. Norms for the older old are now available (Ivnik et al. 1992b).

Summary scores should be used with caution, because information is lost and important discrepancies between individual component scores can be concealed. Nevertheless, they can be convenient and, when one is required, we favor the Delayed Recall weighted raw score over the Immediate Recall weighted raw score because it incorporates a delay and can be expected to be more sensitive to memory impairment in general and age-related memory decline in particular. We prefer the weighted raw scores in some circumstances to the indexes, which can be derived from them, because the former are not age corrected so that an individual's scores can be compared with other individuals of any age.

Finally, we usually use the delayed recall scores rather than a forgetting score calculated by subtracting delayed from immediate recall because we believe that, in most populations, it will be more sensitive to memory impairment without sacrificing specificity to an unacceptable degree. The rationale is as follows: Whatever aspect of memory is involved (encoding, retrieval, rate of forgetting, and so on), delayed recall will be affected. It is true that other disorders (e.g., aphasia) may cause low delayed recall scores by impairing the ability to process the information to be remembered. They can then masquerade as memory impairments, a state of affairs that could be avoided by use of an immediate-recall-minus-delayed-recall criterion that would reveal that the information had not been encoded into memory at the outset. However, as the memoranda on the WMS-R and most other standardized memory tests exceed memory span, moderate memory impairments may affect immediate, as well as delayed, recall and therefore would not be fully reflected in an immediate-recall-minus-delayed-recall measure of forgetting. In community-resident populations, the incidence of false negatives of this kind is likely to exceed the incidence of false positives secondary to inability to adequately process the stimulus material. Further, in clinical evaluations one should never consider any test score in isolation, always remembering that any test, however well designed, can be failed for multiple reasons. When false negatives do occur, there will usually be independent evidence of the responsible disorder to help the clinician interpret the results.

The assessment of memory in the elderly, like neuropsychological evaluation in all other circumstances, therefore involves weighing an individual's current memory function against the level that would be expected for that individual on the basis of age, education, and level of intellectual functioning and against his or her functioning in other cognitive domains. As we acquire more data on the natural history of aging and memory and learn more about the significance of age-inappropriate forgetfulness, we will be better able to set the balance and interpret the results.

Summary and Conclusions

To what extent does our research and review of the recent literature enable us to amplify or modify the generalizations with which we began this chapter? First, the recent evidence, spurred by the provision of psychometric criteria for AAMI, confirms that memory test performance is typically poorer in the elderly than in the young. Age affects delayed recall more than immediate recall, and visuospatial material is typically less well recalled than verbal material. Accordingly, estimates of the prevalence of AAMI vary widely depending on which kind of material and what form of test is used. Our view is that the great majority of elderly people are affected to some degree, but that the decline only reaches significant proportions in a subset, the size of which varies widely depending on the criteria used, and is only perceived as a significant problem by a small minority.

Second, there is sufficient evidence to justify distinguishing age-appropriate and age-inappropriate forms (or levels) of age-related memory decline. The former, of which AAMI is an example, represents a normal age-related phenomenon whereas the latter, the true descendent of benign senescent forgetfulness, is by definition abnormal and, possibly, pathological. Whether age-inappropriate forgetfulness is progressive, whether it can be distinguished from other concepts of mild cognitive decline by virtue of being

specific to memory, and whether it is qualitatively different from normal memory or merely worse is not yet certain. The prevalence of age-inappropriate forgetfulness is also undetermined, but it is certainly less common than the age-appropriate form.

Completely satisfactory diagnostic criteria do not yet exist for AAMI or any other concept of age-related decline in spite of valiant efforts (Blackford and La Rue 1989; Crook et al. 1986a). Improved criteria would take an individual's overall level of intellectual functioning or educational background into account when setting the standard against which to rate memory, distinguish age-appropriate from age-inappropriate decline, make reference to the selectivity of memory impairment, modify the requirement for subjective complaint, and recognize the possibility of a number of comorbidities, rather than impose rigid exclusion criteria. The last might be achieved by assigning a level of probability to the diagnosis much as in the research diagnostic criteria for Alzheimer's disease of the National Institute of Nervous and Communicative Disorders and Stroke and the Alzheimer's Disease and Related Disorders Association (McKhann et al. 1984). Because of the varying sensitivities of different memory tests, it may also be necessary to specify the characteristics of suitable tests, if not actually require that specific, named tests be used.

References

American Psychiatric Association: Diagnostic and Statistical Manual of Mental Disorders, 4th Edition. Washington, DC, American Psychiatric Association, 1994

Baddeley AD: Working Memory. Oxford, England, Clarendon Press, 1986

Bamford KA, Caine ED: Does "benign senescent forgetfulness" exist? Clin Geriatr Med 4:897–916, 1988

Bartus RT, Dean RL, Beer B, et al: The cholinergic hypothesis of geriatric memory dysfunction. Science 217:408–417, 1982

Blackford RC, La Rue A: Criteria for diagnosing age associated memory impairment: proposed improvements from the field. Developmental Neuropsychology 5:295–306, 1989

Bromley DB: Some effects of age on short-term learning and memory. J Gerontol 13:398–406, 1958

Caine ED: Nomenclature and diagnosis of cognitive disorders: a US perspective. Abstract presented at Age Related Cognitive Disorders Conference, Nice, France, June 1992

Caine DB, Eisen A, Meneilly G: Normal aging of the nervous system. Ann Neurol 30:206–207, 1991

Cattell RB: Theory of fluid and crystallized intelligence. Journal of Educational Psychology 54:1–22, 1963

Coffey CE, Wilkinson WE, Parashos IA, et al: Quantitative cerebral anatomy of the aging human brain: a cross-sectional study using magnetic resonance imaging. Neurology 42:527–536, 1992

Craik FIM: Age differences in human memory, in Handbook of the Psychology of Aging. Edited by Birren JE, Schaie KW. New York, Van Nostrand Reinhold, 1977, pp 384–414

Craik FIM: Changes in memory with normal aging: a functional view, in Alzheimer's Disease (Advances in Neurology Series, Vol 51). Edited by Wurtman RJ, Corkin S, Growdon JH, et al. New York, Raven, 1990, pp 202–205

Craik FIM: Memory functions in normal aging, in Memory Disorders: Research and Clinical Practice. Edited by Yanagihara T, Petersen RC. New York, Marcel Dekker, 1991, pp 347–367

Crook TH, Ferris SH: Age associated memory impairment (letter). BMJ 304:714, 1992

Crook TH, Larrabee GJ: Age associated memory impairment: diagnostic criteria and treatment strategies. Psychopharmacol Bull 24:509–514, 1988

Crook TH, Larrabee GJ: A self rating scale for evaluating memory in everyday life. Psychol Aging 5:48–57, 1990

Crook TH, Bartus RT, Ferris SH, et al: Age-associated memory impairment: proposed diagnostic criteria and measures of clinical change-report of a National Institute of Mental Health work group. Developmental Neuropsychology 2:261–276, 1986a

Crook TH, Salama M, Gobert J: A computerized test battery for detecting and assessing memory disorders, in Senile Dementias: Early Detection. Edited by Bes A, Cahn J, Hayer S, et al. London-Paris, John Libby Eurotext, 1986b, pp 79–85

Cullum CM, Butters N, Troster AI, et al: Normal aging and forgetting rates on the Wechsler Memory Scale–Revised. Archives of Clinical Neuropsychology 5:22–30, 1990

Cutler SJ, Grams AE: Correlates of self-reported everyday memory problems. J Gerontol 43:S82–90, 1988

Dawe B, Procter A, Philpot M: Concepts of mild memory impairment in the elderly and their relationship to dementia: a review. International Journal of Geriatric Psychiatry 7:473–479, 1992

Dobbs AR, Rule BG: Adult age differences in working memory. Psychol Aging 4:500–503, 1989

Folstein MF, Folstein SE, McHugh PR: Mini-Mental State: a practical method of grading the cognitive state of patients. Psychiatr Res 12:189–198, 1975

Folstein MF, Anthony JC, Parhad I, et al: The meaning of cognitive impairment in the elderly. J Am Geriatr Soc 33:228–235, 1985

Grober E, Buschke H: Genuine memory deficits in dementia. Developmental Neuropsychology 3:13–36, 1986

Grober E, Buschke H, Crystal H, et al: Screening for dementia by memory testing. Neurology 388:900–903, 1988

Holzer CE, Tischler GL, Leaf PJ, et al: An epidemiological assessment of cognitive impairment in a community population, in Research in Community and Mental Health. Edited by Greenley JR. London, JAL Press, 1984, pp 3–32

Hughes CP, Berg L, Danziger WL, et al: A new scale for the staging of dementia. Br J Psychiatry 140:566–572, 1982

Huppert FA: Memory function in dementia and normal ageing: dimension or dichotomy, in Dementia and Normal Ageing. Edited by Huppert FA, Brayne C, O'Connor D. Cambridge, England, Cambridge University Press (in press)

Ivnik RJ, Malec JF, Smith GE, et al: Mayo's older Americans normative studies: WAIS-R norms for ages 56–97. Clinical Neuropsychologist 6:1–30, 1992a

Ivnik RJ, Malec JF, Smith GE, et al: Mayo's older Americans normative studies: WMS-R norms for ages 56–94. Clinical Neuropsychologist 6:49–82, 1992b

Ivnik RJ, Malec JF, Smith GE, et al: Mayo's older Americans normative studies: updated AVLT norms for ages 56–97. Clinical Neuropsychologist 6:83–104, 1992c

Kahn RL, Zaret SH, Hilbert NM, et al: Memory complaint and impairment in the aged. Arch Gen Psychiatry 32:1569–1573, 1975

Kaszniak AW, Poon LW, Riege W: Assessing memory deficits: an information processing approach, in Clinical Memory Assessment of Older Adults. Edited by Poon LW. Washington DC, American Psychological Association, 1986, pp 168–188

Katzman R, Aronson M, Fuld P, et al: Development of dementing illness in an 80-year-old volunteer cohort. Ann Neurol 25:317–324, 1989

Kesslak JP, Nalcioglu O, Cotman CW: Quantification of magnetic resonance scans for hippocampal and parahippocampal atrophy in Alzheimer's disease. Neurology 41:51–54, 1991

Koss E, Haxby JV, DeCarli C, et al: Patterns of performance preservation and loss in healthy aging. Developmental Neuropsychology 7:99–113, 1991

Kozachuck WE, DeCarli C, Schapiro MB, et al: White matter hyperintensities in dementia of Alzheimer's type and in healthy subjects without cerebrovascular risk factors. Arch Neurol 47:1306–1310, 1990

Kral VA: Neuropsychiatric observations in an old people's home. J Gerontol 13:169–176, 1958

Kral VA: Senescent forgetfulness: benign and malignant. Journal of the Canadian Medical Association 86:257–260, 1962

Kral VA, Cahn C, Mueller H: Senescent memory impairment and its relation to the general health of the aging individual. J Am Geriatr Soc 12:101–113, 1964

Larrabee GJ, Crook TH: Performance subtypes of everyday memory function. Developmental Neuropsychology 5:267–283, 1989

Larrabee GL, Levin HA, High WM: Senescent forgetfulness: a quantitative study. Developmental Neuropsychology 2:373–385, 1986

Larrabee GJ, West RL, Crook TH: The association of memory complaint with computer-simulated everyday memory performance. J Clin Exp Neuropsychol 13:466–478, 1991

Lezak MD: Neuropsychological Assessment, 2nd Edition. New York, Oxford University Press, 1983

McKhann G, Drachman D, Folstein M, et al: Clinical diagnosis of Alzheimer's disease: a Report of the NINCDS-ADRDA work group under the auspices of the Department of Health and Human Services Task Force on Alzheimer's Disease. Neurology 34:939–944, 1984

Morgan DG: Neurochemical changes with aging: predisposition toward age-related mental disorders, in Handbook of Mental Health and Aging, 2nd Edition. Edited by Birren JE, Sloane RB, Cohen GD. New York, Academic Press, 1992, pp 174–199

Morris JC, Heyman A, Mohs RC, et al: The consortium to establish a registry for Alzheimer's disease (CERAD), part I: clinical and neuropsychological assessment of Alzheimer's disease. Neurology 39:1159–1165, 1989

O'Brien JT, Levy R: Age associated memory impairment. BMJ 304:5–6, 1992

O'Brien JT, Beats B, Hill K, et al: Do subjective memory complaints precede dementia? a three-year follow-up of patients with supposed benign senescent forgetfulness. International Journal of Geriatric Psychiatry 7:481–486, 1992

Perlmutter M, Adams C, Berry J, et al: Aging and memory, in Annual Review of Gerontology and Geriatrics, Vol 8. Edited by Schaie KW, Eisdorfer C. New York, Springer, 1987, pp 57–92

Petersen RC, Smith G, Kokmen E, et al: Memory function in normal aging. Neurology 42:396–401, 1992

Poitrenaud J, Malbezin M, Guez D: Self-rating and psychometric assessment of age-related changes in memory among young-elderly managers. Developmental Neuropsychology 5:285–294, 1989

Popkin SJ, Gallagher D, Thompson LW, et al: Memory complaint and performance in normal and depressed older adults. Exp Aging Res 8:141–145, 1982

Poon LW: Differences in human memory with aging: nature causes and clinical implications, in Handbook of the Psychology of Aging, 2nd Edition. Edited by Birren JE, Schaie KW. New York, Van Nostrand Reinhold, 1985, pp 427–462

Poon LW: Clinical Memory Assessment of Older Adults. Washington DC, American Psychological Association, 1986

Press GA, Amaral DG, Squire LR: Hippocampal abnormalities in amnesic patients revealed by high-resolution magnetic resonance imaging. Nature 341:54–57, 1989

Radloff LS: The CES-D Scale: a self-report depression scale for research in the general population. Applied Psychological Measurement 1:385–401, 1977

Raffaele KC, Haxby JV, Schapiro MB: Age-associated memory impairment, in Treatment of Age-Related Cognitive Dysfunction: Pharmacological and Clinical Evaluation. Edited by Racagni G, Medlewicz J. Basel, Switzerland, Karger, 1992, pp 69–79

Raz N, Torres IJ, Acker JD: Age-related shrinkage of the mammillary bodies: in vivo MRI evidence. Neuroreport 3:713–716, 1992

Reisberg B, Ferris SH, Franssen E, et al: Age associated memory impairment: the clinical syndrome. Developmental Neuropsychology 2:401–402, 1986

Rey A: L'examen clinique en psychologie (Clinical examinations in psychology). Paris, Presses Universitaires de France, 1964

Rosen TJ: Age-associated memory impairment: a critique. European Journal of Cognitive Psychology 2:275–287, 1990

Rowe JW, Kahn RL: Human aging: usual and successful. Science 237:143–149, 1987

Salthouse TA, Mitchell RP, Palman R: Memory and age differences in spatial manipulation ability. Psychol Aging 4:480–486, 1989

Salthouse TA, Babcock RL, Shaw RJ: Effects of adult age on structural and operational capacities in working memory. Psychol Aging 118–127, 1991

Schacter DL, Kaszniak AW, Kihlstrom JF: Models of memory and the understanding of memory disorders, in Memory Disorders: Research and Clinical Practice. Edited by Yanagihara T, Petersen RC. New York, Marcel Dekker, 1991, pp 111–134

Scogin F, Storandt M, Lott L: Memory skills training, memory complaints and depression in older adults. J Gerontol 40:562–568, 1985

Seab JP, Jagust WJ, Wong ST, et al: Quantitative NMR measurements of hippocampal atrophy in Alzheimer's disease. Magn Reson Med 8:200–208, 1988

Smith G, Ivnik RJ, Petersen RC, et al: Age-associated memory impairment diagnoses: problems of reliability and concerns for terminology. Psychol Aging 6:551–558, 1991

Spreen O, Strauss E: A compendium of neuropsychological tests. New York, Oxford University Press, 1991

Sunderland A, Harris JE, Baddeley AD: Do laboratory tests predict everyday memory? a neuropsychological study. Journal of Verbal Learning and Verbal Behavior 22:341–357, 1983

Sunderland A, Watts K, Baddeley AD, et al: Subjective memory assessment and test performance in elderly adults. J Gerontol 41:376–384, 1986

Wechsler D: A standardized memory scale for clinical use. J Psychol 19:87–95, 1945

Wechsler D: Wechsler Adult Intelligence Scale. New York, Psychological Corporation, 1955

Wechsler D: Wechsler Adult Intelligence Scale–Revised Manual. New York, Psychological Corporation, 1981

Wechsler D: Wechsler Memory Scale–Revised Manual. San Antonio, TX, Psychological Corporation, 1987

Wilson B, Cockburn J, Baddeley A: The Rivermead behavioural memory test. Reading, England, Thames Valley Test Company, 1985

World Health Organisation: Mental Disorders: Glossary and Guide to their Classification in Accordance with the Ninth Revision of the International Classification of Diseases. Geneva, World Health Organization, 1978

Zarit SH, Cole KD, Guider RL: Memory training strategies and subjective complaints of memory in the aged. Gerontologist 21:158–164, 1981

Zelinski EM, Gilewski MJ: Assessment of memory complaint by rating scales and questionnaires. Psychopharmacol Bull 24:523–529, 1988

Zelinski EM, Gilewski MJ, Thompson LW: Do laboratory tests relate to self assessment of memory ability in the young and old? in New Directions in Memory and Aging: Proceedings of the George A. Talland Memorial Conference. Edited by Poon LW, Fozard JL, Cermak LS, et al. Hillsdale, NJ, Lawrence Erlbaum, 1980, pp 519–544

9

Anatomic Imaging of the Aging Human Brain: Computed Tomography and Magnetic Resonance Imaging

C. Edward Coffey, M.D.

Introduction

Aging is a relatively recent phenomenon in humans. For most of human history, life expectancy was remarkably stable at about 30–40 years (Cutler 1976, 1979). Within the past 150 years, however, advances in medical science (particularly the successful treatment of infectious diseases) have resulted in a dramatic increase in life span, so that men and women born in 1980 can now expect to live for an average 70.0 and 77.5 years, respectively (Rowe and Katzman 1992). As such, the elderly segment of our population is growing; the number of persons 65 years old or older increased eightfold from 1900 (3 million) to 1980 (25 million), and the number of those over age 75 (the so-called old old) has increased elevenfold during that same time period (from 900,000 to 10,000,000) (McFarland 1978).

The continued expansion of the elderly segment of our population and a growing awareness of age-related diseases such as dementia have prompted considerable interest in the study of the aging human brain. Central to this study have been efforts to characterize the spectrum and extent of changes in brain morphology that occur with "normal aging." Such normative data are essential for an understanding of "pathological" brain aging in elderly people (Creasey and Rapoport 1985; DeCarli et al. 1990; Drayer 1988).

Investigations of age-related changes in brain morphology have used two approaches: autopsy studies and brain imaging techniques. Autopsy studies have found consistent age-related reductions in brain weight, brain volume, cortical volume, and regional cortical neuronal number (Creasey and Rapoport 1985; Katzman and Terry 1992; see also Chapter 3). Ventricular dilatation has also been reported, and the variance of measurements of ventricular size appears to increase with age. However, neuropathological measures of brain morphology are subject to sources of error such as selection bias, technical and fixation artifacts, and the influences of premorbid illness and cause of death (which may be different for young versus elderly cohorts). Brain imaging techniques avoid many of these problems and provide an opportunity to examine brain morphology in healthy living subjects, albeit with limited anatomic resolution.

In this chapter, I review imaging studies that have examined the effects of aging on brain anatomy. I begin with a discussion of methodological issues relevant to such investigations, then summarize findings regarding the effects of age on brain ventricular and parenchymal structures. Further, I discuss the potential relationship of these structural brain alterations to age-related changes in cognitive function.

Methodological Issues Relevant to the Imaging Assessment of Age-Related Changes in Brain Structure

Study Design

Imaging studies of brain aging can be designed as either cross-sectional or longitudinal investigations. In cross-sectional studies, a single imaging evaluation is performed at roughly the same time on a group of subjects whose ages differ across a range of interest. Such studies allow for relatively rapid, efficient, and economical acquisition of large amounts of data, and it is not surprising therefore that most investigations to date have used a cross-sectional design. However, cross-sectional studies may be influenced by secular effects (i.e., the possibility that brain size exhibits systematic changes over successive birth cohorts in the general population). For example, successive generations may have, on average, larger parenchymal volumes and smaller ventricular volumes. If such trends actually exist in the population at large and if they are not secondary to secular trends associated with correlates of brain morphology such as cranial size or years of education, an assessment of the true effects of aging on brain size will require longitudinal investigation.

In longitudinal studies, imaging evaluations are repeated on the same group of subjects as they age over time. Such studies are thus free of secular effects, but they are very labor intensive and may suffer from significant attrition effects (i.e., subject dropout may result in a sample at the end of the investigation that is markedly different from that at the beginning). Longitudinal studies may also outlive their usefulness (the period effect); for example, an ongoing study of ventricular size that began in the era of pneumoencephalography would not be of great interest in today's world

Supported in part by Grant MH-41803 from the National Institute of Mental Health, Bethesda, Maryland, and by the Neurosciences Research Center, Medical College of Pennsylvania, Allegheny Campus, Pittsburgh, Pennsylvania.

of high-resolution computed tomography (CT) and magnetic resonance imaging (MRI).

The interpretation of both cross-sectional and longitudinal investigations must also consider the possible influences of "survivor effects" and heterogeneity within the elderly population (Creasey and Rapoport 1985). *Survivor effect* refers to the overrepresentation in study samples of relatively healthy subjects (the survivors) because others with preexisting illnesses may have died before study entry. Relative to younger populations, the elderly exhibit greater heterogeneity in a variety of physiological variables that could indirectly influence brain structure. Both cross-sectional and longitudinal study designs have strengths and limitations: the choice of one approach over the other will depend on available resources and the specific aims of the investigation.

Subject Selection

Brain morphology may be affected by variables in the subject sample that are associated with the aging process (e.g., concomitant medical illnesses), as well as by other variables that are relatively independent of it (e.g., gender, body or head size, handedness, education, socioeconomic status, and psychiatric and drug-use history). These variables must be considered and appropriately controlled before conclusions can be reached about the effects of aging, per se, on brain anatomy. It should also be noted that the apparent effects of age on brain structure may vary depending on the age range of the sample studied. In general, aging effects have been less robust when subjects have been selected from restricted age ranges (Appendixes 9–1, 9–2, and 9–3).

Subject sample. Selection of an appropriate subject sample is obviously a critically important first step in any investigation of aging effects on brain morphology. A sample of healthy volunteers from the community may differ markedly from a sample of medical or psychiatric *patients* with "normal" scans. Although the latter samples provide a convenient and economical source of readily available imaging data, such samples may include individuals with structural brain changes due to causes other than aging. In addition, patient samples are generally less representative of the variability in brain morphology that exists within samples of healthy volunteers. As noted above, such heterogeneity is especially great among the elderly, a finding that may

be related in part to differences between "usual aging" (i.e., no clinically obvious brain disease) and "successful aging" (i.e., minimal decline in neurobiological function in comparison to younger subjects) (Rowe and Kahn 1987).

Thus even within studies that examine healthy community volunteers, considerable variability in brain morphology may exist depending on the relative mix of subjects with usual versus successful aging. Whenever possible, studies should attempt to define the extent to which their subjects fall within these two categories, based in part on thorough medical, neuropsychiatric, and neuropsychological evaluations, as well as on correlative assessments of brain function (e.g., with electroencephalography [EEG], single photon emission computed tomography [SPECT], or positron-emission tomography [PET]). In this chapter, I review only studies that have examined healthy community volunteers.

Gender and body size. Women are smaller (i.e., shorter and lighter) on average than men, and as such their heads and brains also tend to be smaller (Gould 1981). Even within a single-sex study, however, differences in body or head size among subjects may confound apparent age-related differences. Although there is no generally accepted method of correcting for head or body size, this variable may be taken into account either through subject matching (e.g., on height), statistical analysis (e.g., analysis of covariance), or the use of ratio measures (e.g., using intracranial or total brain size as the denominator) (Appendixes 9–1, 9–2, and 9–3).

Handedness. Several studies have demonstrated differences in regional brain size or symmetry between right-handed and left-handed (or non–right-handed) individuals (Kertesz et al. 1992; Witelson 1992). Surprisingly, only a few investigations of the aging brain have specified the handedness of their subjects (Appendixes 9–1, 9–2, and 9–3). This variable should be assessed with continuous quantitative measures (Coffey et al. 1992), and its effects on brain structure should be controlled either statistically or through subject inclusion criteria (e.g., limiting the sample to those subjects with definite motoric lateralization).

Education and socioeconomic status. Recent imaging studies have reported a relationship between brain structure and educational level or socioeconomic class (Andreasen et al. 1990; Pearlson et al. 1989a). This relationship may be an indirect one, however, with both of these variables (and perhaps also IQ) serving as markers for body or head size (Pfefferbaum et al. 1990). Studies of brain aging should assess the potential impact of these variables statistically (Coffey et al. 1992) or attempt to control them through subject matching procedures when appropriate (Pfefferbaum et al. 1990).

Psychiatric and drug use history. Alterations of brain morphology have been described in patients with a variety of psychiatric disorders, including schizophrenia (Pfefferbaum et al. 1990), affective illness (Coffey et al. 1990, 1993), and eating disorders (Laessle et al. 1989). Although some earlier studies failed to specify the psychiatric histories of their subjects, more recent investigations have appropriately excluded patients with such histories (Appendixes 9–1, 9–2, and 9–3). Alcohol and perhaps other drug use may also alter brain structure (Cascella et al. 1991; Lishman 1990), but again studies have varied in the extent to which these factors have been considered (Appendixes 9–1, 9–2, and 9–3). Although more recent investigations of brain aging have generally excluded subjects with substance abuse or dependence, the effects of subclinical drug or alcohol consumption on structural brain aging have not been thoroughly assessed. One major impediment to such efforts has been the inability to obtain reliable and accurate data about the extent of drug use.

Imaging Technique

Imaging modality. Early imaging modalities provided only indirect visualization of the human brain by imaging either the skull (skull radiography), the cerebral vessels (arteriography), or the cerebrospinal fluid (CSF) spaces (pneumoencephalography). More recent developments in computer technology have now made possible in vivo visualization of brain tissue with imaging techniques such as CT and MRI. These techniques differ in their safety, anatomic resolution, and sensitivity to tissue contrast.

X-ray CT images are formed when X rays are passed through the brain from several different directions. Detectors opposite the X-ray source measure the extent to which passage of the X-ray beams has been attenuated by the intervening tissues. Computers relate this information to the density of the various structures (e.g., CSF, bone, gray matter, and white matter) and

then construct a series of tomographic images of the brain and cranium.

X-ray CT is a relatively quick and inexpensive imaging modality, but because subjects are exposed to irradiation (about 2 rad), serial studies in healthy individuals may not be possible. The method is also limited by relatively low spatial and anatomic resolution, partial volume effects (inaccurate averaging of tissue attenuation values), and beam-hardening artifact (false elevation of brain CT values adjacent to the skull). This latter problem limits the precision with which boundaries can be determined for structures adjacent to bone (e.g., the temporal lobes, the apical cortex, or the inferior frontal lobes).

MRI images are formed when the alignment of ions (in medical imaging these are typically protons) in a strong magnetic field is disrupted by a brief radiofrequency pulse. When the pulse is terminated, radiofrequency energy is emitted as the protons become realigned within the magnetic field. Computers relate this emitted radiofrequency energy to various tissue (proton) characteristics, from which a series of planar or three-dimensional images can be constructed. Various imaging sequences may be used to examine different tissue characteristics, resulting in images that are relatively T1- or T2-weighted. In general, T1-weighted images provide greater anatomic resolution, whereas T2-weighted images provide higher contrast and greater sensitivity to pathological tissue changes.

Relative to CT, MRI provides more accurate structural information because of clear differentiation of gray matter, white matter, and CSF; the absence of beam-hardening artifact; and the capability to image in multiple planes, thereby providing optimal views of regional cerebral structures with less volume-averaging artifact (see below). Additionally, MRI has greater sensitivity to detect pathological tissue, particularly hyperintense foci of the subcortical white matter and gray matter nuclei (subcortical hyperintensity) that occur with increasing frequency in elderly people (Coffey and Figiel 1991). Because MRI does not use ionizing radiation, serial studies in healthy subjects are possible.

For these reasons, MRI appears to be uniquely suited to the study of age-related changes in brain morphology. It should be noted however, that accurate assessment of brain structure with MRI may be affected by a number of technical factors, including choice of acquisition sequence parameters (affecting tissue contrast), slice section thickness (adjacent sections that are too thin may result in overlapping profiles and "cross talk" artifact), and magnetic field homogeneity (inhomogeneous fields may result in spatial distortion of objects and object pixel nonuniformity) (Jack et al. 1988). Movement artifact may also be induced by pulsation of blood and CSF, especially in the limbic system where structures lie in close proximity to the ventricles and the carotid arteries—such artifact can be lessened with the use of cardiac-gating and flow-compensated pulse sequences (Pfefferbaum et al. 1990). Careful consideration of these methodological issues is needed to ensure precision of measurement with MRI. Finally, MRI is a more expensive and often more lengthy procedure than CT, and some subjects may be unable to cooperate with the long imaging time, especially if they feel confined by the scanner and develop claustrophobia. In addition, MRI cannot be used in subjects who have a pacemaker or intracranial metallic objects such as surgical clips. Irrespective of whether CT or MRI is employed, the quality of the images collected may be affected by several factors.

Plane of imaging.   The optimal orientation from which to visualize brain anatomy will vary depending on the structure of interest. For example, corpus callosum and medial prefrontal cortex are best seen on midsagittal images, axial images provide a good view of subcortical white matter and gray nuclei (i.e., thalamus and basal ganglia), and coronal sections are required for optimal views of the temporal lobes and limbic structures. With brain CT, the plane of imaging is limited by the patient's position in the scanner: because typically the patient is supine, axial images are produced. With MRI, the plane of imaging can be determined simply by programming the magnetic gradients, making possible images in the coronal, axial, and sagittal planes, irrespective of patient positioning within the scanner.

Once the appropriate imaging plane has been selected, the images must be acquired in a standardized orientation so that valid comparisons across subjects are possible. Proper alignment of acquisition plane is especially critical for studies of brain asymmetry because head tilt can result in artifactual right-left differences. External landmarks (e.g., the canthomeatal line) are relatively quick and easy to establish for orientation, but they may not be consistently related to brain structure (Homan et al. 1987). Such problems may be obviated by use of internal landmarks (e.g., the anterior commissure–posterior commissure line), but

these can be more difficult technically and thus may add to the length of the scanning procedure.

Slice thickness.   Image resolution is affected by section thickness, as each image data point (voxel) in the slice represents an average of slice thickness (mm) raised to the third power. Thus the thinner the section, the higher the resolution. However, with thin sections a greater total scanning time is required to image a given volume, and thin sections are also associated with a reduced signal-to-noise ratio (there is less tissue to produce a signal). Furthermore, slice thickness with MRI is limited by certain technical factors including gradient strength, quantity of radiofrequency energy used for excitation, and the phenomenon of cross-talk artifact. This latter problem can be partially obviated by leaving space between adjacent sections (interscan gap), but this method excludes a given portion of tissue from direct assessment, thereby reducing the accuracy of volume measurements (particularly of small or irregular structures). Section interleaving is another method for reducing cross-talk artifact, but this procedure doubles scanning time.

Phantom calibration.   Verification of the accuracy of imaging data against a known standard (phantom) should be conducted on a regular basis to ensure stability of the imaging hardware. With MRI in particular, image data may be affected by variations in the main magnetic field, the magnetic field gradient systems, and the radiofrequency pulse system.

Head movement artifact.   Involuntary head movement by subjects is another source of artifact that can degrade image quality. Head movement is more likely as the length of the scanning time increases, and it may be especially troublesome in certain clinical circumstances. For example, at least some elderly subjects with arthritic conditions may be unable to lie still for more than a few minutes, making comparisons with younger nonarthritic subjects problematic. Head movement may be reduced by physical restraints (e.g., velcro straps or fitted plastic masks) or the use of sedative medications, but the latter are rarely appropriate for use in nonpatient volunteers.

Methods of Image Analysis

General considerations.   The quality of imaging data is affected by several factors related to the methodology of image analysis. First, measurements can be made on a variety of different forms of imaging data including radiographs, overhead projections of radiographs, photographs of the image, or displays of the original digital image data on computer consoles (Jack 1991). Computerized digital data systems afford the greatest flexibility and permit standardization of window settings across images, thereby providing for greater consistency and accuracy of measurement than is possible from films, where window settings are fixed. Second, the interpretation of brain imaging data will be affected by the criteria used to define the structure of interest. For example, the measured size of the frontal lobes on MRI will vary depending on whether their posterior boundary has been defined by the optic chiasma, the genu of the corpus callosum, or the central sulcus (Coffey et al. 1992; Kelsoe et al. 1988). Anatomic nonuniformity in these landmarks across subjects will also contribute to variability in regional brain measures. Third, the reliability of the measures of brain anatomy will vary with the skill of the rater—both inter- and intra-rater reliabilities should be reported for all raters, using either kappa statistics or intraclass correlation coefficients. Finally, it should be clear from the above that assessment of imaging data requires considerable subjective judgment on the part of the rater. As such, all measurements should be performed by raters who are "blind" to subject data (e.g., age, sex, and diagnostic group) or study hypotheses that could bias such assessments.

Types of measures.   The effects of aging on brain morphology have been assessed with both qualitative and quantitative measures. Qualitative measures consist of various scales to determine the presence and severity of parameters of interest, including, for example, cortical atrophy or ventricular enlargement. Qualitative measures are relatively inexpensive and easy to use, do not require sophisticated technological support, are frequently "clinically relevant," and may show good agreement with more quantitative assessments (Zatz et al. 1982a). Qualitative measures have limited resolution and sensitivity, however, and their accuracy is critically dependent on the skill of the particular rater. For this reason it is often difficult to compare results from different studies, especially when different rating scales have been used.

Quantitative measures of brain size may be either linear (distance measurement), planimetric (area measurement), or volumetric (multisection planimetric). Linear and planimetric measures are relatively quick and inexpensive and are available to researchers who lack sophisticated computerized image processing capabilities. Such measures also correlate reasonably well with volumetric measures, at least for structures of regular shape. For more complicated structures with irregular shapes, however, volumetric measures are much more accurate, especially when the sections are relatively thin (< 5 mm) and contiguous, and when they span the entire extent of the structure of interest. Volumetric measures are also more sensitive than linear and planimetric methods for detecting subtle group differences (Gado et al. 1983; Raz et al. 1987). Finally, volumetric measures are especially important for assessing left-right asymmetries because single-section measures are much more susceptible to the confounding effects of head tilt and patient positioning and because bilateral structures may not be aligned in a perfectly parallel position within the left and right hemispheres. In such situations, the left and right sides of a structure could differ with regard to the particular imaging section on which they appeared larger, in which case left-versus-right comparisons based on a single section clearly would not be representative of any asymmetry in the total volume of that structure.

Among quantitative brain imaging studies, differences exist in the technique used to segment the cranial contents into bone, CSF, white matter, and gray matter compartments. Typically, regions of interest are outlined manually ("trace" technique) and a computer automatically counts the number of pixels within the region. Alternatively, segmentation can be performed automatically by establishing threshold values of pixel intensity for each tissue compartment. These automated procedures should improve substantially test-retest reliability and the speed with which large volumes of imaging data can be analyzed, but they have not yet proved successful at segmenting regions with similar pixel intensity values (e.g., separating amygdala from hippocampus).

Effects of Aging on Brain Structure

Ventricular Size

Brain CT and MRI investigations have consistently demonstrated enlargement of the ventricular system with age (Appendix 9–1). The reported extent of enlargement has varied, however, depending on the way in which ventricular size has been assessed. General estimates from the literature suggest that, over the first nine decades of life, the ventricular-brain ratio (VBR) may increase nonlinearly from 2% to 17% (Barron et al. 1976; Pearlson et al. 1989b; Schwartz et al. 1985; Stafford et al. 1988), the proportion of ventricular fluid volume to brain volume may increase from 2%–4% to 4%–8% (Stafford et al. 1988), and the proportion of ventricular fluid volume to cranial volume may increase from 1%–2% to 2%–4% (Gur et al. 1991; Jernigan et al. 1990; Murphy et al. 1992; Pfefferbaum et al. 1986). These age effects appear to be similar for the lateral and third ventricles (Murphy et al. 1992; Schwartz et al. 1985). In the only longitudinal study, Gado et al. (1983) found a 3.7% increase in the ratio of ventricular volume to cranial volume in 12 elderly subjects followed for 1 year (Appendix 9–1).

In a recently completed study of 76 healthy adult volunteers from our laboratory, we found that increasing age was associated with significantly larger volumes of the lateral ventricles and the third ventricle (Coffey et al. 1992). After adjusting for gender and intracranial size, both lateral ventricular volume and third ventricular volume were found to increase by approximately 3% per year (Figure 9–1). These estimates of ventricular enlargement are comparable with those from previous pathological and quantitative imaging studies (DeCarli et al. 1990; Jernigan et al. 1990; Kaye et al. 1992; LeMay 1984; Pfefferbaum et al. 1986). A significant hemispheric asymmetry (left greater than right) was found in the volumes of the lateral ventricles (similar findings have been reported by others [Zipursky et al. 1990]), but the effects of age were similar for the two hemispheres. Schwartz et al. (1985) and Murphy et al.

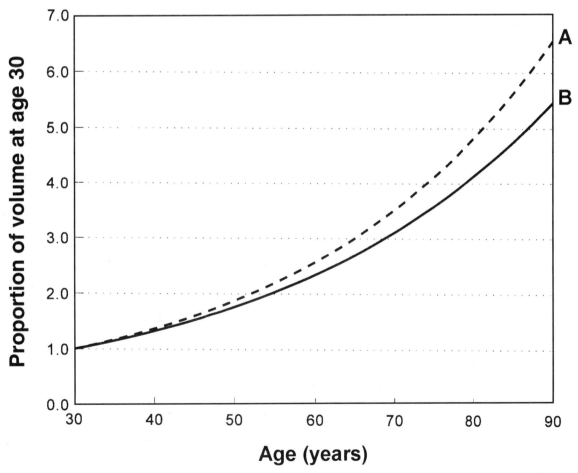

Figure 9–1. Increase in brain ventricular volumes with age, relative to volumes at age 30. Linear regression models for $\log_e$ (volume), controlling for the effects of gender and intracranial size, indicated that volume increased exponentially with age for both the lateral ventricles (*line A*) and the third ventricle (*line B*). The rate of volume increase was similar for each region (3.2% per year and 2.8% per year, respectively).
Source. From Coffey et al. 1992.

(1992) have likewise observed no laterality effects, but Gur et al. (1991) found that the ratio of ventricular CSF volume to cranial volume was more pronounced in the left hemisphere than in the right, a difference they attributed primarily to elderly men.

Blinded ratings of lateral ventricular enlargement were also performed in our study (Coffey et al. 1992) to provide a "clinical context" within which to interpret the volumetric changes. We found that the frequency of at least mild lateral ventricular enlargement (Table 9–1) also increased significantly with age, in agreement with numerous imaging and postmortem studies (Creasey and Rapoport 1985; DeCarli et al. 1990). The odds of at least mild lateral ventricular enlargement

were found to be 0.10 at age 40 and increased by approximately 7.7% per year to 2.22 at age 80. This ventriculomegaly was typically rated as mild in severity however, and more than one-half (54%) of our elderly subjects did not meet criteria for lateral ventricular enlargement (Table 9–1). These findings are consistent with the increased variation in ventricular size with age that others (Creasey and Rapoport 1985; DeCarli et al. 1990) have observed. Thus although ventricular volume increased with age, it appears that "clinically rated" ventricular enlargement is not an inevitable consequence of advancing age.

In our study (Coffey et al. 1992), the effects of age on lateral ventricular enlargement were no different

Table 9–1. Ratings of cortical atrophy, lateral ventricular enlargement, and subcortical hyperintensity

	Age (years)					
Rating score	30–39	40–49	50–59	60–69	70–79	> 80
Cortical atrophy[a]						
0	6(60%)	6(67%)	2(18%)	3(18%)	3(13%)	
1	3(30%)	2(22%)	7(64%)	7(41%)	6(25%)	1(17%)
2 (mild)	1(10%)	1(11%)	2(18%)	7(41%)	12(50%)	4(67%)
3 (moderate)					3(13%)	1(17%)
4 (severe)						
Lateral ventricular enlargement						
0	8(80%)	6(67%)	5(46%)	8(47%)	3(13%)	
1		2(22%)	4(36%)	4(24%)	7(29%)	
2 (mild)	2(20%)	1(11%)	2(18%)	2(12%)	11(46%)	2(33%)
3 (moderate)				3(8%)	3(13%)	4(66%)
4 (severe)						
Subcortical hyperintensity[b]						
Deep white matter						
0	8(80%)	5(56%)	4(36%)	7(44%)	2(8%)	1(17%)
1	1(10%)	3(33%)	5(46%)	7(44%)	15(63%)	2(33%)
2	1(10%)	1(11%)	1(9%)	1(6%)	7(29%)	1(17%)
3			1(9%)	1(6%)		2(33%)
Periventricular white matter						
0						
1	10(100%)	9(100%)	9(82%)	15(94%)	20(83%)	4(67%)
2			2(18%)	1(6%)	4(17%)	2(33%)
3						
Basal ganglia						
0	10(100%)	8(89%)	10(91%)	15(94%)	20(83%)	4(67%)
1 (present)		1(11%)	1(9%)	1(6%)	4(17%)	2(33%)
Thalamus						
0	10(100%)	9(100%)	10(91%)	15(94%)	23(96%)	5(83%)
1 (present)			1(9%)	1(6%)	1(4%)	1(17%)
Pons						
0	10(100%)	9(100%)	11(100%)	10(63%)	15(63%)	5(67%)
1 (present)				6(37%)	9(37%)	1(33%)

[a]See Figure 9–2 for examples of the visual standards used for the ratings of cortical atrophy.
[b]See Figures 9–4 and 9–5 for examples of the visual standards used for the ratings of subcortical hyperintensity.
Source. From Coffey et al. 1992.

for men than for women. In an early study using CT, Zatz et al. (1982a) also found no sex differences regarding the effects of age on ventricular size. Similarly, Yoshii et al. (1988) found that the correlations between age and ratings of lateral ventricular enlargement on MRI were similar in men and women, and Gur et al. (1991) found no sex differences in the slope of the regression line with age for ventricular CSF volume on MRI. Although Grant et al. (1987) reported that men, but not women, exhibited a significant age-related increase in ventricular volume on MRI, this apparent gender difference was not tested.

Brain Atrophy

Generalized brain atrophy. The effects of age on brain size have been assessed with visual estimates (qualitative ratings) of sulcal enlargement, quantitative measurements of CSF spaces, and quantitative measurements of total and regional brain size. Age has been found to be significantly correlated with visual ratings of sulcal enlargement (Coffey et al. 1992; Jacoby et al. 1980; Yoshii et al. 1988) (Appendix 9–2). The single exception to this observation is the report of Laffey et al. (1984), which limited investigation to elderly subjects only.

In our study of 76 healthy adults (Coffey et al. 1992), the odds of a rating of at least mild cortical atrophy were found to increase by approximately 8.9% per year such that, by age 68, subjects had a 50% chance of having acquired cortical atrophy. In spite of this predicted high frequency, the cortical atrophy present in our subjects was typically rated as mild (Figure 9–2). Moderately severe cortical atrophy was uncommon (four [9%] of 46 elderly subjects), and none of our subjects exhibited severe cortical atrophy (Table 9–1). These data suggest that although brain volume declines with age (see below), cortical atrophy (like ventricular enlargement) 1) is not an inevitable correlate of normal aging and 2) when present, is typically mild in severity and therefore relatively unlikely to be considered "clinically significant."

Quantitative studies of sulcal CSF spaces have consistently demonstrated increased CSF volume with age (Appendix 9–2), the only exception being a relatively small study of older adults (Tanna et al. 1991). Estimates of sulcal and cisternal volume range from 1 ml at the second decade of life to 40 ml at the ninth decade (Zatz et al. 1982a). Over the same age span, the proportion of sulcal CSF volume to cranial volume increases from approximately 3% to approximately 10% (Gur et al. 1991; Jernigan et al. 1990; Murphy et al. 1992). The age-related increase in sulcal CSF volume is not linear, however, and appears to be greatest after age 60 (Pfefferbaum et al. 1986; Zatz et al. 1982a). Variability in the measures of sulcal CSF volume also increases substantially with age (Pfefferbaum et al. 1986; Zatz et al. 1982a). In the only longitudinal study, Gado et al. (1983) found that the ratio of sulcal volume to cranial volume increased by an average of 13% in 12 elderly subjects followed over 1 year.

Quantitative investigations that directly measure brain size have consistently found reduced total brain volume with age (Appendix 9–3). The only negative study attempted to estimate brain volume from a single brain section (Yoshii et al. 1988). (It should also be noted that these same subjects did exhibit age-related cortical atrophy as determined from ratings of sulcal enlargement.) Over the first nine decades of life, the ratio of cerebral volume to cranial volume appears to decrease from approximately 93% to approximately 82% (Coffey et al. 1992; Jernigan et al. 1990; Tanna et al. 1991), and brain volume may decrease from an average of approximately 1,200–1300 ml to approximately 1,100–1,200 ml (Coffey et al. 1992; Gur et al. 1991; Murphy et al. 1992).

Regional brain atrophy. Significant age-related reductions have been observed for total gray matter volume (Lim et al. 1992; Schwartz et al. 1985) and cortical gray matter volume (Jernigan et al. 1991), as well as for specific gray matter structures such as the anterior diencephalon (Jernigan et al. 1991), caudate nucleus (Jernigan et al. 1991; Krishnan et al. 1990; Murphy et al. 1992), lentiform nucleus (McDonald et al. 1991; Murphy et al. 1992; Schwartz et al. 1985; negative findings reported by Jernigan et al. 1991), and hippocampus (Golomb et al. 1993; Jack et al. 1992). Conflicting findings have been reported for the thalamus (Jernigan et al. 1991; Murphy et al. 1992; Schwartz et al. 1985). Some (Jernigan et al. 1991; Jack et al. 1992) but not all (Coffey et al. 1992, see below) studies have suggested that age-related atrophy may be especially prominent in mesial temporal lobe structures. Total cerebral white matter volume does not appear to change significantly with age (Jernigan et al. 1991; Lim et al. 1992; Schwartz et al. 1985), but we (Parashosh et al, in press) and others (Doraiswamy et al. 1991) have observed age-related reductions in total and regional areas of the corpus callosum.

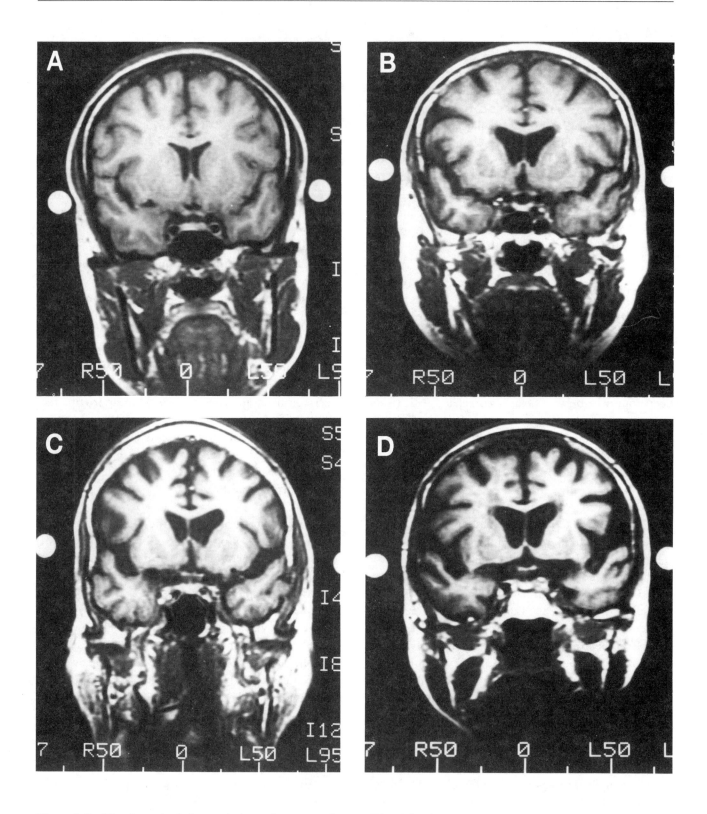

Figure 9–2. Visual standards for cortical atrophy score ratings on T1-weighted coronal magnetic resonance images (repetition time = 500 milliseconds, echo time = 20 milliseconds). *Panel A:* Grade 0, 1 = none, borderline. *Panel B:* Grade 2 = mild cortical atrophy. *Panel C:* Grade 3 = moderate cortical atrophy with widening of the interhemispheric fissure. *Panel D:* Grade 4 = severe cortical atrophy, with widening of almost all sulci. This subject also exhibits moderately severe enlargement of the lateral ventricles.

Source. Reprinted from Coffey CE: "Structural Brain Abnormalities in the Depressed Elderly," in *Brain Imaging in Affective Disorders.* Edited by Hauser P. Washington, DC, American Psychiatric Press, 1991, pp. 92–93. Used with permission.

In our investigation of 76 adult volunteers (Coffey et al. 1992), increasing age was associated with a statistically significant decrease in the total volumes of the cerebral hemispheres, the frontal lobes, the temporal lobes, and the amygdala-hippocampal complex. Although significant hemispheric asymmetries (left less than right) were present in the volumes of the frontal lobes and the amygdala-hippocampal complex (similar anatomic asymmetries have been reported by others [Bear et al. 1986; Chui et al. 1980; Kertesz et al. 1992; LeMay and Kido 1978; Suddath et al. 1989; Weinberger et al. 1982; Weis et al. 1989]), the effects of age were similar for the two hemispheres.

Our data extend previous imaging studies by suggesting that the relative rate of change in cerebral volume with age may differ among individual regions (Figure 9–3). Cerebral hemisphere volume, for example, declined at a rate of about 0.23% per year, a rate that agrees closely with previous postmortem (Davis and Wright 1977; Miller et al. 1980) and MRI studies (Appendix 9–3). In contrast, the rate of volume decrease for the frontal lobes (0.55% per year) was twice as great, indicating that this region may be particularly prone to volume loss associated with aging. This observation is consistent with previous neuropathological studies demonstrating that the frontal lobes are disproportionately affected by age-related changes such as volume loss, thinning of cortical laminae, widening of superficial sulci, and alterations in neuronal cell populations (Haug 1985; Katzman and Terry 1992). These data, taken together with findings from our study, may suggest a neuroanatomic substrate for age-related

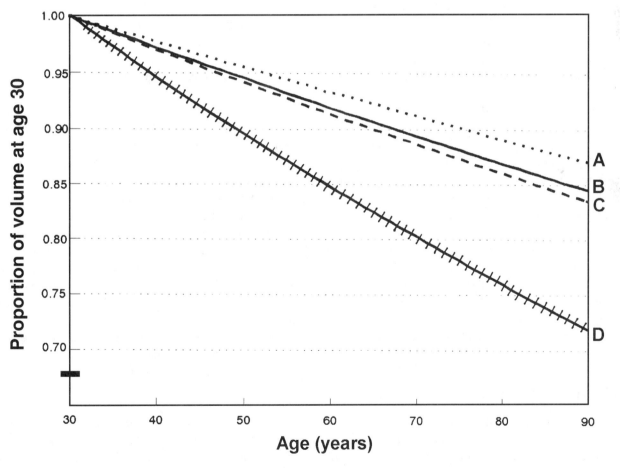

Figure 9–3. Decrease in regional cerebral volumes with age, relative to regional volumes at age 30. Linear regression models for $\log_e$ (volume), controlling for the effects of gender and intracranial size, indicated that volume decreased exponentially with age in the cerebral hemispheres (*line A*), the temporal lobes (*line B*), the amygdala-hippocampal complex (*line C*), and the frontal lobes (*line D*). It is apparent that the rate of change in brain volume with age was substantially greater for the frontal lobes (0.55% per year) than for the other regions (range of 0.23% to 0.30% per year). For example, relative to the cerebral hemispheres, frontal lobe volume decreased at a rate of 0.32% per year ($P < .004$).
Source. From Coffey et al. 1992.

changes in frontal lobe function present in neuropsychological (Mittenberg et al. 1989) and brain metabolic imaging (Alavi 1989; Warren et al. 1985) studies of aging humans. The rates of volume loss for the temporal lobes (0.28% per year) and the amygdala-hippocampal complex (0.30% per year) were similar to that for the cerebral hemispheres.

In our study, the effects of age on cerebral atrophy were comparable for men and women (i.e., there were no significant age-by-sex interactions in the statistical models of parenchymal brain volume or cortical atrophy). Although this finding must be interpreted cautiously given the relatively small number of men examined ($n = 25$), our observations are in agreement with the previous postmortem investigation (Miller et al. 1980) and the majority of imaging studies (Appendixes 9–2 and 9–3) that have examined gender effects. Gur et al. (1991), however, found that sulcal CSF volume was greater for elderly subjects (55 years and older) and for men. Condon et al. (1988) found that men, but not women, exhibited a significant negative correlation between age and the ratio of total brain volume to intracranial volume, but these correlations were not statistically compared.

In addition, our data indicated that the rates of age-related changes in regional cerebral volume were greater for ventricular regions (about 3% per year) than for the parenchymal regions described above (0.23% to 0.55% per year). This finding suggests that ventricular enlargement may provide a more sensitive index of brain aging than does cortical atrophy. It has been assumed that age-related ventricular enlargement occurs by ex vacuo expansion that results from shrinkage of periventricular structures. Current work is underway in our laboratory to examine whether age-related changes in the size of these structures (e.g., caudate and thalamic nuclei) are indeed related to the increase in ventricular volume that accompanies aging.

Subcortical Hyperintensity

Numerous MRI studies have suggested that aging is associated with an increased prevalence and severity of subcortical hyperintensity (foci of increased signal on T2-weighted images) (Appendix 9–4). Many of these reports are difficult to compare, however, because of differences in subject populations, scanning techniques, and lesion definition and grading (Coffey and Figiel 1991). The frequency and severity of subcortical hyperintensity observed in our study of healthy adults

(Coffey et al. 1992) were in close agreement with previous reports that have used similar definitions and grading techniques (Fazekas 1989). Subcortical hyperintensity was present in the deep white matter in 48 subjects (64.0%), in the periventricular white matter in nine (12.0%), in the basal ganglia in 9 (12.0%), in the thalamus in 4 (5.3%), and in the pons in 16 (21.3%) (Table 9–1 and Figures 9–4 and 9–5). Our findings confirmed that increasing age is associated with a significantly higher risk of subcortical hyperintensity—the odds of subcortical hyperintensity increased by 5% to 9% per year, depending on the anatomic region involved (Figure 9–6).

A growing body of neuropathological evidence is beginning to help define the pathophysiological significance of subcortical hyperintensity (Coffey and Figiel 1991). Periventricular hyperintensities in the form of caps or rims (Figure 9–4, *panel A*) are common in healthy individuals and do not appear to constitute pathology. Histological studies suggest that periventricular caps and rims likely reflect increased water content resulting from various combinations of factors, including a loose network of axons with low myelin content, a patchy loss of ependyma with astrocytic gliosis ("ependymitis granularis"), and the normal convergence of flow of interstitial fluid within the periventricular region (Sze et al. 1986). For the more severe changes of subcortical hyperintensity, however (Figures 9–4, *panel C,* and 9–5, *panel C*), a spectrum of histologic changes may be present that range from vascular ectasia and dilated perivascular spaces to edema and demyelination to frank lacunar infarctions. It has been suggested that these more severe changes are a consequence of chronic brain hypoperfusion stemming from some combination of advancing arteriosclerosis, hypertensive vascular disease, chronic recurrent hypotension, cerebral amyloid angiopathy, the presence of "senile" arteriolar hyaline lesions, age-related thickening of meninges, and impaired autoregulation of cerebral circulation associated with aging. Thus as conceptualized by Awad et al. (1986), subcortical hyperintensity in otherwise healthy older subjects may reflect "wear and tear" of brain parenchyma that accompanies aging and chronic cerebrovascular disease.

Other Brain Imaging Parameters

Intracranial calcification. Punctate calcification appears as an area of increased density on CT, but leaves a signal void on MRI. Intracranial calcification may occur in association with many pathological conditions and may also be noted as an incidental finding commonly involving the pineal gland, dura, habenula, petroclinoid ligament, choroid plexus, basal ganglia, and major cerebral vessels (Rhea and DeLuca 1983). Clinical experience and some research suggests that "physiological calcification" of these various structures increases with age (Cohen et al. 1980; Modic et al.

1980), but little systematic information is available in nonclinical elderly samples.

Brain tissue characteristics.   Conflicting data exist on whether increasing age is associated with alterations in CT attenuation values (Hounsfield unit) of the subcortical white matter (Cala et al. 1981; Schwartz et al. 1985; Zatz et al. 1982b). However, patchy areas of decreased

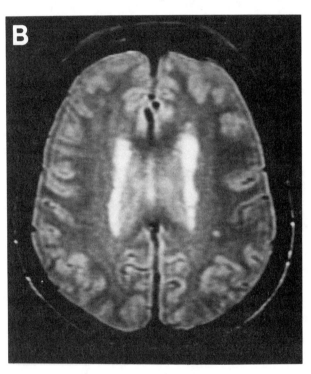

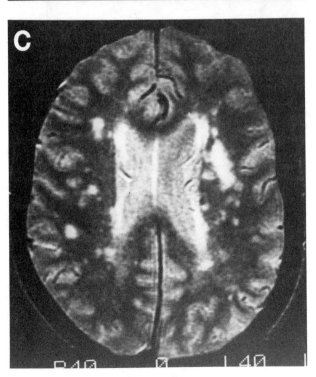

Figure 9–4.   Visual standards for ratings of hyperintensity in the periventricular white matter on T2-weighted magnetic resonance images (repetition time = 2,500 milliseconds; echo time = 80 milliseconds). *Panel A:* Grade 1 = "caps" at anterior tips of frontal horns. *Panel B:* Grade 2 = "halo" along border of lateral ventricles. *Panel C:* Grade 3 = irregular extension of hyperintensity into the deep white matter.
Source.   Reprinted from Coffey CE: "Structural Brain Abnormalities in the Depressed Elderly," in *Brain Imaging in Affective Disorders.* Edited by Hauser P. Washington, DC, American Psychiatric Press, 1991, pp. 94–95. Used with permission.

attenuation in the subcortical white matter do occur with increasing frequency on CT of the elderly (Coffey and Figiel 1991). Such changes likely reflect the effects of hypoperfusion to subcortical structures and are the CT scan equivalent of subcortical hyperintensity on MRI (Coffey and Figiel 1991). Increasing age has also been reported to be associated with regional brain changes in T1 and T2 relaxation time estimates on MRI

(Agartz et al. 1991; Breger et al. 1991), but such data must be considered preliminary given a number of methodological issues (Drayer 1989).

Brain iron.   High-field-strength (1.5 tesla) MRI can be used to visualize brain nuclei that are rich in iron. On heavily "T2-weighted" images, brain iron produces reduced signal intensity (the paramagnetic properties

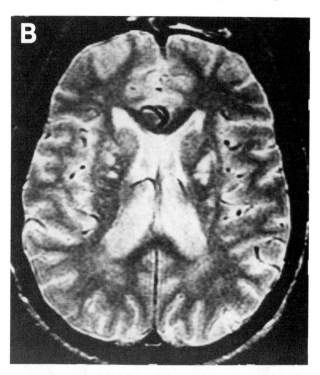

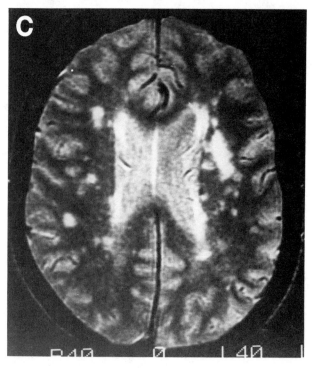

Figure 9–5.   Visual standards for ratings of hyperintensity in the deep white matter on T2-weighted magnetic resonance images (repetition time = 2,500 milliseconds; echo time = 80 milliseconds). *Panel A:* Grade 1 = punctate foci. *Panel B:* Grade 2 = small confluence of foci. *Panel C:* Grade 3 = large confluent areas of signal hyperintensity. *Source.*   Reprinted from Coffey CE: "Structural Brain Abnormalities in the Depressed Elderly," in *Brain Imaging in Affective Disorders.* Edited by Hauser P. Washington, DC, American Psychiatric Press, 1991, pp. 96–97. Used with permission.

of iron accelerate T2 relaxation time) that correlates with the distribution of iron staining in postmortem brains (Coffey et al. 1989; Sachdev 1993). Nuclei of the extrapyramidal system are especially rich in iron, and aging is associated with increased deposition of iron in these regions. These age-related changes are maximal during development and early adulthood, yet apparently do not occur in older people (Pujol et al. 1992).

Magnetic resonance spectroscopy. Magnetic resonance spectroscopy is a noninvasive technique capable of measuring the metabolism and chemical composition of brain tissue (Keshavan et al. 1991). Age-related findings have been reported for magnetic resonance spectroscopy in animals (Pettegrew et al. 1990), but this technique has not yet been applied to the systematic study of "normal or usual" aging in humans. Preliminary efforts are under way to explore the role of

magnetic resonance spectroscopy in age-related conditions such as dementia and cerebrovascular disease (Dager and Steen 1992; Keshavan et al. 1991).

Magnetic resonance imaging of cerebral blood flow. Because of its sensitivity to flow-related phenomena, MRI can be used to image in remarkable detail the extracranial and intracranial vasculature—a form of noninvasive angiography (Ståhlberg et al. 1992). This technique may also permit quantitative measurements of blood flow velocity and volume, and possibly of CSF hydrodynamics as well. Measurement of brain perfusion with MRI may also be possible within the next several years, permitting noninvasive assessment of brain functional activity comparable to that obtained with PET or SPECT. Such techniques would have obvious applications to the study of normal and abnormal brain aging.

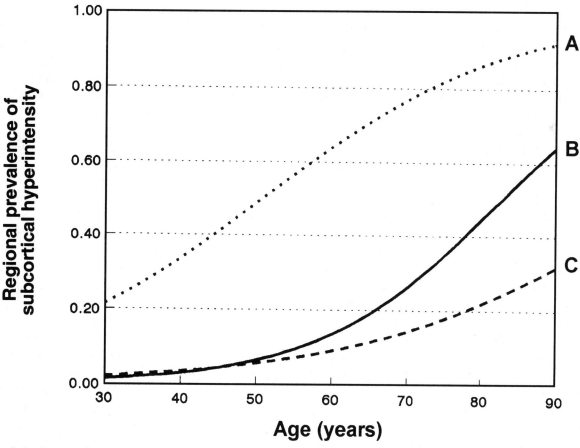

Figure 9–6. Increase in the regional prevalence of subcortical hyperintensity with age. Logistic regression models indicated that the risk of subcortical hyperintensity increased significantly with age in the deep white matter (*line A*) and pons (*line B*), but not in the periventricular white matter or basal ganglia (*line C*). The odds of subcortical hyperintensity increased by approximately 6.3% per year in the deep white matter and by 8.1% per year in the pons.
Source. From Coffey et al. 1992.

Neuropsychological Correlates of Age-Related Changes in Brain Structure

Despite a relatively large literature on the relationship between cognitive functioning and brain structure in patients with dementia, only a few studies have examined such relationships in nonpatient samples of healthy adult volunteers, and results have been conflicting. Earnest et al. (1979) performed neuropsychological testing (Trail Making Test, the Digit Symbol and Block Design subtests of the Wechsler Adult Intelligence Scale [WAIS; Wechsler 1955], and the Visual Reproduction subtest of the Wechsler Memory Scale [Wechsler 1945]) in 59 subjects who had been scanned by CT 1 year earlier (Appendixes 9–1 and 9–2). After adjustments for age, the only significant findings were negative correlations between the Digit Symbol Test and linear ($r = -.40$) and planimetric ($r = -.30$) measures of lateral ventricular size. In a sample of elderly subjects, Soininen et al. (1982) found a negative correlation between a composite neuropsychological test score and linear measures of ventricular size and Sylvian fissure size on CT, but the effects of age were not controlled.

Jacoby et al. (1980) found no significant correlations (after adjustments for age) between a test of memory and orientation and ratings of cortical atrophy, ratings of ventricular enlargement, or planimetric measures of ventricular size on CT scan films of elderly subjects (Appendixes 9–1 and 9–2). Pearlson et al. (1989b) likewise found no significant correlations between the VBR on CT and scores on the Mini-Mental State Exam (MMSE; Folstein et al. 1975), the Boston Naming Test (Kaplan et al. 1978), or a 10-word adaptation of the Rey Auditory-Verbal Learning Test (Rey 1964). Similarly, Matsubayashi et al. (1992) observed no correlations between the VBR on MRI and any of four neuropsychological test measures (MMSE, Hasegawa Dementia Scale [Hasegawa 1974], a visuospatial cognitive performance test, and a test of manual dexterity). Although Stafford et al. (1988) observed a significant negative correlation ($r = -.54$) between a discriminant function related to CSF fluid volume on CT (Appendix 9–2) and a discriminant function related to neuropsychological measures of naming and abstraction ability, the effects of subject age on this correlation were apparently not partialled out. Similarly, Kaye et al. (1992) observed a negative correlation between the sum of performance (but not verbal) scale

scores on the WAIS and ventricular volume on CT, but not after adjustments for the effects of age. Sullivan et al. (1993) found no relationship between scores on 10 neuropsychological tests (MMSE, Trail Making Tests A and B, and 7 subtests of the WAIS-R [Information, Digit Span, Vocabulary, Digit Symbol, Picture Completion, Block Design, and Object Assembly]) and CT scan estimates of total ventricular volume, third ventricular volume, and CSF sulcal volume (Sylvian fissure and vertex, frontal, and parieto-occipital sulci). Finally, two recent MRI investigations have observed relations between IQ and total and regional brain volumes in relatively young samples (Andreasen et al. 1993; Willerman et al. 1991).

A somewhat larger literature exists with respect to the relation between cognition and changes in subcortical white matter (Appendix 9–5), but again results are conflicting and the studies are difficult to compare given methodological differences. In a recent study from our laboratory (Tupler et al. 1992), we examined the relationship between subcortical hyperintensity on MRI and two specific neuropsychological instruments—the Benton Facial Recognition Test (Benton et al. 1983) and the WAIS-R Digit Symbol. The former was chosen because it has yielded the highest level of significance of any test reported to be associated with subcortical hyperintensity, and the latter because it has been reported to be related to subcortical hyperintensity by two independent groups (Appendix 9–5). In addition, both the Benton Facial Recognition Test and the Digit Symbol subtest of the Wechsler Adult Intelligence Scale–Revised (WAIS-R; Wechsler 1981) were favored a priori, because subcortical pathology might be expected to disrupt visuospatial perception and visuomotor execution, respectively.

We found that performance on both tests was highly related to age and education, but not to the presence of subcortical hyperintensity. The majority of our subjects had relatively mild findings of subcortical hyperintensity, however, and it thus remains possible that more severe changes might be associated with cognitive dysfunction in otherwise healthy adults (e.g., see Matsubayashi et al. 1992; Steingart et al. 1987). In addition, an issue not addressed by our study was whether subcortical hyperintensity might be associated with cognitive changes in patients with various medical, neurological, or psychiatric illnesses (Coffey and Figiel 1991). In this regard, we have previously reported that subcortical hyperintensity is more common in patients with severe depression (Coffey et al. 1990; 1993), and correlative studies are currently under way to determine whether the cognitive impairment that frequently afflicts this population might be associated with these brain changes.

Summary

Modern computer-based imaging technologies provide an excellent opportunity to examine in vivo the spectrum and extent of changes in brain morphology that occur with normal aging. Such data are essential for an understanding of pathological brain aging in the elderly. The interpretation of these imaging studies must include careful consideration of a plethora of methodological issues that can obscure, confound, or modify apparent aging effects. Although studies vary in the extent to which such factors have been controlled, there is general agreement in the literature that increasing age is associated with 1) nonlinear increases in lateral and third ventricular volume; 2) increasing sulcal CSF volume; 3) decreasing brain volume, especially of the frontal lobes and of cortical and subcortical gray matter structures; 4) increasing variability in measures of brain size; and 5) increasing frequency and severity of subcortical hyperintensity on MRI. Further study is needed to characterize in greater detail the effects of "usual versus successful" aging on global and regional brain structure, and the relationship of such age-related changes to cognitive function in elderly people.

References

Agartz I, Sääf J, Wahlund LO, et al: T₁ and T₂ relaxation time estimates in the normal human brain. Radiology 181:537–543, 1991

Alavi A: The aging brain. J Neuropsychiatry Clin Neurosci 1 (suppl 1):S51–S60, 1989

Almkvist O, Wahlund LO, Andersson-Lundman G, et al: White-matter hyperintensity and neuropsychological functions in dementia and healthy aging. Arch Neurol 49:626–632, 1992

Andreasen NC, Ehrhardt JC, Swayze VW, et al: Magnetic resonance imaging of the brain in schizophrenia: the pathophysiologic significance of structural abnormalities. Arch Gen Psychiatry 47:35–44, 1990

Andreasen NC, Flaum M, Swayze V, et al: Intelligence and brain structure in normal individuals. Am J Psychiatry 150:130–134, 1993

Austrom MG, Thompson RF, Hendrie HC, et al: Foci of increased T₂ signal intensity in MR images of healthy elderly subjects: a follow-up study. J Am Geriatr Soc 38:1133–1138, 1990

Awad IA, Johnson PC, Spetzler RF, et al: Incidental subcortical lesions identified on magnetic resonance imaging in the elderly, II: post mortem correlations. Stroke 17:1090–1097, 1986

Barron SA, Jacobs L, Kinkel WR: Changes in size of normal lateral ventricles during aging determined by computerized tomography. Neurology 26:1011–1013, 1976

Bear D, Schiff D, Saver J, et al: Quantitative analysis of cerebral asymmetries: fronto-occipital correlation, sexual dimorphism and association with handedness. Arch Neurol 43:598–603, 1986

Benton AL, Hamsher KdeS, Varney NR, et al: Contributions to Neuropsychological Assessment: A Clinical Manual. New York, Oxford University Press, 1983

Boone KB, Miller BL, Lesser IM, et al: Neuropsychological correlates of white-matter lesions in healthy elderly subjects. Arch Neurol 49:549–554, 1992

Brant-Zawadzki M, Fein G, Van Dyke C, et al: MR imaging of the aging brain: patchy white-matter lesions and dementia. AJNR 6:675–682, 1985

Breger RK, Yetkin FZ, Fischer ME, et al: T₁ and T₂ in the cerebrum: correlation with age, gender, and demographic factors. Radiology 181:545–547, 1991

Cala LA, Thickbroom GW, Black JL, et al: Brain density and cerebrospinal fluid space size: CT of normal volunteers. AJNR 2:41–47, 1981

Cascella NG, Pearlson G, Wong DF, et al: Effects of substance abuse on ventricular and sulcal measures assessed by computerized tomography. Br J Psychiatry 159:217–221, 1991

Chui C, Damasio AR: Human cerebral asymmetries evaluated by computed tomography. J Neurol Neurosurg Psychiatry 43:873–878, 1980

Coffey CE: Structural brain abnormalities in the depressed elderly, in Brain Imaging in Affective Disorders. Edited by Hauser P. Washington, DC, American Psychiatric Press, 1991, pp 94–95

Coffey CE, Figiel GS: Neuropsychiatric significance of subcortical encephalomalacia, in Psychopathology and the Brain. Edited by Carroll BJ, Barrett JE. New York, Raven, pp 243–264, 1991

Coffey CE, Figiel GS, Djang WT, et al: Subcortical hyperintensity on magnetic resonance imaging: a comparison of normal and depressed elderly subjects. Am J Psychiatry 147:187–189, 1990

Coffey CE, Alston S, Heinz ER, et al: Brain iron in progressive supranuclear palsy: clinical, magnetic resonance imaging, and neuropathological findings. J Neuropsychiatry Clin Neurosci 1:400–404, 1989

Coffey CE, Wilkinson WE, Parashos IA, et al: Quantitative cerebral anatomy of the aging human brain: a cross-sectional study using magnetic resonance imaging. Neurology 42:527–536, 1992

Coffey CE, Wilkinson WE, Weiner RD, et al: Quantitative cerebral anatomy in depression: a controlled magnetic resonance imaging study. Arch Gen Psychiatry 50:7–16, 1993

Cohen CR, Duchesneau PM, Weinstein MA: Calcification of the basal ganglia as visualized by computed tomography. Neuroradiology 134:97–99, 1980

Condon B, Grant R, Hadley D, et al: Brain and intracranial cavity volumes: in vivo determination by MRI. Acta Neurol Scand 78:387–393, 1988

Creasey H, Rapoport SI: The aging human brain. Ann Neurol 17:2–10, 1985

Cutler RG: Evolution of longevity in primates. Journal of Human Evolution 5:169–202, 1976

Cutler RG: Evolution of human longevity: a critical overview. Mech Ageing Dev 9:337–754, 1979

Dager SR, Steen RG: Applications of magnetic resonance spetroscopy to the investigation of neuropsychiatric disorders. Neuropsychopharmacology 6:249–266, 1992

Davis PJM, Wright EA: A new method for measuring cranial cavity volume and its application to the assessment of cerebral atrophy at autopsy. Neuropathol Appl Neurobiol 3:341–358, 1977

DeCarli C, Kaye JA, Horwitz B, et al: Critical analysis of the use of computer-assisted transverse axial tomography to study human brain in aging and dementia of the Alzheimer type. Neurology 40:872–883, 1990

Doraiswamy PM, Figiel GS, Husain MM, et al: Aging of the human corpus callosum: magnetic resonance imaging in normal volunteers. J Neuropsychiatry Clin Neurosci 3:392–397, 1991

Drayer BP: Imaging of the aging brain, part I: normal findings. Radiology 166:785–796, 1988

Drayer BP: Basal ganglia: significance of signal hypointensity on T2 weighted MR images. Radiology 173:311–312, 1989

Earnest MP, Heaton RK, Wilkinson WE, et al: Cortical atrophy, ventricular enlargement and intellectual impairment in the aged. Neurology 29:1138–1143, 1979

Fazekas F: Magnetic resonance signal abnormalities in asymptomatic individuals: their incidence and functional correlates. Eur Neurol 29:164–168, 1989

Folstein MF, Folstein SE, McHugh PR: Mini-Mental State: a practical method of grading the cognitive state of patients. Psychiatr Res 12:189–198, 1975

Gado M, Hughes CP, Danziger W, et al: Aging, dementia, and brain atrophy: a longitudinal computed tomography study. AJNR 4:699–702, 1983

George AE, deLeon MJ, Kalnin A, et al: Leukoencephalopathy in normal and pathologic aging, 2: MRI of brain lucencies. AJNR 7:567–570, 1986

Golomb J, de Leon MI, Kluger A, et al: Hippocampal atrophy in normal aging: an association with recent memory impairment. Arch Neurol 50:967–973, 1993

Gould SJ: The Mismeasure of Man. New York, WW Norton, 1981

Grant R, Condon B, Lawrence A, et al: Human cranial CSF volumes measured by MRI: sex and age influences. Magn Reson Imaging 5:465–468, 1987

Gur RC, Mozley PD, Resnick SM, et al: Gender differences in age effect on brain atrophy measured by magnetic resonance imaging. Proc Natl Acad Sci U S A 88:2845–2849, 1991

Hasegawa K: An investigation of dementia rating scale for the elderly (in Japanese). Psychiatric Med 16:965–969, 1974

Harrell LE, Duvall E, Folks DG, et al: The relationship of high-intensity signals on magnetic resonance images to cognitive and psychiatric state in Alzheimer's disease. Arch Neurol 48:1136–1140, 1991

Haug H: Are neurons of the human cerebral cortex really lost during aging? a morphometric examination, in Senile Dementia of the Alzheimer Type. Edited by Traber J, Gispen WH. Berlin, Springer-Verlag, 1985, pp 150–163

Hendrie HC, Farlow MR, Austrom MG, et al: Foci of increased T_2 signal intensity on brain MR scans of healthy elderly subjects. AJNR 10:703–707, 1989

Homan RW, Herman J, Purdy P: Cerebral localization in international 10-20 system electrode placement. Electroencephalogr Clin Neurophysiol 66:376–382, 1987

Hunt Al, Orrison WW, Yeo RA, et al: Clinical significance of MRI white matter lesions in the elderly. Neurology 39:1470–1474, 1989

Jack CR: Brain and cerebrospinal fluid volume: measurement with MR imaging. Radiology 178:22–24, 1991

Jack CR, Gehring DC, Sharbrough FW, et al: Temporal lobe measurement from MR images: accuracy and left-right asymmetry in normal persons. J Comput Assist Tomogr 12:21–29, 1988

Jack CR, Petersen RC, O'Brien PC, et al: MR-based hippocampal volumetry in the diagnosis of Alzheimer's disease. Neurology 42:183–188, 1992

Jacoby RJ, Levy R, Dawson JM: Computed tomography in the elderly, I: the normal population. Br J Psychiatry 136:249–255, 1980

Jernigan TL, Press GA, Hesselink JR: Methods of measuring brain morphologic features on magnetic resonance images: validation and normal aging. Arch Neurol 47:27–32, 1990

Jernigan TL, Archibald SL, Berhow MT, et al: Cerebral structures on MRI, part I: localization of age-related changes. Biol Psychiatry 29:55–67, 1991

Kaplan EF, Goodglass H, Weintraub S: The Boston Naming Test. New York, E Kaplan & H Goodglass, 1978

Katzman R, Terry R: Normal aging of the nervous system, in Principles of Geriatric Neurology. Edited by Katzman R, Rowe JW. Philadelphia, PA, FA Davis, 1992, pp 18–58

Kaye JA, DeCarli C, Luxenberg JS, et al: The significance of age-related enlargement of the cerebral ventricles in healthy men and women measured by quantitative computed x-ray tomography. J Am Geriatr Soc 40:225–231, 1992

Kelsoe JR, Cadet JL, Pickar D, et al: Quantitative neuroanatomy in schizophrenia: a controlled magnetic resonance imaging study. Arch Gen Psychiatry 45:533–541, 1988

Kertesz A, Polk M, Black SE, et al: Anatomical asymmetries and functional laterality. Brain 115:589–605, 1992

Keshavan MS, Kapur S, Pettegrew JW: Magnetic resonance spectroscopy in psychiatry: potential, pitfalls, and promise. Am J Psychiatry 148:976–985, 1991

Kozachuk WE, DeCarli C, Schapiro MB, et al: White matter hyperintensities in dementia of Alzheimer's type and in healthy subjects without cerebrovascular risk factors: a magnetic resonance imaging study. Arch Neurol 47:1306–1310, 1990

Krishnan KR, Husain MM, McDonald WM, et al: In vivo stereological assessment of caudate volume in man: effect of normal aging. Life Sci 47:1325–1329, 1990

Laessle RG, Krieg JC, Fichter MM, et al: Cerebral atrophy and vigilance performance in patients with anorexia nervosa and bulimia nervosa. Neuropsychobiology 21:187–191, 1989

Laffey PA, Peyster RG, Nathan R, et al: Computed tomography and aging: results in a normal elderly population. Neuroradiology 26:273–278, 1984

LeMay M: Radiologic changes of the aging brain and skull. AJR 143:383–389, 1984

LeMay M, Kido DK: Asymmetries of cerebral hemispheres on computed tomograms. J Comput Assist Tomogr 2:471–476, 1978

Levine R, Hudgins P, Risch SC, et al: Lowered attention capacity in young, medically healthy men with magnetic resonance brain hyperintensity signals. Neuropsychiatry, Neuropsychology, and Behavioral Neurology 6:38–42, 1993

Lim KO, Zipursky RB, Watts MC, et al: Decreased gray matter in normal aging: an in vivo magnetic resonance study. J Gerontol 47:B26–B30, 1992

Lishman WA: Alcohol and the brain. Br J Psychiatry 156:635–644, 1990

Matsubayashi K, Shimada K, Kawamoto A, et al: Incidental brain lesions on magnetic resonance imaging and neurobehavioral functions in apparently healthy elderly. Stroke 23:175–180, 1992

McDonald WM, Husain M, Doraiswamy PM, et al: A magnetic resonance image study of age-related changes in human putamen nuclei. Neuroreport 2:41–44, 1991

McFarland D: The aged in the 21st century: a demographer's view, in Aging into the 21st Century: Middle Ages Today. Edited by Jarvik LF. New York, Gardner, 1978, pp 5–25

Meese W, Kluge W, Grumme T, et al: CT evaluation of the CSF spaces of healthy persons. Neuroradiology 19:131–136, 1980

Miller AKH, Alston RL, Corsellis JA: Variation with age in the volumes of grey and white matter in the cerebral hemispheres of man: measurements with an image analyzer. Neuropathol Appl Neurobiol 6:119–132, 1980

Mirsen TR, Lee DH, Wong CJ, et al: Clinical correlates of white-matter changes on magnetic resonance imaging scans of the brain. Arch Neurol 48:1015–1021, 1991

Mittenberg W, Seidenberg M, O'Leary DS, et al: Changes in cerebral functioning associated with normal aging. J Clin Exp Neuropsychol 11:918–932, 1989

Modic MT, Weinstein MA, Rothner AD, et al: Calcification of the choroid plexus visualized by computed tomography. Radiology 135:369–372, 1980

Murphy DGM, DeCarli C, Schapiro MB, et al: Age-related differences in volumes of subcortical nuclei, brain matter, and cerebrospinal fluid in healthy men as measured with magnetic resonance imaging. Arch Neurol 49:839–845, 1992

Parashos IA, Coffey CE: Anatomy of the aging human brain, in The Psychiatry of Old Age: An International Textbook. Edited by Copeland JRM, Abou-Saleh MT, Blazer DG. Sussex, England, Wiley (in press)

Parashos IA, Wilkinson WE, Coffey CE: Magnetic resonance imaging of the corpus callosum: predictors of size in normal adults. J Neuropsychiatry Clin Neurosci (in press)

Pearlson GD, Kim WS, Kubos KL, et al: Ventricle-brain ratio, computed tomographic density, and brain area in 50 schizophrenics. Arch Gen Psychiatry 46:690–697, 1989a

Pearlson GD, Rabins PV, Kim WS, et al: Structural brain CT changes and cognitive defects in elderly depressives with and without reversible dementia ("pseudodementia"). Psychol Med 19:573–584, 1989b

Pettegrew JW, Panchalingam K, Withers G, et al: Changes in brain energy and phospholipid metabolism during development and aging in the Fischer 344 rat. J Neuropathol Exp Neurol 49:237–249, 1990

Pfefferbaum A, Zatz LM, Jernigan TL: Computer-interactive method for quantifying cerebrospinal fluid and tissue in brain CT scans: effects of aging. J Comput Assist Tomogr 10:571–578, 1986

Pfefferbaum A, Lim KO, Rosenbloom M, et al: Brain magnetic resonance imaging: approaches for investigating schizophrenia. Schizophr Bull 16:453–476, 1990

Pujol J, Junquè C, Vendrell P, et al: Biological significance of iron-related magnetic resonance imaging changes in the brain. Arch Neurol 49:711–717, 1992

Rao SM, Mittenberg W, Bernardin L, et al: Neuropsychological test findings in subjects with leukoaraiosis. Arch Neurol 46:40–44, 1989

Raz S, Raz N, Weinberger DR, et al: Morphological brain abnormalities in schizophrenia determined by computed tomography: a problem of measurement. Psychiatry Res 22:91–98, 1987

Rey A: L'Examen Clinique En Psychologie. Paris, Press Universitaires de France, 1964

Rhea JT, DeLuca SA: Benign intracranial calcification. American Family Physician 27:151–152, 1983

Rowe JW, Kahn RL: Human aging: usual and successful. Science 237:143–149, 1987

Rowe JW, Katzman R: Principles of geriatrics as applied to neurology, in Principles of Geriatric Neurology. Edited by Katzman R, Rowe JW. Philadelphia, PA, FA Davis, 1992, pp 3–17

Sachdev P: The neuropsychiatry of brain iron. J Neuropsychiatry Clin Neurosci 5:18–29, 1993

Schmidt R, Fazekas F, Offenbacher H, et al: Magnetic resonance imaging white matter lesions and cognitive impairment in hypertensive individuals. Arch Neurol 48:417–420, 1991

Schwartz M, Creasey H, Grady CL, et al: Computed tomographic analysis of brain morphometrics in 30 healthy men, aged 21 to 81 years. Ann Neurol 17:146–157, 1985

Shah SA, Doraiswamy PM, Husain MM, et al: Assessment of posterior fossa structures with midsagittal MRI: the effects of age. Neurobiol Aging 12:371–374, 1991

Soininen H, Puranen M, Riekkinen PJ: Computed tomography findings in senile dementia and normal aging. J Neurol Neurosurg Psychiatry 45:50–54, 1982

Stafford JL, Albert MS, Naeser MA, et al: Age-related differences in computed tomographic scan measurements. Arch Neurol 45:409–415, 1988

Ståhlberg F, Ericsson A, Nordell B, et al: MR imaging, flow and motion. Acta Radiol 33:179–200, 1992

Steingart A, Hachinski VC, Lau C, et al: Cognitive and neurologic findings in subjects with diffuse white matter lucencies on computed tomography scan (leuko-araiosis). Arch Neurol 44:32–35, 1987

Suddath RC, Casanova MF, Goldberg TE, et al: Temporal lobe pathology in schizophrenia: a quantitative magnetic resonance imaging study. Am J Psychiatry 146:464–472, 1989

Sullivan EV, Shear PK, Mathalon D, et al: Greater abnormalities of brain cerebrospinal fluid volumes in younger than in older patients with Alzheimer's disease. Arch Neurol 50:359–373, 1993

Sze G, DeArmond SJ, Brant-Zawadzki M, et al: Foci of MRI signal (pseudolesions) anterior to the frontal horns: histologic correlations of a normal finding. American Journal of Radiology 147:331–337, 1986

Tanna NK, Khon MI, Horwich DN, et al: Analysis of brain and cerebral fluid volumes with MR imaging: impact on PET data correction for atrophy. Radiology 178:123–130, 1991

Tupler LA, Coffey CE, Logue PE, et al: Neuropsychological importance of subcortical white matter hyperintensity. Arch Neurol 49:1248–1252, 1992

Warren LR, Butler RW, Katholi CR, et al: Age differences in cerebral blood flow during rest and during mental activation measurements with and without monetary incentive. J Gerontol 40:53–59, 1985

Wechsler D: A standardized memory scale for clinical use. J Psychol 19:87–95, 1945

Wechsler D: Wechsler Adult Intelligence Scale. New York, Psychological Corporation, 1955

Wechsler D: Wechsler Adult Intelligence Scale–Revised Manual. New York, Psychological Corporation, 1981

Weinberger DR, Luchins DR, Morihisa MD, et al: Asymmetrical volumes of the right and left frontal and occipital regions of the human brain. Ann Neurol 11:97–100, 1982

Weis S, Haug H, Holoubec B, et al: The cerebral dominances: quantitative morphology of the human cerebral cortex. Int J Neurosci 47:165–168, 1989

Willerman L, Schultz R, Rugledge JN, et al: In vivo brain size and intelligence. Intelligence 15:223–228, 1991

Witelson SF: Cognitive neuroanatomy: a new era. Neurology 42:709–713, 1992

Yoshii F, Barker WW, Chang JY, et al: Sensitivity of cerebral glucose metabolism to age, gender, brain volume, brain atrophy and cerebrovascular risk factors. J Cereb Blood Flow Metab 8:654–661, 1988

Zatz LM, Jernigan TL, Ahumada AJ: Changes in computed cranial tomography with aging: intracranial fluid volume. AJNR 3:1–11, 1982a

Zatz LM, Jernigan TL, Ahumada AJ: White matter changes in cerebral computed tomography related to aging. J Comput Assist Tomogr 6(1):19–23, 1982b

Zipursky RB, Lim KO, Pfefferbaum A: Volumetric assessment of cerebral asymmetry from CT scans. Psychiatry Research: Neuroimaging 35:71–89, 1990

Appendix 9–1 Aging and Brain Ventricular Size

Study	Subjects	Imaging and measurement technique	Findings
Barron et al. 1976	135 volunteers 9 months to 90 years old Equal sex distribution in all age groups (8 males, 7 females per decade) No history of neurological disease; psychiatric history not reported Handedness not specified	Computed tomography (CT) Planimetric determination of VBR by single rater (average of 3 measurements) from Polaroid photograph	Age associated with increased ventricular-brain ratio (VBR) Increased variability in VBR with age Gender and laterality effects not reported
Earnest et al. 1979	59 volunteer retirees 60–99 years old 11 males; 48 females Living independently and free of neurological disease Handedness not specified	CT Linear and planimetric measures of ventricular size at three different levels, from photographs No additional data provided	Subjects 80 years or older ($n = 29$) had larger ratio of ventricular size to intracranial size than did younger subjects ($n = 30$)
Jacoby et al. 1980	50 healthy elderly volunteers 62–88 years old 10 males; 40 females No history of significant psychiatric or neurological illness Handedness not specified	CT Ratings (small, normal, enlarged) of ventricular size from films by single blinded rater (rater reliability not reported) Planimetric determination of ventricular-skull ratio and Evans' ratio[a] from films by single rater (average of three measurements) with established reliability	8 (16%) subjects were rated as having "enlarged" lateral ventricles No significant correlation between age and ventricular-skull ratio or Evans's ratio Gender and laterality effects not reported
Meese et al. 1980	160 healthy volunteers 1–71 years old 10 males and 10 females in each decade No additional data provided	CT Linear measurements from four axial slices (no additional details provided)	Apparent age-related changes in some measures of ventricular size, but these changes not analyzed statistically
Cala et al. 1981	115 volunteers 15–40 years old 62 males; 53 females No history of migraine, head trauma, or excessive alcohol intake (no additional details provided) All but 8 subjects right-handed	CT (two different scanners) Planimetric measurement of ventricular-skull ratio at level of frontal horns (no additional details provided) Axial slices, 13 mm thick	No relationship between age and ventricular-skull ratio
Zatz et al. 1982a	123 volunteers 10–90 years old 49 males; 74 females No history of neurological or major medical disease; psychiatric history not reported Handedness not specified	CT Volume measurement derived from computer-assisted pixel segmentation technique (ASI-II program) Axial Slices ($n = 9$), 10 mm thick with 10-mm interscan gap	Age significantly associated with increased ventricular volume (males = females), even after controlling for intracranial volume Increased variability of ventricular size with age
Soininen et al. 1982	85 volunteers: 53 from community and 32 from nursing home Mean ±SD age = 75 ± 7 years No neurological disease (no additional details provided)	CT Linear measurements (from films?) of ventricular and sulcal size Axial slices ($n = 8$ to 12), 8 mm thick No additional details provided	Age correlated with ratios of ventricular width to skull width (frontal horn index and cella media index)

(continued)

Appendix 9–1 Aging and Brain Ventricular Size *(continued)*

Study	Subjects	Imaging and measurement technique	Findings
Gado et al. 1983	12 elderly volunteers 64–81 years old 9 males; 3 females No additional clinical data provided	CT Volume measurement derived from computer-assisted pixel segmentation technique (7 axial slices, 8 mm thick) Linear measurements from axial images ($n = 7$) Number of raters and rater reliabilities not specified	During 1-year follow-up, ratio of ventricular volume to cranial volume increased significantly by an average of 3.7% No significant changes in linear measures of ventricular size (VBR, third ventricular ratio, frontal horn ratio)
Laffey et al. 1984	212 elderly volunteers 65–89 years old 110 males; 102 females No evidence of alcoholism, dementia, or neurological illness	CT Qualitative rating (6-point scale) of ventricular enlargement from films by two experienced radiologists with established reliabilities	Age associated with increased ventricular size Laterality and gender effects not reported
Schwartz et al. 1985	30 healthy male volunteers 21–81 years old No history of major medical, neurological, or psychiatric illness Handedness not specified	CT Volume measurement derived from computer-assisted segmentation technique (ASI-II program) Axial slices ($n = 7$) starting from the plane of the inferior orbito-meatal line (10 mm thick, 7-mm interscan gap)	Age correlated with areas and volumes of lateral and third ventricles, even after adjusting for height and intracranial area Age correlated with VBR Increased variability of ventricular size with age No laterality effects
Pfefferbaum et al. 1986	57 health volunteers 20–84 years old 27 males; 30 females No additional data provided	CT Volume measurement derived from computer-assisted segmentation technique (modification of Gado et al. 1983) Contiguous axial slices ($n = 5$) starting at the level of the superior roof of the orbits	Age associated with increased ratio of ventricular volume to cranial volume Increased variability in ventricular volume with age Gender and laterality effects not reported
Pearlson et al. 1989b	31 healthy volunteers (all 60 years or older); mean ±SD age = 68.3 ± 1.2 years 15 males; 16 females No major medical, neurological, or psychiatric illness Handedness not specified	CT Planimetric determination of VBR from films by one of two raters, each with established reliabilities	Age correlated with VBR Gender and laterality effects not reported
Stafford et al. 1988	79 healthy male volunteers 31–87 years old No severe medical or psychiatric illness Handedness not specified	CT Volume measurement derived from computer-assisted segmentation technique (ASI-II program) Axial slices ($n = 3$) at mid-, high-, and supraventricular levels	Age associated with increased ratio of ventricular volume to brain volume Laterality effects not reported

(continued)

Appendix 9–1   Aging and Brain Ventricular Size *(continued)*

Study	Subjects	Imaging and measurement technique	Findings
Kaye et al. 1992	107 health volunteers 64 males (21–90 years old); 43 females (23–88 years old) No major medical, neuro-logical, or psychiatric illness Handedness not specified	CT Volume measurement derived from computer-assisted segmentation technique (ASI-II program) Axial slices, 10 mm thick, 7-mm interscan gap	Age associated with increased ventricular volume in both genders (about 20% per decade); precipitous increases were observed beginning in the fifth decade in males and in the sixth decade in female
Sullivan et al. 1993	114 healthy volunteers 21–82 years old (mean ±SD = 51.2 ± 17.7 years) 84 males; 30 females No history of major medical, neurological, or psychiatric illness 90% right-handed	CT Volume measurements derived from computer-assisted segmenta-tion technique (modification of Gado et al. 1983) Axial slices ($n = 10$), 10 mm thick	Age correlated with total and third ventricular volume, even after adjustments for head size No gender effects No correlation between age-related changes in third ventricular volume and performance on 10 neuropsychological tests
Grant et al. 1987	64 healthy volunteers 18–64 years old 25 males; 39 females No history of neurological disease; psychiatric history not reported Handedness not specified	Magnetic resonance imaging (MRI) (0.15 tesla) Mathematically derived estimate of ventricular volume from signal intensity measurements made on single sagittal slice (number of raters not specified)	Age associated with increased ventricular volume in males, but not females; however, this apparent gender difference was not tested statistically Laterality effects not reported No control for size of brain or head
Yoshii et al. 1988	58 healthy volunteers 21–81 years old 29 males; 29 females Neurological and psychiatric histories not reported Handedness not specified	MRI (1.0 tesla) Blinded global ratings (4-point scale) of lateral ventricular en-largement from inversion recovery films (axial slices [n unspecified], 10 mm thick, 3-mm interscan gap) Numbers of raters and rater reliabilities not specified	Age correlated with ratings of lateral ventricular enlargement (males = females) Laterality effects not reported
Jernigan et al. 1990	58 healthy volunteers 8–79 years old 35 males; 23 females Excluded neurological, psy-chiatric, or medical (e.g., diabetes mellitus and heart disease) illness Handedness not specified	MRI (1.5 tesla) Volume estimates (one of two raters) derived from computer-assisted pixel classification of multiple spin-echo axial images (5 mm thick, 2.5-mm interscan gap)	Age associated with increased ratio of ventricular cerebrospinal fluid (CSF) volume to cranial volume Gender and laterality effects not reported
Gur et al. 1991	69 healthy volunteers 18–80 years old 34 males; 35 females No neurological or psychiatric illness 66 dextrals; 3 sinistrals	MRI (1.5 tesla) Volume measurements (any two of four raters) derived from seg-mentation technique based on two-feature pixel classifica-tion of multiple spin-echo axial images (5 mm thick, contiguous)	Ratio of ventricular CSF volume to cranial volume greater for elderly subjects (over age 55 years; males = females) Laterality effects (left greater than right) of age were present in elderly males

(continued)

Appendix 9–1   Aging and Brain Ventricular Size *(continued)*

Study	Subjects	Imaging and measurement technique	Findings
Tanna et al. 1991	16 healthy volunteers 52–86 years old 5 males; 11 females No evidence of major medical, neurological, or psychiatric illness Handedness not specified	MRI (1.5 tesla) Volume measurements (one of two raters with established reliabilities) derived from segmentation techniques based on two-feature pixel classification of multiple spin-echo axial images (5 mm thick, 2.5-mm interscan gap)	Age significantly correlated with ratio of ventricular CSF volume to total CSF plus total brain volume Gender and laterality effects not reported
Coffey et al. 1992	76 healthy volunteers 36–91 years old 25 males; 51 females No lifetime evidence of neurological or psychiatric illness All right-handed	MRI (1.5 tesla) Volume measurements (one of three raters with established reliabilities) using computer-assisted trace methodology of T1-weighted coronal images ($n = 30$ to 35, 5 mm thick, contiguous) Blinded clinical ratings (5-point scale) of lateral ventricular enlargement from films (average score of two experienced raters)	Age associated with increased volumes of the third (2.8% per year) and lateral (3.2% per year) ventricles, after adjustment for gender and intracranial area Age associated with increased odds (7.7% per year) of at least mild lateral ventricular enlargement, from 0.10 at age 40 to 2.22 at age 80 No gender or laterality effects
Murphy et al. 1992	27 healthy males 19–92 years old No major medical, neurological, or psychiatric illness Handedness not specified	MRI (0.5 tesla) Blinded volume measurements using computer-assisted trace methodology of proton density axial images ($n = 36$, 7 mm thick, contiguous) Rater reliabilities established, but number of raters not specified	Compared with young males (less than 60 years old; $n = 10$), older males ($n = 17$) had larger ratios of lateral ventricular volume to intracranial volume and of third ventricular volume to intracranial volume No laterality effects
Matsubayashi et al. 1992	73 healthy volunteers 59–83 years old 24 males; 49 females No history of major medical, neurological, or psychiatric illness	MRI (0.5 tesla) Planimetric determination of VBR (no additional details provided)	Age correlated with VBR

[a]Evans's ratio = maximum width of frontal horns of lateral ventricle divided by the maximum internal diameter of skull.
Source.   Adapted from Parashos and Coffey, in press.

Appendix 9–2   Aging and Brain Cerebrospinal Fluid Spaces

Study	Subjects	Imaging and measurement technique	Findings
Earnest et al. 1979	59 volunteer retirees 60–99 years old 11 males; 48 females Living independently and free of neurological disease	Computed tomography (CT) Linear measurement of 4 largest sulci (no additional details provided)	The sum of the widths of the 4 largest sulci was greater in subjects 80 years old (mean ±SD = 4.0 ± 1.1 mm; $n = 29$) than in younger subjects (mean ±SD = 2.9 ± 0.7 mm; $n = 30$)
Meese et al. 1980	160 volunteers 1–71 years old;10 males and 10 females in each decade No additional data provided	CT Linear measurements of sulcal width from 4 axial slices (no additional details provided)	Apparent age-related changes in some measures, but these changes not analyzed statistically
Cala et al. 1981	115 volunteers 15–40 years old 62 males; 53 females No history of migraine, head trauma, or excessive alcohol intake (no additional details provided) All but 8 subjects right-handed	CT (2 different scanners) Ratings (5-point scale) of cortical atrophy (no additional details provided) Axial slices, 13 mm thick	Age apparently associated with increased frequency of mild (grade 2) atrophy of frontal lobes and cerebellar vermis, but no statistical analysis reported
Zatz et al. 1982a	123 volunteers 20–90 years old 49 males; 74 females No history of neurological or major medical disease; psychiatric history not reported Handedness not specified	CT Volume measurement derived from computer-assisted pixel segmentation technique (ASI-II program) Axial slices ($n = 9$), 10 mm thick, 10-mm interscan gap	Age associated with increased sulcal (cerebrospinal fluid [CSF]) volume, even after controlling for intracranial volume
Soininen et al. 1982	85 volunteers, 53 from community and 32 from nursing home Mean ±SD age = 75 ± 7 years No neurological disease (no additional details provided)	CT Linear measurements (from films?) of sulcal size Axial slices ($n = 8$–12), 8 mm thick No additional details provided	Age correlated with mean width of four largest sulci
Gado et al. 1983	12 volunteers 64–81 years old 9 males; 3 females No additional clinical data provided	CT Volume measurements derived from computer-assisted pixel segmentation technique; number of raters and rater reliabilities not specified Axial slices ($n = 7$), 8 mm thick	During 1-year follow-up, ratio of sulcal volume to cranial volume increased significantly by an average of 13%
Schwartz et al. 1985	30 healthy male volunteers 21–81 years old No history of major medical, neurological, or psychiatric illness Handedness not specified	CT Volume measurements derived from computer-assisted pixel segmentation technique (ASI-II program) Axial slices ($n = 7$) starting from the plane of the inferior orbitomeatal line (10 mm thick, 7-mm interscan gap)	Age correlated with CSF volume (ventricular plus basal cisterns), even after controlling for intracranial volume Increased variability of CSF volume with age

(continued)

Appendix 9–2   Aging and Brain Cerebrospinal Fluid Spaces *(continued)*

Study	Subjects	Imaging and measurement technique	Findings
Pfefferbaum et al. 1986	57 healthy volunteers 20–84 years old 27 males; 30 females No additional data provided	CT Volume measurements derived from computer-assisted segmentation technique (modification of Gado et al. 1983) Single axial slice (8 mm thick) approximately 48 mm from the level of the superior roof of the orbits	Age associated with increased ratio of sulcal CSF volume to cranial volume Increased variability of sulcal CSF volume ratio with age
Sullivan et al. 1993	114 healthy vounteers 21–82 years old (mean ±SD = 51.2 ± 17.7 years) 84 males; 30 females No history of major medical, neurological, or psychiatric illness 90% right-handed	CT Volume measurements derived from computer-assisted segmentation technique (modification of Gado et al. 1983) Axial slices ($n = 10$), 10 mm thick	Age correlated with CSF volume in Sylvian fissure and in vertex, frontal, and parieto-occipital sulci No gender effects No correlation between age-related changes in sulcal/fissure CSF volume and performance on 10 neuropsychological tests
Grant et al. 1987	64 volunteers 18–64 years old 25 males, 39 females No history of neurological disease; psychiatric history not reported Handedness not specified	Magnetic resonance imaging (MRI) (0.15 tesla) Mathematically derived estimate of CSF volume from signal intensity measurements made on single sagittal slice (number of raters not specified)	Age associated with increased total (ventricular plus cisternal) cranial CSF volume (males = females)
Jernigan et al. 1990	58 healthy volunteers 8–79 years old 35 males; 23 females No history of neurological, psychiatric, or medical (diabetes mellitus, heart disease) illness Handedness not specified	MRI (1.5 tesla) Volume estimates (one of two raters) derived from computer-assisted pixel classification of spin-echo axial images (5 mm thick, 2.5-mm interscan gap)	Age associated with increased ratio of sulcal CSF volume to cranial volume Gender differences not examined
Gur et al. 1991	69 healthy volunteers 18–80 years old 34 males; 35 females No neurological or psychiatric illness 66 dextrals; 3 sinistrals	MRI (1.5 tesla) Volume measurements (any two of four raters) derived from segmentation technique based on 2-feature pixel classification of multiple spin-echo axial images (5 mm thick, contiguous)	Age correlated with CSF volume For ratio of sulcal CSF volume to cranial volume, age effects greater for males than for females
Tanna et al. 1991	16 healthy volunteers 52–86 years old 5 males; 11 females No evidence of major medical, neurological, or psychiatric illness Handedness not specified	MRI (1.5 tesla) Volume measurements (one of two raters) derived from segmentation techniques based on 2-feature pixel classification of spin-echo axial images (5 mm thick, 2.5-mm interscan gap)	Trend (nonsignificant) for age to be associated with increasing ratio of sulcal CSF volume to total CSF plus total brain volume

(continued)

Appendix 9–2 Aging and Brain Cerebrospinal Fluid Spaces *(continued)*

Study	Subjects	Imaging and measurement technique	Findings
Murphy et al. 1992	27 healthy males 19–92 years old No major medical, neurological, or psychiatric illness Handedness not specified	MRI (0.5 tesla) Blinded volume measurements derived from semi-automated pixel segmentation of proton density axial images ($n = 36$, 7 mm thick, contiguous) Rater reliabilities established, but number of raters not specified)	Compared with young males (less than 60 years old; $n = 10$), older males ($n = 17$) had larger ratios of peripheral CSF volume (total CSF volume minus ventricular volumes) to intracranial volume
Lim et al. 1992	14 healthy male volunteers 8 were young (21–25 years old); 6 were elderly (68–76 years old) No evidence of significant medical or psychiatric illness Handedness not specified	MRI (1.5 tesla) Blinded volume measurements, derived from semi-automated pixel segmentation of intermediate and T2-weighted axial imaging ($n = 8$, 5 mm thick, 2.5 mm-interscan gap)	Compared with younger males, older males had higher percentage of CSF volume to intracranial volume (8% versus 20.1%)

Source. Adapted from Parashos and Coffey, in press.

Appendix 9–3   Aging and Brain Atrophy

Study	Subjects	Imaging and measurement technique	Findings
Jacoby et al. 1980	50 healthy elderly volunteers 62–88 years old 10 men; 40 women No history of significant psychiatric or neurological illness Handedness not specified	Computed tomography (CT) Ratings (4-point scale) of cortical atrophy from films by single blinded rater; five regions rated (frontal, parietal, temporal, insular, and occipital) and scores summed	Age correlated with total cortical atrophy score Gender and laterality effects not reported
Laffey et al. 1984	212 elderly volunteers 65–89 years old 110 men; 102 women No evidence of alcoholism, dementia, or neurological illness	CT Rating (6-point scale) of sulcal widening from films by two experienced radiologists with established reliabilities	No association between age and cortical atrophy ratings
Schwartz et al. 1985	30 healthy male volunteers 21–81 years old No history of major medical, neurological, or psychiatric illness Handedness not specified	CT Volume measurements derived from computer-assisted segmentation technique (ASI-II program) Axial slices ($n = 7$) starting from the plane of the inferior orbitomeatal line (10 mm thick, 7-mm interscan gap)	Age negatively correlated with volume of gray matter and with volume of gray plus white matter, after adjustment for intracranial volume Subjects more than 60 years old ($n = 11$) had smaller volumes of thalamus, lenticular nuclei, and total gray matter than younger subjects ($n = 19$) No laterality effects
Condon et al. 1988	40 volunteers 20–60 years old 20 men; 20 women No additional details provided	Magnetic resonance imaging (MRI) (0.15 tesla) Volume measurement (two raters) derived from computer-assisted pixel segmentation of contiguous sagittal slices (variable slice thickness and number)	Age negatively correlated with ratio of total brain volume to intracranial volume in men, but not women; however, correlations within men and within women not statistically compared
Yoshii et al. 1988	58 volunteers 21–81 years old 29 men; 29 women Neurological and psychiatric histories not reported Handedness not specified	MRI (1.0 tesla) Mathematically derived estimate of brain volume from inversion recovery films, based on planimetric area measurement made on single slice (10 mm thick) at level of foramen of Monro Blinded global ratings of cortical atrophy from films (axial slices [number unspecified], 10 mm thick, 3-mm interscan gap) Number of raters and rater reliabilities not specified	No correlation between age and brain volume Age significantly correlated with ratings of cortical atrophy, for both men and women
Jernigan et al. 1990, 1991	58 healthy volunteers 8–79 years old 35 men; 23 women No history of neurological, psychiatric, or medical illness (diabetes mellitus, heart disease) Handedness not specified	MRI (1.5 tesla) Volume estimates (one of two raters) derived from computer-assisted pixel classification of multiple spin-echo axial images (5 mm thick, 2.5-mm interscan gap)	Age negatively correlated with ratios of cerebral volume to cranial volume and gray matter volume to cranial volume Among gray matter structures, age negatively correlated with ratios of cortical gray matter volume to cranial volume, caudate volume to cranial volume, and diencephalon volume to cranial volume

(continued)

Appendix 9–3 Aging and Brain Atrophy *(continued)*

Study	Subjects	Imaging and measurement technique	Findings
Jernigan et al. *(continued)*			No correlation between age and ratio of white matter volume to cranial volume Laterality effect not reported
Gur et al. 1991	69 healthy volunteers 18–80 years old 34 men; 35 women No neurological or psychiatric illness 66 dextrals, 3 sinistrals	MRI (1.5 tesla) Volume measurements (any two of four raters) derived from segmentation technique based on 2-feature pixel classification of multiple spin echo axial images (5 mm thick, contiguous)	Age negatively correlated with whole brain volume for men and women
Tanna et al. 1991	16 healthy volunteers 52–86 years old 5 men; 11 women No evidence of major medical, neurological, or psychiatric illness Handedness not specified	MRI (1.5 tesla) Volume measurements (one of two raters with established reliabilities) derived from segmentation techniques based on 2-feature pixel classification of multiple spin-echo axial images (5 mm thick, 2.5-mm interscan gap)	Negative correlation of age with ratio of total brain volume to total cerebrospinal fluid plus total brain volume Gender and laterality effects not reported
Coffey et al. 1992	76 healthy volunteers 36–91 years old 25 men; 51 women No lifetime history of neurological or psychiatric illness All right-handed	MRI (1.5 tesla) Volume measurements (one of three raters with established reliabilities) using computer-assisted trace methodology of T1-weighted coronal images ($n = 30$–35, 5 mm thick, contiguous) Blinded clinical ratings (5-point scale) of "cortical atrophy" (average score of two raters)	Increasing age associated with decreasing total volumes of the cerebral hemispheres (0.23% per year), the frontal lobes (0.55% per year), the temporal lobes (0.28% per year), and the amygdala-hippocampal complex (0.30% per year) Increasing age associated with increasing odds (8.9% per year) of "cortical atrophy," from 0.08 at age 40 to 2.82 at age 80 No gender or laterality effects
Krishnan et al. 1990	39 healthy volunteers 24–79 years old 17 men; 22 women No evidence of major medical, neurological, or psychiatric illness	MRI (1.5 tesla) Stereological measurement (one of two raters) of axial slices (variable number, 5 mm thick, 2.5-mm interscan gap) from intermediate and T2-weighted films	Age negatively correlated with total caudate volume (men = women) Caudate volume was less in subjects older than 50 years ($n = 22$) No adjustments for cranial size
McDonald et al. 1991	36 healthy volunteers (subjects also included in Kirshnan et al. 1990 [*above*]) 24–79 years old 13 men; 23 women No evidence of major medical, neurological, or psychiatric illness	MRI (1.5 tesla) Same as Kirshnan et al. 1990 (*above*)	Age negatively correlated with total putamen volume (men = women; left = right), but no adjustments for cranial size
Doraiswamy et al. 1991	36 healthy volunteers (overlap with subjects in McDonald et al. 1991 and Kirshnan et al. 1990 [*above*]) 26–79 years old 16 men; 20 women	MRI (1.5 tesla) Area measurement of T1-weighted midsagittal image using computer-assisted trace methodology Rater reliabilities not reported	Age negatively correlated with corpus callosum area in men, but not women

(continued)

Appendix 9–3   Aging and Brain Atrophy *(continued)*

Study	Subjects	Imaging and measurement technique	Findings
Doraiswamy *(continued)*	No evidence of major medical, neurological, or psychiatric illness		
Shah et al. 1991	36 healthy volunteers (overlap with subjects in Doraiswamy et al. 1991; McDonald et al. 1991; and Krishnan et al. 1990 [*above*]) 26–79 years old 16 men; 20 women No evidence of major medical, neurological, or psychiatric illness	MRI (1.5 tesla) Computer-assisted area measurements from T1-weighted mid-sagittal film by single rater with established intra-rater reliability	Increasing age associated with decreasing midbrain area, after adjusting for gender and cerebral volume No age affects on areas of pons, medulla, anterior cerebellar vermis, posterior cerebellar vermis, or fourth ventricle
Murphy et al. 1992	27 healthy men 19–92 years old No major medical, neurological, or psychiatric illness Handedness not specified	MRI (0.5 tesla) Blinded volume measurements using computer-assisted trace methodology of proton density axial images ($n = 36$, 7 mm thick, contiguous) Tracing of subcortical nuclei performed after image contrast was enhanced by histogram equalization method Rater reliabilities were established but number of raters not reported	Older men (more than 60 years old, $n = 17$) had smaller ratios of total, left, and right hemisphere volume to intracranial volume than younger men ($n = 10$) Older men had smaller ratios of total caudate volume to intracranial volume and total lenticular nuclei volume to intracranial volume than younger men; no difference in ratio of total thalamus volume to intracranial volume Reductions in caudate and lenticular volumes also found when the volumes were normalized to total brain volume, suggesting a differential effect of aging on these structures Older men exhibited a greater right than left asymmetry in lenticular nuclei; the reverse true in younger men
Jack et al. 1992	22 healthy elderly volunteers Mean ±SD age = 76.3 ± 11.3 years 10 men, 12 women No major medical or neurological illness; no depression Handedness not specified	MRI (1.5 tesla) Volume estimates (single rater) derived from computer-assisted pixel classification of T1-weighted coronal images (4 mm thick, contiguous) Intra-rater reliabilities not reported	Age associated with decreased ratio of hippocampal volume to intracranial volume and of anterior temporal lobe volume to intracranial volume Laterality effects not reported
Golomb et al. 1993	154 healthy elderly volunteers 55–88 years old 73 males; 81 females No evidence of active medical, neurological, or psychiatric illness	CT ($n = 51$ subjects); MRI ($n = 81$); both CT and MRI ($n = 22$) Blinded ratings (4-point scale) of hippocampal atrophy as defined by dilatation of transverse choroidal fissure on films	Subjects with hippocampal atrophy (rating of 2 or greater in either hemisphere; $n = 50$) significantly older than those without atrophy More men (41%) than women (25%) with hippocampal atrophy

(continued)

Appendix 9–3 Aging and Brain Atrophy *(continued)*

Study	Subjects	Imaging and measurement technique	Findings
Golomb et al. *(continued)*	Handedness not specified	Inter-rater reliabilities established, but number of raters not reported	After controlling for age, education, and WAIS vocabulary score, subjects with hippocampal atrophy performed worse on recent verbal memory portion of the Guild Memory Scale; no group differences were observed in immediate verbal memory, digit span, or recall of designs
Lim et al. 1992	14 healthy male volunteers 8 were young (21–25 years old) and 6 were elderly (68–76 years old) No evidence of significant medical or psychiatric illness Handedness not specified	MRI (1.5 tesla) Blinded volume measurements derived from semi-automated pixel segmentation of intermediate and T2-weighted axial images ($n = 8$, 5 mm thick, 2.5-mm interscan gap)	Compared to younger men, older men had lower percentage of gray matter volume to intracranial volume (49.7% vs. 38.7%) There was no group difference in percentage of white matter volume to intracranial volume (47.2% vs. 41.2%)
Parashos et al., in press	80 healthy volunteers (overlap with subjects in Coffey et al. 1992) 30–91 years old 28 men; 52 women No lifetime history of neurological or psychiatric illness All right-handed	MRI (1.5 tesla) Blinded area measurements using computer-assisted trace methodology of T1-weighted midsagittal image (5 mm thick), made by single rater with established rater reliabilities	Increasing age associated with smaller total and regional callosal areas, especially of anterior regions No gender effects

Note. WAIS = Wechsler Adult Intelligence Scale (Wechsler 1955).
Source. Adapted from Parashos and Coffey, in press.

Appendix 9–4   Aging and Subcortical Hyperintensity

Study	Subjects	Imaging and measurement technique	Findings
George et al. 1986	47 volunteers Two age groups: older than 45 years (*n* = 35, gender not reported), and 46–78 years old (*n* = 12, 8 males and 4 females) No other clinical information reported	Magnetic resonance imaging (MRI) (0.3 tesla) Determination (present or absent) of SH from T2-weighted axial slices (no additional rater information provided)	Subcortical hyperintensity (SH) present in 8 out of 9 (89%) subjects older than 46 years, but in none of the 35 younger subjects
Hendrie et al. 1989	27 elderly volunteers 63–86 years old 10 males; 17 females No significant medical or neurological illness; psychiatric history not reported	MRI (1.5 tesla) Consensus ratings of SH (4-point scale) from T2-weighted axial slices by two raters with established reliabilities	Mean age increased with severity of SH
Fazekas 1989	87 healthy volunteers 31–93 years old 40 males; 47 females No neurological or psychiatric illness	MRI (1.5 tesla) Ratings of SH (4-point scale) from T2-weighted axial slices (additional rater information not reported)	The incidence and severity of SH increased with age and with the presence of risk factors for vascular disease
Kozachuk et al. 1990	30 healthy volunteers Two age groups: less than 45 (29 ± 6 years old, 7 males and 3 females) and older than 45 (72 ± 12 years old, 11 males and 9 females) No medical, neurological, or psychiatric illness	MRI (0.5 tesla) Rating (4-point scale) by 2 blinded neurologists with established interrater reliability T2-weighted axial slices (*n* = 15, 7 mm thick, contiguous)	Age correlated with SH ratings in the older group only
Jernigan et al. 1991	58 healthy volunteers 8–79 years old 35 males; 23 females Excluded neurological, psychiatric, or medical (diabetes mellitus, heart disease) illness	MRI (1.5 tesla) Volume estimates (one of two raters) derived from computer-assisted pixel classification of spin-echo axial images (5 mm thick, 2.5-mm interscan gap)	Age associated with increased volume of SH in both cortical and subcortical regions
Matsubayashi et al. 1992	73 healthy elderly volunteers 59–83 years old 24 males; 49 females No major medical, neurological, or psychiatric illness	MRI (0.5 tesla) Rating (4-point scale) of periventricular SH on T2-weighted axial slices (no additional details reported)	Subjects with highest SH rating (*n* = 19) significantly older than the other groups
Boone et al. 1992	100 healthy volunteers 45–83 years old 36 males; 64 females No major medical, neurological, or psychiatric illness	MRI (1.5 tesla) Computer-assisted area measurements of SH from T2-weighted axial sections by single rater (additional rater information not reported)	Age greater in those subjects with the largest lesion areas
Almkvist et al. 1992	23 healthy elderly volunteers All older than 75 years 9 males; 14 females No major medical, neurological, or psychiatric illness	MRI (0.02 tesla) Area measurements of SH from T2-weighted axial sections by single blinded rater (reliabilities not reported)	No correlation between age and SH area

(continued)

Appendix 9–4 Aging and Subcortical Hyperintensity *(continued)*

Study	Subjects	Imaging and measurement technique	Findings
Coffey et al. 1992	76 healthy volunteers 36–91 years old 25 males; 51 females No history of neurological or psychiatric illness All right-handed	MRI (1.5 tesla) Consensus ratings of SH from intermediate and T2-weighted axial films (4-point scale) by two blinded raters with established reliabilities	Increasing age associated with increased odds of SH in the deep white matter (6.3% per year) and pons (8.1% per year)

Source. Adapted from Parashos and Coffey, in press.

Appendix 9–5 Published Studies of Neuropsychological Test Performance in Healthy Subjects With Imaging Changes in Subcortical White Matter

Study	Subjects	Imaging and measurement technique	Findings
Brant-Zawadzki et al. 1985	14 elderly volunteers 59–81 years old 6 males; 8 females No medical conditions "associated with cognitive loss" (psychiatric histories not examined)	Magnetic resonance imaging (MRI) (0.35 tesla) Standardized severity ratings (5-point scale) of white matter hyperintensity made by 2 raters (inter-rater agreement not given) from intermediate and T2-weighted scans	No statistical analysis of neuropsychological test data (10 tests) conducted. One of the 10 subjects with a hyperintensity rating of 1 or less scored in the "demented range" on the Wechsler Memory Scale (Russell revision) and Wechsler Adult Intelligence Scale–Revised (WAIS-R) Block Design. One of the 4 subjects with a hyperintensity rating of 2 or greater had impaired performance on WAIS-R Picture Arrangement.
Steingart et al. 1987	105 elderly volunteers 59–91 years old 56 males; 49 females No evidence of dementia or stroke; psychiatric history not examined	Computed tomography (CT) Determination of presence of leukoaraiosis by single blinded rater	Subjects with leuko-araiosis ($n = 9$) had lower scores on the Extended Scale for Dementia than did subjects without the finding ($n = 96$), even after controlling for age, sex, education, and presence of infarct (analysis of covariance).
Rao et al. 1989	50 healthy middle-aged volunteers 25–60 years old 11 males; 39 females No evidence of major medical, neurological, or psychiatric illness	MRI (1.5 tesla) Presence of leuko-araisosis on intermediate and T2-weighted scans (no description of rating methodology provided)	Relative to subjects without leuko-araiosis ($n = 40$), subjects with the finding ($n = 10$) performed significantly worse on 3 of 45 neuropsychological tests (t-tests): Benton Facial Recognition Test ($P < .01$), Brown-Peterson Interference Test (18-second delay [$P < .03$]), and the President's Test ($P < .04$).
Hunt et al. 1989	46 elderly volunteers Mean ±SD = 78.2 ± 4.6 years old 17 males; 29 females No evidence of major medical illness (psychiatric histories not examined)	MRI (1.5 tesla) Single blinded rater determined number (4-point scale) and size (3-point scale) of white matter hyperintensity changes from intermediate and T2-weighted scans Severity score derived from multiplying number by size, summed across 5 brain regions	When controlling for age, a nonsignificant regression coefficient was obtained between total severity of white matter hyperintensity and composite neuropsychological performance in five "domains" derived from 21 tests. No apparent difference in neuropsychological performance between subjects with more or less than the median number of white matter lesions (statistical analysis not conducted).
Hendrie et al. 1989	27 elderly volunteers 63–86 years old 10 males; 17 females No evidence of medical or neurological illness (psychiatric history not examined)	MRI (1.5 tesla) Standardized rating by two blinded raters of severity (4-point scale) of white matter hyperintensity from T2-weighted films	No differences (statistical analysis not described) between the four severity categories of white matter hyperintensity on three cognitive measures (Mini-Mental State Exam [MMSE], CAMCOG, and WAIS Digit Symbol).

(continued)

Appendix 9–5 Published Studies of Neuropsychological Test Performance in Healthy Subjects With Imaging Changes in Subcortical White Matter *(continued)*

Study	Subjects	Imaging and measurement technique	Findings
Austrom et al. 1990	26 elderly volunteers (same subjects as in Hendrie et al. 1989, retested 18 months later) No change in health status since original testing 18 months earlier	Not reported, but presumably same data as reported in Hendrie et al. 1989	Subjects without white matter hyperintensity at baseline ($n = 11$) showed a significant improvement on the WAIS Digit Symbol test, whereas subjects with white matter hyperintensity tended to have lower scores at follow-up. Neither group showed significant changes in MMSE or CAMCOG scores.
Schmidt et al. 1991	32 healthy volunteers 22–49 years old 25 males; 7 females Most receiving medication for hypertension, but otherwise no evidence of major medical, neurological, or psychiatric illness	MRI (1.5 tesla) Blinded determination of white matter lesions from intermediate and T2-weighted films (no description of rating methodology provided)	No differences (t-tests) between subjects with ($n = 12$) and without ($n = 20$) white matter lesions on a computerized test of vigilance and reaction time, a test of visual attention (d2 test), and a test of learning and memory (Lern- und Gedächtnistest).
Mirsen et al. 1991	39 elderly volunteers Mean ±SD = 73.2 ± 5.8 years old 20 males; 19 females 3 subjects with infarcts; an indeterminate number with no evaluation (medical, neurological, or psychiatric), apart from cognitive testing, which was normal	MRI (1.5 tesla) Blinded determination by 2 raters of presence of periventricular hyperintensity and severity (5-point scale) of leuko-araiosis on T1- and T2- weighted films (interrater agreement ranged from 56% to 88%)	Nonsignificant correlations between presence of either periventricular hyperintensity or leuko-araiosis and performance on the Extended Scale for Dementia.
Harrell et al. 1991	25 healthy elderly volunteers Mean ±SD = 65.6 ± 6.9 years old Gender breakdown not reported No history of significant medical, neurological, or psychiatric illness	MRI (0.5 or 1.5 tesla) Standardized severity ratings (6-point scale) of white matter hyperintensity by a single blinded rater from T1- and T2-weighted scans	Nonsignificant correlations between severity of either periventricular or deep white matter hyperintensity and 2 cognitive screening instruments (MMSE and Mattis Dementia Rating Scale).
Almkvist et al. 1992	23 healthy elderly (more than 75 years old) volunteers 9 males; 14 females No history of significant medical, neurological, or psychiatric illness	MRI (0.02 tesla) Computer-assisted volumetric measurements of subcortical hyperintensity by single blinded rater (no intra-rater reliability reported)	No relationship between total or regional volumes of subcortical hyperintensity and performance on 24 neuropsychological tests.
Matsubayashi et al. 1992	73 healthy elderly volunteers 59–83 years old 24 males; 49 females No history of major medical, neurological, or psychiatric illness	MRI (0.5 tesla) Standardized severity ratings (4-point scale) of periventricular hyperintensity by single blinded rater (intrarater agreement not reported)	Subjects with periventricular hyperintensity ratings of 3 or greater ($n = 19$) performed less well on all neuropsychological test measures (MMSE, Hasegawa Dementia Scale, a visuospatial cognitive performance test, and a test of manual dexterity) than did subjects ($n = 54$) with less severe ratings, even after controlling for age effects.

(continued)

Appendix 9–5   Published Studies of Neuropsychological Test Performance in Healthy Subjects With Imaging Changes in Subcortical White Matter *(continued)*

Study	Subjects	Imaging and measurement technique	Findings
Boone et al. 1992	100 healthy volunteers 45–83 years old 36 males; 64 females No major medical, neuro-logical, or psychiatric illness	MRI (1.5 tesla) Computer-assisted area measure-ments of subcoritcal hyper-intensity from T2-weighted axial sections by single rater (additional rater information not reported)	Subjects ($n = 6$) with lesion areas greater than 10 cm^2 performed less well on measures of frontal lobe ability (Auditory Consonant Trigrams, Wisconsin Card Sort Test, and Stroop Test), attention (Digit Span), and speed of in-formation-processing (Digit Symbol, Stroop test).
Tupler et al. 1992	66 healthy volunteers 45–89 years old 24 males; 42 females No evidence of past or present neurological or psychiatric illness	MRI (1.5 tesla) Consensus ratings (4-point scale) of severity of white matter hyper-intensity from axial scans by 2 blinded raters with established reliabilities	Two neuropsychological tests were selected a priori: the Benton Facial Recognition Test and the Digit Symbol. After adjustments for age and education, neither test was associated with subcortical hyperintensity.
Levine et al. 1993	127 healthy nonelderly volunteers 50 males (35.2 ± 11.8 years old); 77 females (43.3 ± 8.4 years old) No history of significant medical, neurological, or psychiatric illness	MRI (0.5 tesla) Presence of subcortical hyperinten-sity determined by three "experienced neuroradiologists" from intermediate and T2-weighted axial scans (no additional data provided)	Among subjects with subcortical hyperintensity (5 males and 7 females), males (but not females) exhibited impaired attention on a dichotic listening task, relative to subjects without subcortical hyperintensity.

Source.   Adapted from Tupler et al. 1992.

10

Functional Neuroimaging: Positron-Emission Tomography in the Study of Cerebral Blood Flow and Glucose Utilization in Human Subjects at Different Ages

Pietro Pietrini, M.D.
Stanley I. Rapoport, M.D.

Senectus enim insanabilis morbus est.

Seneca, *Epistolae,* 108

Introduction

That aging is invariably associated with changes in body and mind has been known since the ancient days. The Roman philosopher Seneca wrote that "aging in fact is an incurable disease." Although advances in health care during the past decades have improved the quality of life of older people and have softened Seneca's statement, it remains true that the human body and mind undergo inevitable modifications during aging, even in the absence of evident disease.

As far as the brain is concerned, many cognitive, neurochemical, histological, and morphological changes are known to accompany aging. Neuropsychological tests, for example, have shown that some cognitive features including perceptual speed, memory span, and associative memory (referred to as *fluid intelligence*) usually decline with age, whereas others including verbal comprehension, general information, and arithmetic skills (referred to as *crystallized intelligence*) remain intact (Horn 1975). This suggests that a large part of cognitive processing, related to the ability to cope with the environment, is preserved in older people (Creasey and Rapoport 1985). Long before the development of the cognitive sciences, the French essayist Montaigne (1580) provided a clear description of the phenomenon:

> Since I was 20 years of age, I am certain that my mind and body have deteriorated more than they have developed. It is likely that knowledge and experience increase with aging, but activity, alertness, strength and other important qualities nevertheless decline.

Different experimental approaches have been used to examine the functional neurological correlates of these alterations. In the past decade, the introduction of sophisticated imaging techniques like positron-emission tomography (PET) has made it possible to visualize cerebral metabolism and blood flow in vivo and to investigate metabolic and flow correlates of brain function and structure in relation to human aging. In this chapter, we describe these and earlier related techniques and examine how functional neuroimaging has helped to elucidate aging of the human brain.

Historical Background: Kety-Schmidt and Xenon-133 Techniques

Noninvasive measurements of brain function have been sought since the beginning of modern medicine. Normally, the brain produces the energy necessary for its functioning through oxidation of glucose. Although comprising only 2% of body weight in the adult, the human brain consumes about 20% of glucose consumed by the body as a whole (Sokoloff 1959). Neurons require energy in the form of adenosine triphosphate (ATP) to maintain their membrane potentials through activation of calcium/potassium membrane pumps, to support their electrical activity and for synthetic processes. Accordingly, the regional cerebral metabolic rate for glucose (rCMRglc) will represent largely the functional and baseline metabolic activity of neurons in a given region. Furthermore, because regional cerebral blood flow (rCBF) normally is coupled with rCMRglc (Roy and Sherrington 1890), the earliest clinical investigations by Kety and Schmidt (1948) were designed to determine in vivo average cerebral blood flow (CBF), so as to examine global brain functional activity. The technique chosen was based on the Fick principle, which relates arterial delivery of a chemically inert substance, its brain uptake, and its removal by the venous system. This method did not provide regional information and was invasive because it required a carotid artery injection and internal jugular sampling of nitrous oxide, a freely diffusible and nonmetabolizable substance. Initial studies with the Kety-Schmidt technique confirmed that global CBF and the cerebral metabolic rate for oxygen ($CMRO_2$) were correlated. Both rapidly decreased from childhood to adolescence, followed by a more gradual, but progressive, decline throughout the adult life span (Kety 1956).

Subsequent modifications of the original method led to the clearance technique that used the γ-emitting isotope xenon-133 (^{133}Xe) (Obrist et al. 1967, 1975; Risberg 1980). With this method, it was possible to quantify rCBF in regions of the cerebral cortex, following inhalation or intracarotid artery injection of ^{133}Xe and, when using extracranial scintillation crystals, to record and localize radioactivity. Although the ^{133}Xe methods were an improvement over the Kety-Schmidt technique, their limited spatial resolution and inability to examine subcortical structures restricted investigations to large areas of the lateral surface of the cerebral cortex. Studies performed with ^{133}Xe consistently indicated an age-related decline of cortical blood flow (Naritomi et al. 1979; Obrist 1978).

In addition to technical limitations, methodological restrictions affected conclusions obtained with the Kety-Schmidt and ^{133}Xe clearance techniques. Most studies did not select optimally healthy subjects, blurring distinctions between effects of healthy aging and of age-related brain disease on CBF. Thus subjects were recruited from hospitalized patients having so-called minor elective surgery (Scheinberg et al. 1953) or minor illness (Schieve and Wilson 1953) or even from patients with a history of convulsive disorder (Kennedy [in Kety 1956]). Patients with a history of psychosis, mental deterioration, or other degenerative processes often were included, and study conditions frequently were uncontrolled. With the exception of the study by Melamed et al. (1980), ^{133}Xe measurements were not performed with subjects in the "resting state" (i.e., with eyes covered and ears plugged with cotton to minimize sensory stimulation). As vision and hearing acuities on average decline with age, observed age-related flow reductions in subjects not studied in the resting state may be due in part to these extrinsic changes, rather than to reduced intrinsic brain functional activity (see below) (Rapoport 1983).

PET

During the past decade, PET has facilitated the noninvasive investigation of brain functional activity in awake human subjects, not only in the cerebral cortex, but also in subcortical structures, with progressively better spatial and temporal resolutions. A number of positron-emitting compounds have been used to study various aspects of brain integrity and function, including neurotransmitter metabolism. It is now possible to determine rCBF, rCMRglc, and the regional cerebral metabolic rate for oxygen (rCMRO2) in regions of the human brain smaller than 3 mm in diameter (Jagust et al. 1990). Radiolabeled transmitters (e.g., [^{18}F]fluoro-L-dopa) and transmitter receptors (e.g., serotonin receptors) can also be studied with PET. PET scans can be repeated, thus allowing brain functional patterns to be evaluated in the same subject under different test conditions (e.g., resting state versus sensory stimulation), before and after drug administration, or in longitudinal studies of aging.

Basic Principles of PET Technology

PET uses unstable nuclides that have an excess of protons in their nucleus and thus emit *positrons,* antimatter electrons with the same mass as an electron but with a positive charge. Once emitted, a positron has the kinetic energy to travel a few millimeters within tissue, until it meets an unbound electron. Because the two particles have opposite charge, they annihilate each other and, following the law of conservation of energy, emit two γ ray photons of 511 kiloelectron volts (KeV) energy at 180° to each other (Horwitz 1990) (Figure 10–1). The γ photons are detected by rings of radiation detectors which surround the subject's head and measure the number of photons originating from all the angles within the brain. Through a computer reconstruction algorithm based on a transmission scan, it is possible to identify where the annihilation event took place and where the positron was emitted (with an approximation of a few millimeters due to the distance traveled by the positron before the event of annihilation), as well as the quantity of radiation emitted from that site.

Cerebral glucose metabolism. By using PET with [^{18}F]fluoro-2-deoxy-D-glucose (FDG), an analog of glucose labeled with fluorine-18, it is possible to visualize and measure the uptake of FDG by neural cells in different brain regions in an awake subject. FDG reaches the brain through blood flow and, like glucose, can be transported bidirectionally across cerebral capillaries by a monosaccharide transport system. Once inside brain cells, FDG is phosphorylated to FDG-6-phosphate (FDG-6-P) by the enzyme hexokinase. Unlike glucose-6-P, however, FDG-6-P cannot be transformed into fructose-6-P and is not further metabolized by glycolytic pathway enzymes. As brain phosphatase activity is low, FDG-6-P remains essentially trapped inside brain cells, virtually unchanged during the duration of the study (Sokoloff 1982) (Figure 10–2).

The quantity of FDG-6-P that has accumulated in a brain region during 45 minutes after FDG injection is measured by PET and is a function of the rate of phosphorylation of glucose to glucose-6-P by hexokinase, the first reaction in the glycolytic pathway, and the integral of FDG in blood to which the brain is exposed. At a steady state with regard to unlabeled concentrations, the net rate of any step in a pathway equals the net rate of the overall pathway; thus the net rate of glucose phosphorylation estimated with FDG represents the net flux of glucose through the entire glycolytic pathway. Sokoloff et al. (1977) elaborated an operational equation to calculate rCMRglc from 1) the quantity of FDG-6-P within brain, 2) the ratio of the integrated plasma activity of FDG to cold plasma glucose concentration during 45 minutes, and 3) a "lumped constant" to correct for the use of FDG instead of the natural glucose ("isotope effect") (Huang et al. 1980).

rCBF. rCBF can be assessed by using PET and water labeled with oxygen-15 (^{15}O). Water is an excellent flow indicator because it is almost freely diffusible at physiological flow rates and can quickly equilibrate between brain and blood. Immediately after an intravenous injection of a bolus of 30–40 millicurie of radiolabeled water, a dynamic acquisition PET scan is obtained to measure local cerebral radioactivity during the subsequent 4 minutes. Radioactivity concurrently is monitored in the blood through an indwelling arterial line connected to an automatic counter. Using this method, it is possible to determine absolute rCBF values, expressed in ml/100 g tissue per minute.

In a variant of this procedure, the subject continuously inhales ^{15}O-labeled carbon dioxide, which in the lung gives rise to ^{15}O-labeled water. When a steady state is reached, and the rate of delivery of radioactive water to the brain equals its rate of removal by venous washout, measured brain radioactivity is directly proportional to the constant input function, which is a function of rCBF (Frackowiak and Lammertsma 1985).

Because the ^{15}O in water has a rapid radioactive decay (half-life = 2.02 minutes), multiple studies only

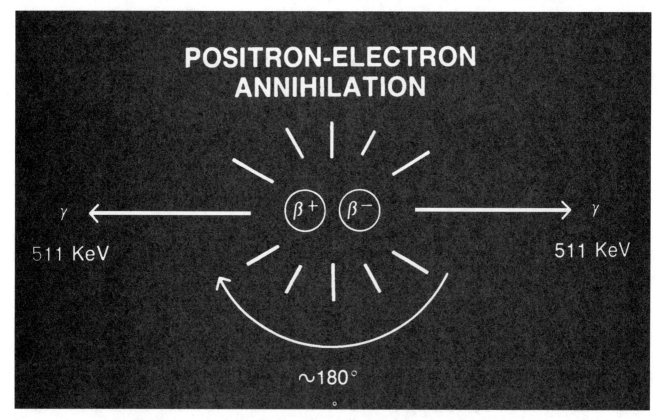

Figure 10–1.   Positron-emission tomography (PET). Following the annihilation of a positron (β^+) with an electron ($\beta-$), two γ rays are emitted in diametrically opposite directions. These γ rays are detected by the PET machine, and their local site of origin and intensity are reconstructed. KeV = kiloelectron volt.

8–12 minutes apart can be performed sequentially in the same subject. This makes it possible to evaluate rCBF repeatedly in a single sitting, while the subject is in the resting state or performing any of several tasks. By subtracting baseline rCBF from task rCBF, regions that are specifically and significantly activated during the task can be identified. In such studies, global CBF frequently is corrected for arterial blood partial pressure of carbon dioxide ($PaCO_2$), which should be measured. (A detailed description of the physical and technical aspects of PET goes far beyond the aims of this review; for more information, see Holcomb et al. 1989; Mazziotta and Phelps 1986.)

PET Studies in Healthy Aging

rCBF and Oxygen Consumption

PET has allowed researchers to overcome many of the limitations of earlier techniques and to obtain more reliable information about relations among regional cerebral metabolism, rCBF, and age. Results with regard to rCBF and $rCMRO_2$ are summarized in Table 10–1, which shows that, in general, studies performed in the resting state demonstrated lesser changes than those in which visual and/or auditory stimulation was uncontrolled.

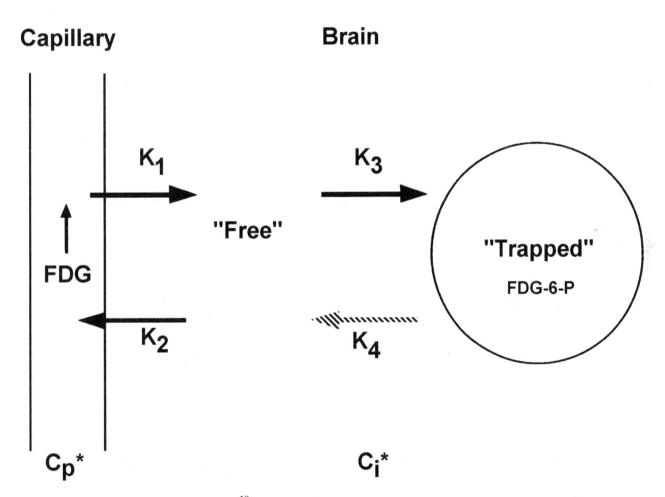

Figure 10–2.   Fluorodeoxyglucose model. [^{18}F]fluoro-2-deoxy-D-glucose (FDG) reaches the brain via blood and is transferred across brain capillaries and into cells with an influx rate constant equal to K_1. Once inside cells, FDG is phosphorylated to FDG-6-P by the enzyme hexokinase, at a rate equal to K_3. FDG-6-P remains essentially trapped intracellularly because the rate of dephosphorylation, K_4, is quite slow due to a low brain activity of the enzyme glucose-6-P phosphatase. K_2 is the rate constant for efflux of FDG from cells to blood. $C_p^* =$ the concentration of FDG in plasma; $C_i^* =$ concentration in brain.
Source.   Reprinted from Grady CL, Rapoport SI: "Cerebral Metabolism in Aging and Dementia," in *Handbook of Mental Health and Aging.* Edited by Birren J, Sloane RB, Cohen G. San Diego, CA, Academic Press, 1992, pp. 201–228. Used with permission.

In accord with conclusions from a majority of studies performed with the ^{133}Xe technique, initial PET studies using the "steady state" ^{15}O inhalation method supported a decrease of rCBF with aging. Frackowiak and colleagues (Frackowiak and Gibbs 1983; Frackowiak et al. 1984) found a 28% reduction in mean gray matter rCBF in a group of 14 older subjects compared with 18 young subjects, not studied in the resting state. The regression between rCBF and age was statistically significant and had a slope of -4.9 ml/100 g per minute per decade. rCMRO$_2$ in gray matter was significantly decreased by 19% in the older subjects, but failed to show a significant regression with age. White matter showed no rCBF group difference. The tendency of the oxygen extraction rate (OER) (i.e., the ratio of rCMRO$_2$ to rCBF) to be elevated in the elderly group, if confirmed, could be an early sign of hemodynamic decompensation (Frackowiak et al. 1984). An age-associated decline in rCBF in temporosylvian, medial frontal, and medial occipitovisual regions also was demonstrated in 19 "hospitalized patients with nonacute illness," using low-resolution PET in subjects with eyes closed, but ears unobstructed (Lebrun-Grandie et al. 1983).

In a later study, the same group (Pantano et al. 1984) examined 27 "healthy hospitalized patients" 19 to 76 years old and found a significant linear decline with age of gray matter rCBF (3.2 ml/100 g per minute per decade) but not of rCMRO$_2$. When the younger (less than 50 years old) and older (more than 55 years old) subjects were compared, both mean rCBF and rCMRO2 were decreased significantly in the older

Table 10–1. Summary of principal studies and of methods and techniques used with positron-emission tomography (PET) relating regional cerebral bloold flow (rCBF) and regional cerebral metabolic rate for oxygen (rCMRO$_2$) in human subjects to age

Study	Subjects	PET procedure	Results and comments
Lebrun-Grandie et al. 1983	Hospitalized patients with nonacute illness 14 men; 5 women 19–76 years old	Oxygen-15 Steady state ECAT (FWHM 19 mm) Eyes closed; ears open Measured attenuation	rCBF declined with age in temporosylvian, medial frontal, and medial occipitovisual regions. No age effect on CMRO$_2$.
Frackowiak and Gibbs 1983	18 young (24–43 years old) 14 older (49–74 years old)	Oxygen-15 Steady state ECAT II (FWHM 17 mm)	Gray matter: 19% CMRO$_2$ and 28% rCBF reductions; -0.5 ml/100 ml per minute per year.
Pantano et al. 1984	Healthy hospitalized patients 19 men; 8 women 19–76 years old	Oxygen-15 Steady state ECAT II (FWHM 17 mm)	CMRO$_2$ significantly reduced in the older group; rCBF: -0.32 ml/100 ml per minute per year.
Yamaguchi et al. 1986	Healthy subjects; no medications 17 men; 5 women 26–64 years old (14 younger than 50; 8 older than 50)	Oxygen-15 Steady state HEADTOME III (FWHM 8.2 mm)	Gray matter CMRO$_2$: linear negative correlation with age; no difference in rCBF, OER, or CBV.
Itoh et al. 1990	Healthy volunteers 17 men; 11 women 50–85 years old	Oxygen-15 Steady state ECAT II (FWHM 17 mm) Calculated attenuation	No change with age; CMRO$_2$ and rCBF were not related to brain atrophy as measured by CT.
Leenders et al. 1990	Patients' relatives and hospital staff 18 men; 16 women 22–82 years old No CT or MRI scan	Oxygen-15 Steady state ECAT II (FWHM 17 mm) Eyes closed; ears open No face mask Measured attenuation	rCBF, CBV, and CMRO$_2$ decreased significantly in the frontal cortex and insular matter. OER increased in some areas.

(continued)

group (by - 18% and - 17%, respectively). Decreases were mostly in frontal, temporosylvian, and parieto-occipital cortical areas. White matter rCBF and rCMRO$_2$ did not differ between groups. Although the OER was age invariant, no correction for a possible difference in cerebral blood volume (CBV) was performed.

Takada et al. (1992) in an inadequately described study also reported a significant linear decline with age for CMRO$_2$ but not for rCBF, and only in the association neocortex of the left hemisphere. Significant age reductions of rCBF in the frontal cortex and insular gray matter and of rCMRO$_2$ and regional cerebral blood volume (rCBV) in white matter and in many cortical areas were reported in healthy subjects between 22 and 82 years old with eyes closed, but ears unobstructed (Leenders et al. 1990). Rates of decline approximated 0.5% per year. In addition, OER significantly increased with age in some cortical regions.

In contrast to these results, no age difference in mean rCBF, OER, or CBV was noted in 22 healthy volunteers, whereas mean gray rCMRO$_2$ significantly decreased with age (Yamaguchi et al. 1986). A slight increase of PaCO$_2$ and a decrease of hematocrit observed in the older subjects could have tended to elevate rCBF in this study, masking an age-related decrease.

Structural changes, such as enlargement of the cerebrospinal fluid (CSF) spaces and cortical atrophy, have been claimed to be responsible for intrinsic (by reducing the number of neurons in the gray matter) and apparent (by increasing partial volume effects of CSF or white matter) age declines in rCBF. However,

Table 10–1. Summary of principal studies and of methods and techniques used with positron-emission tomography (PET) relating regional cerebral blood flow (rCBF) and regional cerebral metabolic rate for oxygen (rCMRO$_2$) in human subjects to age (*continued*)

Study	Subjects	PET procedure	Results and comments
Martin et al. 1991	Healthy subjects; no medications 15 men; 15 women 30–85 years old	Oxygen-15 Steady state ECAT 931/8/12 Eyes closed; ears open Measured attenuation	No change in global CBF; decrease in limbic and association areas.
Takada et al. 1992	Healthy volunteers 15 men; 17 women 27–67 years old	Oxygen-15 Steady state PET scanner: ? Eyes closed; sensory stimulation or deprivation	CMRO$_2$ significantly decreased in bilateral putamen, left temporal, frontal, and parietal cortices. rCBF decreased only in the left superior temporal cortex. Methodology poorly described.
Burns and Tyrrell 1992	Patients' healthy relatives 6 men; 8 women 51–85 years old No careful medical screening	Oxygen-15 Steady state ECAT 931/8/12	CMRO$_2$ significantly decreased in the parietal lobe.
Marchal et al. 1992	Healthy volunteers 14 men; 11 women 20–68 years old Careful medical screening At least 7-year education	Oxygen-15 Steady state LETI TTV03 (FWHM 8 mm) Stereotactic frame Eyes closed; ears open Measured attenuation	CMRO$_2$ decreased in 24/31 cortical gyri (−6% per decade); rCBF decreased in 10/31 gyri.
Grady et al. 1992	Healthy volunteers 11 men (mean age ±SD = 27 ± 4 years) 9 men (mean age ±SD = 72 ± 7 years) Careful medical screening No medications	Oxygen-15 water iv bolus Scanditronix PC1024-7B (FWHM 6 mm) Resting state versus activation Measured attenuation	Young and older subjects have different patterns of activation in the extrastriate cortex during visual processing.

Note. CMRO$_2$ = cerebral metabolic rate for oxygen; FWHM = full width at half maximum [in millimeters]; OER = oxygen extraction rate; CBV = cerebral blood volume; CT = computed tomography; MRI = magnetic resonance imaging. ECAT, ECAT II, HEADTOME III, LETI TTVO3, and Scanditronix PC1024-7B are different PET scanners (whose properties are described in the respective studies).

despite evidence of progressive cortical atrophy by x-ray computed tomography (CT), no significant decrease in rCBF or $rCMRO_2$ was detected in healthy subjects between the ages of 50 and 85 (Itoh et al. 1990). Magnetic resonance imaging (MRI) of the brain and exact coregistration of MRI structural images with functional PET images would be required to demonstrate the extent that atrophy influences PET measurements in the elderly.

With high-resolution PET and a sophisticated method of anatomical localization (the statistical parametric map [SPM]), Martin et al. (1991) recently reported a significant age-related decline in rCBF in limbic regions and in bilateral temporal, parietal, and frontal association cortices, more in the left than right hemisphere. These changes, in subjects studied with eyes closed and ears unobstructed, were unrelated to differences in global CBF and thus were thought to represent an age-related redistribution of rCBF.

As illustrated in Table 10–1, PET studies relating rCBF and $rCMRO_2$ to age have differed technically and methodologically, and it is not surprising therefore that results have been inconsistent and have not led to firm conclusions. Early PET investigations used low-resolution scanners, with limited anatomical definition of cortical and subcortical structures and significant error due to "partial voluming" (see below). Subjects ranged from "healthy hospitalized patients" (Pantano et al. 1984) or "hospitalized patients with nonacute illness" (Lebrun-Grandie et al. 1983) to carefully screened healthy volunteers (Marchal et al. 1992), and cognitive evaluation was rarely carried out. Dementing processes, such as Alzheimer's disease, can have an insidious onset and progress for years before becoming clinically evident. For example, in early stages of Alzheimer's disease, in subjects with only a memory deficit, abnormal rCMRglc has been demonstrated in association neocortices and precedes additional cognitive deficits that later appear (Grady et al. 1988; Haxby et al. 1990). To date, all aging studies have been cross-sectional, and the possibility cannot be ruled out that some reported age-related differences reflected sampling bias from surviving subjects (Martin et al. 1991).

Marchal et al. (1992) attempted to control for some of these variables by studying 25 optimally healthy, carefully screened volunteers between the ages of 20 and 68 studied with eyes closed and ears unobstructed. High-resolution PET and stereotactic positioning of the head were used. A significant decline in rCBF was detected only in two frontal gyri, perhaps be-

cause of the large coefficient of variation in the other regions (up to 32%). However, a significant age-related decrease of $rCMRO_2$ was seen throughout the cerebral cortex, except for the orbitofrontal gyrus, hippocampal, and lateral occipital regions. $rCMRO_2$ declined by 6% per decade. No significant relation was shown between whole-cortex $rCMRO_2$ and gender, cortical atrophy, or head size; subcortical structures, the cerebellum, and white matter showed no significant age-dependent change.

In summary, data from numerous studies relating rCBF and $rCMRO_2$ to age are somewhat contradictory. In studies of subjects not in the resting state, age-dependent reductions are of the order of 20%–25%. The functional significance of these changes is not clear. In some studies, largest reductions were reported in cortical association regions, which subserve cognitive functions that decline even in healthy elderly people. These association areas appeared relatively recently during primate evolution, usually are the latest to myelinate, and may be selectively vulnerable to age-related degenerative processes such as Alzheimer's disease (Rapoport 1988, 1990). In subjects not studied in the resting state, age-reductions could have reflected reduced visual and auditory acuities (Creasey and Rapoport 1985; Grady et al. 1984). A reduced rCBF in older people also might be caused by subclinical cerebrovascular disease, as atherosclerotic brain lesions are more frequent in the elderly and 50% of brains show such lesions after age 50 (Moossy 1971). Atherosclerotic vascular disease (Dastur et al. 1963) and hypertension (Meyer et al. 1985; Salerno et al. 1992), whose prevalence also increases with age, have been shown to be accompanied by reduced rCBF and/or rCMRglc.

rCMRglc

PET studies of rCMRglc and human aging also have led to conflicting results, but in general studies outside of the resting state have demonstrated greater declines than those within it (Table 10–2). Kuhl et al. (1982) found a gradual age decline in rCMRglc in 40 healthy subjects between 18 and 78 years old, who were studied with eyes open and ears unplugged. The rate of decline was 0.43% per year (a net of 26% in the above age range), with no hemispheric preference. The ratio of rCMRglc in the frontal cortex to rCMRglc in the parietal cortex, an index of "hyperfrontality" (Ingvar 1979), fell with age, suggesting a selective effect on the frontal lobe. Chawluk et al. (1987) reported a comparable 0.26% per year decline in rCMRglc in healthy subjects studied outside of the resting state. In contrast, other studies found no significant age-associated reduction in rCMRglc (de Leon et al. 1983; Duara et al. 1983, 1984) or a decrease in only a small number of brain regions (Hoffman et al. 1988). The study by deLeon et al. (1983) was performed on subjects with eyes closed and ears unobstructed, whereas the study by Duara et al. (1983, 1984) was conducted on patients in the resting state (eyes covered and ears plugged with cotton). These differences in methodology may have obscured actual age-related differences.

Factors Influencing PET Studies of Aging

As in the cases of rCBF and rCMRO2, the question of whether rCMRglc declines with age has no conclusive answer. Methodological issues and technical limitations noted above probably contributed to discrepancies in the various studies (Table 10–3). This chapter is not the place to discuss these issues in detail (for an excellent review, see Horwitz 1990), but some deserve brief mention.

What we determine with PET, using the FDG or ^{15}O water isotopes, are absolute values and correlated

Table 10–2. Summary of principal studies and of methods and techniques used with positron-emission tomography (PET), relating regional cerebral metabolic rate for glucose (rCMRglc) in human subjects to age

Study	Subjects	PET procedure	Results and comments
Kuhl et al. 1982	17 men; 23 women 18–78 years old	ECAT II (FWHM 17 mm) Eyes and ears open Calculated attenuation	Generalized decrease in rCMRglc (0.43%/ year); frontal cortex more affected.
de Leon et al. 1983	14 young men (mean age ±SD = 26 ± 5 years) 21 older men (mean age ±SD = 67 ± 7 years)	PETT III (FWHM 15 mm) Eyes closed; ears open No attenuation correction	No change with age.
Hawkins et al. 1983	7 men; 1 woman 18–68 years old	NeuroECAT (FWHM 12 mm) Eyes and ears open	FDG rate constants do not change with age; no rCMRglc change with age.
Duara et al. 1983, 1984	40 healthy male volunteers 21–83 years old Careful medical screening	ECAT II (FWHM 17 mm) Eyes and ears covered Measured attenuation	No change with age.
Horwitz et al. 1986	15 young men (20–32 years old) 15 elderly men (64–83 years old) (Data from Duara 1984)	ECAT II (FWHM 17 mm) Eyes and ears covered Analysis of cerebral functional intercorrelations	Decreased number of correlations between frontal and parietal areas and within the parietal lobes bilaterally in the older subjects.
Chawluk et al. 1987	21 young (mean age 27 years) 23 old (mean age 63 years) Subjects with medical illness included	PETT V (FWHM 16.5 mm) Eyes and ears open Calculated attenuation	rCMRglc was reduced in frontal, parietal, and temporal regions. No difference between subjects with and without cardiovascular or minor noncardiovascular disease.
Schlageter et al. 1987	49 healthy male volunteers 21–83 years old	ECAT II (FWHM 17 mm) Eyes and ears covered CT scan for cerebral atrophy correction	No change with age; cerebral atrophy negatively correlates with rCMRglc.
Hoffman et al. 1988	Healthy volunteers 22 men; 14 women 21–74 years old	NeuroECAT (FWHM 12 mm) Eyes and ears open	Significant rCMRglc reductions only in some frontal areas. No effects of handedness or sex.
Grady et al. 1990	Healthy volunteers 23 men; 37 women 20–90 years old Careful medical screening	Scanditronix PC1024-7B (FWHM 6 mm) Eyes and ears covered Measured attenuation	12% decline in global CMRglc over 60-year age range.

Note. CMRglc = cerebral metabolic rate for glucose; FWHM = full width at half maximum [in millimeters]; FDG = [^{18}F]-fluoro-2-deoxy-D-glucose. ECAT II, PETT III, NeuroECAT, PETT V, and Scanditronix PC1024-7B are different PET scanners (whose properties are described in the respective studies).

patterns of cerebral metabolism and blood flow. Unlike CT or MRI measurements of dimensions of brain structures, which are invariant over years except with progressive neurodegenerative or cerebrovascular disease (Luxenberg et al. 1987), PET examines variable and often uncontrolled states of cerebral functional activity and anxiety (Gur et al. 1987). Differences in sensory input during a scan can induce dramatic variations in rCMRglc or rCBF. Indeed, hemispheric CMRglc was shown to increase by about 20% when young subjects were scanned with their eyes open and ears plugged, compared with the condition of eyes closed and ears plugged (resting state) (Mazziotta et al. 1982). With eyes covered but ears not plugged, on the other hand, CMRglc was increased by 40% above the resting state values, increasing the complexity of visual stimulation–elevated rCMRglc in visual association areas (Phelps et al. 1981). Metabolic and flow responses to different sensory stimuli are unlikely to be age invariant, as visual and auditory acuities, and even proprioception, decline with age (Creasey and Rapoport 1985; Grady et al. 1984). Thus reported age differences in PET measures in subjects not in the resting state could partly reflect reduced sensory acuity rather than only intrinsic age-related reduced activity. To date, resting state studies like those by Duara et al. (1983, 1984) on healthy subjects provide the best estimate of the actual age decline in intrinsic (sensory-independent) brain functional activity.

Other factors, such as anxiety and stress during a scan, may interfere with cerebral metabolism and should be taken into consideration. Although minimally invasive, PET is stressful to some subjects, as it involves arterial catheterization, frequent blood sampling, a restraint to minimize head movement, resting in place for perhaps longer than 1 hour, and some sensory deprivation. Gur et al. (1987) reported an inverted U–shaped relation between rCBF and anxiety; rCBF increased with increasing anxiety up to a point and then decreased with additional anxiety. Swedo et al. (1989) also reported a direct correlation between anxiety during PET and rCMRglc in prefrontal areas. However, when using a 4-grade scale to rate anxiety, Duara et al. (1983, 1984) failed to show a significant correlation with rCMRglc.

Subject selection is particularly important in studies of functional activity with regard to human aging. In many such PET studies, there was no attempt to exclude subjects with cardiovascular risk factors or clinical disorders that might affect the brain. Only a few studies (Duara et al. 1983, 1984; Marchal et al. 1992) performed careful clinical, laboratory, and neuropsychological testing to rule out organic or mental abnormalities that might interfere with functional measurements. Although this approach has been criticized as selecting for "supernormals" who, especially in the elderly, may not represent a "normally distributed" population, for the issue at hand we believe that such selection is appropriate. Less restrictive selection to obtain a sample more representative of the "normal pop-

Table 10–3. Factors contributing to variability in results from positron-emission tomography (PET) studies[a]

PET technique
Low-resolution (17 mm) versus high-resolution (6 mm) PET scanners.
Up to 25% coefficient of variation with low-resolution PET scanners to measure a potential 15%–30% change in regional cerebral metabolic rate for glucose (rCMRglc) over an adult age span of 60 years.

Brain atrophy
"Partial volume effect" may artificially reduce regional cerebral blood flow (rCBF) and rCMRglc values.

Health screening
Selection of "too healthy" elderly subjects ("supernormals").
Inclusion of subjects with (sub)clinical vascular disorders or with subtle cognitive deterioration.

Experimental procedure
Sensory input: eyes covered and ears plugged ("resting state" versus eyes closed and ears open versus eyes and ears open).
Resting state versus cognitive activation (e.g., performing a neuropsychological task).
Calculated versus individually measured radiation attenuation by head tissues and skull.

Anxiety and stress during PET examination
High levels of stress or anxiety may affect frontal lobe metabolism.

Gender
Effect of hormone cycle in female subjects.

[a]See Tables 10–1 and 10–2.

ulation" might be adopted if many hundreds of subjects of both sexes and of different ages could be studied in the same PET facility with the same procedure. Then one would have enough subjects to statistically partial out effects of confounding variables and risk factors (e.g., cardiovascular risk factors, history of psychiatric or medical disorders, and mental status during examination) on the results. Additional variability may derive from gender differences (Baxter et al. 1987; Yoshii et al. 1988) and, within females, from fluctuations in plasma levels of sex hormones linked to the menstrual cycle (Baxter et al. 1987; Horwitz 1990), as has been shown in rat studies (Nehlig et al. 1985).

Finally, technical aspects related to PET instrumentation have contributed to variability between PET centers. Tomographs with different spatial resolutions ranging from 6 to 17 mm full width at half maximum (FWHM) have been used to measure cerebral metabolism and flow. The degree of recovery of radioactivity in a brain region depends on the relation between regional volume and scanner resolution, and only high-resolution PET machines are appropriate for examining small regions.

In this regard, age-associated brain atrophy (de Leon et al. 1984; Schwartz et al. 1985; Zatz et al. 1982) is an additional complication. Due to partial voluming, atrophy can reduce recovery by the scanner of radioactivity from a given region. Attempts to correct for atrophy have been made, but to date absolute superimposition of anatomy obtained by MRI or CT, on PET data, and exact region-by-region atrophy corrections have not been achieved. Measurements of CSF spaces, principally of the volume of the lateral ventricles derived by CT or MRI, have been used to correct PET values (Alavi et al. 1985; Herscovitch et al. 1986; Schlageter et al. 1987).

Schlageter et al. (1987) studied 49 healthy men between 21 and 83 years old with CT and PET. When global CMRglc (which included gray and white matter and ventricular CSF) was corrected for lateral ventricular volume, the correlation coefficient with age changed from − 0.29 to − 0.04, indicating that the calculated age decline in resting glucose utilization could be almost entirely accounted for by partial voluming due to brain atrophy. During initial PET research on aging in our laboratory (Duara et al. 1983, 1984), a low-resolution PET tomograph (ECAT II; FWHM = 17 mm) was used to study subjects in the resting state. Global gray CMRglc, assessed in 77 optimally healthy subjects between 20 and 90 years old, showed a nonsig-

nificant 7% decrease over this age range (Figure 10–3, *panel A*) (Grady et al. 1990). Subsequently, we used a Scanditronix PC-1024-7B scanner (6 mm in plane res-

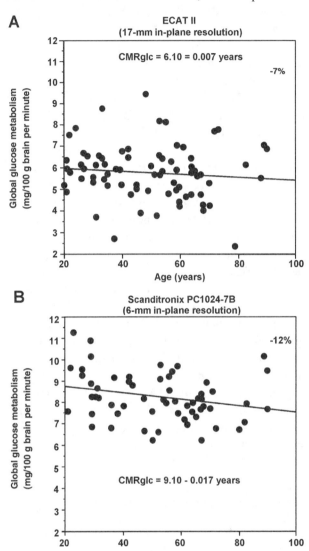

Figure 10–3. Global gray matter cerebral metabolic rate for glucose (CMRglc) as a function of age in 77 healthy men studied with a low-resolution ECAT II PET scanner (*panel A*) and in 60 healthy men studied with a high-resolution Scanditronix PC1024-7B machine (*panel B*). Regression analyses demonstrated an insignificant 7% decrease in cerebral metabolic rate for glucose (CMRglc) over a 70-year range in *panel A*, but a statistically significant 12% decline in *panel B*. Data from the high-resolution scanner had a smaller coefficient of variation than data obtained with the low-resolution scanner.
Source. Reprinted from Grady CL, Rapoport SI: "Cerebral Metabolism in Aging and Dementia," in *Handbook of Mental Health and Aging.* Edited by Birren J, Sloane RB, Cohen G. San Diego, CA, Academic Press, 1992, pp. 201–228. Used with permission.

olution), under the same resting state conditions. The more recent data obtained from 60 healthy subjects show a statistically significant 12% age decrease in global gray CMRglc (Figure 10–3, *panel B*). The slope of the regression lines in Figure 10–3 do not differ significantly (-0.01 versus -0.02 mg glucose/100 g brain per minute per year), but as the slope with the high-resolution Scanditronix scanner had a much smaller coefficient of variation than that with the lower-resolution ECAT scanner, the former reached statistical significance. The 12% decline obtained with the high-resolution scanner likely represents a maximum age decrement in intrinsic global brain functional activity in optimally healthy subjects studied in the resting state. Even this decrement may be too large an estimate of the intrinsic reduction in brain functional activity, as it was not corrected exactly for age-related atrophy.

In summary, despite the many studies that have been carried out to ascertain the effects of age on rCMRglc, the exact relation is not yet known. As for rCBF and rCMRO2, evidence suggests that an age-dependent reduction in rCMRglc, if present, is modest and of the order of 12% for a 60-year range. In view of the many possible confounding factors that can affect measurements, and given the fact that several technical advances have recently been introduced, a renewed effort to quantitate age-related in vivo measures of brain functional activity, and to understand how these measures reflect changes in cognition and behavior, should prove fruitful.

New Experimental Approaches

We recently initiated an experimental paradigm to assess the role of sensory activation and to determine the extent to which age-related declines in visual and auditory acuities (Creasey and Rapoport 1985; Grady et al. 1984) might influence rCMRglc and rCBF. We are using a double FDG injection technique (Brooks et al. 1987; Chang et al. 1987) and the ^{15}O water technique to study the same subjects in the resting state and during sensory activation during the same session. As the two sets of studies are performed less than 1 hour apart, with the subject remaining in the tomograph, variance arising from differences in mental status, head positioning, or experimental procedure is minimized. Our subjects were young (mean age ±SD: 24 ± 2 years; age range 22–26) and older (mean age ±SD: 65 ± 5 years; age range 60–74) optimally healthy men, carefully screened by medical history, clinical exami-

nation, neuropsychological examination, laboratory blood tests, electrocardiogram, electroencephalogram (EEG), audiologic test, visual acuity measurement, and head MRI, as previously described (Duara et al. 1983, 1984). All were drug free for at least 2 weeks before the scan and did not smoke, drink an alcoholic beverage or coffee, or eat caffeine-containing food, for at least 24 hours before the scan.

Partial voluming was minimized by using a high-resolution Scanditronix PC2048-15B scanner that can simultaneously examine 15 brain slices. Attenuation of radiation by brain and skull was corrected for by a transmission scan. Radioactivity was assessed in plasma by removing arterial blood via a radial artery catheter. During the same session, two measurements each of rCBF and rCMRglc were obtained, one when the subject was in the resting state, the other while he watched and listened to a projected documentary color movie. Resting state and activation were alternated randomly, and young and old subjects were studied alternately as well. Anxiety during an examination was rated by a subjective measure (0 = absent; 3 = severe) (Duara et al. 1983) and by administering a State Anxiety Questionnaire (Spielberger 1968) after the scans. Each subject was asked to remain awake during the resting state measurements and told that he was to be given a questionnaire on the content of the movie during the stimulation scan. Although the EEG was not recorded during PET, the attending physician periodically checked that the subject was awake. All studies were performed during mid-to-late morning.

Effects of age, stimulus condition (resting versus activation), and age per condition were analyzed by analysis of variance (ANOVA). Preliminary data from 6 young (22–26 years old) and 5 older (60–74 years old) subjects demonstrated significant bilateral increases of absolute and normalized rCBF and rCMRglc values during sensory activation, in occipital regions of both age groups (Figure 10–4, *panel A*). Significant age and age-per-condition effects were shown in frontal regions, where rCBF and rCMRglc were lower in the old than young subjects in the resting state. Sensory activation increased these parameters in the young subjects but decreased them in the older subjects, thereby increasing differences between the two age groups (Figure 10–4, *panel B*). In both groups, rCBF was correlated with rCMRglc more during sensory activation then in the resting state.

These results indicate an age-related decline in rCBF and rCMRglc even in the resting state, mainly in frontal regions. The effect is enhanced by sensory stimulation (Pietrini et al. 1992). Such enhancement may account for differences in the literature between sensory stimulation and resting state studies. The meaning

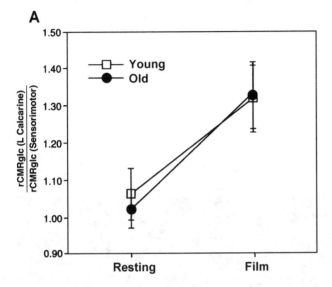

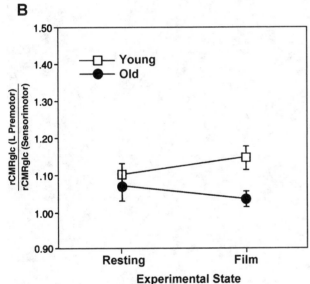

Figure 10–4. Values of regional cerebral metabolic rate for glucose (rCMRglc) normalized to the sensorimotor rCMRglc value (rCMRglc/sensorimotor rCMRglc) (mean ±SD) in a primary visual cortical area (left calcarine, *panel A*) and in a frontal cortical area (left premotor, *panel B*), in young and old subjects scanned while in the "resting state" (eyes covered and ears plugged) and while watching a film. As compared to the resting state, sensory stimulation increased normalized glucose metabolism in the primary visual cortex equally in the young and old subjects. However, metabolism was increased in young subjects and was reduced in old subjects in the premotor cortex in response to stimulation.
Source. From Pietrini et al. 1992.

of the differential effects of sensory stimulation on rCBF and rCMRglc in frontal areas, between old and young subjects, is not clear and needs to be confirmed in a larger sample.

Another way to examine age-related differences in functional activity by means of PET is to examine the overall pattern of brain glucose metabolism, in the resting state or during activation, by using a correlational or multivariate analysis. Thus despite the fact that the subjects studied by Duara et al. (1983, 1984) in the resting state showed no age-related declines in rCMRglc, they did demonstrate clear age differences in their correlation patterns (Horwitz et al. 1986).

Correlation coefficients between pairs of rCMRglc values are thought to indicate functional associations between the two brain regions (Clark et al. 1984; Horwitz et al. 1984; Metter et al. 1984). The fundamental assumption of the correlation method applied to PET rCMRglc data is that if two brain regions (A and B) are functionally coupled, so that neuronal activity in one region depends on activity in the other, a plot of rCMRglc in region A against rCMRglc in region B across subjects, using normalized parameters such as rCMRglc/CMRglc, will demonstrate a statistically significant correlation. Conversely, if two regions show a significant correlation between their normalized rCMRglc parameters, these two regions are assumed to be functionally coupled.

Horwitz et al. (1986) compared pair-wise correlations of normalized resting state metabolic rates between a group of 15 young healthy subjects (20–32 years old) and a group of 15 elderly optimally healthy subjects (64–83 years old). In the young group, a large number of statistically significant positive correlations were demonstrated within and between the frontal and parietal lobes, a smaller number within and between the temporal and occipital lobes, and only a few such correlations were found between the frontal-parietal and the temporal-occipital domains. The older group, although demonstrating the same general pattern of correlations, had fewer significant correlations between frontal and parietal areas and between regions within the parietal lobes than did the younger group. This evidence of loss of functional integration among regions of the parietal lobe corresponded to measured deficits in cognitive performance subserved by parietal structures (Grady et al. 1990).

More recently, Grady et al. (1992) used ^{15}O water to show that, while performing certain visual tasks during PET with equivalent mean accuracies and reaction times, healthy old subjects (*n* = 9; mean age = 72 ± 7 [SE] years), as compared with healthy young subjects (*n* = 11; mean age = 27 ± 4 years), activated different network components within their brain. In the healthy young subjects, the occipitotemporal cortex was selectively activated during an object-recognition task (face matching) as compared with a control task, whereas the occipitoparietal cortex was activated during a spatial-location (dot-location) task (Figure 10–5). The old subjects activated the same regions as did the young, but in addition demonstrated significant increases in rCBF in occipital-temporal cortex during the spatial task and in superior parietal cortex during the object-recognition task, increases which were not evident in the young subjects. Taken together, the resting state

correlation analyses of Horwitz et al. (1986) and the stimulation study of Grady et al. (1992) suggest that healthy aging is associated with a reorganization of network integrity and network processing efficiency in the brain and that such reorganization can be explored in detail with functional imaging techniques and new methods of multivariate data analyses, during tasks related to vision, audition, memory, attention, language, and other cognitive processes.

PET in Geriatric Neuropsychiatry

Although the focus of this chapter is the aging process in healthy humans, it may be useful to mention briefly

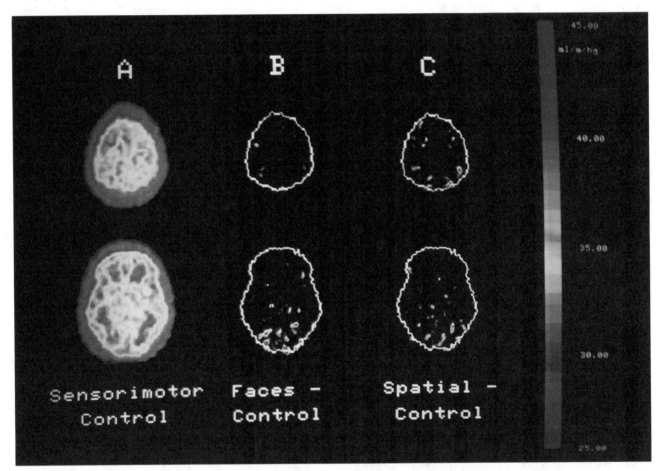

Figure 10–5. Positron-emission tomography (PET) scan images from a young healthy subject, obtained using oxygen-15 water during different neuropsychological tasks. Pictures are taken parallel and 45 mm (*bottom*) and 90 mm (*top*) above the inferior orbitomeatal line. The pictures in *column A* show the pattern of regional cerebral blood flow (rCBF) during a sensorimotor control task. Pictures in *column B* and *column C* are obtained by subtracting the sensorimotor control task rCBF pattern from the rCBF pattern obtained during a faces-matching task and a spatial-location task, respectively. Thus only the areas selectively activated during either task are shown. During face matching, there was a selective activation of the occipitotemporal regions (*column B*), whereas during a spatial location task the occipitoparietal cortex was activated (*column C*). (See text for further explanation.) The color bar on the right side shows rCBF in ml/100 g tissue per minute. For each individual picture, the right side corresponds to the right side of the brain, and the left to the left side.

the PET studies of neuropsychiatric disorders that may affect the elderly, such as dementia and depression.

Alzheimer's disease is the most common cause of dementia, accounting for up to 80% of all cases, followed by vascular diseases (4%–10%) and other diseases, including Pick's dementia (Chui 1989). Alzheimer's disease is characterized by a progressive, global, and irreversible deterioration of cognitive functions, which initially presents with memory problems and, later in the course of the disease, with language, mathematical, visuospatial, and personality decline. Many studies have been conducted with PET to investigate the patterns of cerebral glucose metabolism associated with the different stages of disease in Alzheimer patients. In agreement with autopsy studies that demonstrated an unequal distribution of neuropathological markers in the brain of Alzheimer's disease patients, PET with FDG in the resting state showed reduced rCMRglc values mostly in the association neocortical areas, with a relative sparing of primary neocortical and subcortical regions, at least until the latest stages of the disease (Duara et al. 1986; Grady and Rapoport 1992; Kumar et al. 1991).

As shown in Figure 10–6, the reduction in rCMRglc usually appears in the parietal and temporal neocortical areas, to extend subsequently to most of the neocortical mantle (severe stage), with only a relative preservation of the sensorimotor and primary visual cortices (Duara et al. 1986; Grady and Rapoport 1992; Kumar et al. 1991). The topographic distribution of reduced rCMRglc may be different in individual patients (i.e., some patients may show a greater involvement of the left hemisphere, whereas others may show a predominance of the right hemisphere). Interestingly, these heterogeneous reductions in neocortical rCMRglc precede and predict later nonmemory impairments of cognitive functions thought to involve the neocortex and are correlated with heterogeneous patterns of nonmemory impairments in individual patients (Grady et al. 1988; Haxby et al. 1990). In other words, patients with predominant left-hemisphere hypometabolism will have a greater language impairment compared with visuospatial function, and those with disproportionate right-hemisphere hypometabolism will show a greater impairment of visuoconstructive abilities (Haxby et al. 1985).

Depression in elderly patients often represents a clinical dilemma because its symptoms may resemble those of a dementia process. The term *depressive pseudodementia* was proposed to indicate those cases of depression that, for the coexistence of cognitive impairment, were mistakenly diagnosed as dementia (Kiloh 1961). The importance of early diagnostic differentiation between the two conditions should be emphasized because antidepressive treatments may actually worsen cognitive impairment because of their anticholinergic effects, and an undiagnosed depression may become a life-threatening condition (Dolan et al. 1992). In this light, PET could represent not only a new research tool, but also a diagnostic aider.

Baxter et al. (1989) found that depressive patients had decreased lateral left prefrontal lobe rCMRglc in comparison with matched healthy control subjects. In addition, both bipolar and unipolar depressive patients had significantly lower normalized caudate rCMRglc. Reduced rCMRglc values increased to normal values when patients returned to the euthymic state. The finding of a reduced rCMRglc in prefrontal areas and in the caudate nucleus of depressed patients is of particular interest because an independent study in patients with Parkinson's disease showed reduced inferior orbitofrontal and caudate rCMRglc only in those patients who had depression in addition to the motor symptoms, whereas metabolism was normal in those with motor symptoms only (Mayberg et al. 1990). Further, these regions are not affected in early Alzheimer's disease and thus they could contribute to differentiating the two processes.

Summary

New techniques for functional neuroimaging, as well as new accompanying mathematical models for interpretation of multivariate data, have made it possible to quantitate, localize, and interpret in vivo measures of brain functional activity. Studies to date indicate that absolute and normalized values of rCBF, rCMRglc, and rCMRO$_2$, particularly in the frontal lobe, are minimally affected by the aging process and that the net decline in intrinsic brain functional activity between ages 20 and 70 for these parameters does not exceed about 12% in the resting state. Even this value may be too high, because it reflects partial voluming due to age-related brain atrophy. Larger declines reported in the literature, when obtained under conditions of sensory stimulation, likely are due in part to age-related reductions in visual and auditory acuities.

Age differences in cognition and behavior may be better related to demonstrable and clear differences in integration of brain functional activity, rather than to differences in absolute or normalized values of rCBF, rCMRglc, and rCMRO2. Such differences deserve to be explored in more detail by utilizing multivariate correlation or path analysis approaches. Horwitz et al. (1986) demonstrated clear age differences in correlated metabolic activity obtained in the resting state, which are more robust than the observed differences in absolute or normalized metabolic values. Furthermore, the stimulation approach initiated by Grady et al. (1992), especially if it is utilized parametrically with tasks of continuously varying difficulty (Rapoport and Grady 1993), should prove useful for examining which brain networks actually are used during given cognitive process, as well as how network strategies may change with age.

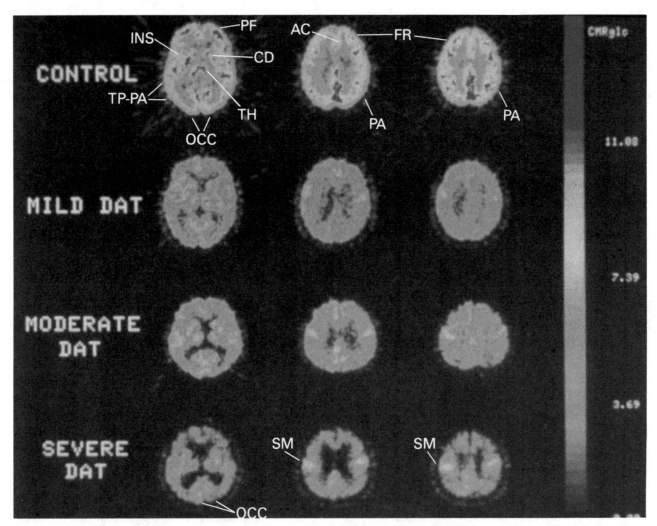

Figure 10–6. Positron-emission tomography (PET) scan images from a healthy control subject (69 years old), a patient with mild dementia (53 years old), a patient with moderate dementia (63 years old), and a patient with severe dementia (72 years old). All subjects are women. Scans were obtained using a Scanditronix PC1024-7B positron tomograph (full width half maximum [FWHM] 6 mm). For each subject, three horizontal brain slices taken parallel and above the inferior orbitomeatal line are shown: 45 mm (*left*), 70 mm (*middle*), and 90 mm (*right*). For each individual picture, the right side corresponds to the right side of the brain, and the left to the left side. In comparison to the healthy control subject, reduction of regional cerebral metabolic rate for glucose (rCMRglc) can be appreciated in the association cortical areas of the patients with dementia. In the early stages of disease, primary cortical areas and subcortical structures are not affected. With progression of disease, the deficit becomes gradually worse and in the patient with severe dementia of the Alzheimer type (DAT) only primary sensorimotor areas show a relative sparing. The color scale indicates rCMRglc in mg/100 g of tissue per minute. INS = insula; TP-PA = temporoparietal cortex; OCC = occipital cortex; TH = thalamus; CD = caudate nucleus; PF = prefrontal cortex; PA = parietal cortex; AC = anterior cingulate; FR = frontal cortex; SM = sensorimotor cortex.
Source. Adapted from Grady and Rapoport 1992.

References

Alavi A, Leonard JC, Chawluk J, et al: Correlative studies of the brain with positron emission tomography, nuclear magnetic resonance, and x-ray computed tomography, in Cerebral Blood Flow and Metabolism Measurement. Edited by Hartmann A, Hoyer S. Berlin, Springer-Verlag, 1985, pp 523–539

Baxter LR, Mazziotta JC, Phelps ME, et al: Cerebral glucose metabolic rates in normal human females versus normal males. Psychiatry Res 21:237–245, 1987

Baxter LR, Schwartz JC, Mazziotta JC, et al: Reduction of prefrontal cortex glucose metabolism common to three types of depression. Arch Gen Psychiatry 46:243–250, 1989

Brooks RA, Di Chiro G, Zukerberg BW, et al: Test-retest studies of cerebral glucose metabolism using fluorine-18 deoxyglucose: validation of method. J Nucl Med 28:53–59, 1987

Burns A, Tyrrell P: Association of age with regional cerebral oxygen utilization: a positron emission tomography study. Age Ageing 21:316–320, 1992

Chang JY, Duara R, Baker W, et al: Two behavioral states studied in a single PET/FDG procedure: theory, method, and preliminary results. J Nucl Med 28:852–860, 1987

Chawluk JB, Alavi A, Jamieson DG, et al: Changes in local cerebral metabolism with normal aging: the effects of cardiovascular and systemic health factors (abstract). J Cereb Blood Flow Metab 7 (suppl 1):S411, 1987

Chui HC: Dementia: a review emphasizing clinicopathologic correlation and brain-behavior relationships. Arch Neurol 46:806–814, 1989

Clark CM, Kessler R, Buchsbaum MS, et al: Correlational methods for determining regional coupling of cerebral glucose metabolism: a pilot study. Biol Psychiatry 19:663–678, 1984

Creasey H, Rapoport SI: The aging human brain. Ann Neurol 17:2–10, 1985

Dastur DK, Lane MH, Hansen DB, et al: Effects of aging on cerebral circulation and metabolism in man, in Human Aging: A Biological and Behavioral Study (Publication No 986). Edited by Birren JE, Butler RN, Greenhouse SW, et al. Bethesda, MD, US Department of Health, Education and Welfare, 1963, pp 59–76

de Leon MJ, Ferris SH, George AE, et al: Computed tomography and positron emission transaxial evaluations of normal aging and Alzheimer's disease. J Cereb Blood Flow Metab 3:391–394, 1983

de Leon MJ, George AE, Ferris SH, et al: Positron emission tomography and computed tomography assessments of the aging human brain. J Comput Assist Tomogr 8:88–94, 1984

Dolan RJ, Bench CJ, Brown RG, et al: Regional cerebral blood flow abnormalities in depressed patients with cognitive impairment. J Neurol Neurosurg Psychiatry 55:768–773, 1992

Duara R, Margolin RA, Robertson-Tchabo EA, et al: Cerebral glucose utilization, as measured with positron emission tomography in 21 healthy men between the ages of 21 and 83 years. Brain 106:761–775, 1983

Duara R, Grady CL, Haxby JV, et al: Human brain glucose utilization and cognitive function in relation to age. Ann Neurol 16:702–713, 1984

Duara R, Grady CL, Haxby JV, et al: Positron emission tomography in Alzheimer's disease. Neurology 36:879–887, 1986

Frackowiak RSJ, Gibbs JM: Cerebral metabolism and blood flow in normal and pathologic aging, in Functional Radionuclide Imaging of The Brain. Edited by Magistretti PL. New York, Raven, pp 305–309, 1983

Frackowiak RSJ, Lammertsma AA: Clinical measurement of cerebral blood flow and oxygen consumption, in Positron Emission Tomography. Edited by Reivich M, Alavi A. New York, Alan R Liss, 1985, pp 153–181

Frackowiak RSJ, Wise RJS, Gibbs JM, et al: Positron emission tomographic studies in aging and cerebrovascular disease at Hammersmith hospital. Ann Neurol 15 (suppl):S112–118, 1984

Grady CL, Rapoport SI: Cerebral metabolism in aging and dementia, in Handbook of Mental Health and Aging. Edited by Birren J, Sloane RB, Cohen G. San Diego, CA, Academic Press, 1992, pp 201–228

Grady CK, Grimes AM, Pikus A, et al: Alterations in auditory processing of speech stimuli during aging in healthy subjects. Cortex 20:101–110, 1984

Grady CL, Sonies B, Haxby J, et al: Cerebral metabolic asymmetries predict decline in language performance in dementia of the Alzheimer type (DAT) (abstract). J Clin Exp Neuropsychol 10:39, 1988

Grady CL, Horwitz B, Schapiro MB, et al: Changes in the integrated activity of the brain with healthy aging and dementia of the Alzheimer's type, in Aging Brain and Dementia. New Trends in Diagnosis and Therapy. Edited by Battistin L, Gerstenbrand F. New York, Wiley-Liss, 1990, pp 355–370

Grady CL, Haxby JV, Horwitz B, et al: Dissociation of object and spatial vision in human extrastriate cortex: age-related changes in activation of regional cerebral blood flow measured with [15-O] water and positron emission tomography. Journal of Cognitive Neuroscience 4:23–34, 1992

Gur RC, Gur RE, Resnick SM, et al: The effect of anxiety on cortical cerebral blood flow and metabolism. J Cereb Blood Flow Metab 7:173–177, 1987

Hawkins RA, Mazziotta JC, Phelps ME, et al: Cerebral glucose metabolism as a function of age in man: influence of rate constants in the fluorodeoxyglucose method. J Cereb Blood Flow Metab 3:250–253, 1983

Haxby JV, Duara R, Grady CL, et al: Relations between neuropsychological and cerebral metabolic asymmetries in early Alzheimer's disease. J Cereb Blood Flow Metab 5:193–200, 1985

Haxby JV, Grady CL, Koss E, et al: Longitudinal study of cerebral metabolic asymmetries and associated neuropsychological patterns in early dementia of the Alzheimer type. Arch Neurol 47:753–760, 1990

Herscovitch P, Auchus AP, Gado M, et al: Correction of positron emission tomography data for cerebral atrophy. J Cereb Blood Flow Metab 6:120–124, 1986

Hoffman JM, Guze BH, Hawk TC, et al: Cerebral glucose metabolism in normal individuals: effects of aging, sex and handedness (abstract). Neurology 38 (suppl 1):167, 1988

Holcomb HH, Links J, Smith C, et al: Positron emission tomography: measuring the metabolic and neurochemical characteristics of the living human nervous system, in Brain Imaging: Applications in Psychiatry. Edited by Andreasen N. Washington, DC, American Psychiatric Press, 1989, pp 235–370

Horn JL: Psychometric studies of aging and intelligence, in Genesis and Treatment of Psychologic Disorders in the Elderly: Aging, Vol 2. Edited by Gershon S, Raskin A. New York, Raven Press, 1975, pp 19–23

Horwitz B: Quantification and analysis of positron emission tomography metabolic data, in Positron Emission Tomography in Dementia. Edited by Duara R. New York, Wiley-Liss, 1990, pp 13–70

Horwitz B, Duara R, Rapoport SI: Intercorrelations of glucose metabolic rates between brain regions: applications to healthy males in a state of reduced sensory input. J Cereb Blood Flow Metab 4:484–499, 1984

Horwitz B, Duara R, Rapoport SI: Age differences in intercorrelations between regional cerebral metabolic rates for glucose. Ann Neurol 19:60–67, 1986

Huang SC, Phelps ME, Hoffman EJ, et al: Non-invasive determination of local cerebral metabolic rate of glucose in man. Am J Physiol 238:E69–E82, 1980

Ingvar DH: "Hyperfrontal" distribution of the cerebral grey matter flow in resting wakefulness; on the functional anatomy of the conscious state. Acta Neurol Scand 60:12–25, 1979

Itoh M, Hatazawa J, Miyazawa H, et al: Stability of cerebral blood flow and oxygen metabolism during normal aging. Gerontology 36:43–48, 1990

Jagust WJ, Eberling JL, Baker MG, et al: Hippocampal glucose metabolism in Alzheimer's disease (abstract book, vol I, p. 283). Paper presented at the annual meeting of the Society for Neurosciences, St. Louis, MO, October–November, 1990

Kety SS: Human cerebral blood flow and oxygen consumption as related to aging. Res Publ Assoc Res Nerv Ment Dis 35:31–45, 1956

Kety SS, Schmidt CF: The nitrous oxide method for quantitative determination of cerebral blood flow in man: theory, procedure and normal values. J Clin Invest 27:475–483, 1948

Kiloh LG: Pseudo-dementia. Acta Psychiatr Scand 37:336–350, 1961

Kuhl DE, Metter EJ, Riege WH, et al: Effects of human aging on patterns of local glucose utilization determined by the [18F]fluorodeoxyglucose method. J Cereb Blood Flow Metab 2:163–171, 1982

Kumar A, Schapiro MB, Grady CL, et al: High-resolution PET studies in Alzheimer's disease. Neuropsychopharmacology 4:35–46, 1991

Lebrun-Grandie P, Baron JC, Soussaline F, et al: Coupling between regional blood flow and oxygen utilization in the normal human brain: a study with positron emission tomography and oxygen 15. Arch Neurol 40:230–236, 1983

Leenders KL, Perani D, Lammertsma AA, et al: Cerebral blood flow, blood volume and oxygen utilization: normal values and effect of age. Brain 113:27–47, 1990

Luxenberg JS, Haxby JV, Creasey H, et al: Rate of ventricular enlargement in dementia of the Alzheimer type correlates with rate of neuropsychological deterioration. Neurology 37:1135–1140, 1987

Marchal G, Rioux P, Petit-Taboue MC, et al: Regional cerebral oxygen consumption, blood flow, and blood volume in healthy human aging. Arch Neurol 49:1013–1020, 1992

Martin AJ, Friston KJ, Colebatch JG, et al: Decreases in regional cerebral blood flow with normal aging. J Cereb Blood Flow Metab 11:684–689, 1991

Mazziotta JC, Phelps ME: Positron emission tomography studies of the brain, in Positron Emission Tomography and Autoradiography: Principles and Applications for the Brain and Heart. Edited by Phelps ME, Mazziotta JC, Schelbert HR. New York, Raven, 1986, pp 493–580

Mazziotta JC, Phelps ME, Carson RE, et al: Tomographic mapping of human cerebral metabolism: sensory deprivation. Ann Neurol 12:435–444, 1982

Mayberg HS, Starkstein SE, Sadotz B, et al: Selective hypometabolism in the inferior frontal lobe in depressed patients with Parkinson's disease. Ann Neurol 28:57–64, 1990

Melamed E, Lavy S, Bentin S, et al: Reduction in regional cerebral blood flow during normal aging in man. Stroke 11:31–35, 1980

Metter EJ, Riege WH, Kuhl DE, et al: Cerebral metabolic relationships for selected brain regions in healthy adults. J Cereb Blood Flow Metab 4:1–7, 1984

Meyer JS, Rogers RL, Mortel KT: Prospective analysis of long-term control of mild hypertension on cerebral blood flow. Stroke 16:985–990, 1985

Montaigne ME de: De l'Age (1580), in Les Essais, Vol 1, Chapter 27. Paris, Editions Garnier, 1952, pp 360–363

Moosy J: Cerebral atherosclerosis: intracranial and extracranial lesions, in Pathology of The Nervous System, Vol 1. Edited by Minckler J. New York, McGraw-Hill, 1971, pp 1423–1432

Naritomi H, Meyer JS, Sakai F, et al: Effects of advancing age on regional cerebral blood flow: studies in normal subject with risk factors for atherothrombotic stroke. Arch Neurol 36:410–416, 1979

Nehlig A, Porrino LJ, Crane AM, et al: Local cerebral glucose utilization in normal female rats: variations during the estrous cycle and comparison with males. J Cereb Blood Flow Metab 5:393–400, 1985

Obrist WD: Noninvasive studies of regional cerebral blood flow in aging and dementia, in Alzheimer's Disease: Senile Dementia and Related Disorders: Aging, Vol 7. Edited by Katzam R, Terry RD, Bick KL. New York, Raven, 1978, pp 213–217

Obrist WD, Thompson HK, King CH, et al: Determination of regional cerebral blood flow by inhalation of 133-xenon. Circ Res 20:124–135, 1967

Obrist WD, Thompson HK Jr, Wang HS, et al: Regional cerebral blood flow estimated by 133-xenon inhalation. Stroke 6:245–256, 1975

Pantano P, Baron JC, Lebrun-Grandie P, et al: Regional cerebral blood flow and oxygen consumption in human aging. Stroke 4:635–641, 1984

Phelps ME, Mazziotta JC, Kuhl DE, et al: Tomographic mapping of human cerebral metabolism: visual stimulation and deprivation. Neurology 31:517–529, 1981

Pietrini P, Horwitz B, Grady CL, et al:: A positron emission tomography study of cerebral glucose metabolism (rCMRglc) and blood flow (rCBF) in normal human aging. Gerontologist 32 (special issue II):242, 1992

Rapoport SI: Brain in aging and dementia, in Medicine for The Laymen Series (National Institutes of Health Publication No 83-2625). Bethesda, MD, US Department of Health and Human Services, Public Health Service, 1983, pp 1–33

Rapoport SI: Brain evolution and Alzheimer's disease. Rev Neurol (Paris) 144:79–90, 1988

Rapoport SI: Integrated phylogeny of the primate brain, with special reference to humans and their diseases. Brain Res Rev 15:267–294, 1990

Rapoport SI, Grady CL: Parametric in vivo brain imaging during activation to examine pathological mechanisms of functional failure in Alzheimer disease. Int J Neurosci 70:39–56, 1993

Risberg J: Regional cerebral blood flow measurements by 133-Xe-inhalation: methodology and application in neuropsychology and psychiatry. Brain Lang 9:9–34, 1980

Roy CS, Sherrington CS: On the regulation of blood supply of the brain. J Physiol (London) 11:85–108, 1890

Salerno JA, Mentis MJ, Grady CL, et al: Positron emission tomographic studies of brain function in older men with chronic essential hypertension (abstract). J Am Geriatric Soc 10:SA13, 1992

Scheinberg P, Blackburn I, Rich M, et al: Effects of aging on cerebral circulation and metabolism. Arch Neurol Psych 70:77–85, 1953

Schieve JF, Wilson WP: The influence of age, anesthesia and cerebral arteriosclerosis on cerebral vascular activity to CO_2. Am J Med 15:171–174, 1953

Schlageter NL, Horwitz B, Creasey H, et al: Relation of measured brain glucose utilization and cerebral atrophy in man. J Neurol Neurosurg Psychiatry 50:779–785, 1987

Schwartz M, Creasey H, Grady CL, et al: CT analysis of brain morphometrics in 30 healthy men, aged 21 to 81 years. Ann Neurol 17:146–157, 1985

Sokoloff L: The action of drugs on the cerebral circulation. Pharmacol Rev 11:1–85, 1959

Sokoloff L: The radioactive deoxyglucose method, theory, procedure and application for the measurement of local cerebral glucose utilization in the central nervous system, in Advances in Neurochemistry, Vol 4. Edited by Agranoff BW, Aprison MH. New York, Plenum, 1982, pp 1–82

Sokoloff L, Reivich M, Kennedy C, et al: The [14C]-deoxyglucose method for the measurement of local cerebral glucose utilization: theory, procedure and normal values in the conscious and anesthetized albino rat. J Neurochem 28:897–916, 1977

Spielberger CD: 20-item State Anxiety Questionnaire: Manual. Palo Alto, CA, Consulting Psychologist Press, 1968

Swedo SE, Schapiro MB, Grady CL, et al: Cerebral glucose metabolism in childhood-onset obsessive compulsive disorder. Arch Gen Psychiatry 45:518–523, 1989

Takada H, Nagata K, Hirata Y, et al:: Age-related decline of cerebral oxygen metabolism in normal population detected with positron emission tomography. Neuroradiological Research 14 (suppl 2):128–131, 1992

Yamaguchi T, Kanno I, Uemura K, et al: Reduction in regional cerebral metabolic rate of oxygen during human aging. Stroke 6:1220–1228, 1986

Yoshii F, Barker WW, Chang JY, et al: Sensitivity of cerebral glucose metabolism to age, gender, brain, volume, brain atrophy, and cerebrovascular risk factors. J Cereb Blood Flow Metab 8:654–661, 1988

Zatz LM, Jernigan TL, Ahumada AJ Jr: Changes on computed cranial tomography with aging: intracranial fluid volume. AJNR 3:1–11, 1982

11

Quantitative Electroencephalography: Neurophysiological Alterations in Normal Aging and Geriatric Neuropsychiatric Disorders

Andrew Leuchter, M.D.
Daniel Holschneider, M.D.

Introduction

Electroencephalography (EEG) is the oldest form of functional brain imaging. It has several advantages over newer forms of functional imaging, such as positron-emission tomography (PET) or single photon emission computed tomography (SPECT): EEG is noninvasive, inexpensive, and portable, and it can provide images based on less than 1 second of data. It also provides direct information about the functional integrity of fiber tracts, without the risk of exposure to ionizing radiation.

The central limitation of EEG has been difficulty in relating potentials measured at the scalp surface to underlying brain physiology (Nunez 1981). Although most of the brain's energy metabolism is devoted to the production of electrical gradients and signals, brain electrical activity traditionally has been only a dim reflection of brain perfusion, metabolism, or structural integrity.

Over the past several years, there have been significant advances in our understanding of the relationship between brain energy metabolism, structure, and electrical signal production. Driven by widespread availability of inexpensive microcomputers, quantitative EEG (qEEG) has supplanted conventional EEG in research laboratories and many clinical settings. Studies correlating alterations in electrical activity with changes in perfusion and metabolism, or with structural disease, have significantly advanced methods for qEEG signal analysis. New algorithms have established qEEG as a reliable, noninvasive method of brain imaging with significant clinical utility. In this chapter, we review the history of EEG and qEEG and discuss their potential uses in geriatric neuropsychiatry.

History of EEG

EEG was popularized in the early 20th century by Hans Berger, a psychiatrist who demonstrated changes in the EEG with arousal, anxiety, and other emotions and activities. Enthusiasm for EEG was supported by Berger's study of the EEGs of institutionalized patients (Berger 1937), many of whom showed distinct abnormalities (particularly diffuse slowing).

Berger's suppositions about the information contained in brain electrical activity were correct, but his technology was inadequate to decode the complex information embedded in the EEG signal. Berger used a double-coil galvanometer whose oscillations moved a mirror, thereby deflecting a beam of light that traced the EEG signal on photographic paper (Gloor 1969). Grass and Gibbs performed qEEG analysis in 1938, but their mechanical Fourier transform (using a rotating drum) was too cumbersome and unreliable to process large volumes of data or multiple channels simultaneously. The development of techniques through pen-and-ink recorders, and then mechanical frequency analyzers, did not provide the tools necessary to decode the complex information contained in the EEG. As a result, researchers struggled with a central irony: although most of the brain's energy metabolism was devoted to the production of electrical potentials, researchers could not realize Berger's dream of studying brain processes, and particularly cognitive functions, using EEG. As a result, the applications for EEG in neuropsychiatry have traditionally been limited.

Conventional EEG in Geriatric Neuropsychiatry

Indications for Conventional EEG

There are several clinical applications for the conventional EEG in psychiatric practice, primarily in the evaluation of disorders at the interface between psychiatry and neurology. First, the EEG is useful for distinguishing healthy elderly subjects from those with possible dementia. The EEG of a healthy elderly subject may differ little from that of a healthy young adult (Hubbard et al. 1976; Hughes and Cayaffa 1977; Katz

The authors appreciate the assistance of Robert Lufkin of the Department of Radiology, UCLA School of Medicine, who provided the magnetic resonance image, and of Ismael Mena, of the Division of Nuclear Medicine, and Bruce Miller, of the Department of Neurology, Harbor-UCLA Medical Center, who provided the single photon emission computed tomography image. The authors also wish to thank John Mazziotta and Michael Phelps of the Division of Nuclear Medicine, Department of Radiology, as well as Lewis Baxter, Barry Guze, and Gary Small of the Department of Psychiatry, UCLA School of Medicine, who supplied the positron-emission tomography image, and Vernita Hughes, who provided expert assistance in the preparation of the manuscript and figures. This work was supported by grant MH 40705 from the National Institute of Mental Health (to AL). Additional support was provided by the UCLA Alzheimer's Disease Center grant P30 AG10123 from the National Institute on Aging, and the UCLA/VAMC Multicampus Geriatric Training grant (to DH).

and Horowitz 1982; Matejcez 1979). Most reports, however, suggest that healthy elderly people show slight changes beginning in the fifth or sixth decades, including a decrease of 0.5–1.0 Hz in the mean frequency of the posterior dominant ("alpha") rhythm (Busse 1983; Kanowski 1971; Obrist and Busse 1965; Roubicek 1977), decreased reactivity of the posterior dominant rhythm to eye opening (decreased alpha blocking) (Andermann and Stoller 1961), increased theta slow-wave activity (Gibbs and Gibbs 1951; Obrist 1979), and focal slowing, primarily in the left anterior temporal region.

Focal slowing has been reported in 17%–59% of healthy elderly subjects (Helmchen et al. 1967; Hughes and Cayaffa 1977; Katz and Horowitz 1982; Obrist and Busse 1965; Otomo and Tsubaki 1966; Soininen et al. 1982; Torres et al. 1983; Visser et al. 1987), but if normal it should be intermittent and never exceed 25% of the EEG recording. Similarly, although the posterior dominant rhythm may slow somewhat, it should remain above 8 Hz in the waking state (Obrist 1979; Oken and Kaye 1992). Some researchers have noted a slight increase in beta activity with aging (Gibbs et al. 1950; Matousek et al. 1967; Mundy-Castle 1951; Obrist 1954). Other researchers have found a decline in beta activity in normal elderly subjects after the sixth decade (Busse and Obrist 1965; Obrist 1976; Schlagenhauff 1973; Wang and Busse 1969), although the pattern of this decline varies in different studies (Busse and Obrist 1965; Schlagenhauff 1973; Wang and Busse 1969).

These findings contrast with those from patients with dementia. EEG abnormalities in dementia were first reported by Berger (1937), who described gross slowing of the dominant frequency. For almost 40 years after Berger's initial reports, EEG studies of dementia described decreases in the frequency, quantity (Stoller 1949), and reactivity of the alpha rhythm (Andermann and Stoller 1961; Dejaiffe et al. 1964), as well as an excess of theta and delta activity (McAdam and Robinson 1956; Weiner and Schuster 1956). Early reports suggested that only patients with moderately advanced dementia could be distinguished from healthy elderly subjects, as normal EEGs were the rule in patients with the early stages of dementia (E. B. Gordon and Sim 1967; Loeb 1980; Weiner and Schuster 1956). More recently, however, it has been shown that a majority of patients with dementia have abnormal EEGs and that fully half of individuals with equivocal impairment (Mini-Mental State Exam scores greater than 24) show abnormalities (Leuchter et al. 1993). The high preva-

lence of abnormalities even in the early stages of the illness increases the diagnostic usefulness of the test.

Conventional EEG is a nonspecific indicator of the type of dementia. Focal abnormalities are reported to be more common in patients with vascular dementia (74% of patients) than those with primary degenerative dementia (19% of patients) (Dejaiffe et al. 1964; Harrison et al. 1979; Logar et al. 1987; Roberts et al. 1978), but this finding is of limited diagnostic usefulness. Furthermore, some patients will have both illnesses, and their coexistence can be difficult to detect (Ettlin et al. 1989). Bilateral paroxysmal activity occurs in approximately 25% of patients with either vascular or primary degenerative dementia (Dejaiffe et al. 1964; Fortin 1966; Liddell 1958). Bifrontal, repetitive sharp waves or triphasic waves are seen in a high percentage of patients with Creutzfeldt-Jakob disease in early stages of the illness (Abbott 1959; Burger et al. 1972; Chiofalo et al. 1980; E. B. Gordon and Sim 1967), but also are seen in various toxic or metabolic dementias. The increase in focal abnormalities seen in vascular dementias; the low-amplitude, background activity of Huntington's disease (Margerison and Scott 1965; Oltman and Friedman 1961; Scott et al. 1972); and the well-preserved, posterior-dominant background rhythm of Pick's disease (Groen and Endtz 1982; Tissot et al. 1975) are characteristic for groups of patients, but have not proven sufficiently specific to allow confident diagnostic classification of individual subjects.

The abnormalities found in patients with dementia have not only diagnostic, but also prognostic, significance. The degree of EEG slowing is the single best predictor of 1-year mortality in patients with dementia (Kazniak et al. 1979).

The EEG is of limited use for distinguishing between depression and dementia: many patients who have cognitive complaints and a primary diagnosis of depression also have abnormal EEGs (Leuchter et al. 1993). An abnormal EEG may identify, however, a subgroup of depressed patients with structural brain disease. Factors associated with aging such as hypertension (Visser 1991), atherosclerosis (Obrist 1963), or diabetes (Mooradian et al. 1988; Pramming et al. 1988) may cause subclinical cerebrovascular insufficiency and both structural and functional brain changes (Giaquinto and Nolfe 1988; Obrist et al. 1963; Visser 1991; Visser et al. 1987). These structural changes (as defined by hyperintensity on T2-weighted magnetic resonance imaging [MRI] images) have been associated both with late-life depression (Leuchter 1994) and EEG abnormalities (Oken and Kaye 1992). In some instances, these abnormalities may portend the development of a dementing illness (Liston 1979). Although an abnormal EEG is not specific for dementia, it may identify the patients at greatest risk for functional decline and therefore is a useful part of the dementia evaluation.

A second illness in which the EEG has a useful diagnostic role is delirium. Excessive slowing is seen almost universally in patients with delirium (Engel and Romano 1959), making EEG a useful physiological tool to support the diagnosis. More importantly, EEG may be used to monitor recovery, as the degree of slowing is an indicator of the severity of the encephalopathy and slowing resolves in response to effective interventions (Brenner 1991; Romano and Engel 1944). In cases in which the intervention is costly or poses significant risk to the patient or in which the mental status examination is equivocal or difficult to perform (e.g., in a patient on a ventilator or with aphasia), such physiological testing may be useful for monitoring the resolution of the delirium. Distinguishing patients with depression or the changes of normal aging from those with delirium has been reported not to be problematic because of the severity of the abnormalities commonly seen in delirium (Brenner 1991; Engel and Romano 1959; Rabins and Folstein 1982).

A third application for EEG is the study of patients with possible seizure disorders. Episodic dissociation, confusion, or behavioral outbursts may uncommonly be due to a seizure disorder. In such situations, a resting-state EEG may be useful for detecting interictal abnormalities that would be indicative of the seizure disorder. Alternatively, long-term observation with ambulatory or telemetered EEG with video monitoring may be necessary to capture an episode of behavioral disturbance and the attendant changes in brain electrical activity.

The reported use of EEG in clinical psychiatry varies considerably, but probably is low. The nationwide rate of use recently was reported at 2.8%; older patients and those diagnosed with organic mental disorders have a somewhat higher use rate (8%) (Olfson 1992). In university-affiliated hospitals, the rate may be as high as 33%. It is unclear how often the EEG would be useful in the assessment of psychiatric conditions. Although some investigators have concluded that the EEG seldom affects clinical decision making, the high rate of abnormality among patients with organic mental disorders suggests greater utility.

Limitations of Conventional EEG

There are at least three factors that limit the applications of conventional EEG in psychiatric practice. First, the EEG is a complex test that is not readily subject to interpretation by most physicians. At least some degree of training is necessary to develop proficiency at test interpretation, which is based largely on pattern recognition. Skill at identification of abnormalities, and in distinguishing abnormalities from artifact, must be developed.

Even among skilled interpreters, there is a second inherent problem of the limited reliability of qualitative interpretation. Different electroencephalographers (or a single electroencephalographer on different occasions) yield different interpretations of the same test a disturbingly high proportion of the time (Woody 1966, 1968).

Third, it is not clear when a possible abnormality is detected, whether it truly reflects a brain disturbance. For example, excessive slow-wave activity in the EEG is a common finding in organically impaired elderly subjects and suggests the presence of either dementia or delirium. There are no well-established guidelines, however, for determining when slow-wave activity is excessive. Electroencephalographers may differ on how much slow-wave activity is acceptable at any given age. Even with general agreement, it is difficult to standardize such agreement between physicians (particularly those who do not work in the same facility), and to determine the sensitivity and specificity of the qualitative finding of "excessive slowing" in detecting brain disease. This lack of standardization also has hampered research efforts.

---

qEEG

qEEG analysis minimizes or even eliminates some of the limitations of conventional EEG. In this section, after a brief discussion of the technical aspect of qEEG, we discuss the clinical applications of the technique.

Description of the qEEG Technique

Conventional EEG rapidly is yielding to qEEG, in which on-line digitization of the signal and recordings onto magnetic or optical media replace analog pen-and-ink recordings. As short a time as 10 years ago, quantitation commonly was performed with a roomful of costly minicomputers. Starting in the mid-1980s, coincident with the wide availability of low-cost microcomputers, qEEG began to flourish and now is performed by academic and community-based physicians.

qEEG data are sampled at rates of at least 100 points per channel per second, and the analog waveforms may be displayed from these digital data either through a polygraph interface on paper or on a high-resolution video display terminal. Either of these display methods allows for conventional EEG interpretation of the digital recording. Commonly, the analog wave forms are displayed real-time as they are collected on the video display terminal, so the technician may monitor the recording and annotate it appropriately.

Once digital data are recorded, the data may be transformed from the domain of amplitude versus frequency in which they are recorded, to the domain of energy (or "power") versus frequency band (Figure 11–1). The process of this transformation is known as *spectral analysis* and commonly is achieved by process-

ing the data through an algorithm known as *Fourier transformation*. This algorithm is based on the assumption that the complex waveform of the EEG may be modeled as the summation of a series of sinusoidal waveforms of different amplitudes and frequencies. A segment (or epoch) is decomposed into a series of simpler sine wave components, and the power at each frequency band for that epoch may be calculated from the characteristics of the sine wave at that frequency. Power may be calculated for frequencies up to half the value of the sampling rate (this is the so-called Nyquist frequency).

Power estimates may be calculated for a second or even less of data, although the representative nature of such a small epoch for that individual's resting brain electrical activity is questionable. Commonly, the power in a series of frequency bands (the so-called power spectrum) is calculated for 20–30 seconds of data, either as discrete, smaller epochs averaged together or as a single epoch.

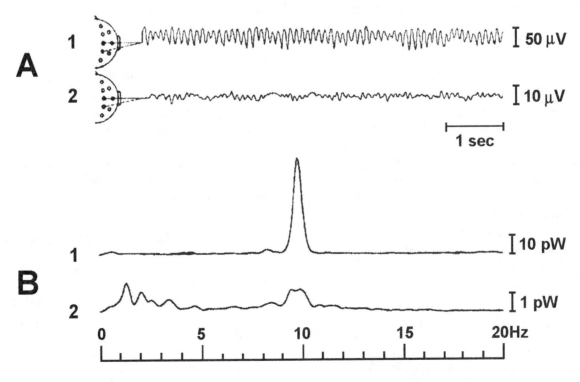

Figure 11–1. Spectral analysis. *Panel A: 1)* Posterior dominant rhythm from a "normal" subject, showing a sinusoidal 10-Hz rhythm. *2)* Posterior dominant rhythm from an "abnormal" subject such as might be seen in a patient with dementia. Although there is some retained 10-Hz activity, there are abundant intermixed slow waves. *Panel B: 1)* Spectral analysis of the signal from the "normal" subject, showing a peak of power at 10 Hz. *2)* Spectral analysis of the signal from the "abnormal" subject, showing peaks of power in the delta (0–4 Hz), theta (4–8 Hz), and alpha (8–12 Hz) ranges.
Source. Reprinted from Spehlmann R: *EEG Primer.* New York, Elsevier Science, 1981, p. 124. Copyright 1981 by Elsevier Biomedical Press. Used with permission.

qEEG overcomes several of the limitations of conventional EEG. Because it yields quantitative, reproducible measurements of the frequency content of any segment of EEG, it provides much more reliable information regarding the amount of slow-wave activity in a record. These quantitative estimates not only minimize errors in judgment, but they also yield reproducible estimates that may be compared over time in a single individual.

The qEEG procedure also provides information that is not accessible from the visual inspection of the conventional recording. For example, qEEG can reliably measure the proportion of the total power that is in any given frequency band (so-called relative power, measured as a percent of total power). This measure is particularly useful because it normalizes for the wide fluctuations in total power across individuals and may detect subtle shifts in brain function in an individual over time.

Another product of the Fourier transform is coherence, or synchronization of electrical activity from different regions within an individual. Coherence is analogous to a correlation coefficient between the signals recorded at two locations, and is computed from the following formula:

$$C_{xy}(\lambda) = \frac{|S_{xy}(\lambda)|^2}{S_x(\lambda) \bullet S_y(\lambda)}$$

in which the square of the cross-spectrum is divided by the product of the spectra of the individual channels (Leuchter et al. 1992). Although electroencephalographers commonly speak of "synchronized" or "desynchronized" electrical activity in a record, this usually refers simply to the visual presence or absence of well-regulated sinusoidal activity in the alpha band. This is different from coherence, which is a quantitative measure of whether signals at multiple locations are rising and falling in a time-locked manner in any frequency band.

Evoked Potentials

In an attempt to standardize qEEG information, some investigators have controlled variability by recording electrical activity while the subjects are exposed·to repetitive visual, auditory, or other stimuli. These so-called evoked potentials (EPs) or event-related potentials (ERPs) are multicomponent waves of positive and negative potentials that result when the EEG signal from the scalp is averaged for a specified time

interval following a stimulus. EP components are labeled usually according to their polarities ("P" for positive; "N" for negative) and according to their latency from time of the stimulus (in milliseconds [msec]); some components are labeled according to their presumed function (e.g., contingent negative variation).

EPs are classified as to the type of triggering physical stimuli used. Visual evoked potentials (VEPs) commonly are generated in response to simple flashes of light or to reversal of background and foreground colors in complex patterns (e.g., a checkerboard). Auditory evoked potentials (AEPs) are generated in response to a series of clicks or tones that may be constant or vary unpredictably over time. Somatosensory evoked potentials (SSEPs) are generated as a result of the electrical stimulation of a peripheral nerve.

After stimulation of a sense organ, it takes approximately 20 msec for the electrical signal to reach the cortex. EPs recorded with short latencies of 20–80 msec are termed *stimulus bound* or *exogenous* as they are believed to represent obligate responses of the nervous system generated in spinal cord or brain stem structures. Perhaps of greater interest for geriatric neuropsychiatry are EPs with medium to long latencies, termed *endogenous* or *cognitive* potentials, thought to represent responses of higher centers (including primary or association cortex). These potentials are sensitive to psychological variables, such as the subjects' motivation, attention, or intention, and less sensitive to characteristics of the eliciting stimulus. Certain endogenous EPs are indicative of the subject's "cognitive set" or preparation for a motor response or cognitive task and may be recorded even in the absence of an associated physical stimulus.

qEEG and EP Changes With Normal Aging

qEEG studies of normal aging reveal some differences from conventional EEG studies. There is agreement that there is slight slowing of the posterior dominant rhythm by 0.5–1.0 Hz, although by definition it must remain above 8 Hz (Busse 1983; Duffy et al. 1984a; Oken and Kaye 1992), and decreased alpha blocking (Duffy et al. 1984a). There is disagreement, however, regarding increases in slow-wave power, with several studies finding that delta and theta power do not increase with normal aging (Duffy et al. 1984a; Katz and Horowitz 1982; Leuchter et al., in press a; Matejcez 1979; Williamson et al. 1990). The finding in some qEEG studies that slow-wave power does not increase with aging probably reflects health status of the subjects as discussed above (Oken and Kaye 1992). qEEG studies further indicate that increased temporal slow-wave power with aging may reflect underlying pathology, as it is inversely related to performance on memory testing (Rice et al. 1991).

Studies of beta power suggest that it increases with aging until the seventh decade, when decreases may occur (Duffy et al. 1984a; Williamson et al. 1990). The effects of health status on beta power have not been addressed, but augmented beta power has been seen during cognitive tasks including states of focused arousal (Sheer 1975, 1976, 1984) and performance on problem-solving tasks (Loring et al. 1985; Spydell and Sheer 1982). Retained beta activity may be an indicator in the elderly of preserved cognitive function.

Investigators have reported consistent changes in long-latency EPs with aging. During development, the P300 decreases in latency until approximately the second decade. Using auditory stimuli, Goodin et al. (1978a) were the first to describe increased P300 latency in the elderly. The effects of age were strongest for the P300, with other components showing relatively small changes in latency. Since then, similar observations have been by made by others using AEPs, VEPs, and SSEPs (Beck et al. 1980; Brown et al. 1983; Pfefferbaum et al. 1984a; Picton et al. 1984; Syndulko et al. 1982). It now is widely accepted that P300 latency increases between 0.9 and 1.8 msec/year (Hillyard and Picton 1987; Polich 1991); this increase is believed to occur independently of any change in motor reaction time. Some investigators have found that the relationship between P300 latency and age is best described by a linear function (Pfefferbaum et al. 1984a; Picton et al. 1984; Polich et al. 1985; Squires et al. 1980; Syndulko et al. 1982), whereas others (Brown et al. 1983; Mullis et al. 1985) have reported a curvilinear relationship with greater annual latency increases for elderly subjects. Some have described increasing frontal distribution of the P300 (Pfefferbaum et al. 1984a; Smith et al. 1980). Others (Maurer et al. 1988; Picton et al. 1984) have been unable to replicate this finding with increasing age (Figure 11–2, *panel A*).

There is no similarly consistent effect reported for P300 amplitude and aging (Brown et al. 1983; Beck et al. 1980; Ford et al. 1982a, 1982b; Goodin et al. 1978a; Picton et al. 1984, 1986; Snyder and Hillyard 1976). Correcting waveforms for latency variability may abolish any of the differences in amplitude attributed to age (Pfefferbaum et al. 1984a).

Detection of Dementia

There is general agreement that qEEG is useful for detecting the presence of a dementing illness (Duffy et al. 1984b; Nuwer 1988; Prichep et al. 1983). Few studies, however, have systematically compared conventional EEG interpretation with qEEG for the detection of dementing illness. Brenner et al. (1986) compared 35 patients with clinically diagnosed dementia of the Alzheimer type (DAT), 23 patients with major depressive episodes, and 61 healthy control subjects. They found that qEEG offered "modest gains" in sensitivity over conventional EEG for the detection of moderate dementia (an increase from 57% to 66%), with essentially equal specificity (95% and 93%, respectively). They improved sensitivity using qEEG methods, despite collecting data from only four pooled qEEG channels from the parasagittal regions, and relying on mean frequency as the sole parameter studied. Furthermore, the fact that minutes of qEEG data could achieve greater sensitivity than conventional EEG, with equal specificity and using less physician time for test interpretation, suggests an advantage of qEEG over conventional EEG for routine evaluations.

Most studies use several types of qEEG measures (absolute power, relative power, and spectral ratios) and use linear combinations of these to discriminate subjects with from those without dementia. These measures are complementary: they are additive in detection of abnormality and yield different regional information regarding the distribution of the abnormalities (Leuchter et al., in press a). Duffy et al. (1984b) found increases in theta and/or delta activity, as well as decreases in beta activity, that were maximal in both temporal regions in early-onset DAT patients and in the frontal regions in late-onset DAT patients when compared with control subjects. Retrospective subject classification by discriminant function analysis using a combination of evoked response and electroencephalographic features correctly discriminated 95.8% of early-onset patients and 90% of late-onset patients from their respective control subjects. Breslau et al. (1989) have similarly found large differences between subjects with late-onset DAT and their elderly control subjects in temporal delta activity. A number of studies have shown increased delta and theta power and decreased alpha and beta power, as well as decreased mean frequency in dementia (Brenner et al. 1986; Coben et al. 1985; Giaquinto and Nolfe 1986; Penttilä et al. 1985; Stigsby et al. 1981; Visser et al. 1985; Vitiello and Prinz 1987). Leuchter et al. (1987) found large differences between dementia subjects (with either DAT or multi-infarct dementia [MID]) and control subjects in spectral ratios, which combine high-frequency and low-frequency power in a single measure. Using spectral ratios, as well as coherence variables, these researchers accurately classified more than 90% of subjects into their correct diagnostic group.

Most studies suggest that there is a positive linear relationship between slowing of the average EEG frequency and the degree of cognitive impairment in dementia (Johannesson et al. 1979; Miyasaka et al. 1978; Rae-Grant et al. 1987). There has been considerable uncertainty, however, concerning how early in the course of dementia qEEG may be useful for detecting disease. The answer to this question depends, to a great extent, on which measures are assessed. Gordon (see E. B. Gordon 1968; E. B. Gordon and Sim 1967) reported that changes in alpha power preceded increased slow-wave power as a manifestation of disease, whereas others (Berg et al. 1984; Coben et al. 1983a; Johannesson et al. 1977, 1979) reported that either increases in

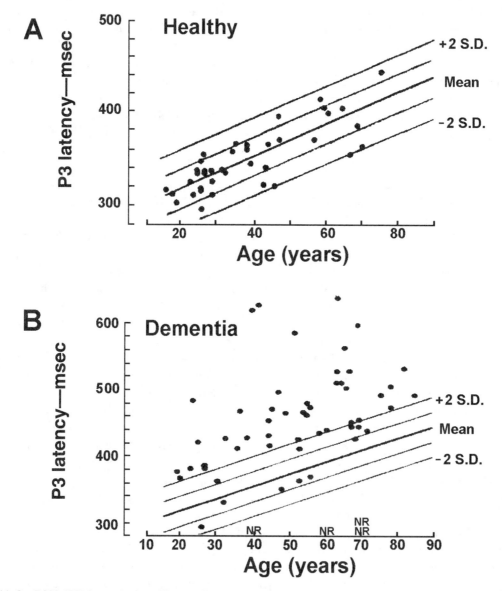

Figure 11–2. P300 (P3) latencies in milliseconds (msec) from the rare-tone evoked potential waveforms as a function of age for individual healthy subjects (*panel A*) and individual dementia patients (*panel B*). Also shown are regression lines 1 and 2 SD from the mean, derived from the data for healthy subjects. NR = individual patients out of the groups for whom no P300 latency could be elicited.

Source. Adapted from Squires et al. 1980. Copyright 1992 by the American Psychological Association. Used with permission.

theta power or decreases in beta power were the earliest changes. The highest sensitivity (24%) and specificity (100%) were reported with percentage theta (Coben et al. 1990). Similar sensitivities (range 20% to 36%) and specificities (range 93% to 100%) have been reported by others using a variety of EEG measures in varying scalp locations (Brenner et al. 1986; John et al. 1988; Prichep et al. 1983). In a recent, unpublished study, we found sensitivity and specificity of greater than 70% for detecting dementia in subjects with Mini-Mental State Exam (MMSE; Folstein et al. 1975) scores of 24 and above; for MMSE scores below 24, this increased to greater than 80%.

qEEG appears to be of greater use for distinguishing depression from dementia than conventional EEG. Pollock and Schneider (1990) reviewed studies performed over the preceding decade and found that more than half found increases in both alpha and beta power in depression; these investigators themselves (Pollock and Schneider 1989) found that increased alpha activity persisted after recovery from depression. Other specific qEEG findings in depression have included right temporal slowing, increased frontal beta power (Schatzberg et al. 1986), and increased left frontal alpha power (Davidson 1988). The increased delta power (Brenner et al. 1986; John et al. 1988; Visser et al. 1985) and decreased beta power in dementia (Brenner et al. 1986; Visser et al. 1985) appear particularly helpful in separating patients with dementia from those with depression alone. Because no single feature appears to be robust for the diagnosis of depression, several investigators have used a multivariate statistical approach to the diagnosis of depression (John et al. 1977, 1988; Shagass et al. 1984) and have reported overall accuracy in classification of 60%–90%. The stability of these multivariate methods for diagnosis remains to be verified.

Several investigators have attempted to use short-latency EPs for the diagnosis of dementia (Coben et al. 1983b; Harkins 1981; Visser et al. 1976). Prolonged flash VEP latency and increased amplitude (Coben et al. 1983b; Visser et al. 1976; Wright et al. 1984), as well as some changes in brain stem AEPs (Harkins 1981) and SSEPs (Huisman et al. 1985), have been reported in patients with dementia. However, the differences in the exogenous potentials between dementia subjects and control subjects are too small or inconsistent to permit definitive classification.

Most of the research on the late components of EPs in dementia has been focused on the P300 peak

(Figure 11–2). It has been established that P300 latency is prolonged in dementia. Goodin et al. (1978b) first reported an abnormally large increase in the P300 latency in a group of patients with dementia of different etiologies; they also noted that the increase in latency correlated with severity of dementia as assessed by the MMSE. Although these findings have been confirmed by several laboratories, prevalence of reported "abnormal" latency varies from 13% to 83%, with most studies reporting that 70%–80% of dementia patients have prolonged P300 latency (Brown et al. 1982, 1983; E. Gordon et al. 1986; Patterson et al. 1988; Squires et al. 1980; Syndulko et al. 1982) (Figure 11–2, *panel B*).

The usefulness of P300 latency alone is limited for several reasons. First, there is the wide variability in the prevalence of the abnormality. Pfefferbaum et al. (1984a, 1984b) used both auditory and visual EP paradigms to compare 77 subjects with dementia of different etiologies (MMSE score less than 25) with 66 control subjects. They reported that fewer than 30% of the dementia patients had P300 latencies that were at least two standard deviations greater than that expected for their age. This low specificity reflects in part the particular paradigm used to elicit the P300 component, as well as the variability in normal P300 latency in the control subjects. The increases in P300 latency in mild dementia have been reported to be too small to be clinically useful (Leppler and Greenberg 1984; Polich et al. 1986; Syndulko et al. 1984).

Second, P300 latency has been shown to be prolonged in other conditions, and has been reported in up to 12% of depressed and 13% of schizophrenic patients (E. Gordon et al. 1986). Furthermore, an increased P300 latency is seen with dementia in a variety of conditions such as alcohol abuse, Huntington's disease, Parkinson's disease, Down's syndrome, scopolamine-induced "dementia," and others (Calloway et al. 1985; Hansch et al. 1982; Lukas 1990; Pfefferbaum et al. 1979; Rosenberg et al. 1985; St. Clair et al. 1985). DAT patients cannot be distinguished from other dementias on the basis of P300 amplitude or latency (Brown et al. 1982; Polich et al. 1986).

P300 latency measures are useful in certain clinical situations and as a component of a broader neurophysiological evaluation. Measurement of P300 latency may be useful as a component of an overall evaluation when there is a specific diagnostic question of dementia versus depression or delirium (Goodin 1990; Pfefferbaum et al. 1990), although it probably is of little use for specifying the type of dementia (Pfefferbaum et al. 1990).

In combination with measures of power and/or coherence, this EP measure may add greater sensitivity to the qEEG evaluation of dementia.

Diagnosis and Assessment of Delirium

qEEG offers substantial advantages over conventional EEG in the examination of subjects with delirium. Although Engel and Romano (1959) demonstrated that EEG slowing is almost invariably present in delirium and that grossly excessive slowing suggests the presence of delirium instead of or in addition to dementia (Brenner 1991; Rabins and Folstein 1982), it is difficult to determine the severity of slowing by visual inspection.

Examination of a series of subjects with delirium indicates that qEEG can be used to successfully quantitate the magnitude of slow-wave power. qEEG detects significant changes in the amount of slow-wave power in the course of a delirium when the conventional EEG shows equivocal change, and decreases in slow-wave power may actually precede improvements in mental status (Leuchter and Jacobson 1991). qEEG indices are strongly correlated with not only the severity of delirium, but also the length of delirium and hospitalization (Koponen 1991; Koponen et al. 1989).

Although it has been suggested that the severity of slowing may differ between subjects with delirium or dementia, recent studies indicate that it may be practical to differentiate these two groups based on qEEG. Koponen et al. (1989) found that delirious subjects with concomitant dementia had more severe slowing than those without dementia. Jacobson et al. (1993a) reported that several qEEG indices were useful for distinguishing delirium from dementia. Follow-up work from this group has indicated that distinct qEEG measures of absolute and relative power indices are sensitive to the progression of dementia or the development of delirium, suggesting that qEEG may be particularly helpful for identifying the onset of delirium as a complication of dementia (Jacobson et al. 1993b).

EPs have also been used recently in the assessment of delirium, primarily in patients with hepatic or renal encephalopathy (some of whom are elderly). Some investigators have reported abnormal latencies of brain stem auditory evoked potential (BAEPs) (Chu and Yang 1987; Pierelli et al. 1985; Rossini et al. 1984), whereas others have not (Trzepacz et al. 1989; Yang et al. 1986). More consistent results have been obtained with SSEPs, for which changes in latency correlate with severity of encephalopathy (Trzepacz et al. 1989; Yen and Liaw 1990), and with VEPs (Casellas et al. 1985; Kuba et al. 1983; Levy et al. 1987; Levy et al. 1990; Pierelli et al. 1985; Rossini et al. 1981; Zeneroli et al. 1984).

In hepatic encephalopathy, there are changes in both SSEP and VEP latency during progressive stages of encephalopathy (Davies et al. 1991). In a recent review of the clinical usefulness of qEEG methods including spectral analysis, EEG, SSEPs, BAEPs, VEPs, and P300, van der Rijt and Schalm (1992) found that the highest percentage of abnormalities in patients with subclinical hepatic encephalopathy was detected by flash VEPs (25%–46%, 95% confidence interval). The auditory and pattern reversal P300 shows an increase in latency and may be used for the detection of milder disease, although its applications are limited as it requires more patient participation than short-latency EPs (Sandford and Saul 1988).

Little work has been done using EP topographic mapping in hepatic encephalopathy, and this holds considerable promise for the future. Researchers led by Matos and Paiva (Matos 1988; Paiva et al. 1988) have reported that 73%–75% of liver disease patients without clinical signs of encephalopathy show abnormal VEP topographic maps.

Limitations of qEEG

Quantitation of the power in different frequency bands has been touted as more "objective" and as minimizing variability in interpretation. It is true that qEEG yields more reliable and reproducible measurements of brain activity and is more likely to detect subtle focal or generalized alterations in brain function (Jerrett and Corsak 1988; Nuwer et al. 1987). Quantitation alone does not, however, indicate whether activity is normal or abnormal; traditionally, these determinations are made based on statistical comparison of data from an individual to a normal base value and determining whether the individual is beyond the "cutoff" for normality. Thus qEEG does not eliminate the confounding problem that slowing increases both with age and emergence of organic brain disease. It does, however, allow the clinician to be more precise regarding the amount of slowing and whether this appears to be excessive for the patient's age. The most common method for establishing base values is building a "normative data base" by collecting data from individuals who are in good health and not receiving any medications that might influence brain electrical activity.

Stratification of normative data by age and gender may be additionally helpful in determining whether changes in an individual's record are indicative of abnormality. Commonly, when the amount of slow-wave power at a given site is two standard deviations from the mean of a group of control subjects, this is interpreted as abnormal.

This statistical data base approach can be useful for the interpretation of an individual's data, but has significant limitations. First, it is not clear how much deviation from a group of age-matched control subjects is acceptable for any given EEG measure. Some patterns of brain activity are very different from the patterns seen on most EEGs, and would be two standard deviations from a normal mean, but are a recognized "normal variant" (e.g., the low-voltage fast recording without any posterior dominant rhythm). Second, there are instances in which a persistent focal increase in slow-wave power is significant and indicative of abnormality, but may be less than two standard deviations from the mean for that subject's age group. Such a focal increase may be especially significant if it is progressive over time. Third, a small but consistent deviation at many or all recording sites could be highly significant clinically and indicative of brain dysfunction, even if less than two standard deviations. Finally, a highly significant difference (i.e., four standard deviations) at a single recording site may need to be interpreted with caution because, with multiple tests at multiple recording sites in multiple frequency bands, false positive results may occur.

There are several different approaches to increasing confidence in the comparisons between a patient and a normative data base. Some researchers have proposed looking at multiple independent segments of data from within a recording session (Duffy 1990; Duffy et al. 1992). An alternative is to examine a subject using multiple modalities, such as resting EEG and EPs. If a brain area appears abnormal in multiple independent samples of data, obtained under different recording paradigms, this could increase confidence that a finding is valid (Duffy 1988). Of course, because the abnormality is not detected on all occasions or under all conditions does not necessarily mean it is not "real"; it simply may be episodic or state dependent.

An alternative to the normative data base model is to compare a given individual to their own baseline. When the first recording is performed in the premorbid condition, this may be the ideal method for assessment of brain electrical activity. Both the absolute intensity of power in any given frequency band, as well as the proportional distribution of power across frequency bands, may be examined, and a determination may be made whether there has been a change from the individual's baseline. This method is particularly applicable to the study of patients with delirium, in whom multiple studies over a short period of time may be indicated, or for the long-term follow-up of patients with dementia. Unfortunately, normal baseline studies rarely are available, so this method is of little help in interpreting the initial study of a patient with possible dementia or delirium. Furthermore, there may be significant fluctuations in patients' brain electrical activity with changes in state, so that it still is difficult to determine whether subtle changes are indicative of abnormality or are within the normal range.

At present, qEEG is considered an adjunct to conventional EEG in the study of psychiatric illnesses (American Psychiatric Association Task Force on Quantitative Electrophysiological Assessment 1991). This is understandable, as there are clinical situations in which conventional EEG offers some advantages over qEEG. Very fast transient EEG activity lasting only milliseconds is not easily detected through quantitative analysis, because it accounts for a very low proportion of the total power in a recording epoch. Therefore, an area of focal damage that is producing transient disturbances, such as rare epileptiform spikes, will not be detected by spectral analysis unless it also is producing a disproportionate amount of slow- or fast-wave power. There are computer programs currently available to scan qEEG data for the presence of epileptiform spikes or other specific abnormalities, but these are not yet widely accepted.

qEEG is sensitive to the proportion of energy in any given frequency band, but is much less sensitive to specific wave morphology; in other words, it is less sophisticated at pattern recognition. Thus rhythmic triphasic waves would not be readily distinguished from frontally predominant intermittent rhythmic delta activity or from continuous polymorphic delta activity in the frontal region. Though pattern recognition might lead the electroencephalographer to suspect either a particular metabolic encephalopathy or focal structural lesion with one or the other of these patterns, the frequency spectra might look remarkably similar.

The unique advantages of visual pattern interpretation indicate that there always will be a role for conventional electroencephalography, although as artificial intelligence algorithms for pattern recognition develop, conventional EEG may evolve into "computer-assisted EEG."

New Methods for Interpreting qEEG

qEEG interpretation traditionally has lacked the face and construct validity that is shared by other methods of brain imaging. A clinician can view a [^{18}F]2-deoxy-D-glucose positron-emission tomography (FDG-PET) scan and gain insights about brain metabolism, a [^{99m}Tc]*d,l*-hexamethylpropyleneamineoxime single photon emission tomography (HMPAO-SPECT) scan and assess brain perfusion, or MRI and study brain structure. The clinician viewing qEEG maps, however, examines quantities called *power* and *amplitude* that in and of themselves have no clear physiological meaning. It is easily overlooked that PET, SPECT, and MRI images represent electromagnetic emission data that are processed through complex algorithms, and that the so-called images are a secondary form of information derived from a complex matrix of numbers. Information on metabolism, blood flow, and structure are only a small portion of the masses of electromagnetic emission data recorded by these scanners, albeit the most relevant portions for clinical purposes. Research has allowed physicians to derive the relevant "signal" from the abundant "noise" concerning other aspects of brain function and structure and display a "meaningful" quantity.

To develop qEEG as a robust method of functional imaging, what has been missing is a method for translating surface-recorded electrical activity into images with immediate clinical relevance. One method for performing this translation would be to examine known brain diseases (e.g., stroke and tumors) with qEEG and other imaging methods, to identify the electrical equivalent of hypoperfusion, hypometabolism, or a structural lesion. By comparing qEEG with other measures of brain function, researchers now are deciphering brain electrical activity by examining lesions with multiple forms of brain imaging.

Neurophysiology of EEG Abnormalities

To translate qEEG signals into clinically relevant images, some researchers have examined lesions presumed to cause cortical deafferentation. This strategy takes advantage of the true strength of qEEG: its ability to monitor the activity and integrity of afferent and efferent fibers that are responsible for integrating elec-

trical activity of different brain areas. Examination of fiber tract damage holds promise as a neuropsychiatric framework for interpreting qEEG, because damage to associative pathways has long been known to lead to complex neuropsychiatric disturbances (Geschwind 1965). Furthermore, damage to the pyramidal cells (the origin and terminations of long fiber pathways) has been implicated in illnesses ranging from schizophrenia (Benes et al. 1991; Christison et al. 1989; Conrad et al. 1991) to DAT (Lewis et al. 1987; Morrison et al. 1986; Pearson et al. 1985).

There is ample evidence from studies of both animals and humans indicating that pathological slow waves in the EEG are caused by partial deafferentation of pyramidal cells of the cerebral cortex (Steriade et al. 1990). Complete destruction of cortex does not cause excessive slowing, but instead leads to electrical silence; only through partial deafferentation of the cortex or nonlethal damage to cortical neurons do pathological slow waves develop (Gloor et al. 1977) (Figure 11–3). Deafferentation can be the result of pri-

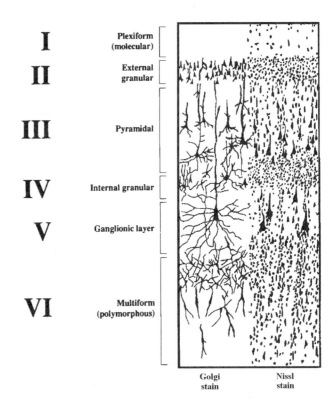

Figure 11–3. Schematic representation of the layers of the cerebral cortex (showing association cortex). Partial deafferentation of the large pyramidal cells in layers II and III is the cause of pathological slow waves in the electroencephalogram.

mary neuronal disease or of a brain insult (e.g., a stroke) secondarily affecting nerve function.

Deafferentation can occur at any level: direct damage to the cortex, undercutting of the cortex by white matter lesions, or damage to the cortically projecting basal forebrain neurons all can cause an increase in cortically recorded slow waves. Research suggests that deafferentation can be structural (e.g., through permanent physical damage) or functional (e.g., through reversible toxic damage) (Steriade et al. 1990). This finding explains the similar patterns of increased slowing caused by either DAT or administration of atropine: the former process causes loss of the origins of cortically projecting cholinergic afferents from the basal forebrain, whereas the latter inhibits firing of the cortically projecting afferent cells (Buzsàki et al. 1988; Detari et al. 1987; Schaul et al. 1981; Steriade et al. 1990). The mechanism of slow waves that accompany metabolic derangements such as hypoxia, hypoglycemia, or other toxic states has not been established, but these conditions also may be caused by dysfunction of cells projecting to the cortex or of the cortical pyramidal cells themselves.

Detection of Deafferented Cortex: The Cordance Method

A specific measure of cortical deafferentation could be very useful clinically. Such a measure could potentially indicate which slow waves were pathological and even in the absence of grossly excessive slowing suggest that pathology exists. Based on the knowledge that surface-recorded EEG should be sensitive to cortical deafferentation, we (Leuchter et al., in press b; in press c) studied subjects with large white matter lesions that presumably undercut and partially deafferented cerebral cortex. These areas appeared to be hypoperfused on SPECT scanning and hypometabolic on PET, findings consistent with deafferentation. Such areas showed a characteristic qEEG pattern: although the deafferented cortex produced less slow-wave power on an absolute basis than did other cortical areas, it produced greater slow-wave power on a relative basis compared with other brain areas.

This finding of decreased absolute but increased relative slow-wave power over white matter lesions was termed *discordance*. Though not all white matter lesions were sufficient to cause discordance, the presence of discordance was associated reliably with areas that were found to be hypoperfused due to stroke or the pres-

ence of brain degeneration (i.e., DAT). The opposite indicator state, called *concordance,* was associated reliably with states of high perfusion, and appears to be an indicator of cortex that is functioning normally. For example, in patients with DAT, discordance is seen over the parietal regions and other areas that are hypometabolic (Figure 11–4). These areas are known to be deafferented by the degenerative processes of DAT, in which the pyramidal cells of laminae II and III that project corticocortical afferents die selectively (Morrison et al. 1986). Concordance is seen over the central brain areas, particularly the area of the motor strip, which is known to be relatively spared by the neuropathological changes of DAT.

Figure 11–5 shows brain maps from a 76-year-old woman with a frontal lobe degeneration, whose HMPAO-SPECT scan (Figure 11–5, *panel A*) shows profound frontal hypoperfusion, with relatively preserved perfusion posteriorly. The cordance maps (Figure 11–5, *panel B*) show frontal discordance, with concordance maximal posteriorly (Figure 11–5, *panel C*).

The concordance and discordance indicators (known jointly as *cordance*) show promise for detecting pathological changes, even in cognitively intact subjects. In a subject with depression and white matter lesions under the frontal cortex (Figure 11–6) that are more prominent on the left, the discordance map shows bifrontal discordance worse on the left, even in the absence of excess slowing on conventional EEG or absolute or relative power mapping.

Cordance may have wide applicability for the study not only of mental disorders, but also of cognitive functions. Preliminary data from our unpublished study suggest that cordance detects areas of high and low perfusion even within the normal range. Cordance, therefore, may be a powerful method for detecting areas of activation and inactivation associated with tasks.

Disconnection Between Brain Areas: The Role of Coherence

Another example of the usefulness of the deafferentation model of qEEG lies in the ability of this model to detect damage to afferent and efferent fibers linking two brain regions. This deafferentation is measured through qEEG coherence, which has proved useful in detecting differences between DAT and MID subjects. Traditionally, differential diagnosis between these disorders has relied on detection of focal abnormalities, which reportedly are more common among subjects with MID. This finding is not sufficiently prevalent, however, to be of diagnostic usefulness (Dejaiffe et al. 1964; Harrison et al. 1979; Logar et al. 1987; Roberts et al. 1978). Although several investigators found differences in spectral analysis performed in the resting state (Leuchter et al. 1987) or during verbal tasks (Loring et al. 1985) to be useful in distinguishing between these two types of dementia, qEEG overall was of limited use in differentiating between DAT and MID (Leuchter et al., in press a; Logar et al. 1987).

Electrographic coherence has been used with greater success to distinguish DAT from MID patients. As discussed above, coherence is a measure of synchronization of brain electrical activity between regions. Coherence appears to be a reliable measure of the functional connections between brain areas, monitoring interactions between cortical areas while subjects are at rest or engaged in a relevant cognitive task (Busk and Galbraith 1975; Davis and Wada 1974; O'Connor and Shaw 1978; Shaw et al. 1977, 1978; Tucker et al. 1986). Two previous studies of subjects with DAT and MID have shown that these conditions have different effects on coherence between brain regions, with increased coherence between some brain regions and decreased coherence between others relative to control subjects (Leuchter et al. 1987; O'Connor et al. 1979).

Coherence has been thought to be mediated by either corticocortical or corticosubcortical fibers linking brain areas, but until recently researchers have failed to identify any specific fiber tracts that mediate coherence or to use coherence to detect specific types of disconnection. Coherence now has been shown to detect different types of disconnection in the aging brain. The two most common types of dementia (DAT

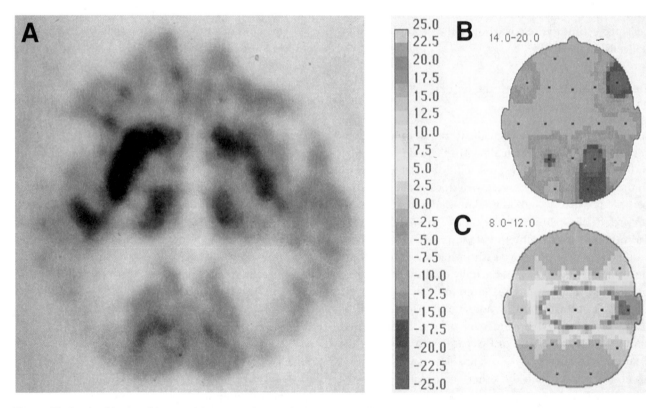

Figure 11–4. An 88-year-old man with progressive confusion, memory loss, social withdrawal, and agitation, who was diagnosed with dementia of the Alzheimer type (DAT). His positron-emission tomography (PET) scan showed biparietal hypometabolism, as well as focal right temporal hypometabolism (*panel A*). The cordance map shows three prominent areas of beta discordance, at the right and left parietal and right temporal electrodes, that have a strong spatial association with the three areas of hypometabolism (*panel B*). There is significant alpha concordance over the frontocentral region bilaterally, in the general area of the motor strip (*panel C*); this area commonly has the highest metabolism in subjects with DAT. The PET scan shows the brain as viewed from below, whereas the cordance map shows it viewed from above (i.e., right and left are reversed in the two pictures).

or MID) have been hypothesized, on the basis of neuropathological data, to affect different types of brain connections: DAT causes selective disconnection of long corticocortical fibers, whereas MID causes more diffuse disconnection of corticosubcortical white matter networks. We (Leuchter et al. 1992) have shown that coherence detects these different types of disconnection and may be used to detect successfully high proportions of subjects with DAT or MID (Figures 11–7 and 11–8).

Given the ubiquitous nature of white matter disease in geriatric patients with depression, dementia, or those without illness, the concept of disconnection may have applications for the study of other groups of elderly subjects. An area that is particularly vulnerable to white matter changes is the periventricular region (Bowen et al. 1990), in which high-signal lesions may be seen in 60%–100% of asymptomatic control subjects (Leuchter 1994). These periventricular fibers are critical components of the networks that subserve higher cortical functions, containing the projections of the prefrontal cortical neurons and the visual associa-

tion pathways. We (Leuchter et al., in press d) have shown that there is an association between the presence of periventricular damage seen on MRI and decreased coherence in the frontal and visual networks of connections. The association between these two measures is stronger than the association between white matter disease and clinical diagnosis, suggesting that the degree and type of disconnection may be a useful model for categorizing cognitive impairment among elderly subjects, even those who do not meet all criteria for dementia.

Morrison and colleagues (Hof et al. 1990; Morrison et al. 1991) have highlighted the heterogeneity in types of disconnection among DAT patients and have found that those with greater visuospatial difficulty (Balint's syndrome) show greater neuropathological disruption of the visual association pathways. The strong associations between performance on neuropsychological tests and coherence in relevant brain regions (particularly visuospatial function and visual system coherence) (J. J. Dunkin, S. Osato, A. F. Leuchter, unpublished data, February 1994) suggest that co-

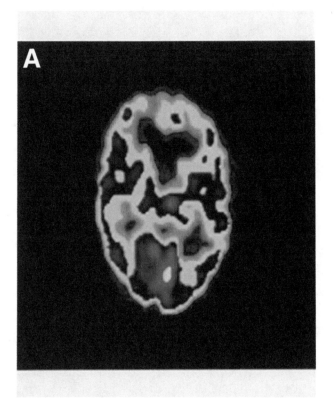

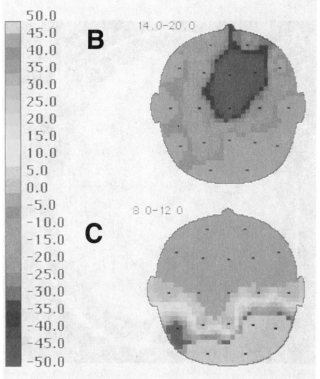

Figure 11–5. A 76-year-old woman with a progressive dementia that presented primarily with delusions, personality changes, and difficulties with complex tasks. A dementia with frontal lobe features, such as Pick's disease, was diagnosed; the diagnosis was supported by a single photon emission computed tomography (SPECT) scan showing frontal hypoperfusion (*panel A*). She also showed frontal discordance in the beta band (*panel B*). Concordance was seen in the alpha band over areas that showed high perfusion (*panel C*).

herence may be useful for characterizing the distribution of pathology among patients with dementia.

Recent results indicate that coherence also may be important as an indicator of outcome in elderly patients with dementia or depression. We recently have shown that low baseline coherence is associated with poorer functional status at 2-year follow-up in patients with dementia (Leuchter et al., in press e) and with poorer outcome and increased mortality in patients with depression (Leuchter et al., in press f).

Deafferentation in Ascending Pathways: The Role of EPs

A third type of afferent connection that can successfully be characterized with qEEG comprises the sensory input pathways. Detection of a brain-generated waveform in response to peripheral sensory input (either stimulation of peripheral nerves, visual flash stimulation, or auditory stimulation) monitors the function of sensory pathways. These pathways have been hypothesized to be of interest in several mental illnesses. Braff and Geyer (1990) and Freedman et al. (1983) have hypothesized that these potentials are of significant interest for psychiatry as a measure of "sensory gating" in patients with psychosis. As discussed above, Goodin et al. (1978b) found that the long-latency potentials (particularly the P300) are useful measures of higher cortical functions.

The clinical utility of EPs has been limited because of both a lack of specificity for changes observed and absence of a clear physiological correlate for these changes. Recent results suggest, however, that many of the changes observed in EPs reflect changes in afferent fiber function and structure. Some of the most compelling evidence for EPs changing in response to afferent damage has been seen in patients with dementia. Several researchers (Abbruzzese et al. 1984; Kato et al. 1990) have shown a delayed central conduction time for SSEPs in patients with MID, but not those with DAT. This finding is consistent with the fact that MID subjects have central white matter demyelination (which

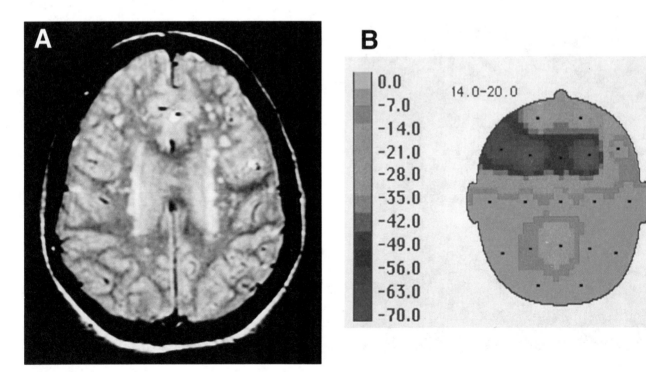

Figure 11–6. An 80-year-old woman with symptoms of severe depression, anxiety, and depersonalization, who was diagnosed as having a major depressive episode. Magnetic resonance imaging (MRI) revealed several patches of white matter disease under the frontal lobes, separated from the anterior ventricular horns with the more severe disease adjacent to the left anterior horn (*panel A*). The two frontal lesions are associated with beta discordance, with the cortex overlying the larger lesions on the left showing broader and more intense discordance (*panel B*). MRI and cordance maps with opposite right-left orientations (as described in Figure 11–4).

delays conduction of impulses), whereas DAT subjects do not have such demyelination.

Using the deafferentation model, investigators have used EPs to localize damage to brain structures. Mauguiere and Ibanez (1990) studied a series of patients with strokes in a variety of subcortical (either thalamus or subcortical white matter) and cortical locations, to determine if lesion location explained losses of specific SSEPs. These investigators found that damage to specific afferent pathways (confirmed by MRI) was associated with loss of specific EP components and with the particular symptoms that patients reported. These investigators concluded that alterations in specific EP components represented states of "hemispheric deafferentation." This finding may have implications for studies of sensory gating using EPs in psychiatric patients.

Of greater direct relevance to geriatric neuropsychiatry are the changes in latency and amplitude of the P300 and other long-latency EPs, that are now well established in schizophrenia (Barrett et al. 1986; Morstyn et al. 1983). These also have been reported in schizophrenic children (Erwin et al. 1986) and relatives of schizophrenic subjects (Blackwood et al. 1991; Saitoh et al. 1984). Some evidence has suggested significant P300 asymmetry, with lower amplitude potentials specifically over the left temporal region (McCarley et al. 1993; Morstyn et al. 1983); other investigators, however, were unable to confirm this asymmetry and suggested that it might represent a medication effect (Pfefferbaum et al. 1984b). Recent work by McCarley et al. (1993), however, has indicated that these EP abnormalities are associated with specific damage to the left superior temporal gyrus and that left-sided abnor-

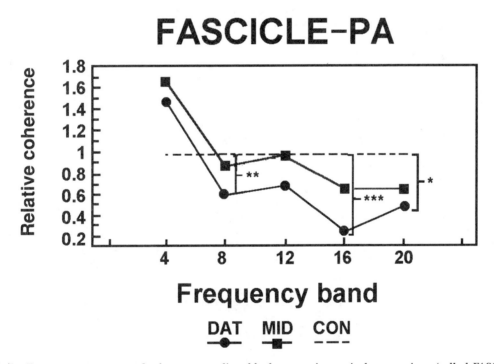

Figure 11–7. Frequency spectrum of coherence mediated by long corticocortical connections (called *FASCICLE-PA measure*, because it is similar to the distribution of fibers of the superior longitudinal fasciculus). Coherence is displayed for the dementia of the Alzheimer type (DAT) (*circles*) and multi-infarct dementia (MID) (*squares*) groups as a proportion of the mean value for the control (CON) group (*broken line*). Mean value for the control group is standardized to 1 in each frequency band, and indicated by the dotted line across the middle of the figure. Frequency bands are displayed across the bottom of the figure, with numbers representing the center frequency of each band (i.e., *4* represents the 2- to 6-Hz band; *8* represents the 6- to 10-Hz band; and so on).
*Difference between DAT and control subjects, $P < .05$.
**Difference between DAT and control subjects, $P < .01$.
***Difference between DAT and control subjects, $P < .005$.
Source. From Leuchter AF, Newton TF, Cook IA, et al: "Changes in Brain Functional Connectivity in Alzheimer-Type and Multi-Infarct Dementia." *Brain* 115:1543–1561, 1992. Copyright 1992 by Oxford University Press. Used with permission.

malities are associated not only with reduced P300 amplitude over the left hemisphere, but also with positive symptoms. McCarley et al. (1991) hypothesized that the P300 abnormalities seen in schizophrenic patients may represent the results of neuronal excitotoxicity on the pyramidal cells of the left hippocampus. They proposed that both psychotic symptoms and neuroleptic responsiveness reflect alteration in response in efferent fibers from the hippocampus, once again emphasizing the potential usefulness of the afferent fiber model of neurophysiology.

Future of qEEG

qEEG offers a unique contribution to the armamentarium of imaging technologies. There are several powerful imaging technologies, such as PET or SPECT, that directly measure the metabolism or perfusion of brain tissue; these techniques provide little or no information about damage to pathways that bring information into the central nervous system or that transfer information between critical brain areas. qEEG complements these techniques by assessing fiber system function. In some situations, qEEG using the cordance method may be the preferred method for assessing perfusion and metabolism. Because it is noninvasive, does not expose the patient to ionizing radiation, and does not require costly equipment, cordance would be ideal for patients who require long-term, frequent, or even bedside monitoring.

For similar reasons, qEEG has a variety of uses in the research setting. Researchers can observe brain

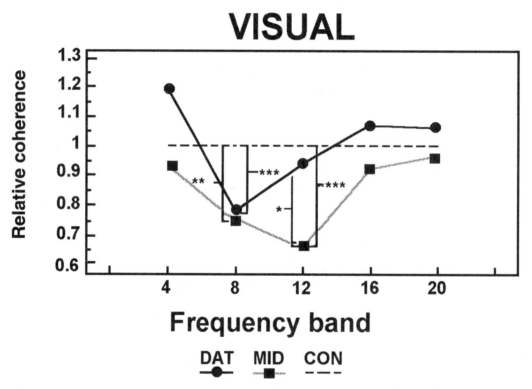

Figure 11–8. Frequency spectrum of coherence mediated by networks of short corticocortical and corticosubcortical conections (called *VISUAL measure*, because it is similar to the projctors of the visual pathway). Coherence is displayed for the dementia of the Alzheimer type (DAT) (*circles*) and multi-infarct dementia (MID) (*squares*) groups as a proportion of the mean value for the control (CON) group (*broken line*). Mean value for the control group is standardized to 1 in each frequency band and indicated by the dotted line across the middle of the figure. Frequency bands are displayed across the bottom of the figure, with numbers representing the center frequency of each band (i.e., *4* represents the 2- to 6-Hz band, *8* represents the 6- to 10-Hz band, and so on).
[*]Difference between DAT and control subjects, $P < .05$.
[**]Difference between DAT and control subjects, $P < .01$.
[***]Difference between DAT and MID subjects, $P < .05$.
Source. From Leuchter AF, Newton TF, Cook IA, et al: "Changes in Brain Functional Connectivity in Alzheimer-Type and Multi-Infarct Dementia." *Brain* 115:1543–1561, 1992. Copyright 1992 by Oxford University Press. Used with permission.

function to assess drug effects, monitor the course of illness, determine prognosis, or screen novel treatments in a cost-effective manner. Multivariate analysis of qEEG measures, using several sensory modalities of EPs or cognitive activation tasks, may improve diagnostic accuracy. The correlation of anatomic and physiological measures of brain function obtained from MRI, SPECT, and PET, with qEEG measurements, holds great promise for the future.

In the next few years, conventional EEG and qEEG probably will evolve into independent and complementary diagnostic tests. The clinician interested in detecting epileptiform abnormalities, or some other transient brain electrical activity, will request a conventional EEG. Clinicians interested in assessing global brain function, detecting focal brain dysfunction, or assessing cerebral perfusion or metabolism will request qEEG alone.

A conventional EEG in addition to a qEEG study will yield marginally more information than the quantitative study alone, at least until computer-assisted, pattern-recognition algorithms develop further. As pressures for medical cost containment mount, however, clinicians in all specialties likely will more heavily use diagnostic tests that are computer-based and that therefore require less physician time. Just as computers have reduced the physician time required for electrocardiogram interpretation, qEEG will eventually eliminate much of the physician time required for EEG interpretation. qEEG in many places still is a relatively costly procedure. As computer prices decline and qEEG systems become more widely available, however, qEEG will become a highly cost-effective means of imaging the brain.

Summary

EEG is an important tool in the evaluation of cerebral function and brain disease in geriatric patients. EEG findings rarely are pathognomonic for a specific diagnosis, but provide information that is consistent with (e.g., slowing in DAT or delirium), supportive of (e.g., triphasic waves in Creutzfeldt-Jakob disease), or highly suggestive of (e.g., anterior temporal spike-and-wave foci in a seizure disorder) the presence of a particular illness.

In the clinical practice of geriatric neuropsychiatry, the conventional EEG is sensitive to the presence of an encephalopathy, but it remains a nonspecific indicator of the type of dysfunction. EEG is a useful physiological tool to confirm the diagnosis and severity of delirium and for monitoring response to treatment, but lacks specificity in differentiating between dementia and mild-to-moderate states of delirium.

qEEG overcomes many of the limitations of conventional EEG. It yields more reliable and reproducible measurements of brain activity, and is more sensitive for detecting subtle focal or generalized alterations in brain function. qEEG measures such as absolute power, relative power, and spectral ratios provide information that is not accessible from visual inspection of the conventional recording. These measures yield different functional and regional information regarding abnormality and thus are complementary and additive in the detection of brain dysfunction.

Another product of qEEG analysis are EPs: multicomponent waves of positive and negative potentials that result when the EEG signal from the scalp is averaged for a specified time interval following a repetitive stimulus. EPs may be useful as supportive evidence in the diagnosis of dementia, depression, or delirium, but probably are of little use for specifying the type of dementia.

Quantitation of the power in different frequency bands is more "objective" than conventional EEG interpretation and therefore minimizes variability in test interpretation. Standard qEEG does not, however, overcome all the limitations of conventional EEG. For example, despite the greater precision of qEEG in power determinations, the nature of the power changes observed with normal aging still share some of the features of emerging organic brain disease. Normative data bases of age-matched control subjects are useful for describing the range of normality, but are of limited use for determining that a clinically significant abnormality exists in patients with mild excesses of slowing. In the absence of a consensus definition of what constitutes a statistically significant excess of slowing, comparison of serial studies from a patient over time remains the most reliable method for determining if abnormalities exist.

Recent research suggests that qEEG can provide information that is specific for the detection and diagnosis of different organic mental syndromes. New algorithms appear to be sensitive and specific for the detection of cortical deafferentation, through monitoring dysfunction in different types of fiber tracts. Coherence, a measure of the synchronization of electrical activity between different cortical regions, has proved useful in distinguishing DAT and MID subjects and in detecting fiber tract dysfunction associated with periventricular white matter changes on MRI. Cordance, a measure of cortical deafferentation in a single brain region, has strong associations with direct measures of perfusion or metabolism. Cordance appears to reliably detect areas of hypoperfusion caused by stroke or brain degeneration (i.e., Alzheimer's disease). EPs have also been useful in examining deafferentation of ascending sensory pathways. Multivariate analysis of qEEG measures holds great promise for improving diagnostic accuracy.

Currently, qEEG is considered an adjunct to conventional EEG. Conventional EEG remains more sensitive for detecting very fast transient EEG activity, as well as specific wave morphology, and is the modality of choice for the evaluation of possible seizure disorders. As more sophisticated algorithms for interpreting neurophysiological signals are developed and validated, conventional EEG and qEEG may evolve into independent clinical tests.

References

Abbott J: The EEG in Jakob-Creutzfeldt's disease. Electroencephalogr Clin Neurophysiol 11:184–185, 1959

Abbruzzese G, Reni L, Cocito L, et al: Short-latency somatosensory evoked potentials in degenerative and vascular dementia. J Neurol Neurosurg Psychiatry 47:1034–1037, 1984

American Psychiatric Association Task Force on Quantitative Electrophysiological Assessment: Quantitative electroencephalography: a report on the present state of computerized EEG techniques. Am J Psychiatry 148:961–964, 1991

Andermann K, Stoller A: EEG patterns in hospitalized and non-hospitalized aged. Electroencephalogr Clin Neurophysiol 13:319, 1961

Barrett K, McCallum WC, Pocock PV: Brain indicators of altered attention and information processing in schizophrenic patients. Br J Psychiatry 148:414–420, 1986

Beck EC, Swanson C, Dustman RE: Long latency components of the visually evoked potential in man: effects of aging. Exp Aging Res 6:523–545, 1980

Benes FM, McSparren J, Bird ED, et al: Deficits in small interneurons in prefrontal and cingulate cortices of schizophrenic and schizoaffective patients. Arch Gen Psychiatry 48:996–1001, 1991

Berg L, Danziger WL, Storandt M, et al: Predictive features in mild senile dementia of the Alzheimer's type. Neurology 34:563–569, 1984

Berger H: On the electroencephalogram of man: twelfth report. Archiv für Psychiatrie und Nervenkrankheiten 106:165–187, 1937

Blackwood DRH, St Clair DM, Muir WJ, et al: Auditory P300 and eye tracking dysfunction in schizophrenic pedigrees. Arch Gen Psychiatry 48:899–909, 1991

Bowen B, Barker W, Lowenstein D, et al: MR signal abnormalities in memory disorder and dementia. American Journal of Neuroradiology 11:283–290, 1990

Braff DL, Geyer MA: Sensorimotor gating and schizophrenia: human and animal model studies. Arch Gen Psychiatry 47:181–188, 1990

Brenner RP: Utility of electroencephalography in delirium: past views and current practice. Int Psychogeriatr 3:211–229, 1991

Brenner RP, Ulrich RF, Spiker DG, et al: Computerized EEG spectral analysis in elderly normal, demented, and depressed subjects. Electroencephalogr Clin Neurophysiol 64:483–492, 1986

Breslau J, Starr A, Sicotte N, et al: Topographic EEG changes with normal aging and SDAT. Electroencephalogr Clin Neurophysiol 72:281–289, 1989

Brown WS, Marsh JT, La Rue A: Event-related potentials in psychiatry: differentiating depression and dementia in the elderly. Bulletin of the Los Angeles Neurological Societies 47:91–107, 1982

Brown WS, Marsh JT, LaRue A: Exponential electrophysiological aging: P300 latency. Electroencephalogr Clin Neurophysiol 55:277–285, 1983

Burger LJ, Rowan J, Goldenshon E: Creutzfeldt-Jakob disease. Arch Neurol 26:428–433, 1972

Busk J, Galbraith G: EEG correlates of visual-motor practice in man. Electroencephalogr Clin Neurophysiol 38:415–422, 1975

Busse EW, Obrist W: Pre-senescent electroencephalographic changes in normal subjects. J Gerontol 20:315–320, 1965

Busse EW: Electroencephalography, in Alzheimer's Disease: The Standard Reference. Edited by Resiberg B. New York, Free Press, 1983, pp 231–236

Buzsáki G, Bickford R, Armstrong D, et al: Electric activity in the neocortex of freely moving young and aged rats. Neuroscience 26:735–744, 1988

Calloway E, Halliday R, Naylor H, et al: Effects of oral scopolamine on human stimulus evaluation. Psychopharmacology 85:133–138, 1985

Casellas F, Sagalés T, Calzada MD, et al: Visual evoked potentials in hepatic encephalopathy. Lancet 1:394–395, 1985

Chiofalo N, Fuentes A, Galvez S: Serial EEG findings in 27 cases of Creutzfeldt-Jakob disease. Arch Neurol 37:143–145, 1980

Christison GW, Casanova MF, Weinberger DR, et al: A quantitative investigation of hippocampal pyramidal cell size, shape, and variability of orientation in schizophrenia. Arch Gen Psychiatry 6:1027–32, 1989

Chu N-S, Yang S-S: Brainstem auditory evoked potentials in different types of hepatic diseases. Electroencephalogr Clin Neurophysiol 67:337–339, 1987

Coben LA, Danziger WL, Berg L: Frequency analysis of the resting awake EEG in mild senile dementia of Alzheimer type. Electroencephalogr Clin Neurophysiol 55:372–380, 1983a

Coben LA, Danziger WL, Hughes CP: Visual evoked potentials in mild senile dementia of the Alzheimer's type. Electroencephalogr Clin Neurophysiol 55:121–130, 1983b

Coben LA, Danziger W, Storandt M: A longitudinal EEG study of mild senile dementia of Alzheimer type: changes at 1 year and at 2.5 years. Electroencephalogr Clin Neurophysiol 61:101–112, 1985

Coben LA, Chi D, Synder AZ, et al: Replication of a study of frequency analysis of the resting awake EEG in mild and probable Alzheimer's disease. Electroencephalogr Clin Neurophysiol 75:148–154, 1990

Conrad AJ, Abebe T, Austin R, et al: Hippocampal pyramidal cell disarray in schizophrenia as a bilateral phenomenon. Arch Gen Psychiatry 48:413–417, 1991

Davidson RJ: EEG measures of cerebral asymmetry: conceptual and methodological issues. Int J Neurosci 39:71–89, 1988

Davies MG, Rowan MJ, Feely J: EEG and event related potentials in hepatic encephalopathy. Metab Brain Dis 6:175–186, 1991

Davis A, Wada J: Hemispheric asymmetry: frequency analysis of visual and auditory evoked responses to non-verbal stimuli. Electroencephalogr Clin Neurophysiol 37:1–9, 1974

Dejaiffe G, Constantinidis J, Rey-Bellet J, et al: Corrélations électrocliniques dans les démences de l'age avancé. Acta Neurol Belg 64:677–707, 1964

Detari L, Vanderwolf CH: Activity of cortically projecting and other basal forebrain neurons during large slow waves and cortical activation in anesthetized cat. Brain Res 437:1–8, 1987

Duffy F: Clinical decision making in quantified electroencephalographic analysis, in Statistics and Topography in Quantitative EEG. Edited by Samson-Dollfus D. Rouen, France, Elsevier Press, 1988, pp 9–26

Duffy FH: Quantified neurophysiology with mapping: statistical inference, exploratory and confirmatory data analysis. Brain Topogr 3:3–12, 1990

Duffy FH, Albert MS, McAnulty G, et al: Age-related differences in brain electrical activity in healthy subjects. Ann Neurol 16:430–438, 1984a

Duffy FH, Albert MS, McAnulty G: Brain electrical activity in patients with presenile and senile dementia of the Alzheimer type. Ann Neurol 16:439–448, 1984b

Duffy FH, Jones K, Bartels P, et al: Unrestricted principal components analysis of brain electrical activity: issues of data dimensionality, artifact, and utility. Brain Topogr 4:291–307, 1992

Engel G, Romano J: Delirium, a syndrome of cerebral insufficiency. Journal of Chronic Diseases 9:260–277, 1959

Erwin RJ, Edward R, Tanguay PE, et al: Abnormal P300 responses in schizophrenic children. Journal of the American Academy of Child Psychiatry 25:615–622, 1986

Ettlin TM, Staehelin H, Kischka U, et al: Computed tomography, electroencephalography, and clinical features in the differential diagnosis of senile dementia. Arch Neurol 46:1217–1220, 1989

Folstein MF, Folstein SE, McHugh PR: Mini-Mental State: A practical method for grading the cognitive state of patients for the clinician. J Psychiatr Res 12:189–198, 1975

Ford JM, Duncan-Johnson CC, Pfefferbaum A, et al: Expectancy for events in old age: stimulus sequence effects on P300 and reaction time. J Gerontol 37:696–704, 1982a

Ford JM, Pfefferbaum A, Tinklenberg JR, et al: Effects of perceptual and cognitive difficulty on P3 and RT in young and old adults. Electroencephalogr Clin Neurophysiol 54:311–321, 1982b

Fortin A: La signification clinique du tracé EEG de la maladie de Alzheimer. Acta Neurol Belg 66:106–115, 1966

Freedman R, Adler LE, Waldo MC, et al: Neurophysiological evidence for a defect in inhibitory pathways in schizophrenia: comparison of medicated and drug-free patients. Biol Psychiatry 18:537–51, 1983

Geschwind N: Disconnexion syndromes in animals and man, part I. Brain 88:237–294, 1965

Giaquinto S, Nolfe G: The EEG in the normal elderly: a contribution to the interpretation of aging and dementia. Electroencephalogr Clin Neurophysiol 63:540–546, 1986

Giaquinto S, Nolfe G: The electroencephalogram in the elderly: discrimination from demented patients and correlation with CT scan and neuropsychological data: a review, in The EEG of Mental Activities. Edited by Giannitrapani M. Basel, Switzerland, Karger, 1988, pp 50–65

Gibbs FA, Gibbs EL: Changes with age awake, in Atlas of Electroencephalography. Edited by Gibbs FA, Gibbs EL. Reading, MA, Addison-Wesley, 1951, pp 82–88

Gibbs E, Lorimer F, Lennox W: Clinical correlates of exceedingly fast activity in the electroencephalogram. Diseases of the Nervous System 11:323–326, 1950

Gloor P (ed): Hans Berger on the electroencephalogram of man. Electroencephalogr Clin Neurophysiol 25 (suppl 28):37–320, 1969

Gloor P, Ball G, Schaul N: Brain lesions that produce delta waves in the EEG. Neurology 27:326–333, 1977

Goodin D: Clinical utility of long latency "cognitive" event-related potentials (P3): the pros. Electroencephalogr Clin Neurophysiol 76:2–5, 1990

Goodin D, Squires K, Henderson B, et al: Age-related variations in evoked potentials to auditory stimuli in normal human subjects. Electroencephalogr Clin Neurophysiol 44:447–458, 1978a

Goodin DS, Squires KC, Starr A: Long latency event-related components of the auditory evoked potential in dementia. Brain 101:635–648, 1978b

Gordon E, Kraiuhin C, Harris A, et al: The differential diagnosis of dementia using P300 latency. Biol Psychiatry 21:1123–1132, 1986

Gordon EB: Serial EEG studies in presenile dementia. Br J Psychiatry 114:779–780, 1968

Gordon EB, Sim M: The EEG in presenile dementia. J Neurol Neurosurg Psychiatry 30:285–291, 1967

Groen JJ, Endtz LJ: Hereditary Pick's disease: second re-examination of a large family and discussion of other hereditary cases with particular reference to electroencephalography and computerized tomography. Brain 105:443–459, 1982

Hansch EC, Syndulko K, Cohen SN, et al: Cognition in Parkinson disease: an event-related potential perspective. Ann Neurol 11:599–607, 1982

Harkins SW: Effects of presenile dementia of the Alzheimer's type on brainstem transmission time. Int J Neurosci 15:165–170, 1981

Harrison MJ, Thomas DJ, Du-Boulay GM, et al: Multi-infarct dementia. J Neurol Sci 40:97–103, 1979

Helmchen H, Kanowski S, Künkel H: Die Altersabhängigkeit der Lokalisation von EEG-Herden. Archiv für Psychiatrie und Nervenkrankheiten 209:474–483, 1967

Hillyard SA, Picton TW: Electrophysiology of cognition, in Handbook of Physiology, 5th Edition. Edited by Mountcastle VB, Plum F, Geiger SR. Bethesda, MD, American Physiology Society, 1987, pp 519–584

Hof PR, Bouras C, Constantinidis J, et al: Selective disconnection of specific visual association pathways in cases of Alzheimer's disease presenting with Balint's syndrome. J Neuropathol Exp Neurol 49:168–184, 1990

Hubbard O, Sunde D, Goldensohn ES: The EEG in centenarians. Electroencephalogr Clin Neurophysiol 40:407–417, 1976

Hughes JR, Cayaffa JJ: The EEG in patients at different ages without organic cerebral disease. Electroencephalogr Clin Neurophysiol 42:776–784, 1977

Huisman UW, Posthuma J, Visser SL, et al: The influence of attention on visual evoked potentials in normal adults and dementia. Clin Neurol Neurosurg 87:11–16, 1985

Jacobson S, Leuchter A, Walter D: Conventional and quantitative EEG in the diagnosis of delirium among the elderly. J Neurol Neurosurg Psychiatry 56:153–158, 1993a

Jacobson S, Leuchter AF, Walter D, et al: Serial quantitative EEG among elderly subjects with delirium. Biol Psychiatry 34:135–140, 1993b

Jerrett S, Corsak J: Clinical utility of topographic EEG brain mapping. Clin Electroencephalogr 19:134–143, 1988

Johannesson G, Brun A, Gustafson I, et al: EEG in pre-senile dementia related to cerebral blood flow and autopsy findings. Acta Neurol Scand 56:89–103, 1977

Johannesson G, Hagberg B, Gustafson L, et al: EEG and cognitive impairment in presenile dementia. Acta Neurol Scand 59:225–240, 1979

John ER, Karmel BZ, Corning WC, et al: Neurometics: numerical taxonomy identifies different profiles of brain functions within groups of behaviorally similar people. Science 196:1393–1410, 1977

John ER, Prichep LS, Fridman J, et al: Neurometrics: computer-assisted differential diagnosis of brain dysfunctions. Science 239:162–169, 1988

Kanowski S: EEG und Alterpsychiatrie. Nervenarzt 42:347–355, 1971

Kato H, Sugawara Y, Ito H, et al: White matter lucencies in multi-infarct dementia: a somatosensory evoked potentials and CT study. Acta Neurol Scand 81:181–183, 1990

Katz RI, Horowitz GR: Electroencephalogram in the septuagenarian: studies in a normal geriatric population. J Am Geriatr Soc 3:273–275, 1982

Kazniak AW, Garron D, Fox J, et al: Cerebral atrophy, EEG slowing, age, education, and cognitive functioning in suspected dementia. Neurology 29:1273–1278, 1979

Koponen H: Delirium in the elderly: a brief overview. Int Psychogeriatr 3:177–179, 1991

Koponen H, Partanen J, Paakkonnen A, et al: EEG spectral analysis in delirium. J Neurol Neurosurg Psychiatry 52:980–985, 1989

Kuba M, Peregrin J, Vit F, et al: Pattern-reversal visual evoked potentials in patients with chronic renal insufficiency. Electroencephalogr Clin Neurophysiol 56:438–442, 1983

Leppler JG, Greenberg HJ: The P3 potential and its clinical usefulness in the objective classification of dementia. Cortex 20:427–433, 1984

Leuchter AF: Brain structural and functional correlates of late-life depression, in Diagnosis and Treatment of Depression in Late-Life: Results of the NIH Consensus Development Conference. Edited by Schneider L, Reynolds CF, Lebowitz B, et al. Washington, DC, American Psychiatric Press, 1994, pp 117–130

Leuchter AF, Jacobson S: Quantitative measurement of brain electrical activity in delirium. Int Psychogeriatr 3:231–247, 1991

Leuchter AF, Spar J, Walter D, et al: Electroencephalographic spectra and coherence in the diagnosis of Alzheimer's-type and multi-infarct dementia. Arch Gen Psychiatry 44:993–998, 1987

Leuchter AF, Newton TF, Cook IA, et al: Changes in brain functional connectivity in Alzheimer-type and multi-infarct dementia. Brain 115:1543–1561, 1992

Leuchter AF, Daly K, Rosenberg-Thompson S, et al: The prevalence of electroencephalographic abnormalities among patients with possible organic mental syndromes. J Am Geriatric Soc 41:605–611, 1993

Leuchter AF, Cook IA, Newton TF, et al: Regional differences in brain electrical activity in dementia: use of spectral power and spectral ratio measures. Electroencephalogr Clin Neurophysiol (in press a)

Leuchter AF, Cook IA, Lufkin RB, et al: Cordance: a new method for assessment of cerebral perfusion and metabolism using quantitative electroencephalography. Neuroimage (in press b)

Leuchter AF, Cook IA, Mena I, et al: Assessment of cerebral perfusion using quantitative EEG cordance. Psychiatry Res (in press c)

Leuchter AF, Dunkin JJ, Lufkin RB, et al: The effect of white-matter disease on functional connections in the aging brain. J Neurol Neurosurg Psychiatry (in press d)

Leuchter AF, Simon SL, Daly KA, et al: Neurophysiologic correlates of outcome in elderly psychiatric patients, I: cross-sectional and longitudinal assessment of patients with dementia. Am J Geriatr Psychiatry (in press e)

Leuchter AF, Simon SL, Daly KA, et al: Neurophysiologic correlates of outcome in elderly psychiatric patients, II: two-year follow-up of patients with depression. Am J Geriatr Psychiatry (in press f)

Levy LJ, Bolton RP, Losowsky MS: The use of VEP in delineating a state of subclinical encephalopathy. J Hepatol 5:211–217, 1987

Levy LJ, Bolton RP, Losowsky MS: The visual evoked potential in clinical hepatic encephalopathy in acute and chronic liver disease. Hepatogastroenterology 37 (suppl 2):66–73, 1990

Lewis D, Campbell M, Terry R, et al: Laminar and regional distributions of neurofibrillary tangles and neuritic plaques in Alzheimer's disease: a quantitative study of visual and auditory cortices. J Neurosci 7:1799–1808, 1987

Liddell DW: Investigations of EEG findings in presenile dementia. J Neurol Neurosurg Psychiatry 21:173–176, 1958

Liston E: Clinical findings in presenile dementia. J Nerv Ment Dis 167:337–342, 1979

Loeb C: Clinical diagnosis of multi-infarct dementia, in Aging of the Brain and Dementia. Edited by Amaducci L, Davison AN, Antuono P. New York, Raven, 1980, pp 251–260

Logar C, Grabmair W, Schneider G, et al: EEG-Veränderungen bei seniler Demenz vom Alzheimer Typ. Zeitschrift EEG-EMG 18:214–216, 1987

Loring DW, Sheer DE, Largen JW: Forty hertz EEG activity in dementia of the Alzheimer's type and multi-infarct dementia. Psychophysiology 22:116–121, 1985

Lukas SE, Mandelson SH, Kourii E, et al: Ethenol-induced alteration in EEG alpha activity and apparent source of the auditory P300 evoked response potential. Alcohol 7:471–477, 1990

Matos L, Paiva T, Cravo M: Multimodal evoked potentials in subclinical hepatic encephalopathy, in Advances in Ammonia Metabolism and Hepatic Encephalopathy. Edited by Soeters PB, Wilson JHP, Meijer AJ, et al. Amsterdam, Elsevier Science, 1988, pp 373–381

Margerison JH, Scott DF: Huntington's chorea: clinical EEG and neuropathological findings. Electroencephalogr Clin Neurophysiol 19:314, 1965

Matejcez M: Pharmaco-encephalography: the value of quantified EEG. Psychopharmacology and Pharmacopsychiatry 12:126–136, 1979

Matousek M, Volavka J, Roubicek J, et al: EEG frequency analysis related to age in normal adults. Electroencephalogr Clin Neurophysiol 23:162–167, 1967

Mauguiere F, Ibanez V: Loss of parietal and frontal somatosensory evoked potentials in hemispheric deafferentation, in New Trends and Advanced Techniques in Clinical Neurophysiology. Edited by Rossini P, Mauguiere F. New York, Elsevier Science, 1990, pp 274–285

Maurer K, Ihl R, Dierks T: Topographie der P300 in der Psychiatrie, II: Kognitive P300-felder bei Demenz. Zeitschrift EEG-EMG 19:26–29, 1988

McAdam W, Robinson RA: Senile intellectual deterioration and the electroencephalogram: a quantitative correlation. Br J Psychiatry 102:819–825, 1956

McCarley RW, Faux SF, Shenton ME, et al: Event-related potentials in schizophrenia: their biological and clinical correlates and a new model of schizophrenic pathophysiology. Schizophr Res 4:209–231, 1991

McCarley R, Shenton M, O'Donnell B, et al: Auditory P300 abnormalities and left posterior superior temporal gyrus volume reduction in schizophrenia. Arch Gen Psychiatry 50:190–198, 1993

Miyasaka M, Nakano T, Ohmori K, et al: The mental deterioration in the aged and the computerized EEG analysis. Folia Psychiatrica et Neurologica Japonica 32:95–108, 1978

Mooradian AD, Perryman K, Fitten J, et al: Cortical function in elderly non-insulin dependent diabetic patients: behavioral and electrophysiologic studies. Arch Intern Med 148:2369–2372, 1988

Morrison J, Scheerr S, Lewis D, et al: The laminar and regional distribution of neocortical somatostatin and neuritic plaques: the implications for Alzheimer's disease as a global neocortical disconnection syndrome, in The Biological Substrates of Alzheimer's Disease. Edited by Scheibel A, Wechsler A, Brazier M. Orlando, FL, Academic Press, 1986, 115–131

Morrison JH, Hof PR, Bouras C: An anatomic substrate for visual disconnection in Alzheimer's disease. Ann N Y Acad Sci 640:36–43, 1991

Morstyn R, Duffy FH, McCarley RW: Altered P300 topography in schizophrenia. Arch Gen Psychiatry 40:729–734, 1983

Mullis RJ, Holcomb PJ, Diner BC, et al: The effects of aging on the P3 component of the visual event-related potential. Electroencephalogr Clin Neurophysiol 62:141–149, 1985

Mundy-Castle AC: Theta and beta rhythm in the electroencephalograms of normal adult. Electroencephalogr Clin Neurophysiol 3:477–486, 1951

Nunez P: Electric Fields in the Brain: The Neurophysics of EEG. New York, Oxford University Press, 1981

Nuwer MR: Quantitative EEG, II: frequency analysis and topographic mapping in clinical settings. J Clin Neurophysiol 5:45–85, 1988

Nuwer MR, Jordan SE, Ahn SS: Evaluation of stroke using EEG frequency analysis and topographic mapping. Neurology 37:1153–1159, 1987

O'Connor K, Shaw J: Field dependence, laterality and the EEG. Biol Psychology 6:93–109, 1978

O'Connor KP, Shaw JC, Ongley CO: The EEG and differential diagnosis in psychogeriatrics. Br J Psychiatry 135:156–162, 1979

Obrist WD: The electroencephalogram of normal aged adults. Electroencephalogr Clin Neurophysiol 6:235–244, 1954

Obrist WD: The electroencephalogram of healthy aged males, in Human Aging: A Biological and Behavioral Study. Edited by Birren JE, Butler RN, Greenhouse SW, et al. Washington, DC, US Government Printing Office, 1963, pp 79–93

Obrist WD: Problems of aging, in Handbook of Electroencephalography and Clinical Neurophysiology. Edited by Remond A. Amsterdam, Elsevier, 1976, pp 275–292

Obrist WD: Electroencephalographic changes in normal aging and dementia, in Brain Function in Old Age: Bayer Symposium VII. Edited by Hoffmeister F, Müller C. Berlin, Springer-Verlag, 1979, pp 102–111

Obrist WD, Busse EW: The electroencephalogram in old age, in Applications of Electroencephalography in Psychiatry. Edited by Wilson WP. Durham, NC, Duke University Press, 1965, pp 185–205

Obrist WD, Sokoloff L, Lassen NA, et al: Relation of EEG to cerebral blood flow and metabolism in old age. Electroencephalogr Clin Neurophysiol 15:610–619, 1963

Oken BS, Kaye JA: Electrophysiologic function in the healthy, extremely old. Neurology 42:519–526, 1992

Olfson M: Utilization of neuropsychiatric diagnostic tests for general hospital patients with mental disorders. Am J Psychiatry 149:1711–1717, 1992

Oltman JE, Friedman S: Comments on Huntington's chorea. J Med Genet 3:298–314, 1961

Otomo E, Tsubaki T: Electroencephalography in subjects sixty years and over. Electroencephalogr Clin Neurophysiol 20:77–82, 1966

Patterson JV, Michalewski HJ, Starr A: Latency variability of the components of auditory event-related potentials to infrequent stimuli in aging, Alzheimer type dementia, and depression. Electroencephalogr Clin Neurophysiol 71:450–460, 1988

Paiva T, Fred A, Nunes-Leitao J: EEG and VER mapping in some metabolic disease, in Statistics and Topography in Quantitative EEG. Paris, Elsevier Science, 1988, pp 237–241

Pearson R, Esiri M, Hiorns R, et al: Anatomical correlates of the distribution of the pathological changes in the neocortex in Alzheimer disease. Proc Natl Acad Sci U S A 82:4531–4534, 1985

Penttilä M, Partanen JV, Soininen H, et al: Quantitative analysis of occipital EEG in different stages of Alzheimer's disease. Electroencephalogr Clin Neurophysiol 60:1–6, 1985

Pfefferbaum A, Horvath TB, Roth WT, et al: Event-related potential changes in chronic alcoholics. Electroencephalogr Clin Neurophysiol 47:637–647, 1979

Pfefferbaum A, Ford JM, Wenegrat BG, et al: Clinical application of P3 component of event-related potentials, I: normal aging. Electroencephalogr Clin Neurophysiol 59:85–103, 1984a

Pfefferbaum A, Wenegrat BG, Ford JM, et al: Clinical application of the P3 component of event-related potentials, II: dementia, depression and schizophrenia. Electroencehpalogr Clin Neurophysiol 54:104–124, 1984b

Pfefferbaum A, Ford JM, Kraemer C: Clinical utility of long latency "cognitive" event-related potentials (P3): the cons. Electroencephalogr Clin Neurophysiol 76:6–12, 1990

Pierelli F, Pozzessere G, Sanarelli L, et al: Electrophysiological study in patients with chronic hepatic insufficiency. Acta Neurol Belg 85:284–291, 1985

Picton TW, Stuss DT, Champagne SC, et al: The effects of age on human event-related potentials. Psychophysiology 21:312–325, 1984

Picton TW, Cherri AM, Champagne SC, et al: The effects of age and task difficulty on the late positive component of the auditory evoked potential. Electroencephalogr Clin Neurophysiol 38:132–133, 1986

Polich J: P300 in the evaluation of aging and dementia, in Event-Related Brain Research. Edited by Brunia CHM, Mulder G, Verbaten MN. New York, Elsevier Science, 1991, pp 304–323

Polich J, Howard L, Starr A: Aging effects on the P300 component of the event-related potential from auditory stimuli: peak definition, variation, and measurement. J Gerontol 40:721–26, 1985

Polich J, Ehlers CL, Otis S, et al: P3 latency reflects the degree of cognitive decline in dementing illness. Electroencephalogr Clin Neurophysiol 63:138–144, 1986

Pollock VE, Schneider LS: Topographic electroencephalographic alpha in recovered depressed elderly. J Abnorm Psychol 3:268–273, 1989

Pollock VE, Schneider LS: Quantitative, waking EEG research on depression. Biol Psychiatry 27:757–780, 1990

Pramming S, Thorsteinsson B, Stigsby B, et al: Glycaemic threshold for changes in electroencephalograms during hypoglycaemia in patients with insulin dependent diabetes. British Medical Journal of Clinical Research 296:665–667, 1988

Prichep L, Mont FG, John ER, et al: Neurometric electroencephalographic characteristics of dementia, in Alzheimer's Disease: The Standard Reference. Edited by Reisberg B. New York, Macmillan, 1983, pp 252–257

Rabins P, Folstein MF: Delirium and dementia: diagnostic criteria and fatality rates. Br J Psychiatry 140:149–153, 1982

Rae-Grant A, Blume W, Lau C, et al: The electroencephalogram in Alzheimer-type dementia. Arch Neurol 44:50–54, 1987

Rice D, Buchsbaum M, Hardy D, et al: Focal left temporal slow EEG activity is related to a verbal recent memory deficit in a non-demented elder population. J Gerontology 4:144–151, 1991

Roberts M, McGeorge AP, Caird FI: Electroencephalography and computerized tomography in vascular and nonvascular dementia in old age. J Neurol Neurosurg Psychiatry 41:903–906, 1978

Romano J, Engel G: Delirium, I: electroencephalographic data. Arch Neurol Psychiatry 51:356–377, 1944

Rosenberg C, Nudleman K, Starr A: Cognitive evoked potentials (P300) in early Huntington's disease. Arch Neurol 42:984–987, 1985

Rossini PM, Pirchio M, Treviso M, et al: Checkerboard reversal pattern and flash VEPs in dialyzed and nondialyzed subjects. Electroencephalogr Clin Neurophysiol 52:435–444, 1981

Rossini PM, diStefano E, Febbo A, et al: Brainstem auditory evoked responses in patients with chronic renal failure. Electroencephalogr Clin Neurophysiol 57:507–514, 1984

Roubicek J: The electroencephalogram in the middle-aged and elderly. J Am Geriatr Soc 25:145–152, 1977

Saitoh O, Niwa S, Hiramatsu K, et al: Abnormalities in late positive components of event-related potentials may reflect a genetic predisposition to schizophrenia. Biol Psychiatry 19:293–303, 1984

Sandford NL, Saul RE: Assessment of hepatic encephalopathy with visual evoked potentials compared with conventional methods. Hepatology 8:1094–1098, 1988

Schatzberg AF, Elliot GR, Lerbinger JE, et al: Topographic mapping in depressed patients, in Topographic Mapping of Brain Electrical Activity. Edited by Duffy FH. Boston, MA, Butterworths, 1986, pp 389–391

Schaul N, Lueders H, Sachdev K: Generalized, bilaterally synchronous bursts of slow waves in the EEG. Arch Neurol 38:690–692, 1981

Schlagenhauff RE: Electroencephalogram in gerontology. Clin Electroencephalogr 4:153–163, 1973

Scott DF, Heathfield KWG, Toone B, et al: The EEG in Huntington's chorea: a clinical and neuropathological study. J Neurol Neurosurg Psychiatry 35:97–102, 1972

Shagass C, Romer RA, Straumanis JJ, et al: Psychiatric diagnostic discriminations with combinations of quantitative EEG variables. Br J Psychol 144:581–592, 1984

Shaw JC, O'Connor K, Ongley C: The EEG as a measure of cerebral functional organization. Br J Psychiatry 130:260–264, 1977

Shaw JC, O'Connor K, Ongley C: EEG coherence as a measure of cerebral functional organization, in Architectonics of the Cerebral Cortex. Edited by Brazier MAB, Petsche H. New York, Raven, 1978, pp 245–255

Sheer DE: Biofeedback training of 40 Hz EEG activity and behavior, in Behavior and Brain Electrical Activity. Edited by Burch N, Altschuler H. New York, Plenum, 1975, pp 325–362

Sheer DE: Focused arousal and 40 Hz EEG, in The Neuropsychology of Learning Disabilities. Edited by Knight RM. Baltimore, MD, University Park Press, 1976, pp 71–87

Sheer DE: Focused arousal, 40 Hz EEG, and dysfunction, in Self-Regulation of the Brain and Behavior. Edited by Elbert T, Rockstroh B, Lutzenberger W, et al. New York, Springer-Verlag, 1984, pp 64–84

Smith DBD, Michalewski HJ, Brent GA, et al: Auditory averaged evoked potentials and aging: factors of stimulus, task. Electroencephalogr Clin Neurophysiol 49:217–230, 1980

Snyder E, Hillyard SA: Long-latency evoked potentials to irrelevant, deviant stimuli. Behav Biol 16:319–331, 1976

Soininen H, Partanen VJ, Helkala EL, et al: EEG findings in senile dementia and normal aging. Acta Neurol Scand 65:59–70, 1982

Spehlmann R: EEG Primer. New York, Elsevier Science, 1981

Spydell JD, Sheer DE: Forty hertz EEG activity in Alzheimer's type dementia. Psychophysiology 20:313–319, 1982

Squires KC, Chippendale TJ, Wrege KS, et al: Electrophysiological assessment of mental function in aging and dementia, in Aging in the 1980s. Edited by Poon LW. Washington, DC, American Psychological Association, 1980, pp 125–134

St. Clair D, Blackwood D, Christine JE: P3 and other long latency auditory evoked potentials in presenile dementia Alzheimer type and alcoholic Korsakoff syndrome. Br J Psychiatry 147:702–706, 1985

Steriade M, Gloor P, Llinas R, et al: Basic mechanisms of cerebral rhythmic activities. Electroencephalogr Clin Neurophysiol 76:481–508, 1990

Stigsby B, Johanneson G, Ingvar DH: Regional EEG analysis and regional cerebral blood flow in Alzheimer's and Pick's diseases. Electroencephalogr Clin Neurophysiol 51:537–547, 1981

Stoller A: Slowing of the alpha-rhythm of the electroencephalogram and its association with mental deterioration and epilepsy. Journal of Mental Science 95:972–984, 1949

Syndulko K, Hansch MA, Cohen SN, et al: Long-latency event-related potentials in normal aging and dementia, in Clinical Applications of Evoked Potentials in Neurology. Edited by Courjon J, Maugiere F, Revol M. New York, Raven, 1982, pp 279–285

Syndulko K, Cohen SN, Pettler-Jennings P, et al: P300 and neurocognitive function in neurologic patients, in Evoked Potentials, II: The Second International Evoked Potentials Symposium. Edited by Nodar RH, Barber C. Boston, MA, Butterworths, 1984, pp 441–445

Tissot R, Constantinidis J, Richard J: La Maladie de Pick. Paris, Masson, 1975

Torres F, Faoro A, Loewenson R, et al: The electroencephalogram of elderly subjects revisited. Electroencephalogr Clin Neurophysiol 56:391–398, 1983

Trzepacz PT, Sclabassi RJ, Van Thiel DH: Delirium: a subcortical phenomenon? J Neuropsychiatry 1:283–290, 1989

Tucker D, Roth D, Bair T: Functional connections among cortical regions: topography of EEG coherence. Electroencephalogr Clin Neurophysiol 63:242–250, 1986

van der Rijt CCD, Schalm SW: Quantitative EEG analysis and evoked potentials to measure (latent) hepatic encephalopathy. J Hepatol 14:141–142, 1992

Visser SL: The electroencephalogram and evoked potentials in normal aging and dementia, in Event-Related Brain Research. Edited by Brunia CHM, Mulder G, Verbaten MN. New York, Elsevier Science, 1991, pp 289–303

Visser SL, Stan FC, Van Tilburg W, et al: Visual evoked response in senile and presenile dementia. Electroencephalogr Clin Neurophysiol 40:385–392, 1976

Visser SL, Van Tilburg W, Hooijer C, et al: Visual evoked potentials (VEPs) in senile dementia (Alzheimer type) and in non-organic behavioral disorders in the elderly: comparison with EEG parameters. Electroencephalogr Clin Neurophysiol 60:115–121, 1985

Visser SL, Hooijer C, Jonker C, et al: Anterior temporal focal abnormalities in EEG in normal aged subjects: correlations with psychopathological and CT brain scan findings. Electroencephalogr Clin Neurophysiol 66:1–7, 1987

Vitiello MV, Prinz PN: Sleep and EEG studies in Alzheimer's disease, in Alzheimer's Disease: Advances in Basic Research and Therapies. Edited by Wurtman RJ, Corkin SH, Growdon JH. Cambridge, MA, Center for Brain Sciences and Metabolism Charitable Trust, 1987, pp 625–634

Wang H, Busse E: EEG of healthy old persons: a longitudinal study, I: dominant background activity and occipital rhythm. J Gerontol 24:419–426, 1969

Weiner H, Schuster DB: The electroencephalogram in dementia: some preliminary observations and correlations. Electroencephalogr Clin Neurophysiol 8:479–488, 1956

Williamson PC, Merskey H, Morrison S, et al: Quantitative electroencephalographic correlates of cognitive decline in normal elderly subjects. Arch Neurol 47:1185–1188, 1990

Woody RH: Intra-judge reliability in clinical EEG. J Clin Psychol 22:150–154, 1966

Woody RH: Inter-judge reliability in clinical EEG. J Clin Psychol 24:251–256, 1968

Wright CE, Harding GFA, Orwin A: Presenile dementia: the use of the flash and pattern VEP in diagnosis. Electroencephalogr Clin Neurophysiol 57:405–415, 1984

Yang S-S, Chu N-S, Liaw YF: Brainstem auditory evoked potentials in hepatic encephalopathy. Hepatology 6:1352–1355, 1986

Yen CL, Liaw YF: Somatosensory evoked potentials and number connection test in the detection of subclinical hepatic encephalopathy. Hepatogastroenterology 37:332–334, 1990

Zeneroli ML, Pinelli G, Gollini G, et al: Visual evoked potential: a diagnostic tool for the assessment of hepatic encephalopathy. Gut 25:291–299, 1984

Neuropsychiatric Aspects of Psychiatric Disorders in the Elderly

Section Editor
Godfrey D. Pearlson, M.D.

Chapter 12

Mood Disorders

Chapter 13

Late-Life–Onset Psychoses

Chapter 14

Anxiety Disorders

Chapter 15

Substance Abuse

Chapter 16

Sleep Disorders in Late Life:
A Biopsychosocial Model for Understanding
Pathogenesis and Intervention

Chapter 17

Pain

Chapter 18

Delirium

12

Mood Disorders

Marsden H. McGuire, M.D.
Peter V. Rabins, M.D., M.P.H.

Introduction

In this chapter, we 1) provide an overview of neuropsychiatric conditions affecting elderly people in which mood disturbances occur, 2) review the biological and structural features of the central nervous system (CNS) that correlate with "primary" (or "idiopathic") mood disorders in elderly people, and 3) discuss difficult conceptual areas in the neuropsychiatry of mood disorders affecting the elderly population such as the syndrome of depression-induced cognitive impairment. We also intend this chapter to be practical, as it contains information about the appropriate evaluation and treatment of elderly patients with mood disturbances.

Definitions

Mood refers to a sustained emotional state that modulates a person's perception of himself or herself and his or her surroundings. Although patients describe their moods in a great variety of terms, clinicians tend to use a limited list of descriptors in an effort to achieve consistency and reliability. Examples of these descriptors include dysphoric, euphoric, irritable, elevated, expansive, and euthymic.

Affect refers to the observable expression of a person's emotional state and is described in terms of appropriateness for the situation, degree of stability, and congruence with the patient's self-reported mood. In major depression, for example, the range of affect is often restricted and the affect itself blunted or flat.

Mood and affect usually vary in parallel fashion but may diverge. Both need to be assessed in a neuropsychiatric evaluation. Whereas the distinction between mood and affect is generally appreciated in clinical practice, as well as in the literature, the terms *mood disorder* and *affective disorder* are sometimes used synonymously.

Mood Symptoms and Syndromes

Mood *symptoms* are ubiquitous. The language of emotion is found in the most common of ritualized greetings (e.g., "How are you feeling?") and the most sublime of poetic expressions. At times, however, mood interferes with usual functioning and becomes associated with particular thoughts, feelings, beliefs, and behaviors. This cluster of signs and symptoms is then recognizable as a specific mood syndrome with a characteristic course.

Mood *syndromes,* in contrast, have no pathognomonic features. When present, they may reflect an underlying delirium or dementia. However, an altered mood that persists for days or weeks in spite of environmental change and in the absence of cognitive impairment or a fluctuating level of consciousness is strong presumptive evidence that a mood syndrome is present. Often, the direction of mood change is clear; however, the patient with an irritable mood or "mixed" mood state (in which elements of euphoria and depression coexist or rapidly alternate) can present a confusing picture.

The distinction between mood symptoms and mood syndromes may have particular relevance to the elderly population, as the Epidemiologic Catchment Area (ECA) study found higher rates of depressive symptoms, but lower rates of major depression, in respondents older than 65 compared with those younger than 65 (Romanoski et al. 1992; Weissman et al. 1991).

In addition to a prolonged period of altered mood, other signs and symptoms are required to make a diagnosis of a syndromic mood disorder. These include changes in a person's ability to experience pleasure, degree of self-confidence, interest in surroundings, and sense of mental and physical vitality. Typically, the direction of these changes is down in depressive disorders and up in mania. Changes in self-attitude are common in mood disorders; despair, guilt, worthlessness, and hopelessness are seen in depression, whereas a feeling of invincibility occurs in mania. Motor activity is frequently affected; in mania it is increased, whereas in depression both restlessness and a slowing or scarcity of movement can be seen. Biologically driven behaviors such as eating and sleeping may be adversely affected and difficulties with memory and concentration are often present. Hallucinations can occur and are usually auditory; their content tends to be self-deprecating or hopeless in depression and laudatory in mania. Delusions may be present and are usually "mood-congruent" (i.e., consonant with the direction of mood change). In depression, the predominant themes of delusions are self-deprecating, hopeless, or nihilistic, and in mania, self-aggrandizing. Suicidal ideation or urges, which frequently accompany depression, are of particular concern in the elderly population, which has the highest rate of completed suicide of any age group. In DSM-IV (American Psychiatric Association 1994) each mood syndrome is defined (in part) by a checklist of symptoms, a minimum number of which must be present to make a diagnosis (see Table 12–1 for the checklist for major depression).

The mood syndromes of DSM-III-R (American Psychiatric Association 1987) included bipolar disorder, major depression, dysthymia, cyclothymia, and adjustment disorder with depressed mood. Bipolar disorder, major depression, and, to a lesser extent, all the other mood disorders are distinguished by their phenomenology, epidemiology, course, and responses to treatment. In turn, each of these disorders is a heterogeneous category made up of various subtypes. Bipolar disorder, for example, is made up of bipolar I (at least one manic episode and usually one or more depressed episodes), bipolar II (at least one hypomanic and one depressed episode), and rapid cycling subtypes. Major depression occurs in many varieties including "melancholia," in which social withdrawal, sleep or appetite disturbance, and diurnal mood variation are prominent features. Any of these subtypes can in turn be characterized by the presence or absence of psychotic

features (i.e., hallucinations, delusions, or catatonia) and may occur in a seasonal pattern. Cyclothymia (alternating bouts of hypomania and mild to moderate depression) and dysthymia (persistent mild to moderate depression) are controversial mood syndromes that resemble personality disorders in their chronicity. These disorders further differ from bipolar disorder and major depression in that no studies have linked them to neuropsychiatric conditions affecting the elderly population.

Minor depression is a mood syndrome that may be of special importance in the elderly population. For example, Blazer et al. (1989) identified six clusters of depressive symptoms, one of which—characterized by multiple depressive complaints, cognitive impairment, and a lack of association with any of the currently defined depressive syndromes—was unique to the population over age 60. The concurrence of cognitive impairment and depression suggests an association with neuropsychiatric disease.

Emotional incontinence and emotional lability are two important mood syndromes typically seen in elderly patients with neurological conditions. They are not listed in DSM-IV because they are rarely seen in patients without some degree of brain injury.

Emotional incontinence describes a syndrome in which there is a sudden expression of emotion, either laughter or crying, that is not experienced by the patient as accompanied by the emotion usually associated with that affect (Poeck 1969). Other characteristics of emotional incontinence are its rapid onset and precipitation by a minor or inconsequential stimulus. It is almost always associated with signs of pseudobulbar palsy (increased jaw jerk, spastic cranial nerve VII function, and heightened gag reflex), that is, bilateral involvement of corticobulbar fibers. The dissociation between mood and affect seen in emotional incontinence suggests that the control of emotional expression is predominantly in the brain stem, whereas the experience of mood is grounded elsewhere, most likely in the limbic system (Poeck 1969). Tricyclic antidepressants are effective in treating emotional incontinence (Robinson et. al. 1993; Schiffer et al. 1985). In the elderly, emotional incontinence is most commonly seen in individuals with bilateral stroke. Progressive supranuclear palsy and multiple sclerosis are other common causes.

Emotional lability refers to frequent wide swings in mood. These mood swings are said to come on less quickly than do the changes of emotional inconti-

Table 12–1. Symptoms of major depressive episode

1. Depressed mood: most of the day, nearly every day, as indicated either by subjective account or observation by others

2. Markedly diminished interest or pleasure in all, or almost all, activities most of the day, nearly every day (as indicated either by subjective account or observation by others of apathy most of the time)

3. Significant weight loss when not dieting or weight gain (e.g., more than 5% of body weight in a month) or decrease or increase in appetite nearly every day

4. Insomnia or hypersomnia nearly every day

5. Psychomotor agitation or retardation nearly every day (observable by others, not merely subjective feelings of restlessness or being slowed down)

6. Fatigue or loss of energy nearly every day

7. Feelings of worthlessness or excessive or inappropriate guilt (which may be delusional) nearly every day (not merely self-reproach or guilt about being sick)

8. Diminished ability to think or concentrate, or indecisiveness, nearly every day (either by subjective account or as observed by others)

9. Recurrent thoughts of death (not just fear of dying), recurrent suicidal ideation without a specific plan, or a suicide attempt or a specific plan for committing suicide

Note. Adapted from criterion A in DSM-IV (American Psychiatric Association 1994).

nence, but the validity of this distinction is unclear. Emotional lability is usually precipitated by an upsetting environmental event and appears as an emotional overreaction. This contrasts with the precipitation by a minor or inconsequential stimulus seen in emotional incontinence. Emotional lability can follow lesions in any area of the brain. It is unclear whether a greater amount of tissue destruction or a specific location (e.g., frontal lesions) increases its occurrence.

Classification, Differential Diagnosis, and Treatment of Mood Disorders in the Elderly Population

The classification of mood symptoms in the elderly population is evolving, and no current system is fully satisfactory. Differences of opinion have resisted resolution for several decades, and data can be cited to support many of the positions taken in these debates.

The search for causes of secondary mood disorders requires that the examiner consider the possibility that such a cause might exist. All patients should have a physical examination to search for the specific etiologies discussed in the next section. Careful history taking can identify individuals at risk for secondary mood disorders and direct appropriate gathering of data and ordering of laboratory tests. The clinical interview should always include a thorough family history with a focus on psychiatric (e.g., mood disorder and dementia), neurogenetic (e.g., Huntington's disease and movement disorder), and structural brain disease (e.g., stroke and Parkinson's disease).

The physical examination can suggest specific etiologies of mood disorder in elderly patients. Findings suggestive of endocrine disease (e.g., hyper- or hypothyroidism or Cushing's disease) should prompt a careful search for these etiologies. The finding of focal abnormalities on neurological examination suggests a primary brain lesion (e.g., stroke, tumor, or abscess). The stigmata of alcoholism suggests the coexistence of alcoholism and a secondary mood disorder. A finding of enlarged lymph nodes, a history of high-risk behavior, and evidence on history or examination of illnesses that are associated with immunosuppression suggest the possibility of human immunodeficiency virus (HIV) infection.

No standard laboratory battery has been demonstrated to be cost effective and efficient in identifying individuals with secondary depression. Most clinicians would suggest that all elderly patients with depression have a screening battery including a complete blood count, serum chemistries (including tests of renal and liver function, calcium, phosphate, and electrolytes), thyroid function tests, and a serological test for syphilis. Some would add a B_{12} level to this list. A computed tomography (CT) or magnetic resonance imaging (MRI) scan should be ordered when cognitive disorder is present, a brain lesion is suspected by history, or a focal neurological abnormality is present on the physical examination. The MRI is more sensitive for identifying small vascular disease lesions, but lacks specificity. Conversely, a CT scan is less sensitive but more specific. Although data on the utility of neuroimaging studies in the diagnosis of neuropsychiatric causes of depression is lacking, the practice of many clinicians is to order an imaging study for any individual with an onset of depression or mania after age 65.

Neuropsychiatric Disorders Presenting With Mood Symptoms in the Elderly Population

Alzheimer's Disease

Alzheimer's disease is an age-related dementing illness with a variably progressive course. The neuropathological lesions of Alzheimer's disease include cortical and limbic neuronal loss, intracellular neurofibrillary tangles, and extracellular amyloid-containing plaques. Cortical atrophy and sulcal widening are prominent, with the most affected region being the temporoparietal areas. Mesial temporal loss, with perihippocampal tissue loss and temporal horn enlargement, is also prominent. The etiology of Alzheimer's disease is unknown.

Cummings and Victoroff (1990) separated the affective syndromes seen in Alzheimer's disease into four main groups: depression, elation, emotional lability (including catastrophic reactions), and anxiety. Estimates of the prevalence of depression in Alzheimer's disease vary from none to 86% (Burns 1991). Most studies have found a prevalence of 17% to 29% (Teri and Wagner 1992; Fischer et al. 1990). Among the factors that underlie this variation in prevalence rates are the criteria used to diagnose depression, the level of cognitive impairment required to make a diagnosis of dementia, the number and reliability of informants, and the method of case finding. Mania-like symptoms are seen in 3%–17% of cases of Alzheimer's disease

(Bucht and Adolfsson 1983; Burns et al. 1990; Sim and Sussman 1962). Catastrophic behavior has been directly observed in about half of Alzheimer's disease patients (Swearer et al. 1988). In one study (Rabins et al. 1982), 77% of patients had family members who reported such incidents. We are unaware of any reliable estimates of the prevalence of anxiety, either alone or concomitant with depression, in Alzheimer's disease patients.

Depression in Alzheimer's disease can be difficult to identify for several reasons. First, the behavioral manifestations of depression (i.e., psychomotor agitation or slowing, insomnia, weight loss, anhedonia, and impaired insight) can occur in patients without depression (Cummings and Victoroff 1990). Second, depression-induced cognitive impairment can resemble the cognitive deficits of Alzheimer's disease (for a further discussion of this topic, see Chapter 20). Third, the scales used to assess depression in Alzheimer's disease patients were, in many cases, developed for a population without dementia. Recently developed scales may correct this problem. The Cornell Scale for Depression in Dementia (Alexopoulos et al. 1988) reliably differentiates between depressed and nondepressed dementia patients. The Hamilton Rating Scale for Depression (Hamilton 1960) appears to respond to changes in the depressive symptoms of Alzheimer's disease patients (Greenwald et al. 1989; Lazarus et al. 1987), and the Sunderland Dementia Mood Assessment Scale (Sunderland et al. 1988) may be sensitive to changes in the depressive symptoms of Alzheimer's disease patients.

The relationship between depression and dementia is complex. Depression in dementia patients generally resembles "idiopathic" depression, although in one study (Greenwald et al. 1989) depressed patients with Alzheimer's disease had more self-pity, more rejection sensitivity, more anhedonia, and fewer neurovegetative symptoms than did comparison subjects without dementia. Depression may be the presenting symptom of a dementia, a point made by Alzheimer (1898 [cited in Forstl and Howard 1991]) almost a century ago. A careful clinical assessment might identify such patients. For example, Reding et al. (1985b) found that 13 of 16 elderly depressed patients who had developed dementia 3 years after assessment first had had signs of neurological disease during their initial depression. In several studies of patients with both disorders, the degree of cognitive impairment correlated inversely with severity of depressive symptoms (Burns et al. 1990; Fischer et al. 1990; Pearson et al. 1989; Teri

and Wagner 1992). However, Rovner and Morris (1989) found cognitive deficits to be more severe in depressed patients with Alzheimer's disease than in nondepressed comparison subjects with dementia alone, suggesting that the cognitive deficits of depression and dementia are additive. Of particular interest, new cognitive deficits arising in the course of a depressive episode may fail to resolve even after the resolution of the mood symptoms (Reifler et al. 1986). The mechanism by which an irreversible dementing process might accelerate during a depressive episode, or arise de novo after it, is unknown.

Neuropathological differences have been found between the brains of depressed and nondepressed patients with Alzheimer's disease. The brains of depressed patients with Alzheimer's disease have significantly fewer locus ceruleus neurons than do those of nondepressed Alzheimer subjects (Chan-Palay and Asan 1989; Zweig et al. 1988) and significantly more degenerative changes (i.e., plaques, tangles, neuronal loss, extraneuronal pigment astrocytosis, and Lewy bodies) in the locus ceruleus and substantia nigra (Zubenko et al. 1988). CNS measurements of serotonin, 5-hydroxyindoleacetic acid (5-HIAA), and norepinephrine are lower in depressed than in nondepressed Alzheimer patients, presumably as a result of specific cell loss in brain stem nuclei (Zubenko et al. 1988, 1990; Zweig et al. 1988). Burns (1991) proposed that a norepinephrine deficit might lead to target cell receptor supersensitivity and upregulation and thereby precipitate a depressive episode. He also suggested that the dementing process might guard against severe depression by the loss of these target cells.

Genetic predisposition may contribute to the development of depression in Alzheimer's disease. Pearlson et al. (1990) found that depressed Alzheimer patients are more likely to have positive family histories of depression than those without depression even when the proband had no past history of depression.

The treatment of depression in Alzheimer's disease is similar to the treatment of "idiopathic" major depression. In a double-blind trial, Reifler et al. (1989) demonstrated that imipramine was effective for the treatment of major depression and milder depressive symptoms in Alzheimer patients, although improvement was also noted in the placebo-treated group. Citalopram, a serotonin reuptake inhibitor, has recently been shown by Gottfries et al. (1992) to be effective in treating depression in Alzheimer patients, as well as in diminishing agitation, anxiety, irritability, and restlessness. However, this study was not fully double blind. Other antidepressant therapies have been investigated but, to our knowledge, not by sufficiently rigorous studies to recommend their use over current therapies for depressed elderly patients without dementia. In general, highly anticholinergic medications such as amitriptyline and imipramine should be avoided in patients with dementia because of the dependence of cognition on cholinergic integrity. Pharmacotherapy is more likely to be effective if there are fewer initial cognitive impairments, fewer sleep problems, and greater severity of depressive symptoms (C. F. Reynolds et al. 1986). Nonpharmacological approaches may also be effective. For example, behavioral techniques have been shown to decrease Beck Depression Inventory (BDI; Beck 1978) rating scores in depressed Alzheimer patients (Teri and Wagner 1992).

Parkinson's Disease

Parkinson's disease is an age-related neurological illness of uncertain etiology that commonly presents with tremor, rigidity, and bradykinesia. The neuropathology of Parkinson's disease includes mild cortical and subcortical neuronal loss with the greatest diminution in the dopamine-containing neurons that project from the substantia nigra to the striatum.

The prevalence of depression in Parkinson's disease patients varies from 4% to 70%, with most studies reporting a severe depression rate of 35%–50% (Cummings 1986, 1992). Longitudinal studies (Brown and Wilson 1972; Mayeux et al. 1988) have demonstrated that Parkinson's disease patients tend to segregate into depressed and nondepressed groups with minimal crossover from one group to the other in follow-up.

Mood symptoms may precede motor changes in Parkinson's disease. Mayeux et al. (1981) found that 43% of 26 depressed Parkinson patients had an episode of depression prior to developing motor symptoms. This finding suggests that the depression of Parkinson's disease is not merely a psychological reaction. Comparative studies generally support the concept that depression in Parkinson's disease is an expression of, rather than a response to, the illness. Parkinson patients have higher rates of depression than do heterogeneous groups of chronically medically ill patients (Horn 1974; Robins 1976; Singer 1974; Warburton 1967) including paraplegic patients with a similar degree of physical disability (Horn 1974).

The measurement of depression in Parkinson's disease is made difficult by the high prevalence of somatic symptomatology in nondepressed Parkinson patients. Nevertheless, Levin et al. (1988) showed that somatic items on the BDI cluster with mood rather than motor symptoms, and Starkstein et al. (1990c) found these items to be predictive of future depressive episodes.

The depression experienced by Parkinson patients has several distinguishing features. In comparison to patients with "idiopathic" depression, Parkinson patients are more dysphoric and pessimistic and less guilty and self-blaming (Brown and Wilson 1972; Huber et al. 1990; Levin et al. 1988). Anxiety and suicidal ideation are more prevalent in depressed Parkinson patients, although attempted suicide is less frequent (Cummings 1992; Robins 1976). Cognitive deficits (especially those involving the frontal lobe) are more prevalent in depressed than in nondepressed Parkinson patients (Cummings 1992; Starkstein et al. 1989a; Taylor et al. 1986). In depressed Parkinson patients, the severity of cognitive deficits appears to correlate with the severity of the depressive symptoms (Starkstein et al. 1990b). Depression may manifest differently in early- (before age 55) and late-onset forms of Parkinson's disease. Starkstein et al. (1989a) showed that early-onset Parkinson's disease patients had a higher rate of major depression (43% versus 10%), greater cognitive impairment, a higher rate of abnormal movements, more "on-off" episodes, and more left-hemisphere involvement.

The relationship between the mood and motor features of Parkinson's disease has been closely examined, but remains poorly understood. Several investigators have found that patients with (predominantly) right-body hemi-parkinsonism have higher rates of depression than do patients with left-sided symptoms (Baxter et al. 1989; Cummings 1992; Direnfeld et al. 1984; Starkstein et al. 1990b). In reviewing the literature, Cummings (1992) noted an association of depression with gait and postural difficulties (which are dopamine agonist responsive conditions) but not with tremor (which is less dopamine agonist responsive). Similarly, the "on-off" phenomenon (in which patients "switch" between an "on" phase with relatively good mobility and an "off" phase with poor mobility) is a dopamine agonist responsive condition that can be accompanied by parallel mood changes (Cummings 1992; Nissenbaum et al. 1987). Depression has also been associated with greater degrees of bradykinesia, rigidity, and overall motor disability in Parkinson patients (Huber et al. 1988, 1990).

Several biological correlates have been postulated in depressed Parkinson patients. The dexamethasone suppression test (DST) is more often abnormal in depressed than in nondepressed Parkinson patients. However, the evidence to date suggests that it is not a sufficiently specific or sensitive measure to serve as a useful marker of depression (Frochtengarten et al. 1987; Kostic et al. 1990; Mayeux et al. 1986). In several studies (Mayeux et al. 1986, 1988), the cerebrospinal fluid serotonin metabolite 5-HIAA was lower in depressed Parkinson patients than in euthymic control subjects with Parkinson's disease. However, there was no correlation between 5-HIAA levels and severity of depression. In addition, many of the nondepressed patients had low 5-HIAA values. Rapid-eye-movement latency is shorter in depressed versus nondepressed Parkinson patients (Kostic et al. 1991). Finally, Chan-Palay and Asan (1989) showed that depressed Parkinson patients with dementia had greater cell loss in the locus ceruleus than did Parkinson patients with dementia who were not depressed.

A model for depression in Parkinson's disease that emphasizes regional brain changes was recently offered by Cummings (1992). He noted that the frontal lobes of patients with Parkinson's disease have diminished input from subcortical nuclei (via connections between the substantia nigra, caudate, thalamus, and prefrontal cortex). The results of this diminished input includes impairments of 1) dopamine-mediated reward mechanisms (possibly leading to anhedonia), 2) prefrontal lobe function (leading to cognitive symptoms of depression; e.g., low self-esteem and hopelessness), and 3) the ability to adapt to stress (leading to dysphoria). Consistent with this model, Mayberg et al. (1990) demonstrated in a positron-emission tomography (PET) study that depressed Parkinson patients exhibit a selective hypometabolic deficit of the caudate and orbitofrontal cortex. This pattern was distinct from the left dorsal ventrolateral frontal cortical deficit seen in "idiopathic" depression (Baxter et al. 1989).

Successful treatment of depression in Parkinson's disease may improve motor symptoms, but the treatment of motor symptoms does not appear to affect depressed mood. Electroconvulsive therapy (ECT) improves both mood and motor symptoms, but the latter benefit is short lived (see Chapter 30). In reviewing double-blind studies of antidepressant therapy in depressed patients with Parkinson's disease, Cummings (1992) noted that imipramine, desipramine, and bupropion are effective (Goetz at al. 1984; Latinen 1969; Strang 1965) with response rates of 42% to 60%. In addition, 15%–54% of subjects in these studies also experienced some improvement of movement disorder. However, standardized assessments of both mood and motor symptoms were not used. Using structured ratings, Andersen et al. (1980) found nortriptyline to be effective for mood, but not for movement symptoms. Psychostimulants and dopamine agonists have not been shown to alleviate depressive symptoms in Parkinson patients. Selegiline, a monoamine oxidase inhibitor (MAOI), improves depressed mood in Parkinson patients when used alone (Ruggieri et al. 1986) or in conjunction with levodopa (Birkmayer et al. 1983). The transplantation of fetal tissue into the brains of Parkinson patients improves motor symptoms in some patients, but does not change baseline BDI scores (Goetz et al. 1990).

Mania in Parkinson's disease is rare. The few reported cases in the literature are associated with preexisting bipolar disorder, recent onset of antidepressant therapy, a positive family history of affective disorder (Shulman et al. 1992), or postencephalitic parkinsonism. Its treatment is similar to that of "idiopathic" mania, but special care is needed in the administration of neuroleptic compounds because they can exacerbate the motor symptoms of Parkinson's disease.

Stroke

Stroke is an age-related acute injury to the brain caused by thrombosis, embolism, or hemorrhage of the cerebrovascular system. Risk factors besides older age include hypertension, diabetes mellitus, cardiovascular disease, African-American race, smoking, and alcohol consumption. The manifestations of stroke depend on the pathophysiology of the lesion (thrombotic, embolic, or hemorrhagic) and its location (anterior cerebral artery, middle cerebral artery, or posterior circulation). The mood complications of stroke include depression, emotional incontinence, irritability, anxiety, mania, and mood lability.

Estimates of the prevalence of poststroke depression range from 5% to 60%. This variation reflects differences in subject characteristics (including age), the populations under study, diagnostic criteria, and timing of the assessment. In a hospital-based study, Robinson et al. (1987) found that 25% of stroke patients met DSM-III criteria (American Psychiatric Association

1980) for major depression (minus the duration requirement) and 20% had "minor depression" (which they defined as equivalent to dysthymia minus the duration requirement) during the initial poststroke period. At 2-year follow-up, there were no cases of major depression, but 14% still had "minor depression." Lower prevalence rates (11%) of poststroke depression were reported in a community-based study (House et al. 1990).

Poststroke depression may have features that distinguish it from depression in other settings. In one study, Federoff et al. (1991) found that poststroke depression patients had more generalized anxiety, more frequent ideas of reference, and greater cognitive impairment than did depressed medically ill control subjects. When the DSM-III criteria for major depression were restricted to exclude patients who endorsed the nonspecific symptoms of depression associated with medical illness, the prevalence of poststroke depression fell only slightly (from 25% to 22%). Thus misidentification of somatic complaints as depressive symptoms do not seem to result in falsely high rates of depression after stroke.

The status of poststroke "minor depression" has been controversial. Some investigators consider it phenomenologically distinct from poststroke major depression (Starkstein and Robinson 1989), but other investigators have noted that the distribution of depressive symptoms in this group resembles that of elderly control subjects without mood disorder (House et al. 1991).

Lesion location has been shown to have specific linkages with poststroke mood symptoms and syndromes. Depression is more common following left-hemisphere than right-hemisphere stroke. Further, in patients with left cortical lesions, proximity to the frontal pole correlates with increasing severity of depression. This correlation has been found in patients with bilateral lesions (Lipsey et al. 1983), right-handedness (Robinson et al. 1984), left-handedness (Robinson et al. 1985), combined cortical and subcortical lesions (Starkstein et al. 1987, 1988a), and reversed brain symmetry (i.e., larger left than right frontal lobes and larger right than left occipital lobes) (Starkstein et al. 1991a). However, not all investigators have found such robust associations between left-sided lesions and depression (House et al. 1990), and some have found none (Eastwood et al. 1989; Ebrahim et al. 1987; Sinyor et al. 1986; Wade et al. 1987). Depression after right-sided lesions is associated with a positive family history

of depression and parietal lobe lesion location (Starkstein et al. 1989b).

Lesion size may be an important determinant of poststroke mood. House et al. (1989) suggested that emotional lability was more common after large lesions. Further, Starkstein et al. (1988b) found poststroke depression to be linked with increased third ventricle-to-brain ratio (VBR) and lateral VBR. They suggested that elevated VBR may predate stroke and be a risk factor for the development of poststroke depression. Lesion size may also correlate with cognitive impairment (Starkstein et al. 1988b).

Poststroke depression is associated with a higher rate of cortisol nonsuppression by dexamethasone, but sensitivity and specificity are too low to make the DST a useful diagnostic marker (Lipsey et al. 1985; Reding et al. 1985a). A diminished growth hormone response to desipramine has been reported in poststroke depressed patients (Barry and Dinan 1990), suggesting that measures of α-adrenergic receptor function may serve as a biological marker in this population.

Poststroke mania, anxiety, and mood lability are less well studied than depression. Mania in poststroke populations is relatively infrequent. It usually occurs after right-sided strokes affecting the cortical limbic areas and subcortical nuclei (Robinson et al. 1988). On the other hand, poststroke anxiety is common. Starkstein et al. (1990a) studied 98 poststroke patients and found 6 to have a "pure" anxiety syndrome, 23 to have mixed anxiety and depression, and 24 to have depression alone. Cortical lesions are associated with mixed anxiety and depression, whereas basal ganglia lesions are associated with depression (Starkstein et al. 1990a). Finally, 10%–20% of poststroke patients have significant mood lability (House et al. 1989).

The etiology of poststroke mood disorders remains obscure. Robinson et al. (1984) noted that the norepinephrine-containing and serotonin-containing neurons project from brain stem nuclei through the median forebrain bundle and into the frontal cortex. They hypothesized that anterior cortical strokes lead to massive neurotransmitter depletion and depression. Projections from the basal ganglia to the frontal cortex that are interrupted by subcortical or cortical lesions may lead to similar results. Why left-sided lesions should result in higher rates of depression than right-sided lesions is not clear. One possible explanation was suggested by Mayberg et al. (1988): in a PET study of poststroke patients, those with left-sided lesions had lower compensatory serotonin receptor upregulation than did those with right-sided lesions. These investigators also found that left temporal cortex spiperone binding to serotonin receptors was inversely related to the likelihood of being depressed.

The treatment of poststroke mood disorders is similar in principle to that of "idiopathic" mood conditions. We are aware of only two double-blind studies that examined the efficacy of pharmacological treatments in this setting. Lipsey et al. (1984) reported that nortriptyline provided a significant antidepressant benefit, but their study was affected by a drop-out rate of one-third. Reding et al. (1986) demonstrated the effectiveness of trazodone, but only in patients with a positive DST result. Studies of other agents have been less rigorously designed, but suggest some benefits. Methylphenidate was effective in 8 of 10 patients in a case series reported by Lazarus et al. (1992). ECT has been shown to be safe and effective for patients with poststroke depression (Murray et al. 1986).

Vascular Dementia

Vascular dementia (multi-infarct dementia) is a common, age-related source of cognitive impairment in elderly individuals. Recently, Skoog et al. (1993) reported that one-third of the 85-year-old individuals in a community survey had dementia, half of which were likely to be of vascular origin.

The estimated prevalence of depression in multi-infarct dementia varies from 19% to 27% (Fischer et al. 1990). This range is similar to the range for depression in Alzheimer's disease. However, Cummings et al. (1987) noted that "depression is more uniformly accepted as an accompaniment of multi-infarct dementia [than of dementia of the Alzheimer type]." Studies comparing these conditions have yielded inconclusive results. Reding et al. (1985b) demonstrated more cases of depression in an Alzheimer group than in a comparison group with multi-infarct dementia, whereas Cummings et al. (1987) found a higher prevalence of depression in patients with multi-infarct dementia. Fischer et al. (1990) were unable to find any significant difference in rates of depression between these groups.

The increased prevalence of white matter hyperintensities (which may indicate underlying vascular pathology) noted in elderly depressive patients by Coffey et al. (1989) may predict the development of dementia. However, this assertion remains unproved. The mechanism by which multi-infarct dementia leads to depressive symptomatology is unknown, but depression may result from the same regional and biochemical deficits involved in the genesis of depression in other neuropsychiatric conditions.

Mania is observed in multi-infarct dementia (as well as in many other organic causes of cerebral disturbance), but we are unaware of any prevalence estimates in the literature. Specific treatment for mood disorders in the setting of vascular dementia have not been developed.

Other Disorders

Huntington's disease.   Huntington's disease is an autosomal dominant degenerative disorder that usually presents in the mid-life years with chorea, dementia, personality changes, and mood symptoms. The primary neuropathological lesion is atrophy and neuronal loss in the caudate nuclei.

The prevalence of mood disorder in Huntington's disease is approximately 40%, with cases tending to cluster within some families (Folstein et al. 1983). Approximately 75% percent of patients with mood disorder have depressive symptoms only, whereas the remainder have a mixture of depressive and manic symptoms. Mood symptoms may precede the onset of dementia or movement disorder by up to 5 years (Minski and Guttman 1938), and their frequency increases in late-onset cases (Folstein et al. 1983). However, mood symptoms do not appear to increase in frequency or severity over the course of the illness. Although the irritability, aggression, apathy, uncharacteristic sexual behaviors, and impaired judgment seen in some Huntington patients may falsely suggest the presence of a mood disorder (Folstein 1989), these disturbances may also be amplified when a mood disorder is present.

Biological correlates of mood disorder in Huntington's disease relating specifically to aging have not been identified. We are not aware of studies demonstrating the superior efficacy of particular antidepressant or antimanic therapies in patients with Huntington's disease.

Cardiovascular disease.   A number of authors have noted that the presence of cardiovascular disease significantly increases fatality rates among depressed elderly patients. Rabins et al. (1985) reviewed these findings and found that 75% of elderly depressed patients who were deceased within 1 year had a discharge diagnosis of cardiovascular disease. They reviewed possible causal connections between cardiovascular disease and depression and recommended that prospective studies be conducted to clarify the risks of one condition leading to the other.

Head trauma.   Elderly people are especially prone to falling and therefore to head trauma (see Chapter 24). The estimated prevalence of depressive symptoms for all ages after brain injury ranges from 6% to 39% after mild injury and 10% to 77% after severe injury (Silver et al. 1992). The incidence and severity of depression appears to be related to the extent of neuropsychological impairment (Dikmen and Reitan 1977) and to right-hemisphere damage in the case of penetrating injuries to the brain (Silver et al. 1992). Mania has been reported after traumatic brain injuries but less frequently than depression (Silver et al. 1992). Starkstein et al. (1991b) demonstrated that injuries to the basal region of the right temporal lobe and to the right orbitofrontal area (in subjects with a family history of mood disorder) are predisposing factors for posttraumatic mania.

Metabolic.   Cobalamin (vitamin B_{12}) deficiency has been cited as a cause of neuropsychiatric disturbances in elderly patients. Lindenbaum et al. (1988) found that 2 of 40 subjects with a depressive disorder had reversal of their symptoms apparently in response to vitamin replacement. Folic acid deficiency has also been linked to depression in patients of all ages (Carney 1967; E. H. Reynolds et al. 1970). Elderly people may be especially vulnerable to vitamin deficiencies because of their increased risk of poor nutrition.

Endocrine.   Hypothyroidism is common in the elderly and may cause or contribute to symptoms of depression. Lishman (1987) described the typical picture as "one of mental lethargy, general dulling of the personality and slowing of all cognitive functions" (p. 433). The usual mood change is one of apathy with frequent irritability. This clinical picture often resolves with the correction of the thyroid deficit alone. If it does not, a trial of antidepressant therapy is warranted. Similarly, hyperthyroidism can induce (or exacerbate) the affective, cognitive, and behavioral features of mania. Correcting the thyroid disturbance may be sufficient to normalize the patient's psychiatric condition.

Medications.   Elderly people may be at particularly high risk for mental status (including mood) changes induced by the use of over-the-counter and prescribed medications (see Chapter 29). The list of medications causing these effects is long. Antihypertensives, barbiturates, guanethidine, levodopa, steroids, and indomethacin are reported causes of depression, whereas decongestants, steroids, antidepressants, levodopa, and sympathomimetics have been implicated as causes of mania (Stoudemire 1987). Thus taking a comprehensive medication history is paramount.

Miscellaneous.   Other neuropsychiatric conditions associated with mood disorder in the elderly populations include alcoholism, endocrine disorders not mentioned above (e.g., Cushing's disease, Addison's disease, hypo- and hypercalcemia, and hypoglycemia), epilepsy, tumor, mental retardation, infection, collagen-vascular diseases, multiple sclerosis, and delirium. However, their treatment is, for the most part, the same as that in younger age groups.

Neuropsychiatric Aspects of "Idiopathic" Mood Disorder in Elderly Patients

In this section, we address the elements of "idiopathic" mood disorder of interest from a neuropsychiatric standpoint. Most of the discussion concerns depression because of the relative infrequency of manic-like symptoms and bipolar disorder in the elderly.

Epidemiology

In the ECA study, the 1-year prevalence of major depression peaked in the fourth decade at 3.9% and declined to 0.9% after age 65 (Weissman et al. 1991). In addition, the same study found that lifetime prevalence of major depression decreased with age. There are several plausible explanations for these reported declines in the prevalence of depression in late life: increasingly stressful living conditions since the end of World War II that have increased the incidence of depression among the young; a lower likelihood of elderly subjects being able to remember depressive symptoms (recall bias); higher mortality from depression that has decreased the number of depressed people living to old age; and greater stigma of mental illness among the elderly leading to underreporting of depressive symptoms.

The prevalence of late-onset mania in the general population is unknown. Young (1992) reviewed the status of new-onset mania in elderly subjects and found existing data on changing incidence over the life span to be inconclusive. However, he noted that several studies suggested an increased rate of index admissions in elderly men with no such increase noted in elderly women. Data from retrospective studies indicate the mean age at onset to be in the fifth and sixth decades.

Biological Markers

Few studies of the neurochemistry and neuropathology of depression in the elderly have yielded robust results. Even fewer studies suggest the presence of a "trait-dependent" marker (i.e., an enduring genetic, biochemical, or metabolic measure predictive of the illness) for mood disorder. A key difficulty is the current inability to determine whether alleged markers are crucial to the genesis of the disorder or whether they are merely epiphenomena. However, several trends can be noted.

Elevated plasma cortisol levels have been reported in depressed elderly patients compared with depressed younger patients (Ferrier et al. 1988) and nondepressed elderly control subjects (Schliefer et al. 1989). Post-DST cortisol levels in depressed elderly patients seem to correlate with measures of depression severity (Molchan et al. 1990) and with cognitive decline during the illness (Siegal et al. 1989). Skare et al. (1990) pooled data from 27 articles on the use of the DST in elderly patients and demonstrated its failure to discriminate between patients with major depression, Alzheimer's disease, and vascular dementia. Although abnormal hypothalamic-pituitary-adrenal (HPA) function normalizes after recovery from depression in elderly patients as it does in younger patients (Goodwin and Jamison 1990), it is unclear if the same changes occur in elderly patients with depression. Finally, lymphocyte proliferation rates and T4 lymphocyte counts appear to be selectively decreased in elderly patients with depression (Darko et al. 1988; Schleifer et al. 1989).

Platelet imipramine binding is decreased in depressed elderly patients (Schneider et al. 1985), and its specificity as a marker for depression may increase with age (Nemeroff et al. 1988). Crow et al. (1984) found decreased platelet imipramine binding in the brains of depressed elderly patients who went on to commit suicide. Ferrier and McKeith (1991) reviewed the status of neurochemical correlates of mood disorder in elderly subjects. They concluded that serotonin, subtype 2 (S_2), receptor density may be increased in the frontal cortices of depressed elderly patients, but could not reach consensus regarding serotonin (subtype 1 [S_1]), adrenergic (α and β), dopaminergic, cholinergic, or neuropeptide receptor density changes. McKeith et al. (1987) demonstrated an elevation in S_2 receptor density in the frontal cortices of patients who had a history of major depression and then died of "natural causes." This suggests, but does not prove, that elevated S_2 receptor density is a trait-dependent marker for depression in the elderly population.

Francis et al. (1993) found that intraventricular concentrations of 5-HIAA were significantly lower in patients with severe and prolonged depression than in control subjects with dementia or other neurological and psychiatric illnesses. This finding provides a biochemical rationale for treatments that selectively enhance CNS serotonergic activity (e.g., serotonin reuptake inhibitors).

Little work has been done to investigate the biological correlates of late-onset mania in elderly patients. However, late-onset cases are associated with a lower rate of positive family history for mood disorder than are early-onset cases (Glasser and Rabins 1984; Shulman and Post 1980). Late-onset cases have also been associated retrospectively with an increased frequency of "organic" conditions such as medical illness and drug treatment (Krauthammer and Klerman 1978). Stone (1989) found that 22 of 92 inpatients with late-onset mania were reported to have "organic cerebral impairment," whereas Dhingra and Rabins (1991) found higher than expected rates of cognitive impairment in elderly manic patients followed for 5 years. Thus late-onset mania appears to be a heterogeneous condition. This fact, in addition to the rarity of late-onset mania, makes problematic any efforts to search for an single underlying cause.

Neuroimaging

CT imaging of elderly patients with mood disorders has yielded much conflicting data. Difficulties stem from uncertainty about how CT images change with "normal" aging, varying definitions of the structures being measured, differing study methodologies, heterogeneous subject samples, and variable equipment and measuring techniques.

VBR is the most common CT measure used in studies of elderly patients; it increases in dementia and in normal aging (Beats 1991) but with considerable overlap. However, Laffey et al. (1984) and Bird et al. (1986) found that 85% of nondepressed elderly patients had normal CT results when subjects with dementia, alcoholism, and neurological illnesses were excluded.

Most studies have concluded that VBR increases in depression, but not to the degree found in Alzheimer's disease (Pearlson et al. 1989). Alexopoulos et al. (1992), however, reported findings on a group of elderly depressed patients with VBRs approximating those of nondepressed Alzheimer's disease patients. A finding which might reconcile these discrepant findings is the observation of Bird et al. (1986) that more than half the elderly subjects who seemed well at the study onset, but who were noted to have increased VBRs, developed depression (without cognitive impairment) by the 2.5-year follow-up.

In depressed elderly patients, increased VBR correlates with the degree of reversible cognitive impairment during the depressive disorder (Kellner et al. 1986; Pearlson et al. 1989). VBR is larger in patients with late-onset depression (Alexopoulos 1989; Jacoby and Levy 1980) and endogenous features. Larger VBR predicts increased mortality at 2-year follow-up (Jacoby and Levy 1980). Alexopoulos (1989) reported an association of increased VBR with elevated post-DST plasma cortisol levels and with a diminished clinical response to nortriptyline. He also found that larger lateral ventricle posterior horn size was associated with a positive response to ECT treatments.

In spite of the consistency of these findings, the status of VBR measurement remains controversial because longitudinal studies have failed to demonstrate that increases in VBRs last beyond the depressive episode. Explanations for the increased VBRs seen in currently or recently depressed patients include atrophy from weight loss and fluid shifts secondary to treatment with lithium or tricyclic antidepressants (Nasrallah et al. 1989).

Jacoby et al. (1983) found the brain "density," (i.e., CT attenuation numbers) of elderly depressed patients to be significantly lower than that of nondepressed control subjects. Furthermore, these lower measurements approximated the values obtained for Alzheimer patients. This group and Pearlson et al. (1989) found the greatest decreases in brain density in patients who exhibited cognitive impairment during their depressive episodes.

MRI has surpassed CT as the study of choice for examining the fine structure of the brain. However, as with CT, technical and methodological differences between studies make the drawing of general conclusions difficult. White matter lesions are areas of signal hyperintensity in the periventricular and deep white matter regions in some MRI scans of the brain. These lesions have been noted in some "normal" subjects and in association with a wide variety of medical conditions (Beats 1991). The genesis of white matter lesions is controversial and is most likely multifactorial. Their presence is clearly associated with hypertension and aging. In one study of nondepressed elderly patients (Matsubayashi et al. 1992), the number of white matter lesions correlated inversely with performance on a number of neuropsychological measures. Coffey et al. (1993) showed that depressed elderly patients referred for ECT had significantly more white matter lesions than did control subjects, even after controlling for the presence of CNS vascular disease.

In depressed elderly patients, white matter lesions have been found to correlate with psychotic features (Lesser et al. 1991), late-onset, referral for ECT, lack of response to pharmacotherapy, and an increased likelihood of developing Alzheimer's disease when cognitive impairment is present during the depression (Coffey et al. 1988). Coffey et al. (1993) showed that lesion location affects the likelihood of an elderly person developing a mood disorder. In their sample, 40% of 35 depressed patients had lesions of the thalamus and basal ganglia (compared with 5% of 22 nondepressed elderly control subjects). Similarly, Rabins et al. (1991) found more basal ganglia lesions in depressed elderly patients, whereas Husain et al. (1991) found smaller putamen size in subjects with major depression.

Other changes noted on MRI scans of depressed (versus nondepressed) elderly subjects include increased lateral and third ventricle size, greater cortical sulcal atrophy (Coffey et al. 1993; Rabins et al. 1991), enlarged Sylvian fissures, increased temporal horn size (Rabins et al. 1991), and smaller frontal lobe volumes (Coffey et al. 1993). Rabins et al. (1991) found no difference in any of these measures between the delusional and nondelusional patients in their study. They also reported that the degree of cortical sulcal atrophy correlated with the age at onset of depression.

To date, studies using PET and single photon emission computed tomography (SPECT) have not focused on elderly subjects. However, these functional studies are of great potential value because of their ability to measure specific receptor categories and to detect changes in metabolic activity at sites throughout the brain (thereby allowing hypotheses about "neural networks" to be tested). One finding of interest is the specific orbitofrontal hypometabolic deficit noted in depressed Parkinson's disease patients (Mayberg et al. 1989, 1990). This pattern differs from the left dorsal ventrolateral frontal-cortical deficit noted by Baxter et al. (1989) in PET scans of nonelderly patients with "idiopathic" depression. It remains unclear if these differences are related to age or whether they reflect different etiologies of depression.

Depression-Induced Cognitive Impairment

Reports of coexisting disorders of mood and cognition date back to ancient Egyptian medical writings (Loza and Milad 1990). Among the terms used to describe this co-occurrence are *pseudodementia, dementia syndrome of depression, coexisting dementia and depression, cognitive-affective disorder, delirious mania, depressive stupor,* and *organic affective syndrome.* The term *depression-induced cognitive disorder* (Rabins and Pearlson, in press) is used here to refer to cognitive impairment that is secondary to a primary mood disorder. It occurs most frequently in the elderly.

Long-term follow-up studies of patients with disorders of both cognitive and mood impairment have demonstrated approximately equal percentages of a primary dementing illness or a primary mood disorder (Reding et al. 1986; C. F. Reynolds et al. 1986). However, the longest term follow-up (Kral 1983) suggested that a significant majority of patients (91%) eventually develop dementia.

The predominant cognitive impairment in depression-induced cognitive disorder is memory disorder. Free recall memory (i.e., demonstrated by the ability to recall a set of objects after a time delay) is impaired in both depression-induced cognitive impairment and irreversible dementia, whereas recognition memory (i.e., demonstrated by the ability to correctly identify items from a list that includes previously presented items and a set of distractor items the subject had not been previously exposed to) is intact in depression-induced cognitive impairment and impaired in irreversible dementia.

CT attenuation numbers in patients with depression-induced cognitive impairment are lower than those in patients with major depression and normal cognition (Pearlson et al. 1989). This suggests that depression-induced cognitive impairment reflects underlying structural brain disease. Parallel findings were reported by Abas et al. (1990), who found a positive correlation between the degree of depression-induced

cognitive slowing and the degree of ventricular enlargement. The hypothesis that depression-induced cognitive impairment reflects physiological abnormalities in the CNS has been further strengthened by the correlation between cognitive performance and cerebral blood flow in a group of cognitively normal depressed subjects (Silfverskiöld and Risberg 1989).

Treatment

The treatment of depression in elderly patients is a topic too large to consider fully here. However, several points deserve special attention. First, the standard treatments for mood disorder in younger patients also appear to be effective in elderly patients. Salzman et al. (1993) reviewed the literature for all pharmacological studies of antidepressant therapy in elderly patients and found that only 33 of 400 reports dealt exclusively with patients over age 65 and none were controlled and double blind. They concluded that recommendations made for the "elderly" (i.e., those over age 65) were based on data derived from studies of younger patients. In the mixed-age (i.e., including patients above and below age 65) studies, several reports provided useful information, though none compared the results of therapy in patients by age group. For example, Ather et al. (1985) showed that trazadone and amitriptyline provided greater antidepressant benefit in elderly subjects than diazepam and that trazadone worked more quickly and caused fewer side effects than amitriptyline. Finch and Katon (1989) demonstrated a robust response in elderly patients to lithium augmentation of antidepressant therapy. In placebo-controlled double-blind studies, methylphenidate (Kaplitz 1975) and doxepin (Lakshmanan et al. 1986) were effective in chronically medically ill patients. In a controlled study of antidepressant therapy of patients over the age 75, Katz et al. (1989) demonstrated that nortriptyline was effective in 12 of 30 patients at doses of 25–50 mg/day, but "severe" side effects occurred in many individuals. Although none of these studies include data on serotonin reuptake blockers or MAOIs, case reports testifying to the efficacy of these agents abound. The enzyme monoamine oxidase increases with age, suggesting that drugs that inhibit its function might be particularly useful in elderly patients.

The second point to be made is that elderly patients need to be monitored for the side effects of medications even more closely than do younger patients. Drug interactions are more common in elderly patients because they are taking more medications. In addition, the pharmacokinetics of some antidepressant drugs are altered in elderly patients. Dawling et al. (1980) demonstrated that nortriptyline has an elimination half-life that is two to three times longer in elderly subjects. Idiosyncratic side effects may also more common. Methylphenidate may be particularly useful in treating depression in extremely old patients because it has fewer problematic side effects (Gurian and Rosowsky 1990). Of the nonpharmacological treatments of severe depression in the elderly population, ECT seems to be the most effective (see Chapter 30).

The treatment of late-onset mania has not been studied in sufficient detail to make definitive statements about treatment recommendations. Lithium seems to be of at least equal efficacy in late-onset as in early-onset cases. We are unaware of any well-designed studies of continuation therapy of lithium in elderly patients. Acute toxicity may appear at lithium levels considered low or "therapeutic" in younger patients (Foster et al. 1977; Van der Velde 1971). The pharmacotherapy of acute manic episodes in elderly patients with neuroleptics is complicated by the high likelihood of extrapyramidal side effects. As with depression, ECT is a safe and effective treatment of mania in the elderly.

Summary

Several major points can be made about the neuropsychiatric foundations of mood disorders in the elderly:

1. The prevalence of organic syndromes affecting mood increases over the life span. Thus an underlying neuropsychiatric condition should be suspected in all mood disturbances of new onset in elderly patients.
2. The phenomenology (i.e., signs and symptoms) of "idiopathic" and "secondary" mood disorders affecting elderly patients are essentially identical. Thus the history, physical examination, and ancillary testing are essential tools in the search for potential neuropsychiatric causes of a mood disturbance in an elderly person.
3. Converging lines of evidence suggest that the left frontal lobe plays an essential role in the genesis of "idiopathic" and secondary depression. Modest evidence from similar studies also suggests a role for the basal ganglia.
4. Evidence from neuropathological and functional

imaging studies suggests that disruption of cortical and subcortical tracts (from stroke, demyelination, or neuronal degeneration) impairs norepinephrine and serotonin neurotransmission and may increase the likelihood of a mood disturbance (usually depression). Because there are age-related decrements in these neurotransmitter systems (as well as an increase in monoamine oxidase), the concordance of disease-induced and age-related changes in these systems puts the elderly at special risk for developing mood disorders.

5. The treatments that are effective for "idiopathic" mood syndromes are also useful in treating secondary mood syndromes. Removal of the causative agent (e.g., medications or endocrine dysfunction) is sometimes an effective treatment for secondary mood symptoms, but is not always possible. Lower doses of medication are often appropriate in elderly patients. Side effects from medication are more likely to limit therapy in elderly patients than in younger ones. Finally, ECT is an effective treatment for severe depression or mania in elderly patients, and its side effects are often better tolerated than pharmacological therapy.

References

Abas MS, Sahakian J, Levy R: Neuropsychological deficits and CT scan changes in elderly depressives. Psychol Med 20:507–520, 1990

Alexopoulos GS: Biological abnormalities in late-life depression. Journal of Geriatr Psychiatry 22:25–34, 1989

Alexopoulos GS, Abrams RC, Young RC, et al: Cornell Scale for Depression in Dementia. Biol Psychiatry 23:271–284, 1988

Alexopoulos GS, Young RC, Shindledecker RD: Brain computed tomography findings in geriatric depression and primary degenerative dementia. Biol Psychiatry 31:591–599, 1992

American Psychiatric Association: Diagnostic and Statistical Manual of Mental Disorders, 3rd Edition. Washington, DC, American Psychiatric Association, 1980

American Psychiatric Association: Diagnostic and Statistical Manual of Mental Disorders, 3rd Edition, Revised. Washington, DC, American Psychiatric Association, 1987

American Psychiatric Association: Diagnostic and Statistical Manual of Mental Disorders, 4th Edition. Washington, DC, American Psychiatric Association, 1994

Andersen J, Aabro E, Gulmann N, et al: Anti-depressive treatment in Parkinson's disease. Acta Neurol Scand 62:210–219, 1980

Ather SA, Anker SI, Middleton RSW: A double blind evaluation of trazadone in the treatment of depression in the elderly. Br J Clin Pract 39 (May):192–199, 1985

Barry S, Dinan TG: Alpha-2 adrenergic receptor function in post-stroke depression. Psychol Med 20:305–309, 1990

Baxter LR, Schwartz JM, Phelps ME: Reduction of prefrontal cortex glucose metabolism common to three types of depression. Arch Gen Psychiatry 46:243–250, 1989

Beats BC: Structural imaging in affective disorder. International Journal of Geriatric Psychiatry 6:419–422, 1991

Beck AT: Depression Inventory. Philadelphia, PA, Philadelphia Center for Cognitive Therapy, 1978

Bird JM, Levy R, Jacoby RJ: Computed tomography in the elderly: change over time in the normal population. Br J Psychiatry 148:80–86, 1986

Birkmeyer W: Deprenyl (selegiline) in the treatment of Parkinson's disease. Acta Neurol Scand Suppl 95:103–106, 1983

Blazer D, Woodbury M, Hughes DC, et al: A statistical analysis of the classification of depression in a mixed community and clinical sample. J Affect Disord 16:11–20, 1989

Brown GL, Wilson WP: Parkinsonism and depression. South Med J 65:540–545, 1972

Bucht G, Adolfsson R: The comprehensive psychopathological rating scale in patients with dementia of the Alzheimer type and multi-infarct dementia. Acta Psychiatr Scand 68:263–270, 1983

Burns A: Affective symptoms in Alzheimer's disease. International Journal of Geriatric Psychiatry 6:371–376, 1991

Burns A, Jacoby R, Levy R: Psychiatric phenomena in Alzheimer's disease, III: disorders of mood. Br J Psychiatry 157:81–86, 1990

Carney MWP: Serum folate values in 423 psychiatric patients. BMJ 4:512–516, 1967

Chan-Palay V, Asan E: Alterations in catecholamine neurons of the locus ceruleus in senile dementia of the Alzheimer type and in Parkinson's disease with and without dementia and depression. J Comp Neurol 187:373–392, 1989

Coffey CE, Figiel GS, Djang WT: Leukoencephalopathy in elderly depressed patients referred for ECT. Biol Psychiatry 24:143–161, 1988

Coffey CE, Figiel GS, Djang WT: Subcortical white matter hyperintensity on magnetic resonance imaging: clinical and neuroanatomic correlates in the depressed elderly. J Neuropsychiatry Clin Neurosci 1:135–144, 1989

Coffey CE, Wilkinson WE, Weiner RD, et al: Quantitative cerebral anatomy in depression: a controlled magnetic resonance imaging study. Arch Gen Psychiatry 50:7–16, 1993

Crow TJ, Cross AJ, Cooper SJ, et al: Neurotransmitter receptors and monoamine metabolites in the brains of patients with Alzheimer-type dementia and depression and suicides. Neuropharmacology 23:1561–1569, 1984

Cummings JL: Subcortical dementia: neuropsychology, neuropsychiatry and pathophysiology. Br J Psychiatry 149:682–687, 1986

Cummings JL: Depression and Parkinson's disease: a review. Am J Psychiatry 149:443–454, 1992

Cummings JL, Victoroff JI: Noncognitive neuropsychiatric syndromes in Alzheimer's disease. Neuropsychiatry, Neuropsychology, and Behavioral Neurology 3:140–158, 1990

Cummings JL, Miller B, Hill MA, et al: Neuropsychiatric aspects of multi-infarct dementia and dementia of the Alzheimer type. Arch Neurol 44:389–393, 1987

Darko DF, Lucus AH, Gillin JC, et al: Age, cellular immunity and the HP axis in major depression. Prog Neuropsychopharmacol Biol Psychiatry 12:713–720, 1988

Dawling S, Chrome P, Braithwaite R: Pharmacokinetics of single oral doses of nortriptyline in depressed elderly hospital patients and young healthy volunteers. Clin Pharmacokinet 5:394–401, 1980

Dhingra U, Rabins PV: Mania in the elderly: a 5–7 year follow-up. J Am Geriatr Soc 39:581–583, 1991

Dikmen S, Reitan RM: Emotional sequelae of head injury. Ann Neurol 2:492–494, 1977

Direnfeld LK, Albert ML, Volicer L, et al: Parkinson's disease: the possible relationship of laterality to dementia and neurochemical findings. Arch Neurol 41:935–941, 1984

Eastwood MR, Rifut SL, Nobbs H, et al: Mood disorder following cerebrovascular accident. Br J Psychiatry 154:195–200, 1989

Ebrahim S, Bauer D, Nouri F: Affective illness after stroke. Br J Psychiatry 151:52–56, 1987

Federoff JP, Starkstein SE, Parikh RM, et al: Are depressive symptoms non-specific in patients with acute stroke? Am J Psychiatry 148:1172–1176, 1991

Ferrier JN, McKeith IG: Neuroanatomical and neurochemical changes in affective disorders in old age. International Journal of Geriatric Psychiatry 6:445–451, 1991

Ferrier IN, Pascual J, Charlton BG, et al: Cortisol, ACTH and dexamethasone concentrations in a psychogeriatric population. Biol Psychiatry 23:252–266, 1988

Finch EJL, Katon CLE: Lithium augmentation in the treatment of refractory depression in old age. International Journal of Geriatric Psychiatry 4:41–46, 1989

Fischer P, Simamyi M, Danielczyk W: Depression in dementia of the Alzheimer type and in multi-infarct dementia. Am J Psychiatry 147:1484–1487, 1990

Folstein SE: Huntington's Disease: A Disorder of Families. Baltimore, MD, Johns Hopkins University Press, 1989

Folstein SE, Abbott MH, Chase GA, et al: The association of affective disorder with Huntington's disease in a case series and in families. Psychol Med 13:537–542, 1983

Forstl H, Howard R: Recent studies on dementia senilis and brain disorders caused by atheromatous vascular disease (by A. Alzheimer, 1898). Alzheimer Dis Assoc Disord 5:257–264, 1991

Foster JR, Geshell WJ, Goldfarb AJ: Lithium treatment in the elderly, I: clinical usage. J Gerontol 32:299–302, 1977

Francis PT, Pangalos MN, Stephens PH, et al: Ante-mortem measurements of neurotransmission: possible implications for pharmacotherapy of Alzheimer's disease and depression. J Neurol Neurosurg Psychiatry 56:80–84, 1993

Frochtengarten ML, Villares JCB, Maluf E, et al: Depressive symptoms and the dexamethasone suppression test in Parkinsonian patients. Biol Psychiatry 22:386–389, 1987

Glasser M, Rabins P: Mania in the elderly. Age Ageing 13:210–217, 1984

Goetz GG, Tanner CM, Klawans HL: Bupropion in Parkinson's disease. Neurology 34:1092–1094, 1984

Goetz GG, Tanner CM, Penn RD, et al: Adrenal medullary transplant to the striatum of patients with advanced Parkinson's disease: one year motor and psychomotor data. Neurology 40:273–276, 1990

Goodwin FK, Jamison KR: Manic-depressive Illness. New York, Oxford University Press, 1990

Gottfries CG, Karlsson I, Nyth AL: Treatment of depression in elderly patients with and without dementia disorders. Int Clin Psychopharmacol 6 (suppl 5):55–64, 1992

Greenwald BS, Kramer-Ginsberg E, Marin DB, et al: Dementia with coexistent major depression. Am J Psychiatry 146:1472–1478, 1989

Gurian B, Rosowsky E: Low-dose methylphenidate in the very old. J Geriatr Psychiatry Neurol 3:152–154, 1990

Hamilton M: A rating scale for depression. J Neurol Neurosurg Psychiatry 23:56–62, 1960

Horn S: Some psychological features in Parkinsonism. J Neurol Neurosurg Psychiatry 37:27–31, 1974

House A, Dennis M, Molyneux A, et al: Emotionalism after stroke. BMJ 289:992–994, 1989

House A, Dennis M, Warlow C, et al: Mood disorders after stroke and their relation to lesion location. Brain 113:1113–1129, 1990

House A, Dennis M, Mogridge L, et al: Mood disorders in the first year after stroke. Br J Psychiatry 158:83–92, 1991

Huber SJ, Paulson GW, Shuttleworth EC: Depression in Parkinson's disease. Neuropsychiatry, Neuropsychology, and Behavioral Neurology 1:47–51, 1988

Huber SJ, Freidenberg DL, Paulson GW, et al: The pattern of depressive symptoms with progression of Parkinson's disease. J Neurol Neurosurg Psychiatry 53:275–278, 1990

Husain MM, McDonald WM, Doraiswamy PM, et al: A magnetic resonance imaging study of putamen nuclei in major depression. Psychiatry Research: Neuroimaging 40:95–99, 1991

Jacoby RJ, Levy R: Computed tomography in the elderly, III: affective disorder. Br J Psychiatry 136:270–275, 1980

Jacoby RJ, Dolan RJ, Baldy R, et al: Quantitative computed tomography in elderly depressed patients. Br J Psychiatry 143:124–127, 1983

Kaplitz SE: Withdrawn apathetic geriatric patients responsive to methylphenidate. J Am Geriatr Soc 23:271–276, 1975

Katz IR, Simpson GM, Jethanardani V, et al: Steady-state pharmacokinetics of nortriptyline in the frail elderly. Neuropsychopharmacology 2:229–236, 1989

Kellner CH, Rubinow DR, Post RM: Cerebral ventricular size and cognitive impairment in depression. J Affect Disord 10:215–219, 1986

Kostic VS, Covickovic-Sternic N, Belsac-Bubasirevic L, et al: Dexamethasone suppression test in patients with Parkinson's disease. Mov Disord 5:23–26, 1990

Kostic VS, Susic V, Praedborski S, et al: Sleep EEG in depressed and non-depressed patients with Parkinson's disease. J Neuropsychiatry Clin Neurosci 3:176–179, 1991

Kral V: The relationship between senile dementia, Alzheimer's type, and depression. Can J Psychiatry 28:304–306, 1983

Krauthammer C, Klerman GL: Secondary mania: manic syndromes associated with antecedent physical illness or drugs. Arch Gen Psychiatry 35:1333–1339, 1978

Laffey PA, Payster RG, Nathan R, et al: Computed tomography and ageing: results in a normal elderly population. Neuroradiology 26:273–278, 1984

Lakshmanan M, Mion LC, Frengley JD: Effective low dose tricyclic antidepressant treatment for depressed geriatric rehabilitation patients: a double-blind study. J Am Geriatr Soc 34:421–426, 1986

Latinen L: Desipramine in treatment of Parkinson's disease. Acta Neurol Scand 45:109–113, 1969

Lazarus LW, Newton N, Cohler B, et al: Frequency and presentation of depressive symptoms in patients with primary degenerative dementia. Am J Psychiatry 144:41–45, 1987

Lazarus LW, Winemiller DR, Lingam VR, et al: Efficacy and side effects of methylphenidate for post-stroke depression. J Clin Psychiatry 53:447–449, 1992

Lesser IM, Miller BL, Boone KB, et al: Brain injury and cognitive function in late-onset psychotic depression. J Neuropsychiatry Clin Neurosci 3:33–40, 1991

Levin BE, Llabie MM, Weiner WJ: Parkinson's disease and depression: psychometric properties of the Beck Depression Inventory. J Neurol Neurosurg Psychiatry 51:1401–1404, 1988

Lindenbaum J, Healton EB, Savage DG, et al: Neuropsychiatric disorders caused by cobalamin deficiency in the absence of anemia or macrocytosis. N Engl J Med 318:1720–1727, 1988

Lipsey JR, Robinson RG, Pearlson GD, et al: Mood change following bilateral hemisphere brain injury. Br J Psychiatry 143:366–373, 1983

Lipsey JR, Robinson RG, Pearlson GD, et al: Nortriptyline treatment of post-stroke depression. Lancet 1:297–300, 1984

Lipsey JR, Robinson RG, Pearlson GD: Dexamethasone suppression test and mood following stroke. Am J Psychiatry 142:318–323, 1985

Lishman WA: Organic Psychiatry: The Psychological Consequences of Cerebral Disorder, 3rd Edition. Oxford, England, Blackwell Scientific, 1987

Loza N, Milad G: Notes from ancient Egypt. International Journal of Geriatric Psychiatry 5:403–405, 1990

Matsubayashi K, Shimada K, Kawamoto A, et al: Incidental brain lesions on magnetic resonance imaging and neurobehavioral functions in the apparently healthy elderly. Stroke 23:175–180, 1992

Mayberg HS, Robinson RG, Wong DF, et al: PET imaging of cortical S2 serotonin receptors after stroke: lateralized changes and relationship to depression. Am J Psychiatry 145:937–943, 1988

Mayberg HS, Starkstein SE, Bolduc P, et al: Frontal lobe hypometabolism in depressed non-demented patients with Parkinson's disease (abstract). J Cereb Blood Flow Metab 9 (suppl 1):S346, 1989

Mayberg HS, Starkstein SE, Sadzot B, et al: Selective hypometabolism in the interior frontal lobe in depressed patients with Parkinson's disease. Ann Neurol 28:57–64, 1990

Mayeux R, Stern Y, Rosen J, et al: Depression, intellectual impairment and Parkinson's disease. Neurology 3:645–650, 1981

Mayeux R, Stern Y, Williams JBW, et al: Clinical and biochemical features of depression in Parkinson's disease. Am J Psychiatry 143:756–759, 1986

Mayeux R, Stern Y, Sano M, et al: The relationship of serotonin to depression in Parkinson's disease. Mov Disord 3:237–244, 1988

McKeith IG, Marshall EF, Ferrier IN, et al: 5-HT receptor binding in post-mortem brain from patients with affective disorder. J Affect Disord 13:67–74, 1987

Minski L, Guttman E: Huntington's chorea: a study of thirty-four families. Journal of Mental Science 84:21–96, 1938

Molchan SE, Hill JL, Mellow AM, et al: The dexamethasone suppression test in Alzheimer's disease and major depression: relationship to dementia severity, depression and CSF monoamines. Int Psychogeriatr 2:99–122, 1990

Murray BB, Shea V, Conn DK: Electroconvulsive therapy for post-stroke depression. J Clin Psychiatry 47:258–260, 1986

Nasrallah HA, Coffman JA, Olson SC: Structural brain imaging findings in affective disorders: an overview. J Neuropsychiatry Clin Neurosci 1:21–26, 1989

Nemeroff CB, Knight DL, Krishnan KRR, et al: Marked reduction in the number of platelet tritiated imipramine binding sites in geriatric depression. Arch Gen Psychiatry 45:919–923, 1988

Nissenbaum H, Qunn NP, Brown RG, et al: Mood swings associated with the "on-off" phenomenon in Parkinson's disease. Psychol Med 17:899–904, 1987

Pearlson GD, Rabins PV, Kim WS, et al: Structural brain changes and cognitive deficits in elderly depressives with and without reversible dementia ("pseudodementia"). Psychol Med 19:573–584, 1989

Pearlson GD, Ross CA, Lohr WD, et al: Association between family history of affective disorder and the depressive syndrome of Alzheimer's disease. Am J Psychiatry 147:452–456, 1990

Pearson J, Teri L, Nefler B, et al: Functional status and cognitive impairment in Alzheimer's disease patients with and without depression. J Am Geriatr Soc 39:1117–1121, 1989

Poeck K: Pathophysiology of emotional disorders associated with brain damage, in Handbook of Clinical Neurology, Vol 3: Disorders of Higher Nervous Activity. Edited by Vinken PJ, Bruyn GW. Amsterdam, North-Holland Publishing, 1969, pp 343–367

Rabins PV, Pearlson GD: Depression induced cognitive impairment, in Dementia. Edited by Burns A, Levy R. London, Chapman and Hall, in press

Rabins PV, Mace NL, Lucas MJ: The impact of dementia on family. JAMA 248:333–335, 1982

Rabins PV, Harvis K, Koven S: High fatality rates of late-life depression associated with cardiovascular disease. J Affect Disord 9:165–167, 1985

Rabins PV, Pearlson GD, Aylward E, et al: Cortical magnetic resonance imaging changes in elderly inpatients with major depression. Am J Psychiatry 148:617–620, 1991

Reding MJ, Orto LA, Willenski P: The dexamethasone suppression test: an indicator of depression in stroke but not a predictor of rehabilitation outcome. Arch Neurol 42:209–212, 1985a

Reding MJ, Haycox J, Blass J: Depression in patients referred to a dementia clinic. Arch Neurol 42:894–896, 1985b

Reding MJ, Orto LA, Winter SN, et al: Antidepressant therapy after stroke: a double blind trial. Arch Neurol 43:763–765, 1986

Reifler BV, Larson E, Teri L: Dementia of the Alzheimer's type and depression. J Am Geriatr Soc 34:855–859, 1986

Reifler BV, Teri L, Raskind M, et al: Double-blind trial of imipramine in Alzheimer's disease patients with and without depression. Am J Psychiatry 146:45–49, 1989

Reynolds CF, Kupfer DJ, Hoch CC, et al: Two-year follow-up of elderly patients with mixed depression and dementia. J Am Geriatr Soc 34:793–799, 1986

Reynolds EH, Preece JM, Bailey J, et al: Folate deficiency in depressive illness. Br J Psychiatry 117:287–292, 1970

Robins AH: Depression in patients with Parkinsonism. Br J Psychiatry 128:141–145, 1976

Robinson RG, Kubos KL, Starr LB, et al: Mood disorders in stroke patients: importance of location of lesion. Brain 107:82–93, 1984

Robinson RG, Lipsey JR, Bolla-Wilson K, et al: Mood disorder in left-handed stroke patients. Am J Psychiatry 142:1426–1429, 1985

Robinson RG, Bolduc PL, Price TR: Two-year longitudinal study of post-stroke mood disorders: diagnosis and outcome at one and two years. Stroke 18:837–843, 1987

Robinson RG, Boston JD, Starkstein SE, et al: Comparison of mania with depression following brain injury. Am J Psychiatry 145:172–178, 1988

Robinson RG, Rajesh RM, Lipsey JR, et al: Pathological laughing and crying following stroke: validation of a measurement scale and a double-blind treatment study. Am J Psychiatry 150:286–293, 1993

Romanoski AJ, Folstein MF, Nestadt G, et al: The epidemiology of psychiatrist-ascertained depression and DSM-III depressive disorders. Psychol Med 22:629–655, 1992

Rovner BW, Morris RK: Depression and Alzheimer's disease, in Depression and Coexisting Disease. Edited by Robinson RC, Rabins PV. New York, Igate Shoin Medical, 1989, pp 202–212

Ruggieri S, Stocchi F, Devoro A, et al: The role of MAO-B inhibitors in the treatment of Parkinson's disease. J Neural Transm Suppl 22:227–233, 1986

Salzman C, Schneider L, Lebowitz B: Antidepressant treatment of very old patients. American Journal of Geriatric Psychiatry 1:21–29, 1993

Schiffer RB, Herndon RM, Rudick RA: Treatment of pathologic laughing and weeping with amitriptyline. N Engl J Med 312:1480–1482, 1985

Schleifer SJ, Keller SE, Bond RB, et al: Major depressive disorder and immunity. Arch Gen Psychiatry 46:81–87, 1989

Schnieder LS, Severson JA, Sloane RB: Platelet [3H] imipramine binding in depressed elderly patients. Biol Psychiatry 20:1232–1234, 1985

Shulman KI, Post F: Bipolar affective disorder in old age. Br J Psychiatry 136:26–32, 1980

Shulman KI, Tohen M, Satlin A, et al: Mania compared with unipolar depression in old age. Am J Psychiatry 149:341–345, 1992

Siegal B, Gurevich D, Oxenkrug GF: Cognitive impairment and cortisol resistance to dexamethasone suppression in elderly depression. Biol Psychiatry 25:229–234, 1989

Silfverskiöld P, Risberg J: Regional cerebral blood flow in depression and mania. Arch Gen Psychiatry 46:253–259, 1989

Silver JM, Hales RE, Yudofsky SC: Neuropsychiatric aspects of traumatic brain injury, in The American Psychiatric Association Textbook of Neuropsychiatry, 2nd Edition. Washington, DC, American Psychiatric Association, 1992, pp 363–395

Sim M, Sussman I: Alzheimer disease: it's natural history and differential diagnosis. J Nerv Ment Dis 135:489–499, 1962

Singer E: The effect of treatment with levodopa on Parkinson patients' social functioning and outlook on life. Journal of Chronic Diseases 27:581–594, 1974

Sinyor D, Jacques P, Laloupek DG, et al: Post-stroke depression and lesion location: an attempted replication. Brain 109:537–546, 1986

Skare S, Pew B, Dysken M: The dexamethasone suppression test in dementia: a review of the literature. J Geriatr Psychiatry Neurol 3:124–138, 1990

Skoog I, Nilsson L, Palmertz B, et al: A population based study of 85 year olds. N Engl J Med 328:153–158, 1993

Starkstein SE, Robinson RG: Affective disorders and cerebral vascular disease. Br J Psychiatry 154:170–182, 1989

Starkstein SE, Robinson RG, Price TR: Comparison of cortical and sub-cortical lesions in the production of post-stroke mood disorders. Brain 110:1045–1059, 1987

Starkstein SE, Boston JD, Robinson RG: Mechanisms of mania after brain injury: 12 case reports and review of the literature. J Nerv Mental Dis 176:87–100, 1988a

Starkstein SE, Robinson RG, Price TR: Comparison of patients with and without post-stroke major depression matched for size and location of lesion. Arch Gen Psychiatry 45:247–252, 1988b

Starkstein SE, Preziosi TJ, Berthier ML, et al: Depression and cognitive impairment in Parkinson's disease. Brain 112:1141–1153, 1989a

Starkstein SE, Robinson RG, Honig MA, et al: Mood changes after right hemisphere lesions. Br J Psychiatry 155:79–85, 1989b

Starkstein SE, Cohen BS, Federoff P, et al: Relationship between anxiety disorders and depressive disorders in patients with cerebrovascular injury. Arch Gen Psychiatry 47:246–251, 1990a

Starkstein SE, Preziosi TJ, Bolduc PL, et al: Depression in Parkinson's disease. J Nerv Mental Dis 178:27–31, 1990b

Starkstein SE, Preziosi TJ, Forrester AW, et al: Specificity of affective and autonomic symptoms of depression in Parkinson's disease. J Neurol Neurosurg Psychiatry 53:275–278, 1990c

Starkstein SE, Bryer JB, Berthier ML, et al: Depression after stroke: the importance of cerebral hemisphere assymetries. J Neuropsychiatry Clin Neurosci 3:276–285, 1991a

Starkstein SE, Federoff P, Berthier ML, et al: Manic-depressive and pure manic states after brain lesions. Biol Psychiatry 29:149–158, 1991b

Stone K: Mania in the elderly. Br J Psychiatry 155:220–224, 1989

Stoudemire GA: Selected organic mental disorders, in American Psychiatric Press Textbook of Neuropsychiatry. Washington, DC, American Psychiatric Association, 1987, pp 130–131

Strang RR: Imipramine in treatment of Parkinsonism: a double-blind placebo study. BMJ 2:33–34, 1965

Sunderland T, Alterman IS, Yount D, et al: A new scale for the assessment of depressed mood in demented patients. Am J Psychiatry 145:955–959, 1988

Swearer JM, Drachmann DA, O'Donnell BF, et al: Troublesome and disruptive behaviors in dementia. J Am Geriatr Soc 36:784–790, 1988

Taylor AE, Saint-Cyr JA, Lang AE: Frontal lobe dysfunction in Parkinson's disease. Brain 109:845–883, 1986

Teri L, Wagner A: Alzheimer's disease and depression. J Consult Clin Psychol 60:379–391, 1992

Van der Velde CD: Toxicity of lithium carbonate in elderly patients. Am J Psychiatry 127:1075–1077, 1971

Wade DR, Legh-Smith JE, Herew RA: Depressed mood after stroke: a community study of its frequency. Br J Psychiatry 151:200–205, 1987

Warburton JW: Depressive symptoms in Parkinson patients referred for thalotomy. J Neurol Neurosurg Psychiatry 30:368–370, 1967

Weissman MM, Bruce ML, Leaf PJ, et al: Affective disorders, in Psychiatric Disorders in America. Edited by Robins LN, Regier DA. New York, Free Press, 1991, pp 53–80

Young RC: Geriatric mania. Clin Geriatr Med 8:387–398, 1992

Zubenko GS, Moosy J: Major depression in primary dementia: clinical and neuropathological correlates. Arch Neurol 45:1182–1186, 1988

Zubenko GS, Moosy J, Koop U: Neurochemical correlates of major depression in primary dementia. Arch Neurol 47:209–214, 1990

Zweig RM, Ross CA, Hedreen JC, et al: The neuropathology of aminergic nuclei in Alzheimer's disease. Ann Neurol 24:233–242, 1988

13

Late-Life–Onset Psychoses

Godfrey D. Pearlson, M.D.
Richard G. Petty, M.D.

Introduction

Late-life–onset psychosis is a fascinating but heterogeneous and insufficiently explored syndrome. To examine it objectively, one should put aside commonly held notions, such as that most cases of late-life–onset psychosis represent coarse brain disease (e.g., Alzheimer's disease or microvascular pathology) or that early- and late-life–onset schizophrenia merely represent opposite tails of age distribution of the same syndrome.

Late-life–onset psychosis is a common condition, accounting for up to 10% of admissions to psychiatric hospitals for patients over age 60 (Bridge and Wyatt 1980a, 1980b; Kay and Roth 1961; Roth 1955; Siegel and Goodman 1987). It is feasible that all psychoses, including late-life–onset forms, represent a final common expression of diverse etiopathologies. This diversity is likely to be especially marked in late-life–onset conditions, a viewpoint argued by Holden (1987) and Post (1966). In part, this may be related to a general increase in age-related biological heterogeneity (Jeste and Caligiuri 1991), as well as to the emergence in late life of several neurodegenerative disorders in which psychotic symptoms are common.

Late-life–onset psychosis is a disorder classically defined on the basis of clinical phenomenology, but clinicians also define cases, somewhat inconsistently, on the basis of pathological entities (e.g., Alzheimer's disease) and etiologic descriptions (e.g., amphetamine psychosis). Two useful, but competing, approaches to defining the syndrome are 1) to cast the net broadly (i.e., include all patients with onset of delusions and hallucinations for the first time in late life) and 2) to examine a more narrowly defined group of patients who have late-life–onset delusions and hallucinations, but in the clear absence of an affective syndrome, progressive cognitive impairment, or obvious organic cause. This more restricted syndrome is closer to what has been termed *late-life–onset schizophrenia*, or *late paraphrenia*.

Depending on which of these approaches is chosen and which age at onset is used, mixtures of patients will emerge with differing etiopathologies, genetics, brain changes, and responses to treatment (Jeste et al. 1988a, 1988b, 1991). The emergence of such heterogeneous patient mixtures is precisely what has occurred with studies of such patients, resulting in a lack of clarity. As late-life–onset psychosis likely comprises a heterogeneous group of etiopathologies, even the narrowly defined group referred to above, which has been assumed by many to be most similar to early-onset schizophrenia, may well exhibit significantly more heterogeneity than would be found among a comparable group of early onset schizophrenic patients, a point made recently (Rabins and Pearlson, in press). (The full range of conditions commonly included under the broad umbrella of "late-life–onset psychosis" is discussed in the section "Diagnostic Diversity and Classification of Late-Life–Onset Psychosis" below.)

Historical Background

Use of the term *paraphrenia* (or *late paraphrenia*) is potentially problematic because of the weight of historical debates dragged in its wake. Kraepelin (1919) used this term to describe a group of chronic paranoid psychoses distinguished not by age at onset, but clinically by preservation of personality with lack of long-term deterioration and cross-sectionally by prominent elaborate delusions and hallucinations occurring in clear consciousness. Mayer (1921) followed up a large series of Kraepelin's patients and demonstrated that deterioration occurred over the long term in most such patients. The use of the term *paraphrenia* was, therefore, deleted from the following edition of Kraepelin's textbook (Kraepelin 1926). Both Bleuler (1943) and Kraepelin (1903–1904) felt that late-life–onset cases of schizophrenia closely resembled, phenomenologically, more typical early-onset cases.

Roth revived the term in his descriptions of patients with "late paraphrenia" (i.e., elderly patients with vivid and paranoid delusions and multiple hallucinations occurring in clear consciousness, with maintenance of emotional responsiveness over time) (Roth 1955; Roth and Morrisey 1952). He demonstrated that the clinical course of "late paraphrenia" was different from that of both affective disorder and dementia with onset in late life in its cross-sectional symptomatic presentation, response to treatment, and outcome; in later studies (Tomlinson et al. 1968), he demonstrated that it differed neuropathologically from dementia. Patients with "senile psychoses" (mainly Alzheimer's disease), delirious states, and arteriosclerotic psychoses (presumably multi-infarct dementia) showed a 30%–

Supported in part by National Institutes of Health Grant MH43326 (to GDP).

50% death rate at 6-month follow-up. Late paraphrenic patients, who constituted approximately 10% of Roth's total group of elderly, hospitalized psychotic patients, showed a 6-month follow-up death rate of less than 5%.

Confusingly, though some authors have remained faithful to the original definition of *late paraphrenia,* others have retained the term, but significantly broadened the concept to include patients with earlier onset (e.g., after age 45) or all late-life onset psychoses.

Epidemiology and Prevalence

In a review of the literature, Harris and Jeste (1988) estimated that 13% of hospitalized schizophrenic patients have onset of the syndrome in their 50s, 7% in their 60s, and 3% in their 70s or later. Prevalence rates of late-life–onset schizophrenia in previous studies are frequently complicated by the unselected nature of the patient populations (see Harris and Jeste 1988). Social isolation and suspiciousness associated with the syndrome may also tend to minimize the true prevalence of the disorder. Reviews by Almeida et al. (in press) and Naguib and Levy (1991) show that prior epidemiological surveys of schizophrenia in the elderly have mainly surveyed hospital populations. For example, the studies of Roth and Morrisey (1952), Kay and Roth (1961), and Blessed and Wilson (1982) showed that about 10% of elderly patients admitted to psychiatric hospitals have a later-life–onset schizophrenic syndrome. A small number of community-based studies in the United States and United Kingdom have depicted late-life–onset schizophrenia rates varying from

1% to 4% in elderly individuals. Holden's study (1987) of a community case register in the United Kingdom showed rates of 17–25 per 100,000 surveyed. Obviously, prevalence rates vary depending on the inclusion or exclusion criteria, perhaps most significantly the issue of possible organic etiology.

Clinical Picture and Phenomenology: Old Versus Young Schizophrenic Patients

The best documented clinical descriptions of patients with late-life–onset schizophrenia remain the classic summaries of Kay and Roth (1961). The phenomenology of late-life–onset psychosis and its relationship to "classic" early-onset cases has engendered debates for nearly a century. As mentioned above, Kraepelin stated in the 7th edition of his textbook (Kraepelin 1903–1904) that late-life–onset schizophrenic cases "cannot be at all separated from juvenile forms" (p. 213). However, some contrasts in phenomenological features in course between early- and late-life–onset cases have also frequently been commented on (e.g., Harris and Jeste 1988; Harris et al. 1988; Kolle 1931; Mayer-Gross 1932). Some of these differences are summarized in Table 13–1.

Phenomenologically, in cases of "late paraphrenia" (i.e., more narrowly defined late-life–onset schizophrenia), persecutory delusions are the most common, but delusions of multiple types are often seen. Auditory hallucinations are most commonly seen, but hallucinations in multiple modalities are frequently reported, as are Schneiderian first-rank symptoms (Marneros and

Table 13–1. Comparison of symptoms among late-life–onset, young early-onset, and elderly early-onset schizophrenia patients

Symptoms	Young early-onset schizophrenic patients	Late-life–onset schizophrenic patients	Elderly early-onset schizophrenic patients
Hallucinations	80% (Pearlson et al. 1989)	Present in 94%; more vivid in multiple modalities (Kay and Roth 1961; Pearlson et al. 1989)	100% (Pearlson et al. 1989)
Delusions	69% (Pearlson et al. 1989)	98% (Pearlson et al. 1989) especially persecutory (also Kay and Roth 1961)	100% (Pearlson et al. 1989)
Schneiderian first-rank symptoms	50% (Pearlson et al. 1989)	35% (Pearlson et al. 1989); thought insertion and withdrawal rarer than early-onset schizophrenia (Grahame 1984; Holden 1987)	41% (Pearlson et al. 1989)
Formal thought disorder	52% (Pearlson et al. 1989)	Rare (5.6%) (Pearlson et al. 1989); similar (Bleuler 1943; Gabriel 1978; Huber et al. 1975)	55% (Pearlson et al. 1989)
Negative symptoms	22% (Pearlson et al. 1989)	Rarer (e.g., Bleuler 1943; Castle and Howard 1992; Pearlson et al. 1989)	23% (Pearlson et al. 1989)

Deister 1984; Pearlson et al. 1989). Thought disorder and negative symptoms are relatively rare (Bleuler 1943; Castle and Howard 1992; Pearlson and Rabins 1988; Pearlson et al. 1989).

Pathoplastic age-associated features may mold the symptomatic expression. For example, "partition" delusions (i.e., delusions that people, gas, electricity, or some other force enters the patient's home through the walls [partitions] from a neighbor's apartment), which are said to be common in late-life–onset schizophrenia, may be influenced in content rather than form by the isolation and homeboundness commonly seen in elderly people. Castle and Murray (1991) argued that the schizophrenia-like illness occurring for the first time in elderly people, predominantly women, represents a form of affective disorder. Although interesting (and further discussed in this chapter), this assertion remains essentially unproven. However, few studies have contrasted late-life–onset schizophrenic patients with groups of affective disorder patients or other relevant comparison populations, such as early-onset schizophrenic patients grown old and young early-onset schizophrenic patients (some exceptions being Pearlson et al. 1989; Rabins et al. 1984).

Until recently, clinical phenomenology has been the major classificatory tool for schizophrenia researchers. This limitation has put psychiatrists at a disadvantage (comparable to that of cardiologists before electrocardiograms, chest X rays, nuclear medicine cardiac scans, and enzyme studies). Interpreting reasons behind the phenomenological differences between early- and late-life–onset schizophrenic patients, especially the differences in thought disorder and negative symptoms, is difficult. Is this, for example, a completely different illness, the same illness occurring in an older person, or only a case of similar clinical abnormalities occurring in an older brain assailed by neurodegenerative changes and mimicking what is most usually a neurodevelopmental disorder? (After reviewing further evidence, we attempt to address such questions in the "Conclusions" section below.).

Diagnostic Diversity and Classification of Late-Life–Onset Psychosis

Scope of the Disorder

If, as noted in the introduction, one uses a broad definition of late-life–onset psychosis patients, the follow-ing mixture of patient groups is likely to be included (Table 13–2):

1. **Elderly early-onset schizophrenic patients.** Such patients are frequently encountered, as schizophrenia is not a fatal illness. Because it is unresolved whether early- and late-life–onset cases represent the same disorder, verification of age at onset must be carefully sought from available relatives or other informants and by examination of prior medical records.

2. **Patients with late-life–onset schizophrenia ("late paraphrenia").** As discussed in the introduction, nomenclature for this group has been especially confusing. In general, the term *late paraphrenia* (Roth 1955) has been applied to a more circumscribed group consisting of patients who have the onset in late life (i.e., over age 60) of a syndrome that clinically closely resembles early-onset schizophrenia. There is a long debate in the British literature (e.g., Almeida et al. 1992) between those psychiatrists who view these patients as having late-life–onset classic schizophrenia (e.g., Grahame 1984) and those who have emphasized its heterogeneity (e.g., Holden 1987). DSM-IV (American Psychiatric Association 1994) uses the term "late-onset" schizophrenia for patients meeting criteria for schizophrenia, with symptomatic onset (including prodrome) after age 45.

3. **Patients with paranoid psychoses without hallucinations.** Unlike those with late-life–onset schizophrenia, in which hallucinations are vivid and often in multiple modalities, these patients corre-

Table 13–2.   Groups included in a broad classification of "late-life–onset psychosis" patients

Elderly early-onset schizophrenia patients

Patients with late-life–onset schizophrenia ("late paraphrenia")

Patients with paranoid psychoses without hallucinations

Psychotic affective patients

Cerebrovascular disease patients:
  Classic multi-infarct dementia with psychotic symptoms "Multi-infarct disease"

Alzheimer's disease patients with psychotic symptoms

Patients with psychoses of miscellaneous causes with and without defined neuropathology
  Patients in delirious and toxic states
  Patients with extremes of paranoid or schizoid personality types

spond to those with "persistent delusional disorders" with late onset, as described by DSM-IV, and to earlier descriptions in the literature by researchers such as Kay and Roth (1961) and Holden (1987). Anecdotally, such patients do not later develop hallucinations and tend to respond poorly to neuroleptic medications. If such is the case, this disorder seems rather remote from late-life–onset schizophrenia.

4. **Psychotic affective patients.** Elderly patients with mood-incongruent delusions and hallucinations are often encountered (Kay et al. 1976). They correspond to individuals with the late-life–onset of psychosis described as the "affective group" by Holden (1987), and, as discussed in Chapter 12, family history and phenomenology of prior episodes may aid differential diagnosis.

5. **Cerebrovascular disease patients.** *Classic multi-infarct dementia* is not infrequently accompanied by psychotic symptoms. Cummings (1985) reported that approximately 50% of patients with multi-infarct dementia have delusions. We propose below that the number of patients with *"multi-infarct disease"* (see below) is significantly larger than previously estimated, with the larger prevalence now revealed through the increasing clinical application of magnetic resonance imaging (MRI) and single photon emission computed tomography (SPECT). It is becoming clear that an unknown, but significant, percentage of patients with late-life–onset psychosis manifests imaging changes consistent with cerebrovascular disease, not necessarily accompanied by cognitive deficits and hence not meeting criteria for multi-infarct dementia. This accounts for our use of the term *multi-infarct disease.* Case series have been described by Miller et al. (1991, 1992) and Lesser et al. (1992).

6. **Alzheimer's disease patients with psychotic symptoms.** Patients with Alzheimer's disease often manifest secondary delusions and hallucinations (e.g., Rubin 1992). The patient described in Alzheimer's original case report had delusional beliefs, and the characteristics of hallucinating and delusional Alzheimer's patients have recently been described in review articles by Wragg and Jeste (1989) and Burns et al. (1990a, 1990b). Delusions in Alzheimer's disease tend to be rather fragmentary and impersistent. Careful follow-up of late-life–onset psychosis patients is therefore necessary to identify those with emerging dementia syndromes.

7. **Patients with psychoses of miscellaneous causes with and without defined neuropathology.** Cerebral infections, tumors, Parkinson's disease, stroke, head injury, and other causes can all be associated with late-life emergence of hallucinations and delusions in clear consciousness (e.g., Signer 1992). *Delirious and toxic states* (e.g., anticholinergic delirium, alcohol withdrawal, hypothyroidism, and amphetamine psychosis) can manifest with similar symptomatology. Finally, *extremes of paranoid or schizoid personality types* (e.g., those described by Post [1966] and Holden [1987]) can be mistaken for cases of late-life–onset psychosis if only cross-sectional information is available.

A Classificatory and Investigational Scheme

With so many possible syndromes encompassing diverse etiopathologies, yet sharing common clinical features, it is clear that prior studies have often been alluding to diverse patient groups. We (Rabins and Pearlson, in press) used a multiaxial approach to classification using genetics, epidemiology, risk factors, phenomenology, course, treatment response, neuropathology, and biological markers. To evaluate patients thoroughly, to proceed from a common reference point, and to rule out other diagnoses, for a particular patient, the following information in Table 13–3 should ideally be gathered.

Risk Factors for Late-Life–Onset Schizophrenia

As shown in many review articles (Almeida et al., in press; Harris and Jeste 1988; Pearlson and Rabins 1988; Pearlson et al. 1989), multiple risk factors associated with more narrowly defined late-life–onset schizophrenia have been enumerated (Table 13–4).

Genetic

As regards family history of schizophrenia, Kay (1972) showed that the percentage of affected first-degree relatives for late-life–onset schizophrenia patients (3.4%) was intermediate between that of early-onset schizophrenia patients (5.8%) and that of the known risk (1%) in the general population. As reviewed by Castle and Howard (1992) and by us (Pearlson and Rabins 1988), there are problems in the assessment of family history rates, however. Prior studies have often not used standardized instruments such as family history, research diagnostic criteria, or an adoption study design. Informants for late-life–onset diseases are often dead or unavailable or may have died before the age of clinical risk, if the illness "breeds true" as has been suggested by some authors. The evidence overall is consistent with the notion that late-life–onset psychosis is partly genetically determined; however, much remains to be clarified.

Sex

Female sex appears to be a very robust risk factor, even when the relative excess of older women is corrected for. The excess of female patients in late-life–onset cases has variously been reported as 6- to 20-fold (Herbert and Jacobson 1967; Kay and Roth 1961). Although some authors (e.g., Pearlson and Rabins 1988) believe that this sex effect represents a shift in the female incidence of schizophrenia to late life (Lewine 1981, 1985), others (e.g., Castle and Murray 1991) have argued otherwise.

Table 13–3. Information (both clinical and laboratory) to be gathered in cases of late-life–onset psychosis

---

Family history (e.g., of early- or late-onset schizophrenia, affective disorder, and Alzheimer's disease)

Complete past psychiatric history (especially prior affective episodes)

Medical history, including history of stroke, transient ischemic attacks, and an assessment of vascular risk factors, using standardized instruments

Premorbid level of functioning

Premorbid personality

Current medications

Current detailed cognitive functioning

Current social supports

Sensory screening examination

History of present illness, especially age at onset of psychosis, relative to other known comorbid states (e.g., Alzheimer's disease)

Complete physical and neurological examination

Routine laboratory tests for reversible causes of dementia (e.g., B_{12} and folate levels and syphilis serology)

Standardized neuroimaging studies, especially magnetic resonance imaging (MRI) and single photon emission computed tomography (SPECT), both to rule out coarse brain disease (e.g., obvious strokes and tumors) and to quantify extent of nonspecific changes (e.g., subcortical white matter hyperintensities)

Sensory Deficits

Sensory deficits, especially auditory and visual declines, which are more common in late life, have been reported in many studies to be a relative risk factor for late-life–onset schizophrenia. Cataracts and conductive deafness are the most common causes. Some authors (e.g., Eastwood et al. 1981) have stated that psychotic symptoms respond favorably to treatment of the deafness. Findings related to sensory deficits have been reported by multiple authors (e.g., Cooper and Porter 1976; Cooper et al. 1974; Naguib and Levy 1987; Pearlson et al. 1989; Post 1966). Conductive deafness seems to be a risk factor rather specific to late-life–onset schizophrenia, with prevalence being significantly higher than in late-life–onset affective patients (e.g., Cooper et al. 1974). As reviewed by us (Pearlson and Rabins 1988), sensory impairment can be associated with reduced social contact and lead, therefore, to social isolation, suspiciousness, and liability to misinterpret environmental events. In an individual who is already predisposed to develop late-life–onset schizophrenia, sensory impairment may therefore encourage symptomatic formation. Sensory deficits may thus in part account for the higher rates of social isolation reported in late-life–onset schizophrenia patients. Kay and Roth (1961) reported sensory impairments rates three times higher among late-life–onset schizophrenia patients than those among elderly affective disorder patients.

Premorbid Personality

Another factor undoubtedly contributing to social isolation is the abnormal premorbid personality (mainly paranoid or schizoid) identified by multiple researchers as preceding late-life–onset psychosis (Kay 1972;

Table 13–4. Risk factors associated with late-life–onset schizophrenia

---

Family history of schizoprenia

Female sex

Sensory deficits (primarily auditory and visual)

Social isolation

Abnormal premorbid personality

Never married/no children

Human leukocyte antigen (HLA) subtypes

Lower social class

Kay and Roth 1961; Herbert and Jacobson 1967; Pearlson et al. 1989; Post 1966). Kay and Roth (1961) and Post (1966), but not our team (Pearlson et al. 1989), found that women with late-life–onset schizophrenia were significantly more likely to have never married or had children. This observation has been reported less often in United States studies. If the finding is valid, low marriage rates may be related to the abnormal premorbid personalities seen in such patients.

It remains to be determined whether the abnormal premorbid personality traits described in late-life–onset schizophrenia represent a forme fruste of a schizophrenic disorder of a longstanding nature, significantly predating emergence of overt clinical symptoms, or a "risk factor" as classically understood. Other, miscellaneous factors have been explored, such as association with human leukocyte antigens (HLA) (Naguib et al. 1987). Post (1966) showed that many late-life–onset schizophrenic patients tended to have lower socioeconomic status.

Wong et al. (1984), using positron-emission tomography (PET) to measure dopamine, subtype 2 (D_2), receptors, showed age-related decreases in the estimated number of D_2 receptors, in agreement with postmortem studies (e.g., Seeman et al. 1987). The PET data suggested that healthy men possess more D_2 receptors, but lose them at an accelerated rate with normal aging, compared with women. Hence, older women are left with a relative excess of D_2 receptors compared with men of the same age. If, as some (e.g., Pearlson and Coyle 1983) have suggested, schizophrenia is indeed related to an excess of D_2 receptors, the relative excess of D_2 receptors in young men and in elderly women may explain the classic age-related sex expression differences for schizophrenia (i.e., the fact that schizophrenia is usually expressed by men at a significantly earlier age than by women). Seeman (1981, 1986) has speculated that estrogens have "neuroleptic-like" effects on D_2 receptors, which would be lost following menopause. Similar changes in sex preponderance are not seen with early versus late-life affective disorder (e.g., Weisman 1987). A recent PET study (Pearlson et al. 1993) offered preliminary support for D_2 receptor increases in late-life–onset schizophrenia.

Brain Changes in Late-Life–Onset Schizophrenia

Compared with their respectively age-matched healthy control groups, individuals with late-life–onset psycho-sis have a significantly higher prevalence of identifiable brain abnormalities than do young individuals with similar symptoms (Miller et al. 1991). This observation is a rather general one, however. Many late-life–onset psychosis patients do not have a specific lesion or an etiology for their brain change, and lesions reported in many recent studies apparently do not share common localization or represent a single well-defined pathology. The reported prevalence of such brain changes varies, as might be expected for such a heterogeneous syndrome as late-life–onset psychosis. Some studies have carefully excluded all patients with probably organic pathology (e.g., Krull et al. 1991; Naguib and Levy 1987). Such series of screened patients have generally reported a smaller number of nonspecific brain changes (e.g., white matter hyperintensities) on MRI scans. Nevertheless, given the above caveat, new and potentially important information has emerged from structural and functional brain imaging study of patients with late-life–onset psychosis in recent years (Table 13–5). It is clear that demonstrably altered brain structure and/or function is a predisposing factor in a proportion of such cases and that this proportion is far higher than was suspected before modern neuroimaging methods. Reported changes fall into three broad categories; global structural changes, white matter hyperintensities on MRI, and cerebral blood flow changes documented on SPECT scans.

Structural Change

Several studies have demonstrated increased ventricular-to-brain ratio (VBR) in late-life–onset schizophrenia patients compared with age-matched healthy control subjects. For computed tomography (CT), such studies include Burns et al. (1989), Naguib and Levy (1987), Rabins et al. (1987), and us (Pearlson et al. 1987). Howard et al. (1992a, 1992b) found lateral VBR (as well as third ventricular changes) to be no different from that for control subjects. Rabins et al. (1987) found late-life–onset schizophrenia patients to have VBRs greater than those of control subjects, but smaller than those of Alzheimer's disease patients with psychotic symptoms. Similarly, Krull et al. (1991), assessing VBRs on MRI scans, found values in late-life–onset schizophrenia patients to be intermediate between those of control subjects and Alzheimer's disease patients. Howard et al. (1992a; see also, Almeida et al. 1992) found late-life–onset schizophrenia patients without Schneiderian first-rank symptoms to have ventricular and sulcal enlargement more comparable to that seen in Alzheimer's disease patients; in contrast, late-life–onset schizophrenia patients with first-rank symptoms were more comparable to elderly control subjects.

MRI studies in general have been less convincing in showing ventricular enlargement in late-life–onset psychosis subjects. For example, Miller et al. (1991) found no differences between patients and control subjects; we reported a similar finding (Pearlson et al. 1991). We (Pearlson et al. 1993) also reported significant third ventricular enlargement in late-life–onset psychosis patients in an MRI study, whereas Burns et al. (1989) found no cortical atrophy compared with control subjects using CT. Overall, there is some evidence for moderate cortical and subcortical changes in late-life–onset psychosis, but less so for "late paraphrenic" patients and in MRI studies.

Many studies have now reported an excess of white matter abnormalities or "unidentified bright objects" (UBOs) in late-life–onset schizophrenia patients compared with healthy control subjects (Figure 13–1). Such studies include Miller et al. (1986), Miller and Lesser (1988), Breitner et al. (1990), Lesser et al.

(1991, 1992), and Miller et al. (1991). Although there have been some suggestions of localized patterns in such studies, a general review of the changes reported (including periventricular white matter hyperintensities, probable subcortical vascular lesions, and white matter hyperintensities) does not convince one that they are either uniform in nature or clearly localized to particular brain regions.

For example, Breitner et al. (1990) reported on 8 late-life–onset paranoia patients, all of whom had significant white matter hyperintensities and 7 of whom had vascular lesions in pons or basal ganglia. Lesser et al. (1992) reported that 6 of 12 geriatric patients with DSM-III-R psychotic disorder not otherwise specified (American Psychiatric Association 1987) had large confluent white matter lesions. Miller et al. (1991) examined 24 late-life–onset psychosis patients. Temporal lobe white matter hyperintensities occurred six times more frequently among these patients than in control subjects, whereas frontal and occipital hyperintensities were found four times more frequently. Significant excess of basal ganglia and cortical abnormalities was also reported in these subjects. Flint et al. (1991) examined 16 patients with late-life–onset paranoia or paraphrenia. Five of the 16 subjects had "silent cerebral in-

Table 13–5.   Structural and functional abnormalities reported in early-onset and late-life–onset psychosis patients

Abnormality	Early-onset schizophrenia patients	Late-life–onset schizophrenia patients	Late-life–onset depression patients
Increased ventricular-brain ratio on CT or MRI	Johnstone et al. 1976; Pearlson et al. 1987; Weinberger et al. 1979	Howard et al. 1992a, 1992b; Naguib and Levy 1987; Rabins et al. 1987	Pearlson et al. 1987; Rabins et al. 1991
Third ventricular enlargement	Boronow et al. 1985	Pearlson et al. 1989 Breitner et al. 1990; Flint et al. 1991; Kohlmeyer 1988; Miller et al. 1986 (but not Krull et al. 1991)	Coffey et al. 1989, 1990; Krishnan et al. 1988; Zubenko et al. 1990
White matter abnormalities on MRI			
Cortical atrophy on CT or MRI	Gur et al. 1991; Pfefferbaum et al. 1988	Howard et al. 1992a, 1992b (but not Burns et al. 1989; Pearlson et al. 1993 [as CSF %])	Pearlson et al. 1987
Blood flow abnormalities on SPECT	Gur et al. 1985; Matthew et al. 1988	Miller et al. 1992	
Increased dopamine, subtype 2, receptor B_{max} on PET	Tune et al. (in press); Wong et al. 1986a, 1986b, 1986c		
rCBF abnormalities during provocative tasks	Weinberger et al. 1988		

Note.   CT = computed tomography; MRI = magnetic resonance imaging; CSF = cerebrospinal fluid; SPECT = single photon emission computed tomography; B_{max} = measure of receptor density; PET = positron-emission tomography; rCBF = regional cerebral blood flow.

farction," especially those with paranoia (i.e., delusional patients without hallucinations). Krull et al. (1991) carefully screened their population of 11 late-life–onset psychosis patients to attempt to eliminate those most likely to have a diagnosis of organic cerebral disorder. In 9 remaining such patients, they found no increase in white matter disease compared with Alzheimer patients or healthy control subjects.

Functional Changes

SPECT studies. Several SPECT studies now agree in showing a relative excess in late-life–onset psychosis patients of multiple areas of reduced cerebral blood flow. For example, in a diagnostically mixed group of such patients Lesser et al. (1993) showed that approximately 75% had SPECT scan abnormalities of this type. Miller et al. (1992) also demonstrated cerebral blood flow abnormalities suggestive of cerebrovascular disease in a proportion of late-life–onset psychosis patients. Further, 83% of the late-life–onset psychosis patients, versus 27% of the control subjects, had one or more small temporal or frontal areas of hypoperfusion.

PET studies. We (Pearlson et al. 1993) compared 13 neuroleptic-naive, late-life–onset schizophrenia patients (clinical onset after age 55) with 17 control subjects. Two PET scans were obtained in each subject to estimate caudate D_2 receptor density using the method previously described by Wong et al. (1986a, 1986b, 1986c). The second scan was preceded by the administration of unlabeled haloperidol to demonstrate binding under conditions of D_2 receptor blockade (Figure 13–2), and D_2 receptor B_{max} (receptor density) values were calculated using a four-compartment model.

To account for variation in B_{max} values with age and sex (the control subjects were younger), a regression equation was calculated in the control subjects and a predicted B_{max} was then computed for each schizophrenic subject based on the control regression equation. Residual values were then determined by subtraction of the observed B_{max} minus the predicted B_{max}. Standardized residual B_{max} values for schizophrenic subjects showed significant increases from zero, suggesting that B_{max} values were elevated in this group of schizophrenic subjects, even when age and sex were taken into account. This finding is similar to reports of elevated B_{max} values for D_2 receptors in drug-naive, early-onset schizophrenia patients reported by the same group (Wong et al. 1986a), although not by others using a different method (Farde et al. 1987).

There are some caveats with many of the above neuroimaging studies. First, a proportion of patients in many of the reports had clinical evidence of cerebro-

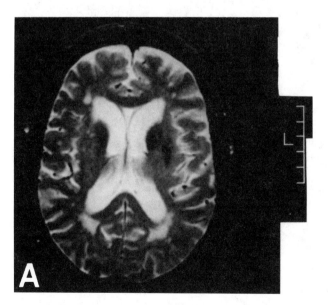
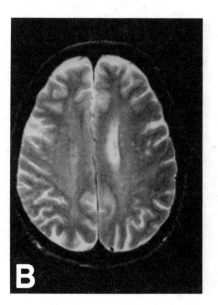

Figure 13–1. T2-weighted 5-mm axial magnetic resonance images of a 71-year-old woman with first onset of schizophrenic syndrome at age 69 (*panel A:* widest portion of lateral ventricles; *panel B:* centrum semiovale). Periventricular, subcortical, and cortical hyperintensities are visible. Ventricular enlargement is also evident (in *panel A*).

vascular disease and would unequivocally be diagnosed as having organic psychiatric syndromes. The Flint et al. (1991) and Miller et al. (1986) studies in fact identified a proportion of patients whose stroke was first diagnosed by the neuroimaging studies. Many of the changes described in the structural and blood flow studies above are nonspecific—in the sense of being unlocalized in the brain and occurring in association with other late-life–onset disorders, such as late-life–onset depression (e.g., Coffey et al. 1990)—and are not clearly associated with a particular neuropathology. Most of the reported series are small, and usually there was no follow-up to determine whether or not these patients later clinically expressed dementia syndromes. Neuropathological confirmation was lacking for most of the cases scanned. Late-life–onset psychosis patients are generally representative of an unselected series, possibly representing a referral bias in which more cases are likely to have organic factors. Most of the imaging car-

ried out has been semi- or nonquantitative. Populations have generally been diagnostically heterogeneous, including not only patients with late-life–onset schizophrenia, but also those with late-life–onset delusional disorder and late-life–onset psychosis not otherwise specified and control subjects have not always been appropriately screened or matched to patients on age, sex, race, or IQ. Nevertheless, much useful information is emerging, and study designs are gradually improving.

Neuropathology

Tomlinson et al. (1968) found no excess of plaques and tangles in late-life–onset schizophrenia patients compared with age-matched control subjects. Kay and Roth (1961) found limited cerebral lesions (mainly consisting of small strokes) in a percentage of patients with late-life–onset schizophrenia. They interpreted

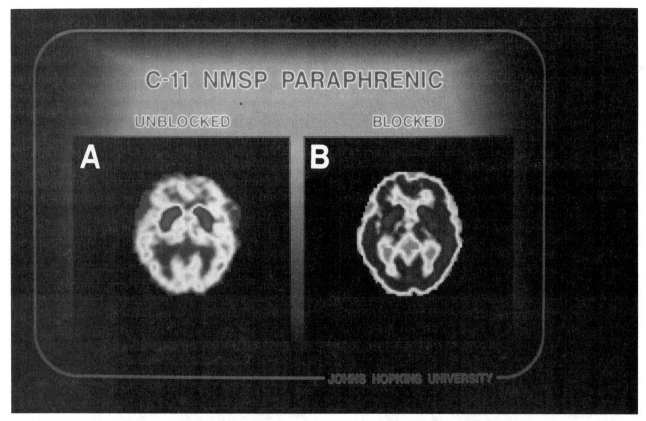

Figure 13–2. Transaxial positron-emission tomography (PET) images through basal ganglia in a never-medicated patient with late-life–onset schizophrenia (paraphrenia). *Panel A:* Uptake before blockade with oral neuroleptic, with high basal ganglia uptake relative to cortex. *Panel B:* A second scan in same subject, taken 4 hours after pretreatment with unlabeled oral haloperidol. Dopamine, subtype 2 (D_2), receptors are blocked by the cold ligand, revealing consequently lower basal ganglia activity.
Source. Photograph courtesy of D. Wong, Department of Radiology, Johns Hopkins University, Baltimore, Maryland.

these lesions as having often been present years before the onset of psychotic symptoms. This observation contrasts with the studies of Bleuler (1943) who found cerebral lesions in a proportion of late-life–onset schizophrenia patients, which he believed had appeared years after the onset of their psychotic symptoms. This vascular neuropathology, however, is in accord with several recent studies (Flint et al. 1991; Holden 1987; Miller et al. 1986) that have reported on association between stroke and the onset of psychotic symptoms in elderly patients. Such cases appear to be associated with mild cognitive loss, a greater propensity to manifesting visual hallucinations, fewer overall hallucinations, and fewer Schneiderian first-rank symptoms and are thus less typically "schizophrenic." Overall, neuropathological studies are few, and clear conclusions are hard to draw. Imaging studies and neuropathology suggest a role for cerebrovascular disease in some patients—a theme expanded in the "Conclusions" section below.

Neuropsychological Testing in Late-Life–Onset Psychosis

Miller et al. 1991 compared 21 late-life–onset psychosis patients (over age 45) with an equal number of individually matched (on education, age, and sex) healthy control subjects. The psychotic patients showed an overall decrement in cognitive functioning. After correction for multiple comparisons, several frontal measures and a verbal memory task showed significant impairment of the psychotic patients. The authors felt that this was a pattern similar to that identified by previous researchers in early-onset schizophrenia. Naguib and Levy (1987) tested 43 late paraphrenic subjects and found cognitive differences from healthy control subjects. These patients were later followed by Hymas et al. (1989), who tested 42 patients with "late paraphrenia" and attempted to exclude those with obvious early dementias. Mild neuropsychological deficits were present at the onset of illness and tended to progress somewhat with time, but not to frank dementia.

Overall, patients seen in our own clinic tend to be poorly educated and from rural backgrounds, with low average estimated premorbid IQ. It is especially hard in such cases to document deterioration from an uncertain but low premorbid level of functioning. Our review of the literature suggests that patients with late-life–onset psychosis tend to perform worse on stan-

dardized tests than do matched control subjects, but if patients with obvious organic factors are excluded, the remaining patients do not have obvious dementia and most do not develop diagnosable dementing illnesses at follow-up.

Treatment and Treatment Response

Differential diagnosis needs first to be confirmed. The mainstay of treatment of late-life–onset psychosis has been neuroleptic drugs, but lack of insight into illness and suspiciousness can result in variable medication compliance. Late-life–onset psychosis patients tend not to seek treatment. The psychiatrist is often involved late in the illness, offering treatment to an uncooperative patient (e.g., see, Almeida et al., in press; Post 1984). As might be expected, medication compliance, depot medication, and use of a community psychiatric nurse for outpatients all favorably affect treatment response (Howard and Levy 1992).

Despite the paucity of well-organized, double-blind crossover treatment trials, several open trials of neuroleptics have shown substantial improvement in a subgroup of well-characterized, late-life–onset psychosis patients. Four studies over a 25-year period are summarized in Table 13–6.

Clinical improvement overall seems most likely to occur in late-life–onset psychosis patients whose phenomenology most resembles that of early-onset schizophrenia. We (Pearlson et al. 1989) found that patients with poor medication response tend to be characterized by schizoid premorbid traits; we also found no effect on response of presence of first-rank symptoms, positive family history of schizophrenia, or sex. Holden (1987) found that patients with poor clinical response were characterized by an absence of auditory halluci-

Table 13–6. Results of neuroleptic treatment in late-life–onset psychosis

Study	Complete remission	Partial remission	No improvement	N patient
Post 1966	60.5%	31%	8.5%	71
Rabins et al. 1984	57%	28.5%	14.5%	34
Pearlson et al. 1989	48%	28%	24%	54
Howard and Levy 1992	27%	31%	42%	64

nations or affective features. This is similar to the situation in younger people with schizophrenia, in which florid hallucinations, prominent affective features, and an acute onset (especially if associated with some precipitating event) are all associated with a good prognosis. Flint et al. (1991) similarly found patients with paranoid delusions alone to respond poorly to neuroleptic agents.

Although both early- and late-life–onset schizophrenia patients tend to respond to neuroleptics with amelioration of positive symptoms, factors affecting interpretation of studies in late-life–onset patients include differential symptom patterns in late- versus early-onset forms of schizophrenia and different pharmacodynamics in young versus old patients. Treatment with neuroleptic medications in elderly patients must be tempered by knowledge of differential responsiveness, which depends in part on age-related changes in body size and composition (e.g., increased proportion of adipose tissue and decreased renal function) (for a review, see Tran-Johnson et al. 1992). There are also pharmacokinetic changes (e.g., trend for higher plasma neuroleptic levels at same doses compared with younger patients) and pharmacodynamic changes, including increased sensitivity to therapeutic and toxic effects (possibly due to altered density and affinity of relevant cerebral receptors) (see Branchey et al. 1978). The differential side effect profile of older patients includes higher risk of tardive dyskinesia, falls, anticholinergic side effects with low-potency neuroleptics (including delirium, worsening of glaucoma, cardiac abnormalities, and urinary outflow obstructions), and worsening of preexisting parkinsonian syndromes. Knowledge of individual patients' existing medical illness and other medications is therefore necessary (see Table 13–2).

Course and Prognosis

Although there is a paucity of long-term follow-up studies, investigators agree that the course of late-life–onset schizophrenia is a chronic one (Herbert and Jacobson 1967; Kay and Roth 1961). Fish (1960) emphasized the poor prognosis of the condition, but Roth (1955) offered more optimism, stating that mortality was much less than in comparably aged dementia or depression patients. It is clear, however, that a subgroup of late-life–onset psychosis patients do develop dementia. Again, because heterogeneous samples

have been followed in many studies, the relative proportions of subjects with clear-cut dementing illnesses presenting with psychotic symptoms are unknown.

Based on chart review only, Kay and Roth (1961) found that 12% of their late-life–onset paraphrenia patients had developed dementing illnesses at 10-year follow-up. Holden (1987) found that 35% of his patient group had dementia at 3-year follow-up. Craig and Bregman (1988) followed a select group of treatment-resistant, late-life–onset psychosis patients and found that 10 of 15 had dementia. Lesser et al. (1989) and Miller et al. (1991) found that, as a group, their 24 late-life–onset psychosis patients had mild cognitive abnormalities when initially evaluated; on follow-up, many of these patients had developed classic dementia syndromes such as Alzheimer's or Pick's disease. Finally, Hymas et al. (1989) found that nearly half of their 42 late-life–onset psychosis patients showed evidence of cognitive decline at 4-year follow-up, especially those with low cognitive scores at entry. Only 2 of the patients, however, met diagnostic criteria for dementia.

The inconsistency of results obtained in different studies is difficult to explain, but probably relates to ascertainment bias. The key point is that in all studies there has been a significantly higher incidence of dementia in patients found to have late-life–onset psychosis than would be found in a comparable population of elderly individuals. Overall, the long-term outcome of late-life–onset psychosis depends on a more clear division of these patients into diagnostic subgroups as suggested above.

Multi-Infarct Disease and Its Relationship to Late-Life–Onset Psychosis

Our hypothesis concerning multi-infarct disease and its relationship to late-life–onset psychosis is a straightforward one: that microvascular disease in elderly patients can be associated with new onset of major psychiatric disorders, including schizophrenia, in the absence of dementia. Thus we draw a distinction between multi-infarct *disease* and multi-infarct *dementia*.

Evidence for this conjecture derives from several sources. The observed excess of UBOs in both late-life–onset depression and late-life–onset schizophrenia on MRI and the patchy areas of reduced cerebral blood flow on SPECT suggest vascular pathology in patients with these syndromes. It appears from many studies (e.g., Breitner et al. 1990; Miller and Lesser 1988;

Miller et al. 1986) that patients with white matter lesions on MRIs tend to have higher numbers of vascular risk factors. Various hypotheses can be generated from these observations. The most nonspecific is that any form of "brain damage" in late life renders an individual more likely to express major psychiatric syndromes and such "damage" subsumes a collection of common etiologies for several late-life–onset major psychiatric illnesses. Alternatively, and far more specifically, the observed white matter abnormalities on MRI and SPECT may represent a single pathophysiological outcome (i.e., cerebral microvascular disease) that is a highly specific risk factor for late-life–onset schizophrenia. This seems unlikely, however, as similar changes are reported for late-life–onset depressive syndromes (Coffey et al. 1988). In addition, confirmation of the vascular etiology and/or pathology of the changes seen on cerebral imaging studies is still lacking.

From a consideration of the same observations, Guze and Szuba (1992) offered an alternative interpretation. They suggested that these neuroimaging findings are a function of normal age-related brain changes, but "beyond a critical threshold, they may increase vulnerability" to late-life–onset major psychiatric illnesses, in combination with other risk factors. Such additional risk factors could include family history of a particular disorder and the anatomic site of the brain findings (e.g., Rabins et al. 1991). These combined vulnerabilities determine the final form of the illness (e.g., late-life–onset schizophrenia, late-life–onset depression, multi-infarct dementia, or a senile-onset movement disorder). If UBOs and white matter lesions are of vascular origin, the above suggestions taken to their logical conclusion would place many cases of late-life–onset psychosis and depression in a continuum of pathology with multi-infarct dementia.

Conclusions

Late-life–onset psychosis is clearly a heterogeneous and understudied syndrome. Much that is vital to comprehend is still unknown, for example, how best to subdivide the condition meaningfully and, for each resulting separate syndrome, how to determine its precise prevalence and find its important pathophysiological underpinnings. Also remaining obscure are the syndrome's precise relationship to early-onset schizophrenia, response to treatment, and long-term outcome.

Although neuroimaging has the potential to provide important insights into the underlying pathophysiology, the numbers of subjects studied in most recent studies have been small, and there is a great need for large-scale longitudinal studies with suitable comparison patients (e.g., patients with late-life–onset affective disorders or elderly patients with early-onset schizophrenia). Finally, neuropathological examination is ultimately needed to clarify the nature of the underlying brain processes.

More narrowly defined cases of late-life–onset schizophrenia (or late paraphrenia) appear both more clinically homogeneous and most phenomenologically similar to early-onset schizophrenia. Even when more narrowly defined, late-life–onset psychosis appears to be a more diverse syndrome than early-onset schizophrenia, and neurodegenerative changes play a larger etiologic role than formerly envisioned. Evidence suggests that neurodegenerative and neurodevelopmental changes likely contribute to late-life–onset psychosis, but because the relative importance of each is unknown in most cases it is too soon to settle the question of whether early- and late-life–onset schizophrenia are essentially the same condition (a theme discussed by both Almeida et al. [in press] and us [Rabins and Pearlson, in press]). Perhaps the clearest parallel is with late-life–onset depressive illness (see Chapter 12). There, too, one finds a genetic risk for the appropriate illness (albeit a diminished one compared with early-onset forms of the disease), evidence in some subjects of nonspecific brain changes (identified by neuroimaging techniques), and a likely heterogeneous mixture of delayed "true" cases and "organic phenocopies." Neuroimaging clearly has the potential to help "biotype" the syndrome and to clarify the question of diversity. However, documenting the choice of index and comparison patients, as well as of control subjects, is critical in this endeavor, as some neuroimaging studies have cast their recruitment net broadly, whereas others have excluded cases with likely "organic" associations.

Returning to the theme of affective illness, we believe that Castle and Murray's viewpoint (1991) that late-life–onset cases of schizophrenia in fact represent affective disorder is unlikely. Our opinion is based on recent observations that late-life–onset schizophrenia and affective disorder comparison patients have different patterns of atrophy on the CERAD (Consortium to Establish a Registry for Alzheimer's Disease; Morris et al. 1989) MRI rating scale (Aylward et al. 1993; Rabins et al., in press) and differ phenomenologically (Rabins et al. 1984). Also the types of abnormal premorbid personality reported in late-life–onset schizophrenia and affective disorder differ, the risks of family members being affected with affective disorder versus schizophrenia appear to be different in the two groups, and the syndromes respond to different types of treatment.

So far, interactions between the various risk factors reported for late-life–onset schizophrenia, as well as the ability to separate necessary from sufficient associations, lack the development of an encompassing theory. As we have stated (Pearlson et al. 1993), the etiology and timing of the structural changes in late-life–onset schizophrenia are unknown. They could be primarily initiated in late life, or alternatively, depend on age-related brain changes unmasking a preexisting (perhaps genetic) vulnerability. If a developmental origin, similar to that proposed for early-onset cases (Weinberger 1987), is also applicable to some cases of late-life–onset schizophrenia (e.g., as we have suggested [Pearlson and Rabins 1988]), a vital point to address is why symptomatic onset has been delayed to the senium. In this chapter, we have reviewed evidence that such possible precipitants for late-life–onset psychosis could include neuronal loss due to usual aging and vascular or age-related functional changes, especially those affecting females, such as postmenopausal estrogen loss and thus alterations in the relative balance of dopamine D_2 receptors in basal ganglia. The role of late-life brain abnormalities and the relative contributions of neurodegenerative processes versus brain damage secondary to stroke or microvascular disease remain to be elucidated. Cerebrovascular pathology is likely to prove an important etiologic factor for a significant proportion of late-life–onset major psychiatric illnesses, including psychosis.

References

Almeida OP, Howard R, Förstl H, et al: Should the diagnosis of late paraphrenia be abandoned? (editorial). Psychol Med 2:11–14, 1992

Almeida OP, Howard R, Förstl H, et al: Coming to terms with late paraphrenia, in Functional Psychiatric Disorders in the Elderly. Edited by Chiu E. Cambridge, England, Cambridge University Press (in press)

American Psychiatric Association: Diagnostic and Statistical Manual of Mental Disorders, 3rd Edition, Revised. Washington, DC, American Psychiatric Association, 1987

American Psychiatric Association: Diagnostic and Statistical Manual of Mental Disorders, 4th Edition. Washington, DC, American Psychiatric Association, 1994

Aylward EH, Pearlson GD, Rabins PV: Differences in early and late onset schizophrenia (letter). Am J Psychiatry 150:846–849, 1993

Blessed G, Wilson D: The contemporary natural history of mental disorder in old age. Br J Psychiatry 141:59–67, 1982

Bleuler M: Late schizophrenic clinical pictures (in German). Fortschr Neurol Psychiatr 15:259–290, 1943

Boronow J, Pickar D, Ninan PT: Atrophy limited to third ventricle only in chronic schizophrenic patients: report of a controlled series. Arch Gen Psychiatry 40:266–271, 1985

Branchey M, Lee J, Amen R, et al: High and low-potency neuroleptics in elderly psychiatric patients. JAMA 239:1860–1862, 1978

Breitner JCS, Husain MM, Figiel GS, et al: Cerebral white matter disease in late-onset paranoid psychosis. Biol Psychiatry 28:266–274, 1990

Bridge TP, Wyatt RJ: Paraphrenia: paranoid states of late life, I: European research. J Am Geriatr Soc 27:193–200, 1980a

Bridge TP, Wyatt RJ: Paraphrenia: paranoid states of late life, II: American research. J Am Geriatr Soc 27:201–205, 1980b

Burns A, Carrick J, Ames D, et al: The cerebral cortical appearance in late paraphrenia. International Journal of Geriatric Psychiatry 4:31–34, 1989

Burns A, Jacoby R, Levy R: Psychiatric phenomena in Alzheimer's disease, I: disorders of thought content. Br J Psychiatry 157:72–76, 1990a

Burns A, Jacoby R, Levy R: Psychiatric phenomena in Alzheimer's disease, II: disorders of perception. Br J Psychiatry 157:76–81, 1990b

Castle DJ, Howard R: What do we know about the aetiology of late-onset schizophrenia? European Psychiatry 7:99–108, 1992

Castle DJ, Murray RM: The neurodevelopmental basis of sex differences in schizophrenia. Psychol Med 21:565–575, 1991

Coffey CE, Figiel GS, Djang WT, et al: Leukoencephalopathy in elderly depressed patients referred for ECT. Biol Psychiatry 24:143–161, 1988

Coffey CE, Figiel GS, Djang WT, et al: White matter hyperintensity on magnetic resonance imaging: clinical and neuroanatomic correlates in the depressed elderly. J Neuropsychiatry Clin Neurosci 1:135–144, 1989

Coffey CE, Figiel GS, Djang, WT, et al: Subcortical hyperintensity on magnetic resonance imaging: a comparison of normal and depressed elderly subjects. Am J Psychiatry 47:187–189, 1990

Cooper AF, Porter R: Visual acuity and occular pathology in the paranoid and affective psychoses of later life. J Psychosomatic Res 20:107–114, 1976

Cooper AF, Kay DWK, Curry AR, et al: Hearing loss in paranoid and affective psychoses of the elderly. Lancet 2:851–861, 1974

Craig TJ, Bregman Z: Late onset schizophrenia-like illness. J Am Geriatr Soc 36:104–107, 1988

Cummings J: Organic delusions: phenomenology, anatomical correlations and review. Br J Psychiatry 145:184–197, 1985

Eastwood MR, Corbin S, Reed M: Hearing impairment and paraphrenia. J Otolaryngol 10:306–308, 1981

Fish F: Senile schizophrenia. Journal of Mental Science 106:938–946, 1960

Flint AJ, Rifat SL, Eastwood MR: Late-onset paranoia: distinct from paraphrenia? International Journal of Geriatric Psychiatry 6:103–109, 1991

Gabriel D: Die Langfristige Entwicklung der Spatchziophrenien. Basel, Karger, 1978

Grahame PS: Schizophrenia in old age (late paraphrenia). Br J Psychiatry 145:493–495, 1984

Gur RE, Bur RC, Skolnik BE, et al: Brain function in psychiatric disorders, III: regional cerebral blood flow in unmedicated schizophrenics. Arch Gen Psychiatry 42:329–334, 1985

Gur RE, Mozley PD, Resnick SM, et al: Magnetic resonance imaging in schizophrenia, I: volumetric analysis of brain and cerebrospinal fluid. Arch Gen Psychiatry 48:407–412, 1991

Guze BH, Szuba MP: Leukoencephalopathy and major depression: a preliminary report. Psychiatry Research: Neuroimaging 45:169–175, 1992

Harris MJ, Jeste DV: Late-onset schizophrenia: an overview. Schizophr Bull 14:39–55, 1988

Harris MJ, Cullum CM, Jeste DV: Clinical presentation of late-onset schizophrenia. J Clin Psychiatry 49:356–360, 1988

Herbert ME, Jacobson S: Late paraphrenia. Br J Psychiatry 113:461–469, 1967

Holden NL: Late paraphrenia or the paraphrenias? a descriptive study with a 10 year follow-up. Br J Psychiatry 150:635–639, 1987

Howard R, Levy R: Which factors affect treatment response in late paraphrenia? International Journal of Geriatric Psychiatry 7:667–672, 1992

Howard RJ, Förstl H, Almeida O, et al: Computer-assisted CT measurements in late paraphrenics with and without Schneiderian first-rank symptoms: a preliminary report. International Journal of Geriatric Psychiatry 7:35–38, 1992a

Howard RJ, Förstl H, Almeida O, et al: First-rank symptoms of Schneider in late paraphrenia: cortical structural correlates. Br J Psychiatry 160:108–109, 1992b

Huber G, Gross A, Schuttler R: Late schizophrenia. Archiv Psychaitrische Nervenkranken 221:53–66, 1975

Hymas N, Naguib M, Levy R: Late paraphrenia: a follow-up study. International Journal of Geriatric Psychiatry 4:23–29, 1989

Jeste DV, Caligiuri MP: Biological research in geriatric psychiatry (editorial). Biol Psychiatry 30:855–856, 1991

Jeste DV, Harris MJ, Pearlson GD, et al: Late-onset schizophrenia: studying clinical validity. Psychosis and Depression in the Elderly 11:1–13, 1988a

Jeste DV, Harris JM, Zweifach M: Late-onset schizophrenia. Psychiatry 56:1–8, 1988b

Jeste DV, Manley M, Harris MJ: Psychoses, In Comprehensive Review of Geriatric Psychiatry. Edited by Sadavoy J, Lazarus L, Jarvik L. Washington, DC, American Psychiatric Press, 1991, pp 353–368

Johnstone E, Crow T, Frith C, et al: Cerebral ventricular size and cognitive impairment in chronic schizophrenia. Lancet 2:924–926, 1976

Kay DWK: Schizophrenia and schizophrenia-like states in the elderly. Br J Hosp Med 8:369–379, 1972

Kay DWK, Roth M: Environmental and hereditary factors in the schizophrenias of old age ("late paraphrenia") and their bearing on the general problem of causation in schizophrenia. Journal of Mental Science 107:649–686, 1961

Kay DWK, Cooper AF, Garside RF, et al: The differentiation of paranoid from affective psychoses by patients' premorbid characteristics. Br J Psychiatry 129:207–215, 1976

Kohlmeyer K: Periventrikuläre Dichteminderungen des Grosshirnhemispherenmarks in Computertomogrammen von neuropsychiatrischen Patienten in der zweiten Lebenshälfte: diagnostische Bedeutung und Pathogenese. Fortschr Neurol Psychiatr 56:279–287, 1988

Kolle K: Die Primare Verucktheit. Leipzig, Thieme, 1931

Kraepelin G: Psychiatrie: Ein Lehrbuch für Studierende und Artzte, 7th Edition. Leipzig, Barth, 1903–1904

Kraepelin E: Dementia praecox and paraphrenia (1919), in Text-Book of Psychiatry, 8th Edition. Translated from the German by Barclay RM. Edited by Robertson GM. Huntington, NY, Krieger, 1971

Kraeplin E: Psychiatrie: Ein Lehrbuch für Studierende und Arizie, 9th Edition. Leipzig, Barth, 1926

Krishnan KRR, Goli V, Ellinwood EH, et al: Leukoencephalopathy in patients diagnosed as major depressive. Biol Psychiatry 23:519–522, 1988

Krull AJ, Press G, Dupont R, et al: Brain imaging in late-onset schizophrenia and related psychoses. International Journal of Geriatric Psychiatry 6:651–658, 1991

Lesser IM, Miller BL, Boone KB, et al: Psychosis as the first manifestation of degenerative dementia. Bulletin of Clinical Neurosciences 54:59–63, 1989

Lesser IM, Miller BL, Boone KB, et al: Brain injury and cognitive function in late-onset psychotic depression. J Neuropsychiatry Clin Neurosci 3:33–40, 1991

Lesser IM, Jeste DV, Boone KB, et al: Late-onset psychotic disorder, not otherwise specified: clinical and neuroimaging findings. Biol Psychiatry 31:419–423, 1992

Lesser IM, Miller BL, Swartz JR, et al: Brain imaging in late-life schizophrenia and related psychoses. Schizophr Bull 19:773–782, 1993

Lewine RJ: Sex differences in schizophrenia: timing or subtypes? Psychol Bull 90:432–444, 1981

Lewine RJ: Schizophrenia: an amotivational syndrome in men. Can J Psychiatry 30:316–318, 1985

Marneros A, Deister A: The psychopathology of "late schizophrenia." Psychopathology 17:264–274, 1984

Matthew RJ, Wilson WH, Tant SR, et al: Abnormal resting regional cerebral blood flow patterns and their correlates in schizophrenia. Arch Gen Psychiatry 45:542–549, 1988

Mayer W: On paraphrenic psychoses. Zeitschrift für die Gesamte Neurologie und Psychiatrie 71:187–206, 1921

Mayer-Gross W: Die Schizophrenie. Berlin, Springer, 1932

Miller BL, Lesser IM: Late-life psychosis and modern neuroimaging. Psychiatr Clin North Am 11:33–46, 1988

Miller BL, Benson FD, Cummings JL, et al: Late-life paraphrenia: an organic delusional system. J Clin Psychiatry 47:204–207, 1986

Miller BL, Lesser IM, Boone KB, et al: Brain lesions and cognitive function in late-life psychosis. Br J Psychiatry 158:76–82, 1991

Miller BL, Lesser IM, Mena I, et al: Regional cerebral blood flow in late-life–onset psychosis. Neuropsychiatry, Neuropsychology, and Behavioral Neurology 5:132–137, 1992

Morris JC, Heyman A, Mohs RC, et al: The consortium to establish a registry for Alzheimer's disease (CERAD), part I: clinical and neuropsychological assessment of Alzheimer's disease. Neurology 39:1159–1165, 1989

Naguib M, Levy R: Late paraphrenia: neuropsychological impairment and structural brain abnormalities on computed tomography. International Journal of Geriatric Psychiatry 2:83–90, 1987

Naguib M, Levy R: Paraphrenia, in Psychiatry in the Elderly. Edited by Jacoby R, Oppenheimer C. Oxford, England, Oxford University Press, 1991, pp 758–778

Naguib M, McGuffin P, Levy R, et al: Genetic markers in late paraphrenia: a study of HLA antigens. Br J Psychiatry 150:124–127, 1987

Pearlson GD, Coyle JT: The dopamine hypothesis and schizophrenia, in Neuroleptics: Neurochemical, Behavioral and Clinical Perspectives, Vol 3: CNS Pharmacology. Edited by Coyle JT, Enna S. New York, Raven, 1983, pp 297–327

Pearlson GD, Rabins PV: The late onset psychoses: possible risk factors. Psychiatr Clin North Am 11:15–33, 1988

Pearlson GD, Garbacz DJ, Tompkins RH, et al: Lateral cerebral ventricular size in late onset schizophrenia, in Schizophrenia and Aging. Edited by Miller NE, Cohen GD. New York, Guilford, 1987, pp 246–248

Pearlson GD, Kreger L, Rabins PV, et al: A chart review study of late-onset and early onset schizophrenia. Am J Psychiatry 146:1568–1574, 1989

Pearlson GD, Barta PE, Tune LE, et al: Quantitative MRI and PET in late life onset schizophrenia, in American College of Neuropsychopharmacology, Abstracts of Panels and Posters, 30th Annual Meeting, Caribe Hilton, San Juan, Puerto Rico. Nashville, TN, ACNP Secretariat, 1991, p 56

Pearlson, GD, Tune LE, Wong DF, et al: Quantitative D_2 dopamine receptor PET and structural MRI changes in late onset schizophrenia: a preliminary report. Schizophr Bull 19:783–795, 1993

Pfefferbaum A, Zipursky RB, Lim KO, et al: Computed tomographic evidence for generalized sulcal and ventricular enlargement in schizophrenia. Arch Gen Psychiatry 45:633–640, 1988

Post F: Persistent Persecutory States of the Elderly. London, Pergamon, 1966

Post F: Schizophrenic and paranoid psychoses, in Handbook of Studies on Psychiatry and Old Age. Edited by Kay DWK, Burrows W. Amsterdam, Elsevier Science, pp 291–302, 1984

Rabins PV, Pearlson GD: Late onset paranoid disorders: issues requiring answers (b): paraphrenia or schizophrenia? in Functional Psychiatric Disorders in the Elderly. Edited by Chiu E. Cambridge, England, Cambridge University Press (in press)

Rabins P, Pauker S, Thomas J: Can schizophrenia begin after age 44? Compr Psychiatry 25:290–295, 1984

Rabins PV, Pearlson GD, Jayaram G, et al: Elevated VBR in late-onset schizophrenia. Am J Psychiatry 144:1216–1218, 1987

Rabins PV, Pearlson GD, Aylward EH, et al: Cortical magnetic resonance imaging changes in elderly inpatients with major depression. Am J Psychiatry 148:617–620, 1991

Rabins PV, Aylward EH, Lavrisha M, et al: MRI measures using the CERAD scale in elderly depressed and schizophrenic patients. Psychiatry Research Neuroimaging (in press)

Roth M: The natural history of mental disorder in old age. Journal of Mental Science 101:281–301, 1955

Roth M, Morrissey J: Problems in the diagnosis and classification of mental disorders in old age. Journal of Mental Science 98:66–80, 1952

Rubin EH: Delusions as part of Alzheimer's disease. Neuropsychiatry, Neuropsychology, and Behavioral Neurology 5:108–113, 1992

Seeman MV: Gender and the onset of schizophrenia: neurohumoral influences. Psychiatry Journal of the University of Ottawa 6:136–137, 1981

Seeman MV: Current outcome in schizophrenia: women vs. men. Acta Psychiatr Scand 73:609–617, 1986

Seeman PF, Bzowej NH, Guan HC, et al: Human brain dopamine receptors in children and aging adults. Synapse 1:399–404, 1987

Siegel CE, Goodman AB: Mental illness among the elderly in a large state psychiatric facility: a comparison with other age groups, in Schizophrenia and Aging. Edited by Miller NE, Cohen GD. New York, Guilford, 1987, pp 23–34

Signer SF: Psychosis in neurologic diseases: Capgras symptom and delusions of reduplication in neurologic disorders. Neuropsychiatry, Neuropsychology, and Behavioral Neurology 5:138–143, 1992

Tomlinson BE, Blessed G, Roth M: Observations on the brains of non-demented old people. J Neurol Sci 7:331–343, 1968

Tran-Johnson TK, Krull AJ, Jeste DV: Late life schizophrenia and its treatment: pharmacologic issues in older schizophrenic patients. Clin Geriatr Med 8:401–410, 1992

Tune LE, Wong DF, Pearlson GD, et al: Elevated dopamine D_2 receptor density in 23 schizophrenic patients: a PET study with 11C-N-methylspiperone. Psychiatry Research Neuroimaging (in press)

Weinberger DR: Implications of normal brain development for the pathogenesis of schizophrenia. Arch Gen Psychiatry 44:660–669, 1987

Weinberger DR, Torrey EF, Neophytides AN, et al: Lateral cerebral ventricular enlargement in chronic schizophrenia. Arch Gen Psychiatry 36:735–739, 1979

Weinberger DR, Berman KF, Illowsky BP: Physiological dysfunction of dorsolateral prefrontal cortex in schizophrenia. Arch Gen Psychiatry, 45:609–615, 1988

Weisman MM: Advances in psychiatric epidemiology: rates and risks for major depression. Am J Public Health 77:445–451, 1987

Wong DF, Wagner HN, Dannals RF, et al: Effects of age on dopamine and serotonin receptors measured by positron emission tomography in the living human brain. Science 226:1393–1396, 1984

Wong DF, Wagner HN Jr, Tune LE, et al: Positron emission tomography reveals elevated D$_2$ dopamine receptors in drug-naive schizophrenics. Science 234:1558–1563, 1986a

Wong DF, Gjedde J, Wagner HN Jr: Quantification of neuroreceptors in the living human brain, I: irreversible binding of ligands. J Cereb Blood Flow Metab 6:177–146, 1986b

Wong DF, Gjedde J, Wagner HN Jr, et al: Quantification of neuroreceptors in the living human brain, II: assessment of receptor density and affinity using inhibition studies. J Cereb Blood Flow Metab 6:147–153, 1986c

Wragg R, Jeste DV: An overview of depression and psychosis in Alzheimer's disease. Am J Psychiatry 146:577–587, 1989

Zubenko GS, Sullivan P, Nelson JP, et al: Brain imaging abnormalities in mental disorders of late life. Arch Neurol 47:1107–1111, 1990

14

Anxiety Disorders

Javaid I. Sheikh, M.D.

Introduction

Anxiety is a normal human emotion in the elderly, as in the young, with adaptive value in that it helps one anticipate and prepare for noxious events. This normal emotion, however, can be considered pathological when it becomes unjustifiably excessive and maladaptive, as in morbid anxiety in clinical situations. This morbid anxiety usually manifests itself in the form of a multitude of cognitive, behavioral, and physiological symptoms, whereas the mental content of such anxiety may range from excessive worrying about everyday concerns regarding job and relationships to episodes of intense anxiety and fear (panic attacks). I use the term *anxiety* in this chapter to refer to such clinically significant or morbid anxiety, unless specified otherwise. Anxiety disorders are diagnostic entities comprising various constellations of signs and symptoms of anxiety combined with criteria regarding their intensity and duration, as described in DSM-IV (American Psychiatric Association 1994). Table 14–1 lists some examples of multidimensional symptoms that might be experienced by patients with various anxiety disorders.

Anxiety disorders are some of the most frequent but least studied of psychiatric illnesses in elderly patients. For example, an analysis of the Epidemiologic Catchment Area (ECA) data by Blazer et al. (1991) indicated a 6-month prevalence of 19.7% for all anxiety disorders in the 65 or older age group, with phobias the most common psychiatric syndrome in elderly women and the second most common in elderly men. Systematic studies of anxiety disorders in elderly subjects, however, remain scant. In this chapter, I begin

with a description of the classification of anxiety disorders based on DSM-IV, summarize findings of phenomenology of anxiety disorders in elderly patients from the literature, discuss manifestations of anxiety in certain medical illnesses, present a systematic way of assessing anxiety in the elderly and differentiating it from depression, and summarize treatment methods particularly suited to geriatric anxiety.

Classification of Anxiety Disorders

DSM-IV describes operationally defined, phenomenologically oriented diagnostic criteria for various anxiety disorders. A list of various anxiety disorders based on DSM-IV classification appears in Table 14–2.

Epidemiological Studies

Epidemiological studies of anxiety disorders in elderly patients have been few and far between. Studies of anxiety syndromes in the elderly performed before the introduction of DSM-III (American Psychiatric Association 1980) were mostly conducted in the United Kingdom and have tended to categorize anxiety and depression into a mixed, anxious-depressive neurosis following the tradition at that time (Bergmann 1971; Post 1972). It is difficult to discern the prevalence of different anxiety disorders based on those studies.

Data from the ECA study (Myers et al. 1984) can

Table 14–1. Multidimensional symptoms of anxiety

Cognitive	Behavioral	Physiological
Nervousness	Hyperkinesis	Tachycardia
Apprehension	Repetitive motor acts	Palpitations
Racing thoughts	Stiffness	Chest tightness
Worry	Phobias	Dry mouth
Fearfulness	Pressured speech	Hyperventilation
Irritability	Startle response	Paresthesias
Distractibility		Lightheadedness
		Sweating
		Urinary frequency

Source. Reprinted from Sheikh JI: "Clinical Features of Anxiety Disorders," in *The Psychiatry of Old Age.* Edited by Copeland JM, Abou-Saleh MT, Blazer DG. Chichester, England, Wiley, 1993a, p. 107.1. Used with permission.

Table 14–2. DSM-IV anxiety disorders

Panic attack
Agoraphobia
Panic disorder
  With agoraphobia
  Without agoraphobia
Agoraphobia without history of panic disorder
Specific phobia (simple phobia)
Social phobia (social anxiety disorder)
Obsessive-compulsive disorder
Posttraumatic stress disorder
Acute stress disorder
Generalized anxiety disorder
Anxiety disorder due to a general medical condition
Substance-induced anxiety disorder
Anxiety disorder not otherwise specified

Source. From American Psychiatric Association 1994.

be considered a first step toward investigating the true prevalence of anxiety disorders in the elderly population. These figures indicate that phobias are the most common psychiatric disorder in elderly women and the second most common in elderly men. Some other recent studies have reported prevalence data of anxiety disorders in the elderly using a computerized program, AGECAT, which is an algorithm for assembling information at interview (Kay 1988). The rate of anxiety disorders is around 2%, though it appears that 50%–75% of elderly cases with clinical levels of anxiety were diagnosed as depression (Copeland et al. 1987; Kay 1988). Kay (1988) suggested that, if diagnosed independently, the prevalence of anxiety disorders would be doubled.

In a comparison of the ECA data between age groups of 45–64 (middle-aged) and 65 or older (older-aged), Blazer et al. (1991) documented the 6-month and lifetime prevalence in the Duke Community Sample for all anxiety disorders excluding posttraumatic stress disorder (PTSD). Their analysis also showed that both 6-month and lifetime prevalences of all anxiety disorders decline somewhat from the middle-aged to the older-aged group, but still stands at a formidable combined prevalence of 19.7% for the 6-month period and 34.05% for the lifetime for all anxiety disorders (Table 14–3). It also appears that people in the older-aged group are more likely to use outpatient mental health services or benzodiazepines when they do report symptoms of generalized anxiety. The authors suggested the possibility of underreporting due to a higher threshold for reporting generalized anxiety

Table 14–3. Prevalence of anxiety disorders by age

Diagnosis	6 months		Lifetime	
	45–64	65+	45–64	65+
Simple phobia	13.29	9.63	18.11	16.10
Social phobia	2.04	1.37	3.18	2.64
Agoraphobia	7.30	5.22	9.40	8.44
Panic disorder	1.10	0.04	2.04	0.29
Obsessive-compulsive disorder	2.01	1.54	3.33	1.98
Generalized anxiety disorder	3.10	1.90	6.70	4.60

Note. From the Duke Epidemiologic Catchment Area Community Sample.
Source. Reprinted from Blazer D, George LK, Hughes D: "The Epidemiology of Anxiety Disorders: An Age Comparison," in *Anxiety in the Elderly.* Edited by Salzman C, Lebowitz BD. New York, Springer, 1991, p. 21. Used with permission.

symptoms in the older-aged group and a tendency to seek assistance when that threshold is reached.

In conclusion, it appears that anxiety symptoms and disorders are among the most common psychiatric ailments experienced by older adults and the least studied in that age group.

Phenomenology of Anxiety Disorders in the Elderly Population

As noted above, empirical studies of the phenomenology of anxiety disorders are scant. However, recent data shed some light on panic disorder and phobias in elderly patients (Lindesay 1991; Luchins and Rose 1989; Sheikh et al. 1988). Panic disorder is usually a chronic syndrome with frequent recurrences and remissions. Preliminary investigations suggest that many older patients with onset of panic attacks in early life seem to continue with their symptomatology in later life, with many of them receiving inadequate or no treatment over the years (Sheikh et al. 1991). It also appears that though it may not be very common for panic disorder to appear de novo in old age, it does occur (Luchins and Rose 1989; Sheikh et al. 1988).

Data from ongoing research in our program also suggest some phenomenological differences in early-(onset before age 55) versus late-onset (onset at age 55 or older) panic disorder patients. In a survey of 1,746 volunteers wanting to participate in various treatment programs for panic disorder in our research project (Sheikh et al. 1991), 520 subjects reported a history of spontaneous panic attacks. Of these, 445 subjects were younger than 55 and the remaining 75 were 55 or older. The latter group was further subdivided into those reporting the age at onset of their first panic attack before 55 (*n* = 57) and those reporting it at age 55 or older (*n* = 18). These subjects were asked to rate on a scale of 0 to 4 how they would most typically behave in 10 situations: 0 = can do without anxiety; 1 = can do with mild anxiety; 2 = can do with severe anxiety; 3 = can do only with extreme terror; and 4 = cannot do under any circumstances. The 10 situations were 1) shopping alone in a large department store; 2) being alone at home for 2 days; 3) driving a car alone 10 miles on a freeway; 4) walking alone away from home for 1 mile; 5) shopping alone in a large grocery store; 6) being alone in crowded places like a movie theater or church; 7) crossing busy streets alone; 8) eating a complete meal alone at a restaurant; 9) using public transportation alone; 10) waiting in long lines at banks or the department of motor vehicles.

As shown in Figure 14–1, patients with late-onset panic attacks reported significantly less avoidance compared with the early-onset groups, both young and old. In addition, the group with late-onset panic attacks also reported fewer symptoms during panic attacks. These initial findings were recently reconfirmed in our program (Sheikh 1993b) in subjects who were diagnosed as having panic disorder using a Structured Clinical Interview for DSM-III-R (American Psychiatric Association 1987) (SCID; Spitzer et al. 1987). It thus appears that patients with late-onset panic disorder report fewer panic symptoms and less avoidance than those

with early-onset panic disorder. In-depth studies are currently under way to test these findings in larger samples of patients, as well as to study the medical and psychiatric comorbidity in these patients.

Epidemiologic data (Blazer et al. 1991) indicate that phobic disorders are chronic and persisting in old age. Clinical experience suggests that public speaking may seem less frightening and eating in public more bothersome to elderly people than to younger people. Fear of crime seems to be particularly prevalent in the elderly population, especially in an urban setting. In a survey of elderly people in an English urban setting, Clarke and Lewis (1982) reported that 66% of their sample stated that they did not go out after dark for

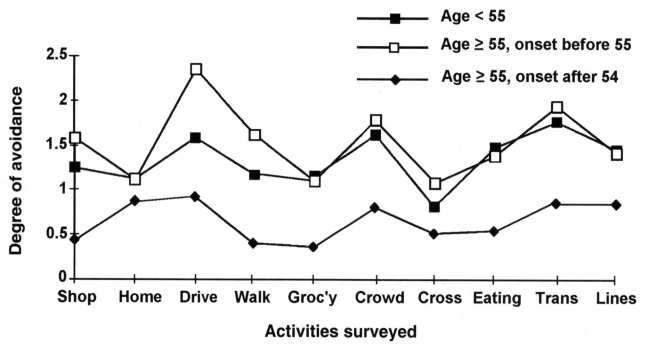

Figure 14–1. Avoidance patterns in individuals with early-onset compared with late-onset panic disorder. Shop = shopping alone in a large department store; Home = being alone at home for 2 days; Drive = driving a car alone on a freeway-like highway; Walk = walking alone away from home for 1 mile; Groc'y = shopping alone in a large grocery store; Crowd = being alone in a crowded place (e.g., theater or church); Cross = crossing busy streets alone; Eating = eating a complete meal alone in a restaurant; Trans = using public transportation alone; Lines = waiting in a long line.
Source. Reprinted from Sheikh JI: "Anxiety Disorders and Their Treatment," in *Clinics in Geriatric Medicine: Psychiatric Disorders in Late Life,* Vol. 8, No. 2. Edited by Alexopoulos GS. Philadelphia, PA, WB Saunders, 1992b, p. 423. Used with permission.

fear of victimization and 15% reported that this fear was a primary concern. There is also a suggestion of nocturnal neurosis in the elderly as a result of fear of crime (Cohen 1976). Elderly people thus appear to be the most anxious group about crime, though they are apparently the least likely to be victimized (Clarke and Lewis 1982). In a recently reported study, Lindesay (1991) indicated that phobic disorders in elderly patients are associated with considerably higher psychiatric and medical morbidity compared with control subjects. Further, 17 of 28 agoraphobic subjects in Lindesay's study reported the onset of their symptomatology after age 65, and despite increased rates of contact with primary care services, none was receiving any specific treatment for their phobic disorders. These findings tend to confirm the assertion that anxiety disorders in the elderly population tend to remain undiagnosed and untreated.

Neurobiology of Anxiety in Elderly Individuals

Most recent work investigating neurobiology of anxiety has been performed in younger populations and its relevance to the elderly population remains unknown at present. In this section, I summarize literature on the neurobiology of anxiety and discuss relevance of age-related changes in various neurotransmitter systems to phenomena of anxiety and fear in elderly individuals.

Attempts to discern neurobiology of anxiety date back to empirical work by Cannon (1929) in cats, suggesting that central discharges, possibly thalamic in origin, are the harbinger of fear and anxiety. Increasing evidence during the last several years has pointed to locus coeruleus in the midbrain, containing approximately half of central norepinephrine neurons, as the harbinger of states of fear and panic. For example, Redmond and Huang (1979) documented central noradrenergic activation in anxiety and fear states and suggested that the locus coeruleus is implicated in such emotions. Charney and Heninger (1985) reported a greater number of yohimbine-induced anxiety symptoms in panic patients compared with control subjects, as well as a blunting of yohimbine response after treatment with alprazolam, supporting the hypothesis of noradrenergic activation due to locus coeruleus discharge in panic attacks. Simson and Weiss (1988) also suggested that locus coeruleus plays a key role in the

"fight or flight" response mediated via activation of central noradrenergic system.

As for the normal age-related changes in noradrenergic functioning in older populations, Sunderland et al. (1991) summarized findings from several studies suggesting that there is a decline of such function in old age, including a decrease in the number of locus coeruleus neurons, a decreased norepinephrine content in many brain areas, and an increase in monoamine oxidase (type B) levels. These findings support the phenomenological research documenting a milder symptomatology in late-onset panic disorder (Sheikh et al. 1991). Unlike studies of noradrenergic system, those of serotonergic system in younger anxiety disorder patients, as well as in nonanxious elderly patients, have yielded mixed and nonconclusive results (Sunderland et al. 1991).

Since the report by Pitts and McClure (1967) that an infusion of 10 mg/kg body weight of 0.5 M racemic sodium lactate produced panic symptoms in 13 out of 14 anxiety neurotic patients (panic disorder by present criteria) and in only 2 out of 16 control subjects, various investigators have reproduced this finding (Kelly et al. 1971; Liebowitz et al. 1984). It is now well accepted that lactate infusion produces panic attacks in about 70% of panic disorder patients. The underlying mechanism for induction of panic attacks with sodium lactate remains unclear. However, various postulates include sodium lactate being a nonspecific stimulant producing uncomfortable somatic sensations or a conversion of lactate to bicarbonate and CO_2, with CO_2 crossing the blood-brain barrier and producing a transient intracerebral hypercapnia leading to stimulation of brain stem chemoreceptors. Other techniques for successful induction of panic include caffeine administration, which may block adenosine receptors (Boulenger et al. 1984); yohimbine, which may challenge locus coeruleus activation due to its α_2-adrenergic antagonism (Charney et al. 1982); and inhalation of 5% CO_2 (Gorman et al. 1989). No reports of panic induction in elderly patients are described in the literature, and it is not clear whether such methods will be safe to use in this population. Availability of neuroimaging techniques has recently provided an impetus for carrying out more specific studies to delineate neurobiological basis of anxiety disorders. For example, Reiman et al. (1989) have documented increased parahippocampal activity during panic attacks provoked by lactic acid, as well as significant blood flow increases bilaterally in the temporal poles.

Of the various theoretical models of anxiety based on neurobiological findings, two seem to be the most popular at present. The first is a complex schema espoused by Gray (1982) of the central role of a "Behavioral Inhibition System" in the manifestations of anxiety, which involves neuroanatomical structures of septohippocampal system and noradrenergic, serotonergic, and GABAergic[1] neurotransmitter systems in a rather complicated relationship. The second model is that of Gorman et al. (1989), who have proposed a neuroanatomical hypothesis for panic disorder locating the acute panic attack in the brain stem, anticipatory anxiety in the limbic system, and phobic avoidance in the prefrontal cortex. Relevance of such theorizing to elderly patients is unknown at present. In summary, it appears that unlike with depression, which may be predisposed to by neurobiological changes of normal aging, such a relationship does not seem to exist with anxiety.

Anxiety and Medical Illness

Anxiety is quite commonly associated with medical illness either as an expected response to a physical stressor or a manifestation of physiological changes occurring as a result of a medical illness that may produce anxiety or possibly coincidentally. In some cases, such comorbidity may confound the clinical picture for both the primary care physician and the psychiatrist. A list of such conditions is presented in Table 14–4. The clinical picture of anxiety in the more common of these medical illnesses is briefly described below.

Cardiovascular Illness

Panic attacks can be simulated by both angina pectoris and myocardial infarction with symptoms consisting of palpitations, dyspnea, chest tightness, sweating, and a fear of dying. Such episodes in older age group patients should always prompt a thorough investigation of the cardiac status of the patient, except perhaps in ones in whom a diagnosis of panic disorder is well established. The relationship of panic disorder and mitral valve prolapse remains unclear, with some of the studies suggesting a higher rate of association than in control subjects (Gorman et al. 1981; Kantor et al. 1980) and others questioning such evidence (Margraf et al. 1988; Mazza et al. 1986).

Dietary Causes

Caffeine intake in the form of coffee, tea, and sodas can produce anxiety-like symptoms in doses as little as 200 mg (one cup = 150 mg) (Victor et al. 1981). It has also been implicated in precipitating full-blown panic attacks (Charney et al. 1985; Lee 1985; Uhde et al. 1984). A history of caffeine use should be obtained in patients with symptoms of anxiety to rule out any temporal relationship. A decrease in daily caffeine consumption in some cases can be a simple and effective intervention.

Table 14–4.	Physical disorders often presenting with anxiety

Cardiovascular	**Hematologic**
Myocardial infarction	Anemia
Paroxysmal atrial tachycardia	**Immunologic**
Mitral valve prolapse	Systemic lupus erythematosus
Dietary	**Neurological**
Caffeine	Central nervous system (CNS) infections
Vitamin deficiencies	CNS masses
Drug-related	Toxins
Akathisia	Temporal lobe epilepsy
Anticholinergic toxicity	Postconcussion syndrome
Antihypertensive side effects	**Pulmonary**
Digitalis toxicity	Chronic obstructive lung disease
Withdrawal syndromes	Pneumonia
Alcohol	Hypoxia
Sedative-hypnotics	
Endocrinologic	
Insulinoma	
Hypoglycemia	
Hypo- or hyperthyroidism	
Hypo- or hypercalcemia	
Pheochromocytoma	
Carcinoid syndrome	
Hypothermia	
Cushing's disease	
Hyperkalemia	

Source. Reprinted from Jenike MA: *Handbook of Geriatric Psychopharmacology.* Littleton, MA, PSG Publishing, 1985, p. 98. Used with permission.

---

[1] GABA = γ-aminobutyric acid.

Drugs

For common cold and allergic conditions, elderly people commonly use over-the-counter preparations that may produce anxiety-like symptoms due to their adrenergic agents like ephedrine or pseudoephedrine. Prescription drugs that can produce anxiety include amphetamines, bronchodilators like isoproterenol and theophylline, and some calcium channel blockers like verapamil, nifedipine, and diltiazem. A careful history of drug intake should thus be a part of the clinical assessment of anxiety in elderly patients.

Akathisia, a common side effect of neuroleptics, is a subjective sense of restlessness often indistinguishable from anxiety. It can also closely resemble agitation due to a tendency in patients with both conditions to pace around. Inquiring about drug history can give a clue into its temporal relationship with drug intake. Alcohol withdrawal is a well-recognized cause of anxiety and agitation among hospitalized patients (Lerner and Fallen 1985). Sedative-hypnotic withdrawal, however, might be somewhat underestimated as a cause of anxiety syndromes in older populations in which hypnotic usage is quite frequent (Schweizer et al. 1989). Clinicians should inquire about any such usage at the beginning of the hospitalization and cover with appropriate medications.

Endocrine Causes

Unlike younger populations, in whom two-thirds or more of hyperthyroid patients may meet DSM-III criteria for an anxiety disorder (Kathol et al. 1986), patients over age 60 have hyperthyroidism more insidious in presentation, sometimes labelled as "apathetic" as opposed to the "anxious or agitated" hyperthyroidism of younger people (Hurley 1983). Hypo- and hyperparathyroidism, hypo- and hyperpituitarism, hypoglycemia, diabetes mellitus, and Cushing's syndrome can also be associated with anxiety-like symptoms (Popkin and Mackenzie 1980).

Neurological Causes

Many neurological disorders are associated with symptoms of anxiety or a diagnosable anxiety disorder. In a comprehensive review of psychiatric presentations of medical illnesses, Hall (1980) suggested that neurological disorders are among major contributors to medical causes of anxiety and contended that cerebral vascular insufficiency may be the most common neurological cause of anxiety.

Although association of depression with Parkinson's disease is now considered a generally accepted fact, the presence of anxiety in this illness has only recently received attention from researchers. In one study (Stein et al. 1990), 9 (38%) out of 24 subjects (mean age = 58) with idiopathic Parkinson's disease had a clinically significant anxiety disorder. Another study (Schiffer et al. 1988) found that 12 of 16 patients with Parkinson's disease met the criteria of a present or past diagnosis of either panic disorder or generalized anxiety disorder. In a more recent study, Henderson et al. (1992) documented a picture of mixed anxiety-depression in 38% of 164 Parkinson's disease patients (mean age = 67) compared to 8% in 150 age-matched healthy spouse control subjects. It also appears that left-sided Parkinson's disease may be associated with greater degree of anxiety and depression (Fleminger 1991). There is some speculation that high prevalence of anxiety disorders in patients with Parkinson's disease may be due to a loss of normally existing dopaminergic inhibition of locus coeruleus (Iruela et al. 1992). Finally, one has to be mindful that the drug treatment of Parkinson's disease itself may produce symptoms of anxiety (Cummings 1991).

Although both depression and anxiety can be consequences of a stroke, Robinson and Starkstein (1990) reported that co-morbid major depression and generalized anxiety disorder are associated with cortical lesions, whereas depression alone is associated with subcortical lesions. Anxiety-like symptoms and agitated behaviors are also quite common in dementing disorders (Teri et al. 1988).

Anxiety remains one of the most disturbing symptoms in a small percentage of postconcussion syndrome patients (Leigh 1979). Temporal lobe epilepsy can mimic panic disorder (Edlund et al. 1987). Other neurological disorders described in the literature as sometimes associated with anxiety include multiple sclerosis, peripheral neuropathy, myasthenia gravis, Huntington's disease, Wilson's disease, closed head injury, and tumors of the brain (Hall 1980).

Pulmonary Causes

Elderly patients at bed rest remain at risk for pulmonary embolism, which might be the most common pulmonary cause of sudden anxiety in such patients. A ventilation-perfusion scan and a phlebogram can be diagnostic. Some reports also suggest an unusually high number of panic disorder cases among patients with chronic obstructive pulmonary disease (Karajgi et al. 1990; Yellowlees et al. 1987).

Evaluation of Anxiety in Elderly Patients

Clinicians need to be aware of potential difficulties in proper assessment of geriatric anxiety. These include a confounding of symptom picture by high medical comorbidity, difficulty of differentiating from depression, falsely high scores on anxiety rating scales due to overendorsement of cardiac and respiratory problems, and a tendency to resist psychiatric evaluation in older cohorts. With these caveats in mind, evaluation of geriatric anxiety is usually accomplished in three major ways: clinical evaluation, assessment by rating scales, and laboratory investigations.

Clinical Evaluation

The clinical evaluation should include a history of presenting symptomatology, past illness (e.g., panic disorder can be characterized by remissions and relapses), medication history (e.g., cold medications and anticholinergic medications), drug and alcohol history (e.g., hypnotic use), and a family history (may be helpful in panic disorder). A mental status examination of anxious elderly may reveal many of the cognitive and behavioral signs and symptoms of anxiety including apprehension, fearfulness, distractibility, hyperkinesis, and startled response. Physiological signs and symptoms including increased pulse rate, rapid breathing, sweating, and trembling should be looked for during the physical examination.

Assessment by Rating Scales

Anxiety rating scales are useful adjuncts to the clinical evaluation of anxiety. These can serve as initial screening devices, can be helpful in assessing severity of symptoms, and can be used as instruments to document effectiveness of various psychological and pharmacological therapeutic interventions. These scales are primarily of two kinds: observer-rated and self-rated. The most commonly used observer-rated scale is the Hamilton Anxiety Rating Scale (HARS; Hamilton 1959). It has 14 items consisting of 89 symptoms measuring psychic and somatic components of anxiety

with each item rated on a scale of 0 ("none") to 4 ("very severe"). A rating of 18 or above is generally considered to be suggestive of clinically significant anxiety. Though HARS is presently the standard in the field as a measure of change in clinical situations and in pharmacological research, published studies in geriatrics are infrequent and seem to indicate limited sensitivity to change with active drug treatment (Kochansky 1979; Salzman 1977). Our own experience suggests that it is cumbersome to go through the list of 89 symptoms and that elderly patients tend to overendorse the somatic items.

The most frequently used self-rated scale is the State-Trait Anxiety Inventory (STAI; Speilberger et al. 1970). The STAI consists of two 20-item scales: the STAI-A-State scale measures anxiety as an emotional state currently; and the STAI-A-Trait scale measures anxiety as a relatively stable personality trait. In clinical situations, STAI-A-State seems preferable as it provides an avenue to measure changes in severity of anxiety in response to therapeutic interventions. Patients are instructed to check the responses correctly describing the intensity of their feelings for each item on a scale of 1 ("not at all") to 4 ("very much so"). Scores of 40 or above are generally considered clinically significant. A modified form for geriatric populations has been described by Patterson et al. (1980). Other commonly used scales include the revised Symptom Checklist–90 (SCL-90-R; Derogatis 1975) and the Beck Anxiety Inventory (Beck et al. 1988). A more detailed discussion of the advantages and disadvantages of various anxiety rating scales in the elderly is available elsewhere (Sheikh 1991).

Laboratory Investigations

Laboratory tests can aid in diagnosing underlying medical conditions producing signs and symptoms of anxiety. A complete blood count, vitamin B_{12} and folate levels, electrocardiogram, thyroid function tests, blood glucose, blood gases, and drug and alcohol screening can be helpful when used appropriately to rule out medical causes of anxiety described earlier and listed in Table 14–4.

Clinical Differentiation Between Anxiety and Depression

Debate about the unresolved and somewhat controversial issue of whether anxiety and depression lie on the same continuum, or whether they are separate conditions, is a recurring theme in the psychiatric literature. Despite recent advances in our knowledge about the phenomenology and biology of these conditions, we do not seem any closer to resolving this controversy. There is some suggestion that the distinction between anxiety and depression is more difficult to make in older populations (Kay 1988). Clinicians working with the elderly encounter this mixed symptom picture frequently. There may be a tendency to treat patients with such mixed pictures symptomatically, leading to polypharmacy. It is helpful to remember that making a distinction between anxiety and depression is of considerable pragmatic value because medications used for these disorders have very different side effect profiles. For example, tricyclic antidepressants may have many undesirable side effects—cardiotoxicity, anticholinergic side effects, and orthostasis—compared with the relatively safer profile of anxiolytics, such as benzodiazepines and buspirone. Table 14–5 summarizes some clinically useful distinctions between anxiety states and depressive syndromes.

Complications of Anxiety Disorders

Physical Illness

The issue of short- and long-term effects of anxiety on physical health remains unresolved. This question may be of particular relevance to the elderly population because of their relatively increased susceptibility to developing physical illness and the possibility that they may accumulate adverse effects of anxiety over many years. A strong association of anxiety states with many medical conditions has been discussed in the literature in the past two decades. For example, researchers have documented association of anxiety with asthma (Alexander 1972), hypertension (Whitehead et al. 1977), and duodenal ulcer (Sandberg and Bliding 1976). Some also believe that anxiety can give rise to potentially lethal arrhythmias (Jenkins 1971) and have suggested the use of diazepam in such cases.

There is also evidence that anxiety might act as a predictor of future morbidity in cancer patients. For example, Carey and Burish (1985) found that in cancer patients receiving chemotherapy, greater treatment gains were found in patients with lower pretreatment anxiety. Such associations cannot be considered causal, however, as the relationship between anxiety and physical functioning is complicated. For example, anxiety seems to contribute to heart disease, whereas heart disease itself increases anxiety (Jenike 1985), thus producing a vicious cycle. Though knowledge about the specific mechanism by which anxiety and autonomic arousal can cause tissue damage is lacking, it is possible that elderly people accumulate deleterious effects of anxiety over many years and are thus at risk for the cumulative adverse effects of anxiety on physical functioning. Of relevance, Nowlin et al. (1973) reported in a prospective study that elevated levels of anxiety predicted the future occurrence of myocardial infarction in older men. Though this study can only be considered preliminary because of the small sample, it is of sufficient importance to warrant attempts at replication. In another survey of older

Table 14–5. Differences between anxiety and depression

Variable	Depression	Anxiety
Symptomatology	Depressed mood Worse in A.M. Lack of energy Terminal insomnia Feelings of guilt and anhedonia more common	Anxious mood Worse in P.M. Agitation Initial insomnia Panic attacks, phobias, and symptoms of autonomic activation more common
Premorbid personality	Usually better adjusted premorbid personalities, except in chronic depression	Usually poorly adjusted personalities with dependent and avoidant traits quite common
Clinical course	Usually a history of regular cycles of depression with intervening periods of remission	Irregularly recurrent with somewhat incomplete periods of remission

Source.   Adapted from Sheikh JI: "Clinical Features of Anxiety Disorders," in *The Psychiatry of Old Age.* Edited by Copeland JM, Abou-Saleh MT, Blazer DG. Chichester, England, Wiley, 1993a, p. 107.4. Used with permission.

adults, Himmelfarb and Murrell (1984) found a significant association of anxiety with the presence of some medical conditions including high blood pressure, kidney or bladder disease, heart trouble, stomach ulcers, hardening of the arteries, stroke, and diabetes. Cause or effect issues aside, such association warrants further studies.

Alcohol Abuse

Several studies have documented unusually high rates of comorbidity between anxiety disorders and alcohol abuse (Chambless et al. 1987; Hesselbrock et al. 1985; Kushner et al. 1990; Ross et al. 1988; Weissman 1988). Boyd et al. (1984) estimated that the risk of alcohol problems in phobic patients is about two-and-a-half times that of the general population, and the risk in patients with panic disorder is more than four times. There is also some evidence from family studies suggesting that perhaps alcoholism and anxiety are on the same spectrum of disorders. For example, one study (Munjack and Moss 1981) found that 26.5% of the first-degree relatives of agoraphobic patients, 20% of the relatives of social phobia patients, and 8.6% of the relatives of mixed simple phobia patients were alcohol abusers. Harris et al. (1983) found that about 10% of the relatives of panic disorder patients and 17.6% of the relatives of agoraphobic patients were alcoholic, as opposed to only 5.4% in the control group. Although a relationship as to the cause and effect between alcoholism and anxiety disorders is not clear at present, there is sufficient evidence from a review of the literature (Kushner et al. 1990) that at least in cases of agoraphobia and social phobia, alcohol problems seem to be related to attempts at self-medication. It also appears that comorbidity is not uniform for all anxiety disorders, and thus generalizations regarding alcoholism in anxiety states as a homogeneous group should be avoided.

Even though none of these studies have looked at this issue with particular reference to the elderly population, one should keep in mind that similar comorbidity with alcoholism can exist in that population also. Considering that older people may be particularly vulnerable to the effects of alcohol because of changes in hepatic metabolism and increased sensitivity of the central nervous system (Atkinson 1989; Liptzin 1991), clinicians need to be alert to inquire about such history in patients with anxiety. Finally, alcohol withdrawal can itself present as severe anxiety, as noted above.

Insomnia

Sleep disturbances are common in patients with anxiety. In a study assessing vegetative signs and symptoms of anxiety, Mathew et al. (1982) found that restless sleep was the only vegetative symptom consistently related to anxiety. On the other hand, anxiety appears to be a common finding in patients with chronic insomnia. Some investigators have looked at differential effects on sleep of various anxiety syndromes. For example, in a study conducted by Reynolds et al. (1983), patients with generalized anxiety disorder were found to have difficulty similar to that of depressed patients in both initiating and maintaining sleep. However, these investigators also found that the shortened rapid-eye-movement (REM) latency and increased percentage of REM sleep found in depressed patients were missing in anxious patients. Other researchers (Insel et al. 1982) have suggested similarities between the sleep of obsessive-compulsive and depressed patients in that both groups seem to have short REM latency compared with that in control subjects. Like patients with generalized anxiety disorder, panic disorder patients frequently complain of difficulty in initiating and maintaining sleep (Sheehan et al. 1980). However, it appears that their REM latencies, though shorter than those of control subjects as a group, still fall within the lower limit of normal, unlike those of depressed patients (Uhde et al. 1984). Finally, it appears that patients with PTSD show a reduced efficiency of sleep with recurrent nightmares and a lower percentage of REM sleep.

It thus appears from the foregoing studies that anxiety disorders can create problems in initiating and maintaining sleep, as well as significantly affect the quality of sleep. The implications of these findings are significant for about five million elderly people in the United States, who have severe sleep problems (Moran et al. 1988). Inquiry into the duration and quality of sleep should be an integral component of any management plans for geriatric anxiety. Such inquiry should take into account the common clinical observation that older people tend to go to bed early and may nap during the day; a seemingly early wake-up time may not be so in reality and the total amount of sleep, including nap time, may be sufficient for many. In cases in which both anxiety and insomnia overlap, it would be prudent to consider treatments beneficial for both, be they nonpharmacological aids to sleep or sedative-hypnotics. (A review of the therapeutic effects and side effects of the latter, along with guidelines for use in an elderly population, are described below).

Increased Mortality of Cardiovascular Origin

In a series of long-term (30–50 years) follow-up studies, Coryell et al. (1982, 1986) documented increased mortality due to cardiovascular disease among men (but not women) patients with panic disorder. Specifically, it appears that men with a panic disorder diagnosis were twice as likely to die compared with expected deaths based on age and sex matching. After a review of causes of death in his sample of men, Coryell (1988) attributed the excess mortality to chronic hyperarousal and exercise intolerance of panic disorder patients and possibly to additional deleterious effects of associated smoking or alcohol abuse. Such findings suggest the need for proper control of panic attacks and associated chronic hyperarousal, as well as for paying attention to managing the associated smoking or alcohol abuse if present.

Management of Geriatric Anxiety

Effective management of geriatric anxiety can be accomplished by using pharmacological and/or psychological treatments. In the following sections, I provide a summary of the advantages and disadvantages of various treatments, as well as recommendations of their usage in specific anxiety disorders.

Pharmacological Treatments

While prescribing any medications to elderly patents, one needs to be aware of age-related physiological changes in absorption, distribution, protein binding, metabolism, and excretion of drugs (see Chapter 29). These changes can significantly alter plasma levels of drugs, lead to excessive accumulation of medications in various body tissues, and make elderly patients particularly prone to toxic effects, even at average dose ranges for the general population. To summarize these changes, drug absorption may be altered due to decreases in splanchnic blood flow, increases in gastric pH, and changes in active and passive transport (Ouslander 1981). An increase in the proportion of body fat with aging may prolong half-life of lipophilic compounds like benzodiazepines by affecting their distribution into tissues and across the blood-brain barrier (Jenike 1989). A reduction in serum albumin may mean more free drug in plasma, especially if there is dietary insufficiency or chronic illness, and a greater chance of toxicity (Greenblatt 1979). A decrease in hepatic metabolism may further increase levels of unmetabolized drug. Finally, a gradual decrease in glomerular filtration rate and renal blood flow to 50% by the age of 70 (compared with the rate at age 40) means slower clearance of drugs and higher chances of toxicity (Papper 1978).

Over the years, numerous compounds have been used as anxiolytics, including alcohol, barbiturates, antihistamines, antidepressants, neuroleptics, betablockers, benzodiazepines, and azapirones. A brief description of different classes of compounds commonly used as anxiolytics these days follows.

Benzodiazepines. These medications have been the most frequently prescribed anxiolytics for the last three decades. Elderly patients are prescribed benzodiazepines at a rate disproportionately high to their percentage in the population (Moran et al. 1988). Table 14–6

Table 14–6. Commonly used anxiolytic benzodiazepines: a summary of pharmacokinetics

Drug	Half-life (hour)	Active metabolites	Daily dose (mg) Adult	Elderly
Alprazolam	12–15	Yes	0.25–2.0	0.125–1
Chlordiazepoxide	7–28	Yes	25–100	5–50
Clonazepam	18–56	Yes	1–8	0.5–4
Clorazepate	30–200	Yes	15–60	7.5–30
Diazepam	20–60	Yes	5–30	2–15
Lorazepam	10–20	None	1–6	0.5–3
Halazepam	15–50	Yes	20–160	20–80
Oxazepam	5–15	None	15–90	10–45
Prazepam	25–200	Yes	20–60	10–20

lists the more commonly used benzodiazepines along with relevant information about their half-lives and the daily doses recommended for elderly patients. Short half-life benzodiazepines such as lorazepam, oxazepam, and temazepam appear preferable in that they are inactivated by direct conjugation in the liver, a mechanism that does not seem to be affected by aging (Moran et al. 1988). In addition, these drugs are relatively less lipophilic and are thus less prone to accumulate in fatty tissues of elderly patients compared with a more lipophilic drug like diazepam. Most other benzodiazepines tend to be metabolized via oxidative pathways into active metabolites, which tend to linger on in elderly patients for long periods of time.

Several studies of elderly patients have documented undesirable side effects of long-acting benzodiazepines (e.g., diazepam, clorazepate, chlordiazepoxide) including drowsiness, fatigue, psychomotor impairment, and cognitive impairment (Boston Collaborative Drug Surveillance Program 1973; Curran et al. 1987; Larson et al. 1987; Pomara et al. 1984, 1991). For example, Rosenbaum (1979) documented that the half-life of diazepam's metabolites increases from 20 hours in a 20-year-old patient to 90 hours in an 80-year-old patient. Alprazolam, a commonly used, intermediate half-life, antipanic medication, has also been shown to have half-lives of more than 21 hours in elderly people compared to 11 hours in young people (Kroboth et al. 1990).

In summary, these studies suggest that short-acting benzodiazepines like oxazepam, lorazepam, and temazepam are preferable in elderly patients, whereas long-acting benzodiazepines like diazepam, clorazepate, and flurazepam appear less desirable in general. Given the probability that, if taken for long periods of time, even short-acting benzodiazepines will tend to accumulate in older people, any use of benzodiazepines in this population should be for specific indications and time limited, preferably to less than 6 months. Table 14–7 lists potential complications of long-term use of benzodiazepines in the elderly.

Buspirone. In double-blind studies (Rickels and Schweizer 1987; Rickels et al. 1982), this anxiolytic medication with partial serotonin-agonist properties has demonstrated efficacy comparable to that of diazepam in patients with generalized anxiety disorder. Its nonaddictive profile, absence of withdrawal symptoms when discontinued (Rickels et al. 1988), and lack of psychomotor impairment even with long-term usage

(Smiley and Moskowitz 1986) seem to be advantages over benzodiazepines in chronic anxiety conditions. Studies in geriatric populations indicate that it is well tolerated, does not cause adverse interactions when coprescribed with other medications (including antihypertensives, cardiac glycosides, and bronchodilators), and is effective for remediation of chronic anxiety symptoms in this population (Napoliello 1986). It also appears that in both acute and chronic dosing, the pharmacokinetics of buspirone in elderly patients are very similar to those in younger patients (Gammans et al. 1989). Such a profile seems to suggest that buspirone may be a particularly desirable anxiolytic for chronic anxiety conditions of elderly patients where long-term use might be indicated. However, in contrast to research data, clinical experience with this medication suggests that a therapeutic response is somewhat inconsistent. It is important to remember that buspirone may take 1–4 weeks before manifesting its therapeutic effects. It might be desirable to combine it initially with a short-acting benzodiazepine that can then be withdrawn after 4 weeks.

Antidepressants. Several researchers have documented the effectiveness of antidepressants, particularly tricyclic imipramine and the monoamine oxidase inhibitor phenelzine, in panic disorder and agoraphobia (Mavissakalian and Michelson 1986; Sheehan et al. 1980; Zitrin et al. 1983). More recently, several studies have demonstrated efficacy of serotonin reuptake inhibitors (SRIs) in panic disorder (Ohrstrom et al. 1992; Schneier et al. 1990). In the same vein, the antidepressants clomipramine (Insel et al. 1983; Thoren et al.

Table 14–7. Potential complications of long-term benzodiazepine use in elderly patients

Excessive daytime drowsiness

Cognitive impairment and confusion

Psychomotor impairment and a risk of falls

Depression

Intoxication (even on therapeutic dosages)

Paradoxical reactions

Amnestic syndromes

Respiratory problems

Abuse and dependence potential

Breakthrough withdrawal reactions

Source. Adapted from Sheikh 1992a. Used with permission.

1980; Volavka et al. 1985), fluoxetine, and sertraline (Chouinard et al. 1990; Greist et al. 1992) have shown efficacy for alleviating symptoms of obsessive-compulsive disorder. There are no placebo-controlled studies of these medications in elderly patients with anxiety disorders, though they are routinely used in clinical settings to manage these syndromes in this population. Our practice is to use one of the SRIs as the first line of treatment in older patients, as they seem to be much better tolerated by the elderly than are tricyclic antidepressants. We tend to begin SRIs at half the starting doses usual for the general population, that is, 25 mg with sertraline (Zoloft), 10 mg with paroxetine (Paxil), and 10 mg with fluoxetine (Prozac), and titrate the dose upward depending on response and/or side effects.

Beta-blockers, antihistamines, and neuroleptics.
Some reports suggest that beta-blockers like propranolol and oxprenolol may be quite suitable for some geriatric patients with anxiety and agitation (Petrie 1983; Petrie and Ban 1981), particularly for agitation of individuals with dementia who are refractory to antipsychotic or benzodiazepine therapy. Propranolol 10 mg bid, to be gradually increased to 20–30 mg bid if no response occurs, is usually sufficient in these cases. Antihistamines like hydroxyzine and diphenhydramine are also used sometimes to manage mild anxiety with varying degree of success. Finally, our clinical experience suggests that low-dose, high-potency neuroleptics like haloperidol and fluphenazine (e.g., haloperidol 0.25–0.5 mg bid) can be quite effective in anxiety and agitation associated with organic brain syndromes. In conclusion, a variety of compounds including benzodiazepines, buspirone, antidepressants, and beta-blockers seem to show effectiveness for various anxiety disorders of the elderly.

Psychological Treatments

Studies suggest that dynamic psychotherapy is of limited therapeutic usefulness in alleviating specific anxiety disorders, other than being helpful as a supportive strategy for the patient (Sheehan et al. 1980; Weiss 1964; Zitrin et al. 1978). As usual, no systematic studies in the elderly population exist, but there is no reason to believe that dynamic psychotherapy will be any more effective for these conditions in this age group.[2]

Relaxation procedures primarily consist of adaptations of the progressive relaxation techniques of Bernstein and Borkovec (1973) and consist of tension-relaxation exercises of different muscle groups from head to toe. *Cognitive restructuring techniques* to overcome anxiety are adaptations from Meichenbaum (1974), Mahoney (1974), Beck et al. (1985), and Clark (1986). These techniques usually consist of information gathering from the patient about fearful cognitions, identifying fearful cognitions, providing alternative cognitions and other coping strategies for stressful situations, and finally application and practice. *Exposure* has been the mainstay for management of phobias in the last two decades (Bandura 1969; Marks 1987; Sherman 1972) and can be either real life (in vivo) to the phobic situation or fantasy exposure (in vitro) using imagery to recreate the phobic situation. Both techniques usually require graded exposure to the feared object or situation over a period of a few weeks, whether in real life or in fantasy. Marks (1987) has contended that in vivo exposure is more efficient even if both were equally effective, because fantasy exposure would ultimately require transfer to real-life situations.

Despite extensive systematic research documenting effectiveness of cognitive-behavior therapy in anxiety disorders of younger populations, such research is in general lacking for elderly populations. One has to settle for inference based on studies in younger groups and hope that these methods will be similarly effective in geriatric patients. There is some indirect evidence from the memory training literature that relaxation techniques can improve performance in anxious elderly patients by possibly reducing their anxiety (Yesavage et al. 1988).

There are also a few case studies that can be instructive as models for cognitive-behavioral treatments of geriatric anxiety. For example, Woods and Britton

---

[2] The cognitive-behavior therapy literature is full of reports describing anxiety management procedures of demonstrated efficacy in a younger population (see Chapter 31). A number of cognitive and behavioral interventions are efficacious for the treatment of generalized anxiety (Barlow 1988; Beck 1988), panic disorder (Barlow and Cerny 1988; Clark 1989; Clark et al. 1985), phobias (Marks 1981, 1987), and obsessive-compulsive disorder (Marks 1981; Rachman and Hodgson 1980) in the general population. These procedures generally fall into three main categories: relaxation training, cognitive restructuring, and exposure.

(1985) described behavioral treatment of a 64-year-old widow who was afraid to leave her apartment. Desensitization treatment began with education and commitment from the patient to work toward getting better. This was followed by other sessions involving relaxation instructions and encouragement to walk increasing distances from home. She improved quite a bit over a period of 5–6 months, as evidenced by self-reports (confirmed by the family) of decreased fear and increased activity and of going out of home alone quite frequently. In another case study, Haley (1983) described an anxious elderly woman calling her niece about 10 times daily. After training by role playing, the niece was able to extinguish her aunt's behavior by refusing to answer more than three calls per day. This method successfully stopped the excessive calling. In another report, Hussian (1981) described successful treatment of four elderly residents in a long-term care facility who had developed severe anxiety related to riding the elevator. The treatment began with relaxation training plus cover imagery followed by education about cognitions, anxiety, and avoidance. This treatment was followed by identification of fearful thoughts related to riding in an elevator and a learning of appropriate coping statements. Finally, the task of riding the elevator was added, and all four subjects responded well and maintained the improvement at a 2-month follow-up.

Cognitive-behavioral treatment should thus be considered as an alternative to pharmacological treatment where the possibility of side effects and drug interactions is high because of intercurrent medical problems and polypharmacy or where compliance with a medication regimen is an issue. Table 14–8 summarizes strategies for effective management of anxiety disorders in elderly patients.

Conclusions and Future Directions

Despite increasing research interest in the area of anxiety in younger age groups, few systematic studies of the phenomenology and treatment of anxiety disorders in elderly patients have been performed. Data from ECA studies suggest that anxiety disorders remain among the most prevalent of all psychiatric disorders in this age group. Geriatric anxiety thus remains woefully underaddressed, with large gaps of knowledge and a relevant information-base predictably inadequate. The following is a list of the knowledge gaps and suggested directions for future research:

1. To begin with, we need more information about the phenomenology of anxiety disorders in the elderly, both in healthy and physically ill populations. This goal can be achieved by designing large-scale surveys of elderly subjects in various settings, including community, outpatient clinics in general medical settings, outpatient mental health clinics, hospitals, and nursing homes. DSM-IV should be used as the guiding principle, but not the limiting factor, in such surveys as there may be differences in phenomenology from the general population.
2. There is a need to carry out validation studies of the existing scales of anxiety using various structured diagnostic interviews as external criteria. These studies may in turn lead to the development of better measures specifically geared toward measuring anxiety in elderly patients.
3. The issue of comorbidity of anxiety disorders with other psychiatric conditions (e.g., alcohol abuse and depression), as well as certain medical illnesses (e.g., ischemic heart disease), needs to be studied.

Table 14–8. Strategies for effective management of anxiety disorder in elderly patients

Disorder	Treatment of choice	Alternative treatments
Panic disorder with or without agoraphobia	Serotonin reuptake inhibitors (e.g., fluoxetine, paroxetine, and sertraline)	Imipramine, phenelzine, and cognitive-behavior therapy (CBT)
Generalized anxiety disorder	Benzodiazepines or buspirone	CBT
Obsessive-compulsive disorder	Serotonin reuptake inhibitors	Clomipramine and CBT
Social phobia		
Generalized	Phenelzine plus CBT	Benzodiazepines
Specific	Beta-blockers plus CBT	Buspirone
Simple (specific) phobia	CBT or benzodiazepines	Beta-blockers
Posttraumatic stress disorder	As indicated	—

4. Studies are needed to examine the differential phenomenology, clinical course, and treatment responses of late-onset versus early-onset anxiety disorders.

5. We need to perform controlled clinical trials of various anxiolytic medications to establish empirically derived guidelines for safety, efficacy, and specificity of these drugs for this population. Such studies are a priority for the field.

6. As mentioned above, behavior therapy literature is replete with reports describing anxiety management procedures of demonstrated efficacy in a younger population. Due to the special vulnerability of elderly patients to side effects of medications, there is clearly a need to study the efficacy of non-pharmacological methods for the management of anxiety in this population.

7. Finally, we have no information about the course and prognosis of various anxiety disorders in elderly patients, and such issues will need to be investigated.

References

Alexander AB: Systematic relaxation and flow rates in asthmatic children: relationship to emotional precipitants and anxiety. J Psychosom Res 16:405–410, 1972

American Psychiatric Association: Diagnostic and Statistical Manual of Mental Disorders, 3rd Edition. Washington, DC, American Psychiatric Association, 1980

American Psychiatric Association: Diagnostic and Statistical Manual of Mental Disorders, 3rd Edition, Revised. Washington, DC, American Psychiatric Association, 1987

American Psychiatric Association: Diagnostic and Statistical Manual of Mental Disorder, 4th Edition. Washington, DC, American Psychiatric Association, 1994

Atkinson R: Aging and alcohol use disorders: diagnostic issues in the elderly. Paper presented at the NIMH/APA DSM-IV Geriatric Workshop, San Francisco, CA, May 1989

Bandura A: Principles of Behavior Modification. New York, Holt, Rinehart & Winston, 1969

Barlow DH: Anxiety and Its Disorders: The Nature and Treatment of Anxiety and Panic. New York, Guilford, 1988

Barlow DH, Cerny JA: Psychological Treatment of Panic (Treatment Manuals for Practitioners Series). New York, Guilford, 1988

Beck AT: Cognitive approaches to panic disorder: theory and therapy, in Panic: Psychological Perspectives. Edited by Rachman S, Maser JD. Hillsdale, NJ, Lawrence Erlbaum Associates, 1988, pp 91–109

Beck AT, Emery G, Greenberg RL: Anxiety Disorders and Phobias: A Cognitive Perspective. New York, Basic Books, 1985

Beck AT, Epstein N, Brown G, et al: An inventory for measuring clinical anxiety: psychometric properties. J Consult Clin Psychol 56:893–897, 1988

Bergmann K: The neuroses of old age, in Recent Developments in Psychogeriatrics, British Journal of Psychiatry, Special Publication No. 6. Edited by Kay DWK, Walk A. Ashford, England, Headley Brothers, 1971

Bernstein DA, Borkovec TD: Progressive Relaxation: A Manual for the Helping Professions. Champaign, IL, Research Press, 1973

Blazer D, George LK, Hughes D: The epidemiology of anxiety disorders: an age comparison, in Anxiety in the Elderly. Edited by Salzman C, Lebowitz BD. New York, Springer, 1991, pp 17–30

Boston Collaborative Drug Surveillance Program: Clinical depression of the central nervous system due to diazepam and chlordiazepoxide in relation to cigarette smoking and age. N Engl J Med 288:277–280, 1973

Boulenger JP, Marangos PJ, Patel J, et al: Central adenosine receptors: possible involvement in the chronic effects of caffeine. Psychopharmacol Bull 20:431–435, 1984

Boyd JH, Burke JD, Greenberg E, et al: Exclusion criteria of DSM-III: a study of co-occurrence of hierarchy-free syndromes. Arch Gen Psychiatry 41:983–989, 1984

Cannon WB: Bodily Changes in Pain, Hunger, Fear, and Rage: An Account of Recent Researches into the Function of Emotional Excitement. New York, Appleton-Century-Crofts, 1929

Carey MP, Burish TG: Anxiety as a predictor of behavioral outcome for chemotherapy patients. J Consult Clin Psychol 53:860–865, 1985

Chambless DL, Cherney J, Caputo GC, et al: Anxiety disorders and alcoholism: a study with inpatient alcoholics. Journal of Anxiety Disorders 1:29–40, 1987

Charney DS, Heninger GR: Noradrenergic function and the assessment of action of antianxiety treatment, I: The effect of long-term alprazolam treatment. Arch Gen Psychiatry 42:458–467, 1985

Charney DS, Heninger GR, Sternberg DE: Assessment of α-2 adrenergic autoreceptor function in humans: Effects of oral yohimbine. Life Sci 30:2033–2041, 1982

Charney DS, Heninger GR, Jatlow PL: Increased anxiogenic effects of caffeine in panic disorder. Arch Gen Psychiatry 42:233–243, 1985

Chouinard G, Goodman W, Greist J, et al: Results of a double-blind placebo controlled trial of a new serotonin uptake inhibitor, sertraline, in the treatment of obsessive-compulsive disorder. Psychopharmacol Bull 26:279–284, 1990

Clark DM: A cognitive approach to panic. Behav Res Ther 24:461–470, 1986

Clark DM: Anxiety states: panic and generalized anxiety, in Cognitive Behavior Therapy for Psychiatric Problems: A Practical Guide. Edited by Hawton K, Salkovskis PM, Kirk J, et al. New York, Oxford University Press, 1989, pp 3–96

Clark DM, Salkovskis PM, Chalkley AJ: Respiratory control as a treatment for panic attacks. J Behav Ther Exp Psychiatry 16:23–30, 1985

Clarke AH, Lewis MJ: Fear of crime among the elderly. British Journal of Criminology 232:49, 1982

Cohen CI: Nocturnal neurosis of the elderly: failure of agencies to cope with the problem. J Am Geriatr Soc 24:86–88, 1976

Copeland JR, Davidson LA, Dewey ME: The prevalence and outcome of anxious depression in elderly people aged 65 and over living in the community, in Anxious Depression: Assessment and Treatment. Edited by Racagnia G, Sneraldi E. New York, Raven, 1987, pp 43–47

Coryell W: Mortality of anxiety disorders, in Classification, Etiological Factors and Associated Disturbances, Handbook of Anxiety, Vol 2. Edited by Noyes R Jr, Roth M, Burrows GD. Amsterdam, Elsevier/North Holland Science, 1988, pp 311–320

Coryell W, Noyes R, Clancy J: Excess mortality in panic disorder: a comparison with primary unipolar depression. Arch Gen Psychiatry 39:701–703, 1982

Coryell W, Noyes R, Hause JD: Mortality among outpatients with anxiety disorders. Am J Psychiatry 143:508–510, 1986

Cummings JL: Behavioral complications of drug treatment of Parkinson's disease. J Am Geriatr Soc 39:708–716, 1991

Curran HV, Allen D, Lader M: The effects of single doses of alprazolam and lorazepam on memory and psychomotor performance in normal humans. Journal of Psychopharmacology 2:81–89, 1987

Derogatis LR: The SCL-90-R. Baltimore, MD, Clinical Psychometric Research, 1975

Edlund MJ, Swan AC, Clothier J: Patients with panic attacks and abnormal EEG results. Am J Psychiatry 144:508–509, 1987

Fleminger S: Left-sided Parkinson's disease is associated with greater anxiety and depression. Psychol Med 21:629–638, 1991

Gammans RE, Westrick ML, Shea JP, et al: Pharmacokinetics of buspirone in elderly subjects. J Clin Pharmacol 29:72–78, 1989

Gorman JM, Fyer AJ, Gliklich J, et al: Mitral valve prolapse and panic disorders: effect of imipramine, in Anxiety: New Research and Changing Concepts. Edited by Klein DF, Rabkin JG. New York, Raven Press, 1981, pp 317–326

Gorman JM, Liebowitz MR, Fyer AJ, et al: A neuroanatomical hypothesis for panic disorder. Am J Psychiatry 146:148–161, 1989

Gray JA: The Neuropsychology of Anxiety. New York, Oxford University Press, 1982

Greenblatt DJ: Reduced serum albumin concentrations in the elderly: a report from the Boston Collaborative Drug Surveillance Program. J Am Geriatr Soc 27:20–22, 1979

Greist J, Chouinard G, DuBoff E, et al: Double-blind comparison of three doses of sertraline and placebo in the treatment of outpatients with obsessive-compulsive disorder. Poster presented at the 18th Collegium Internationale NeuroPsychopharmacologicum Congress, Nice, France, June 1992

Haley WE: A family behavioral approach of the cognitively impaired elderly. Gerontologist 23:18–20, 1983

Hall RCW (ed): Psychiatric Presentations of Medical Illness. New York, Spectrum, 1980

Hamilton M: The assessment of anxiety states by rating. Br J Med Psychol 32:50–55, 1959

Harris EL, Noyes R, Crowe RR, et al: Family study of agoraphobia: report of a pilot study. Arch Gen Psychiatry 40:1061–1064, 1983

Henderson R, Kurlan R, Kersun JM, et al: Preliminary examination of the comorbidity of anxiety and depression in Parkinson's disease. J Neuropsychiatry Clin Neurosci 4:257–264, 1992

Hesselbrock MN, Meyer RE, Keener JJ: Psychopathology in hospitalized alcoholics. Arch Gen Psychiatry 42:1050–1055, 1985

Himmelfarb S, Murrel SA: The prevalence and correlates of anxiety symptoms in older adults. J Psychol 116:159–167, 1984

Hurley JR: Thyroid diseases in the elderly. Med Clin North Am 67:497–516, 1983

Hussian RA: Geriatric Psychology: A Behavioral Perspective. New York, Van Nostrand Reinhold, 1981

Insel TR, Gillin JC, Moore A, et al: The sleep of patients with obsessive-compulsive disorder. Arch Gen Psychiatry 39:1372–1377, 1982

Insel TR, Murphy DL, Cohen RM, et al: Obsessive-compulsive disorder: a double-blind trial of clomipramine and clorgyline. Arch Gen Psychiatry 40:605–612, 1983

Iruela LM, Ibanez-Rojo V, Palanca I, et al: Anxiety disorders and Parkinson's disease (letter). Am J Psychiatry 149:719–720, 1992

Jenike MA: Handbook of Geriatric Psychopharmacology. Littleton, MA, PSG Publishing, 1985

Jenike MA: Anxiety disorders of old age, in Geriatric Psychiatry and Psychopharmacology. Edited by Jenike MA. St. Louis, MO, Mosby Year Book, 1989, pp 248–271

Jenkins CD: Psychological and social precursors of coronary disease. N Engl J Med 284:244–255, 1971

Kantor JS, Zitrin CM, Zeldis SM: Mitral valve prolapse syndrome in agoraphobic patients. Am J Psychiatry 137:467–469, 1980

Karajgi B, Rifkin A, Doddi S, et al: The prevalence of anxiety disorders in patients with chronic obstructive pulmonary disease. Am J Psychiatry 147:200–201, 1990

Kathol RG, Turner R, Delahunt J: Depression and anxiety associated with hyperthyroidism: response to antithyroid therapy. Psychosomatics 27:501–505, 1986

Kay DWK: Anxiety in the elderly, in Biological, Clinical and Cultural Perspectives: Handbook of Anxiety, Vol 1. Edited by Roth M, Noyes JR, Burrows GD. Amsterdam, Elsevier/North Holland Science, 1988, pp 289–310

Kelly D, Mitchell-Heggs SN, Sherman D: Anxiety and the effects of sodium lactate assessed clinically and physiologically. Br J Psychiatry 119:129–141, 1971

Kochansky GE: Psychiatric rating scales for assessing psychopathology in the elderly: a critical review, in Psychiatric Symptoms and Cognitive Loss in the Elderly. Edited by Raskin A, Jarvik L. Washington, DC, Hemisphere, 1979, pp 125–156

Kroboth PD, McAuley JW, Smith RB: Alprazolam in the elderly: pharmacokinetics and pharmacodynamics during multiple dosing. Psychopharmacology 100:477–484, 1990

Kushner MG, Sher KJ, Beitman BD: The relation between alcohol problems and the anxiety disorders. Am J Psychiatry 147:685–695, 1990

Larson EB, Kukull WA, Buchner D, et al: Adverse drug reactions associated with global cognitive impairment in elderly persons. Ann Intern Med 107:169–173, 1987

Lee MA: Anxiety and caffeine consumption in people with anxiety disorders. Psychiatry Res 15:211–217, 1985

Leigh D: Psychiatric aspects of head injury. Psychiatry Digest 40:21–32, 1979

Lerner WD, Fallen HJ: The alcohol withdrawal syndrome. N Engl J Med 313:511–515, 1985

Liebowitz MR, Fyer AJ, Gorman JM, et al: Lactate provocation of panic attacks, I: clinical and behavioral findings. Arch Gen Psychiatry 41:764–770, 1984

Lindesay J: Phobic disorders in the elderly. Br J Psychiatry 159:531–541, 1991

Liptzin B: Masked anxiety: alcohol and drug use, in Anxiety in the Elderly. Edited by Salzman C, Lebowitz BD. New York, Springer, 1991, pp 87–101

Luchins DJ, Rose RP: Late-life onset of panic disorder with agoraphobia in three patients. Am J Psychiatry 146:920–921, 1989

Mahoney MJ: Cognition and Behavior Modification. Cambridge, MA, Ballinger, 1974

Margraf J, Ehlers A, Roth WT: Mitral valve prolapse and panic disorder: a review of their relationship. Psychosom Med 50:93–113, 1988

Marks IM: Cure and Care of Neuroses: Theory and Practice of Behavioral Psychotherapy. New York, Wiley, 1981

Marks IM: Fears, Phobias, and Rituals: Panic, Anxiety, and Their Disorders. New York, Oxford University Press, 1987

Mathew RJ, Swihart AA, Weinman ML: Vegetative symptoms in anxiety and depression. Br J Psychiatry 141:162–165, 1982

Mavissakalian M, Michelson L: Agoraphobia: relative and combined effectiveness of therapist-assisted in vivo exposure and imipramine. J Clin Psychiatry 47:117–122, 1986

Mazza DL, Martin D, Spacavento L, et al: Prevalence of anxiety disorders in patients with mitral valve prolapse. Am J Psychiatry 143:349–352, 1986

Meichenbaum D: Self-instructional strategy training: a cognitive prosthesis for the aged. Hum Dev 17:273–280, 1974

Moran MG, Thompson TL II, Nies AS: Sleep disorders in the elderly. Am J Psychiatry 145:1369–1378, 1988

Munjack KJ, Moss HB: Affective disorder and alcoholism in families of agoraphobics. Arch Gen Psychiatry 38:869–871, 1981

Myers JK, Weissman MM, Tischler GL, et al: Six-month prevalence of psychiatric disorders in three communities: 1980–1982. Arch Gen Psychiatry 41:959–967, 1984

Napoliello MJ: An interim multicenter report on 677 anxious geriatric outpatients treated with buspirone. Br J Clin Pract 40:71–73, 1986

Nowlin JB, Williams R, Wilkie F: Prospective study of physical and psychological factors in elderly men who subsequently suffer acute myocardial infarction (AMI). Clin Res 21:465, 1973

Ohrstrom JK, Judge R, Manniche PM, et al: Paroxetine in the treatment of panic disorder, paper presented at the annual meeting of the American College of Neuropsychopharmacology, San Juan, Peruto Rico, December 1992

Ouslander JG: Drug therapy in the elderly. Ann Intern Med 94:711–722, 1981

Papper S: Clinical Nephrology. Boston, MA, Little, Brown, 1978

Patterson RL, Sullivan MJ, Spielberger CD: Measurement of state and trait anxiety in elderly mental health clients. Journal of Behavior Assessment 2:89–96, 1980

Petrie WM: Drug treatment of anxiety and agitation in the aged. Psychopharmacol Bull 19:238–246, 1983

Petrie WM, Ban TA: Propranolol in organic agitation (letter). Lancet 1:324, 1981

Pitts FN Jr, McClure JN: Lactate metabolism in anxiety neurosis. N Engl J Med 227:1329–1336, 1967

Pomara N, Stanley B, Block R, et al: Diazepam impairs performance in normal elderly subjects. Psychopharmacol Bull 20:137–139, 1984

Pomara N, Deptula D, Singh R, et al: Cognitive toxicity of benzodiazepines in the elderly, in Anxiety in the Elderly. Edited by Salzman CL, Lebowitz BD. New York, Springer, 1991, pp 175–196

Popkin MK, Mackenzie TB: Psychiatric presentations of endocrine dysfunction, in Psychiatric Presentations of Medical Illness. Edited by Hall RCW. New York, Spectrum, 1980, pp 139–156

Post F: The management and nature of depressive illness in late life: a follow through study. Br J Psychiatry 121:393–404, 1972

Rachman SJ, Hodgson R: Obsessions and Compulsions. Englewood Cliffs, NJ, Prentice-Hall, 1980

Redmond DE, Huang HY: New evidence for a locus coeruleus-norepinephrine connection with anxiety. Life Sci 25:2149–2162, 1979

Reiman EM, Raichle ME, Robins E, et al: Neuroanatomical correlates of a lactate-induced anxiety attack. Arch Gen Psychiatry 46:493–500, 1989

Reynolds CF, Shaw DH, Newton TF, et al: EEG sleep in outpatients with generalized anxiety: a preliminary comparison with depressed outpatients. Psychiatry Res 8:81–89, 1983

Rickels K, Schweizer EE: Current pharmacotherapy of anxiety and panic, in Psychopharmacology: The Third Generation of Progress. Edited by Meltzer HY. New York, Raven, 1987, pp 1193–1203

Rickels K, Weisman K, Norstad N, et al: Buspirone and diazepam in anxiety: a controlled study. J Clin Psychiatry 43:81–86, 1982

Rickels K, Schweizer EE, Csanalosi I, et al: Long-term treatment of anxiety and risk of withdrawal: prospective comparison of clorazepate and buspirone. Arch Gen Psychiatry 45:444–450, 1988

Robinson RG, Starkstein SE: Current research in affective disorders following stroke. J Neuropsychiatry Clin Neurosci 2:1–14, 1990

Rosenbaum J: Anxiety, in Outpatient Psychiatry: Diagnosis and Treatment. Edited by Lazare A. Baltimore, MD, Williams & Wilkins, pp 252–256, 1979

Ross HE, Glasser FB, Germanson T: The prevalence of psychiatric disorders in patients with alcohol and other drug problems. Arch Gen Psychiatry 45:1023–1031, 1988

Salzman C: Psychometric rating of anxiety in the elderly, in Proceedings of a Conference on Anxiety in the Elderly. Co-sponsored by Roche Laboratories, University of Arizona College of Medicine, Tucson, AZ, November 1977, pp 5–21

Sandberg B, Bliding A: Duodenal ulcer in army trainees during basic training. J Psychosom Res 20:61–74, 1976

Schiffer RB, Kurlan R, Rubin A, et al: Evidence for atypical depression in Parkinson's disease. Am J Psychiatry 145:1020–1022, 1988

Schneier FR, Liebowitz MR, Davies SO, et al: Fluoxetine in panic disorder. J Clin Psychopharmacol 10:119–121, 1990

Schweizer E, Case WG, Rickels K: Benzodiazepine dependence and withdrawal in elderly patients. Am J Psychiatry 146:529–531, 1989

Sheehan DV, Ballenger JC, Jacobsen G: Treatment of endogenous anxiety with phobic, hysterical, and hypochondriacal symptoms. Arch Gen Psychiatry 37:51–59, 1980

Sheikh JI: Anxiety rating scales for the elderly, in Anxiety in the Elderly. Edited by Salzman C, Lebowitz BD. New York, Springer, 1991, pp 251–265

Sheikh JI: Problems associated with long-term benzodiazepine use in the elderly, in Psychopharmacological Treatment Complications in the Elderly. Edited by Shamoian CA. Washington, DC, American Psychiatric Press, 1992a, pp 71–87

Sheikh JI: Anxiety disorders and their treatment, in Clinics in Geriatric Medicine: Psychiatric Disorders in Late Life, Vol 8, No 2. Edited by Alexopoulos GS. Philadelphia, PA, WB Saunders, 1992b, pp 411–426

Sheikh JI: Clinical features of anxiety disorders, in The Psychiatry of Old Age. Edited by Copeland JM, Abou-Saleh MT, Blazer DG. Chichester, England, Wiley, 1993a, pp 107.1–107.5

Sheikh JI: Is late-onset panic disorder a distinct syndrome? Paper presented at the annual meeting of the American Psychiatric Association, San Francisco, CA, May 1993b

Sheikh JI, Taylor CB, King RJ, et al: Panic attacks and avoidance behavior in the elderly. Presented at the annual meeting of the American Psychiatric Association, Montreal, Canada, May 1988

Sheikh JI, King RJ, Taylor CB: Comparative phenomenology of early onset versus late-onset panic attacks: a pilot survey. Am J Psychiatry 148:1231–1233, 1991

Sherman PW: Real life exposure as a primary therapeutic factor in desensitization treatment of fear. J Abnorm Psychol 79:19–28, 1972

Simson PE, Weiss JM: Altered activity of locus coeruleus in an animal model of depression. Neuropsychopharmacology 1:287–295, 1988

Smiley A, Moskowitz H: Effects of long-term administration of buspirone and diazepam on driver steering control. Am J Med 80 (suppl 3B):22–29, 1986

Spielberger C, Gorsuch R, Lushene R: STAI Manual for the State-Trait Anxiety Inventory. Palo Alto, CA, Consulting Psychologists Press, 1970

Spitzer RL, Williams JBW, Gibbon M: Structured Clinical Interview for DSM-III-R—Patient Version (SCID-P, 4/1/87). New York, New York State Psychiatric Institute, 1987

Stein MB, Heuser IJ, Juncos JL, et al: Anxiety disorders in patients with Parkinson's disease. Am J Psychiatry 147:217–220, 1990

Sunderland T, Lawlor B, Martinez R, et al: Anxiety in the elderly: neurobiological and clinical interface, in Anxiety in the Elderly. Edited by Salzman C, Lebowitz BD. New York, Springer, 1991, pp 105–129

Teri L, Larson EB, Reifler B: Behavioral disturbance in dementia of Alzheimer type. J Am Geriatr Soc 36:1–6, 1988

Thoren P, Asberg M, Cronholm B, et al: Clomipramine treatment of obsessive-compulsive disorder, I: a controlled clinical trial. Arch Gen Psychiatry 37:1281–1285, 1980

Uhde TW, Roy-Byrne P, Gillin JC, et al: The sleep of patients with panic disorder: a preliminary report. Psychiatry Res 12:251–259, 1984

Victor BS, Lubersky M, Greden F: Somatic manifestations of caffeinism. J Clin Psychiatry 42:185–188, 1981

Volavka J, Neziroglu F, Yaruya-Tobias JA: Clomipramine and imipramine in obsessive-compulsive disorder. Psychiatry Res 14:83–91, 1985

Weiss E: Agoraphobia in the Light of Ego Psychology. New York, Grune & Stratton, 1964

Weissman MM: Anxiety and alcoholism. J Clin Psychiatry 49 (suppl):17–19, 1988

Whitehead WE, Blackwell B, DeSilva H, et al: Anxiety and anger in hypertension. J Psychosom Res 21:383–389, 1977

Woods RT, Britton PG: Clinical Psychology With the Elderly. Rockville, MD, Aspen, 1985

Yellowlees PM, Alpers JH, Bowden JJ, et al: Psychiatric morbidity in patients with chronic airflow obstruction. Med J Aust 146:305–307, 1987

Yesavage JA, Sheikh JI, Tanke ED, et al: Response to memory training and individual differences in verbal intelligence and state anxiety. Am J Psychiatry 145:636–639, 1988

Zitrin CM, Klein DF, Woerner MG: Behavior therapy, supportive psychotherapy, imipramine, and phobias. Arch Gen Psychiatry 35:307–316, 1978

Zitrin CM, Klein DF, Woerner MG, et al: Treatment of phobias, I: comparison of imipramine hydrochloride and placebo. Arch Gen Psychiatry 40:125–138, 1983

15

Substance Abuse

Roland M. Atkinson, M.D.
Linda Ganzini, M.D.

Introduction

Although the first papers on geriatric alcoholism and drug addiction were published 40 years ago, geriatricians and addiction experts alike have only recently acknowledged that significant substance abuse occurs in older people. Espoused in several influential papers in the 1960s, the view that these disorders were seldom seen after middle age was not challenged for decades (Atkinson et al. 1992). Lifelong alcoholic and drug-addicted individuals presumably either died prematurely or recovered spontaneously, and late-onset addiction was said to be rare. Trained to this view, clinicians often overlook these disorders in elderly patients. In addition, symptoms of substance abuse in older individuals may mimic symptoms of other medical and behavioral disorders, leading to misdiagnosis. Finally, elderly patients, particularly, tend to underreport drinking problems, and clinicians also are less likely to record these problems and to make appropriate referrals in this population (Atkinson et al. 1992; Curtis et al. 1989). In this chapter, we address substance abuse in elderly individuals. We begin with an overview of the terms and concepts used in the field, as well as the risk factors involved for substance abuse in late life. We then discuss the general principles or assessment and management of these disorders. Finally, we present special sections on alcohol, prescription drugs, illicit drugs, and tobacco dependence.

Table 15–1.   Definitions of some terms used in the substance abuse field

Psychoactive: Any chemical—alcohol, therapeutic agent, industrial compound, or illicit drug—with important effects on the central nervous system.

Substance: A psychoactive that typically is associated with a substance use disorder. The term includes alcohol; opioids; sedative-hypnotics and antianxiety agents of the barbiturate and benzodiazepine types; psychomotor stimulants, especially amphetamines and cocaine; tobacco products; and certain over-the-counter psychoactives. The terms *chemical* and *drug* in this context are synonymous with substance (e.g., "chemical dependence" or "drug abuse").

Use: Appropriate medical or social consumption of a psychoactive in a manner that minimizes the potential for dependence or abuse.

Heavy use: Use of a substance in greater quantity than the usual norms, but without obvious negative social, behavioral, or health consequences. Heavy alcohol or tobacco users may be dependent on the substance.

Misuse: Use of a prescribed drug in a manner other than directed. The term can mean overuse, underuse, improper dose sequencing, or lending or borrowing another person's medication, with or without harmful consequences.

Problem use: Use of a substance in a manner that induces negative social, behavioral, or health consequences. A "problem" user may or may not meet criteria for substance dependence or abuse, although many do. Alcohol "problems" or drug "problems" are categories that often have been used by epidemiologists in community prevalence surveys.

Abuse: Abuse of a substance is defined in DSM-IV (American Psychiatric Association 1994) as "a maladaptive pattern of substance use leading to clinically significant impairment or distress, as manifested by one (or more) of the following, occurring within a 12-month period: 1) recurrent substance use resulting in a failure to fulfill major role obligations at work, school, or home (e.g., repeated absences or poor work performance related to substance use; substance-related absences, suspensions, or expulsions from school; neglect of children or household); 2) recurrent substance use in situations in which it is physically hazardous (e.g., driving an automobile or operating a machine when impaired by substance use); 3) recurrent substance-related legal problems (e.g., arrests for substance-related disorderly conduct); 4) continued substance use despite having persistent or recurrent social or interpersonal problems caused or exacerbated by the effects of the substance (e.g., arguments with spouse about consequences of intoxication, physical fights); and [with the exclusion criterion that] the symptoms have never met the criteria for substance dependence for this class of substance." (pp. 182–183). *Harmful use* (ICD-10; World Health Organization 1988) approximates abuse in definition. Both imply milder severity of substance involvement than in substance dependence.

Dependence: Dependence on a substance is defined by explicit diagnostic criteria, such as those listed in DSM-IV or ICD-10 (see Table 15-2). Serious and persistent involvement in the heavy use of the substance is the rule. These approaches set aside the older distinction between *physical dependence* and *psychological dependence,* which are now viewed as differing manifestations of similar disorders. The terms *alcoholism* and *addiction* are usually used as synonyms for dependence on alcohol and other drugs, respectively.

Substance use disorder: A clinical condition in which substance abuse or substance dependence can be diagnosed.

Substance abuse, chemical dependence, and addictions: These terms are often used to refer to the entire professional-scientific field.

General Terms and Concepts in the Field of Substance Abuse

Table 15–1 lists the definitions of substance abuse terms used in this chapter. The development and promulgation (beginning in 1980) of explicit criteria for diagnosis of substance use disorders has aided epidemiological and clinical research. Two currently used sets of criteria for substance dependence, the fundamental behavioral disorder underlying most sub-

stance-related problems, are listed in Table 15–2. (For further general information on substance abuse, see Donovan and Marlatt 1988; Kissin and Begleiter 1983a, 1983b; Lowinson et al. 1992; Schuckit 1989.)

Risk Factors for Substance Use Disorders in Later Life

Several distinctions about the nature and risk of substance abuse in younger people have less meaning in

Table 15–2. DSM-IV versus ICD-10 (provisional) criteria for substance dependence

DSM-IV criteria	ICD-10 criteria

1. Tolerance, as defined by either of the following:
  a. A need for markedly increased amounts of the substance to achieve intoxication or desired effect
  b. Markedly diminished effect with continued use of the same amount of the substance
	1. Strong desire or sense of compulsion to take the substance.

2. Withdrawal, as manifested by either of the following:
  a. The characteristic withdrawal syndrome for the substance[a]
  b. The same (or a closely related) substance is taken to relieve or avoid withdrawal symptoms
	2. Subjective awareness of an impaired capacity to control substance taking behavior in terms of onset, termination, or levels of use.

3. The substance is often taken in larger amounts or over a longer period than was intended.	3. Substance used with the intention of relieving withdrawal symptoms and with awareness that this strategy is effective.
4. There is a persistent desire or unsuccessful efforts to cut down or control substance use.	4. Physiological withdrawal state.
5. A great deal of time is spent in activities necessary to obtain the substance (e.g., visiting multiple doctors or driving long distances), use the substance (e.g., chain-smoking), or recover from its effects.	5. Evidence of tolerance such that an increased amount is required to achieve effects originally produced by lesser amounts.
6. Important social, occupational, or recreational activities are given up or reduced because of substance use.	6. Narrowing of personal repertoire of patterns of substance use (e.g., a tendency to use in the same way on weekdays and weekends, whatever social constraints there may be regarding appropriate or safe use).
7. The substance use is continued despite knowledge of having a persistent or recurrent physical or psychological problem that is likely to have been caused or exacerbated by the substance (e.g., current cocaine use despite recognition of cocaine-induced depression, or continued drinking despite recognition that an ulcer was made worse by alcohol consumption).	7. Progressive neglect of alternative pleasures/interests in favor of substance use.
	8. Persisting with use despite clear evidence of overtly harmful consequences (medical, social, and psychological).
	9. Evidence that return to substance use after a period of abstinence leads to more rapid reappearance of other features of dependence than occurs with nondependent individuals.

Note. For either system, at least 3 of the listed criteria must be met in order to make the diagnosis of dependence on a substance.
DSM-IV = Diagnostic and Statistical Manual of Mental Disorders, 4th Edition (American Psychiatric Association 1994);
ICD-10 = International Classification of Diseases, 10th Edition (Provisional Version) (World Health Organization 1988).
[a]Refer to criteria A and B of the criteria sets for "withdrawal" from the specific substances (American Psychiatric Association 1994).

old age. For example, pathophysiological effects of alcohol in many instances can no longer be considered merely transitory "side effects," but have more pervasive consequences because they aggravate preexisting diseases that are more common in later life. When older people continue to drink despite feeling physically unwell or advice to stop, this meets the definition of abusive drinking, even though such drinking may not be associated with socially deviant behavior or the desire to feel intoxicated. Put another way, the distinction between heavy drinking and problem drinking narrows with age. Biomedical manifestations of substance abuse become as important in older patients as the psychosocial manifestations that form the more familiar clinical picture of these disorders in younger patients. The risk factors listed in Table 15–3 reflect this perspective.

Predisposing factors are similar at all ages. Factors that may increase substance exposure and consumption level, and thus set the stage for abuse or dependence in some individuals, include demographics (e.g., gender and ethnicity) (Helzer et al. 1991); chronic illnesses for which controlled substances are often prescribed on a regular basis (Finlayson 1984);

Table 15–3. Risk factors for substance abuse in elderly patients

Predisposing factors
    Family history (alcohol)
    Previous substance abuse
    Previous pattern of substance consumption (individual and cohort effects)
    Personality traits (sedative-hypnotics and anxiolytics)
Factors that may increase substance exposure and consumption level
    Gender (men: alcohol and illicit drugs; women: sedative-hypnotics and anxiolytics)
    Chronic illness associated with pain (opioid analgesics), insomnia (hypnotic drugs), or anxiety (anxiolytics)
    Caregiver overuse of "as-needed" medication (institutionalized elderly individuals)
    Life stress, loss, and social isolation
    Family collusion and drinking partners (alcohol)
    Discretionary time and money (alcohol)
Factors that may increase the effects and abuse potential of substances
    Age-associated drug sensitivity (pharmacokinetic and pharmacodynamic factors)
    Chronic medical illnesses
    Other medications (alcohol-drug or drug-drug interactions)

---

institutionalization in long-term care settings; and several psychosocial factors (see Table 15–3). Factors that may increase the effects of substances also increase their abuse potential. Increasing biological sensitivity to most psychoactive drugs is associated with aging. Findings support a multivariate model: modified drug sensitivity may be based on age-related changes in several biological systems affecting pharmacokinetics and pharmacodynamics (Atkinson and Kofoed 1982; Atkinson et al. 1992). Regular psychoactive drug use can also increase functional impairment caused by a variety of illnesses that are more common in old age (e.g., cognitive, cardiovascular, pulmonary, gastrointestinal, and metabolic disorders). Clinical complications can arise from adverse drug-drug interactions between psychoactive substances and other prescribed medications. These alterations in biological sensitivity to drugs, comorbid medical illness, and medication interactions can lead to biomedical problems at substance consumption rates that would have caused no difficulty earlier in life.

Principles of Assessment and Management

Assessment of Geriatric Substance Use Disorders

General approach.   Denial of substance abuse is common in affected people of all ages, but may be exaggerated in elderly patients because of memory problems, pessimism about recovery, and shame based on a belief that substance abuse is immoral. For these reasons, careful rapport building through repeated contacts; inquiry with relatives, caregivers, and others in the social network; reviews of medical and pharmacy records; and home visitation are especially useful case-assessment methods. The DSM-IV (American Psychiatric Association 1994) and ICD-10 (World Health Organization 1988) dependence criteria offer a reasonable framework for acquiring information in order to establish a clinical diagnosis (Table 15–2).

Special examinations.   Physical and laboratory findings can help establish a diagnosis of alcohol dependence. Toxicological examinations of urine and blood for other suspected substances may be useful to corroborate the history. Neuropsychological evaluation and brain imaging (e.g., computed tomography [CT] and magnetic resonance imaging [MRI]) may help identify complicating brain disorders. Primary dementias and dementias secondary to alcohol or drugs may produce similar initial cognitive or imaging deficits. Insofar as substance-induced deficits either remain static or actually improve with prolonged abstinence (Brandt et al. 1983; Grant et al. 1984; Larson et al. 1984a; Ron 1983), serial psychometric testing may be useful in differential diagnosis.

Clinical Features

Signs and symptoms of substance use disorders.   In old age the signs and symptoms of substance use disorders can be subtle, atypical, or mimic symptoms of other geriatric illness. In mild or circumscribed cases among community-dwelling elderly individuals, episodic alcohol abuse or benzodiazepine dependence may not produce physical signs or complaints and may be easily concealed from others. Moderate alcohol dependence may have a circumscribed clinical presentation of increasingly uncontrolled hypertension or diabetes mellitus, whereas moderate benzodiazepine or alcohol dependence may present with the complaint of forgetfulness. In more severe cases, substance abuse can produce delirium or dementia (American Psychiatric Association 1990; Freund 1987; Ron 1983), which the clinician may incorrectly attribute to other causes. Other serious but nonspecific presenting signs and symptoms (e.g., poor grooming, depression, erratic changes of mood or behavior, malnutrition, bladder and bowel incontinence, muscle weakness or frank myopathy, gait disorders, recurring falls, burns, or head trauma) may be caused by unsuspected alcohol or drug abuse.

Features that may be associated with alcohol or prescription drug dependence.   These features include heavy tobacco use, chronic pain syndromes or insomnia, persistent family discord, a course of inexplicable ups and downs, a pattern of doing well in hospital but poorly at home, and patient or caregiver defensiveness when queried about substance use. When such factors are noted, the clinician needs to be alert to the possibility of underlying substance dependence.

Case Management and Treatment

The goals of substance abuse treatment in the elderly are threefold: 1) stabilization and reduction of substance consumption, 2) treatment of coexisting medical and psychiatric problems, and 3) arrangement of appropriate social interventions. Reducing consumption may be simple and straightforward in mild dependence, especially if the older person is highly cooperative; or it may be very complicated and hazardous, requiring hospital care or a protracted outpatient course, in cases of longstanding or high dose dependence. Treatment of coexisting problems can be a crucial step in curbing substance consumption, especially when chronic pain, chronic insomnia, or a mood disorder has been a major factor sustaining the substance dependence or when serious medical complications of substance abuse are present. Social interventions range from informal plans (e.g., arranging for in-

Table 15–4.   Prevalence of active alcohol problems among older patients in selected clinical settings

Setting (study)	Age cutoff	Sample size	Sex	Frequency of active alcoholism
General medical outpatient clinic (T. V. Jones et al. 1992)	≥ 65	154	Both	4%
Acute medical inpatient wards (Schuckit et al. 1980)	≥ 65	222	Men	6%
Community geriatric outreach mental health team (Reifler et al. 1982)	≥ 60	2,309	Both	9%
Nursing home admissions (Joseph et al. 1992)	> 50[a]	67	Both	11%
Emergency department visitors (Adams et al. 1992)	≥ 65	205	Both	14%
Geriatric psychiatry residential treatment unit (Speer and Bates 1992)	≥ 55	128	Both	23%

[a]Mean age 67 years, SD ± 8.

creased visitation by loved ones or enrollment in a senior activity program or day center) to major formal interventions (e.g., admission to a senior substance abuse program or to residential care).

Alcohol Use Disorders and Alcohol-Associated Organic Mental Disorders

Epidemiology

A majority of people over age 60 continue to drink beverage alcohol (Atkinson 1990). Reported community prevalence rates for heavy use (6% to 14%) and problematic use (1% to 17%) of alcohol by older people vary depending on the population sampled (Atkinson 1990). Representative reports of the prevalence of *active* alcoholism in elderly cohorts from various clinical settings are summarized in Table 15–4. Teetotalers are more common among older women than older men. Men are between two and six times more likely than women to have clinically documented alcohol problems (Atkinson 1990). Indeed, prevalence data support the conclusion that alcoholism now constitutes a public health problem of moderate proportion in men in their 60s and early 70s. Cross-sectional studies have shown a decline in the prevalence of alcohol use and abuse with age (Liberto et al. 1992). There is some real decline, accounted for by both premature deaths of early-onset alcoholics and moderation or cessation of drinking over time by surviving alcoholics (Liberto et al. 1992) and social drinkers (Adams et al. 1990). But many drinkers maintain steady consumption levels into later life (Glynn et al. 1985; Gordon and Kannel 1983). Because younger birth cohorts tend to have increasingly higher rates of alcohol consumption and alcoholism (reviewed in Atkinson et al. 1992), the prevalence of alcohol problems in old age may increase, especially among women, for birth cohorts entering their 60s in the 1990s and beyond.

Alcohol Use and Abuse

Early- versus late-onset alcohol problems. Although onset of alcoholism after age 45 was long thought to be rare, recent findings from community (Eaton et al. 1989) and clinical samples (Atkinson 1992; Atkinson et al. 1990) offer evidence that late-onset alcoholism is not uncommon. Late-onset alcohol problems are often milder and more circumscribed than those beginning earlier in life. Compared with alcoholism of long duration, late-onset problems tend to resolve "spontaneously" (i.e., without formal treatment) (Moos et al. 1991) and may be more amenable to treatment (Atkinson, in press; Atkinson et al. 1993; Schonfeld and Dupree 1991).

Reactive drinking. Older alcoholics (late-onset alcoholism, late relapse in early-onset alcoholics after years of sobriety, or recent increase in lifelong heavy drinking) may report major losses as precipitants of increased drinking. In addition, excess discretionary time (boredom) in persons lacking the capacity or resources to use time productively and other subtle but enduring strains may lead to increased alcohol consumption. Both social and solitary drinking may be promoted in certain retirement settings (Alexander and Duff 1988).

Therapeutic use and health maintenance value of alcohol. The use of small amounts of beverage alcohol has been advocated as a social adjuvant in elder residential care facilities (reviewed in Atkinson and Kofoed 1984). Similarly, alcohol is often touted as an appetite stimulant: in healthy elderly persons caloric intake and blood levels of some micronutrients may increase with alcohol intake, though other micronutrient levels decrease (Jacques et al. 1989). Several cautions apply, however. The list of potentially hazardous interactions of alcohol with chronic medical disorders and medications is lengthy. Clinicians who advise outpatients to use alcohol should beware that in the residential studies discussed above the quantity of alcohol consumed was regulated and its use within a social context was assured. Iatrogenic alcohol use disorders do occur. Alcohol as an "aid" for sleep is discussed below.

Protective value against coronary heart disease. An intriguing epidemiological finding is the association of regular, but moderate, alcohol use (up to two drinks per day) with lower morbidity and mortality from coronary artery disease in men, when compared with heavy alcohol users and abstainers. This U- or J-shaped relationship appears to be quite robust.

It is, of course, unsurprising that heavy alcohol use is associated with increasing coronary artery disease. The puzzling question is why teetotalers should have higher morbidity and mortality than moderate drinkers. Alcohol elevates plasma levels of high-density lipo-protein (HDL) cholesterol, including a subfraction (HDL$_3$) with antiatherogenic activity, but apparently it does not elevate the most antiatherogenic subfraction (HDL$_2$) (Davidson 1989). Alcohol also reduces blood platelet aggregation and has other anticoagulant effects, although under some circumstances alcohol also increases selected hemostatic processes (Davidson 1989).

Another interpretation is that the heterogeneous abstainer group includes subgroups at high risk for coronary artery disease (e.g., former heavy drinkers) (Atkinson et al. 1992). Unfortunately many reported studies were not designed to account for this possibility, including the one study of elderly subjects reported to date (Scherr et al. 1992). Recent studies that have closely examined abstainers report conflicting findings, that is, that risk for coronary artery disease in the abstainer group was either greater (Shaper et al. 1988) or not greater (Klatsky et al. 1990) than risk in the moderate drinking group. The alcohol-protective hypothesis in coronary artery disease must be questioned further before acceptance (Davidson 1989).

Clinical Features and Course of Alcohol Use Disorders

Primary and associated features: screening and diagnosis. There is no evidence that the elderly population differs from other age groups in the primary manifestations of alcohol dependence (Table 15–2). Even though several of the criteria for alcohol dependence (i.e., those related to social consequences) have questionable relevance in elderly people (Atkinson 1990), preliminary testing suggests that the criteria are adequate to establish a diagnosis in this age group (Atkinson and Tolson 1992). The CAGE test is an effective screening device for alcoholism in the elderly (Beresford 1992b; Buchsbaum et al. 1992), as is the MAST-G, a version of the Michigan Alcoholism Screening Test designed for geriatric patients (F. C. Blow, unpublished data, June 1992; Joseph et al. 1992). Several characteristic laboratory abnormalities accompanying many cases of geriatric alcohol dependence are listed in Table 15–5.

Complications. Alcohol-associated organic mental disorders and psychiatric comorbidities are considered separately below. Alcohol-related liver disease, when present, carries a poor prognosis if drinking continues (Woodhouse and James 1985). Hypoglycemia, hyperuricemia, hypertriglyceridemia, osteoporosis, anemias, congestive heart failure, aspiration pneumonia, and accidental hypothermia can also be caused or aggravated by alcohol dependence. Alcohol problems are found in 7%–30% of older suicides (Blazer 1982; Conwell et al. 1990; Martin and Streissguth 1982). The association of alcoholism with suicide may be stronger in late-middle–aged men than in women or elderly men (Conwell et al. 1990). Functional impairment ranges from mild to very severe, presenting in extreme cases as "senile squalor" or "Diogenes syndrome" (Droller 1964; Kafetz and Cox 1982; MacMillan and Shaw 1966; Wattis 1981).

Course. The span from onset of the first alcohol problem to date of entry into current treatment can be as long as 50 years. Over this course, drinking may have been steady, progressive, or fluctuating. In some cases, sober periods of 10 years or more occur between prob-

Table 15–5. Frequency of laboratory abnormalities in elderly and younger alcoholic inpatients

Blood tests	Results[a] Patients > 65 years[b] n	Patients > 65 years[b] %	Younger patients[b] n	Younger patients[b] %
MCH increased	213	71	123	57**
AST increased	214	56	123	42*
GGT increased	123	55	101	48
MCV increased	213	44	124	17**
Glucose increased	206	32	124	36
Uric acid increased	201	21	123	< 1**
Albumin decreased	186	17	115	3**
Akaline phosphatase increased	213	11	123	15
Triglycerides increased	191	16	122	19
Phosphorus increased	198	9	124	11

Note. MCH = mean corpuscular hemoglobin; AST = aspartate aminotransferase; GGT = γ-glutamyltransferase; MCV = mean corpuscular volume.
[a] n = number of patients tested in each age group; % = percent of patients tested in the age group who had an abnormal value.
[b] Older patients: n = 216; mean age 69.6 years; age range from 65 to 83 years. Younger patients: n = 125; mean age 44.3 years; age range 19 to 64 years.
** $P < .01$, using Wilcoxon two-sample rank sum test to compare age groups for proportion having an abnormal value.
* $P < .05$.
For others, $P > .3$.
Source. Adapted from Hurt et al. 1988.

lem drinking episodes. Cross-sectional surveys of problem drinking that are further stratified for age after 60 show steadily declining prevalence with age, and generally rates after age 85 are negligible. Mortality rates are very high when active drinking continues in the face of frank dementia (Simon et al. 1968).

Alcohol-Associated Organic Mental Disorders

Alcohol-associated organic mental disorders are listed in Table 15–6 and described in standard texts on neuropsychiatry (Lishman 1987; Yudofsky and Hales 1992). Here, we highlight selected features of these disorders that have special relevance to geriatric alcoholism and geriatric neuropsychiatry.

Aging and alcohol neurotoxicity.   Alcohol is a potent neurotoxin, aside from any effects of associated malnutrition. An age-associated increase in central nervous system (CNS) sensitivity to alcohol has been demonstrated in studies of humans and animals (reviewed in Wood et al. 1984; York 1983), including a few behavioral studies of nonalcoholic humans measuring memory (M. K. Jones and Jones 1980) and body sway and hand dexterity (Vogel-Sprott and Barrett 1984) after single alcohol doses. Some studies of cognitive functioning of "social drinkers" have suggested that alcohol consumption level is correlated with performance decrements in memory, learning, or problem solving when subjects are tested in the sober state. This effect tends to be most evident in older subjects (Parker and Noble 1977, 1980). However, these findings have been challenged as influenced by several confounding factors, such as innate aptitude for the measured task and test anxiety (Delin and Lee 1992; Emmerson et al. 1988). Regional cerebral blood flow (rCBF) is also reduced in otherwise healthy elderly volunteers, proportional to reported alcohol consumption level (Meyer et al. 1984).

There is a sizable literature on the neuropsychology of alcoholism, and this information sheds light on the complicated relationship of aging to chronic alcohol effects on CNS functioning. Findings vary with the function assessed and the instrument used to assess it (Ryan and Butters 1986). One of two general models tends to fit typical neuropsychological findings relating age, alcoholism, and performance. Some findings suggest that chronic alcoholism "ages" performance (i.e., error scores of an alcoholic individual at any age are equivalent to scores of a nonalcoholic individual who

is perhaps 5 to 15 years older ["premature aging" model]). In contrast, other neuropsychological measures show small, if any, effects of alcohol consumption on performance in younger alcoholics, but increasingly greater effects in older alcoholics ("increased vulnerability to alcohol with age" model).

Three general conclusions can be made regarding this body of research. First, in either model it is *age*, more than *duration* of alcoholism, that appears to determine the degree of alcohol neurotoxic effect on performance. Second, when neuropsychologists speak of premature aging, they refer merely descriptively to measured performance, not necessarily the mediating mechanisms of CNS activity. The pathology may be different in alcoholism than in normal aging, even though the neuropsychological performance may be

Table 15–6.   Alcohol-associated organic mental disorders

Disorders manifest primarily by altered mental status
  Alcohol intoxication
    Simple intoxication
    Idiosyncratic intoxication
    Alcohol blackout
  Alcohol withdrawal syndromes
    Uncomplicated alcohol withdrawal ("tremulous syndrome")
    Alcohol hallucinosis
    Alcohol withdrawal seizures ("rum fits")
    Alcohol withdrawal delirium (delirium tremens—"DTs")
  Wernicke-Korsakoff syndrome
    Wernicke's encephalopathy
    Alcohol amnestic disorder (Korsakoff's psychosis)
  Other cognitive disorders related to alcohol
    Neurotoxicity
    Alcoholic dementia
    Focal alcoholic cognitive deficits
  Alcohol associated insomnia
  Alcohol associated mood disorder
Disorders manifest primarily by focal neurological findings
  Alcoholic peripheral polyneuropathy
  Alcoholic cerebellar degeneration
  Alcohol-associated movement disorder (Parkinson's)
Rare neurological disorders associated with chronic alcoholism
  Marchiafava-Bignami disease
  Nutritional amblyopia
  Central pontine myelinosis
Disorders associated with chronic alcoholism but not with alcohol neurotoxicity
  Hepatic encephalopathy
  Acquired hepatocerebral degeneration
  Trauma-induced acute and chronic subdural hematoma

similar (Freund 1984; Ryan and Butters 1986). Third, although performance deficits may be subtle and of questionable clinical significance in some cases (Willenbring 1988), more severe deficits result in impaired psychosocial functioning (Horvath 1975) and can compromise alcoholism treatment (McCrady and Smith 1986; Walker et al. 1983).

Cortical atrophy (cortical shrinkage and/or ventricular dilation seen on CT and MRI scans) also occurs in individuals with chronic alcoholism (Besson et al. 1981, 1989; Carlen et al. 1978, 1986; Lishman 1987; Pfefferbaum et al. 1988; Ron 1983). rCBF is reduced in individuals with chronic alcoholism, and age-associated decrements in rCBF become more pronounced in alcoholics (i.e., chronic alcoholism also "ages" rCBF) (Meyer et al. 1984). The relationship of rCBF and imaging changes to neuropsychological performance is unclear. Basic mechanisms that might account for alcohol-aging interactions in the CNS include neuron loss and damage (Samorajski et al. 1984), reduced dendritic connections (Ryan and Butters 1986), neuron membrane changes (Wood et al. 1984; York 1983), and reduced activity in both catecholaminergic (Carlsson et al. 1980; Mair and McEntee 1983; McEntee and Mair 1978; Wilcox 1984) and cholinergic (Butters 1985; Freund 1984; Hodges et al. 1991) neuronal systems. Despite fragmentary information, a pattern has emerged in animal studies that is comparable to neuropsychological and rCBF findings in humans: chronic alcohol administration tends to produce changes in several of these neuronal systems similar to those seen at an older age in non–alcohol-treated control animals.

Alcohol intoxication and withdrawal. Elderly people show increased intoxication after a standard alcohol load, compared with younger people. Factors that may contribute to this phenomenon include 1) age-associated pharmacokinetic factors (e.g., increased peak blood alcohol level) related to reduced volume of distribution (Vestal et al. 1977; Vogel-Sprott and Barrett 1984) and perhaps to absorption (Beresford 1992a) of alcohol; 2) age-associated increases in CNS sensitivity as reviewed above; 3) potentiation of alcohol CNS effects by medications; 4) comorbid organic mental disorders; and 5) comorbid medical disorders (e.g., those that influence circulation, hepatic function, and tissue metabolism).

Anecdotal reports suggest that alcohol withdrawal is both less severe and less complicated in elderly patients. However, compared with younger cohorts reported elsewhere (Atkinson 1988), major alcohol withdrawal disorders were equally common in a large series of patients 65 or older who were admitted to an inpatient alcohol treatment unit (Finlayson et al. 1988). In a study of alcoholic men who had recently consumed very high volumes of alcohol, an older cohort (age 58–77) demonstrated more severe withdrawal symptoms and required more sedative medications to control withdrawal, even though the older group consumed somewhat less alcohol than did the younger patients (age 21–33) before admission (Liskow et al. 1989). The findings further indicated that duration of alcoholism and prior history of complicated alcohol withdrawal, rather than age, might have explained these group differences in withdrawal severity. On the other hand, age itself may also play a role; animal studies have demonstrated age-associated increases in both dependence liability (Ritzmann and Melchior 1984) and alcohol withdrawal (Samorajski et al. 1984; Wood et al. 1984).

Slowly resolving cognitive deficits following alcohol withdrawal. Cognition is often impaired in recently detoxified alcoholic patients of all ages (Cutting 1978), but deficits are greater in older patients (Grant et al. 1984). Impairment immediately after prolonged drinking bouts is probably multifactorial, representing the effects of chronic alcohol neurotoxicity, residual alcohol intoxication, depression, hepatic and metabolic dysfunction (Schafer et al. 1991), alcohol withdrawal, sedative medication used to treat withdrawal (Liskow et al. 1989), and in some cases comorbid drug abuse, such as with cocaine (N. Butters, personal communication, June 1992). The dramatic improvement in cognitive functioning of individuals with chronic alcoholism that typically occurs during the first few weeks of sobriety is attributable to amelioration of all these factors. Improvements in depression and liver dysfunction may be especially important (Schafer et al. 1991). Age, however, is an important predictor of the extent of residual neuropsychological performance deficits after 3–4 weeks of sobriety (Schafer et al. 1991). These lingering deficits may be focal or patchy (i.e., they may affect only one or a few specific cognitive functions) or may be sufficiently widespread to fulfill diagnostic criteria for dementia (Ryan and Butters 1986). DSM-IV offers no diagnostic category for the focal abnormalities (apart from the characteristic amnestic disorder of Korsakoff's syndrome), inspiring terms such as *atypical organic mental disorder* (Finlayson et al. 1988) or *subacute alcohol-related organic mental disorder* (Grant et al. 1984) to describe them. Because focal and even widespread dysfunction is partially reversible over years of sobriety, workers uneasy about the use of the term *dementia* for such conditions have suggested terms like "reversible alcoholic cognitive deterioration" (Lishman 1987).

Lingering deficits resulting in psychosocial dysfunction occur in up to 9% of mixed-age sober alcoholic patients (Horvath 1975), but they are more commonly found in older patients tested beyond 1 month. In a series of 50 elderly alcoholic male outpatients who were assessed clinically and neuropsychologically 1 to 6 months after their last drink, 16% showed focal deficits, whereas another 6% met criteria for dementia (Atkinson and Tolson 1992). In another series, older patients (50 to 69 years), who were tested between 1 and 59 months after their last drink, performed less well on several measures of memory and visuospatial tasks than did younger patients or age-matched control subjects (Brandt et al. 1983). Resolution of some deficits (e.g., psychomotor skills and short-term memory) can be demonstrated 5 years or more after initiation of abstinence (Brandt et al. 1983). On the other hand, long-term memory tends to remain impaired even after 7 years of abstinence. These differences suggest different mediating mechanisms for reversible and nonreversible functions (Butters 1985; Ryan and Butters 1986). rCBF (Ishikawa et al. 1986) also improves with continued abstinence. Corresponding resolution of imaged brain changes (Carlen et al. 1978, 1986; Ishikawa et al. 1986; Lishman 1987) suggests that "cortical atrophy" seen in early abstinence may be a function of brain fluid abnormality or some other reversible phenomenon (Harper et al. 1988).

Alcoholic dementia and Alzheimer's disease. We do not intend to take up the debate about whether the dementia associated with chronic alcoholism is distinct from the Wernicke-Korsakoff syndrome or a part of it ("continuity theory"); this subject is well addressed in other sources (Heindel et al. 1991; Lishman 1987; Ryan and Butters 1986; Victor et al. 1989; Willenbring 1988). We do wish, however, to address the clinical dilemma that arises in the differential diagnosis of dementia in older patients with heavy drinking histories. This issue has practical significance for the clinician, because the prognosis for alcoholic dementia is different from that for Alzheimer's disease, provided abstinence can be maintained. Family advice, long-term care plans, and expectations will vary substantially depending on presumptive diagnosis.

Confounding of precise dementia diagnosis by alcoholism and heavy drinking history may be a more substantial problem than previously acknowledged. In a British community survey of psychiatric disorders (Saunders et al. 1991), men with heavy drinking histories were 4.6 times more likely to have a dementia diagnosis than were other men. In clinical case series, alcohol-related dementias represent 4% (Larson et al. 1984b; Renvoize et al. 1985) to 10% (Wells 1979) of dementias from all causes. But in more recently established dementia registries, if patients with heavy drinking histories are included with those having histories of alcohol use disorders, the proportion of cases at least partially attributable to alcohol is considerably higher, having been reported in 14 of 65 patients (21.5%) in one series (King 1986) and in 26 of 120 patients (21.7%) in another (D. M. Smith and R. M. Atkinson, "Alcoholic Dementia in an Alzheimer's Registry," unpublished data, October 1992).

Commonly used criteria for primary degenerative dementia of the Alzheimer type prohibit this diagnosis when alcoholism or a history of heavy alcohol consumption is present. On the other hand, there is nothing in the DSM-IV criteria for alcoholic dementia that distinguishes it from dementias of other etiologies: it is, in fact, a diagnosis of exclusion. Further, casting doubt on the entity of alcoholic dementia, some have argued that this disorder is in fact Alzheimer's or multi-infarct dementia coincident with chronic alcoholism (Ryan and Butters 1986). Imaging of the cerebral cortex is not helpful, because changes of early Alzheimer's disease are similar to those seen in chronic alcoholism (Jacoby and Levy 1980; Pfefferbaum et al. 1988; Ron 1983).

Currently efforts are underway to improve differential diagnosis by specifying additional provisional features associated with alcoholic dementia (e.g., Osuntokun et al. 1992). Table 15–7 illustrates one such effort, based on a retrospective study of 120 cases in a dementia registry (D. M. Smith and R. M. Atkinson, "Alcoholic Dementia in an Alzheimer's Registry," unpublished data, October 1992). About half of all cases in the registry could be classified into one of four groups depicted in Table 15–7. Peripheral neuropathy and cerebellar ataxia (common in alcoholic patients with cognitive deficits but not Alzheimer's disease) and anomia (common in neuropsychological assessment of Alzheimer's disease but not alcoholic dementia) varied significantly among groups. Moreover, in contrast with the other groups, the group diagnosed as having "alcoholic dementia" at intake showed no deterioration on serial testing with the Mini-Mental State Exam (MMSE; Folstein et al. 1975) over a 20-month period. This approach to differential diagnosis, if affirmed by prospective studies, may help distinguish more precisely among alcohol-associated dementia, Alzheimer's dementia, and mixed cases. Although imaging of the cortex may not distinguish between alcoholic dementia and Alzheimer patients, careful study of the cerebellar vermis using MRI might be of value in differential diagnosis, because cerebellar atrophy is much more likely to be associated with chronic alcoholism (Ron 1983) than with Alzheimer's disease.

Alcohol-associated insomnia. Insomnia is emphasized because aging and chronic alcohol consumption affect sleep architecture in similar ways: elderly subjects and recently abstinent alcoholic subjects tend to show frequent awakenings, especially from deep slow wave sleep, and reduced rapid-eye-movement (REM) sleep (Dustman 1984; see also Chapter 16). Put another way, sleep of 40-year-old alcoholics in one study (Dustman 1984) more closely resembled the sleep of healthy elderly individuals than the sleep of age-matched healthy control subjects. Sleep in recovering alcoholics improves with abstinence, but slow wave sleep may not reach normal values even after 4 years of abstinence. Advising an older patient to take a drink near bedtime to aid sleep is not warranted; although

sleep latency might be reduced by this practice, if continued over time, late night drinking is likely to exaggerate age-associated alterations of sleep pattern.

Alcohol-associated mood disorder. Depressive *symptoms* are widespread in newly admitted alcoholic patients of all ages, including elderly ones. For example, in a special treatment program for alcoholic male veterans 55 or older, 54% of 135 patients scored 70 or more (T score) on the Depression Scale of the Minnesota Multiphasic Personality Inventory (MMPI) at entry (R. M. Atkinson, unpublished data, January 1990). Depressive symptoms are much more common than diagnosable depressive *disorders*, which occurred in 12% of a large hospitalized series of elderly alcoholic patients (Finlayson et al. 1988). These symptoms resolve in the majority of alcoholics over the first 3–4 weeks of abstinence, without specific antidepressant therapy (e.g., Brown and Schuckit 1988). Residual depression after this time, present in perhaps 6%–15% of patients, suggests a comorbid disorder. But what is the meaning of the early, evanescent depressive symptoms that resolved? The high prevalence of depressive symptoms, as well as evidence that the level and recency of prior alcohol consumption is correlated with depressive symptoms in early abstinence (e.g., Nakamura et al. 1983), supports the inference that this depression may represent an organic mood disorder.

Only 5% of alcoholic men and 15%–25% of alco-

Table 15–7. Alcohol and dementia: neurological and neuropsychological features of 59 patients in a dementia registry

Variable	Alcoholic Dementia ($n = 12$)	Possible AD/alc ($n = 14$)	Possible AD/no alc ($n = 22$)	Probable AD/no alc ($n = 11$)
Ataxia	9/10	8/14	5/21	0/11[a]
Peripheral neuropathy	6/8	11/13	5/20	1/11[a]
Nystagmus	3/6	3/10	0/18	0/9[b]
Anomia	1/12	4/14	15/22	9/11[a]
Frontal cortical atrophy	3/12	2/14	2/22	0/9 (ns)
Mean initial MMSE score	20.8	23.7	19.7	17.3 (ns)
Mean change in MMSE score per month	+ .03	– .27	– .33	– .43[c]

Note. Neurological findings based on standard clinical examination by a neurologist; anomia was assessed by screening measures—the Mini-Mental State Exam (MMSE; Folstein et al. 1975) and Neurobehavioral Cognitive Status Examination (Kiernan et al. 1987). Frontal cortical atrophy based on routine readings of computed tomography scan or magnetic resonance imaging by a neuroradiologist. Serial MMSE scores were available for an average of 20 months.

AD = Alzheimer's disease; alc = history of alcohol consumption of more than 3–4 drinks per day during some previous period; no alc = no history of prior alcohol use; ns = $P > .05$ by χ^2 or analysis of variance (ANOVA) test.

[a]χ^2 $P < .01$.
[b]χ^2 $P < .05$.
[c]ANOVA $P < .01$.

Source. From D. M. Smith, R. M. Atkinson: "Alcoholic Dementia in an Alzheimer's Registry," unpublished data, October 1992.

holic women have a history of depressive disorders predating their alcoholism (Atkinson and Kofoed 1982). Some investigators hypothesize that subclinical chronic depression or a potential depressive diathesis may be manifest by evanescent depressive symptoms in early sobriety, or even by alcoholism itself. As such, this underlying depressive disorder may be a risk factor for relapse of alcoholism (L. F. Jarvik, personal communication, November 1992). This assumption is the rationale for recent trials of antidepressant drug maintenance of alcoholic patients who do not have an obvious comorbid depressive disorder. Also of interest are the findings that a history of prior heavy drinking can be a risk factor for the occurrence (Saunders et al. 1991) and severity (B. L. Cook et al. 1991) of subsequent depressive disorders in elderly individuals.

Alcohol-associated movement disorder (Parkinson type).

A single report (Carlen et al. 1981) described 7 older alcoholic patients (age 53–70) who developed transient parkinsonian symptoms and signs either during alcohol withdrawal or during chronic severe intoxication. Parkinsonism disappeared or improved significantly with reduced alcohol consumption alone. This association is plausible in the light of evidence that alcohol can disrupt striatal dopamine activity (reviewed in Wilcox 1984).

Psychiatric Comorbidity in Alcohol Use Disorders

There are few reports characterizing comorbid psychiatric disorders in elderly alcoholic samples. Active tobacco dependence is highly prevalent in elderly alcoholics (about 70%), recent illicit drug abuse is rare, and active dependence on prescribed sedatives and anxiolytics varies (from 2% to 14%) depending on the cohort studied (Atkinson and Tolson 1992; Blow et al. 1992; Finlayson et al. 1988). Non–substance-related psychiatric comorbidities in clinical data sets vary even more, depending on the cohort and clinical setting where studied. Finlayson et al. (1988) found that comorbid psychiatric diagnoses were made in about half of a sample of elderly patients hospitalized for alcoholism treatment. Dementias (25% of cases) were more common than mood disorders (12%), two thirds of which were major depression (Finlayson et al. 1988). A dissimilar pattern was found in an older alcoholism outpatient clinic cohort examined 1 to 6 months after the last drink (Atkinson and Tolson

1992): only a third of patients had comorbid diagnoses, and minor to moderate mood disorders (14%) were more common than dementia (6%). In a mental health clinic setting, unsurprisingly, alcoholic patients have comorbid schizophrenia or anxiety disorders more often than patients seen in alcohol treatment settings (Blow et al. 1992). In the psychiatric inpatient setting, a common constellation may be concurrent alcohol use, affective, and personality disorders (Speer and Bates 1992). It is not known how these comorbidity rates compare with those in geriatric medical settings.

Management of Alcohol-Related Disorders in Elderly Patients

Intervention.   Once the diagnosis of an alcohol use disorder is established it is important to present the information thoroughly and objectively to the patient and spouse or other relative or caregiver as a basis for urging an appropriate course of action (Atkinson 1985). It is helpful to reassure the patient and family that older alcoholic patients fare as well as or better than younger patients in a variety of alcohol treatment settings (Atkinson, in press).

Management.   In mild cases success can be achieved sometimes simply by offering advice to cut down or abstain, accompanied by informal social interventions as needed. The use of structured patient education and contracting to reduce alcohol intake ("brief intervention") merits study in the elderly (W. L. Adams, personal communication, November 1992). The person with more severe alcoholism should enter an outpatient geriatric alcoholism treatment program if possible. Successful programs have been set up within geriatric centers and general substance abuse programs (reviewed in Atkinson, in press). Family involvement in treatment improves compliance and outcome (Atkinson et al. 1993). Use of deterrent drugs such as disulfiram can be hazardous and is usually unnecessary in the elderly. Other specific treatment principles have been discussed in detail elsewhere (Atkinson 1991, in press).

The most serious cases should be referred to an alcoholism inpatient treatment unit, which is also indicated when outpatient efforts fail. If severe medical or psychiatric complications are present, or major withdrawal is anticipated or is already occurring, initial treatment on an acute medical or general psychiatric inpatient unit is warranted. Patients with dementia or chronic psychosis are best managed in a psychiatric day treatment center or home visitation program. Patients with personality disorders and major mental illness can best be managed individually in a psychiatric outpatient clinic, preferably in conjunction with an alcoholism group. Intractable heavy drinking in the face of dementia or other coexisting major mental disorder may force placement in residential care, where, unfortunately, alcoholic patients are not always welcomed. In a few United States locales, "alcohol free" foster homes and other residential facilities have been established and are staffed by personnel trained to care for recovering alcoholics in an accepting manner.

Benzodiazepine Dependence

Among young polysubstance abusers, benzodiazepine abuse includes behaviors such as consumption of the drug outside of medical supervision, use for euphoriant effects, escalation of the dosage over time, and continued use despite adverse social, economic, or legal consequences. This pattern of abuse is distinctly rare among older people (Busto et al. 1986a; Pinsker and Suljaga-Petchel 1984). However, among elderly patients long-term therapeutic prescribing of benzodiazepines may lead to physical dependence with characteristic symptoms when the drug is discontinued. Three forms of discontinuance phenomena are recognized: 1) recurrence symptoms that include reemergence and persistence of the anxiety symptoms for which the drug was originally prescribed; 2) rebound anxiety, that is, recurrence symptoms that are temporarily worse than before treatment; and 3) a true withdrawal syndrome—signs and symptoms that are time-limited and unlike symptoms of the disorder for which the drug was originally prescribed (American Psychiatric Association 1990). Although discontinuance symptoms occur after stopping a variety of psychotropic agents, the recurrence, rebound, and withdrawal symptoms that follow benzodiazepine cessation are so unpleasant as to promote relapse to drug use in a significant proportion of patients (Roy-Byrne and Hommer 1988).

Epidemiology

Benzodiazepines are prescribed for elderly patients primarily as hypnotics or anxiolytics. In either case,

this class of drugs is recommended for short-term use, but epidemiological studies indicate that courses of therapy are considerably longer in elderly than in younger patients. A large United States survey reported that 80% of younger patients, compared to 56% of older patients, who were prescribed these drugs used them for less than 4 months (Mellinger et al. 1984). A large community-based study from Great Britain found that only 5.4% of elderly benzodiazepine users, compared to 56.6% of young and middle-aged benzodiazepine users, were treated for less than 4 months (Dunbar et al. 1989). Short-term use is more common in young patients whether the drugs are prescribed as anxiolytics or hypnotics (Morgan et al. 1988; Smart and Adlaf 1988). A prospective study confirmed that once a benzodiazepine was prescribed, old age, especially if associated with low educational level, was significantly associated with continued prescriptions (Mant et al. 1988).

A 1979 cross-national survey found that 1.6% of the population had used benzodiazepines for longer than 1 year (Mellinger et al. 1984); 71% of these long-term users were more than 50 years old. They were more likely to report physical health problems than nonusers, and despite use of these psychotropic drugs they reported considerable residual anxiety and depression. A British study (Rodrigo et al. 1988) found that 41% of long-term users were over age 70 and had used benzodiazepines daily for a mean of 5 years. Most had poor physical health, and a third had depressive disorders.

Despite many years of continued benzodiazepine prescription, elderly long-term users rarely exceed recommended dosages or escalate their dosage over time (Busto et al. 1986a; Pinsker and Suljaga-Petchel 1984; Salzman 1991). One United States study found that the average daily dose for elderly outpatients rarely exceeded 4 mg in diazepam equivalents (Pinsker and Suljaga-Petchel 1984). The most popular benzodiazepines in the United States are diazepam, lorazepam, and alprazolam (American Psychiatric Association 1990).

Among institutionalized elderly patients, physician prescription of benzodiazepines is widespread. A survey of one state's Medicaid recipients found that 24% of elderly patients were prescribed a benzodiazepine and that flurazepam, a long half-life hypnotic, was one of the most frequently prescribed psychotropic drugs (Buck 1988). Another survey reported that 28% of 850 residents of intermediate care facilities received a regularly scheduled sedative-hypnotic (Beers et al. 1988).

Of those patients prescribed a benzodiazepine, 30% received a drug with a long half-life. These and other studies in nursing homes have documented poorly advised prescribing practices, such as benzodiazepine prescription in the absence of a mental disorder for which these agents are indicated, use of benzodiazepines with long half-lives (which are more likely to cause toxicity in elderly patients), and use of standing orders for hypnotics as opposed to as-needed prescribing (Beardsley et al. 1989; Beers et al. 1988).

Adverse Effects of Benzodiazepine Use

The most important adverse effects of benzodiazepines in elderly patients include excess daytime sedation, ataxia, and cognitive impairment. Studies have demonstrated that elderly patients have more adverse effects than young patients at similar dosages of these medications, especially patients treated with high dosages of long half-life agents (Greenblatt and Shader 1991). As a person's age increases, regularly administered doses of some of these agents are cleared less rapidly, producing higher steady state serum or plasma drug concentrations (Greenblatt and Shader 1991). However, even when old and young patients have comparable serum or plasma drug concentrations, elderly patients develop more sedation and more psychomotor impairment, possibly indicating an enhanced pharmacodynamic effect (Castleden et al. 1977; Greenblatt and Shader 1991).

After single and multiple doses of benzodiazepines, elderly patients experience substantial impairment in attention, memory, arousal, and psychomotor abilities (Pomara et al. 1991). Among healthy elderly patients, single doses of diazepam as low as 2.5 mg may impair immediate and delayed memory and psychomotor performance (Pomara et al. 1985). Cognitive impairment is also more prolonged in older compared with younger patients after single doses of a benzodiazepine (Nikaido et al. 1990). Elderly medical and surgical inpatients show deterioration in daytime performance after several nightly doses of even short–half-life benzodiazepines such as temazepam (P. J. Cook et al. 1983), and daytime hangover from hypnotics can be especially prominent in frail elderly patients with dementia, hypoalbuminemia, or chronic renal insufficiency (P. J. Cook 1986). Compared with young patients, elderly patients have more daytime balance impairment after nightly hypnotic treatment (Bonnet and Kramer 1981).

In older people, memory improves following discontinuation of chronic benzodiazepine treatment (Golombok et al. 1988), and clinical studies have demonstrated excess cognitive disability and morbidity associated with chronic benzodiazepine use. In a study of drug-induced cognitive impairment, benzodiazepines were the offending agent in 22 out of 35 patients (Larson et al. 1987). Cognitive, psychomotor, and balance impairments induced by benzodiazepines combine to increase the risk of falls and accidents in elderly patients (Kramer and Schoen 1984). The adjusted odds ratio for falls associated with sedative use was 28.3 in one report (Tinetti et al. 1988). Hip fractures in persons over age 65 are more prevalent in persons prescribed benzodiazepines, especially agents with long half-lives, with the relative risk ranging from 1.8 to 3.1 in both nursing home and community dwelling elderly subjects (Ray et al. 1987, 1989). Benzodiazepines probably impair the driving skills of older drivers (American Psychiatric Association 1990).

Among long-term benzodiazepine users, increased brain atrophy on neuroimaging studies has been reported indicating possible permanent CNS damage (Lader et al. 1984). However, this finding was not confirmed in several studies that controlled for confounding variables such as alcohol abuse (Perera et al. 1987; Poser et al. 1983; Rickels 1985).

Discontinuation Phenomena

Types and frequency of symptoms. The reported incidence of benzodiazepine discontinuation symptoms in long-term users (people who have taken them daily for more than 1 year) varies widely from none to 100%, reflecting heterogeneous characteristics of the patient populations and differing measurement and definition of withdrawal syndromes (Bowden and Fisher 1980; Golombok et al. 1987; Laughren et al. 1982; Noyes et al. 1988; Petursson and Lader 1981). Symptoms increase substantially after 8–12 months' daily use but withdrawal symptoms have been reported in patients whose duration of daily use was only 4–6 weeks (Higgitt et al. 1985; Murphy et al. 1984; Rickels et al. 1983). Rebound insomnia may occur after 1 week of hypnotic therapy (Kales et al. 1979).

Symptoms that occur frequently after cessation of long-term benzodiazepines are, for the most part, recurrence and rebound phenomena. These signs and symptoms include anxiety, irritability, insomnia, fatigue, headache, muscle twitching, tremor, sweating, dizziness, and concentration difficulties (American Psychiatric Association 1990; Rickels et al. 1990; Roy-Byrne and Hommer 1988; Schweizer et al. 1990). In a recent well-done study of mixed-age patients, 90% undergoing gradual discontinuation and 100% undergoing abrupt discontinuation experienced at least mild discontinuance symptoms (Rickels et al. 1990; Schweizer et al. 1990). True withdrawal signs and symptoms (which include nausea, loss of appetite, tinnitus, perceptual distortions, hyperacusis, depersonalization, and derealization) are less common than recurrence or rebound symptoms, but develop in 20%–50% of long-term users following discontinuation (Roy-Byrne and Hommer 1988; Schweizer et al. 1990). Withdrawal symptoms generally abate within 2 to 4 weeks of drug cessation, although persistence for months of isolated symptoms such as tinnitus and perceptual distortions has been reported (Busto et al. 1986b; Schweizer et al. 1990). Psychosis, delusions, and convulsions are the most morbid of withdrawal phenomena. These major withdrawal symptoms are reported anecdotally but are rarely seen in controlled benzodiazepine discontinuation trials. Seizures are more common in patients taking higher than therapeutic doses of benzodiazepines, especially high-potency agents (American Psychiatric Association 1990; Noyes et al. 1988). In an analysis of 48 case reports of benzodiazepine withdrawal seizures, only 9 patients were over age 60, suggesting that elderly patients are not disproportionately represented among those experiencing this adverse event (Fialip et al. 1987).

Only two studies have examined discontinuance symptoms in elderly subjects. In one report (Foy et al. 1986), a confusional state following abrupt benzodiazepine withdrawal occurred in 7 of 52 elderly long-term benzodiazepine users prescribed a mean of diazepam 7.75 mg/day. However, in a controlled study (Schweizer et al. 1989), elderly patients reported significantly less severe withdrawal symptoms and were as likely to be benzodiazepine-free as young patients matched for drug dose and duration of benzodiazepine use after gradual drug withdrawal. Withdrawal and other discontinuance symptoms in elderly patients may be attenuated because of lowered prevalence of panic disorders, decreased rate of decline of benzodiazepine plasma levels, or altered functional capacity of neurotransmitter systems (Schweizer et al. 1989).

Other studies have failed to show age-related differences in withdrawal severity, but most excluded patients over age 70 and patients with medical problems (Roy-Byrne and Hommer 1988). The patients who are most likely to develop benzodiazepine dependence because of the likelihood that they will receive long-term prescriptions, namely elderly patients who have multiple chronic medical problems, have received little study. In addition, withdrawal among institutionalized frail elderly has not been systematically studied.

Several studies have reported on the correlates of withdrawal severity among long-term users, though none has focused on the elderly. The following variables were correlated with increased severity of withdrawal in some but not all studies of mixed-age patients: presence of panic disorder, abrupt drug withdrawal, high dosages, short half-life agents, comorbid alcohol problems, and personality pathology (American Psychiatric Association 1990; Busto et al. 1986b, Noyes et al. 1988; Rickels et al. 1990; Roy-Byrne and Hommer 1988; Schweizer et al. 1990; Tyrer 1989).

Clinically, benzodiazepine withdrawal may be overlooked in the elderly. In one study of elderly psychiatric inpatients (Whitcup and Miller 1987), benzodiazepine withdrawal was often not recognized or was misdiagnosed as myocardial infarction, hypertensive crisis, or infection.

Outcome of benzodiazepine withdrawal. Despite evidence that old age is not associated with more severe withdrawal, elderly patients have a poorer outcome following therapeutic attempts to discontinue benzodiazepines. Studies indicate that approximately half of mixed-age patients who participate in a withdrawal protocol successfully complete the program (Busto et al. 1986b; Golombok et al. 1987; Schweizer et al. 1990). Fifty percent to 70% remain benzodiazepine free at follow-up ranging from 10 months to 5 years (Ashton 1987; Golombok et al. 1987; Rickels et al. 1991). However, investigators of one study (Holton et al. 1992)—in which *abstinence* was defined as complete nonuse of benzodiazepines throughout a 5-year period—independently validated the subject's claims of abstinence and reported that only 15% were completely benzodiazepine free during this time period. Older age was associated with both difficulty completing withdrawal protocols and increased likelihood of relapse to benzodiazepine use despite completion of a cessation program (Ashton 1987; Golombok et al. 1987; Holton et al. 1992; Rickels et al. 1991). The mean age of subjects in these follow-up studies was between 40 and 50 years, and the numbers of elderly subjects were small.

People who participate in supervised withdrawal

protocols are more successful at discontinuing these drugs than are those who taper or discontinue drugs more casually. In one program, 73% of 48 subjects who completed a withdrawal protocol were benzodiazepine free at 3-year follow-up compared with 39% of 38 who failed the taper and 14% of 37 who were administratively ineligible for the study (Rickels et al. 1991). The mean age of all subjects in this program was 47 years, and younger age was a significant predictor of benzodiazepine free outcome. Other risk factors for relapse in studies of mixed-aged patients include personality pathology, agents with short half-lives, higher dosages, caffeine intake, and continued psychiatric symptomatology (American Psychiatric Association 1990; Golombok et al. 1987; Holton et al. 1992; Rickels et al. 1991).

Benefits of Long-Term Benzodiazepine Use

The benefit of long-term benzodiazepine treatment has generated considerable debate. There is little support for the long-term use of benzodiazepines as hypnotics because hypnotic efficacy diminishes substantially after several weeks of treatment (American Psychiatric Association 1990). Rebound insomnia after discontinuation is a significant clinical problem, especially with agents that have short half-lives (Kales et al. 1979). Most patients do not develop tolerance to the anxiolytic effects of benzodiazepines (American Psychiatric Association 1990). Patients most likely to receive continued benzodiazepine prescriptions are those with both chronic somatic illness and substantial psychological distress. Several authors have proposed that if these patients receive continued benefit from benzodiazepine treatment, ongoing prescription is appropriate (Uhlenhuth et al. 1988; Woods et al. 1988). Yet very few rigorously designed studies of the efficacy of long-term benzodiazepine prescribing in elderly patients have been published. Most studies have examined elderly institutionalized patients with organic mental syndromes, manifesting agitation as opposed to anxiety syndromes (Salzman 1991). Some prospective studies of younger anxious patients have demonstrated no difference in outcome between those treated with anxiolytic drugs and those treated with psychotherapy (Catalan et al. 1984), and some studies of mixed-age patients who have completed benzodiazepine withdrawal programs have demonstrated that anxiety levels are lower 4–6 weeks after drug cessation than before discontinuation (Rickels et al. 1990).

More research is needed on the appropriate indications for benzodiazepine treatment in elderly patients. The possible benefits of benzodiazepines must be balanced against the increased risks of adverse effects of these medications in old age.

Treatment of Benzodiazepine Dependence

Several interventions may both decrease the severity of benzodiazepine withdrawal and improve the ability to maintain abstinence. There is, however, a paucity of data regarding the effectiveness of these interventions in the elderly.

Withdrawal severity may be lessened, though rarely completely avoided, by a gradual taper schedule (Busto et al. 1986b). The schedule should be titrated as tolerated by the patient, and considerable slowing of the rate of decrease is often required for the last 25% of the taper (Higgitt et al. 1985). Several authors have suggested that taper schedules should last at least 4 weeks, with many patients requiring 2–4 months to tolerate complete withdrawal (Higgitt et al. 1985; Noyes et al. 1988; Schweizer et al. 1990). Switching to a longer–half-life drug with an equivalent potency may decrease withdrawal severity, but this has not been empirically demonstrated (American Psychiatric Association 1990). Adjuvant pharmacological treatments are of limited success. In controlled trials, buspirone and clonidine appeared ineffective in lessening withdrawal severity (Goodman et al. 1986; Lader and Olajide 1987; Schweizer and Rickels 1986). Propranolol has a modest effect on withdrawal severity, but not on the success of the taper (Tyrer et al. 1981), whereas carbamazepine improves outcome without diminishing withdrawal severity (Schweizer et al. 1991). Substitution of phenobarbital with a gradual taper of this agent has been touted as effective especially in cases of mixed benzodiazepine and alcohol abuse (American Psychiatric Association 1990). These studies have not included significant numbers of elderly or medically ill patients who could be expected to have more sedation and ataxia from carbamazepine and phenobarbital and cardiovascular and respiratory complications from propranolol.

Several other interventions have been proposed to improve the long-term success of benzodiazepine discontinuation. A proportion of patients will be able to reduce or discontinue benzodiazepines with only encouragement and support from the prescribing physician (Cormack et al. 1989; Hopkins et al. 1982). Patients who have completed a formal discontinuation program are more likely to be free of benzodiazepines at follow-up than are those who do not participate (Rickels et al. 1991). Pharmacological treatment of the comorbid depressive illnesses found in so many benzodiazepine-dependent elderly patients is recommended. Antidepressants are also an alternative therapy for panic disorder. Cognitive and behavioral therapies, and other nondrug anxiety management techniques have only modest effects on withdrawal severity, but their effect on long-term outcome is not well studied (Higgitt et al. 1985; Roy-Byrne and Hommer 1988; Teare 1984). Most patients who are successfully withdrawn will continue to have significant anxiety, insomnia, and depression (Ashton 1987; Golombok et al. 1987; Higgit 1988; Higgitt et al. 1985).

Prescription Analgesic Drug Abuse

In one community survey, the 2-week prevalence of prescribed narcotic use was 2.1% for elderly women and 2.3% for elderly men (Chrischilles et al. 1990). Abuse of narcotics by the elderly appears rare unless the patient abused opiates when young (Jinks and Raschko 1990). Case series of hospitalized elderly patients indicate that opiate-analgesic dependence was less common than was dependence on antianxiety and sedative-hypnotic agents (Finlayson 1984; Jinks and Raschko 1990; Whitcup and Miller 1987). An audit at one large medical center revealed that although 12,000 narcotic prescriptions were filled, only four patients developed narcotic abuse (Porter and Jick 1980). Low rates of addiction from prescribed opiates are also found in reports from headache clinics and burn centers (Portenoy and Payne 1992).

Old age is associated with the development of various nonmalignant, but painful, chronic conditions (e.g., arthritis and neuropathies) for which narcotics are frequently, though controversially, prescribed. Tolerance and physical dependence can occur even in the absence of abuse (Portenoy and Payne 1992). The degree to which chronic narcotic use causes cognitive impairment remains unknown. One study of middle-aged persons found no evidence of cognitive impairment associated with chronically prescribed narcotics (Hendler et al. 1980). However, studies in elderly subjects, who might be expected to be more sensitive to adverse CNS effects, are lacking.

Illicit Drugs

Illicit drug use by elderly individuals is very uncommon and limited primarily to aging criminals and long-term heroin addicts (Myers et al. 1984). Opioid addicts are the best studied of elderly illicit drug abusers. Elderly narcotic addicts typically have a history of several decades of opiate use (Capel et al. 1972). Many enter methadone maintenance as they get older, but those who do tolerate subsequent narcotic detoxification poorly (Capel and Peppers 1978; Pascarelli 1979). In 1985, 2% of methadone maintenance clients in New York City were over age 60 (Pascarelli 1985). Factors that contribute to the low prevalence of elderly addicts include low incidence of new opioid abuse after age 25 years, high mortality associated with illicit drug use, imprisonment, and increasing abstinence associated with age (Des Jarlais et al. 1985; Ghodse et al. 1985; Harrington and Cox 1979; Maddux and Desmond 1980; Vaillant 1983).

Psychiatric and medical illnesses cause considerable morbidity in elderly addicts. As in younger addicts, elderly addicts experience the medical effects of contaminated needles and impure drugs, which increase their risk of systemic infections including endocarditis, sepsis, skin and CNS abscesses, and hepatitis B (Novick 1992). Of all elderly individuals with acquired immunodeficiency syndrome (AIDS), 3% contracted the human immunodeficiency virus (HIV) through intravenous drug use (Moss and Miles 1987). To some degree the risk of medical complications is mitigated by the tendency of elderly addicts to practice scrupulous hygiene regarding needles and syringes (Capel et al. 1972; Des Jarlais et al. 1985; Pascarelli and Fischer 1974). Long-term heroin addicts develop neuropsychological and neuroimaging abnormalities (caused by cerebral damage from infections, injected foreign substances, and so on) that are likely to further impair their function in the community (Schuckit 1977; Strang and Gurling 1989). Aging opioid-dependent people frequently die from the consequences of alcohol and tobacco dependence (Des Jarlais et al. 1985).

Little information is available regarding the use of other illicit drugs by the elderly. In 1982, the 1-year prevalence of marijuana use in people over age 50 was 1% (J. D. Miller et al. 1983). There are sporadic case reports of cocaine abuse in the elderly, but no systematic studies (Abrams and Alexopoulos 1988). The abuse of most illicit drugs is substantially higher in elderly individuals who are alcohol dependent (N. S. Miller et al. 1991).

Tobacco (Nicotine) Dependence

Epidemiology

Among the elderly population in the United States, tobacco dependence is the most common of all substance use disorders. In 1987, the following national smoking prevalence rates were determined (U.S. Department of Health and Human Services 1989):

- Age 45–64: men 33.5%, women 28.6%
- Age 65–74: men 20.2%, women 18%
- Age 75 or older: men 11.3%, women 7.5%

A survey of four large geographically diverse areas in the United States reported the prevalence of current smoking among people over age 84 as ranging from 4.6% to 10.8% for men and from 1.1% to 4.0% for women (Colsher et al. 1990). The prevalence of tobacco use among adults has declined steadily over the last 25 years. Rates are lower in the elderly as compared with young and middle-aged people because of mortality among smokers (U.S. Department of Health and Human Services 1988b) and more successful smoking cessation. Currently 60% of elderly women and 70% of elderly men who have at any time been tobacco dependent are now abstinent (U.S. Department of Health and Human Services 1988a) and increasing age is correlated with success at quitting (Fiore et al. 1990). Annual smoking cessation rates among the elderly population are 10% (Salive et al. 1992).

Nicotine-Dependence Disorder

Nicotine is the addictive substance in tobacco and regular use of tobacco in any form produces a nicotine-dependence disorder. Similar to heroin or cocaine addiction, nicotine dependence is characterized by pursuit of pleasurable effects from nicotine use, regular and compulsive patterns of use despite knowledge of harmful effects, withdrawal symptoms, tolerance to effects with compensatory increased intake, and craving and relapse with abstinence (Hughes et al. 1987; Jarvik and Schneider 1992; U.S. Department of Health and Human Services 1988a). Nicotine has euphorigenic properties. The primary pleasure-producing ef-

fects of nicotine appear to be mediated by increased dopamine release in brain reward centers (Jarvik and Schneider 1992). Smokers claim, and some objective evidence supports, that nicotine improves motor performance and mood and decreases anxiety (Jarvik and Schneider 1992). There is a paucity of data on how the psychotropic effects of nicotine are modified by age. When tobacco is discontinued, smokers experience a variety of unpleasant mood and physical symptoms that begin within hours of abstinence. Psychological symptoms include irritability, anxiety, depression, and craving. Physiological symptoms include low energy, concentration difficulties, headache, increased appetite, and nonspecific somatic complaints (American Psychiatric Association 1994; Hughes et al. 1986; Jarvik and Schneider 1992). There has been little investigation into age-related changes in the prevalence or severity of these withdrawal symptoms.

Complications and Comorbidities

Tobacco use is the leading preventable cause of death in adults. Smoking increases the risk of a variety of cancers, atherosclerotic disease, chronic obstructive lung disease, peptic ulcer disease, and osteoporosis (Agner 1985; Mellstrom et al. 1982; Rundgren and Mellstrom 1984). Smoking may contribute to malnutrition in frail elderly people by promoting weight loss and impairing sense of taste and smell (Rimer 1988). The metabolism of many prescribed drugs is altered by smoking (Dawson and Vestal 1984). Even in old age, smoking cessation benefits health, increasing life expectancy by 2–4 years (Sachs 1986).

In mixed-aged populations, abusers of cocaine, heroin, and alcohol are likely to be smokers. In a large national survey, the odds ratio (± 95% confidence interval) of an alcoholic ever being a smoker was 5.2 (4.1–6.8) (Glassman et al. 1990). Studies that have concentrated on elderly subjects have demonstrated that elderly smokers are more likely to consume alcohol and that 70% of older alcoholic subjects are current smokers (Atkinson and Tolson 1992; Colsher et al. 1990; Finlayson et al. 1988). Continued smoking in elderly people is associated with increased prevalence of psychiatric symptoms and syndromes. Elderly smokers have higher levels of depression symptoms than never or former smokers (Colsher et al. 1990). Among mixed-aged populations, persons with a lifetime history of major depression are significantly more likely to smoke and to have difficulty quitting (Glassman et al.

1990). The prevalence of smoking in young people with schizophrenia is 88%; however, smoking prevalence has not been examined in elderly cohorts with severe mental illnesses (Hughes et al. 1986).

Smoking Cessation

Ninety percent of all adult smokers who quit do so without a specialized treatment program, typically by stopping abruptly (Fiore et al. 1990). Specialized smoking cessation strategies include behavioral techniques such as aversion therapies (rapid smoking and satiation), cognitive therapies, relaxation training, social support, coping skills training, hypnosis, acupuncture, and group and individualized counseling (Heinold 1984; Rimer 1988; U.S. Department of Health and Human Services 1988a). Rapid smoking may be contraindicated because of increased health risk in some older patients with heart disease, hypertension, or peptic ulcer disease. Multicomponent trials combining two or more of these techniques have the best outcomes with up to 50% abstinence sustained at 1-year follow-up (U.S. Department of Health and Human Services 1988a). Effective interventions for elderly patients may not differ substantially from those generally available, but little investigation has been done comparing efficacy of different methods by age group (Sachs 1986; Atkinson et al. 1992).

In recent years nicotine replacement systems have been introduced to reduce nicotine withdrawal symptoms. Currently in the United States nicotine polacrilex gum and transdermal nicotine are available as pharmacological treatments. Both are significantly more successful than placebo over the short-term (up to 6 months), but more studies are needed to document long-term efficacy. The transdermal patch may be preferable in elderly patients with dental concerns (Jarvik and Schneider 1992).

Summary

In this chapter, we have reviewed the leading substance abuse problems affecting the elderly, with special emphasis on neuropsychiatric features of these disorders. Tobacco, alcohol, and controlled prescription drugs, especially the benzodiazepines, present the greatest substance abuse hazards in old age.

Several aspects of substance abuse in old age can be highlighted. Tobacco, the substance most widely abused by elderly people, does not have prominent deleterious neurotoxic effects, though morbid effects on other organ systems such as the vascular system may result in cognitive impairment. Elderly people are more sensitive than younger people to neurotoxic effects of substances such as alcohol and benzodiazepines. These effects are manifested as both decrements in performance on cognitive testing and functional decline common to frail elderly individuals such as impairments in activities of daily living or falls.

Illicit drug use by elderly people is uncommon, but poorly investigated. The recent decade has produced little new information on the demography, characteristics, or treatment of elderly people who abuse illicit drugs. The increased prevalence of drug abuse in current middle-aged people suggests that illicit substance abuse among elderly people looms as a future public health problem. Information is especially scarce on the neuropsychiatric effects of both licit and illicit opiates.

Fatalism on the part of health care providers regarding substance abuse in old age is misplaced. Studies of alcohol and tobacco dependence suggest that abstinence that could not be achieved in young age may be more successfully achieved in old age. Significant health benefits occur. Treatment of substance abuse may result in either reversing or arresting neuropsychiatric dysfunction and may account for the largest portion of treatable dementias. Further research is needed in specialized age-appropriate treatment for the substance-abusing elderly person.

References

Abrams RC, Alexopoulos GS: Substance abuse in the elderly: over-the-counter and illegal drugs. Hosp Community Psychiatry 39:822–823, 829, 1988

Adams WL, Garry PJ, Rhyne R, et al: Alcohol intake in the healthy elderly: changes with age in a cross-sectional and longitudinal study. J Am Geriatr Soc 38:211–216, 1990

Adams WL, Magruder K, Trued S, et al: Alcohol abuse in elderly emergency department patients. J Am Geriatr Soc 40:1236–1240, 1992

Agner E: Smoking and health in old age: a ten-year follow-up study. Acta Medica Scandinavica 218:311–316, 1985

Alexander F, Duff RW: Social interaction and alcohol use in retirement communities. Gerontologist 28:632–638, 1988

American Psychiatric Association: Diagnostic and Statistical Manual of Mental Disorders, 4th Edition. Washington, DC, American Psychiatric Association, 1994

American Psychiatric Association: Benzodiazepine Dependence, Toxicity, and Abuse. Washington, DC, American Psychiatric Association, 1990

Ashton H: Benzodiazepine withdrawal: outcome in 50 patients. British Journal of Addiction 82:665–671, 1987

Atkinson RM: Persuading alcoholic patients to seek treatment. Compr Ther 11(11):16–24, 1985

Atkinson RM: Alcoholism in the elderly population (editorial). Mayo Clin Proc 63:825–829, 1988

Atkinson RM: Aging and alcohol use disorders: diagnostic issues in the elderly. Int Psychogeriatr 2:55–72, 1990

Atkinson RM: Alcohol and drug abuse in the elderly, in Psychiatry in the Elderly. Edited by Jacoby R, Oppenheimer C. Oxford, England, Oxford University Press, 1991, pp 819–851

Atkinson RM: Late life problem drinkers: frequency and risk factors. Paper presented in symposium on Physiologic and Clinical Research on Aging and Alcohol Use at the annual meeting of the Research Society on Alcoholism, San Diego CA, June 1992

Atkinson RM: Treatment programs for aging alcoholics, in Alcohol and Aging. Edited by Beresford TP, Gomberg ESL. New York, Oxford University Press (in press)

Atkinson RM, Kofoed LL: Alcohol and drug abuse in old age: a clinical perspective. Substance and Alcohol Actions/Misuse 3:353–368, 1982

Atkinson RM, Kofoed LL: Alcohol and drug abuse, In Geriatric Medicine, Vol 2: Fundamentals of Geriatric Care. Edited by Cassell CK, Walsh JR. New York, Springer-Verlag, 1984, pp 219–235

Atkinson RM, Tolson RL: Late onset alcohol use disorders in older men. Research poster presented at the annual meeting of the American Association for Geriatric Psychiatry, San Francisco, CA, February 1992

Atkinson RM, Tolson RL, Turner JA: Late versus early onset problem drinking in older men. Alcoholism (New York) 14:574–579, 1990

Atkinson RM, Ganzini L, Bernstein MJ: Alcohol and substance-use disorders in the elderly, in Handbook of Mental Health and Aging, 2nd Edition. Edited by Birren JE, Sloane RB, Cohen GD. New York, Academic Press, 1992, pp 515–555

Atkinson RM, Tolson RL, Turner JA: Factors affecting outpatient treatment compliance of older male problem drinkers. J Stud Alcohol 54:102–106, 1993

Beardsley RS, Larson DB, Burns BJ, et al: Prescribing of psychotropics in elderly nursing home patients. J Am Geriatr Soc 37:327–330, 1989

Beers M, Avorn J, Soumerai SB, et al: Psychoactive medication use in intermediate-care facility residents. JAMA 260:3016–3020, 1988

Beresford TP: Age comparisons in metabolism and intoxication. Paper presented in a symposium on Physiologic and Clinical Research on Aging and Alcohol Use at the annual meeting of the Research Society on Alcoholism, San Diego, CA, June 1992a

Beresford TP: Remarks on use of the CAGE questionnaire in medical inpatients stratified for age group. Presentation at the Workshop on Alcoholism in the Elderly, American Medical Association (Department of Geriatric Health), Chicago, IL, November 1992b

Besson JAO, Glen AIM, Foreman EI, et al: Nuclear magnetic resonance observations in alcoholic cerebral disorder and the role of vasopressin. Lancet 2:923–924, 1981

Besson JAO, Crawford JR, Parker DM, et al: Magnetic resonance imaging in Alzheimer's disease, multi-infarct dementia and Korsakoff's psychosis. Acta Psychiatr Scand 80:451–458, 1989

Blazer DG: Depression in Late Life. St Louis, MO, CV Mosby, 1982

Blow FC, Cook CAL, Booth BM, et al: Age-related psychiatric comorbidities and level of functioning in alcoholic veterans seeking outpatient treatment. Hosp Community Psychiatry 43:990–995, 1992

Bonnet MH, Kramer M: The interaction of age, performance and hypnotics in the sleep of insomniacs. J Am Geriatr Soc 29:508–512, 1981

Bowden CL, Fisher JG: Safety and efficacy of long-term diazepam therapy. South Med J 73:1581–1584, 1980

Brandt J, Butters N, Ryan C, et al: Cognitive loss and recovery in long-term alcohol abusers. Arch Gen Psychiatry 40:435–442, 1983

Brown SA, Schuckit MA: Changes in depression among abstinent alcoholics. J Stud Alcohol 49:412–417, 1988

Buchsbaum DG, Buchanan RG, Welsh J, et al: Screening for drinking disorders in the elderly using the CAGE questionnaire. J Am Geriatr Soc 40:662–665, 1992

Buck JA: Psychotropic drug practice in nursing homes. J Am Geriatr Soc 36:409–418, 1988

Busto U, Sellers EM, Naranjo CA, et al: Patterns of benzodiazepine abuse and dependence. Br J Addict 81:87–94, 1986a

Busto U, Sellers EM, Naranjo CA, et al: Withdrawal reaction after long-term therapeutic use of benzodiazepines. N Engl J Med 315:854–859, 1986b

Butters N: Alcoholic Korsakoff's syndrome: some unresolved issues concerning etiology, neuropathology and cognitive deficits. J Clin Exp Neuropsychol 7:181–210, 1985

Capel WC, Peppers LG: The aging addict: a longitudinal study of known abusers. Addictive Disease 3:389–403, 1978

Capel WC, Goldsmith BM, Waddell KJ, et al: The aging narcotic addict: an increasing problem for the next decades. J Gerontol 27:102–106, 1972

Carlen PL, Wortzman G, Holgate RC, et al: Reversible cerebral atrophy in recently abstinent chronic alcoholics measured by computed tomographic scans. Science 200:1076–1078, 1978

Carlen PL, Lee MA, Jacob M, et al: Parkinsonism provoked by alcoholism. Ann Neurol 9:84–86, 1981

Carlen PL, Penn RD, Fornazzari L, et al: Computerized tomographic scan assessment of alcoholic brain damage and its potential reversibility. Alcoholism (New York) 10:226–232, 1986

Carlsson A, Adolfsson R, Acquilonius SM, et al: Biogenic amines in human brain in normal aging, senile dementia, and chronic alcoholism, in Ergot Compounds and Brain Function: Neuroendocrine and Neuropsychiatric Aspects. Edited by Goldstein M. New York, Raven, 1980, pp 295–304

Castleden CM, George CF, Marcer D, et al: Increased sensitivity to nitrazepam in old age. BMJ 1:10–12, 1977

Catalan J, Gath D, Edmonds G, et al: The effects of non-prescribing of anxiolytics in general practice, I: controlled evaluation of psychiatric and social outcome. Br J Psychiatry 144:593–602, 1984

Chrischilles EA, Lemke JH, Wallace RB, et al: Prevalence and characteristics of multiple analgesic drug use in an elderly study group. J Am Geriatr Soc 38:979–984, 1990

Colsher PL, Wallace RB, Pomrehn PR, et al: Demographic and health characteristics of elderly smokers: results from established populations for epidemiologic studies of the elderly. Am J Prev Med 6:61–70, 1990

Conwell Y, Rotenberg M, Caine ED: Completed suicide at age 50 and over. J Am Geriatr Soc 38:640–644, 1990

Cook BL, Winokur G, Garvey MJ, et al: Depression and previous alcoholism in the elderly. Br J Psychiatry 158:72–75, 1991

Cook PJ: Benzodiazepine hypnotics in the elderly. Acta Psychiatr Scand Suppl 332:149–158, 1986

Cook PJ, Huggett A, Graham-Pole R, et al: Hypnotic accumulation and hangover in elderly inpatients: a controlled double blind study of temazepam and nitrazepam. BMJ (Clinical Research Edition) 286:100–102, 1983

Cormack MA, Owens RG, Dewey ME: The effect of minimal interventions by general practitioners on long-term benzodiazepine use. J R Coll Gen Pract 39:408–411, 1989

Curtis JR, Geller G, Stokes EJ, et al: Characteristics, diagnosis, and treatment of alcoholism in elderly patients. J Am Geriatr Soc 37:310–316, 1989

Cutting J: The relationship between Korsakoff's syndrome and "alcoholic dementia." Br J Psychiatry 132:240–251, 1978

Davidson DM: Cardiovascular effects of alcohol. West J Med 151:430–439, 1989

Dawson GW, Vestal RE: Smoking, age, and drug metabolism, in Smoking and Aging. Edited by Bosse R, Rose CL. Lexington, MA, Lexington Books, 1984, pp 131–156

Delin CR, Lee TH: Drinking and the brain: current evidence. Alcohol Alcohol 27:117–126, 1992

Des Jarlais DC, Joseph H, Courtwright DT: Old age and addiction: a study of elderly patients in methadone maintenance treatment, in The Combined Problems of Alcoholism, Drug Addiction and Aging. Edited by Gottheil E, Druley KA, Skoloda TE, et al. Springfield, IL, Charles C Thomas, 1985, pp 201–209

Donovan DM, Marlatt GA (eds): Assessment of Addictive Behaviors. New York, Guilford, 1988

Droller H: Some aspects of alcoholism in the elderly. Lancet 2:137–139, 1964

Dunbar GC, Perera MH, Jenner FA: Patterns of benzodiazepine use in Great Britain as measured by a general population survey. Br J Psychiatry 155:836–841, 1989

Dustman RE: Alcoholism and aging: electrophysiological parallels, in Alcoholism in the Elderly: Social and Biomedical Issues. Edited by Hartford JT, Samorajski T. New York, Raven, 1984, pp 201–225

Eaton WW, Kramer M, Anthony JC, et al: The incidence of specific DIS/DSM-III mental disorders: data from the NIMH epidemiologic catchment area program. Acta Psychiatr Scand 79:163–178, 1989

Emmerson RY, Dustman RE, Heil J, et al: Neuropsychological performance of young nondrinkers, social drinkers, and long- and short-term sober alcoholics. Alcoholism (New York) 12:625–629, 1988

Fialip J, Aumaitre O, Eschalier A, et al: Benzodiazepine withdrawal seizures: analysis of 48 case reports. Clin Neuropharmacol 10:538–544, 1987

Finlayson RE: Prescription drug abuse in older persons, in Alcohol and Drug Abuse in Old Age. Edited by Atkinson RM. Washington, DC, American Psychiatric Press, 1984, pp 61–70

Finlayson RE, Hurt RD, Davis LJ, et al: Alcoholism in elderly persons: a study of the psychiatric and psychosocial features of 216 inpatients. Mayo Clin Proc 63:761–768, 1988

Fiore MC, Novotny TE, Pierce JP, et al: Methods used to quit smoking in the United States. JAMA 263:2760–2765, 1990

Folstein MF, Folstein SE, McHugh PR: Mini-Mental State: a practical method for grading the cognitive state of patients for the clinician. J Psychiatr Res 12:189–198, 1975

Foy A, Drinkwater V, March S, et al: Confusion after admission to hospital in elderly patients using benzodiazepines (letter). BMJ (Clinical Research Edition) 293:1072, 1986

Freund G: Neurotransmitter function in relation to aging and alcoholism, in Alcoholism in the Elderly: Social and Biomedical Issues. Edited by Hartford JT, Samorajski T. New York, Raven, 1984, pp 65–83

Freund G: Drug- and alcohol-induced dementias, in Geriatric Clinical Pharmacology. Edited by Wood WG, Strong R. New York, Raven, 1987, pp 95–105

Ghodse AH, Sheehan M, Taylor C, et al: Deaths of drug addicts in the United Kingdom 1967–81. BMJ (Clinical Research Edition) 290:425–428, 1985

Glassman AH, Helzer JE, Covey LS, et al: Smoking, smoking cessation, and major depression. JAMA 264:1546–1549, 1990

Glynn RJ, Bouchard GR, LoCastro JS, et al: Aging and generational effects on drinking behaviors in men: results from the Normative Aging Study. Am J Publ Health 75:1413–1419, 1985

Golombok S, Higgitt A, Fonagy P, et al: A follow-up study of patients treated for benzodiazepine dependence. Br J Med Psychol 60:141–149, 1987

Golombok S, Moodley P, Lader M: Cognitive impairment in long-term benzodiazepine users. Psychol Med 18:365–374, 1988

Goodman WK, Charney DS, Price LH, et al: Ineffectiveness of clonidine in the treatment of the benzodiazepine withdrawal syndrome: report of three cases. Am J Psychiatry 143:900–903, 1986

Gordon T, Kannel WB: Drinking and its relation to smoking, BP, blood lipids, and uric acid. Arch Intern Med 143:1366–1374, 1983

Grant I, Adams KM, Reed R: Aging, abstinence, and medical risk factors in the prediction of neuropsychologic deficit among long-term alcoholics. Arch Gen Psychiatry 41:710–718, 1984

Greenblatt DJ, Shader RI: Benzodiazepines in the elderly: pharmacokinetics and drug sensitivity, in Anxiety in the Elderly: Treatment and Research. Edited by Salzman C, Lebowitz BD. New York, Springer, 1991, pp 131–145

Harper CG, Kril JJ, Daly JM: Brain shrinkage in alcoholics is not caused by changes in hydration: a pathological study. J Neurol Neurosurg Psychiatry 51:124–127, 1988

Harrington P, Cox TJ: A twenty-year follow-up of narcotic addicts in Tucson, Arizona. Am J Drug Alcohol Abuse 6:25–37, 1979

Heindel WC, Salmon DP, Butters N: Alcoholic Korsakoff's syndrome, in Memory Disorders: Research and Clinical Practice. Edited by Yanagihara T, Petersen R. New York, Marcel Dekker, 1991, pp 227–253

Heinold JW: The efficacy of smoking-cessation strategies: does it vary with age? in Smoking and Aging. Edited by Bosse R, Rose CL. Lexington, MA, Lexington Books, 1984, pp 203–220

Helzer JE, Burnam A, McEvoy LT: Alcohol abuse and dependence, in Psychiatric Disorders in America: The Epidemiologic Catchment Area Study. Edited by Robbins LN, Regier DA. New York, Free Press, 1991, pp 81–115

Hendler N, Cimini C, Ma T, et al: A comparison of cognitive impairment due to benzodiazepines and to narcotics. Am J Psychiatry 137:828–830, 1980

Higgitt A: Indications for benzodiazepine prescriptions in the elderly (editorial). International Journal of Geriatric Psychiatry 3:239–243, 1988

Higgitt AC, Lader MH, Fonagy P: Clinical management of benzodiazepine dependence. BMJ 291:688–690, 1985

Hodges H, Allen Y, Sinden J, et al: The effects of cholinergic drugs and cholinergic-rich foetal neural transplants on alcohol-induced deficits in radial maze performance in rats. Behav Brain Res 43:7–28, 1991

Holton A, Riley P, Tyrer P: Factors predicting long-term outcome after chronic benzodiazepine therapy. J Affect Disord 24:245–252, 1992

Hopkins DR, Sethi KBS, Mucklaw JC: Benzodiazepine withdrawal in general practice. J R Coll Gen Pract 32:758–762, 1982

Horvath TB: Clinical spectrum and epidemiological features of alcoholic dementia, in Alcohol, Drugs and Brain Damage. Edited by Rankin JG. Toronto, Canada, Addiction Research Foundation, 1975, pp 1–16

Hughes JR, Hatsukami DK, Mitchell JE, et al: Prevalence of smoking among psychiatric outpatients. Am J Psychiatry 143:993–997, 1986

Hughes JR, Gust SW, Pechacek TF: Prevalence of tobacco dependence and withdrawal. Am J Psychiatry 144:205–208, 1987

Hurt RD, Finlayson RE, Morse RM, et al: Alcoholism in elderly persons: medical aspects and prognosis of 216 inpatients. Mayo Clin Proc 63:753–760, 1988

Ishikawa Y, Meyer JS, Tanahashi N, et al: Abstinence improves cerebral perfusion and brain volume in alcoholic neurotoxicity without Wernicke-Korsakoff syndrome. J Cerebral Blood Flow Metab 6:86–94, 1986

Jacoby RJ, Levy R: Computed tomography in the elderly, II: senile dementia: diagnosis and functional impairment. Br J Psychiatry 136:256–269, 1980

Jacques PF, Sulsky S, Hartz SC, et al: Moderate alcohol intake and nutritional status in nonalcoholic elderly subjects. Am J Clin Nutr 50:875–883, 1989

Jarvik ME, Schneider NG: Nicotine, in Substance Abuse: A Comprehensive Textbook, 2nd Edition. Edited by Lowinson JH, Ruiz P, Millman RB, et al. Baltimore, MD, Williams & Wilkins, 1992 pp 334–356

Jinks MJ, Raschko RR: A profile of alcohol and prescription drug abuse in a high-risk community-based elderly population. Drug Intelligence and Clinical Pharmacy—Annals of Pharmacotherapy 24:971–975, 1990

Jones MK, Jones BM: The relationship of age and drinking habits to the effects of alcohol on memory in women. J Stud Alcohol 41:179–186, 1980

Jones TV, Lindsey BA, Yount P, et al: Alcohol consumption patterns in an elderly ambulatory care population. Poster presented at the annual meeting of the American Geriatrics Society, Washington DC, November 1992

Joseph C, Atkinson R, Ganzini L, et al: Screening for alcohol problems in the nursing home. Poster presented at the annual meeting of the American Geriatrics Society, Washington DC, November 1992

Kafetz K, Cox M: Alcohol excess and the senile squalor syndrome. J Am Geriatr Soc 30:706, 1982

Kales A, Scharf MB, Kales JD, et al: Rebound insomnia: a potential hazard following withdrawal of certain benzodiazepines. JAMA 241:1692–1695, 1979

Kiernan RJ, Mueller J, Langston JW, et al: The Neurobehavioral Cognitive Status Examination: a brief but differentiated approach to cognitive assessment. Ann Intern Med 107:481–485, 1987

King MB: Alcohol abuse and dementia. International Journal of Geriatric Psychiatry 1:31–36, 1986

Kissin B, Begleiter H (eds): The Pathogenesis of Alcoholism: Biological Factors. New York, Plenum, 1983a

Kissin B, Begleiter H (eds): The Pathogenesis of Alcoholism: Psychosocial Factors. New York, Plenum, 1983b

Klatsky AL, Armstrong MA, Friedman GD: Risk of cardiovascular mortality in alcohol drinkers, ex-drinkers and nondrinkers. Am J Cardiol 66:1237–1242, 1990

Kramer M, Schoen S: Problems in the use of long-acting hypnotics in older patients. J Clin Psychiatry 45:176–177, 1984

Lader M, Olajide D: A comparison of buspirone and placebo in relieving benzodiazepine withdrawal symptoms. J Clin Psychopharmacol 7:11–15, 1987

Lader MH, Ron M, Petursson H: Computed axial brain tomography in long-term benzodiazepine users. Psychol Med 14:203–206, 1984

Larson EB, Reifler BV, Canfield C, et al: Evaluating elderly outpatients with symptoms of dementia. Hosp Community Psychiatry 35:425–428, 1984a

Larson EB, Reifler BV, Featherstone HJ, et al: Dementia in elderly outpatients: a prospective study. Ann Intern Med 100:417–423, 1984b

Larson EB, Kukull WA, Buchner D, et al: Adverse drug reaction associated with global cognitive impairment in elderly persons. Ann Intern Med 107:169–173, 1987

Laughren TP, Battey Y, Greenblatt DJ, et al: A controlled trial of diazepam withdrawal in chronically anxious outpatients. Acta Psychiatr Scand 65:171–179, 1982

Liberto JG, Oslin DW, Ruskin PE: Alcoholism in older persons: a review of the literature. Hosp Community Psychiatry 43:975–984, 1992

Lishman WA: Organic Psychiatry, 2nd Edition. Oxford, England, Blackwell, 1987

Liskow BI, Rinck C, Campbell J, et al: Alcohol withdrawal in the elderly. J Stud Alcohol 50:414–421, 1989

Lowinson JH, Ruiz P, Millman RB (eds): Comprehensive Textbook of Substance Abuse. Baltimore, MD, Williams & Wilkins, 1992

MacMillan D, Shaw P: Senile breakdown in standards of personal and environmental cleanliness. BMJ 2:1032–1037, 1966

Maddux JF, Desmond DP: New light on the maturing out hypothesis in opioid dependence. Bull Narc 32:15–25, 1980

Mair RG, McEntee WJ: Korsakoff's psychosis: noradrenergic systems and cognitive impairment. Behav Brain Res 9:1–32, 1983

Mant A, Duncan-Jones P, Saltman D, et al: Development of long term use of psychotropic drugs by general practice patients. BMJ (Clinical Research Edition) 296:251–254, 1988

Martin JC, Streissguth AP: Alcoholism and the elderly: an overview, in Treatment of Psychopathology in the Aging. Edited by Eisdorfer C, Fann WE. New York, Springer, 1982, pp 242–280

McCrady BS, Smith DE: Implications of cognitive impairment for the treatment of alcoholism. Alcoholism (New York) 10:145–149, 1986

McEntee WJ, Mair RG: Memory impairment in Korsakoff's psychosis: a correlation with brain noradrenergic activity. Science 202:905–907, 1978

Mellinger GD, Balter MB, Uhlenhuth EH: Prevalence and correlates of the long-term regular use of anxiolytics. JAMA 251:375–379, 1984

Mellstrom D, Rundgren A, Jagenburg R, et al: Tobacco smoking ageing and health among the elderly: a longitudinal population study of 70-year-old men and an age cohort comparison. Age Ageing 11:45–58, 1982

Meyer JS, Largen Jr JW, Shaw T, et al: Interaction of normal aging, senile dementia, multi-infarct dementia, and alcoholism in the elderly. in Alcoholism in the Elderly: Social and Biomedical Issues. Edited by Hartford JT, Samorajski T. New York, Raven, 1984, pp 227–251

Miller JD, Cisin IH, Gardner-Keaton H, et al: National Survey on Drug Abuse: Main Findings, 1982 (DHHS Publication No ADM-83-1263). Washington, DC, US Government Printing Office, 1983

Miller NS, Belkin BM, Gold MS: Alcohol and drug dependence among the elderly: epidemiology, diagnosis, and treatment. Compr Psychiatry 32:153–165, 1991

Moos RH, Brennan PL, Moos BS: Short-term processes of remission and nonremission among late-life problem drinkers. Alcoholism (New York) 15:948–955, 1991

Morgan K, Dallosso H, Ebrahim S, et al: Prevalence, frequency, and duration of hypnotic drug use among the elderly living at home. BMJ (Clinical Research Edition) 296:601–602, 1988

Moss RJ, Miles SH: AIDS and the geriatrician. Am Geriatr Soc 35:460–464, 1987

Murphy SM, Owen R, Tyrer PJ: Withdrawal symptoms after six weeks' treatments with diazepam (letter). Lancet 2:1389, 1984

Myers JK, Weissman MM, Tischler GL, et al: Six-month prevalence of psychiatric disorder in three communities, 1980 to 1982. Arch Gen Psychiatry 41:959–967, 1984

Nakamura MM, Overall JE, Hollister LE, et al: Factors affecting outcome of depressive symptoms in alcoholics. Alcoholism (New York) 7:188–193, 1983

Nikaido AM, Ellinwood EH Jr, Heatherly DG, et al: Age-related increase in CNS sensitivity to benzodiazepines as assessed by task difficulty. Psychopharmacology 100:90–97, 1990

Novick DM: The medically ill substance abuser, in Substance Abuse: A Comprehensive Textbook, 2nd Edition. Edited by Lowinson JH, Ruiz P, Millman RB, et al. Baltimore, MD, Williams & Wilkins, 1992, pp 657–647

Noyes R Jr, Garvey MJ, Cook BL, et al: Benzodiazepine withdrawal: a review of the evidence. J Clin Psychiatry 49:382–389, 1988

Osuntokun BO, Hendrie HC, Fisher K, et al: The diagnosis of alcohol associated dementia. Research poster presented at the annual meeting of the American Association for Geriatric Psychiatry, San Francisco, CA, February 1992

Parker ES, Noble EP: Alcohol consumption and cognitive functioning in social drinkers. J Stud Alcohol 38:1224–1232, 1977

Parker ES, Noble EP: Alcohol and the aging process in social drinkers. J Stud Alcohol 41:170–178, 1980

Pascarelli EF: An update on drug dependence in the elderly. Journal of Drug Issues 9:47–54, 1979

Pascarelli EF: The elderly in methadone maintenance, in The Combined Problems of Alcoholism, Drug Addiction and Aging. Edited by Gottheil E, Druley KA, Skoloda TE, et al. Springfield, IL, Charles C Thomas, 1985, pp 210–214

Pascarelli EF, Fischer W: Drug dependence in the elderly. Int J Aging Hum Dev 5:347–356, 1974

Perera KMH, Powell T, Jenner FA: Computerized axial tomographic studies following long-term use of benzodiazepines. Psychol Med 17:775–777, 1987

Petursson H, Lader MH: Withdrawal from long-term benzodiazepine treatment. BMJ (Clinical Research Edition) 283:643–645, 1981

Pfefferbaum A, Rosenbloom M, Crusan K, et al: Brain CT changes in alcoholics: effects of age and alcohol consumption. Alcoholism (New York) 12:81–87, 1988

Pinsker H, Suljaga-Petchel K: Use of benzodiazepines in primary-care geriatric patients. J Am Geriatr Soc 32:595–597, 1984

Pomara N, Stanley B, Block R, et al: Increased sensitivity of the elderly to the central depressant effects of diazepam. J Clin Psychiatry 46:185–187, 1985

Pomara N, Deptula D, Singh R, et al: Cognitive toxicity of benzodiazepines in the elderly, in Anxiety in the Elderly: Treatment and Research. Edited by Salzman C, Lebowitz BD. New York, Springer, 1991, pp 175–196

Portenoy RK, Payne R: Acute and chronic pain, in Substance Abuse: A Comprehensive Textbook, 2nd Edition. Edited by Lowinson JH, Ruiz P, Millman RB, et al. Baltimore, MD, Williams & Wilkins, 1992, pp 691–721

Porter J, Jick H: Addiction rare in patients treated with narcotics (letter). N Engl J Med 302:123, 1980

Poser W, Poser S, Rosher D, et al: Do benzodiazepines cause cerebral atrophy? (letter) Lancet 1:715, 1983

Ray WA, Griffin MR, Schaffner W, et al: Psychotropic drug use and the risk of hip fracture. N Engl J Med 316:363–369, 1987

Ray WA, Griffin MR, Downey W: Benzodiazepines of long and short elimination half-life and the risk of hip fracture. JAMA 262:3303–3307, 1989

Reifler B, Raskind M, Kethley A: Psychiatric diagnoses among geriatric patients seen in an outreach program. J Am Geriatr Soc 30:530–533, 1982

Renvoize EB, Gaskell RK, Klar HM: Results of investigations in 150 demented patients consecutively admitted to a psychiatric hospital. Br J Psychiatry 147:204–205, 1985

Rickels K: Clinical management of benzodiazepine dependence (letter). BMJ (Clinical Research Edition) 291:1649, 1985

Rickels K, Case WG, Downing RW, et al: Long-term diazepam therapy and clinical outcome. JAMA 250:767–771, 1983

Rickels K, Schweizer E, Case WG, et al: Long-term therapeutic use of benzodiazepines, I: effects of abrupt discontinuation. Arch Gen Psychiatry 47:899–907, 1990

Rickels K, Case WG, Schweizer E, et al: Long-term benzodiazepine users 3 years after participation in a discontinuation program. Am J Psychiatry 148:757–761, 1991

Rimer B: Smoking among older adults: the problem, consequences and possible solutions, in Surgeon General's Report on Health Promotion for Older Adults. Washington, DC, US Department of Health and Human Services, 1988

Ritzmann RF, Melchior CL: Age and development of tolerance to and physical dependence on alcohol, in Alcoholism in the Elderly: Social and Biomedical Issues. Edited by Hartford JT, Samorajski T. New York, Raven, 1984, pp 117–138

Rodrigo EK, King MB, Williams P: Health of long term benzodiazepine users. BMJ (Clinical Research Edition) 296:603–606, 1988

Ron MA: The alcoholic brain: CT scan and psychological findings. Psychol Med (monograph suppl) 3:1–33, 1983

Roy-Byrne PP, Hommer D: Benzodiazepine withdrawal: overview and implications for treatment of anxiety. Am J Med 84:1041–1052, 1988

Rundgren A, Mellstrom D: The effect of tobacco smoking on the bone mineral content of the ageing skeleton. Mech Ageing Dev 28:273–277, 1984

Ryan C, Butters N: The neuropsychology of alcoholism, in The Neuropsychology Handbook. Edited by Wedding D, Horton A, Webster J. New York, Springer, 1986, pp 376–409

Sachs DPL: Cigarette smoking: health effects and cessation strategies. Clin Geriatr Med 2:337–362, 1986

Salive ME, Cornoni-Huntley J, LaCroix AZ, et al: Predictors of smoking cessation and relapse in older adults. Am J Public Health 82:1268–1271, 1992

Salzman C: Pharmacologic treatment of the anxious elderly patient, in Anxiety in the Elderly: Treatment and Research. Edited by Salzman C, Lebowitz BD. New York, Springer, 1991, pp 149–173

Samorajski T, Person K, Bissell C, et al: Biology of alcoholism and aging in rodents: brain and liver, in Alcoholism in the Elderly: Social and Biomedical Issues. Edited by Hartford JT, Samorajski T. New York, Raven, 1984, pp 43–63

Saunders PA, Copeland JRM, Dewey ME, et al: Heavy drinking as a risk factor for depression and dementia in elderly men. Br J Psychiatry 159:213–216, 1991

Schafer K, Butters N, Smith T, et al: Cognitive performance of alcoholics: a longitudinal evaluation of the role of drinking history, depression, liver function, nutrition, and family history. Alcoholism (New York) 15:653–660, 1991

Scherr PA, LaCroix AZ, Wallace RB, et al: Light to moderate alcohol consumption and mortality in the elderly. J Am Geriatr Soc 40:651–657, 1992

Schonfeld L, Dupree LW: Antecedents of drinking for early and late-onset elderly alcohol abusers. J Stud Alcohol 52:587–592, 1991

Schuckit MA: Geriatric alcoholism and drug abuse. Gerontologist 17:168–174, 1977

Schuckit MA: Drug and Alcohol Abuse, 3rd Edition. New York, Plenum, 1989

Schuckit MA, Atkinson JH, Miller PL, et al: A three-year follow-up of elderly alcoholics. J Clin Psychiatry 41:412–416, 1980

Schweizer E, Rickels K: Failure of buspirone to manage benzodiazepine withdrawal. Am J Psychiatry 143:1590–1592, 1986

Schweizer E, Case WG, Rickels K: Benzodiazepine dependence and withdrawal in elderly patients. Am J Psychiatry 146:529–531, 1989

Schweizer E, Rickels K, Case WG, et al: Long-term therapeutic use of benzodiazepines, II: effects of gradual taper. Arch Gen Psychiatry 47:908–915, 1990

Schweizer E, Rickels K, Case WG, et al: Carbamazepine treatment in patients discontinuing long-term benzodiazepine therapy: effects on withdrawal severity and outcome. Arch Gen Psychiatry 48:448–452, 1991

Shaper AG, Wannamethee G, Walker M: Alcohol and mortality in British men: explaining the U-shaped curve. Lancet 2:1267–1273, 1988

Simon A, Epstein LJ, Reynolds L: Alcoholism in the geriatric mentally ill. Geriatrics 23:125–131, 1968

Smart RG, Adlaf EM: Alcohol and drug use among the elderly: trends in use and characteristics of users. Can J Public Health 79:236–242, 1988

Speer DC, Bates K: Comorbid mental and substance disorders among older psychiatric patients. J Am Geriatr Soc 40:886–890, 1992

Strang J, Gurling H: Computerized tomography and neuropsychological assessment in long-term high-dose heroin addicts. British Journal of Addiction 84:1011–1019, 1989

Teare P: Skills not pills: learning to cope with anxiety symptoms. J R Coll Gen Pract 34:258–260, 1984

Tinetti ME, Speechley M, Ginter SF: Risk factors for falls among elderly persons living in the community. N Engl J Med 319:1701–1707, 1988

Tyrer P: Risks of dependence on benzodiazepine drugs: the importance of patient selection. BMJ 298:102, 104–105, 1989

Tyrer P, Rutherford D, Huggett T: Benzodiazepine withdrawal symptoms and propranolol. Lancet 1:520–522, 1981

US Department of Health and Human Services: The health consequences of smoking: nicotine addiction—a report of the surgeon general (DHSS Pub No CDC-88-8406). Washington, DC, US Government Printing Office, 1988a

US Department of Health and Human Services: State-specific estimates of smoking-attributable mortality and years of potential life lost—United States, 1985. Morbidity and Mortality Weekly Review 37:689–693, 1988b

US Department of Health and Human Services: Tobacco use by adults—United States, 1987. Morbidity and Mortality Weekly Report 38:685–687, 1989

Uhlenhuth EH, DeWit H, Balter MB, et al: Risks and benefits of long-term benzodiazepine use. J Clin Psychopharmacol 8:161–167, 1988

Vaillant GE: The Natural History of Alcoholism. Cambridge, MA, Harvard University Press, 1983

Vestal RE, McGuire EA, Tobin JD, et al: Aging and ethanol metabolism in man. Clin Pharmacol Ther 21:343–354, 1977

Victor M, Adams RD, Collins GH: The Wernicke-Korsakoff Syndrome and Related Neurologic Disorders Due to Alcoholism and Malnutrition (Contemporary Neurology Series, Vol 3). Philadelphia, PA, FA Davis, 1989

Vogel-Sprott M, Barrett P: Age, drinking habits and the effects of alcohol. J Stud Alcohol 45:517–521, 1984

Walker RD, Donovan DM, Kivlahan DR, et al: Length of stay, neuropsychological performance and aftercare: influence on alcohol treatment outcome. J Consult Clin Psychol 52:900–911, 1983

Wattis JP: Alcohol problems in the elderly. J Am Geriatr Soc 29:131–134, 1981

Wells CE: Diagnosis of dementia. Psychosomatics 20:517–522, 1979

Whitcup SM, Miller F: Unrecognized drug dependence in psychiatrically hospitalized elderly patients. J Am Geriatr Soc 35:297–301, 1987

Wilcox RE: Changes in biogenic amines and their metabolites with aging and alcoholism, in Alcoholism in the Elderly: Social and Biomedical Issues. Edited by Hartford JT, Samorajski T. New York, Raven, 1984, pp 85–115

Willenbring ML: Organic mental disorders associated with heavy drinking and alcohol dependence. Clin Geriatr Med 4:869–887, 1988

Wood WG, Armbrecht HJ, Wise RW: Aging and the effects of ethanol: the role of brain membranes, in Alcoholism in the Elderly: Social and Biomedical Issues. Edited by Hartford JT, Samorajski T. New York, Raven, 1984, pp 139–151

Woodhouse KW, James OFW: Alcoholic liver disease in the elderly: presentation and outcome. Age Ageing 14:113–118, 1985

Woods JH, Katz JL, Winger G: Use and abuse of benzodiazepines: issues relevant to prescribing. JAMA 260:3476–3480, 1988

World Health Organization: Mental, behavioural and developmental disorders: clinical descriptions and diagnostic guidelines, in International Classification of Diseases, 10th Edition (1988 draft). Geneva, World Health Organization, Division of Mental Health, 1988

York JL: Increased responsiveness to ethanol with advancing age in rats. Pharmacol Biochem Behav 19:687–691, 1983

Yudofsky SC, Hales RE (eds): The American Psychiatric Press Textbook of Neuropsychiatry, 2nd Edition. Washington DC, American Psychiatric Press, 1992

16

Sleep Disorders in Late Life: A Biopsychosocial Model for Understanding Pathogenesis and Intervention

Charles F. Reynolds III, M.D.
Mary Amanda Dew, Ph.D.
Timothy H. Monk, Ph.D.
Carolyn C. Hoch, Ph.D.

Introduction

The primary challenge posed by the increasing proportion of elderly people in the United States is to increase active life expectancy and compress morbidity. Otherwise, increase in longevity is likely to be associated primarily with prolongation of dependency (Rosenwaike 1985).

Changes in sleep, sleep quality, and daytime alertness in late life have enormous impact on quality of life, level of functioning, and ability to remain independent (Morin and Gramling 1989; Prinz et al. 1990; Wauquier et al. 1992). Hence, preserving the integrity of sleep for as along as possible is a major public health priority, as emphasized by the National Institutes of Health Consensus Development Conference on Sleep Disorders in Late Life (Consensus Development Conference 1990). Although the 6-month prevalence of severe cognitive impairment usually reported within community populations is 4%–6% (Robins et al. 1984), the prevalence of sleep disturbances was even higher in community-resident elderly (a 12%–15% 6-month rate) in the Epidemiologic Catchment Area (ECA) survey (Ford and Kamerow 1989). Furthermore, the ECA analysis showed that persistent sleep disturbance is a significant risk factor for the subsequent development of major depression, as well as a major factor in decisions to seek services from the primary care sector.

Similarly, in the context of sleep, psychiatric morbidity, and quality of life, a longitudinal study of depressed mood and sleep disturbances in the elderly examined the association between frequency of depressed mood and self-reports of four sleep problems over a 3-year period in a random sample of 198 community residents (mean age 72) (Rodin et al. 1988). The authors found a clear, robust association between frequency of depressed mood (independent variable) and severity of sleep symptoms (dependent variable), after controlling for health status, sex, and age. Longitudinal fluctuation in sleep complaints (particularly sleep continuity disturbance and early morning awakening) covaried strongly with intensity of depressive symptoms.

Taken together, these studies suggest that sleep disturbance is a consequence of depressive symptoms (Rodin et al. 1988), as well as a significant correlate of help-seeking behavior and a major risk factor for the subsequent development of syndromal major depression (Ford and Kamerow 1989). Other studies (Pollak et al. 1990; Rabins et al. 1982; Sanford 1975) have shown that sleep-related behaviors often precipitate the decision of families to institutionalize an elderly relative with dementia. Any understanding of how to attenuate the sleep changes and disturbances of usual and pathological aging that would reduce psychiatric morbidity, burden to families, and the rate of institutionalization, even by a single percentage point, would pay for itself many times over. Therefore, the benefits that would accrue from an understanding of how the successful functioning of the aging circadian timekeeping system can be preserved in the face of medical and psychosocial challenges would have an impact not only on elderly patients themselves, but on society as a whole.

To facilitate understanding of this chapter, a brief glossary of key concepts from normal sleep physiology will be useful. Two operating states of the central nervous system characterize sleep: rapid-eye-movement (REM) sleep and non-REM sleep. The deepest level of non-REM sleep, slow-wave sleep, decreases greatly with age, whereas REM sleep tends to remain more stable. The continuity of sleep also tends to diminish with age, resulting in decreased "sleep efficiency" (the ratio of time spent asleep to total recording period). Sometimes, as noted below, decreased sleep efficiency with age is the result of intrinsic sleep pathologies (e.g., sleep-disordered breathing), whereas at other times it may reflect psychopathological processes such as depression. The latter is also often associated with the early onset of REM sleep (so-called short REM latency). The regular alteration of these operating states constitutes the essential ultradian rhythm of sleep, which in turn occurs within a circadian rhythm of sleep and wakefulness.

A Conceptual Framework for Understanding Challenges to Sleep and Circadian Timekeeping in Late Life

We have formalized a model of the multiple factors that challenge successful circadian timekeeping (in-

Supported in part by AG06836 (to THM and CFR), MH37869 (to CFR and CCH), MH00295 (to CFR), and MH30915 (to CRC: DJ Kupfer, PI).

cluding sleep in elderly individuals). The model is based on the results of our own work, as well as other data in the literature, and is shown in Figure 16–1. The model explicitly shows important predictors of, as well as outcomes resulting from, the development of sleep and circadian function in very late life. Thus changes in health and cognitive status and negative life events (particularly those associated with bereavement) are hypothesized to lead to "decay" in sleep and sleep quality. However, the model posits that much of the effect these changes have is not direct, but is instead mediated by two factors: changes in mood (negative shifts in affect balance) and worsening of sleep-disordered breathing. We also hypothesize that characteristics such as sex, stability of social rhythms, social support, nutrition, and physical fitness serve as important moderators, helping to buffer the subject from the effects of medical burden, negative life events, and their mediators. It is noteworthy that the model explicitly recognizes that sleep changes are also likely to influence subsequent adaptation to aging along physical and psychological dimensions. Thus what appear as major predictors in the model may, over time, ultimately be influenced by the very outcomes that they have helped to produce.

Psychosocial and Medical Burden

Medical burden and increasing physical functional limitations, together with other negative life events and difficulties (e.g., financial strain, family member illnesses, and deaths), represent chronic stressors in the model and are among the vulnerability factors most frequently addressed in previous research on the precursors of psychiatric symptoms and disorders (for a review, see George 1989). The specific chronic stressors that have received the most empirical scrutiny in mixed-age samples are job stress, chronic financial strain, and chronic physical illness, with all three being related to increased risk of psychiatric morbidity (George 1989). Similarly, the primary protective factor examined in previous research is social support, including the dimensions of social network, tangible support, and perceived social support. George (1989) concluded that "high levels of social support are asso-

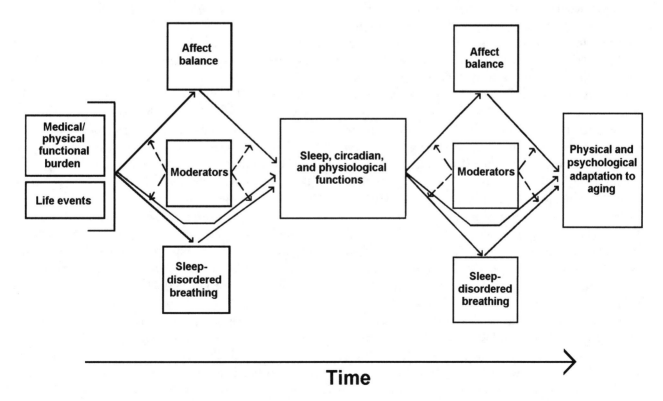

Figure 16–1. Conceptual model of longitudinal relationships of sleep, circadian, and physiological parameters with other key variables. *Solid lines* denote direct effects; *broken lines* denote moderating effects.

ciated with decreased risk of psychiatric morbidity and that perceived support is the dimension most strongly related to mental health outcomes" (p. 215). However, we do not know whether or not support exerts its effects directly on such outcomes or primarily serves to buffer the impact of other stressors (see also Cohen and Wills 1985; George 1989; Kessler and McLeod 1985).

Our own work, as well as that of others (e.g., N. G. Bliwise et al. 1985; Roehrs et al. 1982) provides evidence linking negative affect balance (i.e., depression) and sleep outcomes in late life. Sleep is frequently disturbed among recently bereaved elderly people who have a full depressive syndrome. Sleep efficiency is diminished, REM latency is short, and early slow-wave sleep generation is also reduced, compared with those of nondepressed, recently bereaved subjects and compared with elderly control subjects (Reynolds et al. 1992). These findings are similar to those of Cartwright (1983) in depressed divorcing women. Depressed widows and widowers in our study carried a heavier burden of chronic medical illness than did the control subjects (Reynolds et al. 1992). Similar findings linking stress, depression, and electroencephalographic (EEG) sleep disturbances (including decreased delta sleep and shortened REM latency) were reported by Cartwright and Wood (1991) in a study of middle-aged divorcing spouses. Divorce, like the loss of a spouse through death, can be an occasion for grief. We were able to find one negative report, from Vitiello et al. (1990), who observed that sleep was undisturbed in elderly depressed individuals who have *not* sought health care.

As recently reviewed by D. L. Bliwise (1993), there is now considerable evidence underscoring the general effects (either direct or indirect) of medical illness in the poor sleep of old age (e.g., Ford and Kamerow 1989; Gislason and Almqvist 1987; Morgan et al. 1989). Specific clinical symptoms or disorders have been shown to have negative effects on sleep quality in late life, including nocturia (e.g., Zepelin and Morgan 1981), headache (Cook et al. 1989), gastrointestinal illness (Karacan et al. 1976; Mant and Eyland 1988), bronchitis and asthma (Mant and Eyland 1988), cardiovascular symptoms, and non-insulin-dependent diabetes mellitus (Hyyppa and Kronholm 1989). Chronic pain from conditions like osteoarthritis also disrupts sleep in elderly individuals (Wittig et al. 1982). In addition, elevated autonomic activity (Prinz et al. 1979; Zepelin and McDonald 1987) and a greater susceptibility to external arousal (Roth et al. 1972; Zepelin et al.

1984) may be important predisposing factors to disturbed sleep in very late life.

Neuropsychiatric Burden

In this general context, a study from our group provides evidence linking medical burden and cognitive impairment to sleep. We have reported both increases in sleep-disordered breathing and decreases in sleep continuity and REM sleep in patients with Alzheimer's dementia (Reynolds et al. 1988). These changes appear to be correlated with probability of mortality (Hoch et al. 1989). Similar findings with respect to the loss of REM sleep in Alzheimer's dementia were reported earlier by Prinz et al. (1982) and confirmed by Vitiello et al. (1990). Kripke et al. (1990), Ancoli-Israel et al. (1989), and D. L. Bliwise et al. (1988) have reported high prevalence of sleep apnea with aging and attendant increases in morbidity and mortality. Other data (e.g., He et al. 1988) suggest, however, that sleep-disordered breathing has a stronger relationship to mortality in midlife than in late life.

Burden of Life Events

Life events have received the greatest attention as social risk factors for psychiatric symptoms and disorders, based on two major research strategies: studies of aggregated life events and studies of specific life events (e.g., widowhood). Negative life events are consistently related to increased risk of both psychiatric symptoms and disorders, especially depression, anxiety, and alcohol abuse (Blazer et al. 1987; Brown and Harris 1978). These relationships have been observed in mixed-age samples including older adults.

Findings tend to support the stress buffering hypothesis, which predicts that life events have stronger negative effects on psychiatric outcomes in the absence of adequate social support (Cohen and Wills 1985; Kessler and McLeod 1985). However, as pointed out in George's review (1989), relatively few studies of stress buffering have been based on older samples or have examined other potential buffers. The hypothesized role of social-rhythm stability as a buffer against depression has been suggested in the theoretical context of the social *zeitgebers* hypothesis of depression (Ehlers et al. 1988) and in the empirical context of our EEG sleep studies of bereavement-related, syndromal major depression and subsyndromal depressive symptoms. We have found that depressed widowers and widows are characterized by intermittently lower levels of social rhythm stability, lower volume of social rhythm activity, and lower social support than are nondepressed widows and widowers (Reynolds et al. 1992).

If a stress buffer model of challenges to successful aging is supported by further longitudinal study, then critical points for intervention will have been identified, and the goals for intervention will have been clarified, namely, to maintain stability of positive affect balance, stability of social rhythms, and/or stability of social support and to treat sleep-disordered breathing.

Sleep in Successful Aging

There are now considerable data to support the face validity and clinical utility of conceptualizing sleep, particularly sleep continuity, delta sleep, and REM sleep, as psychobiological markers or correlates of successful aging and adaptation in very late life (Reynolds et al., in press). The concept "successful aging" is borrowed from Rowe and Kahn (1987) and is intended to convey preservation of good mental and physical health, vitality (maintenance of engagement in life), and resilience (ability to bounce back from stressors and setbacks). As elaborated below, successful adaptation in very late life is associated with stable preservation of REM sleep and sleep continuity. Failed adaptation is associated with decrements of sleep continuity and delta sleep and by either a relative increase of REM sleep (e.g., mood disorders) or decrease in REM sleep (e.g., neurodegenerative disorders). The latter, decreased REM sleep generation, has also been shown to be correlated with decreased survival time (Hoch et al. 1989).

In comparing the nocturnal sleep of healthy 80-year-old subjects with that of healthy 60- and 70-year-old subjects (i.e., "old old" versus "young old"), we (Reynolds et al. 1991) have reported stability of sleep efficiency and REM sleep across three decades of late life, but a slight decline of slow-wave sleep in the old old (i.e., decreased total delta wave counts by automated period and amplitude analysis). Women showed better preservation of slow-wave sleep than did men.

In the broader context provided by studies of sleep in pathological aging, we concluded that the stability of REM sleep in successful aging suggests the utility and validity of REM sleep as a marker or correlate of suc-

cessful adaptation in late life (Reynolds et al. 1991). It remains to be shown whether sex-related differences in slow-wave sleep and sleep continuity are stable over time and whether they have significance with respect to subsequent health status and longevity.

Preservation of physical and mental health into late old age is associated with a level of daytime sleepiness no greater than, and perhaps even less than, that seen in young adults (Reynolds et al. 1991). This finding provides additional support for the concept that sleep measures provide a useful psychobiological correlate of successful aging and adaptation in late life.

In our investigation of sleep, mood, and performance responses to acute sleep deprivation in healthy 80- and 20-year-old subjects, we found that sleep continuity and delta sleep were enhanced in both groups on the first recovery night, indicating that sleep changes in very old subjects are at least partially reversible by this procedure. Surprisingly, mood and performance were disturbed by sleep loss to a significantly greater extent among the young subjects, suggesting that acute total sleep loss is a more disruptive procedure for the young than for the elderly who are aging successfully (Brendel et al. 1990). In contrast to healthy elderly patients, older patients with major depression and with probable Alzheimer's dementia show less of the expected physiological hallmarks of recovery sleep after a night of total sleep deprivation (slow-wave sleep rebound and REM sleep rebound), attesting to diminished physiological resilience and plasticity (Reynolds et al. 1987). The reversibility of age-dependent sleep changes needs to be further addressed by identifying factors that support or enhance successful aging.

In a study of the prevalence of sleep-disordered breathing in healthy 80-year-old subjects versus that in healthy 70- and 60-year-old subjects, sleep-disordered breathing increased significantly with advancing age even in the healthy subjects and was more marked in healthy men than in healthy women (Hoch et al. 1990). The clinical correlates of this finding, particularly the increasing medical burden, need to be investigated further.

Although healthy 80-year-old subjects reported worse subjective sleep quality on average than did healthy young adult subjects, and these differences reflect age-related differences in polysomnographic sleep measures, we found that most (68.1%) healthy old-old subjects had sleep quality scores in the range of good sleepers, based on a categorical classification (Buysse et al. 1991). In the proposed model of longitudinal challenges to healthy aging, we expect to see "decay" in sleep quality with increasing medical burden and negative life events, an effect mediated in part by alterations in mood and increases in sleep-disordered breathing, but moderated by stability of social rhythms and social support.

Sleep in Usual Aging: The Impact of Spousal Bereavement on Sleep in Late Life

Given the theoretical interest of negative life events and their potential to disrupt sleep via changes in mood, we reported an investigation of EEG sleep measures in elderly, recently bereaved volunteers stratified by the presence or absence of syndromal major depression (Reynolds et al. 1992). As hypothesized, depressed bereaved subjects had significantly lower sleep efficiency and worse sleep quality, more early-morning awakening, shorter REM latency, greater REM percent, and lower rates of delta wave generation in the first non-REM sleep period (i.e., lower delta sleep ratio) compared with nondepressed, bereaved volunteers. Sleep in the latter group was similar to that of healthy control subjects.

The relevance of these data to the proposed model of challenges to successful aging is that depression (or depressive symptoms) may be an important mediating variable that links negative life events with sleep-circadian outcomes, as well as with changes in perceived sleep quality. With respect to the role of hypothesized moderators (i.e., social support and stability of social rhythms), our data suggested greater stability of psychosocial rhythms and higher levels of perceived social support among nondepressed widows and widowers compared with their depressed counterparts. Testing of the proposed model would help elucidate antecedent-consequent relationships.

Similarly, we have recently investigated the role of psychosocial factors in buffering the impact of major life events on depressive symptoms in our sample of elderly widows and widowers (Prigerson et al. 1993). Our results suggested the importance of subjects' sense of mastery—their feeling of competence in the face of stress—as a predictor of mood response following life stressors. Similar findings have been reported elsewhere in nonelderly samples (e.g., Dew et al. 1990), further supporting the selection of mastery as a potential buffer against the onset of disturbed mood and sleep.

Sleep in Pathological Aging

Given the theoretical interest in the impact of medical burden and cognitive impairment on sleep, we have published the observation that Alzheimer's disease (in contrast to major depression) is associated with deficits in the production of phasic activity during sleep (including REMs, spindles, and K-complexes) and with increased rates of sleep-disordered breathing (Reynolds et al. 1988).

The relevance of this observation to the current model (and to its prediction that sleep outcomes influence subsequent adaptation) is that EEG sleep measures predicted survival status at 2 years in patients with mixed clinical presentations of depression and cognitive impairment (Hoch et al. 1989), with nonsurvivors showing impaired capacity to generate REM sleep and to maintain respiratory control during sleep.

For a comprehensive review of sleep in Alzheimer's dementia and other dementing illnesses, the reader is referred to D. L. Bliwise (in press). Among the major observations and hypotheses in the Bliwise review of sleep in dementing disorders are the following: 1) more is known about sleep physiological changes in Alzheimer's dementia than in other types of dementia, such as those related to Parkinson's disease, Huntington's disease, or progressive supranuclear palsy; 2) impaired respiration during sleep may be more strongly related to multi-infarct dementia than to other forms of dementia; 3) persistence of waking movement disorders of Parkinson's disease into sleep could have a disruptive effect on the sleep of such patients, as does the presence of superimposed depression, whereas adequate treatment of the illness may be associated with improvement in sleep efficiency; 4) increased spindle density is characteristic of Huntington's disease (possibly reflecting dysfunction within corpus striatum), but also diminished sleep efficiency and reduced slow wave sleep (correlating with caudate atrophy), and reduced REMs; and 5) severe diminution of REM sleep is seen in progressive supranuclear palsy (possibly correlating with degenerative changes in pontine tegmentum).

Neurocircuitry and Neurotransmitters in Sleep

Several neurotransmitter systems have been extensively studied in sleep, including serotonin, dopamine, acetylcholine, and noradrenergic systems. (For a systematic review, see Meltzer 1987—particularly the chapters by Jacobs, Bartus, Meltzer, and Janowsky.) Although the data in this area are not easily summarized, two particular observations appear to have relevance to the model proposed in this chapter. First, as reviewed by Meltzer and Lewy (see Meltzer 1987), "decreased serotonergic activity is consistent with many of the changes in mood and somatic function observed in depressed patients, e.g., depressed mood, insomnia, decreased REM latency [and] disturbed circadian rhythms" (p. 515). Second, as reviewed by Janowsky and Risch (see Meltzer 1987), "cholinergic agonists generally cause a shortening of REM latency and an increase in REM density [particularly] in patients with an affective disorder episode or a family history of affective disorder" (p. 529). These observations have led to the hypothesis that sleep changes in depression may reflect neurotransmitter abnormalities, particularly an increased ratio of cholinergic-to-aminergic neurotransmission. Conversely, the decreased capacity for REM sleep generation in Alzheimer's dementia may reflect impairment, loss, and underactivity in cholinergic systems.

Principles of Therapeutic Intervention

We believe that it is important to consider disturbed sleep in late life as symptomatic of underlying causes, with typically more than one factor operating in combination, and that therapy should address causes and related mediating factors (e.g., depression, as proposed in the model described above). Promising avenues of nonpharmacological intervention for persistent insomnia in late life usually address behaviors with a negative effect on sleep (e.g., sleep restriction approaches limit time in bed to enhance sleep efficiency and depth) or help to realign sleep and circadian rhythms with external time cues (e.g., via the use of bright-light exposure). Useful pharmacological approaches tend to be simple, for example, monotherapy of depression, which uses a single medication and avoids the premature use of adjunctive sleeping pills. Further research is strongly needed to address the utility of maintenance medication, such as, low-dose antidepressants or intermittent benzodiazepines, for persistent, idiopathic ("primary") insomnia in late life.

Summary

Successful aging is associated with preservation of sleep quality, ability to maintain daytime alertness, and physiological integrity of nocturnal EEG sleep (Reynolds et al., in press). Failure to adapt is associated with loss of sleep continuity and alterations in the temporal distribution of delta wave activity and by either a relative increase of REM sleep (mood disorders) or a relative decrease in REM sleep (neurodegenerative disorders). The increase in REM sleep that accompanies depression is also correlated with an attendant decrease in positive affect balance and diminished stability of social rhythms. By contrast, diminished capacity for REM sleep generation accompanies neurodegenerative disorders and is a correlate not only of cognitive impairment, but also of early mortality.

Taken together, these findings provide the empirical basis for the model of longitudinal challenges to sleep and circadian timekeeping in late life. The model attempts to account for data at different points along the continuum of aging, from successful, to usual, to pathological aging. Further longitudinal investigations are required to model the hypothesized interrelationships among sleep, aging, and medical and psychosocial variables.

References

Ancoli-Israel S, Klauber MR, Kripke DF, et al: Sleep apnea in female nursing home patients: increased risk of mortality. Chest 96:1054–58, 1989

Blazer DG, Hughes D, George LK: Stressful life events and the onset of a generalized anxiety syndrome. Am J Psychiatry 144:1178–1183, 1987

Bliwise DL: Sleep in normal aging and dementia. Sleep 16:40–81, 1993

Bliwise DL: Sleep in dementing illness, in American Psychiatric Press Review of Psychiatry, Vol 13. Edited by Oldham JM, Riba MB. Washington, DC, American Psychiatric Press (in press)

Bliwise DL, Bliwise NG, Partinen M, et al: Sleep apnea and mortality in an aged cohort. Am J Public Health 78:544–547, 1988

Bliwise NG, Bliwise DL, Dement WC: Age and psychopathology in insomnia. Clinics in Gerontology 4:3–9, 1985

Brendel DH, Reynolds CF, Jennings JR, et al: Sleep-stage physiology, mood, and vigilance responses to total sleep deprivation in healthy eighty year olds and twenty year olds. Psychophysiology 27:677–686, 1990

Brown GW, Harris T: Social Origins of Depression: A Study of Psychiatric Disorder in Women. London, Tavistock, 1978

Buysse DJ, Reynolds CF, Monk TH, et al: Quantification of subjective sleep quality in healthy elderly men and women using the Pittsburgh Sleep Quality Index. Sleep 14:331–338, 1991

Cartwright RD: REM sleep during and after mood-disturbing events. Arch Gen Psychiatry 40:197–201, 1983

Cartwright RD, Wood E: Adjustment disorders of sleep: the sleep effects of a major stressful event and its resolution. Psychiatry Res 39:199–209, 1991

Cohen S, Wills TA: Stress, social support, and the buffering hypothesis. Psychol Bull 98:310–357, 1985

Consensus Development Conference: Diagnosis and Treatment of Sleep Disorders in Late Life. Bethesda, MD, National Institutes of Health, 1990

Cook NR, Evans DA, Funkenstein H, et al: Correlates of headache in a population based cohort of elderly. Arch Neurol 46:1338–1344, 1989

Dew MA, Ragni MV, Nimorwicz P: Infection with human immunodeficiency virus and vulnerability to psychiatric distress. Arch Gen Psychiatry 47:737–744, 1990

Ehlers CL, Frank E, Kupfer DJ: Social zeitgebers and biological rhythms: a unified approach to understanding the etiology of depression. Arch Gen Psychiatry 45:948–952, 1988

Ford DE, Kamerow DB: Epidemiologic study of sleep disturbances and psychiatric disorders: an opportunity for prevention? JAMA 262:1479–1488, 1989

George LK: Social and economic factors, in Geriatric Psychiatry. Edited by Busse E, Blazer DG. Washington, DC, American Psychiatric Press, 1989, pp 203–234

Gislason T, Almqvist M: Somatic diseases and sleep complaints. Acta Medica Scandinavica 221:475–481, 1987

He J, Kryger MH, Zorick FJ, et al: Mortality and apnea index in obstructive sleep apnea: experience in 385 male patients. Chest 94:1–14, 1988

Hoch CC, Reynolds CF, Houck PR, et al: Predicting mortality in mixed depression and dementia using EEG sleep variables. J Neuropsychiatry Clin Neurosci 1:366–371, 1989

Hoch CC, Reynolds CF, Monk TH, et al: Comparison of sleep-disordered breathing among healthy elderly in the seventh, eighth, and ninth decades of life. Sleep 13:502–511, 1990

Hyyppa MT, Kronholm E: Quality of sleep and chronic illnesses. J Clin Epidemiol 42:633–638, 1989

Karacan I, Thornby JI, Anch M, et al: Prevalence of sleep disturbance in a primarily urban Florida county. Soc Sci Med 10:239–244, 1976

Kessler RC, McLeod JC: Social support and mental health in community samples, in Social Support and Health. Edited by Cohen S, Syme SL. New York, Academic Press, 1985, pp 219–240

Kripke DF, Ancoli-Israel S, Mason WJ, et al: Sleep apnea: association with deviant sleep durations and increased mortality, in Sleep Apnea Syndrome: Clinical Research and Treatment. Edited by Guilleminault C, Partinen M. New York, Raven, 1990, pp 9–14

Mant A, Eyland EA: Sleep patterns and problems in elderly general practice attenders: an Australian survey. Community Health Studies 12:192–199, 1988

Meltzer HY (ed): Psychopharmacology: The Third Generation of Progress. New York, Raven, 1987

Morgan K, Healey DW, Healey PJ: Factors influencing persistent subjective insomnia in old age: a follow-up study of good and poor sleepers aged 65–74. Age Aging 18:117–122, 1989

Morin C, Gramling S: Sleep patterns and aging: comparison of older adults with and without insomnia complaints. Psychol Aging 4:290–294, 1989

Pollak CP, Perlick D, Linsner JP, et al: Sleep problems in the community elderly as predictors of death and nursing home placement. Community Health 15:123–135, 1990

Prigerson HG, Frank E, Reynolds CF, et al: Protective psychosocial factors in depression among spousally bereaved elders. American Journal of Geriatr Psychiatry 1:296–309, 1993

Prinz PN, Halter J, Benedetti C, et al: Circadian variation of plasma catecholamines in young and old men: relation to rapid eye movements and slow wave sleep. J Clin Endocrinol Metab 49:300–304, 1979

Prinz PN, Peskind ER, Vitaliano PR, et al: Changes in the sleep and waking EEG's of nondemented and demented elderly subjects. J Am Geriatr Soc 30:86–93, 1982

Prinz PN, Vitiello MV, Raskind MA, et al: Geriatrics: sleep disorders and aging. N Engl J Med 323:520–526, 1990

Rabins PV, Mace NL, Lucas MJ: The impact of dementia on the family. JAMA 248:333–335, 1982

Reynolds CF, Kupfer DJ, Hoch CC, et al: Sleep deprivation as a probe in the elderly. Arch Gen Psychiatry 44:982–990, 1987

Reynolds CF, Kupfer DJ, Houck PR, et al: Reliable discrimination of elderly depressed and demented patients by EEG sleep data. Arch Gen Psychiatry 45:258–264, 1988

Reynolds CF, Monk TH, Hoch CC, et al: EEG sleep in the healthy "old old": a comparison with the "young old" in visually scored and automated (period) measures. J Gerontol (Med Sci) 46:M39–46, 1991

Reynolds CF, Hoch CC, Buysse DJ, et al: EEG sleep in spousal bereavement and bereavement-related depression of late life. Biol Psychiatry 31:69–82, 1992

Reynolds CF, Hoch CC, Buysse DJ, et al: REM sleep in successful, usual, and pathological aging: the Pittsburgh experience 1980–1991. Journal of Sleep Research (in press)

Robins LN, Helzer JE, Weissman MM, et al: Lifetime prevalence of specific psychiatric disorders in three sites. Arch Gen Psychiatry 41:949–958, 1984

Rodin J, McAvay G, Timko C: Depressed mood and sleep disturbances in the elderly: a longitudinal study. J Gerontol 43:45–52, 1988

Roehrs T, Lineback W, Zorick F, et al: Relationship of psychopathology to insomnia in the elderly. J Am Geriatr Soc 30:312–315, 1982

Rosenwaike I: A demographic portrait of the oldest old. Millbank Memorial Fund Quarterly 63:187–205, 1985

Roth T, Kramer M, Trinder J: The effect of noise during sleep on the sleep patterns of different age groups. Canadian Psychiatric Association Journal 1(17):ss197–ss201, 1972

Rowe JW, Kahn RL: Human aging: usual and successful. Science 237:143–149, 1987

Sanford JRA: Tolerance of debility in elderly dependents by supports at home: significance for hospital practice. BMJ 3:471–473, 1975

Vitiello MV, Prinz PN, Avery DH, et al: Sleep is undisturbed in elderly, depressed individuals who have not sought health care. Biol Psychiatry 27:431–440, 1990

Wauquier A, van Sweden B, Lagaay AM, et al: Ambulatory monitoring of sleep-wakefulness in healthy elderly males and females (greater than 88 years): the "senieur" protocol. J Am Geriatr Soc 40:109–114, 1992

Wittig RM, Zorick FJ, Blumer D, et al: Disturbed sleep in patients complaining of chronic pain. J Nerv Ment Dis 170:424–431, 1982

Zepelin H, McDonald CS: Age differences in autonomic variables during sleep. J Gerontol 42:142–146, 1987

Zepelin H, Morgan LE: Correlates of sleep disturbance in retirees (abstract). Sleep Research 10:120, 1981

Zepelin H, McDonald CS, Zammit GK: Effects of age on auditory awakening thresholds. J Gerontol 39:294–300, 1984

17

Pain

James M. Schuster, M.D., M.B.A.
Kenneth L. Goetz, M.D.

Introduction

Pain occurs frequently among geriatric patients (Lavsky-Shulan et al. 1985). Low-back pain is found in approximately 20% of the elderly population, and 300,000 Americans over age 65 have limitations from back or spine problems. Geriatric patients may have both medical problems and psychiatric illnesses that present with pain (Harkins and Warner 1980).

It is often difficult to evaluate pain in elderly patients, who may have multiple medical problems with several resulting painful conditions (Ouslander 1981). Serious medical conditions in older patients may present with nonspecific symptoms. Depression and dementia, which are relatively common among the geriatric population, are associated with physical complaints.

In this chapter, we review the physiology and assessment of pain problems among elderly patients. We also discuss the distinctions between acute and chronic benign pain and the interactions between common psychiatric illnesses and pain problems. We conclude with a review of the role of psychotropic medications, psychotherapies, and other modalities used in the treatment of pain.

Anatomy and Pathophysiology

Ascending Pain Pathways

Pain receptors, or nociceptors, consist of free nerve endings of myelinated A-delta or largely unmyelinated C-fibers located in skin, viscera, and other body tissues. These receptors are activated by mechanical, thermal, or chemical noxious stimuli and have their cell bodies located in the dorsal root ganglia. The cell axons synapse in the dorsal horn, particularly in laminae I, II (substantia gelatinosa), and V. The dorsal horn performs a high degree of sensory processing and modulation of these afferent signals, which, through a series of interneurons, project into the spinothalamic, spinoreticular, and spinomesencephalic tracts, which then transmit the nociceptive information to the brain (Figure 17–1). The lateral portion of the spinothalamic tract (neospinothalamic tract) synapses with neurons in the ventral posterolateral thalamic nucleus, which projects to the somatosensory cortex (Pasternak 1988). This tract consists of large, rapid conduction fibers that are probably used for locating painful im-

pulses in the body. The medial portion (paleospinothalamic tract) connects extensively with the brain stem reticular formation, hypothalamus, medial, intralaminar, and posterior thalamic nuclei, as well as with limbic forebrain and other subcortical structures (Hendler 1982). The medial portion is less somatotopically organized, slower in conduction, and carries a more poorly localized pain sensation than the lateral

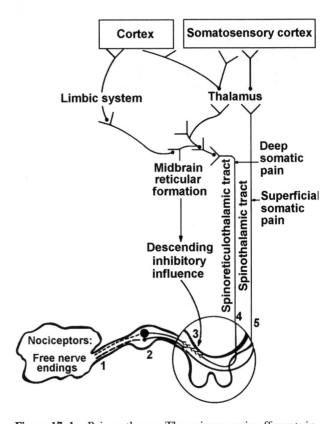

Figure 17–1. Pain pathways. The primary pain afferents in the peripheral nerve (*1*) are dendrites whose cell bodies are in the dorsal root ganglion (*2*). Their axons enter the dorsal horn of the spinal cord and synapse in the substantia gelatinosa (*3*). Deep somatic pain perception requires activation of multiple interneurons in the spinal cord before ascending in the spinoreticulothalamic tract (*4*), whereas superficial somatic pain promptly traverses the spinal cord to the spinothalamic tract (*5*), thalamus, and somatosensory cortex. The deep pain pathways project to the midbrain reticular formation, and then they diffuse through the limbic system and thalamus to the cortex and somatosensory cortex. These pathways allow for the fast specific quality of superficial somatic pain and the diffuse emotional quality of deep somatic pain. The projection to the midbrain reticular formation connects deep somatic pain perception to the endogenous pain control system.
Source. Reprinted from Newton PA: "Chronic Pain," in *Geriatric Medicine.* Edited by Cassel CK, Walsh JR. New York, Springer-Verlag, 1984, p. 237. Used with permission.

tract. This pathway is implicated in mechanisms of chronic pain and may mediate the patient's behavioral responses to pain.

Descending Pathways and the Endogenous Pain Control System

It is clear that the central nervous system can modulate perception of and response to pain. Understanding of the endogenous pain control mechanism developed from two areas of study (see review by Basbaum and Fields 1978). The first was the demonstration of profound analgesia from electrical stimulation of a number of areas of the brain, termed *stimulation-produced analgesia* (SPA) (Mayer and Liebeskind 1974). The areas of the brain implicated include the medial brain stem structures and, in particular, the periaqueductal gray area. Second was the identification of the endogenous opiates, particularly the enkephalins (Pasternak et. al. 1975), as well as the endorphins (Cox et al. 1976). These peptides and the corresponding opiate receptors are found in high concentration in the reticular formation and the periaqueductal gray (Pert et al. 1976). The injection of exogenous opiates in the periaqueductal gray also results in profound analgesia (Pert and Yaksh 1974) suggesting that both SPA and opiate-mediated analgesia operate via similar mechanisms. Both types of analgesia can be blocked by naloxone administration (Adams 1976).

These results led to the hypothesis that opiates moderate analgesia through activation of a descending pain suppression system originating in the brain stem (Basbaum and Fields 1978). Other research indicates that this system originates in the nucleus raphe magnus (NRM) in the medulla and descends through the dorsal lateral funiculus, terminating in the cells of origin of the spinothalamic tract in the dorsal horn of the spinal cord. It presumably has an inhibitory effect on ascending pathways (Basbaum and Fields 1978). The NRM receives rich innervation from the periaqueductal gray and reticular formation; the latter is itself a receiving area for ascending pain pathways. This descending pathway uses the neurotransmitter serotonin, which is strongly implicated in a variety of areas of pain modulation at both spinal and supraspinal levels.

Opiate-induced analgesia and SPA can be abolished using serotonin blockers (Yaksh et al. 1976). Conversely, administration of serotonin precursors potentiates analgesia (Sewel and Spencer 1974). As discussed below, this hypothesis may also explain the efficacy of tricyclic antidepressants and other serotonin-enhancing agents in relieving chronic pain. Furthermore, naloxone completely reverses SPA in the NRM, implicating endorphins as the ultimate mediator of the system (Basbaum and Fields 1978). Additionally, systemically administered opiates appear to act primarily in this descending system, though both endogenous and exogenous opiates probably have some action at the spinal cord level.

In summary, noxious stimuli activate the ascending pain transmission system. This opiate-mediated system stimulates the descending pathways in the periaqueductal gray and reticular formation. The periaqueductal gray receives inputs from multiple brain areas allowing for complex control of pain sensation by various higher cortical areas. These pathways result in stimulation of the serotonergic descending system originating in the NRM. Ultimate inhibition in the dorsal horns probably occurs in the substantia gelatinosa with transmission of substance P between interneurons.

The Gate Theory

The gate theory of pain medication was first proposed by Melzack and Wall (1965) and may represent an alternative means of pain modulation. The theory suggests that proprioceptive fibers inhibit transmission of noxious stimuli in the spinal cord through an intraneuronal "gate" located in the substantia gelatinosa in the dorsal horn. Stimulation of proprioceptive fibers excites these interneurons, which subsequently close the "gate" and inhibit transmission of pain impulses. This model led to a number of therapeutic modalities such as dorsal column stimulation and transcutaneous electrical nerve stimulation (TENS).

This theory has been questioned by research, which has failed to show that either the proprioceptive fibers or the substantia gelatinosa neurons have the physiological properties predicted by the gate theory. In addition, both TENS and dorsal column stimulation have very limited effects, which also suggests that the gate theory may be an overly simplistic model of pain control.

Neurotransmitters

Neurotransmitters other than serotonin have also been implicated in the endogenous pain control system. However, their mechanism of action has not been as well delineated. Dopamine receptor blockade reduces SPA, whereas receptor stimulation potentiates this analgesia (Akil and Liebeskind 1975). Depletion of norepinephrine also potentiates SPA (Akil and Liebeskind 1975). Similar roles for these catecholamines have been implicated through studies of morphine or other opiate-induced analgesia (Mayer and Price 1976). γ-Aminobutyric acid (GABA) and acetylcholine have also been shown to inhibit pain transmission (Willcockson et al. 1984). This work, coupled with our understanding of the descending serotonergic system, may have important implications for the future pharmacotherapy of pain.

Perception and Prevalence of Pain in Elderly Patients

Psychosocial stressors such as bereavement, social isolation, loss of mobility, and increasing dependence on others are common in elderly patients. These difficulties may limit a patient's ability to cope with a new stress such as a painful medical condition. In addition, pain complaints and pain behaviors may provide a means for the patient to obtain care and attention. However, older patients appear to report less pain because of either stoicism or a belief that the pain is a normal result of aging. Whether cognitive deficits add to this underreporting is unclear, as dementia may also decrease the ability to cope with pain. The experience of pain is influenced by a number of factors that go far beyond the noxious stimulus itself.

Biochemical changes in the elderly may affect pain transmissions, though clear differences between age groups have been difficult to candidate. Aging has been associated with increases in monoamine oxidase and subsequent decreases in monoamine neurotransmitter levels (Robinson et al. 1972). Decreases in serotonin may directly affect the pain pathways discussed above. Endorphin levels may decline with age (Moricca and Arcuri 1980), possibly decreasing pain tolerance. At the cellular level, response to inflammation may alter during the aging process and nerve cells themselves may undergo degenerative processes. Whether changes also occur in peripheral nerve conduction or in spinal cord mechanisms in aging patients is still unclear. Studies have evaluated pain threshold and tolerance directly, using various nociceptive stimuli in laboratory settings, and strongly suggest that pain perception among age groups tends to be more similar

than different (Harkins 1988; Harkins and Chapman 1976; 1977; Harkins et al. 1986; Sherman and Robillard 1964). Clinical studies have also found only small and inconsistent differences between age groups, making it difficult to form conclusions about how pain perception changes with age. (Cartwright et al. 1973; Davis et al. 1990; MacDonald et al. 1983; Moss et al. 1991; Sorkin et al. 1990).

Drug usage studies have found analgesic use to decline with age (Faherty and Grier 1984; Portenoy and Kanner 1985). In addition, elderly patients have been shown to obtain significantly more pain relief from fixed narcotic dosages than younger patients (Bellville 1971). Whether these findings represent simple pharmacokinetic differences in elderly patients or prescription biases among physicians is unclear. In Bellville's study (1971), however, no differences in side effects, including sedation, were found between age groups, suggesting that alteration in absorption or distribution may not explain these age-related differences. Clearly, more research in the area of pain perception in the elderly population is needed. However, there is little evidence to support a large difference in pain perception or experience between geriatric patients and younger populations.

Though pain perception or response to treatment may not change with age, the prevalence of pain may be quite high in the geriatric population because of the increased prevalence of medical illnesses commonly associated with pain. These include degenerative disorders, such as rheumatoid and osteoarthritis, as well as neuropathies often associated with chronic medical conditions, such as diabetes. Vascular problems including intermittent claudication and vasculitis occur frequently as do radiculopathies and cervical spondylosis. Other problems such as postherpetic neuralgia and trigeminal neuralgia are almost exclusively found in the elderly population. Pain complicating neoplastic processes would also be expected to occur more often in geriatric patients given that the prevalence of most tumors increases with age. Fractures, particularly of the hip and spine, are also more common in the elderly (Harkins 1988).

The expected high prevalence of pain complaints in the geriatric population, especially chronic degenerative pain, has been confirmed (Crook et al. 1984). Complaints regarding rheumatoid and osteoarthritis dramatically increase with age, whereas headache and backache complaints tend to peak in middle age and then decline (Harkins 1988).

Studies of nursing home populations also suggest that pain problems in geriatric patients are frequent, with prevalence reported between 71% (Ferrell et al. 1990) and 83% (Roy and Thomas 1986). Moss et al. (1991) found 37% of geriatric patients in their last year of life reported pain frequently or all of the time. This prevalence increased to 66% 1 month prior to death.

Psychosocial Factors

Several psychosocial issues affect patients' pain problems. They may include a history of personal deprivation, whether or not the patient is receiving compensation or disability, family responses to the patient, and the patient's own beliefs about his or her coping abilities. Though the impact of these issues varies from one patient to another, assessment of them is important in the formulation of the patient's pain problem.

Many authors believe that patients with chronic, benign pain have often had childhoods in which they were deprived emotionally or physically and that the chronic pain problem is an unconscious attempt to receive special care. Engel (1959) has described psychodynamic and other psychological explanations for "pain prone patients." Others (Adler et al. 1989) have written that such patients have a relatively high incidence of disturbed interpersonal relationships, verbally or physically abusive parents (Reiter et al. 1991), or parents who suffered from illnesses or pain. However, other studies (Tauschke et al. 1991) have found that pain patients have less evidence of poor care in childhood than do other psychiatric patients.

Psychological test results of patients with documented organic pain have significant overlap with those of patients without organic pain, and these distinctions alone cannot be used to differentiate patients (Wade et al. 1992), especially as many patients initially thought to have "nonorganic pain" are eventually diagnosed as having physical disease (Trief et al. 1987). Minnesota Multiphasic Personality Inventory (MMPI) findings (Leavitt 1990) do not clearly distinguish patients with organic pain from those with functional pain. The most common finding is MMPI elevations on the hysteria, depression, and hypochondriasis scales (Chaney 1984; Gamsa and Vikis-Freiberg 1991; Thorvaldsen and Sorenson 1990; Valdes 1989; Wood et al. 1990). Swanson (1984) has posited that chronic pain is an "emotion" and that it is an expression of internal distress like anxiety and depression. Patients' self-confidence may be more important than their particular personality style (M. P. Jensen et al. 1991).

Many patients with chronic pain are on compensation or disability because of their condition. As many as 49% of patients in pain clinics may receive disability benefits (Mendelson 1992). The impact of work-related disability and compensation on pain problems is unclear (Brena and Chapman 1989; Jamison et al. 1988; Leavitt 1990; Mendelson 1986; Weintraub 1992). Psychogenic pain appears frequently among pain patients engaged in litigation (Weintraub 1992). The impact of compensation and disability litigation may be less significant in elderly patients, as many of these patients are no longer employed.

Interactions between patients and their families may also influence how patients cope with pain. Pain patients may present with illness behavior that allows them to avoid responsibilities and increase their use of resources typically provided for those who are ill (Dworkin 1991). Family members can sometimes decrease patients' disabilities by reinforcing "healthy" behaviors and "rewarding" the patient for increased activity. However, the contribution of the family to pain problems remains unclear (Adelman and Shank 1988).

Psychiatric Disorders and Pain

Psychiatric disorders are frequently found among patients with chronic pain. At the same time, pain is a common complaint among psychiatric patients. Clinicians are often asked to determine whether or not patients have a chronic, benign pain problem; a psychiatric disorder; or both. In this section we discuss the relationships between psychiatric disorders and acute and chronic pain.

Mood Disorders

There is a strong relationship between depression and pain, especially chronic pain. Incidence of depression in patients with chronic pain has been reported to be as high as 87% (Lindsay and Wyckoff 1981). Chronic pain occurs frequently in psychiatric patients, including those who present with depressive, anxiety, and somatoform disorders (Chaturvedi and Michael 1986). Studies of depression in pain patients have been criticized because the patients evaluated are often ones who present to chronic pain clinics and have significant disability from their pain.

However, although depression is more common in pain patients who present to a psychiatric clinic than in those who present to other settings, the rates of somatic complaints and anxiety are about the same in all settings (Merskey et al. 1987). Keefe found that depression is also an important predictor of pain behavior in patients presenting for neurosurgical evaluation. A number of theories have been proposed to explain the relationship between depression and pain. Blumer (see Blumer and Heilbronn 1982) has written that chronic pain is a masked depressive state with characteristic premorbid traits, psychodynamic features, genetic history, and response to specific psychodynamic approaches. Depressive symptoms often predate the chronic pain, and the primary psychodynamic issues include a need to be cared for, an inability to verbalize feelings, and a high level of premorbid energy followed by depressive anergia after the onset of the pain. Others (e.g., Krishnan 1985) concur that the occurrence of pain with depression may suggest a genetic vulnerability to depression. There is not a high rate of depression among relatives of nondepressed pain patients (France et al. 1986).

Others (e.g., Rudy et al. 1988) have proposed a cognitive behavioral model to explain the relatively high rate of depression among patients with chronic pain. For example, pain patients who are unsatisfied with their lives and who have low feelings of self-control are more likely to become depressed than are other pain patients. These factors may account for over 68% of the variance in depressed mood.

Depression and pain may also share similar neurotransmitter deficits. Ward et al. (1982) found that depression, anxiety, and urinary 3-methoxy-4-hydroxyphenylglycol (MHPG) all correlate significantly with severity of pain in patients with both pain and depression. Serotonin, norepinephrine, and other biogenic amines may modulate paleospinothalamic tract transmissions and the endogenous pain control system, as well as patients' mood, and therefore alterations in levels of these biogenic amines may lead to both pain and depression.

It may be difficult to view all patients with chronic pain as having "masked depression" and chronic pain as a depressive equivalent (Magni 1987). However, a relatively high percentage of patients with pain have a family history of depression and depressive spectrum disorders. In addition, some of these patients have biological markers, such as abnormal thyrotropin-releasing hormone stimulation tests, decreased rapid-eye-movement latency, and decreased platelet density of tritiated imipramine-binding sites, which are commonly found in patients with major depressive episodes. The results of these studies are equivocal, and many patients with chronic pain do not have depressive symptoms. In fact, endogenous depressive symptoms are unusual in patients with chronic pain (Davidson et al. 1985), even among those with major depressive disorder. Pain is more often associated with atypical depressive symptoms including hyperphagia, weight gain, and rejection hypersensitivity.

Dysthymia and anxiety are the most common psychiatric diagnoses in elderly pain patients. Geriatric patients with dysthymia and atypical depression report pain more frequently than do nondepressed elderly (Magni et al. 1985). Many studies (e.g., Chaturvedi 1987) suggest that patients with pain and depression are more often older and employed than are nondepressed pain patients, though these findings are not uniform (Haythornwaite et al. 1991).

Anxiety Disorders

Anxiety is a common finding in patients with acute and chronic pain. However, the relationship between anxiety and pain is unclear. In some patients, anxiety may exacerbate pain, whereas in others it may serve as a distraction from pain. Postoperative acute pain may be related to underlying preoperative anxiety, anxiety at discharge, and the length of hospital stay (Boeke et al. 1991). In addition, extended hospital stays themselves may contribute to a patient's anxiety.

Patients with chronic back pain have significant elevations in anxiety measured using the State-Trait Personality Inventory (Kinder et al. 1986). Elevation in anxiety appears to correspond with elevations in the hysteria, depression, and hypochondriasis scales on the MMPI. Though anxiety is associated with acute pain, studies have suggested that anxiety decreases some patients' pain sensitivity. Attention to a pain stimulus may increase reported pain (Arntz et al. 1991), whereas anxiety about other issues decreases it (Al Absi and Rokke 1991).

High rates of anxiety occur in patients who present with acute chest or pelvic pain (Grandi et al. 1988; Slocumb et al. 1989). Reviews of patients presenting to an emergency room with atypical chest pain found that about one-third of these patients have panic disorder, whereas about one-fourth have major depression. Patients with chest pain (Beitman and Kushner 1991) and normal or near normal cardiac catheterizations also have about a 33% rate of panic disorder. These rates contrast with the rate of panic disorder of 1%–5% found in general primary care populations. A self-report anxiety rating scale accurately identifies many patients who have chest pain due to panic disorder (Kushner et al. 1989). Patients with organic coronary artery lesions may have panic disorder, but the rate appears to be much lower, about 6%. Panic disorder has been shown to cause electrocardiographically significant changes, whereas panic episodes can also be triggered by chest pain (Katon 1990).

Many elderly patients with atypical chest pain may have new onset of a panic disorder (Beitman et al. 1991). Panic disorder can begin in later life and should be part of the differential diagnosis of atypical pain presentations. Patients with late-onset panic disorder are more likely to have other anxiety symptoms, as well as depression. However, some of the symptoms in the elderly that resemble panic disorder may be caused by medications or other medical problems.

Although there is a correlation between acute chest pain and panic disorder, it is not clear that panic disorder increases other types of pain. One study (Roy-Byrne et al. 1985) found no distinction in pain sensitivity between patients with panic disorder and a control group. There also appeared to be no relationship between frequency of panic attacks and pain, even though patients with panic disorder appeared to be more sensitive to a number of other stimuli.

Somatoform Disorders

Any somatoform disorder can present with pain, including conversion disorder, hypochondriasis, and somatization disorder. However, pain is usually not the only, or even the most prominent symptom of these disorders. The exception is somatoform pain disorder. This disorder is characterized by the presence of prolonged, disabling pain. Although some organic pathology may be present, the pain complaint greatly exceeds the observed physiological factors. The onset of the pain is often temporally related to environmental stimuli and psychological conflict. It may enable the patient to avoid responsibility or to receive emotional support. The pain complaint is not secondary to another psychiatric disorder such as major depression (American Psychiatric Association 1994).

Diagnosis of somatoform pain disorder is difficult. It depends on both the patient's report and the clinician's assessment of the pain; both are subjective. In addition, the symptoms of psychogenic pain disorder appear to overlap significantly with conversion disorder (Stoudemire and Sandhu 1987). Both diagnoses are sometimes used to describe individuals in whom psychological complaints play a significant role in pain problems.

There are many explanations of how psychological conflicts lead to pain. Engel (1959) suggested that pain serves as punishment for some patients with masochistic character structures, that some patients develop pain as a replacement for a loss and that patients' pain location can be determined by unconscious identification with a love object. Roy and Thomas (1986) found that some patients have acute exacerbations of their pain when they face episodes of helplessness or insoluble family problems.

Socioeconomic factors, as well as psychological ones, may differentiate patients with nonorganic chronic pain from those with chronic pain from an organic etiology. Chaturvedi et al. (1984) noted that nonorganic intractable pain is more often found in patients who are younger, unmarried, and more educated than in patients with pain related to a physical illness.

Theories of neurophysiological function also address psychogenic pain. These include the gate theory of pain transmission (discussed above). Patients with somatoform disorders appear to have unusually high levels of autonomic activity (Miller 1984). In addition, an acute pain problem may cause autonomous pain pathways to develop that continue to operate even after the initial stimulus is resolved.

Substance Abuse

Substance abuse is a frequent complication of chronic pain (Finlayson et al. 1986) and is one of the most common psychiatric disorders among patients with chronic pain (Reich et al. 1983). Substance abuse problems are often overlooked by treating physicians, even when there are few physical findings to explain patients' pain.

Patients with chronic pain and substance dependence may not differ in other ways from patients with chronic pain who do not abuse substances, although psychological testing suggests that these patients have considerably more psychopathology than do general medical patients (Finlayson et al. 1986). Family history of substance abuse is not higher in pain patients with substance abuse than in other chronic pain patients. Patients with substance dependence and chronic pain may be especially resistant to psychological interventions typically used with chronic pain patients.

Treatment of patients with both chronic pain and substance abuse should initially focus on treatment of the substance abuse (Finlayson et al. 1986). Though detoxification programs can temporarily decrease substance use, intensive substance abuse treatment programs may provide better results, as these patients often attempt to rationalize their substance use by the presence of pain and use defense mechanisms of denial and minimization. Even if successful treatment of the substance dependence problem does not decrease patients' pain, it may improve both patients' ability to work and their marital relationships.

Organic Mental Disorders

Little has been written about the role of pain in patients with organic mental disorders. It is important to note that patients with cognitive impairment frequently express emotional distress with physical symptoms. In addition, their inability to clearly express themselves can complicate their histories and make evaluations difficult. Careful cognitive and physical evaluations are important as underlying illnesses or medical treatments may contribute to delirium or other cognitive dysfunction.

Acute Versus Chronic Pain

Acute pain can be differentiated from chronic pain using a number of parameters. Temporally, *acute pain* is often defined as pain lasting less than 3 months. It is seen as a self-limited reaction to a clear injury or acute disease process and is expected to diminish with resolution of the illness or trauma. Acute pain is usually associated with significant emotional response, particularly anxiety, and the pain is felt to serve a useful purpose by warning the individual of the noxious process. The pain is typically not associated with "pain behaviors" found in more chronic pain syndromes and is considered a normal response to injury.

Acute pain is associated with a different group of disease processes than is chronic pain. Harkins et al. (1984) included pain associated with "myocardial in-

farction, burns, trauma and surgery as well as pain due to various somatic and visceral disorders" in their definition of *acute pain*. One could add acute herpetic neuralgia, pain during the postoperative period, and possibly acute exacerbations of more chronic degenerative conditions such as arthritis. Acute pain, therefore, must be considered in the differential diagnosis of all geriatric patients presenting with mental status changes of unclear etiology (Newton 1984). Treatment of acute pain does not differ substantially among age groups. However, geriatric pain patients are quite sensitive to both the therapeutic actions and side effects of medications because of the multiple physiological changes that occur in aging patients.

Assessment of Pain in Elderly Patients

Assessment of pain in older adults requires thorough medical and psychiatric evaluations. Geriatric pain patients who seek psychiatric evaluations usually have chronic pain complaints and often have seen multiple physicians before their presentation to the psychiatrist. Because of the complexity of pain problems, multidisciplinary clinics are the best setting for evaluation of many patients (Ferrell et al. 1990). However, psychiatrists often see pain patients in their offices, especially those with chronic pain, and they must be prepared to complete comprehensive differential diagnoses and treatment plans.

Patients with pain must be approached carefully by mental health personnel, as these patients often resent the suggestion that the pain is "in their head." The provider must tell the patient that he or she understands the patient's distress and that he or she will try to help relieve the patient's pain (Erskine et al. 1986). The clinician must also reassure patients who are anxious about discussing their pain or who minimize their pain with a feeling that they must "shoulder the burden" (Forman and Stratton 1991).

Many physical illnesses in elderly individuals, ranging from rheumatoid arthritis to intracerebral tumors, present with pain and must be assessed in initial evaluations. Clinicians should be careful not to prematurely classify patients' symptoms as psychogenic. Presentations of physical illnesses in elderly patients may be atypical (Steel 1978). At the same time, depression may present with physical complaints, and hypochondriasis is not uncommon. Psychiatrists should also thoroughly review patients' past and current medication history.

The physician should evaluate the patient's presenting problems, as well as the impact of these problems on the patient's ability to function. Patients may rationalize that problems due to other illnesses really result from pain (Fordyce 1978a). A detailed assessment that includes verbal and visual pain scales is indicated. Instruments such as the McGill Pain Questionnaire (Herr and Mobily 1991) can be included in the evaluation, although they are time intensive for both the clinician and the patient.

A review of the patient's psychiatric history should include not only formal psychiatric history and treatment, but also the patient's developmental history. Some patients with pain present with significant early-life deprivation, which may have a role in the their pain problems. Assessment of the patient's personality is especially important in cases in which psychosomatic illness is suspected. The psychiatric history must also discuss current or past substance abuse. An extensive history of the patient's work and social status and the impact of his or her pain on these areas is important. Some patients focus their lives around their pain, whereas other patients' families reinforce their pain behaviors. A family history of psychiatric illness, pain, and substance abuse can also play a role in a patient's current presentation. Finally, history should also be obtained from a friend, spouse, or other family member who may add information.

The mental status evaluation must be complete with special emphasis placed on an examination of the patient's mood because of the high rate of depression in this population. The issue of suicide should also be explored as chronic medical illness is a significant risk factor. A thorough cognitive examination is important in elderly patients who often present with organic mental illnesses, including dementia and delirium.

Treatment of Pain

Specific therapeutic interventions follow from a careful assessment of the pain complaint and an established diagnosis. In the geriatric patient careful evaluation is particularly critical. Back pain in a patient with a long history of degenerative arthritis may be the result of a compression fracture, rather than a simple exacerbation of the inflammatory disease. Elderly patients frequently present with more than one chronic process, which often complicates the differential diagnosis of their pain complaints. Psychosocial factors also deserve consideration, but practitioners should assume that any new pain complaint signals a physical process. As with younger patients, aging patients deserve adequate pain management. Undertreatment of pain is particularly problematic in elderly patients as physicians and nurses are often so concerned about overmedicating the elderly that patients receive subtherapeutic dosages of medication.

Once the etiology of the pain has been determined, pain treatment should proceed in a stepwise fashion to minimize excessive medications. Attempts at treating the primary disease process may give as much pain relief as a narcotic or other analgesic medication. For example, in acute herpes zoster, the mainstay of treatment is probably acyclovir or corticosteroids. These measures can also reduce the incidence of chronic postherpetic neuralgia (Galer and Portenoy 1991).

Nonpharmacological therapies and nonnarcotic medications can reduce the incidence of medication side effects. For postoperative pain, neural blockade can often be quite effective, precluding the need for opiates (Kreïtzer et al. 1991). TENS has been effective for this problem and may reduce the likelihood of postoperative complications, such as ileus and atelectases, more frequently seen with narcotic analgesics (Long and Hagfors 1975). Appropriate pain relief can hasten the rehabilitation of the postsurgical elderly patient and decrease pulmonary and other complications.

Pharmacotherapy

Several different classes of medications are used to treat pain. However, drug treatment in elderly patients requires special care (Vestal 1978) as the elderly have high rates of adverse reactions to multiple classes of medications.

Geriatric patients have slower metabolism and excretion of medications than do younger patients, often resulting in higher blood levels with equivalent doses. Changes in gastric and intestinal absorption are coupled with decline in hepatic metabolism and renal excretion. The volume of distribution of drugs may also be altered because of changes in body fat and serum protein binding. Older patients often have multiple disease states that predispose them to problems with medication side effects. Also, they may receive multiple medications, which can lead to untoward medication interactions. Finally, geriatric patients are less compliant than are other patients, possibly because of their high incidence of cognitive impairment. In the aging pain patient, it is particularly important to use short-acting medications to avoid drug accumulation. As with younger patients, routine dosage rather than an as-needed schedule is preferable. This prevents pain from reaching intolerable levels before the medication dosage time and can serve to decrease more chronic pain behavior. However, in geriatric patients, the physician may need to withhold occasional doses to balance untoward side effects, particularly sedation. Though polypharmacy is generally discouraged, use of adjuvant medication may be beneficial in elderly patients to minimize side effects from any one particular class of drugs. The physician should consider the combination of narcotics with nonsteroidal analgesics or the addition of augmenting medications such as hydroxyzine. With the above caveats in mind, the physician should aggressively treat the pain complaint in the aging patient.

Nonnarcotic Analgesics

The mainstay of acute pain management continues to be nonnarcotic analgesic medications. However, the role of nonnarcotic analgesics in the treatment of chronic pain is unclear. They are very effective in inflammatory pain, and, due to their relatively low rate of side effects, it is reasonable to offer them to all pain patients. Patients should receive at least 2-week trials of therapeutic doses (Portenoy 1987).

These agents are peripherally acting analgesics, which decrease inflammation and may also affect pain through other mechanisms such as suppression of endogenous prostaglandin production (Portenoy 1987). Decreases in serum protein in the geriatric patient may increase the free-drug concentration of these medications (Foley 1990). This increase, coupled with prolonged metabolism and excretion (Schlagel and Paulus 1986), necessitates use of somewhat lower dosages to avoid side effects such as gastrointestinal distress, headache, and hepatic and renal toxicity. In addition, careful attention must be paid to interactions with other drugs often taken in this population, such as antihypertensives.

Narcotics

Narcotics are frequently used in the treatment of acute pain, especially postoperative pain and malignant pain, though they are less commonly used with chronic pain because of fears of habituation and addiction and questions about their efficacy. Narcotics decrease pain by binding to opiate receptors and activating descending efferent pathways, which inhibit pain transmission neurons (Basbaum and Fields 1978). They may also activate opiate receptors at the spinal cord level.

Evaluation of the use of opiates for chronic pain of nonmalignant origin is limited (Merry 1991). The effect of opiates in the treatment of chronic pain is often enhanced by the use of appropriate psychotropic medications such as antidepressants (Breivik and Rennemo 1982). Among chronic, benign pain syndromes, those with diffuse, deep pain appear to respond best to opioids (N. H. Jensen 1991).

The narcotic drug class (Table 17–1) includes agonist-antagonist opioids such as pentazocine, as well as pure agonists such as codeine and morphine. Though the agonist-antagonists have been reported to have less habituation potential than pure agonists, there is little evidence to suggest that they have significant advantages over pure agonists in the treatment of acute or chronic pain (Hoskin and Hanks 1991). In addition, they appear to have little role in the treatment of chronic pain. Narcotics require careful monitoring in elderly patients.

Studies have suggested that elderly patients are more sensitive to these medications than are younger patients (Kaiko et al. 1982). In fact, the relation between the effect of narcotics and age appears to be much stronger than other frequently used criteria such as height, weight, and body surface area. Older patients may respond to morphine with 3–4 times the effect of the response of younger patients (Bellville et al.

Table 17–1. Comparison of commonly used opioid analgesics for treatment of pain

Drug	Equivalent dosage (mg)		Half-life (hours)
	im	po	
Agonists			
Morphine	10	60	2–3
Meperidine	75	300	3–4
Hydromorphone	1.5	7.5	2–3
Levorphanol	2	4	12–16
Methadone	10	20	24
Codeine	120	200	3
Mixed agonists-antagonists			
Pentazocine	60	180	2–3
Butorphanol	2	—	2–3

1971; Kaiko 1980). Side effects such as sedation, constipation, urinary retention, and respiratory depression are particularly problematic in the geriatric population. More importantly, the physician needs to be alert to any mental status changes indicative of an impending delirium. These guidelines also apply to using patient-controlled analgesia, which is as effective in the elderly population as in younger groups. As with nonsteroidal analgesics, the risk of side effects is increased when the patient is on multiple other medications. The age-related increased analgesia is primarily related to an increase in duration from decreased clearance, rather than in peak analgesic effect. Elderly patients may need less frequent dosing of narcotics than do younger patients, though there appears to be a wide range of effects within all age groups.

The rate of narcotic addiction in pain patients with organic illnesses and no prior history of substance abuse is reported to be quite low (Marks and Sachar 1973). However, the rate of substance abuse among patients with chronic, benign pain may be more than 30%. Though narcotics should not be withheld from patients who may benefit from them only because of a fear of substance abuse, their risks and benefits should be carefully evaluated before prescription. For patients with chronic, benign pain, narcotics should probably be used only after other modalities have failed.

Antidepressants

Antidepressants are effective in a number of painful conditions. Controlled studies have confirmed that tricyclic antidepressants can assist in the treatment of arthritis (Puttini et al. 1988), tension headaches (Diamond and Baltes 1971), migraine headaches, facial pain (France 1987; Sharav et al. 1987), back pain (Hameroff et al. 1982), and diabetic neuropathy. Studies have also suggested that they are useful in the treatment of neuralgia and phantom limb pain (Urban et al. 1986), as well as malignant pain (Magni et al. 1987). The medications appear to relieve pain in nondepressed pain patients, as well as depressed patients, though they may be most effective in patients with both disorders (Ward et al. 1979). They are often used in conjunction with other medications. They may be least effective in chronic musculoskeletal pain and somatoform disorders (Getto et al. 1987).

The antidepressants are presumed to effect analgesia by increasing central monoamines, especially serotonin. In fact, a serotonin synthesis inhibitor has

been found to prevent the analgesic effect of antidepressants (Tura and Tura 1990). However, antidepressants that primarily affect the noradrenergic system are also useful, and there may be a link between the serotonergic and noradrenergic systems and their effect on pain (Kehoe and Jacisin 1992). Antidepressants may also increase endogenous opioids (Getto et al. 1987).

There is little data about the use of antidepressants with acute pain. Clinical experience suggests that they help patients with significant sleep disturbance. They also seem especially effective for patients with orthopedic injuries.

The most widely used antidepressants in patients with chronic pain are tricyclic antidepressants. Most studies have found them to be more effective than placebo (Stimmel and Escobar 1986). Patients often respond to low doses with diminished pain, as well as improved sleep and mood. Pain relief does not appear to correlate with age (McQuay 1988). The antidepressants most frequently used in the treatment of pain such as amitriptyline, doxepin, and imipramine have significant serotonergic effects. Noradrenergic antidepressants such as desipramine and nortriptyline have historically been believed to be less effective than amitriptyline. However, recent studies suggest that a primarily noradrenergic antidepressant, desipramine, is as effective in pain patients as amitriptyline. It is clearly efficacious in diabetic neuropathy and postherpetic neuralgia (Kishore-Kumar et al. 1990; Max et al. 1991).

Side effects of tricyclic antidepressants include significant anticholinergic effects that can cause or worsen glaucoma, urinary retention, cardiac arrythmias, diverticulosis, and confusion, as well as postural hypotension with secondary gait instability (Cunha 1988). These effects may be especially prominent in elderly patients with rates of confusional episodes of up to 35% among those over age 40 (Davies et al. 1971). Tricyclic antidepressants can also slow cardiac conduction. The use of amitriptyline, the drug predominantly used for chronic pain, may be problematic in elderly patients because of its anticholinergic effects and orthostasis. Nortriptyline is usually better tolerated. Geriatric patients develop higher blood levels from equivalent doses than do younger patients (Nies et al. 1977) and the medications should be used cautiously in this population. However, age alone is not a contraindication to treatment with tricyclic antidepressants.

Monoamine oxidase inhibitors have also been found to be effective in the treatment of pain, especially in the treatment of migraine headaches (Portenoy 1987), though there are relatively few studies available (France 1987). Trazodone is also useful in pain patients, especially in the treatment of sleep disturbance, though some authors have not found it superior to placebo (Davidoff et al. 1987). Among newer antidepressants, maprotiline is effective in pain patients (Lindsay and Olsen 1985), whereas fluoxetine may be no more effective than placebo (Max et al. 1992; Mendel et al. 1986). No information about the effect of sertraline on pain is available. Antidepressants that affect only serotonergic receptors may not be as effective as the tricyclic antidepressants. Antidepressant doses used to treat pain are often lower than those used to treat depression. For example, studies of pain patients using amitriptyline often involve doses of 50–100 mg/day. Improvement of pain may occur within 2 to 3 days, rather than the 2 or more weeks required for the treatment of depressive syndromes. Treatment of concurrent depression probably requires usual antidepressant doses.

Further research is needed to clarify the role of antidepressants in the treatment of pain. Questions that remain unanswered include the mechanisms by which antidepressants treat pain, the most effective dose range, the relative efficacy of different antidepressants, the role of blood level monitoring, the presence of concurrent psychiatric disorders (Magni 1991), and whether adjunctive medications such as lithium are useful. In addition, further evaluation of the efficacy of antidepressants other than tertiary tricyclic antidepressants is required.

Anxiolytics

There has been little study of benzodiazepines in patients with nonmalignant, chronic pain, though they are frequently used for the treatment of acute pain problems such as muscle spasm. There is some evidence that benzodiazepines reduce chronic pain (Hollister et al. 1981; Westbrook et al. 1990), though other studies suggest that they have the contrary effect (King and Strain 1990). Their role, if any, in the treatment of patients with chronic pain remains unclear, except for a few specific syndromes, such as the use of clonazepam for the treatment of trigeminal neuralgia (Walsh 1991).

Side effects of benzodiazepines include dizziness and problems with muscle coordination. In addition, they may slow patients' cognition and contribute to de-

pression or lead to a paradoxical increase in agitation. Side effects may be more prominent in elderly patients, and the medications must be used cautiously in this population. Unless patients have a preexisting history of substance abuse, development of psychological dependence is uncommon (Hollister et al. 1981). Short-acting preparations are preferred in elderly patients to prevent accumulation of the drug.

Antipsychotics

Antipsychotic agents have also been used to treat patients with chronic pain. Patients typically receive concurrent treatment with a tricyclic antidepressant. However, there are few studies of antipsychotics' efficacy among pain patients. Antipsychotics appear to have little effect in acute pain (Judkins 1982) unless there is a concurrent delirium. They appear to be most effective in patients with postherpetic pain and postoperative scar pain (Clarke 1981), though some studies question their benefit (Mendel et al. 1986).

Antipsychotics have multiple side effects, including pseudoparkinsonian effects and the long-term risk of tardive dyskinesia, which is especially problematic in elderly patients. Because of sensitivity to anticholinergic side effects, elderly patients usually best tolerate higher-potency medications such as haloperidol and fluphenazine rather than low-potency medications such as chlorpromazine or thioridazine.

Anticonvulsants

Anticonvulsants can be effective for some chronic pain syndromes, especially neuropathic pain and neuralgias. The medication of choice is usually carbamazepine, which is especially effective for trigeminal neuralgia. Valproate is used for neuropathies, although data supporting its use are equivocal (McQuay 1988). Phenytoin is effective for diabetic neuropathies, trigeminal neuralgia, and phantom limb pain.

The mechanisms by which anticonvulsants help patients with shooting, lancinating pains is unclear (Swerdlow 1984). Though their effects may not be related to their anticonvulsant action (Portenoy 1987), they appear to decrease pain by suppression of paroxysmal or other abnormal neuronal discharges (Portenoy 1987). Patients are usually treated with anticonvulsant doses, though many clinicians use the guidelines of efficacy and side effects to determine the proper dose, rather than focusing on serum levels.

Other Organic Treatment Modalities

TENS is a battery-operated device that delivers low-voltage electrical current through electrodes placed on the skin. Initially, it was believed effective for both acute and chronic pain (Long et al. 1979), although a recent study suggested that it was no more effective than placebo (Deyo et al. 1990).

Biofeedback has been used in a variety of pain syndromes including muscle contraction headaches, migraine headaches, and various other pain problems. A number of techniques are used in biofeedback including electromyograms of various muscles, measurement of skin temperature, and electroencephalogram measurements. Subjects may receive concurrent counseling or relaxation training. Studies of biofeedback techniques suggest that various techniques provide at least moderate relief of pain (Jessup 1989) and may be as effective as relaxation training.

Pain in elderly patients is often associated with degenerative diseases. Local anesthetic blocks may help relieve a number of pain syndromes associated with these illnesses (Carron 1978). They inhibit inflammatory processes and increase mobility. Local soft tissue injections using either local anesthetics or steroid preparations can be valuable in managing acute connective tissue processes such as bursitis or tendinitis. Acupuncture has also been efficacious in some patients, with pain relief of up to 3 weeks (Shifman 1975).

Psychotherapeutic Treatments

A number of nonpharmacological treatments have been used for the treatment of chronic pain. They include hypnosis, guided visual imagery, operant conditioning, relaxation training, and cognitive-behavioral techniques. Typically used as parts of multidisciplinary treatment programs, these modalities are efficacious in some patients, although it is often difficult to predict which patients will derive the greatest benefit.

Probably the most widely used technique is relaxation training. The relaxation response is an integral part of hypnosis and cognitive-behavior therapies, as well as an independent modality. A relaxation response is associated with decreases in sympathetic nervous activity (Sternbach 1986), oxygen consumption, muscle tension, and heart and respiratory rates, and a slight slowing of the background rhythm of the electroencephalogram. It may also decrease vasoconstriction and resulting acidosis (Ross et al. 1988). These re-

sponses appear to extend beyond the period of relaxation itself. The response may occur with progressive relaxation, with hypnosis, or through meditation practices such as yoga. A number of studies (Holroyd and Penzien 1990) have suggested that the relaxation response is more effective than placebo and that the effects of relaxation training can persist for more than year after completion of the initial training.

Hypnosis is quite effective in pain relief and has even served as anesthesia for some patients (Orne and Dinges 1989) in surgical and dental procedures. The ability to be hypnotized varies among individuals and may be slightly lower among elderly patients. It is more effective among patients with organic pain than among those with a significant psychological component. Depression, other psychiatric disorders, and low patient motivation decrease its effectiveness (Orne and Dinges 1989). Patients with chronic, nonmalignant pain may respond best to hypnosis if it is one element of a multimodal treatment plan. Patients who have severe pain may require anesthesia or other medications prior to hypnosis.

In addition to its use as short-term pain relief, hypnosis can also be used as part of a psychotherapeutic process (hypnotherapy). Establishing rapport with the patient is an essential precondition, and the patient's relationship with the therapist appears to correlate with its effectiveness. Self-hypnosis can also be useful and cost effective.

Cognitive-behavioral approaches to pain have evolved from cognitive-behavior therapies for psychiatric disorders, such as anxiety and depression. They focus on patients' thoughts, feelings, and behaviors and involve techniques designed to help patients correct mistaken beliefs (Turk and Meicherbaum 1989). Cognitive-behavior therapy typically consists of a time-limited number of sessions in which attempts are made to increase the patients' coping skills. It often includes an activity program to increase patients' mobility and to decrease their focus on their pain. A variety of cognitive and relaxation techniques help patients view themselves more positively.

Fordyce (1978b) has written at length about behavioral reinforcers of chronic pain. These include direct positive rewards, such as sympathetic attention and permission to assume the sick role, as well as indirect ones, such as the ability to avoid an undesirable job. As distinct from cognitive therapies, which focus on patients' thoughts, more traditional behavior therapies focus on patients' behaviors and assume that patients' thoughts will change as a result of their behavior changes. Though studies of these treatments have methodological difficulties, they suggest that behavior therapies can be quite effective.

Multidisciplinary Treatment

Multidimensional treatment programs appear to have the best results in patients with chronic pain due to multiple emotional, social, and physical factors. Resolution of the pain often requires treatment of associated secondary problems, as well as attention to the initial physical etiology of the pain. A variety of clinicians, including internists, nurses, orthopedists, anesthesiologists, physiatrists, radiologists, psychiatrists, psychologists, and physical and occupational therapists are required (Slater and Good 1991). In addition, as it is difficult to relieve symptoms, rehabilitation programs focus on increasing patients' function. They treat chronic pain as a chronic problem requiring long-term treatment.

Components of multidisciplinary programs include education, physical reconditioning, behavior management, and detoxification. Programs include work with the family to help them ignore pathological behavior and reinforce healthy behavior (Slater and Good 1991). They may also include cognitive-behavior therapies, marital therapy, and vocational counseling.

Treatment of pain is more effective when clinicians in multiple specialties work together in the development and implementation of a treatment plan than if they provide concurrent care without good communication (Lebovits 1991). Pain centers, which facilitate frequent contacts between providers, are most often based in departments of anesthesiology. Coordination of care is improved if a specific physician assumes primary responsibility for the patient and becomes his or her "patient manager" (Bonica 1977). Group conferences of the clinicians involved in assessing and treating specific patients are useful.

Treatment with multiple behavioral modalities appears to be more effective than treatment with psychoeducational groups alone (Hellman et al. 1990). Though behavioral treatment of pain is expensive, even modest success may be cost effective as, otherwise, less than 50% of patients with chronic pain return to work (Slater and Good 1991) or obtain satisfactory relief from surgical or pharmacological treatments. Elderly patients are as likely as younger patients to accept and complete multidisciplinary pain treatment (Sor-

kin et al. 1990), though, in practice, they may not utilize these programs as often as younger patients (Crook et al. 1989). It is not clear whether this decreased utilization is due to physician referral patterns, age-related stoicism, or decreased mobility of elderly patients.

Conclusions and Summary

Pain problems occur frequently among geriatric patients even though the elderly population may not perceive pain differently than younger populations. Pain imposes significant costs in medical morbidity and decreased functioning. Careful evaluations help to clarify the multiple biological and psychosocial factors that contribute to pain in elderly patients. Treatment may involve multiple modalities similar to those used for other patient groups.

Pain often presents with concurrent psychiatric disorders or as a symptom of those disorders. Treatment of the underlying psychiatric disorders can contribute to effective management of the pain problem. Despite their frequency and morbidity, many questions remain about the etiology of chronic pain problems and about the most effective treatments.

Pain is a frequent finding among elderly patients. It is associated with both medical and psychiatric illnesses, which must be assessed in a thorough evaluation. Elderly patients' perception and expression of pain do not differ significantly from those of younger populations. Treatments include a variety of medications, which should be used cautiously in older patients. Many nonpharmacological treatments are also useful. Multidisciplinary clinics are the best settings for the evaluation and treatment of many pain problems.

References

Adams JE: Naloxone reversal of analgesia produced by brain stimulation in the human. Pain 2:161–166, 1976

Adelman A, Shank JC: The association of psychosocial factors with the resolution of abdominal pain. Fam Med 20:266–270, 1988

Adler R, Zlots HC, Minder C: Engel's psychogenic pain and the pain-prone patient: a retrospective, controlled study. Psychosom Med 51:87–101, 1989

Akil H, Liebeskind JC: Monoaminergic mechanisms of stimulation-produced analgesia. Brain Res 94:279–296, 1975

Al Absi M, Rokke PD: Can anxiety help us tolerate pain? Pain 46:43–51, 1991

American Psychiatric Association: Diagnostic and Statistical Manual of Mental Disorders, 4th Edition. Washington, DC, American Psychiatric Association, 1994

Arntz A, Dressen L, Merckelbach H: Attention, not anxiety, influences pain. Behav Res Ther 29:41–50, 1991

Basbaum AI, Fields HL: Endogenous pain control mechanisms: review and hypothesis. Ann Neurol 4:451–462, 1978

Beitman B, Kushner M: Late onset panic disorder "evidence from a study of patients with chest pain and normal cardiac evaluation." Int J Psychiatry Med 21:29–35, 1991

Bellville JW, Forrest Jr WH, Miller E, et al: Influence of age on pain relief from analgesics. JAMA 217:1835–1841, 1971

Blumer D, Heilbronn M: Chronic pain as a variant of depressive disease. J Nerv Ment Dis 170:381–395, 1982

Boeke S, Duivenvoorden H, Verhage F, et al: Prediction of postoperative pain and duration of hospitalization using two anxiety measures. Pain 45:293–297, 1991

Bonica J: Basic principles in managing chronic pain. Arch Surg 112:783–788, 1977

Breivik H, Rennemo F: Clinical evaluation of combined treatment with Methadone and psychotropic drugs in cancer patients. Acta Anaesthesiol Scand Suppl 74:135–140, 1982

Brena SF, Chapman SL: Pain and litigation, in Textbook of Pain. Edited by Wall P, Melzack R. New York, Churchill Livingstone, 1989, pp 1032–1042

Carron H: Relieving pain with nerve blocks. Geriatrics 33:49–57, 1978

Cartwright A, Hockey L, Anderson JL: Life Before Death. Boston, MA, Routledge & Kegan Paul, 1973

Chaney H, Cohn C, Williams S, et al: MMPI results: a comparison of trauma victims, psychogenic pain and patients with organic disease. J Clin Psychol 40:1450–1454, 1984

Chaturvedi S: Depressed and nondepressed chronic pain patients. Pain 29:355–361, 1987

Chaturvedi S, Michael A: Chronic pain in a psychiatric clinic. J Psychosom Res 30:347–353, 1986

Chaturvedi SK, Varma VK, Malhotra A: Non-organic chronic intractable pain: a comparative study. Pain 19:87–94, 1984

Clarke I: Amitriptyline and perphenazine in chronic pain. Anaesthesia 36:210–212, 1981

Cox, BM, Goldstein A, Li CH: Opioid activity of a peptide, B-lipotropin (61-91), derived from B-lipotropin. Proc Natl Acad Sci U S A 73:1821–1823, 1976

Crook J, Rideout E, Browne G: The prevalence of pain complaints in a general population. Pain 18:299–314, 1984

Crook J, Weir R, Tunks E: An epidemiological follow-up survey of persistent pain sufferers in a group family practice and specialty pain clinic. Pain 36:49–61, 1989

Cunha V: Antidepressants: their uses in nonpsychiatric disorders of aging. Geriatrics 10:63–71, 1988

Davidoff O, Guarracini M, Roth E, et al: Trazadone hydrochloride in the treatment of dysesthetic pain in traumatic myelopathy: a randomized, double-blind, placebo-controlled study. Pain 29:151–161, 1987

Davidson J, Krishan R, France R, et al: Neurovegetative symptoms in chronic pain and depression. J Affect Disord 9:213–218, 1985

Davies RK, Tucker GJ, Harrow M, et al: Confusional episodes and antidepressant medication. Am J Psychiatry 128:95–99, 1971

Davis GC, Cortez C, Rubin BR: Pain management in the older adult with rheumatoid arthritis or osteoarthritis. Arthritis Care Research 3:127–131, 1990

Deyo RA, Walsh NE, Martin DC, et al: A controlled trial of transcutaneous electrical nerve stimulation (TENS) and exercise for chronic low back pain. N Engl J Med 322:1627–1634, 1990

Diamond S, Baltes BJ: Chronic tension headache-treated with amitriptyline: a double-blind study. Headache 11:110–116, 1971

Dworkin S: Illness, behavior and dysfunction: review of concepts and application to chronic pain. Can J Physiol Psychopharmacol 69:662–671, 1991

Engel G: "Psychogenic" pain and the pain-prone patient. AJM 26:899–918, 1959

Erskine WAR, Raine ER, Lindegger G: Assessment and management of chronic pain. S Afr Med J 69:621–625, 1986

Faherty BS, Grier MR: Analgesic medication for elderly people post-surgery. Nurs Res 33:369–372, 1984

Ferrell BA, Ferrell BR, Osterweil D: Pain in the nursing home. J Am Geriatr Soc 38:409–414, 1990

Finlayson R, Maruta T, Morse R, et al: Substance dependence and chronic pain: profile of 50 patients treated in an alcohol and drug dependence unit. Pain 26:167–174, 1986

Foley KM: Pain management in the elderly, in Principles Of Geriatric Medicine and Gerontology. Edited by Hazzard WR, Andres R, Bierman EL, et al. New York, McGraw-Hill, 1990, pp 281–295

Fordyce WE: Evaluating and managing chronic pain. Geriatrics 33:59–62, 1978a

Fordyce WE: Learning processes in pain, in The Psychology of Pain. Edited by Sternbach RA. New York, Raven, 1978b, pp 49–72

Forman W, Stratton M: Current approaches to chronic pain in older patients. Geriatrics 46:47–52, 1991

France R: The future for antidepressants: treatment of pain. Psychopathology 20 (suppl 1):99–113, 1987

France RD, Krishnan K, Trainor M: Chronic pain and depression, III: family history of depression and alcoholism in chronic low back pain patients. Pain 24:185–190, 1986

Galer BS, Portenoy RK: Acute herpetic and postherpetic neuralgia: clinical features and management. Mt Sinai J Med 58:257–266, 1991

Gamsa A, Vikis-Freiberg V: Psychological events are both risk factors in and consequences of chronic pain. Pain 44:271–277, 1991

Getto CJ, Sorkness CA, Howell T: Antidepressants and chronic nonmalignant pain: a review. Journal Of Pain and Symptoms Management 2:9–18, 1987

Grandi S, Fava G, Trombini G, et al: Depression and anxiety in patients with chronic pelvic pain. Psychiatr Med 6:1–7, 1988

Hameroff S, Cork R, Scherer K, et al: Doxepin effects on chronic pain, depression and plasma opioids. J Clin Psychiatry 43:22–27, 1982

Harkins SW: Pain in the elderly, in Proceedings of the 5th World Congress on Pain. Edited by Dubner R, Gebhart GF, Bond MR. Amsterdam, Elsevier Science, 1988, pp 355–367

Harkins SW, Chapman CR: Detection and decision factors in pain perception in young and elderly men. Pain 2:253–264, 1976

Harkins SW, Chapman CR: The perception of induced dental pain in young and elderly women. J Gerontol 32:428–435, 1977

Harkins SW, Warner MH: Age and pain. Annual Review Of Gerontology and Geriatrics 1:121–129, 1980

Harkins SW, Kwentus J, Price DD: Pain and the elderly, in Advances in Pain Research and Therapy, Vol 7. Edited by Benedetti C, Chapman CE, Moricca G. New York, Raven, 1984, pp 103–122

Harkins SW, Price DD, Martelli M: Effects of age on pain perception: thermonociception. J Gerontol 41:58–63, 1986

Haythornwaite J, Sieber W, Kerns R: Depression and the chronic pain experience. Pain 46:177–184, 1991

Hellman C, Budd M, Borysenko J, et al: A study of the effectiveness of two group behavioral medicine interventions for patients with psychosomatic complaints. Behav Med 16:165–173, 1990

Hendler N: The anatomy and psychopharmacology of chronic pain. J Clin Psychiatry 43:15–21, 1982

Herr KA, Mobily PR: Complexities of pain assessment in the elderly. Journal of Gerontological Nursing 17:12–19, 1991

Hollister LE, Conley FK, Britt RH, et al: Long-term use of diazepam. JAMA 246-1568–1570, 1981

Holroyd KA, Penzien DB: Pharmacological versus non-pharmacological prophylatis of recurrent migraine headache: a meta-analysis review of clinical trials. Pain 42:1–13, 1990

Hoskin PJ, Hanks GW: Opioid agonist-antagonist drugs in acute and chronic pain states. Drugs 41:326–344, 1991

Jamison RN, Matt DA, Parris WC: Effects of time-limited vs unlimited compensation on pain behavior and treatment outcome in low back pain patients. J Psychosom Res 32:277–283, 1988

Jensen MP, Turner JA, Romano SM: Self-efficacy and outcome expectancies: relationship to chronic pain coping strategies and adjustment. Pain 42:263–269, 1991

Jensen NH: Accurate diagnosis and drug selection in chronic pain patients. Postgrad Med J 67 (suppl 2):52–58, 1991

Jessup BA: Relaxation and Biofeedback, in Textbook of Pain. Edited by Wall P, Melzack R. New York, Churchill Livingstone, 1989, pp 989–1000

Judkins KC: Haloperidol as and adjunct analgesic in the management of postoperative pain. Anaesthesia 37:1118–1120, 1982

Kaiko RF: Age and morphine analgesia in cancer patients with postoperative pain. Clin Pharmacol Ther 78:823–826, 1980

Kaiko RF, Wallenstein SL, Rogers AG, et al: Narcotics in the elderly. Med Clin North Am 66:1079–1089, 1982

Katon W: Chest pain, cardiac disease and panic disorder. J Clin Psychiatry 5 (suppl):27–30, 1990

Kehoe W, Jacisin J: Selecting and monitoring antidepressant medications. American Journal of Pain Management 2:17–26, 1992

Kinder B, Curtiss G, Kalichman S: Anxiety and anger as predictors of MMPI elevations in chronic pain patients. J Pers Asses 50:651–661, 1986

King SA, Strain JJ: Benzodiazepines and chronic pain. Pain 41:3–4, 1990

Kishore-Kumar R, Max M, Schafer S, et al: Desipramine relieves postherpetic neuralgia. Clin Pharmacol Ther 47:305–312, 1990

Kreitzer JM, Reuben SS, Reed AP: Update on postoperative pain management. Mt Sinai J Med 58:240–246, 1991

Krishnan K, France R, Houpt J: Chronic low back pain and depression. Psychosomatics 26:299–301, 1985

Kushner MG, Beitman BD, Beck NE: Factors predictive of panic disorder in cardiology patient with chest pain and no evidence of coronary artery disease: a cross-validation. J Psychosom Res 33:207–215, 1989

Lavsky-Shulan M, Wallace R, Kohout FS, et al: Prevalence and functional correlates of low back pain in the elderly. J Am Geriatr Soc 33:23–28, 1985

Leavitt F: The role of psychological disturbance in extending disability time among compensable back injured industrial workers. J Psychosom Res 34:447–453, 1990

Lebovits AH: Chronic pain: the multidisciplinary approach. Int Anesthesiol Clin 29:1–7, 1991

Lindsay PG, Olsen RB: Maprotoline in pain-depression. J Clin Psychiatry 46:226–228, 1985

Lindsay P, Wyckoff M: The depression-pain syndrome and its response to antidepressants. Psychosomatics 22:571–577, 1981

Long DM, Hagfors N: Electrical stimulation in the nervous system: the current status of electrical stimulation of the nervous system for relief of pain. Pain 1:109–123, 1975

Long DM, Campbell JN, Gucer G: Transcutaneous electrical stimulation for relief of chronic pain. Advances in Pain Research and Therapy. 3:593–599, 1979

MacDonald JB, Baillie J, Williams BO, et al: Coronary care in the elderly. Age Aging 12:17–20, 1983

Magni G: On the relationship between chronic pain and depression when there is no organic lesion. Pain 31:1–21, 1987

Magni G: The use of antidepressants in the treatment of chronic pain. Drugs 42:730–748, 1991

Magni G, Schifano F, Deleo D: Pain as a symptom in elderly depressed patients. Acta Psychiatrica Neurologica Science 215:143–145, 1985

Magni G, Conlon P, Arsie D: Tricyclic antidepressants in the treatment of cancer pain. Pharmacopsychiatry 20:160–164, 1987

Marks RM, Sachar EJ: Undertreatment of medical inpatients with narcotic analgesics. Ann Intern Med 78:173–181, 1973

Max M, Kishore-Kumar R, Schafer S, et al: Efficacy of desipramine in painful diabetic neuropathy: a placebo-controlled trial. Pain 45:3–9, 1991

Max MB, Lynch SA, Muir S, et al: Effects of desipramine, amitriptyline, and fluoxetine on pain in diabetic neuropathy. N Engl J Med 326:1250–1256, 1992

Mayer DJ, Liebeskind JC: Pain reduction by focal electrical stimulation of the brain: an anatomical and behavioral analysis. Brain Res 68:73–93, 1974

Mayer DJ, Price DD: Central nervous system mechanisms of analgesia. Pain 2:379–404, 1976

McQuay HJ: Pharmacological treatment of neuralgic and neuropathic pain. Cancer Surv 7:141–159, 1988

Melzack R, Wall PD: Pain mechanisms: a new theory. Science 150:971–979, 1965

Mendel C, Klein R, Chappell D: A trial of amitriptyline and fluphenazine in the treatment of painful diabetic neuropathy. JAMA 255:637–639, 1986

Mendelson G: Chronic pain and compensation: a review. Journal of Pain and Symptoms Management 1:135–144, 1986

Mendelson G: Compensation and chronic pain. Pain 48:121–123, 1992

Merry AF: Opioids in the treatment of chronic pain of non-malignant origin. N Z Med J 104:520–521, 1991

Merskey H, Lau C, Russell E, et al: Screening for psychiatric morbidity: the pattern of psychological illness and premorbid characteristics in four chronic pain populations. Pain 30:141–157, 1987

Miller L: Neuropsychological concepts of somatoform disorders. Int J Psychiatry Med 14:31–46, 1984

Moricca A, Arcuri E: Pain in the aging patient: a critical approach, in The Aging Brain. Edited by Barbagallo-Sangiorg G, Exton-Smith AN. New York, Plenum, 1980, pp 315–322

Moss, MS, Lawton P, Glicksman A: The role of pain in the last year of life of older persons. J Gerontol 46:51–57, 1991

Newton PA: Chronic pain, in Geriatric Medicine. Edited by Cassel CK, Walsh JR. New York, Springer-Verlag, 1984, pp 236–274

Nies A, Robinson D, Friedman M, et al: Relationship between age and tricyclic antidepressant levels. Am J Psychiatry 134:790–793, 1977

Orne M, Dinges D: Hypnosis, in Textbook of Pain. Edited by Wall P, Melzack R. New York, Churchill Livingstone, 1989, pp 1021–1031

Ouslander JG: Drug therapy in the elderly. Ann Intern Med 95:711–722, 1981

Pasternak GW: Multiple morphine and enkephalin receptors and the relief of pain. JAMA 259:1362–1367, 1988

Pasternak GW, Goodman R, Snyder SH: An endogenous morphine-like factor in mammalian brain. Life Sci 16:1765–1769, 1975

Pert A, Yaksh T: Site of morphine induced analgesia in the primate brain: relation to pain pathways. Brain Res 80:135–140, 1974

Pert CB, Kuhar MJ, Snyder SH: Opiate receptor: autoradiographic localization in rat brain. Proc Natl Acad Sci U S A 73:3729–3733, 1976

Portenoy RK: Drug treatment of pain syndromes. Semin Neurol 7:139–149, 1987

Portenoy RK, Kanner RM: Patterns of analgesic prescription and consumption in a university-affiliated community hospital. Arch Intern Med 145:439, 1985

Puttini PS, Cazzola M, Boccassini L, et al: A comparison of dothiepin versus placebo in the treatment of pain in rheumatoid arthritis and the association of pain with depression. J Int Med Res 16:331–337, 1988

Reich J, Tupin J, Abramowitz S: Psychiatric diagnosis of chronic pain patients. Am J Psychiatry 140:1495–1498, 1983

Reiter R, Shakerin L, Gambone J, et al: Correlation between sexual abuse and somatization in women with somatic and nonsomatic chronic pelvic pain. Am J Obstet Gynecol 165:104–109, 1991

Robinson DS, Nies A, Davis JN, et al: Aging, monoamines, and monoamine oxidase levels. Lancet 1:290–291, 1972

Ross SL, Keefe FS, Gil KM: Behavioral concepts in the analysis of chronic pain, in Chronic Pain. Edited by France RD, Krishnan KRR. Washington DC, American Psychiatric Press, 1988, pp 104–114

Roy R, Thomas M: A survey of chronic pain in an elderly population. Can Fam Physician 32:513–516, 1986

Roy-Byrne P, Uhde TW, Post RM, et al: Normal pain sensitivity in patients with panic disorder. Psychiatry Res 14:75–82, 1985

Rudy TE, Kerns RD, Turk DC: Chronic pain and depression: toward a cognitive-behavioral model. Pain 35:129–140, 1988

Schlagel SE, Paulus H: Non-steroidal and analgesic therapy in the elderly. Clinics in Rheumatic Diseases 12:245, 1986

Sewel R, Spencer PSJ: Modification of the antinociceptive activity of narcotic agonists and antagonists by intraventricular injection of biogenic amines in mice. Br J Pharmacol 51:140–141, 1974

Sharav Y, Singer E, Schmidt E, et al: The analgesic effect of amitriptyline on chronic facial pain. Pain 31:199–209, 1987

Sherman ED, Robillard E: Sensitivity to pain in relationship to age. J Am Geriatr Soc 12:1037–1044, 1964

Shifman AC: The clinical response of 328 private patients to accupunctive therapy. Am J Chin Med 3:165–179, 1975

Slater M, Good A: Behavioral management of chronic pain. Holistic Nurse Practitioner 6:66–75, 1991

Slocumb JC, Kellner R, Rosenfeld RC, et al: Anxiety and depression patients with the abdominal pelvic pain syndrome. Gen Hosp Psychiatry 11:48–53, 1989

Sorkin BA, Rudy TE, Hanlon RB, et al: Chronic pain in old and young patients: differences appear less important than similarities. J Gerontol 45:64–68, 1990

Steel K: Evaluation of the geriatric patient, in Clinical Aspects of Aging. Edited by Reichel W. Baltimore, MD, Williams & Wilkins, 1978, pp 3–12

Sternbach RA: Survey of pain in the United States: the Nuprin pain report. Clin J Pain 2:49–53, 1986

Stimmel GL, Escobar JL: Antidepressants in chronic pain: a review of efficacy. Pharmacotherapy 6:262–267, 1986

Stoudemire A, Sandhu J: Psychogenic/idiopathic pain syndromes. Gen Hosp Psychiatry 9:79–86, 1987

Swanson DW: Chronic pain as a third pathologic emotion. Am J Psychiatry 141:210–214, 1984

Swerdlow M: Anticonvulsant drugs and chronic pain. Clin Neuropharmacol 7:51–82, 1984

Tauschke E, Helmes E, Merskey H: Evidence that defense mechanisms are more related to personality than to symptoms. Br J Med Psychol 64:132–146, 1991

Thorvaldsen P, Sorenson EB: Psychological vulnerability as a predictor for short-term outcome in lumbar spine surgery. Acta Neurochir 102:58–61, 1990

Trief PM, Elliott DJ, Stein N: Functional vs organic pain: a meaningful distinction? J Clin Psychol 43:219–226, 1987

Tura B, Tura SM: The analgesic effect of tricyclic antidepressants. Brain Res 518:19–22, 1990

Turk D, Meicherbaum D: A cognitive-behavioral approach to pain management, in Textbook of Pain. Edited by Wall P, Melzack R. New York, Churchill Livingstone, 1989, pp 1001–1009

Urban B, France R, Steinberger E, et al: Long term use of narcotic/antidepressant medication in the management of phantom limb pain. Pain 24:191–196, 1986

Valdes M, Garcia L, Treserra J, et al: Psychogenic pain and depressive disorders: an empirical study. J Affect Disord 16:21–25, 1989

Vestal RE: Drug use in the elderly: a review of the problems and special considerations. Practical Therapeutics 16:358–382, 1978

Wade JB, Dougherty LM, Hart RP, et al: Patterns of normal personality structure among chronic pain patients. Pain 48:37–43, 1992

Walsh EM: The psychopharmacology of chronic pain. J Psychopharmacol 5:364–369, 1991

Ward NG, Bloom VL, Freidel RO: The effectiveness of tricyclic antidepressants in the treatment of coexisting pain and depression. Pain 7:331–341, 1979

Ward NG, Bloom V, Dworkin S, et al: Psychobiological markers in existing pain and depression: toward a united theory. J Clin Psychiatry 43:32–41, 1982

Weintraub MI: Litigation-chronic pain syndrome-a distinct entity: analysis of 210 cases. American Journal of Pain Management 2:198–204, 1992

Westbrook L, Cicala RS, Wright M: Effectiveness of Alprazolam in the treatment of chronic pain: results of a preliminary study. Clinical Journal of Pain 6:32–36, 1990

Willcockson WS, Chung JM, Hori Y, et al: Effects of iontophoretically released amino acids on primate spinothalamic tract cells. J Neurosci 4:741–750, 1984

Wood D, Wiesner M, Reiter R: Psychogenic chronic pelvic pain: diagnosis and management. Clin Obstet Gynecol 33:179–195, 1990

Yaksh TL, Duchateau JC, Rudy TA: Antagonism by methysergide and cinanserin of the antinociceptive action of morphine administered into the periaqueductal gray. Brain Res 104:367–372, 1976

18

Delirium

Larry Tune, M.D.
Christopher Ross, M.D., Ph.D.

Introduction

Delirium is a common, serious, and often unrecognized neuropsychiatric disturbance in geriatric psychiatry (Beresin 1988; Inouye et al. 1990; Lipowski 1987; McCartney and Palmateer 1985). It is found commonly among elderly patients with multiple medical problems, where it may be undiagnosed by as many as 32% of treating physicians (Francis et al. 1988). It is a cause of increased morbidity and mortality. Most studies estimate the in-hospital fatality rate for elderly delirious patients at 25%–33% (Bedford 1959; Gottlieb et al. 1991; Hodgkinson 1973; Inouye et al. 1990; Levkoff et al. 1986; Trzepacz et al. 1985). Thomas et al. (1986) looked at the effect of delirium on both death rates and prolonged hospital stay and found that the differences between the delirious and nondelirious patients, when fatality rates and length of stay were compared, were both highly significant. Follow-up studies at 1 month and 1 year postdelirium (Rabins and Folstein 1982) have also revealed significantly elevated mortality rates for patients with delirium. In addition, "development of delirium in the hospital is associated with increased morbidity, closer nursing surveillance, higher hospital costs per day, longer hospitalizations, and increased rates of nursing home placement" (Inouye et al. 1990, p. 941).

Diagnosis and Terminology

One major problem in assessing delirium in patients has been the absence of reliable and valid diagnostic criteria and rating instruments (Liptzin et al. 1991). DSM-IV (American Psychiatric Association 1994) has made diagnoses more consistent by providing more explicit criteria. The DSM-IV criteria for delirium are shown in Table 18–1. The central features of the criteria are alteration in attention (clouding of consciousness) and cognitive dysfunction of relatively transient duration. Delirium is distinguished from dementia principally by the alteration in level of consciousness. It is distinguished from mania or depression by the change in consciousness, as well as by cognitive dysfunction (though the latter can be present in affective disorder as well). It is differentiated from extreme fatigue or sleepiness by the cognitive dysfunction. There are also associated features such as changes in sleep-wake cycles and frequent illusions or hallucinations, usually visual, that can help clarify the

diagnosis. Classic descriptions of the cognitive, perceptual, and emotional features of delirium were provided by Wolff and Curran (1935) and by Chedru and Geschwind (1972).

The Mini-Mental State Exam (MMSE; Folstein et al. 1975) (see Table 18–2) is useful in quantitating the severity of cognitive impairment, but it was not designed specifically to distinguish dementia patients from delirium patients. Anthony et al. (1982) found the MMSE to be 87% sensitive and 82% specific for detecting cognitive impairment compared with a psychiatrist's evaluation; however, the false positive ratio was 39%, and the false positives were characterized by low education (less than 9 years) and advanced age.

To define the profile of cognitive changes in different degrees of delirium, Ross et al. (1991) examined subscales of the MMSE in patients with mild delirium (MMSE scores of 20–30), moderate delirium (MMSE scores of 10–20), and severe delirium (MMSE scores of 0–10) (Figure 18–1). Subscales most affected in the mildly delirious patients were calculation, orientation (especially to time), and recall. Subscales relatively preserved in the severely impaired patients were naming and registration. The patterns of these cognitive changes may explain some of the difficulties in diagnosing delirium. Certain subscales of the MMSE are disproportionately affected in mildly impaired patients. These scales include calculation, recall, and orientation. Tests of these functions may be especially

Table 18–1. DSM-IV criteria for delirium

A. Disturbance of consciousness (i.e., reduced clarity of awareness of the environment) with reduced ability to focus, sustain, or shift attention.

B. A change in cognition (such as memory deficit, disorientation, language disturbance) or the development of a perceptual disturbance that is not better accounted for by a preexisting, established, or evolving dementia.

C. The disturbance develops over a short period of time (usually hours to days) and tends to fluctuate during the course of the day.

D. There is evidence from the history, physical examination, or laboratory findings that the disturbance is caused by the direct physiological consequences of a general medical condition.

Source. Reprinted from American Psychiatric Association: *Diagnostic and Statistical Manual of Mental Disorders,* 4th Edition. Washington, DC, American Psychiatric Association, 1994, p. 129. Used with permission.

sensitive for detecting delirium. However, orientation to place is less sensitive than orientation to time. By contrast, basic language function is relatively preserved both in moderately and severely impaired patients, perhaps explaining why delirium may not be noted during ordinary conversations with patients.

Inouye et al. (1990) described a simple, yet effective method, the "Confusion Assessment Method," which incorporates nine operationalized criteria from DSM-III-R (American Psychiatric Association 1987) into an assessment method that can be applied quickly and reliably. This assessment method was found to have a sensitivity of 94%–100%, specificity of 90%–95%, and a value for positive predictive accuracy of 91%–94%. Validation of this method was somewhat tautological, because DSM-III (American Psychiatric Association 1980) criteria were being compared to DSM-III-R criteria.

The electroencephalogram (EEG) is diffusely slowed in delirium, making it the most useful diagnostic test (Brenner 1985). It is helpful, however, to have a previous baseline. For instance, a patient with Alzheimer's disease may have an abnormally slowed EEG at baseline, worsening further in delirium. Conversely, some delirious patients may have only minimal slowing, which would be read as within broad limits of normal without a previous baseline for comparison. In addition (as discussed below), some patients with activated delirium may not have discernible slowing, though this issue has not yet been well studied. Workup of delirium otherwise includes search for the underlying medical cause.

Table 18–2. Mini-Mental State Exam (MMSE)

Patient _____

Examiner _____

Date _____

Maximum score	Score	
		Orientation
5	( )	What is the (year) (date) (day) (month) (season)?
5	( )	Where are we (state) (county) (town) (hospital) (floor)?
		Registration
3	( )	Name 3 objects: 1 second to say each. Then ask the patient all 3 after you have said them. Give 1 point for each correct answer. Then repeat them until he or she learns all 3. Count trial and record. Trials
		Attention and calculation
5	( )	Serial 7s: 1 point for each correct. Stop after 5 answers. Alternately spell "world" backwards.
		Recall
5	( )	Ask for 3 objects repeated above. Give 1 point for each correct answer.
		Language
2	( )	Name a pencil and watch (2 points)
1	( )	Repeat the following: "no ifs, ands, or buts" (1 point)
3	( )	Follow a 3-stage command: "Take a paper in your right hand, fold it in half, and put it on the floor."
1	( )	Read and obey the following: "Close your eyes." (1 point)
1	( )	Write a sentence. Must contain subject and verb and be sensible. (1 point)
		Visual-motor integrity
1	( )	Copy design (2 intersecting pentagons. All 10 angles must be present and 2 must intersect.) (1 point)
		Total score _____
30	( )	Assess level of consciousness along a continuum. Alert _____ Drowsy _____ Stupor _____ Coma _____

Source. Reprinted from Folstein MF, Folstein SE, McHugh PR: "Mini-Mental State: A Practical Method for Grading the Cognitive State of Patients for the Clinician." *Journal of Psychiatric Research* 12:189–198, 1975. Used with permission.

Delirium is often considered a global and nonspecific disorder and function. This characterization may be appropriate for delirium caused by widespread systemic processes such as hypoxia, hypothermia, and acid-base disturbances. However, several important etiologies of delirium such as hepatic, renal, and other encephalopathies and drug-induced delirium may be associated with more limited and specific brain pathophysiology. Involvement of different brain systems may lead to differing phenotypes as described below.

Patients with delirium may differ in their symptoms. Although all delirious patients have clouding of consciousness (alteration of attention) and cognitive dysfunction, there may be other symptoms such as hallucinations, illusions, and delusions (Wolff and Curran 1935). Delirious patients may be agitated, which can result in injury or refusal to cooperate with medical personnel for treatment.

Many observers have suggested that delirious patients differ in their level of alertness. Some patients may be confused and unable to focus attention or to respond to the environment appropriately but, nevertheless, appear relatively alert. Our research group has termed such patients *activated* (Ross et al. 1991). Other patients are similarly confused but appear drowsy or stuporous. We have termed such patients *somnolent*. Lipowski (1989) made a similar distinction between "hyperalert/hyperactive" and "hypoalert/hypoactive" delirium patients.

We (Ross et al. 1991) have studied the phenomenology of patients with either activated or somnolent forms of delirium. In our study, we divided medically ill patients with delirium into somnolent and activated groups on the basis of apparent alertness. Overall, patients were moderately delirious with average MMSE scores of 13.3. There was little difference between the two groups in severity of delirium by MMSE score, Digit Span, or overall severity of clouding of consciousness (Table 18–3): 31% of patients had hallucinations or delusions or both (24% had hallucinations and 18% had delusions). These symptoms, however, were far more common in the activated patients than in the somnolent patients (Table 18–3). Because their cognitive dysfunction was similar (and there was no difference in language subscales on the MMSE), these differences in positive symptoms could not be explained by differences in the patients' ability to report their internal states. Further, these differences on mental status exam were also supported by differences in hallucinatory and delusional psychotic behaviors observed by nurses.

The importance of recognizing psychosis is twofold. First, it may be the cause of agitation (e.g., 55% of agitated patients had psychosis, whereas only 13% of patients who were not agitated had psychosis), and patients may act on their delusions. Second, psychosis can be treatable (as discussed below).

Etiology was related to phenomenology (Ross et al.

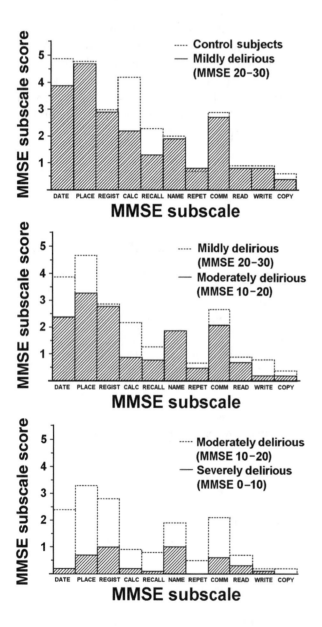

Figure 18–1. Mini-Mental State Exam (MMSE; Folstein et al. 1975) subscales for patients with mild, moderate, and severe delirium compared with control subjects. Orientation to time, calculation (CALC), and recall are most altered in mild delirium. Registration (REGIST), naming (NAME), and following a command (COMM) are most preserved for severe delirium. REPET = repetition.

1991). All of the patients with hepatic encephalopathy were somnolent, whereas fever (the second most common etiology of delirium in this group) was approximately equally likely to cause somnolent or activated delirium. There was a trend for patients with alcohol withdrawal to have activated delirium (3 out of 3), consistent with longstanding clinical observations of patients with delirium tremens as being hyperalert and hallucinated.

There may be clinical utility in differentiating these subtypes of delirium patients. The differentiation may aid in formulating diagnoses. Physicians may not notice the presence of an abnormal mental status in cooperative patients with somnolent delirium. Thus clinical suspicion of delirium in patients who appear sleepy needs to remain high. By contrast, patients with the activated subtype may be appreciated to have abnormal mental status, but may be more likely to be confused with patients who have schizophrenia, hysteria, or other diagnoses. Further, patients with activated delirium may be more likely to injure themselves, refuse treatment, or require close observation. Therefore, recognizing their phenomenology could lead to more timely diagnosis and therapeutic interventions. Furthermore, once the pathophysiologies of different forms of delirium are clarified, it may be found that different subtypes require different treatment.

Table 18–3. Characteristics of patients with somnolent versus activated delirium

Characteristics	Somnolent patients $n = 39$	Activated patients $n = 19$
Age	54.3 ± 18.7	50.4 ± 17.8
MMSE	13.6 ± 7.4	13.2 ± 7.3
Digit span	4.1 ± 2.4	4.6 ± 2.2
Clouding of consciousness (1–10 scale)	5.7 ± 2.4	5.7 ± 2.3
Somnolence (1–10 scale)	5.4 ± 2.3	2.4 ± 2.0[***]
Hallucinations	3%	67%[***]
Illusions	0%	26%[**]
Delusions	3%	50%[***]
Paranoia	0%	20%
Agitation	21%	71%[***]

Note. MMSE = Mini-Mental State Exam (Folstein et al. 1975).
[**]$P < .01$.
[***]$P < .001$.
Adapted from Ross et al. 1991.

Epidemiology

Findings from prevalence studies of delirium have varied greatly. One major contributing factor to this has been the absence of clearly defined, operationalized, diagnostic criteria. In fact, it has only been in the last decade, with the publication of DSM-III and DSM-III-R criteria, that diagnostic criteria for the syndrome have been adequately operationalized to allow cross-study comparisons.

Other problems in establishing meaningful incidence and prevalence figures are large differences in 1) case finding methods; 2) research instruments and techniques; 3) study populations; 4) patient selection criteria (1–4 reviewed in Levkoff et al. 1991); 5) comorbidity—delirium is often found in patients with other etiologies for cognitive impairments (e.g., dementia); and 6) a tendency (partly due to an absence of operationalized criteria) to apply a wide range of diagnostic labels to the syndrome. Liston (1982) identified more than 30 terms that may have been applied to the syndrome of delirium.

Given the broad scope of these problems associated with delirium research, it is not surprising that estimates vary widely. For medical inpatient units, the prevalence varies from 10% to 30%, whereas incidence figures are even more disparate: from 4% to 53.2% (Levkoff et al. 1991). This extreme variation is dramatically diminished with the application of DSM-III criteria. Levkoff et al. (1991) compared five studies (Cameron et al. 1987; Erkinjuntii et al. 1986; Francis et al. 1990; Johnson et al. 1990; Rockwood 1989) in which DSM-III criteria were used to determine prevalence figures for medical inpatients. The prevalence of delirium was 11.3%–16%, and the incidence was 4.2%–10.4%.

Three recent studies of the epidemiology of delirium in elderly patients are particularly noteworthy. The Commonwealth-Harvard study on delirium in elderly patients (Levkoff et al. 1991) investigated patients 65 years or older who were admitted to the Beth Israel Hospital for acute cares over a 1-year period from one of two sources: the Hebrew Rehabilitation Center for the Aged (a local chronic care facility) and a defined community (East Boston). DSM-III criteria were applied prospectively, and well-defined rating instruments were used. Of the 211 community-based elderly subjects, 24.2% satisfied DSM-III criteria for delirium. Of the 114 patients admitted from the chronic care facility, 64.9% were diagnosed as having delirium. In another study, Gottlieb et al. (1991) prospectively determined the incidence and prevalence of delirium in 235 consecutive subjects over age 70 who were admitted to a general medical ward. Using DSM-III criteria, 16% were found to be delirious on admission, and an additional 5% became delirious during their hospital stay. These figures contrast sharply with the estimate of delirium in the community reported in the 1981 East Baltimore Mental Health Survey (part of the Epidemiologic Catchment Area (ECA) program, which found the prevalence of delirium in the population age 55 and over to be 0.4%–1.1% (Folstein et al. 1991).

Neurobiology

Central Arousal Systems

The cardinal symptoms of delirium are disorders of cognition and alterations in arousal and attention. The normal physiology of arousal and attention is still only partially understood, but in the past few years modern pathway tracing techniques and chemical anatomic techniques have allowed the tracing of ascending symptoms likely to be involved in maintenance of normal arousal and attention (see Ross 1991; Saper 1986).

The classic picture of central arousal systems involves the concept of a "reticular activating system" diffusely distributed in the brain stem and projecting multisynaptically to the thalamic intralaminar nuclei (Lindsley et al. 1950; Moruzzi and Magoun 1949). However, studies using modern anatomical techniques (for a review, see Saper 1986) have shown that these so-called nonspecific afferents to the superficial cortex, which are believed to be involved in maintenance of cortical arousal, do not arise exclusively from the thalamus; critical sources of nonspecific cortical afferents may be extrathalamic regions such as basal forebrain, hypothalamus, and more caudal brain stem. Furthermore, these extrathalamic cortical afferent systems contain neurotransmitters, which may relate to the pathophysiology of delirium.

These studies (see Saper 1986) have suggested a differing organization of cortical nonspecific afferents within the thalamus than was previously appreciated. The diffuse innervation of superficial cortex appears now to arise less from the intralaminar nuclei and more from the ventromedial thalamic nucleus, as well as the ventroanterolateral nucleus, the lateral dorsal nucleus, and the posterior and lateral posterior nuclei (Herkenham 1980). Physiological studies of the role of the thalamus in sleep and arousal have yielded contradictory results. Ranson (1939) found little effect of large lesions of the thalamus on sleep and arousal in sleep in the monkey. However, a hereditary condition involving the selective degeneration of certain thalamic nuclei has recently been found to be associated with marked abnormalities of sleep and consciousness (Lugaresi et al. 1986), supporting other clinical observations. There is little knowledge of the neurotransmitters that might be involved in these thalamic projections, so it is at present difficult to relate these projections to the syndrome of delirium.

Basal Forebrain Cholinergic Projections

Cholinergic neurons in the basal forebrain provide widespread topographically organized innervation of layers 1, 3, 5, and 6 of the cerebral cortex (Saper 1984, 1986). Application of acetylcholine within the cortex causes predominantly excitatory responses. This projection may be involved in the generation of cortical and hippocampal EEG rhythms. Basal forebrain cholinergic neurons degenerate in Alzheimer's disease (Coyle et al. 1983). As described below, drugs with anticholinergic properties are important contributors to the problem of delirium in hospitalized patients. It may be that disruption of the function of the basal forebrain cholinergic cortical afferents explains some of the features of anticholinergic delirium. This would be consistent with the fact that patients with Alzheimer's disease, in whom these neurons are already compromised, are unusually sensitive to anticholinergics. However, the fact that under most circumstances Alzheimer's patients do not have changes in consciousness, despite their loss of basal forebrain cholinergic neurons, suggests that abnormalities of other cholinergic neurons such as cholinergic neurons in the brain stem may be more important in delirium.

Hypothalamic-Cortical Projections

Classic physiological experiments suggested early on an important role for the hypothalamus in the regulation of sleep and arousal (Nauta 1946). More recent experiments, such as injections of excitatory amino acid toxins (Jouvet 1988), have suggested a particular role for the posterolateral hypothalamus in regulation of sleep and waking. Although traditional views of the reticular formation assume that the hypothalamus must project through the thalamus to reach the cortex, modern pathway tracing techniques have demonstrated direct hypothalamic projections to the cerebral cortex (Kievet and Kuypers 1975; Saper 1985). The areas that project directly to the cortex are the fields of Forel, the posterior lateral hypothalamic area, and the tuberal lateral and tuberal mammary hypothalamic areas. In fact, the hypothalamus contains more neurons innervating the cerebral cortex than does the basal forebrain. Most suggestive for the pathophysiology of delirium are neurons in this region of hypothalamus containing γ-aminobutyric acid (GABA) and histamine.

Double-label retrograde transport immunocytochemical techniques have been used to demonstrate GABA-synthesizing neurons residing in the posterior hypothalamus and projecting to the cerebral cortex (Vincent et al. 1983). One interesting possibility is that these systems may be involved in the pathophysiology of hepatic encephalopathy. Alterations of GABA or benzodiazepine-like systems in animal models with hepatic encephalopathy are suggested by reports of altered benzodiazepine receptor binding (Baraldi et al. 1984). Benzodiazepine antagonists can ameliorate hepatic encephalopathy in both animal models and patients (Bansky et al. 1985; Baraldi et al. 1984; Bassett et al. 1987). As discussed below, clinical studies in humans have suggested that benzodiazepine antagonists may be helpful in treating hepatic encephalopathy.

Histamine-synthesizing hypothalamic neurons are present in the posterior hypothalamus, are concentrated in the magnocellular nuclei and the tuberal regions (Wada et al. 1991), and project diffusely to the cerebral cortex. Jouvet's group (1988) suggested that histaminergic neurons in the hypothalamus have an arousing function (Lin et al. 1990). It is possible that these neurons may be involved in the delirium caused by anticholinergic drugs (discussed below), because many drugs with anticholinergic properties are also antihistaminergics.

Brain Stem Neuronal Groups

In addition to projections from the hypothalamus and basal forebrain, there are well known monoaminergic nuclei in the pons and midbrain that project diffusely to the cerebral cortex. These include midbrain dopa-minergic groups in the midbrain ventral tegmentum, cholinergic neurons in the rostral pons, noradrenergic neurons in the locus ceruleus, and serotonergic neurons in the raphe complex. Dopaminergic systems have no clear role in the pathophysiology of delirium, but presumably are involved in the response to neuroleptics. Neurons in the locus ceruleus have been implicated in the control of attention and arousal (Foote et al. 1980). Serotonergic neurons have been linked to the visual hallucinations after ingestion of LSD-like hallucinogenic drugs (Glennon et al. 1984; Trulson et al. 1976). Hallucinogens induce an oneiroid state resembling delirium. Further, unlike the characteristic auditory hallucinations of schizophrenia or manic-depressive illness, the hallucinations induced by hallucinogens and seen in delirium tend to be visual.

Pathophysiology

Considering the high prevalence and clinical importance of delirium, there is relatively little known about its pathophysiology. Few studies of cerebral blood flow or metabolic activity have been carried out in delirium. Patients with hepatic encephalopathy have dramatically lower global cerebral metabolic activity compared with control subjects (McDermott and Adams 1954; Posner and Plum 1960). As discussed above, hepatic encephalopathy appears to be a typical somnolent form of delirium. Our group has hypothesized that other patients with the somnolent form of delirium would also have a globally slowed metabolic rate. Interestingly, in one study of patients with alcohol withdrawal delirium, which is characteristic of the activated form of delirium, cerebral blood flow measured by single photon emission computed tomography (SPECT) was normal or even increased (Hemmingsen et al. 1988).

In general, the EEG is slowed in delirium (Romano and Engel 1944), which makes it a very useful diagnostic test, but there may be exceptions in different patients. For instance, slowing is pronounced in hepatic encephalopathy (Parsons-Smith et al. 1957), which we have found to cause the somnolent subtype of delirium (Ross et al. 1991). However, several authors (Isbell et al. 1950; Kennard et al. 1945; Pro and Wells 1977) have suggested that in alcohol or sedative-hypnotic withdrawal delirium, which is more likely to be the activated subtype, the EEG may often exhibit increased low-voltage fast activity. One might make an analogy between these different forms of delirium and different forms of sleep in healthy humans and animals: rapid-eye-movement (REM) sleep and slow-wave sleep are associated with increases and decreases, respectively, of cerebral blood flow and metabolism in specific brain regions, and REM sleep has a low-voltage fast EEG, whereas slow-wave sleep has large slow waves. One might speculate that pathways involved in slow-wave sleep are more important in the pathophysiology of somnolent delirium, whereas those involved in REM sleep are more important in the pathophysiology of activated delirium.

Although many mechanisms may be etiologically relevant to delirium, only a few have been well studied. One of the best-studied hypotheses involves disturbance of cholinergic neurotransmission. As discussed above, the cholinergic system is widely distributed through the brain (Shute and Lewis 1974), including components of the nonspecific cortical afferent system. Cholinergic projections from the nucleus basalis of Meynert to cortex have been shown to be important in memory processes (Kwoonyuen et al. 1990), in aging, and to the pathophysiology of Alzheimer's disease. The cholinergic system is sensitive to a variety of metabolic insults including impairments of oxygenation or glucose utilization, each of which has been shown to impair cholinergic synthesis and/or release (Gibson et al. 1991). Anticholinergic compounds have been shown to impair memory and attention in healthy elderly subjects (Miller et al. 1988) and to impair cognition and to be associated with delirium in situations in which anticholinergic toxicity has been postulated (see below). An animal model of delirium has been developed by treating animals with anticholinergic compounds (Trzepacz et al. 1992). These animals show behavioral impairments suggestive of confusion and EEG slowing and disorganization consistent with human clinical delirium. This model may be useful for testing pharmacological interventions to treat delirium, particularly anticholinergic delirium.

A second animal model of delirium that has been widely studied is that of hepatic encephalopathy. Fulminant hepatic failure can be induced in animals by injection of galactosamine causing behavioral changes and changes in EEG and visual evoked potentials similar to those seen in hepatic encephalopathy (Schafer et al. 1983). Another animal model involves the surgical creation of portacaval shunts. When such animals are given an acute ammonium load, there is stupor accompanied by EEG slowing and decreased cerebral blood flow and metabolism (Gjedde et al. 1978).

It has been suggested that when the liver fails, an endogenous benzodiazepine-like toxin is produced either peripherally or in the brain itself and that this substance binds to cerebral benzodiazepine receptors causing encephalopathy (Basile et al. 1991; Mullen et al. 1987). Consistent with this idea are reports of altered benzodiazepine receptor binding in animal models of hepatic encephalopathy (Baraldi et al. 1984). It has been suggested that a brain neuropeptide called *diazepam-binding inhibitor* (DBI) may be elevated in hepatic encephalopathy and may mediate the syndrome; however, the specificity of these findings is uncertain (Barbaccia et al. 1986; Rothstein et al. 1989). Perhaps the strongest evidence that the benzodiazepine system is involved in hepatic encephalopathy comes from studies of benzodiazepine antagonists. Such antagonists have little effect on healthy animals. However, in animals with experimentally induced hepatic encephalopathy, benzodiazepine antagonists induce behavioral activation, as well as improvement in EEG and visual evoked potential abnormalities (Baraldi et al. 1984; Bassett et al. 1987). Clinical studies in humans have suggested that benzodiazepine antagonists may be helpful in treating human hepatic encephalopathy (Bansky et al. 1985; Grimm et al. 1987).

Etiology and Risk Factors

Etiologies

Among elderly patients, Flint (1956) found that the most frequent etiologies of delirium were cerebrovascular accident, heart failure, and pneumonia. Other causes include drug toxicity, metabolic and electrolyte abnormalities, dementia, cancer, and sensory deprivation or impairments (Table 18–4) (Francis and Kapoor 1990). Many cases are multifactorial; occasionally, no clear etiology may be found.

Risk Factors

Several of the most important studies investigating risk factors for delirium are reviewed in Table 18–5. One of the most common and most widely identified risk factor for delirium is the aging process itself (Beresin 1988; Lipowski 1987, 1989). Lipowski (1989) thought the factors that predisposed elderly people to delirium included "aging processes in the brain, structural brain disease, a reduced capacity for homeostatic reg-

Table 18–4. Common causes of delirium

Metabolic or endocrine

Electrolyte abnormality
(especially Na^+, K^+,
Ca^{++}, and Mg^{++})

Hyperglycemia or
hypoglycemia

Hypoxia or hypercarbia

Liver or kidney failure

Thyroid disorder

Fever

Infection

Sepsis

Pneumonia

Urinary tract infection
or upper respiratory
infection in elderly
patients

Drug toxicity

Anticholinergics

Anticholinergic
psychoactive

medications
(e.g., neuroleptics
and tricyclic
antidepressants)

Lithium

Electroconvulsive
therapy (ECT)

Steroids

Drug or alcohol withdrawal

Central nervous system lesion

Postictal states

Raised intracranial
pressure

Head trauma

Encephalitis or
meningitis

Vasculitis

Multifactorial

ulation and hence for resistance to stress, the impairment of vision and hearing, a high prevalence of chronic diseases, reduced resistance to acute diseases, and age-related changes in the pharmacokinetics and pharmacodynamics of drugs. [Common precipitants were] sleep loss, sensory deprivation, sensory overload, and psychosocial stress occasioned by bereavement or relocation to an unfamiliar environment" (Lipowski 1989, p. 578).

In a study of 229 elderly patients admitted to a general medical service, Francis et al. (1990) identified the following risk factors for delirium in the elderly: abnormal sodium level, severity of illness, dementia, fever or hypothermia, psychoactive drug use, and azotemia. The rate of delirium was 60% when patients had three or more risk factors. In a separate investigation of 91 elderly patients who became delirious following admission to general medical and surgical wards of a tertiary care facility, independent risk factors for in-hospital deliria included prior cognitive impairment, age greater than 80, fracture on admission, symptomatic infection,

Table 18–5. Risk factors for delirium

Study	Patient sample	Age range	Source	Percent delirious	Risk factors
Schor et al. 1992	291 patients not delirious on first evaluation	> 65	Medical and surgical wards	Incidence in hospital = 31.3%	Prior cognitive impairment Age > 80 Fracture on admission Symptomatic infection Male sex Neuroleptic or narcotic use
Michocki and Lamy 1988	46 orthopedic patients	Mean age = 67.5	Orthopedic in-patient unit	26%	Primary aging factors: slower thought and metabolic factors Secondary aging factors: hypoxia, ischemia, sepsis, uremia, fluid electrolyte unbalance, and anemia Tertiary aging factors: psychosocial stress Drug factors: alcohol, antidepressants, sedative, and anticholinergics
Rogers et al. 1989	46 orthopedic patients	Mean age = 67.5	Orthopedic in-patient unit	26%	Drugs: propranolol, flurazepam, scopolamine
Berggren et al. 1987	57 patients with femoral neck fracture	> 64 years	Orthopedic inpatients	44%	History of mental confusion History of anticholinergic drug use
Erkinjuntii et al. 1986	2,000 consecutive patients	≥ 55 years	Medical inpatients	41.4% of patients with dementia 12.4% of patients without dementia	Early postoperative hypoxemia and dementia
Francis et al. 1990	229 elderly patients	≥ 70 years	Medical inpatients	22% overall	Predictors include abnormal sodium level, severe illness, chronic cognitive impairment; fever or hypothermia; psychoactive drug use; azotemia

male sex, and use of either neuroleptics or narcotic an-algesics (Schor et al. 1992).

Dementia and Delirium

One risk factor for delirium in the elderly population is dementia. It is likely that one reason the diagnosis of delirium is missed is the co-occurrence of preexisting cognitive impairment and delirium. In a study of 2,000 consecutive admissions to a general medical service, Erkinjuntii et al. (1986) found that mild to moderate dementia was present in 9.1% of all patients, increasing from 0.8% at age 55 to 31.2% in patients 85 and older. Of the patients with dementia, 41.4% were diagnosed as having delirium on admission, and 24.9% of all delirium patients were found subsequently to have a dementing illness. Delirium patients have more evidence of preexisting brain lesions by imaging than do control subjects, perhaps especially posterior cerebral cortical infarction (Devinsky et al. 1988; Kwoonyuen et al. 1990).

Drug Toxicity

Drug-induced delirium is well recognized (Gosney and Tallis 1984; Report of Royal College of Physicians 1984), and it may be attributed to age-related changes in drug disposition (Greenblatt et al. 1982), to medication errors, and to polypharmacy (Klein et al. 1981). One recent survey (Williamson and Chopin 1980) attributed 10% of geriatric admissions to general medical wards to adverse drug reactions. In a study of 200 consecutive patients over age 60 who presented with the complaint of dementia, Larsen et al. (1985) found that drug toxicity was the most common form of "treatable dementia." There is general agreement that drug toxicity is the most frequent cause of delirium in hospitalized elderly patients (Francis and Kapoor 1990; Lipowski 1989).

One possible mechanism of drug-induced delirium is the accumulation of anticholinergic effects of commonly prescribed medications on a central cholinergic system that declines with age and that is severely impaired by neurodegenerative disease processes common in the elderly population (Blass and Plum 1983; Coffman and Disalver 1988; Francis and Kapoor 1990; Lipowski 1989; Sunderland et al. 1987). This "predisposition" is then coupled with the fact that elderly patients attending general medical clinics tend to take increasing numbers of medications (Klein et al. 1981;

Stewart and Hale 1992), many of which have significant anticholinergic effects (Blazer et al. 1983; Tune et al. 1993). Larsen et al. (1985) found that 11.6% of patients with suspected dementia had drug-related cognitive impairment and that the odds ratio of drug induced dementia increased from 1.0 in patients taking none to one drug to 9.3 in patients taking four to five drugs. Because cross sectional studies of drug use in elderly patients have consistently shown that they typically take 1.7–2.7 prescription drugs, in addition to nonprescription medications, and that these numbers increase with advancing age (Hale et al. 1987; Helling et al. 1987; Stewart and Hale 1992), the risk of drug-induced delirium as a function of increasing age is substantial.

Many commonly prescribed medications not usually associated with anticholinergic toxicity have been found to have anticholinergic activity. The possibility of toxicity, resulting from combinations of many medications with relatively small anticholinergic effects, but whose additive effects are cumulative, must be considered. Recently, 14 of the 25 most commonly prescribed medications in elderly patients were found to have detectable anticholinergic effects (Table 18–6) (Tune et al. 1992). This cumulative effect may be widespread, particularly in nursing home populations (Blazer et al. 1983; Ray et al. 1980) and may occur in up to 16%–35% of elderly patients receiving anticholinergic medications (Lamy 1986; Walker and Brodie 1980). Berggren et al. (1987) found that the use of drugs with anticholinergic effects was significantly associated with postoperative confusion in a cohort of patients undergoing surgery for femoral neck fractures. In a recent investigation of postoperative delirium in a cohort of largely elderly patients in a surgical intensive care unit, the additive anticholinergic effects of a wide variety of medications was associated with the prevalence of delirium (Tune et al. 1993). A few investigators have not found a significant relationship between anticholinergic use and confusion (Seifert et al. 1983).

There is general agreement that physicians are limited in their ability to accurately identify the potential that most medications, singly or in combination, have for inducing cognitive impairments (Morrison and Katz 1989; Stewart and Hale 1992). Although not widely available, serum and plasma anticholinergic drug levels, determined by antimuscarinic anticholinergic radioreceptor assay, have been used by several groups to investigate the relationship between anticholinergic toxicity, primarily from polypharmacy, and toxic and confusional states in elderly patients (Tune and Bylsma 1991). Miller et al. (1988) compared low-dose scopolamine (as a presurgical medication) and placebo in a small group of elderly patients. Even though the dose of scopolamine was very small (0.005 mg/kg body weight), anticholinergic levels were detectable and were significantly associated with impairments in an auditory verbal learning task.

Rovner et al. (1988) studied the relationship between serum anticholinergic drug levels, cognition, and self-care capacity in 22 elderly nursing home residents with dementia. Patients received on average 2.7 drugs per day, resulting in a wide range of anticholinergic drug levels (0.0–9.9 pm/ml; median level = 0.83 pm/ml atropine equivalents). When patients above

and below the median drug level were compared, the higher anticholinergic levels were associated with more impairments in self-care capacity (including dressing, personal hygiene, mobility, toileting, and urinary incontinence). There was a limited, but significant, correlation between anticholinergic drug level and a global self-care score ($r = 0.42$; df = 20; $P = .015$).

Mach et al. (1990) studied a cohort of hospitalized elderly patients with delirium of diverse etiologies and compared them to a cohort of patients who were previously delirious, but in whom the delirium had cleared. Twenty-two of 140 inpatients (ages 62–90) were diagnosed as having delirium. Serum anticholinergic activity was significantly elevated in the delirious patients (anticholinergic level = 30.26 ± 4.7 nM atropine equivalents) compared with that in control subjects (anticholinergic level = 16.91 ± 3.94 nM atropine equivalents; $P < .05$) and with that in patients whose delirium had resolved (anticholinergic level = 19.60 ± 4.03 nM atropine equivalents; $P = .05$).

Tollefson et al. (1991) studied a cohort of 34 randomly selected nursing home residents. Using a randomized, repeated measures design, patients were randomly assigned to an intervention group ($n = 15$; anticholinergics were either discontinued or lowered) and to a control group in which no intervention was made. Patients were administered a battery of tests on inclusion into the study and at 4 weeks postintervention. In the intervention group, several of the neuropsychological test performances improved significantly in direct relationship to decreasing anticholinergic level.

Table 18–6. Anticholinergic drug levels in 25 medications ranked by the frequency of their prescription for elderly patients

Medication[a]	Anticholinergic drug level (ng/ml of atropine equivalents)
1. Furosemide	0.22
2. Digoxin	0.25
3. Dyazide (hydrochlorothiazide and triamterene	0.08
4. Lanoxin[b]	0.25
5. Hydrochlorothiazide	0.00
6. Propranolol	0.00
7. Salicylic acid	0.00
8. Dipyridamole	0.11
9. Theophylline anhydrous	0.44
10. Nitroglycerin	0.00
11. Insulin	0.00
12. Warfarin	0.12
13. Prednisolone	0.55
14. α-Methyldopa	0.00
15. Nifedipine	0.22
16. Isosorbide dinitrate	0.15
17. Ibuprofen	0.00
18. Codeine	0.11
19. Cimetidine	0.86
20. Diltiazem hydrochloride	0.00
21. Captopril	0.02
22. Atenolol	0.00
23. Metoprolol	0.00
24. Timolol	0.00
25. Ranitidine	0.22

[a]Drug concentration = 10^{-8} M.
[b]A digoxin compound.

Treatment

There have been few systematic studies of the management and treatment of delirium. Clearly, the first and critical step is to identify and correct the underlying etiology. Occasionally, the etiology is unclear either because a correct diagnosis cannot be made or because multiple causes can be identified (Cutting 1980; Rabins 1991). Beyond diagnostic issues, it is essential to manage allied behavioral symptoms and to provide an appropriate, supportive environment. Table 18–7 provides a basic checklist of issues relevant to the care and management of the patient with delirium. The patient is disoriented and memory impaired, and a strategy of frequent, shorter interventions is essential. The patient will likely require reassurance and reorientation multiple times through the day. This requires that all caregivers, including the family, be educated about the nature and management of the syndrome. Care must be exercised to ensure that the patient, as much as possible, is not distressed by the environment or the abnormal mental experiences associated with this syndrome. Some patients will be reassured by being told that their confusion is a "side effect" of a transient neuropsychiatric condition. Other patients will be distressed by this information.

The physician should constantly seek psychosocial interventions that minimize the use of medications. For example, moving a patient out of a distressing "high tech" environment (e.g., a surgical intensive care unit), as soon as medically safe, will facilitate in symptomatic improvement. Having family members present to help in reassuring and reorienting the patient can allay the patient's fears. Because many of these "behavioral" techniques are effective, management (or at least involvement in patient management) by a psychiatrist is often essential. Similarly, many delirious patients, especially elderly patients, may be managed better on a psychiatric rather than typical medical floor. The decision regarding the best management venue must be informed by the medical stability of the patient. Many delirious patients, especially elderly patients, do better on psychiatric floors with adequate medical backup than they do on medical floors with psychiatric consultation. General medical measures include prevention and management of possible fluid and electrolyte disturbances, aspiration, malnutrition, decubitus ulcers, and other complications of delirium (Francis and Kapoor 1990).

Of all the pharmacological agents available for short-term management of delirium, haloperidol is most widely used and accepted (Francis and Kapoor 1990; Menza et al. 1988). It should be emphasized that there are few well-controlled studies carefully investigating drugs in the management of delirium. Doses of haloperidol in the range 0.5–2.0 mg, repeated every half hour as needed to suppress agitated behavior, are generally well tolerated even when administered intravenously (Francis and Kapoor 1990). The side effects of haloperidol can mimic or exacerbate symptoms of delirium. Of concern is akathisia, which can easily be confused with agitation associated with delirium. For this reason, care should be taken to examine the patient before treatment (or as soon after as the clinical situation allows) for presence of extrapyramidal symptoms. Should these symptoms occur, the addition of a benzodiazepine to haloperidol may be warranted (Adams et al. 1986; Francis and Kapoor 1990; Menza et al. 1988). Adams et al. (1986) have suggested lorazepam 0.5–1.0 mg iv, repeated hourly as necessary, to ensure adequate sedation.

Neuroleptic malignant syndrome (NMS) is a rare, potentially lethal side effect of neuroleptic administration, associated with change in consciousness, fever, and rigidity. NMS has been described in elderly, delirious patients (Francis and Kapoor 1990). Once again, careful monitoring of the patient's neurological state is essential to identification of possible confounding side effects. Also, the patient should be carefully monitored on a regular basis to ensure that neuroleptics are discontinued as soon as possible. There have been no studies so far comparing the treatment of activated versus somnolent delirium. Haloperidol is often useful for activated delirium; benzodiazepine antagonists might be especially useful for somnolent delirium.

Table 18–7. Management of delirium

A. Pharmacological interventions and physical restraints
1. Avoid physical restraints if possible. Evaluate their need daily. Consider alternatives including the use of sitters and family members to calm the patient.
2. Use lowest possible doses of neuroleptics and/or benzodiazepines.
3. Reassess need for these interventions **at least** daily. The goal is to discontinue neuroleptics as soon as possible.
4. When patients are administered neuroleptics, carefully monitor and document the patient's neurological status for presence of extrapyramidal side effects.

B. Psychosocial aspects (providing a predictable, orienting senvironment)
1. The room should be adequately lit, including the use of night lights in the evening—to decrease illusions (Evans 1987).
2. Avoid excessive stimulation. Keep exposure to chaotic environments (e.g., intensive care units) to a minimum because many delirious patients are hyperresponsive to stimuli.
3. The room should have a large calender and clock.
4. The staff and family should make an effort to remind patient of the day and date **frequently.**
5. If possible, familiar items from home should be brought in.
6. If clinical state allows, provide eyeglasses and hearing aids to patients who had them prior to illness.
7. Encourage **frequent** interactions with staff and family.
8. Consider telling the patient he or she is confused and disoriented.

Summary

Delirium is characterized by reversible alterations in attention ("clouding of consciousness") and cognition. Some "activated" patients have increased levels of arousal and often have hallucinations and delusions, whereas "somnolent" patients have decreased levels of arousal and appear confused and sleepy. The clinical examination remains the mainstay of diagnosis, though slowing of the EEG is a relatively sensitive and specific test, especially for patients with somnolent delirium. The neurobiology of delirium may include relatively specific alteration of ascending pathways with defined neurotransmitters, as well as more diffuse cerebral dysfunction. A number of risk factors have been identified, the most consistent of which are age, comorbid cognitive impairment (notably dementia), and drug toxicity. Drug toxicity may well be reduced by an increased awareness of the cumulative anticholinergic effects of commonly prescribed compounds.

References

Adams F, Fernandez F, Andersson BS: Emergency pharmacotherapy of delirium in the critically ill cancer patient. Psychosomatics 27:33–37, 1986

American Psychiatric Association: Diagnostic and Statistical Manual of Mental Disorders, 3rd Edition. Washington, DC, American Psychiatric Association, 1980

American Psychiatric Association: Diagnostic and Statistical Manual of Mental Disorders, 3rd Edition, Revised. Washington, DC, American Psychiatric Association, 1987

Anthony JC, Niaz LU, von Korff M, et al: Limits of the Mini-Mental State as a screening for dementia and delirium among hospital patients. Psychol Med 12:397–408, 1982

Bansky G, Meier PJ, Zeigler WH, et al: Reversal of hepatic coma by benzodiazepine antagonist (RO15-1788). Lancet 1:1324–1325, 1985

Baraldi M, Zeneroli M, Ventura E, et al: Supersensitivity of benzodiazepine receptors in hepatic encephalopathy due to fulminant hepatic failure in the rat: reversal by a benzodiazepine antagonist. Clin Sci 67:167–175, 1984

Barbaccia ML, Costa E, Ferrero P, et al: Diazepam-binding inhibitor a brain neuropeptide present in human spinal fluid: studies in depression, schizophrenia and Alzheimer's disease. Arch Gen Psychiatry 43:1143–1147, 1986

Basile AS, Hughes RD, Harrison PM, et al: Elevated brain concentrations of 1,4-benzodiazepines in fulminant hepatic failure. N Engl J Med 325:473–478, 1991

Bassett ML, Mullen KD, Skolnick P, et al: Amelioration of hepatic encephalopathy by pharmacologic antagonism of the BABA-benzodiazepine receptor complex in a rabbit model of fulminant hepatic failure. Gastroenterology 93:1069–1077, 1987

Bedford PD: General medical aspects of confusional states in elderly people. BMJ 2:185–188, 1959

Beresin EV: Delirium in the elderly. J Geriatr Psychiatry Neurol 1:127–143, 1988

Berggren D, Gustafson Y, Erikssen B, et al: Postoperative confusion after anesthesia in elderly patients with femoral neck fractures. Anesth Analg 66:497–504, 1987

Blass JP, Plum F: Metabolic encephalopathies in older adults, in The Neurology of Aging. Edited by Katzman R, Terry RD. Philadelphia, PA, FA Davis, 1983, pp 189–219

Blazer DG II, Federspiel CF, Ray WA, et al: The risk of anticholinergic toxicity in the elderly: a study of prescribing practices in two populations. J Gerontol 38:31–35, 1983

Brenner RP: The electroencephalogram in altered states of consciousness. Neurological Clinics 3:615–613, 1985

Cameron DJ, Thomas RI, Mulvihill M, et al: Delirium: a test of the "Diagnostic and Statistics Manual III" criteria on medical inpatients. J Am Geriatr Soc 35:1007–1010, 1987

Chedru F, Geschwind N: Disorders of higher cortical functions in acute confusional states. Cortex 8:395–411, 1972

Coffman JA, Disalver SC: Cholinergic mechanisms in delirium (letter). Am J Psychiatry 145:382–383, 1988

Coyle JR, Price DL, DeLong MR: Alzheimer's disease: a disorder of cortical cholinergic innervation. Science 219:1184–1190, 1983

Cutting J: Physical illness and psychosis. Br J Psychiatry 136:109–119, 1980

Devinsky O, Bear D, Volpe BT: Confusional states following posterior cerebral artery infarction. Arch Neurol 160–163, 1988

Erkinjuntii T, Wikstrom J, Palo J, et al: Dementia among medical inpatients. Arch Int Med 146:1923–1926, 1986

Evans LK: Sundown syndrome in institutionalized elderly. J Am Geriatr Soc 35:101–108, 1987

Flint FJ: Organic basis of confusional states in the elderly. BMJ 2:1537–1539, 1956

Folstein MF, Folstein SE, McHugh PR: Mini-Mental State: a practical method for grading the cognitive state of patients for the clinician. J Psychiatr Res 12:189–198, 1975

Folstein M, Bassett SS, Romanoski A, et al: The epidemiology of delirium in the community: the eastern Baltimore mental health survey. Int Psychogeriatr 3:169–176, 1991

Foote SL, Anton-Jones G, Bloom FE: Impulse activity of locus ceruleus neurons in awake rats and monkeys as a function of sensory stimulation and arousal. Proc Natl Acad Sci U S A 77:3033–3037, 1980

Francis J, Kapoor WN: Delirium in hospitalized elderly. J Gen Intern Med 5:65–79, 1990

Francis J, Strong J, Martin D, et al: Delirium in elderly general medical patients: common but often unrecognized (abstract). Clin Res 36:711A, 1988

Francis J, Martin D, Kapoor WN: A prospective study of delirium in hospitalized elderly. JAMA 263:1097–1101, 1990

Gibson G, Blass JP, Huang H-M, et al: The cellular basis of delirium and its relevance to age related disorders including Alzheimer's disease. Int Psychogeriatr 3:373–395, 1991

Gjedde A, Lockwood AH, Duffy TE, et al: Cerebral blood flow and metabolism in chronically hyperammonemic rats: effect of an acute ammonia challenge. Ann Neurol 3:325–330, 1978

Glennon RA, Titeler M, McKenney JD: Evidence for 5-HT2 involvement in the mechanism of action of hallucinogenic agents. Life Sci 35:2502–2511, 1984

Gosney M, Tallis R: Prescription of contraindicated and interacting drugs in elderly patients admitted to hospital. Lancet 2:564–567, 1984

Gottlieb GL, Johnson J, Wanich C, et al: Delirium in the medically ill elderly: operationalizing the DSM-III criteria. Int Psychogeriatr 3:181–196, 1991

Greenblatt D, Sellers E, Shader RI: Drug disposition in old age. N Engl J Med 306:1081–1088, 1982

Grimm G, Lenz K, Kleinberger G, et al: RO 15-1788 improves coma in 4 out of 5 patients with fulminant hepatic failure: verification by long latency auditory and somatosensory evoked potentials. J Hepatol 4 (suppl 1):S21, 1987

Hale WE, May FE, Marks RG, et al: Drug use in an ambulatory elderly population: a five year update. Drug Intelligence and Clinical Pharmacy 21:530–535, 1987

Helling DK, Lemke JH, Semla TP, et al: Medication use characteristics in the elderly: the Iowa 65+ Rural Health Study. J Am Geriatr Soc 35:4–12, 1987

Hemmingsen R, Vorstrup S, Clemmesen L, et al: Cerebral blood flow during delirium tremens and related clinical states studied with xenon-133 inhalation tomography. Am J Psychiatry 145:1384–1390, 1988

Herkenham M: Laminar organization of thalamic projections to the rat neocortex. Science 207:532–534, 1980

Hodgkinson HM: Mental impairment in the elderly. J Roy Coll Physicians Lond 7:305–317, 1973

Inouye SK, van Dyck CH, Alessi C, et al: Clarifying confusion: the confusion assessment method. Ann Int Med 113:941–948, 1990

Isbell H, Altschul S, Kornetsky CH, et al: Chronic barbiturate intoxication. An experimental study. Arch Neurol Psych 64:1–28, 1950

Johnson JC, Gottlieb GL, Sullivan E, et al: Using DSM-III criteria to diagnose delirium in elderly general medical patients. J Gerontol 45(3):M113–116, 1990

Jouvet M: The regulation of paradoxical sleep by the hypothalamo-hypophysis. Arch Ital Biol 126:259–274, 1988

Kennard MA, Bueding E, Wortis SB: Some biochemical and electro-encephalography changes in delirium tremens. Quarterly Journal of Studies of Alcohol 6:4–14, 1945

Kievet J, Kuypers MGJM: Subcortical afferents to the frontal lobe in the rhesus monkey studied by means of retrograde horseradish peroxidase transport. Brain Res 85:261–266, 1975

Klein LE, German PS, Levine DM: Adverse drug reactions among the elderly: a reassessment. J Am Geriatr Soc 29:525–530, 1981

Kwoonyuen PF, Mandel R, Chen AD, et al: Tetrahydroaminoacridine improves the spatial acquisition deficit produced by nucleus basalis lesions in rats. Exp Neurol 108:221–8, 1990

Lamy P: The elderly and drug interactions. J Am Geriatr Soc 34:586–592, 1986

Larsen EB, Reifler BV, Sumi S, et al: Diagnostic evaluation of 200 elderly outpatients with suspected dementia. J Gerontol 40:536–543, 1985

Levkoff SE, Besdine RW, Wetle T: Acute confusional states (delirium) in the hospitalized elderly. Annual Review of Gerontology and Geriatrics 6:1–26, 1986

Levkoff S, Cleary P, Liptzin B, et al: Epidemiology of delirium: an overview of research issues and findings. Int Psychogeriatr 3:149–167, 1991

Lin JS, Sakai K, Vanni-Mercier G, et al: Involvement of histaminergic neurons in arousal mechanisms demonstrated with H3-receptor ligands in the cat. Brain Res 523:325–330, 1990

Lindsley DB, Schreiner LH, Knowles WB, et al: Behavioral and EEG changes following chronic brain stem lesions in the cat. Electroencephalogr Clin Neurophysiol 2:483–498, 1950

Lipowski ZJ: Delirium: Acute Brain Failure in Man, 2nd Edition. Springfield, IL, Charles C Thomas, 1987

Lipowski ZJ: Delirium in the elderly patient. N Engl J Med 320:578–582, 1989

Liptzin B, Levkoff SE, Cleary PD, et al: An empiric study of diagnostic criteria for delirium. Am J Psychiatry 148:454–457, 1991

Liston EH: Delirium in the aged. Psychiatr Clin North Am 5:49–66, 1982

Lugaresi E, Medori R, Montagna P, et al: Fatal familial insomnia and dysautonomia with selective degeneration of thalamic nuclei. N Engl J Med 315:997–1003, 1986

Mach J, Dysken M, Richards H, et al: Serum anticholinergic activity in hospitalized elderly with delirium (abstract). J Am Geriatr Soc 38:A15, 1990

McCartney JR, Palmateer LM: Assessments of cognitive deficits in geriatric patients. J Am Geriatr Soc 33:467–471, 1985

McDermott WV Jr, Adams RD: Episodic stupor associated with an Eck fistula in human with particular reference to the metabolism of ammonia. J Clin Invest 33:1–9, 1954

Menza MA, Murray GB, Holmes VF, et al: Controlled study of extrapyramidal reactions in delirious, medically ill patients: intravenous haloperidol versus haloperidol plus benzodiazepines. Heart Lung 17:238–241, 1988

Michocki RJ, Lamy PP: A "risk" approach to adverse drug reactions. J Am Geriatr Soc 36:79–81, 1988

Miller P, Richardson JS, Jyu F, et al: Association of low serum anticholinergic levels and cognitive impairment in the elderly presurgical patients. Am J Psychiatry 145:343–345, 1988

Morrison RL, Katz IR: Drug related cognitive impairment: current progress and current problems. Annual Review of Gerontology and Geriatrics 9:232–279, 1989

Moruzzi G, Magoun HW: Brain stem reticular formation and activation of the EEG. Electroencephalogr Clin Neurophysiol 1:455–473, 1949

Mullen KD, Szauter KM, Galloway PG, et al: CSF of patients with hepatic encephalopathy (HE) contains significant benzodiazepine (BX) binding activity: correlation with post mortem cortical BZ binding studies. Hepatology 7:1103, 1987

Nauta WJH: Hypothalamic regulation of sleep in rats: an experimental study. J Neurophysiol 9:285–316, 1946

Parsons-Smith BG, Summerskill WJH, Dawson AM, et al: The electroencephalograph in liver disease. Lancet 2:867–871, 1957

Posner JB, Plum F: The toxic effects of carbon dioxide and acetazolamide in hepatic encephalopathy. J Clin Invest 39:1246–1258, 1960

Pro JD, Wells CE: The use of electroencephalogram in the diagnosis of delirium. Diseases of the Nervous System 38:804–808, 1977

Rabins P: Psychosocial and management aspects of delirium. Int Psychogeriatr 3:309–24, 1991

Rabins PV, Folstein MF: Delirium and dementia: diagnostic criteria and fatality rates. Br J Psychiatry 140:149–153, 1982

Ranson SW: Somnolence caused by hypothalamic lesions in the monkey. Archives of Neurology and Psychiatry 41:1–23, 1939

Ray WA, Federspiel CF, Schaffner W: A study of antipsychotic drug use in nursing homes: epidemiologic evidence suggests misuse. Am J Pub Health 70:485–491, 1980

Report of Royal College of Physicians: Medication for the elderly. J R Coll Physicians Lond 18:7–17, 1984

Rockwood K: Acute confusion in elderly medical patients. J Am Geriatr Soc 37:150–154, 1989

Rogers MP, Liang MH, Daltroy LH, et al: Delirium after elective orthopedic surgery: risk factors and natural history. Int J Psychiatry Med 19:109–121, 1989

Romano J, Engel GL: Delirium, I: electroencephalographic data. Archives of Neurology and Psychiatry 51:356–77, 1944

Ross CA: CNS arousal systems: possible role in delirium. Int Psychogeriatr 3:353–371, 1991

Ross CA, Peyser CE, Shapiro I, et al: Delirium: phenomenologic and etiologic subtypes. Int Psychogeriatr 3(2):135–147, 1991

Rothstein JD, McKhann G, Guarneri P, et al: Cerebrospinal fluid content of diazepam binding inhibitor in chronic hepatic encephalopathy. Ann Neurol 26:57–62, 1989

Rovner B, David A, Blaustein MJ, et al: Self care capacity and anticholinergic drug levels in nursing home patients. Am J Psychiatry 145:378–390, 1988

Saper CB: Organization of cerebral cortical afferent systems in the rat, I: magnocellular basal nucleus. J Comp Neurol 222:313–342, 1984

Saper CB: Organization of cerebral cortical afferent systems in the rat, II: hypothalamocortical projections. J Comp Neurol 237:21–46, 1985

Saper CB: Diffuse cortical projection systems: anatomical organization and role in clinical function, in Handbook of Physiology, Vol 5: The Nervous System. New York, Oxford Univeristy Press, 1986, pp 169–210

Schafer DF, Fowler JM, Munson PJ, et al: Gamma-aminobutyric acid and benzodiazepine receptors in an animal model of fulminant hepatic failure. J Lab Clin Med 102:870–880, 1983

Schor JD, Levkoff SE, Lipsitz LA, et al: Risk factors for delirium in hospitalized elderly. JAMA 267:827–831, 1992

Shute CCD, Lewis PR: The ascending cholinergic reticular system: neocortical, olfactory, and subcortical projections. Brain Res 90:497–520, 1974

Seifert R, Jamieson J, Gardner R Jr: Use of anticholinergics in the nursing home: an empirical study and review. Drug Intelligence and Clinical Pharmacy 17:470–473, 1983

Stewart RB, Hale WE: Acute confusional states in older adults and the role of polypharmacy. Annu Rev Public Health 13:414–430, 1992

Sunderland T, Tariot PN, Cohen RM, et al: Anticholinergic sensitivity in patients with dementia of the Alzheimer type and age-matched controls. Arch Gen Psychiatry 44:418–426, 1987

Thomas R, Cameron DJ, Fahs MC: A prospective study of delirium and prolonged hospital stay. Arch Gen Psychiatry 45:937–940, 1986

Tollefson GD, Montague-Clouse J, Lancaster SP: The relationship of serum anticholinergic activity to mental status performance in an elderly nursing home population. J Neuropsychiatry Clin Neurosci 3:314–319, 1991

Trulson ME, Ross CA, Jacobs BL: Behavioral evidence for the stimulation of CNS serotonin receptors by high doses of LSD. Psychopharmacology Communications, 2:149–164, 1976

Trzepacz PT, Teague GB, Lipowski ZJ: Delirium and other organic mental disorders in a general hospital. Gen Hosp Psychiatry 7:101–106, 1985

Trzepacz PT, Leavitt M, Ciongoli K: An animal model for delirium. Psychosomatics 33:404–415, 1992

Tune L, Bylsma F: Benzodiazepine-induced and anticholinergic induced delirium in the elderly. Int Psychogeriatr 3:397–408, 1991

Tune L, Carr S, Hoag E, et al: Anticholinergic effects of drugs commonly prescribed for the elderly: potential means of assessing risk of delirium. Am J Psychiatry 149:1393–1394, 1992

Tune L, Carr S, Cooper TC, et al: Association of anticholinergic activity of prescribed medications with postoperative delirium. J Neuropsychiatry Clin Neurosci 5:208–210, 1993

Vincent SR, Hokfelt T, Shirboll LR, et al: Hypothalamic gamma aminobutyric acid neurons project to the neocortex. Science 220:1309–1311, 1983

Wada H, Inagaki N, Yamatodani, et al: It the histaminergic neuron system a regulatory center for whole-brain activity? Trends Neurosci 14:415–418, 1991

Walker JI, Brodie HKH: Neuropharmacology of aging, in Handbook of Geriatric Psychiatry. Edited by Busse EW, Blazer DG. New York, Van Nostrand Reinhold, 1980, pp 102–124

Williamson J, Chopin JM: Adverse reactions to prescribed drugs in the elderly: a multicentre investigation. Age Ageing 9:73–80, 1980

Wolff HG, Curran D: Nature of delirium and allied states: the dysergastic reaction. Archives of Neurology and Psychiatry 33:1175–1215, 1935

SECTION

IV

Neuropsychiatric Aspects of Neurological Disease in the Elderly

Section Editor
Jeffrey L. Cummings, M.D.

chapter 19
Nondegenerative Dementing Disorders

chapter 20
Alzheimer's Disease and Frontal Lobe Dementias

chapter 21
Hyperkinetic Movement Disorders

chapter 22
Parkinson's Disease and Parkinsonism

chapter 23
Neuropsychiatric Aspects of Stroke

chapter 24
Traumatic Brain Injury

chapter 25
Neuropsychiatric Aspects of Epilepsy

chapter 26
Neuropsychiatric Aspects of Neoplastic, Demyelinating, Infectious, and Inflammatory Brain Disorders

chapter 27
Neuropsychiatric Aspects of Medical Therapies

19

Nondegenerative Dementing Disorders

William E. Reichman, M.D.

Introduction

Dementia is a syndrome of acquired persistent decline in several realms of intellectual ability. Afflicted individuals display combinations of impaired memory, disturbed language, visuospatial abnormalities, and loss of cognitive abilities such as calculation, abstraction, and problem solving. In concert with these changes, patients may manifest impaired recognition (agnosia) and disturbances in motor planning and sequencing (executive functions deficits).

In addition to the intellectual impairment that characterizes dementia, there is often alteration in the patient's behavior and mood. Neuropsychiatric symptoms such as hallucinations, delusions, anxiety, aggression, and excessively disinhibited or passive behavior commonly occur. Many dementia patients develop sleep-wake cycle abnormalities, alterations in sexual behavior, and dietary changes. Performance in the activities of daily living such as grooming, dressing, eating, toileting, and managing household and personal affairs is universally disturbed in dementia. These clinical features of the syndrome, taken together with any concomitant neurological or medical disability, severely impede the patient's ability to fulfill important vocational, social, and familial obligations. The emotional and financial costs associated with the care of dementia patients has achieved staggering proportions. Dementia has become and will continue to be a major public health concern.

In this chapter, I review the nondegenerative dementing disorders with emphasis on their recognition, underlying pathophysiology, and treatment. Alzheimer's disease and the frontal lobe degenerations are discussed in Chapter 20 and dementia associated with movement disorders is addressed in Chapters 22 and 23.

Nondegenerative Causes of Dementia

The nondegenerative causes of dementia in the elderly population are a heterogeneous group of conditions that include cerebrovascular disease (vascular dementia [VaD]) and other less common states such as hydrocephalus, the dementia syndrome of depression (DOD), infections of the central nervous system, neoplasms, toxic and metabolic encephalopathies, endocrinopathies, and trauma (Table 19–1). Although these individual conditions may alone cause dementia, they may also exacerbate the dementia resulting from degenerative diseases such as Alzheimer's disease or Parkinson's disease.

With the exception of VaD, many of the nondegenerative causes of dementia have been described as "reversible" (Cummings et al. 1980; Rabins 1981). In such cases, implementation of a specific therapy, such as thyroid hormone replacement in hypothyroidism or vitamin B12 supplementation in pernicious anemia, is expected to result in restoration of intellectual function. The proportion of dementia cases that actually fulfill this criterion is unknown. The reversibility of dementia associated with such conditions has been subjected to increasing scrutiny and challenge (Barry and Moskowitz 1988; Clarfield 1988; Larson et al. 1986). Across several studies, potentially reversible conditions comprise approximately 13% of all cases of dementia (Clarfield 1988). Although substantially more research is needed to explore the validity of "reversibility" of dementia, it appears that many of the so-called reversible conditions may be more accurately referred to as "modifiable" (Cummings and Reichman, in press). Treatment of the underlying cause of a nondegenerative dementia may halt or slow the progression of intellectual decline, but not necessarily result in complete restoration of function.

Vascular Dementia

Vascular dementia (VaD) is a clinical syndrome of acquired intellectual and functional impairment resulting from the effects of cerebrovascular disease. VaD is characterized by a wide range of neurological and neuropsychological signs and symptoms reflecting the heterogeneity of responsible lesions. Different causes of VaD demonstrate variability in onset (abrupt or insidious) and course (static, remitting, or progressive) (Roman et al. 1993). Until recently, the lack of estab-

From the Comprehensive Services on Aging (COPSA) Institute for Alzheimer's Disease and Related Disorders, Community Mental Health Center at Piscataway, and the Division of Geriatric Psychiatry, Department of Psychiatry, Robert Wood Johnson Medical School, University of Medicine and Dentistry of New Jersey, Piscataway, New Jersey.

lished diagnostic criteria for VaD hampered effective research into its causes, prognosis, and treatment. The application of different terms to describe dementia resulting from cerebrovascular disease such as *multi-infarct* (MID) or *arteriosclerotic dementia* have been imprecise or misleading. For example, it is now clear that neither multiple large infarctions nor arteriosclerosis is a necessary prerequisite for the development of dementia associated with vascular causes. Whereas multiple large cortical infarctions invariably cause VaD, single, strategically placed lesions; small vessel disease including lacunar infarction; hemorrhage; and hypoperfusion may all cause dementia syndromes (Roman et al. 1993). The contribution of stroke to the cause of dementia in an individual patient remains a matter of clinical judgment (Hachinski 1991). In older patients, it is frequently unclear as to whether identi-

fied cerebrovascular lesions are the sole cause of dementia, are significantly contributing to the clinical features of an underlying neurodegenerative disease ("mixed dementia"), or are neuropsychologically silent (Erkinjuntti and Sulkava 1991). Recently devised diagnostic criteria for research in VaD attempt to provide improved clarity of diagnosis and standardization of nomenclature (Roman et al. 1993) (Table 19–2).

Epidemiology of Vascular Dementia

The lack of an accurate definition for dementia of vascular etiology has confounded attempts to reliably establish the epidemiology of the condition (Kase 1991; Mirsen and Hachinski 1988). In studies of the causes of dementia, the diagnosis may have been established by clinical criteria or neuroimaging data such as computed tomography (CT) or magnetic resonance imaging (MRI). Only a few studies have had confirmatory pathological diagnoses. In some studies, the co-occurrence of stroke and Alzheimer's disease is described as "mixed dementia" or is not addressed. As a result, the percentage of all cases of dementia that are secondary to stroke has varied among studies from 4.5% to 39%. The frequency of VaD is generally quoted in the 12%–20% range (Kase 1991). Despite the methodological limitations of epidemiological surveys, it appears that after Alzheimer's disease, VaD is the second most common cause of dementia in Western societies (Roman 1991).

Clinical Features of Vascular Dementia

The Ischemia Scale (IS) (Hachinski et al. 1975) and subsequent modifications (Loeb and Gandolfo 1983; Small 1985) have enumerated the clinical features of VaD in an attempt to distinguish it from Alzheimer's disease. These general features include all or some of the following: abrupt onset, prior history of stroke, fluctuating course, focal neurological signs, focal neurological symptoms, stepwise deterioration, nocturnal confusion, relative preservation of personality, depression, somatic complaints, emotional lability, hypertension, and associated atherosclerosis. Despite a sensitivity and specificity of 70%–80% in separating VaD from Alzheimer's disease (Chui et al. 1992), the IS is less able to reliably diagnose the co-occurrence of these two conditions in the same individual and may significantly overdiagnose VaD in patients later found to have Alzheimer's disease (Roman et al. 1993).

Table 19–1. Nondegenerative dementing disorders

Vascular dementia

Hydrocephalus

Dementia syndrome of depression and other psychiatric disorders

Infectious disorders
  Neurosyphilis and other spirochetal illnesses (e.g., Lyme disease)
  Acquired immunodeficiency syndrome (AIDS)
  Other viral and prion encephalitides (e.g., Creutzfeldt-Jakob disease)
  Fungal and bacterial infections

Neoplastic conditions
  Primary and metastatic brain tumors
  Meningeal carcinomatosis
  Paraneoplastic dementia

Metabolic and toxic encephalopathies
  Systemic disorders
    Cardiopulmonary failure
    Chronic hepatic encephalopathy
    Chronic uremic encephalopathy
    Anemia
    Endocrinopathy
    Inflammatory conditions
    Porphyria
    Chronic electrolyte disturbances
  Nutritional deficiency (e.g., vitamin B_{12}, folate, and niacin)
  Toxic disorders
    Medication toxicity
    Alcoholic dementia
    Polysubstance abuse
    Heavy metal intoxication

Posttraumatic dementia

Table 19–2. Diagnostic criteria for probable, possible, and definite vascular dementia

I. The criteria for the clinical diagnosis of *probable* vascular dementia include *all* of the following:

1. *Dementia,* defined by cognitive decline from a previously higher level of functioning and manifested by impairment of memory and of two or more cognitive domains (orientation, attention, language, visuospatial functions, executive functions, motor control, and praxis), preferably established by clinical examination and documented by neuropsychological testing; deficits should be severe enough to interfere with activities of daily living not due to physical effects of stroke alone.

    Exclusion criteria: Cases with disturbance of consciousness, delirium, psychosis, severe aphasia, or major sensorimotor impairment precluding neuropsychological testing. Also excluded are systemic disorders or other brain diseases (e.g., Alzheimer's disease [AD]) that in and of themselves could account for deficits in memory and cognition.

2. *Cerebrovascular disease* (CVD), defined by the presence of focal signs on neurological examination (e.g., hemiparesis, lower facial weakness, Babinski's sign, sensory deficit, hemianopsia, and dysarthria) consistent with stroke (with or without history of stroke) and evidence of relevant CVD by brain imaging (computed tomography [CT] or magnetic resonance imaging [MRI]) including multiple large-vessel strokes or a single, strategically placed infarct (angular gyrus, thalamus, basal forebrain, posterior cerebral artery, or anterior cerebral artery territories), as well as multiple basal ganglia and white matter lacunes or extensive periventricular white matter lesions, or combinations thereof.

3. A relationship between the above two disorders, manifested or inferred by the presence of one or both of the following:
    a. Onset of dementia within 3 months after a recognized stroke.
    b. Abrupt deterioration in cognitive functions, or fluctuating, stepwise progression of cognitive deficits.

II. Clinical features consistent with the diagnosis of *probable* vascular dementia include the following:

1. Early presence of a gait disturbance (small-step gait or marchè a petits-pas, magnetic, apraxic-ataxic, or parkinsonian gait).

2. History of unsteadiness and frequent, unprovoked falls.

3. Early urinary frequency, urgency, and other urinary symptoms not explained by urological disease.

4. Personality and mood changes, abulia, depression, emotional incontinence, other subcortical deficits including psychomotor retardation, and abnormal executive function.

III. Features that make the diagnosis of vascular dementia uncertain or unlikely include,

1. Early onset of memory deficit and progressive worsening of memory and other cognitive functions such as language (transcortical sensory aphasia), motor skills (apraxia), and perception (agnosia), in the absence of corresponding focal lesions on brain imaging.

2. Absence of focal neurological signs, other than cognitive disturbance.

3. Absence of cerebrovascular lesions on brain CT or MRI.

IV. Clinical diagnosis of *possible* vascular dementia: May be made in the presence of dementia (Section I) with focal neurological signs, but in the absence of brain imaging confirmation of definite CVD; or in the absence of clear temporal relationship between dementia and stroke; or in patients with subtle onset and variable course (plateau or improvement of cognitive deficits and evidence of relevant CVD).

V. Criteria for diagnosis of *definite* vascular dementia are:

1. Clinical criteria for probable vascular dementia.

2. Histopathological evidence of CVD obtained from biopsy or autopsy.

3. Absence of neurofibrillary tangles and neuritic plaques exceeding those expected for age.

4. Absence of other clinical or pathological disorder capable of producing dementia.

VI. Classification of vascular dementia for research purposes may be made on the basis of clinical, radiological, and neuropathological features, for subcategories or defined conditions such as:

- Cortical vascular dementia
- Subcortical vascular dementia
- Binswanger's disease
- Thalamic dementia

The term *AD with CVD* should be reserved to classify patients fulfilling the clinical criteria for probable AD and who also present clinical or brain imaging evidence of relevant CVD. Traditionally, these patients have been included with vascular dementia in epidemiological studies. The term *mixed dementia* used hitherto should be avoided.

Source. From Roman et al. 1993.

Subtypes of Vascular Dementia

As a result of improved recognition of the clinical and pathological variability produced by cerebrovascular disease, subtypes of VaD have been described (Table 19–3). These subtypes present with variable combinations of motor, sensory, and neuropsychological impairment reflecting the anatomical region disrupted. In addition to clinical features such as hemiparesis and hemisensory loss, afflicted patients may demonstrate parkinsonism, gait instability, urinary incontinence, visual field defects, hemineglect, and pseudobulbar palsy (dysarthria, dysphagia, exaggerated facial and gag reflexes, and pseudobulbar affect). Along with neuropsychological deficits such as impaired memory, language, cognition, and visuospatial ability, patients may also manifest impairment in frontal systems functions (Wolfe et al. 1990). Disturbances of mood, behavior, and perception (hallucinosis) may complicate the clinical course of VaD. In some patients, delusional thinking develops (Cummings et al. 1987).

Multi-infarct dementia.   The cumulative effect of multiple large complete cortical infarctions throughout the distributions of the anterior, middle, or posterior cerebral artery circulations can result in dementia.

Generally, occlusion of these arteries is the consequence of atherosclerotic thrombosis or cardiac embolization. Multi-infarct dementia is typically reported as having an abrupt onset with stepwise progression. The resulting clinical picture is characterized by variable impairment across several areas of intellectual function. Patients may demonstrate "patchiness" of deficits such that while certain intellectual functions are spared, others are significantly affected. As the syndrome progresses, most areas of intellectual function become disturbed. Patients typically manifest neurological signs and symptoms such as dysarthria, hemiparesis, hemisensory loss, visual field disturbances, and pathological reflexes or reflex asymmetries. Disturbances of recognition (agnosia) and praxis (apraxia) are occasionally noted. In many patients, multi-infarct dementia results from a combination of cortical and subcortical infarctions (see below).

Strategic single-infarct dementia.   A solitary infarction may abruptly cause dementia if it occurs in a cortical or subcortical region critical to intellectual functions. Strategically placed single lesions in the distributions of the carotid, anterior, middle, and posterior cerebral arteries give rise to well-recognized dementia syndromes with a variety of neurological and

Table 19–3.   Subtypes of vascular dementia

Subtype	Features
Multi-infarct	Abrupt onset, stepwise progression, "patchy" neuropsychological deficits, pyramidal signs, hemiparesis, hemisensory loss, and impaired memory
Strategic single-infarct	Abrupt onset
Carotid artery	Aphasia (left-sided), visuospatial deficits, and contralateral hemiparesis and hemisensory loss
Anterior cerebral artery	Abulia, dyspraxia, transcortical motor aphasia, dysarthria, apraxia, impaired memory; contralateral hemiparesis and hemisensory loss in lower extremities, and incontinence
Middle cerebral artery	Severe aphasia (left-sided)[a], alexia, agraphia, dyscalculia, psychosis, contralateral pyramidal signs, hemiparesis, hemisensory loss, and visual field deficits
Dominant angular gyrus	Aphasia, alexia, agraphia, impaired verbal memory, visuospatial deficits, right-left disorientation, finger agnosia, and dyscalculia
Posterior cerebral artery	Impaired memory, agnosia, alexia without graphia, visual field deficits, brain stem signs
Branches to thalamic region	Aphasia (left-sided), impaired attention and memory, and variable motor and sensory loss
Hypoperfusion of watershed (borderzone)	Transcortical aphasias, impaired memory, apraxia, and visuospatial deficits
Small-vessel disease	
Lenticulostriate arteries (lacunar state)	Memory loss, psychomotor slowing, apathy, depression, multifocal motor symptoms, parkinsonism, and pseudobulbar palsy
Subcortical arterioles	Memory loss, psychomotor slowing, euphoria, psychosis, symmetric hemiparesis, ataxia supranuclear palsy, incontinence, and parkinsonism (often without tremor)

[a]In the setting of severe aphasia, one cannot adequately determine whether, in fact, dementia exists.

neurobehavioral features (Mahler and Cummings 1991) (Table 19–3).

Hypoperfusion of watershed (borderzone infarction) dementia.   The borderzone regions exist at the borders between the vascular territories of the major cerebral arteries. Reduced cerebral perfusion resulting from cardiac arrest, severe hypotension, or loss of blood volume causes stroke in these cortical areas. The most vulnerable borderzone region appears to be the area between the territories of the middle and posterior cerebral arteries.

Small-vessel disease dementia.   Occlusion of small vessels most prominently causes lesions of subcortical structures such as the basal ganglia, thalamus, internal capsule, and subhemispheric white matter. Disruption of these structures and their connections to the dorsolateral frontal cortex leads to a syndrome called *subcortical dementia*. This state is characterized by psychomotor slowing, dilapidation in cognitive functions, memory impairment, frontal systems dysfunction, and behavioral alterations such as depression and apathy (Cummings 1990). Neurologically, such patients frequently manifest parkinsonism, ataxia, and urinary incontinence.

Lacunar state (*etat lacunaire*) refers to a pattern of infarction in which multiple small lesions in the basal ganglia, thalamus, and internal capsule produce dementia. Neurological signs and symptoms include, but are not limited to, pseudobulbar palsy, gaze abnormalities, psychomotor slowing, and pyramidal and extrapyramidal disorders. Depression, apathy, and emotional lability are frequent accompanying psychiatric features. Dementia often features prominent frontal systems dysfunction (Ishii et al. 1986; Wolfe et al. 1990). Affected patients typically have a history of hypertension.

Ischemic injury of the frontal hemispheric white matter produces a chronic progressive state called *subcortical arteriosclerotic encephalopathy* or *Binswanger's disease* (Babikian and Ropper 1987; Peterson and Summergrad 1989; Summergrad and Peterson 1989). Like lacunar infarction, the signs and symptoms of Binswanger's disease reflect pathology localized to subcortical structures. Disturbances of cortical origin such as agnosia or apraxia are generally absent. Hypertension has been noted in 80% or more of cases (Kinkel et al. 1985). Because the clinical triad of dementia, gait disturbance, and urinary incontinence may be seen in

Binswanger's disease, it is occasionally misdiagnosed as normal-pressure hydrocephalus (NPH) where these features have been considered pathognomonic. As compared with NPH patients, Binswanger's disease patients demonstrate an earlier age at onset, less frequent early gait abnormalities, longer illness duration, and more prominent signs of hypertension and cerebrovascular disease (Gallassi et al. 1991).

Evaluation of Vascular Dementia

After review of the patient's history, the evaluation of VaD includes thorough physical, neurological, and mental status examinations. This approach is complemented by CT or MRI of the brain in order to identify changes consistent with vascular lesions such as gray matter infarctions or ischemic white matter changes.

The frequency of infarctions noted on CT scans of patients given the clinical diagnosis of VaD has varied considerably (from 20% to 86%) (Erkinjuntti and Sulkava 1991). Infarctions appear on CT as regions of lucency. With the advent of MRI, the ability to detect ischemic changes in the subhemispheric white matter has improved, leading to increased speculation regarding their significance. In many intellectually and neurologically intact older patients, MRI may demonstrate patchy and diffuse white matter changes evident as increased signal, especially on T2-weighted images (Almkvist et al. 1992; Boone et al. 1992; Leys et al. 1990). These lesions frequently appear in close proximity to the ventricles and may consist of caps or thickened, irregular rims. These changes have been often referred to as *leukoariosis*. When these lesions are confined to the periventricular region, their clinical significance is unclear (Bondareff et al. 1990). In general, these changes are thought to represent localized areas of demyelination and increased amounts of free water (Zimmerman et al. 1986). In some patients, the periventricular findings are accompanied by single or multiple lesions of the basal ganglia, internal capsule, and thalamus. Large confluent lesions in the subhemispheric white matter may also be noted. Arteriosclerosis may or may not be identified in these subcortical lesions and seems to occur depending on their location (Chimowitz et al. 1992). In general, widespread white matter lesions on neuroimaging are a frequent finding in VaD patients (Figure 19–1) (Erkinjuntti and Sulkava 1991). However, it remains that these lesions have different pathological correlates and may be of variable clinical significance (Chimowitz et al. 1992).

In VaD, functional neuroimaging techniques such as single photon emission computed tomography (SPECT) and positron-emission tomography (PET) (Figure 19–2) demonstrate focal areas of hypoperfusion and hypometabolism, respectively.

Although most cases of VaD occur on the basis of arteriosclerosis in the setting of prominent vascular risk factors, in some patients, stroke may result from inflammatory vasculitis. In these individuals, the clinician often encounters other prominent signs of collagen-vascular disease such as an elevated sedimentation rate and confirmatory serologic abnormalities. Inflammatory diseases such as systemic lupus erythematosus, temporal arteritis, and sarcoidosis have been associated with VaD. Hematologic disorders such as polycythemia, sickle-cell disease, and thrombotic thrombocytopenic purpura may also cause stroke and should be considered when routine blood work is reviewed. Attention to potential embolic sources such as cardiac valvular disease is an important component of the diagnostic assessment.

Treatment of Vascular Dementia

At present, no medication has demonstrated definitive sustained efficacy in preventing, reversing, or modifying the course of VaD. Smoking cessation and optimal control of hypertension or diabetes mellitus have been found to reduce mortality from stroke, but have not yet been sufficiently studied to demonstrate such an effect in VaD (Hier et al. 1989). Some data suggest intellectual improvement with moderately lowered blood pressure in hypertensive patients, but other individuals with VaD may experience further cognitive decline (Meyer et al. 1986). Meyer and colleagues (Meyer et al. 1988, 1989; Wade 1991) have observed therapeutic benefit from cigarette smoking abstinence, aspirin therapy, and surgical interventions such

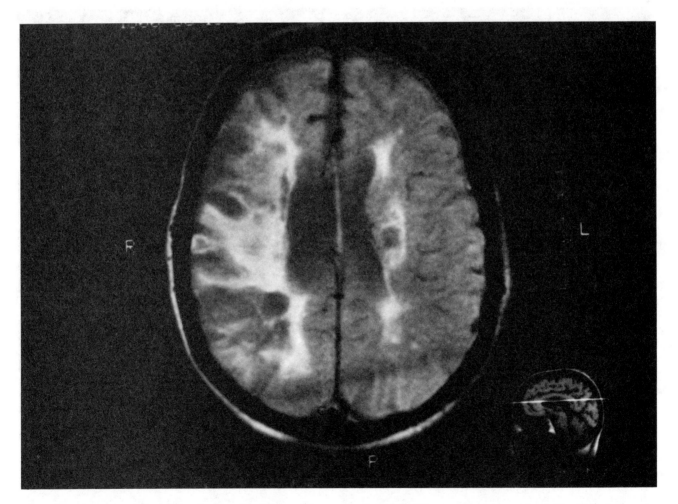

Figure 19–1.   Magnetic resonance image of a patient with vascular dementia. There are large irregular periventricular hyperintensities, as well as large confluent deep white matter hyperintensities.

as endarterectomy and/or cardiac bypass surgery. Though stroke prophylaxis has been shown with the antiplatelet agent ticlopidine, its usefulness for the treatment of VaD is unproven (Gent et al. 1989).

Pharmacological approaches to the treatment of VaD have included vasodilating agents such as dihydroergotamine (Hydergine) and pentoxifylline (Trental) and calcium channel blocking agents. Although data analysis is still preliminary, no agent has demonstrated unequivocal efficacy over placebo.

Hydrocephalic Dementia

The clinical hallmarks of hydrocephalic dementia include dementia, gait instability, and urinary incontinence. Symptoms usually evolve over several months or years. The dementia syndrome has subcortical features including slowness, bradyphrenia, and inattentiveness. Although memory is invariably impaired, patients also appear apathetic and excessively concrete (Benson 1985). NPH is associated with normal intracranial pressure (Adams et al. 1965). The disorder results from impaired absorption of cerebrospinal fluid into the venous circulation at the level of the arachnoid granulations. Although NPH may be idiopathic in occurrence, it may follow cerebral trauma, subarachnoid hemorrhage, encephalitis, or meningitis. Despite its frequent consideration in the differential diagnosis of dementia, NPH is a rare cause of dementia, accounting for less than 2% of cases (Clarfield 1988).

In addition to NPH, other forms of hydrocephalus cause dementia in elderly people. Mass lesions or in-

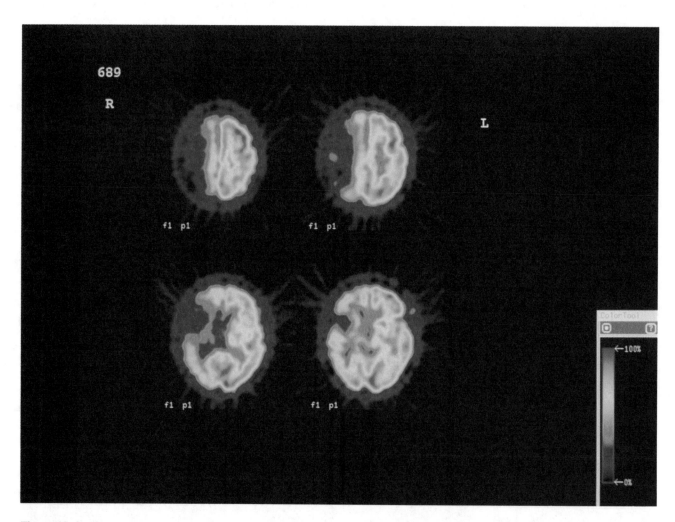

Figure 19–2.   Positron-emission tomography scan of a patient with vascular dementia. There are multiple areas of reduced glucose metabolism.

flammatory conditions such as ependymitis or arachnoiditis can obstruct the normal flow of cerebrospinal fluid (CSF) (obstructive, noncommunicating hydrocephalus). When obstruction due to these causes is relatively acute, the patient demonstrates signs of increased intracranial pressure (headache, papilledema, lethargy, nausea, and emesis) and eventually progresses to somnolence and coma. There may also be bilateral abducens palsies and quadriparesis. When the obstruction is subacute, however, the onset of symptomatology is more gradual and frequently presents as dementia without other neurological signs (Benson 1985).

Ataxia and urinary incontinence associated with hydrocephalic dementia are thought to result from displacement by the enlarging lateral ventricles of those periventricular corticospinal tracts that control lower-extremity and bladder-motor function. Ataxia with hydrocephalus tends to vary in severity and may be accompanied by spasticity of the legs and extensor plantar responses. Difficulty initiating gait is common. Once ambulatory, however, the patient's strides are noted to improve (Fisher 1982).

Whereas ataxia is often a prominent feature of hydrocephalic dementia, urinary incontinence may be mild or only late occurring (Benson 1985). Although frequently cited as a pathognomonic feature of hydrocephalus, urinary incontinence is a common feature of Alzheimer's disease and other dementing disorders and is of limited diagnostic specificity.

Evaluation of Hydrocephalic Dementia

The accurate diagnosis of NPH is often difficult as the characteristic signs and symptoms of the disorder occur in other progressive causes of dementia (Cox et al. 1988). Classically, the radiological appearance of NPH has been reported to consist of ventricular dilatation in the absence of sulcal widening. Although this finding on CT or MRI strengthens the diagnosis of NPH, it is not invariably present. In some cases, elderly dementia patients with clear radiological evidence of NPH may not have the associated features of incontinence or ataxia (Mulrow et al. 1987). Additional diagnostic techniques including radioisotope or CT cisternography are of limited value in improving diagnostic accuracy (Vanneste et al. 1992). Although most patients with NPH may be expected to decline intellectually over time, some may remain stable without additional intervention (Clarfield 1989).

Treatment of Hydrocephalic Dementia

The treatment of hydrocephalic dementia, particularly NPH, involves surgical shunting procedures. Although surgical success rates have been variable, treatment complications have been common (Graff-Radford et al. 1989). Dementia appears to be the symptom of NPH that is least responsive to treatment. Even when the diagnosis is reasonably certain, accurate, consistent predictive tests for surgical outcome are still lacking. In general, those patients best suited for shunt placement are those who initially present with the full clinical triad, have a readily identified cause for NPH, and have had a relatively short duration of symptoms (Clarfield 1989).

Dementia Syndrome of Depression

Pseudodementia has been the term historically applied to describe memory and other cognitive impairments caused by psychiatric disorders such as depression, mania, and schizophrenia (Kiloh 1961). It has been argued that dementia could be "mimicked" or "caricatured" by functional psychiatric illness, implying a hysterical component to the clinical presentation (Wells 1979). Although still controversial, it is now generally accepted that the intellectual deficits that result from psychiatric illness, in particular depression, constitute a "true dementia" that may be modifiable or perhaps reversed with appropriate therapy.

Four essential criteria have been proposed to diagnostically define dementia resulting from functional psychiatric disorders (Caine 1981). First, there must be evidence of a primary psychiatric disorder accompanied by intellectual impairment. Second, the clinical features of the disorder must resemble those noted in degenerative brain disorders with neuropathological confirmation. Third, the intellectual deficit should reverse with psychiatric treatment. Fourth, there must not be evidence of a primary neurodegenerative process that can cause dementia.

Dementia specifically resulting from depressed mood has been aptly termed the *dementia syndrome of depression* (DOD) (Folstein and McHugh 1978). The true prevalence of DOD among the elderly population is unknown, reflecting variability in sampled populations and assessment methods. Across studies, from 2% to 32% of patients evaluated for dementia meet criteria for pseudodementia, of whom 50% to 100% have DOD

(Cummings and Benson 1992). In elderly patients, depression is the psychiatric state most often responsible for dementia. In younger patients, there may be greater variability in the psychiatric causes of intellectual impairment.

The onset of DOD is most typically subacute, occurring in an elderly individual with a personal or family history of depression. As the major depressive episode evolves, intellectual impairment rapidly progresses. Patients appear dysphoric and may complain of poor motivation, anhedonia, and feelings of worthlessness. There may also be heightened levels of anxiety and nihilistic or persecutory delusions. Neurovegetative features of depression are also evident and include disrupted sleep, impaired appetite, anergia, constipation, and impotence. Patients are often hypophonic and appear cognitively and psychomotorically slowed; they may demonstrate diminished affective intensity and range.

The neuropsychological deficits of DOD tend to be variable, and they include some or all of the following: impaired attention and concentration, restricted verbal fluency, memory-retrieval deficits, visuoconstructional disturbances, concreteness, and disrupted calculation ability (Weingartner et al. 1981). Disturbances such as aphasia, apraxia, and agnosia are notably absent. The severity of the patient's underlying depression is highly correlated with the motivation to perform and the level of intellectual impairment (Cohen et al. 1982). The degree of depression is also strongly correlated with the individual's tendency to complain about memory impairment, irrespective of its severity (Kahn et al. 1975; O'Connor et al. 1990). Depressed patients often complain about forgetfulness, as well as indecisiveness, poor concentration, and mental slowing (O'Connor et al. 1990). The degree of awareness and concern verbalized by the typical DOD patient is far greater than that evidenced by the patient with a degenerative cause of dementia such as Alzheimer's disease.

Several studies have documented reduced complaints of impaired memory (Plotkin et al. 1985) and improved intellectual functioning following successful treatment of depression with pharmacotherapy (tricyclic antidepressants and monoamine oxidase inhibitors) or electroconvulsive therapy (Janowsky 1982; Kral and Emery 1989; McAllister and Price 1982). It remains uncertain whether intellectual improvement is complete or whether some deficits persist despite a fully recovered mood (Ames et al. 1990; Greenwald et

al. 1989; Jacoby et al. 1981; Savard et al. 1980).

The long-term prognosis of DOD is also uncertain. Some recent studies suggest that over time, many DOD patients develop a progressive dementia (Ames et al. 1990; Kral 1983; Reding et al. 1985) whereas others, using relatively rigorous criteria for the diagnosis of DOD, have concluded that the risk for developing an irreversible progressive dementia is no greater in patients who have had DOD than in nondepressed elderly patients (Pearlson et al. 1989; Rabins et al. 1984).

Preliminary neuroimaging investigations have demonstrated some structural abnormalities in DOD. In one study (Pearlson et al. 1989), CT scans of DOD patients had ventricle-to-brain ratios that were smaller than those of Alzheimer's patients, but larger than those recorded in depressed, age-matched control subjects without dementia. However, in another series, no significant differences between control subjects and DOD patients were detected with CT (Abas et al. 1990). Elderly patients with late-onset depression have significantly more white matter ischemic changes on MRI than do healthy, age-matched control subjects (Coffey et al. 1990). Whether these lesions predispose to the development of DOD is unknown. In patients with left-hemisphere stroke, concurrent major depression further impairs neuropsychological test performance irrespective of lesion size, lesion location, or other clinical variables (Bolla-Wilson et al. 1989; Robinson et al. 1986).

The diagnosis of DOD rests on the demonstration of a major depressive episode in a patient with secondarily acquired intellectual impairment. The patient must not meet diagnostic criteria for another dementing illness that may cause similar clinical features (especially Parkinson's disease or subcortical cerebrovascular disease). It is also crucial to exclude potentially toxic effects of medications. Centrally acting antihypertensive drugs (reserpine, clonidine, and propranolol) or neuroleptics can disrupt intellectual ability and produce depression, confounding diagnostic accuracy. Final certainty in the diagnosis depends on discriminating improvement in intellectual function with resolution of the mood disorder.

Although less common in elderly patients, dementia has also been noted to secondarily arise from mania or schizophrenic psychosis (Wright and Silove 1988). Manic patients are generally easily distractible and forgetful and exhibit psychomotor agitation. Their mood is grandiose or exceptionally irritable. They may have relatively florid hallucinations or delusions and disturbances of thought processes such as circumstantiality or flight of ideas. Other manic features are variable. Dementia arising solely from the manic phase of bipolar disorder must be distinguished from manic-like behavior encountered in dementia syndromes that disrupt frontal systems. Disorders such as the frontal lobe degenerations, general paresis, alcoholic dementia, cerebral neoplasms, strokes, trauma, and the toxic effects of medications (steroids and levodopa) may cause manic symptoms (secondary mania).

In many schizophrenic patients, dementia has been noted, especially when "negative symptoms" (withdrawal, emotional blunting, loss of reactivity, and apathy) dominate the clinical picture. These features have been correlated with frontal ventricular prominence and sulcal widening (Andreasen et al. 1982). The neuropsychological profile of dementia in schizophrenic patients with prominent negative symptoms has been shown to preferentially, but not exclusively, consist of impaired frontal functions (Breier et al. 1991; Perlick 1992). Less frequently, impaired intellectual ability in schizophrenic subjects may be seen during episodes of psychotic agitation. During such periods, impaired motivation to perform and inattentiveness may underlie the observed deficits. Lastly, a subgroup of elderly schizophrenic subjects demonstrate chronic neuropsychological deficits.

Infectious Disorders

Infectious disorders of the central nervous system are uncommon causes of dementia in the elderly population. Dementia resulting from chronic fungal, helminthic, or protozoan infectious processes most often presents clinically as a chronic confusional state with impaired attention and arousal. Along with features of meningeal irritation, there may be signs of increased intracranial pressure such as papilledema, headache, nausea, and emesis. Seizures and cranial nerve dysfunction may also be evident.

Bacterial infection (meningitis or brain abscess) more often develops as an acute, rapidly progressive clinical state with neuropsychiatric features more reminiscent of delirium than of dementia. Chronic treponemal infections of the nervous system that may cause dementia include neurosyphilis and Lyme disease.

Dementia can be a long-term consequence of viral encephalitis. In herpes simplex encephalitis, severe memory impairment may be a chronic residual feature

reflecting the virus' predilection for the anterior medial temporal cortex. Affected patients may demonstrate aphasia and mild cognitive deficits. Apart from herpes simplex infection, other viral encephalitides can also cause enduring intellectual deficits.

Creutzfeldt-Jakob disease is a rare disorder with onset in the sixth or seventh decade. The disorder, thought to arise from nervous system infection by an unconventional virus, is rapidly progressive, leading to death within several months. Patients manifest progressive dementia with prominent language disturbance, myoclonus, extrapyramidal features, and pyramidal signs. There may also be cerebellar signs, cranial nerve pathology, and choreoathetosis (Brown et al. 1986; Cummings and Benson 1992).

Patients infected with the human immunodeficiency virus (HIV) can have a variety of neuropsychiatric disorders including depression, anxiety, and dementia (Faulstich 1987; Hintz et al. 1990; Perry 1990). Dementia is the most frequent neurological complication of AIDS (Navia and Price 1987). Since early reports of the AIDS epidemic, the tendency of HIV to cause neuropsychological impairment has been well established. Although originally thought to be the result of opportunistic infection, it has been increasingly recognized that dementia may be the direct consequence of HIV infection of the central nervous system (Lunn et al. 1991; Navia et al. 1986). The acquired intellectual impairment directly resulting from HIV infection has been termed the *AIDS dementia complex* (ADC). The disorder may be a presenting manifestation of AIDS (Navia and Price 1987) and has been noted in at least two-thirds of patients who die from an AIDS-related illness (Navia et al. 1986).

ADC has clinical features indicative of subcortical dysfunction including impairment in concentration, forgetfulness, and slowed psychomotor speed. Additionally, patients have poor balance, lower-extremity weakness, hyperreflexia, and an action tremor. Headache, impaired handwriting, and loss of motivation have also been noted frequently (Benson 1987). There may be other associated behavioral features such as depression and hallucinations. In the end stage of AIDS, patients may be incontinent, strikingly apathetic, and mute (Lunn et al. 1991). Though not having AIDS, asymptomatic HIV-infected people may demonstrate subclinical impairment in verbal memory and psychomotor speed (Lunn et al. 1991; Stern et al. 1991).

It remains unclear how HIV enters the central nervous system to produce ADC. One view is that the retrovirus is initially contained within macrophages that cross the blood-brain barrier. With evolving immuno-suppression, the virus replicates within the brain in an uncontrolled fashion (Perry 1990).

Although ADC is most commonly seen in younger age groups, in which risk factors such as homosexuality, intravenous drug use, and prior blood transfusion increase the risk of HIV infection, the disorder may also be seen in the elderly. The diagnosis should be considered in the older patient with any of the above risk factors and a subcortical dementia.

The treatment of ADC involves substantial psychological support for patients and their caregivers augmented by pharmacotherapy. Antiviral therapy, specifically zidovudine (AZT), has been shown to improve intellectual impairment associated with AIDS (Schmitt et al. 1988; Yarchoan et al. 1987). Symptomatic psychotropic, neurological, and analgesic medications are also used where indicated. Specifically, psychotropic agents including psychostimulants for withdrawal and apathy and high-potency neuroleptics for associated psychosis have demonstrated consistent efficacy (Ostrow et al. 1988; Perry 1990).

Neoplasia-Associated Dementia

Primary neoplasms that arise from the brain parenchyma, cerebral blood vessels, pituitary, meninges, and cranial nerves may all sufficiently disrupt neural function to produce dementia. Metastatic lesions from extracranial tumors, granulomas, and lymphomas may all invade the central nervous system to exert profound effects on mentation. The wide variety of cerebral neoplasms that may cause dementia accounts for significant variability in the onset and progression of intellectual impairment and the occurrence of associated neurological signs and symptoms (Rowland 1989).

The clinical features associated with intracranial tumors arise from parenchymal invasion, mass effects, hydrocephalus, vascular occlusion, or any combination of these. Most often, signs and symptoms of intracranial mass lesions arise insidiously and are progressive. Symptoms such as depression, lethargy, apathy, impaired concentration, disturbed memory, and headache may slowly evolve over several weeks to months (Anderson et al. 1990). When other symptoms such as unsteady gait, incontinence, and emesis are noted, a cerebral mass lesion must be strongly suspected. Addi-

tional features consistent with the presence of a brain tumor include papilledema, vasomotor symptoms, focal motor or sensory signs, diplopia, vertigo, and visual field defects (Bannister 1986). Less frequently, the initial manifestations of a cerebral tumor include the abrupt onset of a seizure, focal motor weakness, or hemisensory loss (Adams and Victor 1989).

The pattern of intellectual impairment noted with a cerebral mass lesion is in part a function of neuroanatomic location. Direct pressure effects may cause relatively focal disturbances in language, praxis, or memory. In certain locations, dementia is particularly likely to occur. For example, global intellectual impairment is found in 70% of patients with frontal tumors, whereas language disturbances are particularly prominent with left-temporal masses (Cummings and Benson 1992). Increased intracranial pressure gives rise to altered arousal, attention, and concentration. Tumors disrupting subcortical structures such as the basal ganglia also cause dementia in which there are prominent attentional disturbances and depression. Masses affecting the diencephalic structures may cause dementia associated with personality changes, endocrinologic abnormalities, dietary disturbances, or sleep alterations (Cummings and Benson 1992).

Widespread metastasis to the meninges with dissemination throughout the ventricles has been termed *meningeal carcinomatosis*. Malignant melanoma and carcinomas of the breast, lung, and gastrointestinal tract have been associated with this condition. Affected patients demonstrate signs of increased intracranial pressure, cranial nerve dysfunction, and dementia typified by prominent attention and concentration difficulties (Theodore and Gendelman 1981).

Distant tumors such as occult neoplasms of the lung (oat-cell carcinoma), ovary, or breast may be associated with limbic encephalitis. This disorder has been considered a paraneoplastic condition of unknown pathogenesis. Intellectual impairment is often accompanied by depression and anxiety. There may be impairment of arousal and hallucinatory phenomena. Signs or symptoms of cerebellar dysfunction such as ataxia, nystagmus, tremor, hyporeflexia, dysarthria, and impairment of rapid alternating movements may be noted. Seizures, myopathy, and myeloradiculo-neuropathy have also been documented in this condition (Posner 1989). Although the medial temporal lobe appears to be the site most severely affected, neuronal loss and inflammatory changes have also been discovered throughout the cortex and subcortical regions. Paraneoplastic dementia is an untreatable condition that typically progresses to death within 2 years of onset (Cummings and Benson 1992).

The diagnosis of an intracranial mass is contingent on confirmation by CT or MRI. The addition of contrast enhancement to these procedures increases their sensitivity to detect cerebral neoplasms. These procedures also help to differentiate other dementing conditions such as stroke, cerebral abscess, subdural hematoma, and NPH from brain tumors. Electroencephalography (EEG) may demonstrate diffuse or excessive focal slow-wave activity. CSF examination often reveals a mild leukocytosis with elevated protein and normal glucose levels. (For a more complete discussion of the neuropsychiatric aspects of neoplastic, demyelinating, infectious, and inflammatory diseases of the brain, see Chapter 27.)

Metabolic and Toxic Encephalopathies

Elderly people are particularly vulnerable to the neuropsychiatric effects of systemic illness, nutritional deficiency, and toxin exposure. In most cases, metabolic or toxic derangements of the central nervous system produce acute, time-limited disturbances in cognition and behavior (delirium). However, when the effects persist for an extended period of time, dementia results. The most prominent effects of metabolic and toxic disorders on mentation include fluctuating arousal, impaired attention, and disturbances in memory. Depending on the underlying disorder, other associated neuropsychological deficits may appear. However, severe disturbances of language and the other higher cortical functions such as apraxia and agnosia are uncommon. Motor system abnormalities including tremor, asterixis, and myoclonus often accompany the observed confusional state. EEG shows diffuse slow-wave activity, whereas CT and MRI are generally unrevealing.

Systemic Disorders

Disturbances of the cardiopulmonary, hematologic, hepatic, renal, and endocrinologic systems produce transient or chronic disruptions in intellectual function. Such systemic disorders can cause dementia in the elderly, or, more commonly, contribute to the intellectual impairment caused by other conditions such as Alzheimer's disease or stroke. Diseases such as systemic lupus erythematosus, sarcoidosis, temporal arteritis, and rheumatoid arthritis also cause dementia through inflammation of cerebral vessels leading to stroke.

Nutritional Deficiencies

Deficiency of vitamins such as cyanocobalamin (vitamin B_{12}), folic acid, and niacin have been associated with dementia in elderly patients (Bell et al. 1990a, 1990b). Cyanocobalamin and folic acid are biochemically interrelated vitamins that exert both a separate and concomitant influence on cognition and mood (Bell et al. 1990a). Most often, vitamin B_{12} deficiency leads to impaired memory, psychosis, and depression. Additional neuropsychological impairment is an infrequent finding. Clouding of consciousness appears to be a consistent feature of the alteration in mental status associated with this nutritional cause of dementia (Hector and Burton 1988). The neuropsychiatric manifestations of vitamin B_{12} deficiency and associated neurological deficits such as myelopathy, neuropathy, and seizures may occur in subtle or atypical vitamin B_{12} deficiency states in which hematologic indices and the Schilling test results are normal (Karnaze and Carmel 1990).

The diagnosis of dementia caused by vitamin B_{12} deficiency rests on demonstration of diminished serum cobalamin levels. Diagnostic accuracy may be improved by measurement of pre- and posttreatment serum levels of methylmalonic acid and/or total homocysteine (Lindenbaum et al. 1988).

Replacement therapy of vitamin B_{12} deficiency rarely leads to complete restoration of intellectual function. In some patients, however, supplementation with the deficient vitamin may lead to partial improvement in neuropsychological function (Gross et al. 1986).

It is less clear to what extent isolated folic acid deficiency may cause dementia. Some have speculated that increased levels of folic acid in the elderly cause a variety of neuropsychiatric symptoms, most importantly depression. In general, disruptions in the delicate balance between cyanocobalamin and folic acid probably underlie the emergence of most neuropsychiatric features. The complex relationship between these two vitamins is not completely understood. However, dysfunction in brain cyanocobalamin and folic acid status does appear to have important consequences for neurotransmitter metabolism, particularly those pathways related to serotonergic function (Bell et al. 1990b).

Toxic Disorders

The neuropsychological impairment of chronic alcoholism has been historically considered to be a severe amnestic disorder related to a nutritional deficiency of thiamine (Korsakoff's psychosis). Contemporary research, however, supports the view that along with anterograde and retrograde memory impairment, alcoholism is associated with visuoperceptual and problem-solving disability. Impaired performance of verbal fluency tasks and poor abstract concept formation have also been noted (Butters 1985; Cummings and Benson 1992; Tuck et al. 1984). Improvement of dementia may occur with abstinence, but complete restoration of intellectual function is rare.

Alcohol-associated dementia is more common in the elderly population than in younger alcoholic populations; this finding is independent of the duration of excessive intake (Cummings and Benson 1992). The dementia associated with alcoholism may be in part a product of thiamine deficiency, but is likely also to reflect a direct toxic effect of alcohol. Also largely unexplained is the reversible CT scan finding of enlarged ventricles and widened cortical sulci in the brains of alcoholic patients. The degree of atrophy does not appear to correlate with the severity of intellectual impairment. In elderly alcoholic patients with dementia, the EEG frequently shows abnormal slowing.

Although hemorrhagic lesions of the medial diencephalon have been thought to underlie the memory impairment of alcoholism, evidence has arisen implicating pathology of the nucleus basalis of Meynert and cortical structures (Butters 1985). Postmortem studies of alcoholic patients reveal greater degrees of white matter atrophy than cortical atrophy, implicating a toxic effect of alcohol on myelin (Cummings and Benson 1992).

With aging, the risk of medication toxicity increases as a consequence of alterations in drug metabolism, distribution, binding, and excretion. Aside from excessive dosing or polypharmacy, advancing age may be accompanied by increased sensitivity to the psychotropic effects of various medications (Mahler et al. 1987). Centrally acting antihypertensive agents, anticholinergic drugs, neuroleptics, benzodiazepines, hypnotics, and antidepressants can all impair intellectual function in the susceptible elderly patient.

Posttraumatic Dementia

Elderly people are especially at risk for suffering closed head injury. Physical frailty, disturbances of gait secondary to orthopedic disability, and an increased occurrence of orthostatic hypotension in this population increase the risk of falls and traumatic brain injury. Injury to the brain in this fashion includes hemorrhage, contusion, laceration, or shearing effects. With subtle trauma, older patients have an increased tendency for the bridging veins to rupture and hemorrhage as they course from the cortical surface to the dural sinuses. As a result, subdural collections of blood may form (subdural hematoma), giving rise to altered mentation. The onset of dementia may be subacute or chronic. Affected patients manifest a gradually progressive, chronic confusional state with transient, relatively minor, focal neurological signs that may be mistaken for stroke or tumor.

With chronic subdural hematomas, the collection of blood may be isodense on CT scanning of the brain and thus difficult to detect unless there is obvious shift of the midline structures or obscuring of the cortical sulci. For this lesion, MRI provides significantly improved imaging sensitivity and is the diagnostic procedure of choice (Cummings and Benson 1992). When symptomatic, subdural collections of blood may be surgically evacuated in order to produce some clinical improvement.

Standard Evaluation of Dementia

The standard evaluation of the nondegenerative causes of dementia includes assimilating a thorough history of the patient's present illness with comprehensive attention to cognitive, medical, neurological, and psychiatric features. The interview must review the patient's past medical, educational, social, vocational, and family histories. Any significant exposure of the individual to alcohol, medications, and other potential toxins must be considered. Because the intellectually impaired individual can only rarely provide such comprehensive data accurately, it is recommended that the caregiver be extensively interviewed with and without the patient present. Physical, neurological, and mental status examinations are conducted. A quantifiable screening assessment of the patient's intellectual ability, such as the Mini-Mental

State Exam (MMSE; Folstein et al. 1975), allows the physician to establish a baseline of function for the patient and follow disease course. More extensive neuropsychological assessment may help fully elucidate the patient's deficits.

Several laboratory studies are conducted to augment evaluation of the body's cardiopulmonary, renal, hepatic, endocrinologic, and hematologic systems. When cardiac or pulmonary dysfunction is clinically apparent, electrocardiography, chest radiography, or arterial blood gas determinations may be indicated. Additionally, assays for vitamin B_{12} and folic acid are accompanied by blood tests to detect the presence of systemic infection or inflammation.

The thorough evaluation of dementia requires a neuroimaging study such as CT or MRI of the brain to document the presence of atrophy, mass lesions, stroke, or hydrocephalus. When diagnostic uncertainty is prominent, functional neuroimaging techniques, such as SPECT or PET, if available, can be useful to detect perfusion or metabolic abnormalities characteristic of dementing disorders such as Alzheimer's disease or the frontal lobe degenerations.

When infection or inflammation of the brain parenchyma or meninges is suspected, lumbar puncture is indicated. EEG is an especially useful study to support the presence of seizures or an infectious, toxic, or metabolic encephalopathy. Additionally, EEG studies may be repeated to monitor disease progression or response to treatment (Table 19–4). A diagnostic brain biopsy is infrequently indicated in the evaluation of dementia. The procedure is associated with substantial morbidity and rarely leads to the diagnosis of a reversible condition (Hulette et al. 1992; Kaufman and Catalano 1979). Brain biopsy may be helpful for the diagnosis of Creutzfeldt-Jakob disease (Gajdusek et al. 1977). The comprehensive evaluation of dementia must be augmented by careful surveillance for caregiver anxiety or depression. It is necessary to define any potential causes of excessive burden such as disruptive patient behavior, a lack of familial or social supports, or any financial losses, real or imagined. On establishing a diagnosis, the patient and his or her caregiver must be fully informed and apprised of the prognosis and any potential treatment options. Referral should be made for specialized medical evaluation and care as indicated. Additionally, caregivers often need to be referred for legal counselling and ancillary social services such as home health care, day care, and nursing home care.

Treatment of Dementia: General Considerations

For the nondegenerative dementing disorders, improvement in intellectual function following treatment is often incomplete. Therapies such as resection of a mass lesion, ventricular shunting for NPH, or correction of a metabolic disorder such as vitamin B_{12} deficiency or hypothyroidism often lead to symptomatic improvement, but rarely to complete recovery. The essential requirement for therapy is to halt disease pro-

Table 19–4. Standard evaluation of dementia

History of illness
Review of systems
Past medical history
Medication review
Family history
Psychiatric interview
Physical examination
Neurological examination
Mental status examination (with rating of dementia
  severity)
Laboratory evaluation (mandatory)
  Complete blood count with differential
  Liver function tests
  Serum electrolytes, calcium, phosphorus, and glucose
  High-sensitivity thyroid-stimulating hormone
  Syphilis serology
  Erythrocyte sedimentation rate
  Serum creatinine and blood urea nitrogen
  Urinalysis
  Serum B_{12} and folic acid
Laboratory evaluation (selective)
  Lyme disease antibody titer
  Human immunodeficiency virus titer
  Rheumatologic studies (rheumatoid factor, antinuclear
    antibody titer, and so on)
  Endocrine studies (serum cortisol, parathyroid
    hormone, and so on)
  Arterial blood gas determination
Neuroimaging (mandatory)
  Computed tomography or magnetic resonance imaging
    of the head
Neuroimaging (selective)
  Single photon emission computed tomography
  Positron-emission tomography
Ancillary Studies
  Chest radiograph
  Electrocardiogram
  Electroencephalogram
  Neuropsychological evaluation

gression and minimize disability. In VaD, for example, this generally entails optimal control of risk factors such as hypertension, smoking, and hyperlipidemia.

Although the neuropsychological features of dementia are rarely completely reversible, accompanying neuropsychiatric symptoms such as depression, anxiety, psychosis, sleep disorders, and aggressivity are often successfully treated with a combination of behavioral approaches and pharmacotherapy. The contribution of disruptive behavior to caregiver burden cannot be overemphasized and must receive comprehensive attention.

The nonpharmacological approaches to dysfunctional behavior generally consist of reassurance, distraction, redirection, and structure. Generally, the caregiver should try to respond to the behavior in a calm and direct manner. In the setting of aggressive behavior, caregivers must assure their own safety before attempting to relax the patient. When patients experience hallucinations or verbalize persecutory thoughts such as delusions of theft or infidelity, caregivers should acknowledge the expressed fears and offer calm reassurance and distraction. Wandering behavior should be accommodated whenever possible by providing an open space that is secure and well lit. Exceptionally restless patients or those who frequently

wander must be observed for signs of dehydration and the development of sores on the bottom of the feet.

Disrupted sleep is best treated with improvements in sleep hygiene. This often includes avoiding stimulants and nocturnal fluids, limiting daytime naps, and discouraging all non–sleep-related activities in bed (with the possible exception of sexual relations). A diligent search for coexistent medical conditions that may disturb sleep is also required. (For a fuller discussion of sleep disorders in the elderly, see Chapter 17.)

Augmentation with pharmacotherapy is often necessary to effectively treat disruptive behavior in dementia. Tables 19–5, 19–6, and 19–7 provide guides for the pharmacotherapy of behavioral changes in dementia. (Pharmacotherapy in the elderly is covered more extensively in Chapter 30.) In addition to managing disruptive behavior, treatment of dementia must also include astute attention to the other causes of excessive caregiver burden, such as social isolation and inadequate social and familial supports.

Summary

The nondegenerative causes of dementia in the elderly population include cerebrovascular disease, hy-

Table 19–5. Pharmacotherapy of behavioral changes in dementia—antidepressants

Agent	Dosing guidelines	Side effects
Nortriptyline, desipramine, doxepin	Initiate at 10 mg/day; increase dose by 10 mg/week until treatment response or side effects emerge.	Confusion, sedation, anticholinergic effects, and cardiac conduction delay
Trazodone	Initiate at 50 mg/day; increase dose by 50 mg/week until response or side effects emerge.	Sedation, orthostasis, confusion, and priapism (in males)
Fluoxetine	Initiate at 10 mg/day; increase dose to 20 mg/day after 1 week.	Restlessness, insomnia, anxiety, anorexia, and confusion
Bupropion	Initiate at 75 mg/day; increase dose after 4 days to 150 mg/day; maintain at 300 mg/day maximum.	Insomnia, anxiety, confusion, seizures

Table 19–6. Pharmacotherapy of behavioral changes in dementia—antipsychotics

Agent	Starting daily dose[a]	Relative side effects	
		Parkinsonism	Anticholinergic/sedation
Haloperidol	0.5–1 mg	High	Low
Trifluoperazine	1 mg	Moderate	Moderate
Thiothixene	1 mg	Moderate	Moderate
Thioridazine	10 mg	Low	High

[a]Maintain dosage at lowest possible effective dose; increase as needed every 4–7 days.

Table 19–7.   Pharmacotherapy of behavioral changes in dementia—alternative agents for agitation and aggressivity

Agent	Starting daily dose[a]	Side effects
Carbamazepine[b]	100 mg bid	Sedation, ataxia, dysarthria, bone marrow suppression, and hepatotoxicity
Trazodone	50 mg/day	Sedation, orthostasis, and priapism (in males)
Buspirone	5 mg bid	Dizziness, nausea, and sedation
Clonazepam	0.5 mg bid	Sedation, ataxia, and dysarthria
Fluoxetine	10 mg/day	Restlessness, anxiety, and insomnia
Propranolol[c]	10 mg bid	Sedation, bradycardia, hypotension, depression, and worsening of chronic obstructive pulmonary disease

[a]Dosing will need to be increased for all agents at weekly intervals until response or emergence of side effects.
[b]Monitor serum levels, complete blood count, and liver function tests.
[c]Monitor pulse and blood pressure closely.

drocephalus, psychiatric disorders such as depression, infectious and inflammatory disorders, neoplastic conditions, disorders of the major organ systems, endocrinopathies, nutritional deficiencies, toxic disorders, and trauma. Although any of these conditions may be the primary cause of acquired intellectual impairment, more characteristically, their presence complicates the clinical course of degenerative disorders such as Alzheimer's disease. The standard evaluation of these disorders must be sufficiently broad in scope to detect their occurrence, but should be specifically guided by the data available. Treatment of the nondegenerative dementing disorders is directed at halting progression, restoring intellectual function, managing associated neuropsychiatric features, and relieving caregiver burden. Although such an approach typically leads to symptomatic improvement, only rarely is complete reversal of intellectual deficits accomplished.

References

Abas MA, Sahakian BJ, Levy R: Neuropsychological deficits and CT scan changes in elderly depressives. Psychol Med 20:507–520, 1990

Adams RD, Victor M: Principles of Neurology, 4th Edition. New York, McGraw Hill, 1989

Adams RD, Fisher CM, Hakim S, et al: Symptomatic occult hydrocephalus with "normal" cerebrospinal fluid pressure: a treatable syndrome. N Engl J Med 273:117–126, 1965

Almkvist O, Wahlund LO, Andersson-Lundman G, et al: White-matter hyperintensity and neuropsychological functions in dementia and healthy aging. Arch Neurol 49:626–633, 1992

Ames D, Dolan R, Mann A: The distinction between depression and dementia in the very old. Int J Geriatr Psychiatry 5:193–198, 1990

Anderson SW, Damasio H, Tranel D: Neuropsychological impairments associated with lesions caused by tumor or stroke. Arch Neurol 47:397–405, 1990

Andreasen NC, Olsen SA, Dennert JW, et al: Ventricular enlargement in schizophrenia: relationship to positive and negative symptoms. Am J Psychiatry 139:297–301, 1982

Babikian V, Ropper AH: Binswanger's disease: a review. Stroke 18:2–12, 1987

Bannister R: Brain's Clinical Neurology, 6th Edition. New York, Oxford University Press, 1986

Barry PB, Moskowitz MA: The diagnosis of reversible dementia in the elderly: a critical review. Arch Intern Med 148:1914–1918, 1988

Bell IR, Edman JS, Marby DW, et al: Vitamin B12 and folate status in acute geropsychiatric inpatients: affective and cognitive characteristics of a vitamin nondeficient population. Biol Psychiatry 27:125–137, 1990a

Bell IR, Edman JS, Miller J, et al: Relationship of normal serum vitamin B12 and folate levels to cognitive test performance in subtypes of geriatric major depression. J Geriatr Psychiatry Neurol 3:98–105, 1990b

Benson DF: Hydrocephalic dementia, in Handbook of Clinical Neurology: Neurobehavioral Disorders, Vol 2. Edited by Frederiks JAM. New York, Elsevier Science, 1985, pp 323–333

Benson DF: The spectrum of dementia: a comparison of the clinical features of AIDS/dementia and dementia of the Alzheimer type. Alzheimer Dis Assoc Disord 1:217–220, 1987

Bolla-Wilson K, Robinson RG, Starkstein SE, et al: Lateralization of dementia of depression in stroke patients. Am J Psychiatry 146:627–634, 1989

Bondareff W, Raval J, Woo B, et al: Magnetic resonance imaging and the severity of dementia in older adults. Arch Gen Psychiatry 47:47–51, 1990

Boone KB, Miller BL, Lesser IM, et al: Neuropsychological correlates of white-matter lesions in healthy elderly subjects. Arch Neurol 40:549–554, 1992

Breier A, Schreiber JL, Dyer J, et al: National Institute of Mental Health longitudinal study of chronic schizophrenia: prognosis and predictors of outcome. Arch Gen Psychiatry 48:239–246, 1991

Brown P, Cathala F, Castaigne P, et al: Creutzfeldt-Jakob disease: clinical analysis of a consecutive series of 230 neuropathologically verified cases. Ann Neurol 20:597–602, 1986

Butters N: Alcoholic Korsakoff's syndrome: some unresolved issues concerning etiology, neuropathology, and cognitive deficits. J Clin Exp Neurol 7:181–210, 1985

Caine ED: Pseudo-dementia. Arch Gen Psychiatry 38:1359–1364, 1981

Chimowitz MI, Estes ML, Furlan AJ, et al: Further observations on the pathology of subcortical lesions identified on magnetic resonance imaging. Arch Neurol 49:747–752, 1992

Chui HC, Victoroff JI, Margolin D, et al: Criteria for the diagnosis of ischemic vascular dementia proposed by the State of California Alzheimer's Disease Diagnostic and Treatment Centers. Neurology 42:473–480, 1992

Clarfield AM: The reversible dementias: do they reverse? Ann Intern Med 109:476–486, 1988

Clarfield AM: Normal-pressure hydrocephalus: saga or swamp? JAMA 262:2592–2593, 1989

Coffey CE, Figiel GS, Djang WT, et al: Subcortical hyperintensity on magnetic resonance imaging: a comparison of normal and depressed elderly subjects. Am J Psychiatry 147:187–189, 1990

Cohen RM, Weingartner H, Smallberg SA, et al: Effort and cognition in depression. Arch Gen Psychiatry 39:593–597, 1982

Cox J, Knox J, Brocklehurst G: Normal pressure hydrocephalus (letter). JAMA 36:650, 1988

Cummings JL (ed): Subcortical Dementia. New York, Oxford University Press, 1990

Cummings JL, Benson DF: Dementia: A Clinical Approach, 2nd Edition. Boston, MA, Butterworth-Heinemann, 1992

Cummings JL, Reichman W: The appropriate investigation of dementia, in Challenges in Neurology. Edited by Hachinski V. Philadelphia, PA, FA Davis (in press)

Cummings JL, Miller B, Hill MA, et al: Neuropsychiatric aspects of multi-infarct dementia and dementia of the Alzheimer type. Arch Neurol 44:389–393, 1987

Cummings JL, Benson DF, LoVerme S Jr: Reversible dementia: illustrative cases, definition, and review. JAMA 243:2434–2439, 1980

Erkinjuntti T, Sulkava R: Diagnosis of multi-infarct dementia. Alzheimer Dis Assoc Disord 5(2):112–121, 1991

Faulstich ME: Psychiatric aspects of AIDS. Am J Psychiatry 144:551–556, 1987

Fisher CM: Hydrocephalus as a cause of disturbances of gait in the elderly. Neurology 32:1358–1363, 1982

Folstein MF, McHugh PR: Dementia syndrome of depression, in Alzheimer's Disease: Senile Dementia and Related Disorders. Edited by Katzman R, Terry RD, Bick KL. New York, Raven Press, 1978, pp 87–96

Folstein MF, Folstein SE, McHugh PR: Mini-Mental State: a practical method for grading the cognitive state of patients for the clinician. J Psychiatry Res 12:189–198, 1975

Gajdusek DC, Gibbs CS, Asher DM, et al: Precautions in medical care of, and in handling materials from patients with transmissible virus dementia (Creutzfeldt-Jakob disease). N Engl J Med 297:1253–1258, 1977

Gallassi R, Morreale AN, Montagna P, et al: Binswanger's disease and normal-pressure hydrocephalus. Arch Neurol 48:1156–1159, 1991

Gent M, Blakely JA, Easton JD, et al: The Canadian American Ticlopidine Study (CATS) in thromboembolic stroke. Lancet 1:1215–1220, 1989

Graff-Radford NR, Godersky JC, Jones MP: Variables predicting surgical outcome in symptomatic hydrocephalus in the elderly. Neurology 39:1601–1604, 1989

Greenwald BS, Kramer-Ginsberg E, Marin DB, et al: Dementia with coexistent major depression. Am J Psychiatry 146:1472–1478, 1989

Gross JS, Weintraub NT, Neufeld RR, et al: Pernicious anemia in the demented patient without anemia or macrocytosis: a case for early recognition. J Am Geriatr Soc 34:612–614, 1986

Hachinski VC: Multi-infarct dementia: a reappraisal. Alzheimer Dis Assoc Disord 5(2):64–68, 1991

Hachinski VC, Iliff LD, Zilhka E, et al: Cerebral blood flow in dementia. Arch Neurol 32:632–637, 1975

Hector M, Burton JR: What are the psychiatric manifestations of vitamin B_{12} deficiency? J Am Geriatr Soc 36:1105–1112, 1988

Hier DB, Warach JD, Gorelick PB, et al: Predictors of survival in clinically diagnosed Alzheimer's disease and multi-infarct dementia. Arch Neurol 46:1213–1216, 1989

Hintz S, Kuck J, Peterkin JJ, et al: Depression in the context of human immunodeficiency virus infection: implications for treatment. J Clin Psychiatry 51:497–501, 1990

Hulette CM, Earl NL, Crain BJ: Evaluation of cerebral biopsies for the diagnosis of dementia. Arch Neurol 49:28–31, 1992

Ishii N, Nishihara Y, Imamura T: Why do frontal lobe symptoms predominate in vascular dementia with lacunes? Neurology 36:340–345, 1986

Jacoby RJ, Levy R, Bird JM: Computed tomography and the outcome of affective disorder: a follow-up study of elderly patients. Br J Psychiatry 139:288–292, 1981

Janowsky DS: Pseudodementia in the elderly: differential diagnosis and treatment. J Clin Psychiatry 49:19–25, 1982

Kahn RL, Zarit SH, Hilbert NM, et al: Memory complaint and impairment in the aged. Arch Gen Psychiatry 32:1569–1573, 1975

Karnaze DS, Carmel R: Neurologic and evoked potential abnormalities in subtle Cobalamin deficiency states, including deficiency without anemia and with normal absorption of free Cobalamin. Arch Neurol 47:1008–1012, 1990

Kase CS: Epidemiology of multi-infarct dementia. Alzheimer Dis Assoc Disord 5(2)71–76, 1991

Kaufman HK, Catalano LW: Diagnostic brain biopsy: a series of 50 cases and a review. Neurosurgery 4:129–136, 1979

Kiloh LG: Pseudo-dementia. Acta Psychiatr Scand 37:336–351, 1961

Kinkel WR, Jacobs L, Polachini I, et al: Subcortical arteriosclerotic encephalopathy (Binswanger's disease): computed tomographic, nuclear magnetic resonance and clinical correlations. Arch Neurol 42:951–959, 1985

Kral VA: The relationship between senile dementia (Alzheimer type) and depression. Can J Psychiatry 28:304–305, 1983

Kral VA, Emery OB: Long-term follow-up of depressive pseudodementia of the aged. Can J Psychiatry 34:445–446, 1989

Larson EB, Reifler BV, Sumi SM, et al: Diagnostic tests in the evaluation of dementia: a prospective study of 200 elderly outpatients. Arch Intern Med 146:1917–1922, 1986

Leys D, Soetaert G, Petit H, et al: Periventricular and white matter magnetic resonance imaging hyperintensities do not differ between Alzheimer's disease and normal aging. Arch Neurol 47:524–527, 1990

Lindenbaum J, Healton EB, Savage DG, et al: Neuropsychiatric disorders caused by cobalamin deficiency in the absence of anemia or macrocytosis. N Engl J Med 318:1720–1728, 1988

Loeb C, Gandolfo C: Diagnostic evaluation of degenerative and vascular dementia. Stroke 14:399–401, 1983

Lunn S, Skydsbjerg M, Schulsinger H, et al: A preliminary report on the neuropsychologic sequelae of human immunodeficiency virus. Arch Gen Psychiatry 48:139–142, 1991

Mahler ME, Cummings JL: Behavioral neurology of multi-infarct dementia. Alzheimer Dis Assoc Dis 5:122–130, 1991

Mahler ME, Cummings JL, Benson DF: Treatable dementias. West J Med 146:705–712, 1987

McAllister TW, Price TRP: Severe depressive pseudodementia with and without dementia. Am J Psychiatry 137:1449–1450, 1982

Meyer JS, Judd BW, Tawakina T, et al: Improved cognition after control of risk factors for multi-infarct dementia. JAMA 256:2203–2209, 1986

Meyer JS, McClintic K, Sims P, et al: Etiology, prevention, and treatment of vascular and multi-infarct dementia, in Vascular and Multi-Infarct Dementia. Edited by Meyer JS, Lechner H, Marshall J, et al. Mount Kisco, NY, Futura Publishing, 1988, pp 129–147

Meyer JS, Rogers RL, McClintick K, et al: Randomized clinical trial of daily aspirin therapy in multi-infarct dementia: a pilot study. J Am Geriatr Soc 37:549–555, 1989

Mirsen T, Hachinski V: Epidemiology and classification of vascular and multi-infarct dementia, in Vascular and Multi-Infarct Dementia. Edited by Meyer JS, Lechner H, Marshall J, et al. Mount Kisco, NY, Futura Publishing, 1988, pp 61–75

Mulrow CD, Feussner JR, Williams BC, et al: The value of clinical findings in the detection of NPH. J Gerontol 42:277–279, 1987

Navia BA, Price RW: The acquired immunodeficiency syndrome dementia complex as the presenting or sole manifestation of human immunodeficiency virus infection. Arch Neurol 44:65–69, 1987

Navia BA, Jordan BD, Price RW: The AIDS dementia complex, I: clinical features. Ann Neurol 19:517–524, 1986

O'Connor DW, Pollitt PA, Roth M, et al: Memory complaints and impairment in normal, depressed, and demented elderly persons identified in a community survey. Arch Gen Psychiatry 47:224–227, 1990

Ostrow D, Grant I, Atkinson H: Assessment and management of the AIDS patient with neuropsychiatric disturbances. J Clin Psychiatry 49 (suppl):14–22, 1988

Pearlson GD, Rabins PV, Kim WS, et al: Structural brain CT changes and cognitive deficits in elderly depressives with and without reversible dementia ("pseudodementia"). Psychol Med 19:573–584, 1989

Perlick D: Negative symptoms are related to both frontal and nonfrontal neuropsychological measures in chronic schizophrenia. Arch Gen Psychiatry 49:245–246, 1992

Perry SW: Organic mental disorders caused by HIV: update on early diagnosis and treatment. Am J Psychiatry 147:696–710, 1990

Peterson B, Summergrad P: Binswanger's disease, II: pathogenesis of subcortical arteriosclerotic encephalopathy and its relation to other dementing processes. J Geriatr Psychiatry Neurol 2–4:171–181, 1989

Plotkin DA, Mintz J, Jarvik LF: Subjective memory complaints in geriatric depression. Am J Psychiatry 142:1103–1105, 1985

Posner TB: Paraneoplastic syndromes involving the nervous system, in Neurology and General Medicine. Edited by Aminoff MT. New York, Churchill Livingstone, 1989, pp 342–364

Rabins PV: The prevalence of reversible dementia in a psychiatric hospital. Hosp Community Psychiatry 32:490–492, 1981

Rabins PV, Merchant A, Nestadt G: Criteria for diagnosing reversible dementia caused by depression: validation by 2-year follow-up. Br J Psychiatry 144:488–492, 1984

Reding M, Haycox J, Blass J: Depression in patients referred to a dementia clinic; a three-year prospective study. Arch Neurol 42:894–896, 1985

Robinson RG, Bolla-Wilson K, Kaplan E, et al: Depression influences intellectual impairment in stroke patients. Br J Psychiatry 148:541–547, 1986

Roman GC: The epidemiology of vascular dementia, in Cerebral Ischemia and Dementia. Edited by Hartmann A, Kuschinsky W, Hoyer S. Berlin, Springer-Verlag, 1991, pp 9–15

Roman GC, Tatemichi TK, Erkinjuntti T, et al: Vascular dementia: diagnostic criteria for research studies (report of the NINCDS-AIREN International Work Group). Neurology 43:250–260, 1993

Rowland LP: Merritt's Textbook of Neurology, 8th Edition. Philadelphia, PA, Lea & Febiger, 1989

Savard RJ, Rey A, Post RM: Halstead-Reitan category test in bipolar and unipolar affective disorders: relationship to age and phase of illness. J Nerv Ment Dis 168:297–304, 1980

Schmitt FA, Bigley JW, McKinnis R, et al: Neuropsychological outcome of zidovudine (AZT) treatment of patients with AIDS and AIDS-related complex. N Engl J Med 319:1573–1578, 1988

Small GW: Revised ischemic score for diagnosing multi-infarct dementia. J Clin Psychiatry 46:514–517, 1985

Stern Y, Marder K, Bell K, et al: Multidisciplinary baseline assessment of homosexual men with and without human immunodeficiency virus infection, III: neurologic and neuropsychological findings. Arch Gen Psychiatry 48:131–138, 1991

Summergrad P, Peterson B: Binswanger's disease, I: the clinical recognition of subcortical arteriosclerotic encephalopathy in elderly neuropsychiatric patients. J Geriatr Psychiatry Neurol 2–3:123–133, 1989

Theodore WH, Gendelman S: Meningeal carcinomatosis. Arch Neurol 38:696–699, 1981

Tuck RR, Brew BJ, Britton AM, et al: Alcohol and brain damage. British Journal of Addiction 79:251–259, 1984

Vanneste J, Augustijn P, Davies GAG, et al: Normal-pressure hydrocephalus; is cisternography still useful in selecting patients for a shunt? Arch Neurol 49:366–370, 1992

Wade JPH: Multi-infarct dementia: prevention and treatment. Alzheimer Dis Assoc Disord 5(2):144–148, 1991

Weingartner H, Cohen RM, Murphy DL, et al: Cognitive processes in depression. Arch Gen Psychiatry 38:42–47, 1981

Wells CE: Pseudodementia. Am J Psychiatry 136:895–900, 1979

Wolfe N, Linn R, Babikian VL, et al: Frontal systems impairment following multiple lacunar infarcts. Arch Neurol 47:129–132, 1990

Wright JM, Silove D: Pseudodementia in schizophrenia and mania. New Zealand Journal of Psychiatry 22:109–114, 1988

Yarchoan R, Berg G, Brouwers P, et al: Response of human immunodeficiency-virus-associated neurological disease to 3-azido-3-deoxythymidine. Lancet 1:132–135, 1987

Zimmerman RD, Fleming CA, Lee BCP, et al: Periventricular hyperintensity as seen by magnetic resonance: prevalence and significance. AJR 146:443–450, 1986

20

Alzheimer's Disease and Frontal Lobe Dementias

Bruce L. Miller, M.D.
Linda Chang, M.D.
Grace Oropilla, M.D.
Ismael Mena, M.D.

Introduction

Recently there has been an enormous growth of interest and knowledge regarding dementia. The main cortical dementias are Alzheimer's disease (AD) and frontal lobe dementia (FLD). Both diseases have distinct epidemiological, clinical, and pathological profiles. AD is described as a unitary entity, although it has marked clinical and pathological variability. Eventually it may be possible to identify distinctive subtypes of AD based on etiology or clinical course. The consensus regarding what disease, or diseases, constitutes the FLDs is controversial, with some experts tending to lump patients with Pick's disease, FLD without Pick bodies, and focal anterior cortical degenerations into the same category, whereas others insist that these are each distinct disease entities. As is emphasized in this chapter, one problem with any classification scheme for AD and FLD is that relatively little is known concerning the primary cause of these conditions. This paucity of knowledge regarding etiology leads to a taxonomy that is based largely on clinical and pathological phenomenology. In this chapter, we discuss AD and FLD separately. We address the evolving understanding of the epidemiological, clinical, imaging, chemical, and pathological features of both.

Alzheimer's Disease

Epidemiology

During the final stages of AD, the patient is bedridden and unable to swallow or mobilize, so that death often is secondary to dehydration or sepsis. Therefore, many deaths in end-stage AD patients are coded on death certificates as caused by infection. This problem, along with serious obstacles associated with determining a proper diagnosis, makes ascertainment of the exact prevalence of AD difficult (Hay and Ernst 1987). In addition, the clinical and pathological standards for what constitutes AD are still uncertain, further complicating the determination of prevalence. However, based on the findings from an excellent community-based study (Evans et al. 1989), the prevalence of AD is estimated at around four million in the United States. This estimate indicates that AD is probably the fourth leading cause of death in adults, ranking behind only heart disease, cancer, and stroke (Office of the Technology Assessment Task Force 1988).

The main risk factor for AD is aging, and the prevalence of AD rises with each decade of life. The prevalence of AD is about 6.2% for people over age 65 (Roth 1978), 20% for people over 80 (Mortimer 1983), and 45% for those over 95 (Gottfries 1990). Age-related factors that lead to AD are unknown, but after the age 40, β-amyloid protein builds up in cerebral blood vessels and brain (Vinters and Gilbert 1983; Vinters et al. 1990). This may be central in the pathogenesis of AD, as amyloid is toxic to neurons in cell-culture models (Yankner et al. 1989).

Evaluations of monozygotic twins with AD (Nee et al. 1980, 1987) and patients with Down's syndrome (Ropper and Williams 1980) suggest a strong genetic component to AD. When one twin manifests AD, about 40% of the co-twins also manifest it. However, often there is a long delay between the time of onset for the second twin. This implies both environmental and genetic contributions to AD (Creasey et al. 1989). Further, individuals with Down's syndrome who live beyond age 40 have β-amyloid plaques in the brain, and many also develop dementia. Because Down's syndrome patients have an extra chromosome 21, it was hypothesized that a gene on this chromosome might be key in the pathogenesis of AD. Subsequent studies of families with a strongly inherited form of AD showed that in some, but not others, there was an abnormality on chromosome 21 (St. George-Hyslop et al. 1990; Tanzi et al. 1992).

A complicated picture regarding AD and genetics is beginning to emerge. A small minority of patients with AD have a change in the genetic sequence for the β-amyloid precursor protein on chromosome 21 (Chartier-Harlin et al. 1991). However, this is not present in most individuals with familial AD, nor has it been found in sporadic AD cases (Tanzi et al. 1992). Recent work has pointed, not to 21, but to chromosome 14 (Schellenberg et al. 1992). Despite a growing realization that AD is genetically diverse, these new genetic approaches show promise for delineating molecular mechanisms that can lead to AD.

This work was supported by grants from the Public Health Service AG-10-123-02 (the UCLA Alzheimer's Center), National Institute of Mental Health NH5567-02, and a Fellowship from the French Foundation for Alzheimer Research.

Studies on environmental risks for AD have been disappointing. Some groups have shown small associations between AD and head injury (Graves et al. 1990) or hypothyroidism (Breteler et al. 1991), whereas others found no such association (Paschalis et al. 1990). Recently in Shanghai, China, researchers (Zhang et al. 1990) found a greater prevalence of AD in females from low socioeconomic groups. However, in a study done in Minnesota, this association was not confirmed (Beard et al. 1992). One group suggested that exposure to aluminum (Martyn et al. 1989) was a risk for AD, but this finding needs investigation by others. Although there may be important environmental factors related to AD, these factors still remain unknown.

Cognitive Features

AD is a progressive dementia characterized by a slow decline in memory, language, visuospatial skills, personality, and cognition (Cummings and Benson 1992). Often the first symptom is loss of the ability to learn new information ("amnesia"). Initially, the patient is forgetful and repetitive, losing objects, repeating stories, and missing appointments. Eventually, all learning is lost. Both storage and retrieval are impaired, and, unlike memory problems associated with frontal or subcortical injury, clues do not help the patient remember. AD causes loss of older memories so that recall of movies, history, or events from early life disappears. This helps distinguish AD from Korsakoff's syndrome in which the patient has normal remote memories. The amnesia of AD is due, in part, to injury to the cholinergic septohippocampal tract (Bartus et al. 1982; Whitehouse et al. 1981).

Language declines follow a characteristic progression. Word-finding trouble is first, followed by an anomia, which leads to a fluent aphasia with diminished comprehension (Cummings et al. 1985). Neuropathology is greatest in brain regions just posterior to Wernicke's area (Brun 1987), and a transcortical sensory aphasia often develops. As the disease spreads anteriorly to Wernicke's area, repetition is lost. Finally, the patient becomes mute and unable to comprehend.

Visuospatial deficits are an early clinical finding. Navigating the environment, cooking, and fixing or manipulating mechanical objects in the home are all visuospatial tasks that often are impaired in the first stages of AD. Drawing is abnormal, and one should question the diagnosis of AD if the patient can copy a three-dimensional figure.

Cognition is the ability to manipulate new information (Cummings and Benson 1992), and cognitive changes occur early in AD. This means that calculation, business skills, judgments about wills, and driving are often abnormal. At times, this impairment in cognition can lead to complex legal problems. Parietal and frontal injury both seem to contribute to this aspect of the disease.

The period from onset to death typically takes 7 to 11 years. In some patients, AD progresses with extreme rapidity over several years, whereas in others, it advances slowly over decades. Initially, deficits in higher cortical function predominate, whereas during the middle stages of the disease, the patient often develops behavioral and motor problems. Finally, inability to swallow and movement impairment lead to death.

Neuropsychiatric Features

Subtle personality changes occur in AD, sometimes as an early symptom (Petry et al. 1989; Rubin et al. 1987). Often patients show decreased energy, indifference, egocentricity, impulsivity, or irritability. Social withdrawal and selfishness are seen in some individuals with AD. In contrast to patients with FLD, many AD patients show normal social skills, and profound changes in judgment or behavior are unusual in the early stages.

The true prevalence of depression in AD is controversial, with estimates ranging from none to 57% (Cummings et al. 1987). Major depression is uncommon but many AD patients have brief periods of depressed mood associated with a feeling of inadequacy and hopelessness (Cummings et al. 1987). AD-associated depression is often more modifiable by environmental manipulations than are depressions not associated with AD. As AD progresses delusions, agitation, and even violence can occur. Common delusions relate to theft and infidelity. Hallucinations are less common and can signify a confusional state. The anatomical basis for these psychiatric syndromes is poorly understood, but they may reflect injury to the parietal or limbic cortex (Cummings 1992).

Disorders of sleep, eating, sexual behavior, and psychomotor activity are common. Over 50% of caregivers describe sleep disturbances in the AD patient (Swearer et al. 1988). Electroencephalographic (EEG) telemetry shows more awake time in bed, longer latencies to rapid-eye-movement (REM) sleep, and losses of slow-wave sleep (Prinz et al. 1982). Decreases in appetite are common, although weight gain can occur. Similarly, loss in sexual appetite is more common than increased sexual drive. There is a high prevalence of increased psychomotor activity. Motor restlessness, wandering, agitation, and aggression are behaviors that lead to severe problems for the caregivers. In fact, these behaviors often are precipitating factors in institutionalization. There are various pathological changes in the hypothalamus and ascending catecholaminergic, serotonergic, and cholinergic cortical projection systems that may account for these alterations in behavior.

Differential Diagnosis

Inaccuracy of diagnosis continues to plague AD research and clinical care. In one study (Boller et al. 1989), the diagnosis of two clinicians was compared to findings at pathology. In 63% of cases both clinicians were correct, in 17% of cases one was correct, and in 20% of cases neither was correct. Diagnostic accuracy rarely reaches 95%, and studies with this degree of accuracy usually come from the assessment of groups of highly selected patients for whom diagnosis is more certain (Read et al. 1992; Thal et al. 1991).

AD is overdiagnosed; patients with FLD, Parkinson's disease, diffuse Lewy body disease, and vascular dementias are often incorrectly diagnosed as having AD (Liu et al. 1992). Of great concern, potentially treatable dementias are still reported in postmortem studies from research centers (Joachim et al. 1988).

Ongoing research has helped improve diagnostic accuracy. The National Institute of Neurological and Communicative Disorders and Stroke—Alzheimer's Disease and Related Disorders Association (NINCDS-ADRDA) work group established research criteria for probable and possible AD (McKhann et al. 1984). The Mini-Mental State Exam (MMSE; Folstein et al. 1975)

is a simple and reliable test which allows quantification of the severity of dementia. The Ischemia Scale identifies those patients in whom a vascular contribution to dementia is likely (Hachinski et al. 1975). Use of these clinical tools has helped refine AD diagnosis. Another effective approach has been championed by various researchers (Cummings and Benson 1992; Gustafson 1987; Neary et al. 1988); they have attempted to define the clinical phenomenology that is characteristic of AD compared with the other dementias. Because AD leads to dysfunction in brain regions different from those affected in FLD, and most cases of vascular dementia, a clinical evaluation that focuses on the brain areas that are not functioning properly can be effective in improving diagnosis (Read et al. 1992).

Many metabolic and toxic illnesses cause cognitive impairment, and elderly patients are particularly vulnerable to developing delirium or dementia from systemic insults. Examples of systemic diseases that can lead to a dementia are thyroid disease, hyponatremia, B_{12} deficiency, depression, psychoactive medications, vasculitis, and brain hypoxia from pulmonary disease or arrhythmia (Giombetti and Miller 1990; see also Chapter 26). Primary brain diseases that may mimic AD include brain tumor, stroke, hydrocephalus, syphilis, Lyme encephalopathy, and Whipple's disease. Some of these conditions are treatable, and the dementia can be reversed.

Neuroimaging

Neuroimaging techniques show promise for further improving diagnosis of dementing diseases (Table 20–1). Computed tomography (CT) is valuable because it can identify brain tumors, brain abscesses, and hydrocephalus. It shows many, but not all, previous strokes. AD causes generalized cerebral atrophy, although atrophy also occurs in healthy elderly individuals and in

Table 20–1.   Neuroimaging studies in Alzheimer's disease versus frontal lobe dementia

Study	Alzheimer's disease	Frontal lobe dementia
Computed tomography (CT)	Generalized atrophy	Mild generalized atrophy
Magnetic resonance imaging (MRI)	Decreased brain size	Atrophy, sometimes frontal
Single photon emission computed tomography (SPECT)	Posterior temporal/parietal hypoperfusion	Anterior frontal and temporal hypoperfusion
Positron-emission tomography (PET)	Temporal/parietal hypometabolism	Frontal/temporal hypometabolism
Magnetic resonance spectroscopy (MRS)	Increased phosphomonoesters Increased myoinositol	?

association with many degenerative dementias. This makes atrophy unreliable as a diagnostic marker for AD. Magnetic resonance imaging (MRI) has better resolution than CT and is helpful for defining pathology in the temporal and basal-frontal lobes, brain stem, and white matter—areas that are poorly resolved with CT. Like CT, atrophy on MRI cannot be used to make a presumptive diagnosis of AD. However, quantitative analyses using MRI distinguish most patients with AD from healthy, elderly control subjects by showing reductions in brain size and increases in cerebrospinal fluid in the AD group (DeCarli et al. 1990). MRI is better than CT for defining vascular disease, but some strokes can be missed with this technique. An advantage of MRI is that it delineates white matter disease, a common finding in elderly populations (Boone et al. 1992; Liu et al. 1992). The cause for white matter changes is probably multifactorial, but hypertension is a strong risk factor (Hershey et al. 1987; Salerno et al. 1992). White matter hyperintensities are associated with dementia, but large confluent lesions are necessary before gross cognitive impairment occurs.

The use of positron-emission tomography (PET) and single photon emission computed tomography (SPECT) helps to define dysfunctional brain areas in AD. Studies with PET show marked hypometabolism of glucose in the temporoparietal (TP) cortex and hippocampus—areas where plaques, tangles, and neuronal loss are most intense (Benson et al. 1983). In brain regions in which function is relatively normal, such as motor, sensory, and visual cortex, PET reveals normal metabolic activity. SPECT also shows marked hypoperfusion in the TP area and relatively normal perfusion in the occipital motor and sensory cortex (Jagust et al. 1987; Johnson et al. 1987).

The specificity and sensitivity of PET and SPECT are uncertain. With PET, parkinsonian-dementia patients show TP hypometabolism (Kuhl et al. 1984). With SPECT, TP hypoperfusion occurs with hypoxia, with sleep apnea syndrome, and in some patients with suspected vascular dementia or myotonic dystrophy (Anderson et al. 1991; Miller et al. 1990). Thus TP hypoperfusion is not specific to AD, but most patients with other degenerative dementias do not show this pattern. With PET and SPECT, TP changes occur early. It is unknown whether these changes occur in preclinical stages of AD.

Recent studies with phosphorus-31 (^{31}P) and hydrogen-1 (^{1}H) magnetic resonance spectroscopy (MRS) show promise for AD diagnosis. In an in vivo ^{31}P

MRS study, Brown et al. (1989) found significant increases in phosphomonoesters in AD. This change may reflect attempts of dying neurons to regenerate, leading to a rise in phosphomonoester membrane precursors. In contrast, in patients with subcortical vascular dementia, phosphomonoesters were normal, but phosphocreatine was increased. In this study, ^{31}P MRS showed nearly perfect accuracy in differentiating AD from vascular dementia (Brown et al. 1989).

In vivo ^{1}H MRS has also shown diagnostic promise. In a recent study, Miller et al. (1993a) found decreases in the neuronal marker N-acetyl-L-aspartate. This finding mirrors neuronal losses that are found in the postmortem AD brain. Also there were increases in myoinositol, which is a precursor for phosphatidylinositol triphosphate, an important second messenger in the brain. Postmortem studies have shown that the kinase responsible for phosphorylating inositol is deficient throughout the brain in patients with AD so that the increased myoinositol seen with ^{1}H MRS may reflect the brain's inability to phosphorylate myoinositol (Jolles et al. 1992). Whether this is a primary event in AD pathogenesis or is a nonspecific finding associated with brain degeneration is unknown. However, by combining decreased levels of N-acetyl-L-aspartate and increased levels of myoinositol, we differentiated 9 of 10 AD patients from 11 elderly control subjects. MRS may eventually lead to a better understanding of the pathophysiology of AD, as well as to improved diagnosis.

Neurochemistry

Marked neurochemical changes occur in AD. Decreased cortical acetylcholine synthesis and a deficiency in the enzyme choline acetyltransferase are reliable chemical findings in the AD brain (Francis et al. 1985). Other deficits include losses of somatostatin and serotonin (Bowen and Davison 1986). In contrast, patients with FLD have normal levels of cortical acetylcholine, but decreases in serotonin (Sparks and Markesbery 1991).

Neuropathology

The main neuropathological findings in AD are amyloid plaques, neurofibrillary tangles, and neuronal loss. Minor changes include granulovacuolar degeneration and Hirano bodies (Terry and Katzman 1983). The center of the amyloid plaque consists of a 44–amino-acid protein that is derived from a larger precursor protein, the β-amyloid precursor protein (Glenner and Wong 1984). The precursor protein gene is found on chromosome 21 (St. George-Hyslop et al. 1987). Surrounding the plaque is an area of gliosis and degenerating synapses. Plaques are most densely localized to hippocampus and temporoparietal cortex, areas of the brain in which function is severely impaired. Plaques occur in healthy elderly brains, although their concentration is less dense than in the AD brain (Blessed et al. 1968). β-Amyloid protein is also found in meningeal vessels in patients with AD (Prelli et al. 1988; Vinters et al. 1990).

Neurofibrillary tangles are seen within neurons, and stain positively with antibodies to both tau and ubiquitin (Dickson et al. 1990). Therefore, it is possible that neurofibrillary tangles accumulate due to the abnormal phosphorylation of the neuronal tau protein. Few tangles are seen in the neocortex of healthy elderly individuals, but tangles occur with many dementing conditions including subacute sclerosing panencephalitis, dementia pugilistica, aluminum intoxication, postencephalitic parkinsonism, and the parkinsonian-ALS-dementia[1] complex of Guam (Wisniewski et al. 1979).

Because healthy elderly individuals can have plaques and tangles, the pathological method for diagnosing AD (Khachaturian 1985) uses both the patient's age and the concentration of plaques and tangles to determine diagnosis. For example, to meet research criteria, patients younger than 50 years must have two to five senile plaques per high power field in the cortex, whereas subjects between 50 and 65 must have eight plaques per high power field.

Some AD patients show increases in β-amyloid or β-amyloid precursor proteins within the cerebrospinal fluid (Henriksson et al. 1991; Pardridge et al. 1991). Also, amyloid is deposited in the skin and blood vessels of rectal mucosa in some patients with AD. Unfortunately, because many healthy elderly individuals have similar changes, this technique is not of value for diagnosis (Joachim et al. 1989). In monkeys, periventricular amyloid can be imaged by injecting radioactive antibodies into the lumbar subarachnoid space (Walker 1991). These amyloid tests show promise for improving diagnosis, but, to date, none have shown sufficient sensitivity or specificity to be clinically utilized.

Treatment

The AD patient's family will require advice regarding the dementia, superimposed psychiatric and medical conditions, and psychosocial problems and resources. Many medications have been tried in an attempt to treat the dementia. These include calcium channel blockers, vasodilators, vitamins, anticoagulants, nootropic agents, and acetylcholine precursors. However, none have shown efficacy (Mody and Miller 1990). The value of anticholinesterases is controversial, but, when they do ameliorate the memory deficit, the improvement is modest in degree (Growdon 1992).

Treating superimposed medical conditions can be difficult, as they are often subtle and hard to diagnose. The advanced patient with little or no language cannot communicate, and even small problems such as constipation or a tooth cavity can go unrecognized, leading to serious complications such as bowel obstruction or orofacial abscess. Because patients do not suddenly deteriorate due to AD, when this occurs one should suspect an infection, stroke, myocardial infarction, or drug-induced delirium (Giombetti and Miller 1990).

Drug therapies for AD-associated psychiatric symptoms are often efficacious but also have substantial side effects. Depression responds to antidepressants, but also to placebo (Teri et al. 1991). Violent psychosis is improved with antipsychotics, but these medications are sedating (Devanand et al. 1992). Benzodiazepines rarely help anxiety and may cause a paradoxical increase in agitation. The best therapies for psychiatric symptoms associated with dementia often involve manipulation of the environment. For example, the patient who awakens during the night will sleep during the day. Increasing daytime exercise and eliminating naps is often more effective than a sleeping medication. It is difficult to manage aggressive behaviors in the home, and their presence often means that the patient will require long-term care.

Most families need extensive advice regarding psychosocial issues. The physician will need to know when the patient might benefit from day care and when a nursing home is required. Similarly, families will need advice regarding the nursing homes most appropriate for the patient. Families often benefit from consultation with attorneys. The Alzheimer's Association, a lay

---

[1] ALS = amyotrophic lateral sclerosis.

organization dedicated to helping patients and families of patients with AD, is an excellent community resource for family referrals.

Frontal Lobe Dementias (FLDs)

Nosology

The second major group of cortical degenerative diseases is a cluster of related disorders associated with degeneration of the frontal lobe. The taxonomy connected with FLDs is both confusing and controversial, related in large part to our fundamental lack of knowledge concerning the pathogenesis of these conditions. Compounding this problem, many researchers have described new disease entities (or resurrected diagnoses used in prior decades) to characterize patients with progressive FLD in whom findings at pathology are slightly different from those in patients with classical Pick's disease.

Some of the terms used to describe these patients include *progressive subcortical gliosis* (Neumann and Cohn 1967), *dementia of frontal lobe type* (Neary et al. 1987), *frontal lobe dementia of non-Alzheimer type* (Brun 1987), *dementia lacking distinctive histologic features* (Knopman et al. 1990), and *focal lobar atrophy* (Mesulam 1982; Snowden et al. 1992). Adding further to this confusion is the discovery that some patients with amyotrophic lateral sclerosis (ALS) develop FLD. On postmortem examination of ALS patients, pathological findings in the cortex are often identical to those seen in Pick's disease patients (Sam et al. 1991), or show the findings of Pick's disease except that Pick bodies are absent (Dickson et al. 1986; Mitsuyama 1984).

A compelling argument can be made for continuing to classify each of these diseases as separate entities until more is understood about their pathogenesis. Most investigators feel uncomfortable linking Pick's disease, which has been classified as a distinct illness since 1892 (Pick), with other FLDs in which Pick bodies are absent. However, the clinical, imaging, and pathological features of all the primary FLDs have more similarities than differences, and it is possible they represent a spectrum of diseases with the same etiology.

Epidemiology

The prevalence of FLD is unknown. This reflects a variety of diagnostic problems including confusion with nosology and a tendency toward underdiagnosis. In one study, 18 of 21 patients with a postmortem diagnosis of Pick's disease were misdiagnosed as having AD (Mendez et al. 1993). The best data on prevalence have come from studies in Lund, Sweden, and Manchester, England. In the Swedish study (Gustafson et al. 1990), 20 of 150 (13.3%) patients with presenile dementia had the characteristic pathological findings of FLD including frontal and usually anterior temporal lobe gliosis, spongiosis, and neuronal dropout. Only 4 patients (2.7% of total) had classical Pick's disease, whereas 16 (10.6% of total) had FLD without Pick bodies. In the English study (Neary et al. 1987), 21.9% of 41 patients with a presenile dementia had FLD.

The typical age at onset is the sixth decade, and the duration of illness is approximately 7 years. About 40% of Pick's disease patients have a family history of dementia; often the history suggests a dominantly inherited illness. Other risk factors are ill-defined, although a prior history of alcoholism or electroconvulsive therapy is present at a higher than expected rate in patients with Pick's disease (Mendez et al. 1993). Also, ALS predisposes to one type of FLD.

Clinical Features

Although the varied diseases that produce FLD have slightly different clinical features, similarities between the different entities are far outweighed by differences. Usually, changes in personality precede gross dementia by several years (Miller et al. 1991). The personality changes have been well characterized (Cummings and Duchen 1981; Neary et al. 1987), and many patients are socially withdrawn and apathetic. Sometimes friends are the first to notice that the patient has become withdrawn, passive, and disinterested in social situations. Loss of judgment and insight and behavioral disinhibition are common. Behavioral disinhibition can lead to legal difficulties; patients may be arrested for shoplifting or making sexual advances toward relatives or strangers. Judgment is often severely impaired and disrobing and urinating in public can occur. For example, we (Miller et al. 1991) evaluated a woman with FLD who left an infant grandchild unattended for hours while she went to the store. Rarely do FLD patients show insight into their problems.

The symptoms of apathy and disinhibition can be explained by dysfunction of the frontal lobes. Blumer and Benson (1975) called these the "pseudo-depressed" and "pseudo-psychopathic" personality disorders of frontal lobe dysfunction. Apathy occurs due to medial frontal injury, whereas disinhibition is due to basal-frontal dysfunction (Cummings 1993). Both areas are usually involved in FLD.

There are peculiar behaviors in patients with FLD that are probably attributable to involvement of the anterior temporal lobes. Klüver-Bucy syndrome was described in macaque monkeys after the anterior temporal lobes and amygdala were removed (Klüver and Bucy 1939). These monkeys developed hyperorality, hypersexuality, visual hypermetamorphosis, placidity, and sensory agnosia. In FLD patients, hyperorality can be manifested by compulsive gum chewing or smoking and/or changes in appetite. Massive weight gain can occur, especially in patients who develop an intense craving for sweets. We cared for one patient who attempted to drink 30 cokes a day. Placidity is common and this same patient followed his wife's every movement, ordering whatever she did in restaurants. True hypersexuality is unusual, but sexual changes occur (Miller et al. 1991). In our patient with hyperorality and placidity, the earliest change in personality was a loss of interest in sexual foreplay with his wife.

Other behaviors that may be related to temporal dysfunction include bizarre and remote affect, hyperreligiosity, and development of eccentric ideas. One man complained that making love to his wife who had FLD made him feel like he was with a robot. Intensification of religious ideas may occur. One patient with possible FLD changed from a mild-mannered liberal Democrat to an avid follower of a far–right-leaning politician. Compulsive collecting and ritualistic obsessions related to urination or bowel movements are surprisingly common.

Once cognitive symptoms develop, there is a characteristic pattern of decline. Initially, language output is economical, and as the disease progresses verbal stereotypes such as "let's go, let's go," are seen. Some patients become mute when other cognitive skills are still relatively intact. As in AD, an early language change is difficulty in generating a word list, but unlike in AD, semantic anomia is common. With this rare anomia the patient is not helped by clueing and, when told that an object is a key, the patient might say, "Key, key, I don't know what a key is." Because this type of anomia seems to be associated with anterior temporal involvement, patients with purely frontal pathology do not show the disorder.

Parietal and posterior language functions such as reading, writing, and calculation are relatively normal in the early and even middle stages of FLD. Unlike in AD, visuospatial skills are usually normal, or near normal, and many patients can draw in three dimensions without difficulty. Some patients can draw complex designs and multiply three number integers at a time when they are mute and severely impaired behaviorally. Memory testing often shows that patients can store information, but they have trouble retrieving. Therefore, unlike in AD, memory improves with clues.

Neuropsychological testing shows selective impairment of executive skills in the early stages. This includes perseveration and difficulties in set shifting on the Wisconsin Card Sorting Test, impairments in verbal fluency, poor attention, and response inhibition. Word retrieval, memory, calculation, and pencil-and-paper constructional skills are generally spared relative to executive abilities (Miller et al. 1991).

Motor systems are initially normal. As the disease advances, parkinsonian symptoms including abnormalities of eye movements, tremor, and bradykinesia develop in some patients. A small percentage of patients develop ALS months to years after the onset of their dementia. In the end-stages, patients with FLD are difficult to distinguish from those with AD.

Early on, EEG and CT are usually normal (Gustafson et al. 1990). In one MRI study (Miller et al. 1991), half of eight patients with FLD showed generalized atrophy, one-quarter had normal MRI results, and one-quarter had frontotemporal atrophy. Patients with atrophy tend to be more advanced.

SPECT and PET detect cerebral dysfunction in the frontal and temporal regions even in patients without major cognitive deficits (Table 20–1). SPECT shows frontal and sometimes temporal hypoperfusion in early FLD (Figure 20–1) (Jagust et al. 1989; Neary et al. 1988). In some patients, the temporal lobes are more severely involved than are the frontal regions. Unlike in AD, posterior temporal areas show relatively normal perfusion. With xenon-133 measurements, frontal perfusion usually is below 30 ml/100 gm tissue per minute, whereas parietal and occipital perfusion is in the 35–45 ml/100 gm tissue per minute range (Miller et al. 1991). In patients with advanced disease, hypoperfusion appears posteriorly, although the frontal areas continue to show more severe abnormalities. PET demonstrates frontotemporal hypometabolism (Kamo et al. 1987). Using careful clinical parameters and SPECT, one group (Risberg et al. 1993) achieved diagnostic accuracy of greater than 90% for FLD. SPECT and PET show promise for improving clinical diagnosis; AD and FLD patients can usually be discriminated with these modalities (see SPECT images in Figure 20–2). Table 20–2 compares and contrasts the clinical features of AD and FLD.

Neuropathological Findings

All of the clinical entities described (Table 20–3) show neuropathological similarities. Brain weight is slightly to moderately reduced. Grossly, the brain has mild to severe frontal and/or frontal and anterior temporal atrophy. Neuronal loss, gliosis, and mild-to-moderate spongiform changes are found in the upper layers of the cortex. Gliosis is best seen with stains for glial acid fibrillary protein. Neuronal loss can be so subtle that the pathologist may have difficulty differentiating this from normal cortex. Senile plaques and tangles do not occur beyond what is seen in non-diseased elderly subjects. Further, amygdala and hippocampi show slight neuronal loss. Subcortical structures, such as the substantia nigra, are often abnormal. Severe degeneration of the substantia nigra was observed in 79% of patients with FLD without Pick bodies (Knopman et al. 1990), in 78% of Pick's patients (Kosaka et al. 1991), and in each of three cases of dementia with motor neuron disease (Horoupian et al. 1984).

Distinct Clinical and Pathological Features

Pick's disease. Pick's disease is the best-known and best-studied FLD. The exact prevalence is unknown, but Pick's disease accounts for about 2%–3% of all de-

generative dementias (Gustafson et al. 1990). To date, there is no way to clinically distinguish Pick's disease from FLD without Pick bodies. In the early stages, patients can develop the Klüver-Bucy syndrome (Cummings and Duchen 1981), as opposed to AD, in which this syndrome tends to occur in the later stages (Cummings and Benson 1992). As with the other FLDs, deterioration in personality in Pick's disease contrasts with relatively preserved visuospatial skills (Gustafson 1987). Language disturbances are also common and may consist of semantic anomia, circumlocution, and verbal stereotypies with echolalia (Cummings and Duchen 1981; Miller et al. 1993b). Pick's disease can present as a highly selective language disturbance rather than as a dementia (Pick 1892; Wechsler et al. 1982), though this is more characteristic of the "focal atrophies" (Malamud and Boyd 1940; Mesulam 1982) or "focal lobar atrophy" (Snowden et al. 1992). Neuropsychological tests show mainly frontal lobe dysfunction. These clinical, neuropsychological, and pathological findings have been correlated with metabolic alterations revealed by PET (Kamo et al. 1987).

At autopsy, the brains of Pick's disease patients show circumscribed atrophy of the frontal and/or temporal lobes. Microscopically there is neuronal loss, gliosis, and Pick bodies, which are argentophilic cytoplasmic inclusions within inflated neurons (Corsellis 1976). The cells may be rare, and an extensive search for these lesions may be necessary to achieve diagnosis. Asymmetrical involvement of the frontotemporal lobes is seen in 70% of the patients, and 50% have more left-

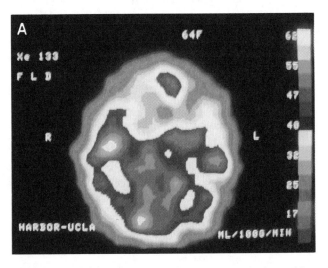
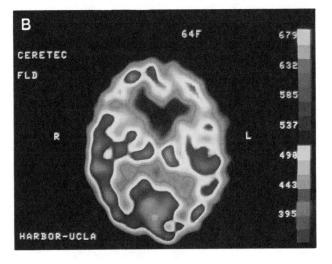

Figure 20–1. *Panel A:* Xenon-133 scan from a patient with early frontal lobe dementia. Note marked decreases in frontal perfusion. *Panel B:* A technetium-99m-labelled hexamethylpropyleneamineoxime (HMPAO) study from the same subject, showing marked frontal hypoperfusion with normal temporoparietal perfusion.

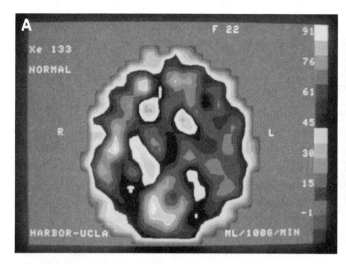
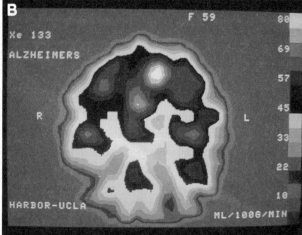
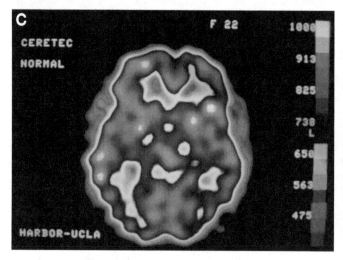
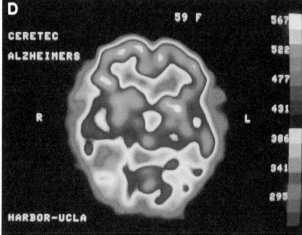

Figure 20–2. *Panel A:* Cerebral blood flow with xenon-133 in an elderly control subject. Cerebral blood flow is color coded to ml/100 gm tissue per minute. Parietotemporal flow is normal. *Panel B:* Xenon-133 scan in a patient with Alzheimer's disease. Note markedly decreased perfusion to the temporoparietal cortex. *Panel C:* High resolution scan of cerebral blood flow in an elderly control subject using technetium-99m-labelled hexamethylpropyleneamineoxime (HMPAO). The scan is color coded, and areas of yellow are 50%–62% of maximal cortical perfusion; areas of green are 40%–50%. Perfusion is symmetrical throughout the cortex. *Panel D:* HMPAO scan showing cerebral blood flow in an Alzheimer patient. Temporoparietal perfusion is approximately 50%–60% of normal (yellow color).

Table 20–2. Clinical differences between Alzheimer's disease and frontal lobe dementias

Clinical variables	Alzheimer's disease	Frontal lobe dementia
Personality	Passive, selfish	Apathetic, disinhibited; sometimes eccentric
Social skills	Spared early	Early deterioration
Klüver-Bucy syndrome	Late	Early
Language	Fluent aphasias	Decreased output, mute
Naming	Lexical anomia	Semantic anomia
Drawing	Impaired early	Relatively spared
Calculation	Impaired early	Relatively spared
Memory	Impaired early, not helped by clues	Variable, helped by clues

sided atrophy (Corsellis 1976; Cummings and Benson 1992). SPECT and PET identify reduced perfusion and metabolism in the frontal and temporal lobes (Kamo et al. 1987; Salmon and Franck 1991), but tissue confirmation with Pick bodies is needed for diagnosis.

Frontal lobe dementia of the non-Alzheimer type and dementia lacking distinctive histologic features. As noted above, the categories, "dementia of the frontal lobe type" (Neary et al. 1988), "frontal lobe dementia of non-Alzheimer type" (Brun 1987), and "dementia lacking distinctive histologic features" (Knopman et al. 1990) seem to be describing the disorders. In the study by Knopman et al. (1990), the authors emphasized memory loss, prominent personality changes, and prominent dysphagia and dysarthria in later stages. Death occurred within 7 years. Fifty percent of the patients had a positive family history of dementia, and cases of ALS were seen rarely in these families. It can be difficult to distinguish FLD from classical Pick's disease at pathology, particularly in patients in whom only the rare Pick cell is seen. Another minor distinction is that with FLD the neuronal loss and gliosis are sometimes more subtle than with classical Pick's disease.

Progressive subcortical gliosis. Neumann and Cohn (1967) described a "new disease entity" for which they coined the term *progressive subcortical gliosis*. Clinically,

---

Table 20–3. Frontal lobe dementias

Primary frontal lobe dementias
  Pick's disease
  Progressive subcortical gliosis
  Frontal lobe dementia of the non-Alzheimer type
  Dementia lacking distinctive histologic features
  Focal lobar atrophy
Secondary frontal lobe dementias
  Vascular dementia (e.g., frontal lobe infarct,
    Binswanger's disease, and lacunar state)
  Alcoholism
  Human immunodeficiency virus (HIV) encephalopathy
  Parkinson's disease
  Huntington's disease
  Creutzfeldt-Jakob disease
  Metachromatic leukodystrophy
  Wilson's disease
  Progressive supranuclear palsy
  Amyotrophic lateral sclerosis (ALS)
  Parkinsonism-ALS-dementia complex of Guam
  Corticobasal degeneration
  Multiple sclerosis

---

their patients showed personality changes including social impropriety, poor judgment, and perseveration. Memory impairment was common. One patient was unable to recognize his family members and had paraphasias; another had "childish behavior" and paranoid delusions. Some developed muscle atrophy before death. Functional neuroimaging studies were not performed, but clinically and pathologically they were similar to patients with FLD.

Pathologically, frontotemporal atrophy of the cortex is seen. Also, neuronal loss with reactive astrocytosis occurs in the cortex, whereas rich gliosis is found in the subcortical areas. Ventral horns and substantia nigra show abnormal gliosis. The presence of muscle atrophy and ventral horn gliosis in patients with progressive subcortical gliosis suggests a possible relationship between this disease and ALS. The prominent pathological feature of these patients is an intense gliosis not seen in classical Pick's disease or FLD of the non-Alzheimer type. However, similar pathological findings in some Pick's disease patients have suggested that this disease might be related to Pick's disease. In fact, the original authors coined the phrase *Pick's disease, type II* (Neumann 1949).

Focal lobar atrophies. Mesulam (1982) described patients with focal left frontotemporal degeneration. Other reports soon followed (Morris et al. 1984). Mesulam described six patients with a progressive aphasia without signs of global dementia. Five began with anomic aphasia, whereas the sixth started with pure word deafness. Most progressed for years with language disturbance, while right-hemisphere functions and memory remained intact. Studies with both SPECT (Mesulam 1982; Snowden et al. 1992) and PET (Chawluk et al. 1986) have shown focal hypoperfusion in the left anterior hemisphere, whereas the right hemisphere shows mild or no hypoperfusion.

Although there are many reports on left frontotemporal degeneration, there is little written concerning the behavioral and neuropsychological changes associated with right frontotemporal degeneration (Tyrrell et al. 1990). The clinical characteristics of five patients with progressive right frontotemporal dysfunction, all of whom differed dramatically on clinical and neuropsychological tests from patients previously studied with left frontotemporal degeneration, have recently been described (Miller et al. 1993b). In these patients there were dramatic changes in personality characterized by remote affect, severe behavioral disinhibition, agitation, hyperreligiosity, and impaired judgment. They showed profound disruption of social conduct. Also they had difficulty recognizing familiar faces and voices, and, surprisingly, some had a semantic anomia. They had less language difficulty and slightly more visuoconstructive problems than did the patients with left frontotemporal involvement. The patients with drawing problems had more right parietal involvement on SPECT.

Patients with progressive aphasia have been examined neuropathologically. In this population the anatomical abnormalities typically are neuronal loss, gliosis, and atrophy localized primarily to the left temporal region, particularly the left-inferior and middle-temporal gyri. These findings mimic those seen in patients with FLD.

Amyotrophic lateral sclerosis. Classically, lesions in ALS are localized to the upper and lower motor neurons; however, more recent studies have shown that other areas of the cortex are often involved (Hudson 1991). Clinically, up to 15% of ALS patients develop mental symptoms (Hudson 1981), and the cognitive changes in these patients often suggest frontal lobe involvement (Hudson 1991; Mitsuyama 1984; Morita et al. 1987). Klüver-Bucy syndrome has been described (Dickson et al. 1986).

ALS patients show deficits in neuropsychological testing (Peavy et al. 1992). Our experience suggests that many patients are neuropsychologically normal, although a few patients show serious deficits in frontal

systems tasks and memory. A minority go on to develop a progressive dementia of the FLD type. In vivo studies with PET, using [^{18}F]fluoro-2-deoxy-D-glucose, have shown generalized hypometabolism, most severe in the sensorimotor cortex and putamen (Dalakas et al. 1987; Hatazawa et al. 1988). Focal frontal and temporal hypometabolism was not reported. Similar patterns have been observed in ALS using SPECT (Figure 20–3). At autopsy, ALS patients show nonspecific neuronal degeneration and gliosis (particularly the upper cortical layers), and sponginess of the neuropil, most severely in the frontal and medial temporal regions (Dickson et al. 1986; Horoupian et al. 1984).

Secondary FLDs. Finally, there are a variety of diseases that cause frontal lobe dysfunction where the major pathology is not at the level of the frontal lobes. Several different mechanisms lead to secondary FLD. One mechanism occurs in patients in whom the primary pathology occurs at the level of the basal ganglia, like patients with Parkinson's disease, Huntington's disease, and Wilson's disease. Because there are extensive connections between the basal ganglia and the frontal lobes, injury to the substantia nigra and neostriatum can cause frontal-lobe–type dysfunction (Cummings 1993). These illnesses can usually be differentiated from primary FLD, as a movement disorder typically is prominent. Also the dementia with these diseases is characterized by marked awareness and concern and mental slowing, in marked contrast to the dementia associated with FLD.

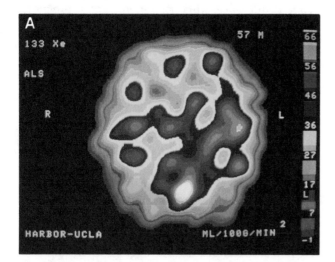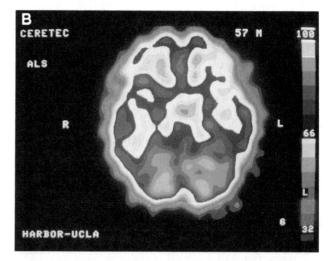

Figure 20–3. *Panel A:* Xenon-133 scan of a patient with amyotrophic lateral sclerosis (ALS). Note mild frontal and temporal hypoperfusion. *Panel B:* Hexamethylpropyleneamineoxime (HMPAO) scan of the same patient, showing frontal and temporal hypopefusion.

A similar mechanism is associated with diseases of subfrontal white matter, which can disconnect the frontal lobes from their subcortical connections. This occurs in some types of vascular dementia such as Binswanger's disease, a few inherited metabolic diseases such as metachromatic leukodystrophy, and a variety of demyelinating illnesses such as multiple sclerosis. These patients can appear clinically similar to those with FLD, although MRI shows extensive white matter lesions not typically present with primary FLD.

With alcoholism, general paresis of the insane, some cases of Creutzfeldt-Jakob disease, and acquired immunodeficiency syndrome (AIDS) dementia, there is a primary attack on the frontal lobes. History, serological testing, and lumbar puncture should differentiate these patients from those with primary FLD. Finally, with some diseases such as corticobasal degeneration, parkinsonian-ALS-dementia complex of Guam, Lewy body dementia, many cases of Creutzfeldt-Jakob disease, and AIDS-dementia, there is involvement of both frontal and subcortical systems. Patients with these diseases can be hard to differentiate from advanced FLD patients in whom both subcortical and frontal lobes are dysfunctional.

Summary

In this chapter, we have outlined the clinical, imaging, and neuropathological characteristics of the two major cortical dementias: AD and FLD. As our knowledge of these conditions advances, and as diagnostic tools are refined, improved diagnosis and a better understanding of pathogenesis will become possible.

References

Anderson TA, Chang L, Giombetti RJ, et al: Abnormal cerebral blood flow in myotonic dystrophy (abstract). Neurology 41 (suppl):420, 1991

Bartus RT, Dean RL 3rd, Beer B, et al: The cholinergic hypothesis of geriatric memory dysfunction. Science 217:408–414, 1982

Beard CM, Kokmen E, Offord KP, et al: Lack of association between Alzheimer's disease and education, occupational status, or living arrangement. Neurology 42:2063–2068, 1992

Benson DF: Progressive Frontal Dysfunction. Paper presented at 2nd International Conference on Frontal Lobe Degeneration of Non-Alzheimer Type. Lund, Sweden, September 1992

Benson DF, Kuhl DE, Hawkins DR, et al: The flourodeoxy-glucose 18F scan in Alzheimer's disease and multi-infarct dementia. Arch Neurol 40:711–714, 1983

Blessed G, Tomlinson BE, Roth M: The association between quantitative measures of dementia and of senile change in the cerebral grey matter of elderly subjects. Br J Psychiatry 117:797–811, 1968

Blumer D, Benson DF: Personality changes with frontal and temporal lobe lesions, in Psychiatric Aspects of Neurological Disease. Edited by Benson DF, Blumer D. New York, Grune & Stratton, 1975, pp 151–170

Boller F, Lopez OL, Moossy J: Diagnosis of dementia: clinico-pathologic correlations. Neurology 39:76–79, 1989

Boone KB, Miller BL, Lesser IM, et al: Neuropsychological correlates of white matter lesions in healthy elderly subjects: a threshold effect. Arch Neurol 49:549–554, 1992

Bowen DM, Davison AN: Biochemical studies of nerve cells and energy metabolism in Alzheimer's disease. Br Med Bull 42:75–80, 1986

Breteler MM, Van Duijn CM, Chandra V, et al: Medical history and the risk of Alzheimer's disease: a collaborative re-analysis of Case Control Studies (EURODEM Risk Factors Research Group). Int J Epidemiol 20 (Suppl 2):S36–S42, 1991

Brown GG, Levine SR, Gorell JM, et al: In vivo 31P NMR profiles of Alzheimer's disease and multiple subcortical infarct dementia. Neurology 39:1423–1426, 1989

Brun A: Frontal lobe degeneration of non-Alzheimer type, I: neuropathology. Archives of Gerontology and Geriatrics 6:193–208, 1987

Chartier-Harlin MC, Crawford F, Houlden H, et al: Early onset Alzheimer's disease by mutation at codon 17 of the beta-amyloid precursor protein gene. Nature 353:844–846, 1991

Chawluk JB, Mesulam MM, Hurtig H, et al: Slowly progressive aphasia without generalized dementia; studies with positron emission tomography. Ann Neurol 19:68–74, 1986

Corsellis JAN: Aging and the dementias, in Greenfield's Neuropathology. Edited by Blackwood W, Corsellis JAN. Chicago, Year Book Medical, 1976, pp 796–848

Creasey H, Jorm A, Longley W, et al: Monozygotic twins discordant for Alzheimer's disease. Neurology 39:1474–1476, 1989

Cummings JL: Psychosis in neurologic disease: neurobiology and pathogenesis. Neuropsychiatry, Neuropsychology, and Behavioral Neurology 5:144–150, 1992

Cummings JL: Frontal-subcortical circuits and human behavior. Arch Neurol 50:873–880, 1993

Cummings JL, Benson DF: Dementia: A Clinical Approach, 2nd Edition. Boston, Butterworth, 1992

Cummings JL, Duchen LW: Kluver-Bucy syndrome in Pick's disease: clinical and pathological correlations. Neurology 31:1415–1422, 1981

Cummings JL, Benson F, Hill MA, et al: Aphasia in dementia of Alzheimer's type. Neurology 35:394–397, 1985

Cummings JL, Miller BL, Hill MA, et al: Neuropsychiatric aspects of multi-infarct dementia and dementia of the Alzheimer type. Arch Neurol 44:389–393, 1987

Dalakas MC, Hatazawa J, Brooks RA, et al: Lowered cerebral glucose utilization in amyotrophic lateral sclerosis. Ann Neurol 22:580–586, 1987

DeCarli C, Kaye JA, Rapoport SI: Critical analysis of the use of computer assisted transverse axial tomography to study human brain in aging and dementia of the Alzheimer type. Neurology 40:884–886, 1990

Devanand DP, Cooper T, Sackeim HA, et al: Low dose oral haloperidol and blood levels in Alzheimer's disease: preliminary study. Psychopharmacol Bull 28:169–173, 1992

Dickson DW, Horoupian DS, Thal LJ: Klüver-Bucy syndrome and amyotrophic lateral sclerosis: a case report with biochemistry morphometics and Golgi study. Neurology 36:1323–1329, 1986

Dickson DW, Wertkin A, Mattiace LA, et al: Ubiquitin immunoelectron microscopy of dystrophic neurites in cerebellar senile plaques of Alzheimer's disease. Acta Neuropathol 79:486–493, 1990

Evans DA, Funkenstein HH, Albert M, et al: Prevalence of Alzheimer's disease in a community population of older persons: higher than previously reported. JAMA 262:2551–2556, 1989

Folstein MF, Folstein SE, McHugh PR: "Mini-mental state": a practical method for grading the cognitive state of patients for the clinician. J Psychiatr Res 12:185–198, 1975

Francis PT, Palmer AM, Sims NR, et al: Neurochemical studies of early onset Alzheimer's disease. N Engl J Med 313:7–11, 1985

Giombetti RJ, Miller BL: Recognition and management of superimposed medical conditions, in Alzheimer's Disease Treatment and Long Term Management. Edited by Cummings JL, Miller BL. New York, Marcel Dekker, 1990, pp 253–261

Glenner GG, Wong CW: Alzheimer's disease: initial report of the purification and characterization of a novel cerebrovascular amyloid protein. Biochem Biophys Res Commun 120:885–890, 1984

Gottfries CG: Neurochemical aspects of dementia disorders. Dementia 1:56–64, 1990

Graves AB, White E, Koepsell TD, et al: The association between head trauma and Alzheimer's disease. Am J Epidemiol 131:491–501, 1990

Growdon JH: Treatment for Alzheimer's disease? N Engl J Med 327:1306–1308, 1992

Gustafson L: Frontal lobe degeneration of non-Alzheimer type, II: clinical picture and differential diagnosis. Archives of Gerontology and Geriatrics 6:209–223, 1987

Gustafson L, Brun A, Risberg J: Frontal lobe dementia of non-Alzheimer type, in Advances in Neurology: Alzheimer's Disease, Vol 51. Edited by Wurtman RJ, Corkin S, Growdon J, et al. New York, Raven Press, 1990, pp 65–71

Hachinski VC, Iliff LD, Zilhka E, et al: Cerebral blood flow in dementia. Arch Neurol 32:632–637, 1975

Hatazawa J, Brooks RA, Dalaas MC, et al: Cortical motor-sensory hypometabolism in amyotrophic lateral sclerosis: a PET study. J Comput Assist Tomogr 12:630–636, 1988

Hay JJ, Ernst RL: The economic costs of Alzheimer's disease. Am J Public Health 77:1169–1175, 1987

Henriksson T, Barbour RM, Braa S, et al: Analysis and quantitation of the beta-amyloid precursor protein in the cerebrospinal fluid of Alzheimer's disease patients with a monoclonal antibody-based immunoassay. J Neurochem 56:1037–1042, 1991

Hershey LA, Modic MT, Greenough G, et al: Magnetic resonance imaging in vascular dementia. Neurology 37:29–36, 1987

Horoupian DS, Thal L, Katzman R, et al: Dementia and motor neuron disease: morphometric, biochemical, and Golgi studies. Ann Neurol 16:305–313, 1984

Hudson AJ: Amyotrophic lateral sclerosis and its association with dementia, parkinsonism and other neurological disorders: a review. Brain 1041:217–247, 1981

Hudson AJ: Dementia and parkinsonism in amyotrophic lateral sclerosis, in Handbook of Clinical Neurology: Diseases of Motor System, Vol 15 (59). Edited by de Jong JMBV. New York, Elsevier Science, 1991, pp 231–240

Jagust WJ, Budinger TF, Reed BR: The diagnosis of dementia with single photon emission computed tomography. Arch Neurol 44:258–262, 1987

Jagust WJ, Reed BR, Seab JP, et al: Clinical-physiological correlates of Alzheimer's disease and frontal lobe dementia. Am J Physiol Imaging 4:89–96, 1989

Joachim CL, Morris JH, Selkoe DJ: Clinically diagnosed Alzheimer's disease: autopsy results in 150 cases. Ann Neurol 24:50–56, 1988

Joachim CL, Selkoe DJ, Hiroshi M: Amyloid B-protein deposition in tissues other than brain in Alzheimer disease. Nature 342:226–230, 1989

Johnson K, Davis KR, Buonanno FS, et al: Comparison of magnetic resonance imaging and Roentgen ray computerized tomography in dementia. Arch Neurol 44:1075–1080, 1987

Jolles J, Bothmer J, Markerink M, et al: Phosphatidylinositol kinase is reduced in Alzheimer's disease. J Neurochemistry 56:2326–2329, 1992

Kamo H, McGeer PL, Harrop R, et al: Positron emission tomography and histopathology in Pick's disease. Neurology 37:439–445, 1987

Khachaturian ZS: Diagnosis of Alzheimer's disease. Arch Neurol 42:1097–1105, 1985

Klüver H, Bucy PC: Preliminary analysis of functions of the temporal lobes in monkeys. Archives of Neurology and Psychiatry 42:547–554, 1939

Knopman DS, Mastri AR, Frey WH, et al: Dementia lacking distinctive histologic features: a common non-Alzheimer degenerative dementia. Neurology 40:251–256, 1990

Kosaka K, Ikeda KK, Kobayashi K, et al: Striato-pallidonigral degeneration in Pick's disease: a clinico-pathological study of 41 cases. J Neurol 238:151–160, 1991

Kuhl DE, Metter EJ, Riege WH: Patterns of local cerebral glucose utilization determined in Parkinson's disease by [18F]fluorodeoxyglucose method. Ann Neurol 15:419–424, 1984

Liu CK, Miller BL, Cummings JL, et al: A quantitative MRI study of vascular dementia. Neurology 42:138–143, 1992

Malamud N, Boyd DA: Pick's disease with atrophy of the temporal lobes. Archives of Neurology and Psychiatry 43:210–222, 1940

Martyn CN, Barker DJ, Osmond C, et al: Geographical relation between Alzheimer's disease and aluminum in drinking water. Lancet 1:59–62, 1989

McKhann G, Drachman D, Folstein MF, et al: Clinical diagnosis of Alzheimer's disease: report of the NINCDS-ADRDA Work Group under the auspices of the Department of Health and Human Services Task Force on Alzheimer's Disease. Neurology 34:939–944, 1984

Mendez MF, Selwood A, Mastri AF, et al: Pick's disease versus Alzheimer's disease: a comparison of clinical characteristics. Neurology 43:289–292, 1993

Mesulam MM: Slowly progressive aphasia without generalized dementia. Ann Neurol 11:592–598, 1982

Miller BL, Mena I, Daly J, et al: Temporal-parietal hypoperfusion with single photon electron computer tomography in conditions other than Alzheimer's disease. Dementia 1:41–45, 1990

Miller BL, Cummings JL, Villanueva-Meyer J, et al: Frontal lobe degeneration: clinical, neuropsychological and SPECT characteristics. Neurology 41:1374–1382, 1991

Miller BL, Moats R, Shonk T, et al: Abnormalities of cerebral myo-inositol in patients with early Alzheimer disease. Radiology 187(2):334–339, 1993a

Miller BL, Chang L, Mena I, et al: Clinical and imaging features of right focal frontal lobe degenerations. Dementia 4:204–213, 1993b

Mitsuyama Y: Presenile dementia with motor neuron disease in Japan: clinico-pathological review of 26 cases. J Neurol Neurosurg Psychiatry 47:953–959, 1984

Mody CK, Miller BL: Unsuccessful treatments, in Alzheimer's Disease Treatment and Long Term Management. Edited by Cummings JL, Miller BL. New York, Marcel Dekker, 1990, pp 69–85

Morita K, Kaiya HK, Ikeda T, et al: Presenile dementia combined with amyotrophy: a review of 34 Japanese cases. Arch Gerontol Geriatr 6:263–277, 1987

Morris JC, Cole M, Banker BQ, et al:: Hereditary dysphasic dementia and the Pick-Alzheimer spectrum. Ann Neurol 16:455–466, 1984

Mortimer JA: Alzheimer's disease and senile dementia: prevalence and incidence, in Alzheimer's Disease. Edited by Reisberg B. New York, New York Free Press, 1983, pp 144–148

Neary D, Snowden JS, Shields RA: Single photon emission tomography using 99mTc-HMPAO in the investigation of dementia. J Neurol Neurosurg Psychiatry 50:1101–1109, 1987

Neary D, Snowden JS, Northen B, et al: Dementia of frontal lobe type. J Neurol Neurosurg Psychiatry 51:353–361, 1988

Nee LE, Polinsky RJ, Eldridge R, et al: A family with histologically confirmed Alzheimer's disease. Arch Neurol 40:203–208, 1980

Nee LE, Eldridge R, Sunderland T, et al: Dementia of the Alzheimer type: clinical and family study of 22 twin pairs. Neurology 37:359–363, 1987

Neumann MA: Pick's disease. J Neuropathol Exp Neurol 8:255–282, 1949

Neumann MA, Cohn R: Progressive subcortical gliosis; a rare form of presenile dementia. Brain 90:405–418, 1967

Office of Technology Assessment Task Force: Confronting Alzheimer's Disease and Other Dementias. Philadelphia, PA, JB Lippincott, 1988

Pardridge WM, Buciak JL, Yang J, et al: Measurement of amyloid peptide precursor of Alzheimer's disease in human blood. Alzheimer Dis Assoc Disord 5:12–24, 1991

Paschalis C, Polychronopoulos P, Lekka NP, et al: The role of head injury, surgical anaesthesia and family history as etiological factors in dementia of the Alzheimer type. Dementia 1:52–55, 1990

Peavy GM, Herzog AG, Rubin NP, et al: Neuropsychological aspects of dementia of motor neuron disease: a report of two cases. Neurology 42:1004–1008, 1992

Perry RH, Irving D, Blessed G, et al: Senile dementia of Lewy body type. J Neurol Sci 95:119–139, 1990

Petry S, Cummings JL, Hill MA, et al: Personality alterations in dementia of the Alzheimer type: a three-year follow up study. J Geriatr Psychiatry Neurol 2:203–207, 1989

Pick A: On the relation between senile atrophy of the brain, in Neurological Classics in Modern Translation. Translated by Schoene WS; edited by Rottenberg DA, Hochberg FH. New York, Hafner Press, 1892, pp 35–40

Prelli F, Castano E, Glenner GG, et al: Differences between vascular and plaque core amyloid in Alzheimer's disease. J Neurochem 51:648–651, 1988

Prinz PN, Vitiliano PP, Vitiello MV, et al: Sleep, EEG, and mental function changes in dementia of the Alzheimer type. Neurobiol Aging 3:361–370, 1982

Read SL, Miller BL, Mena I, et al: SPECT/pathology correlation in dementia (abstract). Neurology 4:316, 1992

Risberg J, Passant U, Warkentin S, et al: Regional cerebral blood flow in frontal lobe dementia of non-Alzheimer type. Dementia 4:186–187, 1993

Ropper AH, Williams RS: Relationship between plaques, tangles, and dementia in Down syndrome. Neurology 30:639–644, 1980

Roth M: The diagnosis of senile and related forms of dementia, in Alzheimer's Disease: Senile Dementia and Related Disorders. Edited by Katzman R, Terry RD, Bick KL. New York, Raven, 1978, pp 337–339

Rubin EH, Morris JC, Berg L: The progression of personality changes in senile dementia of the Alzheimer type. J Am Geriatr Soc 37:721–725, 1987

Salerno JA, Murphy DGM, Horwitz B, et al: Brain atrophy in hypertension: a volumetric magnetic resonance imaging study. Hypertension 20:340–348, 1992

Salmon E, Franck G: Positron emission tomographic study in Alzheimer's disease and Pick's disease. Archives of Gerontology and Geriatrics 1 (suppl):241–247, 1991

Sam M, Gutmann L, Schohet S, et al: Pick's disease: a case clinically resembling amyotrophic lateral sclerosis. Neurology 41:1831–1833, 1991

Schellenberg GD, Bird TD, Wijsman EM, et al: Genetic linkage evidence for a familial Alzheimer's disease locus on chromosome 14. Science 258:668–671, 1992

Snowden JS, Neary D, Man DMA, et al: Progressive language disorder due to lobar atrophy. Ann Neurol 31:174–183, 1992

Sparks DL, Markesbery WR: Altered serotonergic and cholinergic synaptic markers in Pick's disease. Arch Neurol 48:796–799, 1991

St. George-Hyslop PH, Tanzi RE, Polinsky RJ, et al: The genetic defect causing familial Alzheimer's disease maps on chromosome 21. Science 235:885–890, 1987

St. George-Hyslop PH, Haines JL, Farer LA, et al: Genetic linkage studies suggest that Alzheimer's disease is not a single homogeneous disorder. Nature 347:194–197, 1990

Swearer JM, Rachman DA, O'Donnell BF, et al: Troublesome and disruptive behaviors in dementia. J Am Geriatr Soc 36:784–790, 1988

Tanzi RE, Vaula G, Romano DM, et al: Assessment of amyloid beta-protein precursor gene mutations in a large set of familial and sporadic Alzheimer Disease cases. Am J Hum Genet 51:273–282, 1992

Teri L, Reifler BV, Veith RC, et al: Imipramine in the treatment of depressed Alzheimer's patients: impact on cognition. J Gerontol 46:372–377, 1991

Terry RD, Katzman R: Senile dementia of the Alzheimer type. Ann Neurol 14:497–506, 1983

Thal L, Galasko D, Katzman R, et al: Patients assessed at an Alzheimer's center generally have Alzheimer pathology. Neurology 41 (suppl 1):323, 1991

Tyrrell PJ, Warrington EK, Rackowiak RSJ, et al: Progressive degeneration of the right temporal lobe studied with positron-emission tomography. J Neurol Neurosurg Psychiatry 53:1046–1050, 1990

Vinters HV, Gilbert JJ: Cerebral amyloid angiopathy: incidence and complications in the aging brain, II: the distribution of amyloid vascular changes. Stroke 14:924–928, 1983

Vinters HV, Nishimura GS, Secor DL, et al: Immunoreactive A4 and gamma-trace peptide co-localization in amyloidotic arteriolar lesions in the brains of patients with Alzheimer's disease. Am J Pathol 137:233–240, 1990

Walker L: Animal models of cerebral amyloidosis. Bulletin of Clinical Neuroscience 56:86–96, 1991

Wechsler AF, Verity A, Rosenschein S, et al: Pick's disease: a clinical, computed tomographic and histological study. Arch Neurol 39:287–290, 1982

Whitehouse PJ, Price DL, Clark AW, et al: Alzheimer disease: evidence for selective loss of cholinergic neurons in the nucleus basalis. Ann Neurol 10:122–126, 1981

Wisniewski K, Jervis GA, Moretz RC, et al: Alzheimer neurofibrillary tangles in disease other than senile and presenile dementia. Ann Neurol 5:288–294, 1979

Yankner BA, Dawes LR, Fisher S, et al: Neurotoxicity of a fragment of the amyloid precursor associated with Alzheimer's disease. Science 245:417–420, 1989

Zhang M, Katzman R, Salmon D, et al: The prevalence of dementia and Alzheimer's disease in Shanghai, China: impact of age, gender, and education. Ann Neurol 27:428–437, 1990

21

Hyperkinetic Movement Disorders

Joanne M. Wojcieszek, M.D.
Anthony E. Lang, M.D., F.R.C.P.

Introduction

Movement disorders comprise a spectrum of abnormalities, which in broadest terms can be classified as hypokinetic or hyperkinetic (Weiner and Lang 1989). *Hypokinetic* disorders are characterized by significant impairment in the initiation of movement (akinesia) and reduction in the amplitude and speed of movement (bradykinesia), as well as increased muscle tone (rigidity). The most common example of this akinetic-rigid syndrome is Parkinson's disease (see Chapter 22). In contrast, *hyperkinetic* disorders involve excessive motor activity in the form of involuntary movements (or dyskinesias). The common types of dyskinesias include tremor, chorea, dystonia, myoclonus, and tics.

Abnormal movements in elderly patients may occur in a wide variety of primary central nervous system disorders (e.g., neurodegenerative diseases) or systemic illnesses including drug exposure, metabolic disturbances, vascular disease, and hypoxia. When approaching a patient presenting with abnormal movements, a careful history of the onset and course of illness and a detailed physical examination are required. Evaluations should include a remote and current drug history and documentation of family history. It is often necessary to review this information repeatedly or seek additional details from other sources (e.g., other family members or physicians). When assessing a hyperkinetic movement disorder, the physician must first attempt to classify the nature of the dyskinesia. This "what is the dyskinesia?" step is a critical first component of the diagnostic approach to patients with movement disorders. It precedes the classical neurology questions of "where is the lesion?" and "what is the lesion?" Once the dyskinesia is accurately classified using the definitions provided in the following sections, a knowledge of the differential diagnosis of the particular dyskinesia guides the diagnostic evaluation and approach to treatment. Investigations will vary depending on clinical suspicion.

Overview of Basal Ganglia Function

Many of the movement disorders discussed in this chapter are thought to result from dysfunction of the basal ganglia. For this reason, we begin with a brief overview of the anatomy and biochemistry of this region. It should be emphasized that the role of the basal

ganglia in normal motor function is still poorly understood. This obviously compromises our ability to explain the pathophysiology of the movement disorders that occur when these structures are damaged. It should also be emphasized that not all movement disorders are caused by abnormalities of the basal ganglia. For example, tremors are usually caused by lesions outside this region, and the origin of essential tremor, one of the most common movement disorders in elderly patients, is not known. The role of basal ganglia in tic disorders is also not understood. Most forms of myoclonus are probably not caused by dysfunction of the basal ganglia. However, we do know that disturbances in this region result in severe motor deficits, and recent advances in this field have allowed the development of tenable hypotheses to explain the pathophysiology of akinetic-rigid and certain hyperkinetic states.

The basal ganglia primarily consist of the caudate nucleus and putamen (striatum), the internal and external segments of the globus pallidus (GPi and GPe, respectively), the pars reticulata and pars compacta of the substantia nigra (SNr, SNc), and the subthalamic nucleus (STN). The GPi and SNr are functionally the same structure, having been divided by the internal capsule during development.

Although the basal ganglia are involved in the generation and modulation of movement, they influence motor activity indirectly by projecting (via the thalamus) to motor cortices rather than directly interacting with spinal motor neurons. The basal ganglia receive input from all areas of the cerebral cortex. Information is transmitted through the basal ganglia via somatotopically organized pathways (or circuits) that pass through the thalamus before projecting back to many areas of frontal cortex (Alexander and Crutcher 1990). Information from the basal ganglia is delivered to the ventral anterior, ventromedial, and centromedian nuclei of the thalamus before going on to primary motor, premotor, and supplementary motor areas. Other frontal lobe targets of basal ganglia output include the anterior cingulate area, frontal eye fields, and medial and lateral orbitofrontal cortices, which subserve the important roles of the basal ganglia in "limbic," oculomotor, and cognitive processing. At least five different cortical-basal ganglia-cortical loops have been proposed with function depending on the cortical projection areas involved.

The connections between basal ganglia, thalamus, and motor cortex are referred to as "basal ganglia–

thalamocortical" motor circuits (Figure 21–1) (Young and Penney 1988). Cortical areas send excitatory glutamatergic projections to the caudate and putamen (striatum), which serve as the "input" stations of the basal

ganglia. The basal ganglia "output" nuclei include the GPi and the SNr, which exert an inhibitory effect on the thalamus using the neurotransmitter γ-aminobutyric acid (GABA). Within each of the basal ganglia–

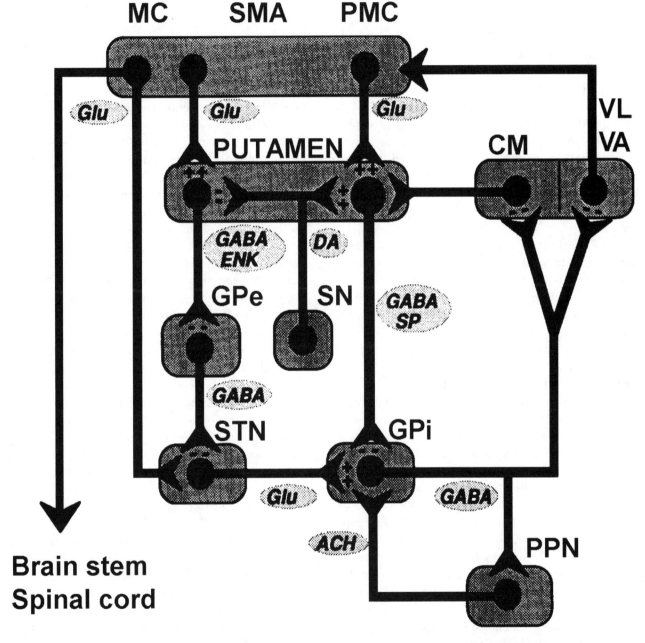

Figure 21–1. Current concept of neuronal connections and neurotransmitters of the basal ganglia, thalamus, and motor cortex. MC = motor cortex; SMA = supplementary motor cortex; PMC = premotor cortex; GPe = globus pallidus externa; GPi = globus pallidus interna (which is functionally similar to the substantia nigra pars reticulata [SNr]); STN = subthalamic nucleus; SN = substantia nigra; CM, VL, and VA = centromedian, ventrolateral, and ventral anterior nuclei of the thalamus, respectively; and PPN = pedunculopontine nucleus. The circled letters represent neurotransmitters. ACH = acetylcholine, GABA = γ-aminobutyric acid, DA = dopamine, ENK = enkephalin, GLU = glutamic acid, and SP = substance P.
Source. Reprinted from Nutt JG: "Dyskinesia Induced by Levodopa and Dopamine Agonists in Patients With Parkinson's Disease," in *Drug-Induced Movement Disorders.* Edited by Lang AE, Weiner WJ. Mount Kisco, NY, Futura Publishing, 1992, p. 296. Used with permission.

thalamocortical circuits is both a "direct" and "indirect" pathway. Information travels through the direct pathway in the following sequence: input from cortex → striatum → GPi/SNr → thalamus → cortex. The striatal efferents (using GABA and substance P) inhibit GPi/SNr which thus disinhibits the thalamus. The overall effect is that thalamocortical input is increased, which is thought to stimulate (using glutamate) cortically mediated motor activity. In the indirect pathway, signals flow as follows: input from cortex → striatum → GPe → STN → GPi/SNr → thalamus → cortex. Activation of the indirect pathway leads to inhibition (using GABA and enkephalin) of GPe, which promotes disinhibition of the STN. The STN provides excitatory drive (using glutamate) to the output nuclei (GPi and SNr). Disinhibition of the STN leads to thalamic inhibition by these output nuclei. The overall postulated result is that cortically initiated movements may be reduced.

The manner in which the nigrostriatal dopaminergic pathway modulates striatal activity is poorly understood. It is currently hypothesized that dopamine has an inhibitory effect on the indirect pathway (possibly involving the dopamine, subtype 2 [D_2], receptors) and an excitatory effect (possibly involving the dopamine, subtype 1 [D_1], receptors) on the direct pathway.

The two pathways by which information is passed from the striatum to the output station of the GPi/SNr appear to have opposing effects, with the direct pathway reinforcing cortical motor activity and the indirect pathway decreasing motor activity. The duelling effects of these pathways may allow the basal ganglia to perform a modulatory function in motor behavior. Alterations in the normal activity of these pathways offer at least a tentative explanation for hyperkinetic and hypokinetic disorders. For example, pathological loss of the normal STN input to the GPi/SNr would be expected to result in disinhibition of thalamic drive to the cortex and the development of hyperkinetic movements. This is exactly what happens with a lesion in the STN, which results in hemiballistic movements on the opposite side of the body. Parkinsonism, on the other hand, would result from pathologically decreased activity of the direct pathway and/or increased activity of the indirect pathway. Experimental studies in animals provide supportive evidence for these changes (DeLong 1990).

In the remainder of this chapter, we review the hyperkinetic movement disorders seen in older pa-

tients. Where possible we discuss the pathophysiology of the hyperkinesia in the light of the circuitry described above. The behavioral changes that commonly occur in these patients, either as a primary component of the disorder or secondary to the resulting disability, are highlighted.

Tremor

Tremor is defined as involuntary rhythmic oscillatory movement that can result from alternating or synchronous contraction of antagonist muscles. Tremor can be an exaggeration of a normal physiological process, can occur as an isolated monosymptomatic illness, or can be part of a variety of neurological disorders. Tremor is usually classified according to the circumstances in which it occurs. A rest tremor is seen with the body part in complete repose. Maintenance of a posture, such as extending the arms parallel to the floor, elicits a postural tremor. Kinetic tremor (or intention tremor) is seen during volitional movement. Other important descriptive qualities of tremor include the frequency, amplitude, and topographic distribution (e.g., face or lower extremities).

Rest tremor is most commonly a sign of Parkinson's disease or its drug-induced counterpart, but sometimes may be seen in other conditions. Approximately 75% of patients with Parkinson's disease exhibit a 4- to 6-Hz rest tremor, which usually begins unilaterally in the upper or lower extremity. The well-recognized appearance of a "pill-rolling" tremor of the arm is characteristic of Parkinson's disease and results from rhythmic extension-flexion of the wrist, pronation-supination of the forearm, and grasping movements of the fingers. Many Parkinson patients also have an 8- to 12-Hz postural tremor of the arms that is clinically indistinguishable from essential tremor. (For further discussion of Parkinson's disease, see Chapter 22.)

Unlike the close association between rest tremor and Parkinson's disease, postural and kinetic tremors occur in a wide range of disorders. Pathological postural and kinetic tremors in elderly individuals are most often caused by essential tremor or is a side effect of medications. Table 21–1 provides a summary of the various causes of tremor in elderly people.

All of us have a low-amplitude 10- to 12-Hz physiological tremor that can sometimes be seen in the outstretched fingers when the arms are extended. Physiological tremor can be accentuated by a variety of emotional and metabolic factors such as stress, fatigue, thyrotoxicosis, and hypoglycemia or as a result of drugs including caffeine, sympathomimetics, tricyclic antidepressants, and steroids.

Essential Tremor

Essential tremor is one of the most common movement disorders, occurring more frequently with advancing age. It is often inherited as an autosomal dominant trait, but the expression is variable. When a

---

Table 21–1. Classification and differential diagnosis of tremor in elderly patients

Rest tremor
Parkinson's disease
Other parkinsonian syndromes (less commonly)
Midbrain ("rubral") tremor: the rest tremor is less prominent than the postural tremor, which is less prominent than the kinetic tremor
Essential tremor—only if severe: rest tremor much less severe than the postural and kinetic tremors

Postural tremor (typically with terminal accentuation)
Physiological tremor
Exaggerated physiological tremor
  Stress, fatigue, and emotion
  Endocrine: hypoglycemia, thyrotoxicosis, pheochromocytoma, and steroids
  Drugs and toxins: Beta agonists, dopamine agonists, lithium, tricyclic antidepressants, neuroleptics, theophylline, caffeine, valproic acid, amphetamines, alcohol withdrawal, mercury, lead, arsenic, and others
Essential tremor
Primary writing tremor
With other central nervous system disorders
  Parkinson's disease and other akinetic-rigid syndromes
  Idiopathic dystonia including focal dystonias
  With peripheral neuropathy
Cerebellar tremor

Kinetic tremor
Disease of cerebellar "outflow" (dentate nucleus and superior cerebellar peduncle): vascular, tumor, acquired hepatocerebral degeneration, drugs, toxins (e.g., mercury), multiple sclerosis, and others

Miscellaneous rhythmical movement disorders
Psychogenic tremor
Orthostatic tremor
Rhythmical myoclonus (segmental myoclonus—such as palatal myoclonus and spinal myoclonus)
Asterixis
Clonus
Epilepsia partialis continua

Source. Adapted from Weiner and Lang 1989.

---

positive family history is elicited, the disorder is referred to as *familial tremor,* and when it appears for the first time after age 65 it has been called *senile tremor.* Essential tremor is a slowly progressive disorder that usually begins as an 8- to 10-Hz postural tremor of the hands. There may be involvement of the tongue, head, voice, or trunk with less common involvement of the legs. The tremor typically persists during action and worsens at endpoints (terminal accentuation). In more severely affected patients, the tremor may also be present at rest. The wider amplitude and more severe forms tend to have slower frequencies (4–6 Hz) and are more often seen in older individuals.

For many patients the tremor does not produce major symptoms, and only a small percentage of essential tremor patients are thought to seek medical attention. For some patients, however, the tremor interferes with handwriting, eating, drinking, and fine manipulations, as well as being a source of social embarrassment. With time there is often an increase in the amplitude of the tremor, which further compromises the ability to perform discrete movements. Although it is often preceded by the prefix "benign," essential tremor can be quite disabling (Koller et al. 1986). In some patients, notably those with prominent head tremor, embarrassment plays a major role in disability. Some patients become social recluses because of their concern about what others think of their appearance. Stress and anxiety typically increase tremors, accentuating the problem. Reactive depression may be a consequence in some individuals.

A clinical feature of both diagnostic and therapeutic significance is that most essential tremor patients note dramatic reduction in tremor after ingesting alcohol. The judicious use of small amounts of alcohol before meals and important events is not contraindicated, and surprisingly the risk of alcohol abuse among these patients is low (Koller 1983a). For patients who require treatment, the two most effective drugs for essential tremor are primidone and propranolol or other β-adrenergic blockers (mainly those with peripheral β2-adrenergic antagonist properties). Acute vestibulocerebellar side effects are common in response to primidone, even when given in low doses (50–62.5 mg/day). These may be more common in elderly patients and can be very disabling and protracted. For this reason, some neurologists briefly admit elderly patients to the hospital to initiate primidone therapy. Many elderly patients cannot take beta-blockers because of cardiac or pulmonary disease. Alternative treatments such as alprazolam and phenobarbital also may not be well tolerated. Other second-line drugs include clonazepam and carbonic anhydrase inhibitors. Drug contraindications, intolerance, and poor efficacy leave a significant number of elderly essential tremor patients with persistent disability from their tremor. Occasionally, there is a role for stereotactic thalamotomy or high-frequency thalamic stimulation in patients with disabling, drug-resistant tremor.

The physiological basis for essential tremor is unknown, but it is thought to be due to an abnormal oscillation of a central nervous system "pacemaker" (the location of which is uncertain) that is influenced by peripheral reflex pathways. No neurotransmitter or structural abnormalities have been identified as yet.

Other Tremors

Primary writing tremor is a tremor that is induced almost exclusively by writing. It is characterized predominantly by pronation-supination movements of the forearm at 5–7 Hz. Because many such patients have an associated mild postural tremor, primary writing tremor may be related to essential tremor. However, the task specificity and response in some patients to anticholinergics suggest that it may be more akin to dystonic "writer's cramp."

Patients with orthostatic tremor develop rapid rhythmic contractions of the legs and sometimes the buttocks within a few minutes of assuming a standing position. Walking, sitting, or lying will cause the tremor to cease. Most patients respond to clonazepam, primidone, or propranolol.

Cerebellar disease most commonly causes slow, irregular tremor of the head and trunk (titubation) when the patient is upright. Cerebellar tremor of the limbs is typically absent at rest and during the initial stages of motion, but becomes symptomatic through the course of and at the end of action. The term *intention tremor* has been used to describe the increase in tremor as the limb approaches a precise destination. This is not specific to cerebellar tremor and is common to most forms of postural tremor.

Lesions in the midbrain involving the superior cerebellar peduncle and possibly the substantia nigra near the red nucleus result in midbrain tremor or "rubral" tremor. This type of tremor is present at rest, increases with maintenance of posture, and increases still further with action. It is believed to result from interruption of the connections between cerebellar dentate nuclei and the thalamus. A lesion anywhere in this outflow pathway may cause such a tremor (thus the term *cerebellar outflow tremor*). Additional involvement of the dopaminergic nigrostriatal pathway may contribute to the tremor. Demyelinative lesions in multiple sclerosis are the most common cause of midbrain tremor overall, whereas posterior circulation stroke accounts for most cases in elderly patients. Other features of midbrain or diencephalic dysfunction typically accompany the tremor in this setting. Sometimes the onset of tremor may be delayed for weeks after a brain stem event (e.g., stroke or head injury). Medications are often not effective for this tremor type. Stereotactic thalamotomy may be useful in patients with severe debility; however, the disabling proximal component of the tremor is often resistant to this approach.

Numerous drugs can produce tremor (Table 21–1). As indicated above, often this is an accentuation of normal physiological tremor. Any patient who develops tremor acutely or subacutely after initiation of a new medication should be suspected of having a drug-induced tremor regardless of whether tremor is a recognized side effect. Some individuals may have a further predisposition to develop tremor from medications by virtue of underlying disorders such as essential tremor or subclinical Parkinson's disease. For example, we have seen the development of pronounced mixed postural and resting tremor in patients with pre-existing essential tremor who are treated with neuroleptic drugs. A number of medications used in psychiatric practice are capable of causing tremor. Tricyclic antidepressants may accentuate physiological tremor; however, this rarely poses a management problem. Tremor is an extremely common side effect of lithium therapy, which occasionally requires treatment with beta-blockers or primidone.

Neuroleptic drugs may cause a postural tremor or a parkinsonian resting tremor. One variant of the latter is a tremor of the perinasal and oral region known as the *rabbit syndrome*. Neuroleptic-induced parkinsonian tremor typically subsides on drug withdrawal. Patients who require ongoing neuroleptic therapy who have sufficiently bothersome or disabling tremor require therapy with anticholinergics or amantadine. However, because of the frequency of cognitive and psychiatric side effects, anticholinergics should be avoided in patients over 65 and are contraindicated in patients with known cognitive disturbance. Other considerations include a change to a less-potent neuroleptic or to an atypical agent such as clozapine.

Chorea

The term *chorea* is derived from the Greek word for dance. Choreic movements are brief, jerky, purposeless involuntary movements that occur in random sequence. They can involve the distal or proximal limbs, face, or trunk. The movements may be brisk and abrupt as in Sydenham's chorea or more slow and flowing as in Huntington's disease. The various causes of chorea in elderly patients are listed in Table 21–2. Because the types of chorea most frequently encountered in psychiatric practice include Huntington's disease and tardive dyskinesia, these topics are emphasized in the following discussion.

Huntington's Disease

Huntington's disease is a progressive hereditary disorder characterized by chorea, personality disturbances, and dementia. The prevalence of Huntington's disease in North America ranges from 4 to 8 per 100,000 (Harper 1991). Symptoms usually appear insidiously between 35 and 40 years of age. Typically, both the movement disorder and the mental changes are present at the onset of the disease, but one may precede the other by a period of years.

Movement disorders.   Initial involuntary movements usually involve the upper limbs and face with "fidgeting" of the hands, shrugging of the shoulders, grimacing of the face, or pursing of the lips. With time, more obvious and generalized choreic movements develop. Patients often try to incorporate these movements into normal purposeful acts, such as raising the hand to the head as if to smooth the hair. The chorea is increased by mental concentration, emotional stimuli, performance of complex motor tasks, and walking.

There is early impersistence of motor tasks such as the inability to sustain tongue protrusion or hand grip ("milkmaid grip"). Oculomotor disturbances are invariably present and include slowed pursuit and saccadic eye movements. Initially patients may be unable to rapidly direct their gaze in a given direction (i.e., generate a saccade) without blinking their eyes or thrusting their head. Later, gaze palsies may be pronounced. Other prominent findings include decreased fine motor coordination, dysarthria, dysphagia, orolingual apraxia (inability to perform tasks such as licking the lips or sucking an imaginary straw),

Table 21–2.   Causes of chorea in elderly patients

Hereditary causes
  Huntington's disease
  Benign hereditary chorea (typically childhood onset)
  Neuroacanthocytosis

Other central nervous system degenerations
  Olivopontocerebellar atrophy
  Machado-Joseph disease
  Kufs disease
  Dentatorubropallidoluysian atrophy

Aging-related causes
  Spontaneous orofacial dyskinesias
  "Edentulous orodyskinesia"
  "Senile chorea" (probably several etiologies)

Drug-induced causes
  Neuroleptics, metoclopramide, flunarizine, cinnarizine, antiparkinsonian drugs, amphetamines, methylphenidate, tricyclic antidepressants, monoamine oxidase inhibitors, lithium, estrogens (including estrogen creams for atrophic vaginitis), steroids, antihistamines, α-methyldopa, anticonvulsants (phenytoin, ethosuximide, carbamazepine, and phenobarbital), benzodiazepines, digoxin, methadone, and toluene

Metabolic causes
  Hyperthyroidism
  Hypoparathyroidism
  Hypo- and hypernatremia, hypomagnesemia, hypocalcemia
  Hypo- and hyperglycemia (latter may cause hemichorea or hemiballism)
  Acquired hepatocerebral degeneration, Wilson's disease

Infectious causes
  Encephalitides
  Subacute bacterial endocarditis
  Creutzfeldt-Jakob disease

Toxins
  Alcohol intoxication and withdrawal, anoxia, carbon monoxide, manganese, mercury, toluene, and thallium

Immunological causes
  Systemic lupus erythematosus
  Recurrence of Sydenham's chorea
  Primary anticardiolipin antibody syndrome

Vascular causes
  Infarctions usually involving striatum, subthalamic nucleus region
  Hemorrhage
  Arteriovenous malformation
  Polycythemia rubra vera
  Migraine

Tumors

Trauma: subdural hematoma

Miscellaneous: including paroxysmal choreoathetosis

Source. Adapted from Lang 1992a.

and manual apraxia. The gait takes on a dancing, stuttering character, which may be associated with lateral swaying or decreased arm swing. As the disease progresses, postural stability becomes impaired and axial chorea may throw the patient off balance. Later, dystonia and rigidity often become superimposed on the chorea. Involuntary movements may become so severe that routine activities of daily living are impossible. Importantly, apraxia and bradykinesia also contribute greatly to later motor disability.

Neuropsychological and psychiatric features.   Early mental disturbances in patients with Huntington's disease include personality and behavioral changes such as irritability, apathy, depression, decreased work performance, violence, impulsivity, and emotional lability. Intellectual decline usually follows the personality changes. The neuropsychological profile characteristically includes a type of memory disturbance, suggesting an impairment of information retrieval. Patients often have difficulty recalling information on command, but are able to give the correct answer in a multiple choice format. Other deficits in memory include loss of detailed recollections equally severe across all decades of a patient's life. There is difficulty with organization, planning, and sequencing even when all the necessary information is available (Caine et al. 1978). Other prominent abnormalities include visuospatial deficits, dyscalculia, impaired judgment, and ideomotor apraxia (the inability to perform previously learned tasks in the context of intact elementary motor function) (Brandt and Butters 1986). As the disease advances there are more global intellectual deficits.

A wide range of psychiatric disturbances are seen in Huntington's disease. Thirty-eight percent of patients have an affective disorder. Depression is the most common psychiatric symptom and does not appear to be simply a reaction to fatal illness. Evidence for this is the fact that mood disorders are not randomly distributed but occur in subsets of families with Huntington's disease (Peyser and Folstein 1990). Ten percent of patients develop mania. Psychosis is less common. Suicide accounts for 5.7% of deaths in patients with Huntington's disease, and 25% of all patients attempt suicide at least once (Farrer 1986).

Course.   The duration of Huntington's disease from onset to death is typically 15–20 years. Death is often caused by pneumonia, trauma, or suicide. In 10% of patients, the disease begins before age 20. Juvenile-

onset Huntington's disease is commonly an akinetic-rigid disorder (the Westphal variant). The predominant signs are bradykinesia, rigidity, dementia, seizures, and cerebellar disturbance often with little or no chorea. This form of Huntington's disease is rapidly progressive and the duration of illness is shorter than the adult-onset type. Occasionally the akinetic-rigid variant is seen in adults either de novo or developing after a choreic presentation.

Twenty-five percent of patients have late-onset Huntington's disease, which is usually defined as the onset of motor manifestations after age 50. One study of this population of patients (Myers et al. 1985) revealed that the average onset of chorea was 57.5 years and the average age at the time of diagnosis was 63 years. The clinical features are similar to those of the typical adult-onset variety, but the rate at which motor signs progress appears to be slower and the patients often demonstrate much milder cognitive changes.

Genetics.   Huntington's disease is inherited as an autosomal dominant trait with complete penetrance. Thus all people who inherit the gene will develop symptoms of the disease if they do not die prematurely. The Huntington gene has been localized to the short arm of chromosome 4 (Gusella et al. 1983). It has been found to contain an expanded and unstable CAG trinucleotide repeat. The normal gene contains between 11 and 34 copies of the CAG repeat unit, whereas the repeat length extends from 37 to 86 repeat units on the Huntington's chromosome (Gusella et al. 1993). Juvenile-onset patients usually inherit the gene from their fathers, whereas elderly patients are more likely to have inherited the gene from their mothers (Myers et al. 1983). This suggests that other factors influence the expression of the Huntington's disease gene. A younger age at onset is associated with longer trinucleotide repeat lengths.

Diagnosis.   A diagnosis of Huntington's disease can be made with confidence when a patient has dominantly inherited chorea and dementia with onset in adult life. Until the recent discovery of the genetic defect, the diagnosis was always a clinical one. There are no definite biochemical or radiological markers for Huntington's disease. Routine imaging demonstrates atrophy of the striatum (caudate and putamen) most easily appreciated as enlargement of the frontal horns of the lateral ventricles (Figure 21–2). In elderly patients this may be a less useful diagnostic feature unless it is very pronounced, given the normal reduction in brain mass with age and the occurrence of atrophy in other disorders that might be confused with Huntington's disease. [18F]fluorodeoxyglucose positron-emission tomography (PET) demonstrates striatal hypometabolism even before atrophy is seen on computed tomography (CT) or magnetic resonance imaging (MRI). However, this is a nonspecific finding, which may be seen in other disorders combining striatal degeneration and chorea (e.g., neuroacanthocytosis). The PET abnormalities in Huntington's disease may develop close to the time that symptoms begin, which means that this technique is probably not helpful in the evaluation of persons at risk for Huntington's disease.

Until recently, the most sensitive method for detecting gene carriers had been genetic linkage analysis. The discovery of DNA markers closely linked to the Huntington's disease gene allowed prediction of a patient's chances of developing the disease (with up to 95% reliability) if enough affected family members were available for testing. It is now possible to evaluate the CAG repeat length in an individual patient. Repeat

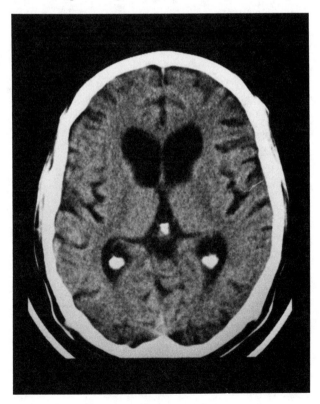

Figure 21–2. Computed tomography scan of a patient with Huntington's disease. Note the enlarged frontal horns with loss of the lateral indentation of the frontal horns reflecting the atrophy of the caudate nucleus.

lengths of greater than 38–40 are diagnostic of the disorder. Problems arise in cases with repeat lengths in the 34–38 unit range (Gusella et al. 1993). In addition, a small number of symptomatic patients have repeat lengths in the normal range. Further studies are required to resolve these confounding issues. The ethics of predictive testing have been extensively discussed as no treatment is currently available (Huggins et al. 1990). A carefully designed counseling service is a necessary component of any presymptomatic or diagnostic testing program.

Difficulties in diagnosis often arise when the family history is negative. It may be necessary to interview several relatives on more than one occasion to be certain of the family history. Some families deny the presence of cognitive or psychiatric disease in other family members. Patients should be asked about extramarital conception. If the affected parent had late-onset Huntington's disease, the diagnosis may have been missed for a variety of reasons. The symptoms may have been so mild as to go unnoticed, or the parent may have died before clinically apparent symptoms developed. Further, physicians may fail to consider the possibility of Huntington's disease in elderly patients, preferring to label the problem as "senile chorea" due to the minimal cognitive or behavioral changes. Still, the likelihood of Huntington's disease in a patient with typical clinical features and negative family history is at least 75% (Bateman et al. 1992). The availability of CAG repeat length analysis will now allow a definitive diagnosis in many patients with Huntington's disease who lack a clear family history.

The differential diagnosis of Huntington's disease in the elderly patient includes various degenerative, systemic, and drug-related conditions including tardive dyskinesia (Table 21–2). One important source of confusion is the patient treated with neuroleptics for a psychiatric presentation of Huntington's disease. The subsequent development of a movement disorder may then be mistaken for a complication of the drug therapy rather than an important clue to the underlying neurological diagnosis. A knowledge of the clinical differences between the movement disorders of Huntington's disease and the abnormal movements typically seen in tardive dyskinesia will help avoid this confusion (Table 21–3).

Pathology and neurochemistry.	At autopsy, the Huntington's disease brain is usually atrophic. Coronal sections reveal dramatic shrinkage of the caudate heads with resultant dilatation of the lateral ventricles. The gross appearance of the brain is a reflection of neuronal loss in the striatum with less severe changes in the globus pallidus and thalamus. Cortical volume may be reduced by as much as 20%, reflecting cell loss primarily in layers 3, 5, and 6 (Sotrel et al. 1991). Microscopically, there is preferential loss of small and medium-sized spiny neurons. Many neurotransmitters and their synthesizing enzymes are decreased as a result of the striatal cell loss. The most marked deficiencies include GABA, glutamic acid decarboxylase, acetylcholine, choline acetyltransferase, substance P, and enkephalin (J. B. Martin and Gusella 1986).

Striatal neurons are not uniformly affected in Huntington's disease (Reiner et al. 1988). In early and middle stages of Huntington's disease, somatostatin-neuropeptide-Y–containing interneurons and cholinergic interneurons are relatively spared, but these constitute only a small fraction of the total striatal neuron population. The majority of striatal neurons project to other areas and contain a variety of neuropeptides. It is this group of neurons that undergo early and progressive degeneration in Huntington's disease.

Striatal GABA/enkephalin neurons projecting to the GPe and substance P neurons projecting to the substantia nigra are preferentially depleted in early Huntington's disease (Figure 21–1). The resulting disinhibition of the GPe results in enhanced inhibition of the STN. This diminishes the excitatory drive of the STN to the GPi, in turn reducing the normal inhibitory output of the basal ganglia to the thalamus. The final result is thought to be disinhibition of excitatory thalamocortical efferents, which possibly results in excessive abnormal involuntary movements (Reiner et al. 1988).

In the later stages of Huntington's disease, there is a loss of the "direct" inhibitory substance P and GABA striatal projections to the GPi/SNr. This promotes more inhibition of the thalamus, and the resulting reduction of excitatory thalamocortical drive correlates with the late signs of rigidity and bradykinesia.

By the late stages of Huntington's disease, all striatal projection neurons are affected either from the primary degenerative process or as a result of transsynaptic degeneration. The mechanism of neuronal loss is not known, but the current hypothesis suggests that an endogenous excitotoxin (possibly glutamate) contributes in some way to the premature death of striatal neurons. Neurons possessing the *N*-methyl-D-aspartate (NMDA) glutamate receptor appear to be especially vulnerable to injury (Young et al. 1988). Future approaches to preventative therapy for Huntington's disease may involve NMDA receptor antagonists.

The dementia of Huntington's disease has been classically ascribed to primary striatal dysfunction. Evidence for this is the proven correlation between severity of cognitive impairment and degree of caudate and not cortical atrophy (Bamford et al. 1989; Starkstein et al. 1988), as well as earlier PET demonstration of glucose hypometabolism in the striatum but not in the cortex (Hayden et al. 1986; Weinberger et al. 1988;

Table 21–3.   Clinical features that help distinguish tardive dyskinesia (TD), oromandibular dystonia (OMD), and Huntington's disease (HD)

Feature	TD	OMD	HD
Forehead chorea	0	+	+++
Blepharospasm	+	++++	+/−
Movements of mouth	++++	++++	+
Platysma	+/−	++++	+/−
Nuchal muscles	+	+++	+/−
Trunk, arms, and legs	+++	0	+++
Stereotyped nature of movements	++++	++	0
Flowing movements	0	0	+++
Akathisia	+++	0	0
Marching in place	+++	0	0
Truncal rocking	+++	0	+
Dysarthria	+/−	+++	++++
Facial apraxia	0	0	+++
Impersistence of tongue protrusion	0	0	+++
Oculomotor defects	0	0	+++
Respiratory dyskinesia	++	+/−	+
Gait disorder	+	0	+++
Postural instability	0	0	+++
Dementia	+	0	+++
Effect of			
Talking or chewing	Decrease	Increase	+/−
Tongue protrusion to command	Decrease	+/−	+/−
Antidopaminergics	Decrease	Decrease	Decrease
Anticholinergics	Increase	Decrease	+/−
Effect on			
Talking or chewing	+	++++	+
Swallowing	0	++	++++

Note.   ++++ = Extremely common or marked; +++ = common or frequent; ++ = often; + = occasional; +/− = rarely present or variable; 0 = usually absent.
Source.   From S. Fahn, personal communication, July 1992.

Young et al. 1986). However, many of the features of Huntington's disease dementia are suggestive of "prefrontal" disturbance, and recent PET studies have shown diffuse abnormalities in cortical function with early frontal involvement in addition to striatal changes (Kuwert et al. 1990; W. R. W. Martin et al. 1992). Anatomically the caudate connects primarily with the frontal association cortices, so it is to be expected that caudate degeneration may lead to frontal lobe dysfunction. The high prevalence of affective disturbance is also not surprising given the rich connections between the striatum and the limbic system.

Treatment.   Management of Huntington's disease requires a team approach involving a wide variety of medical, paramedical, and social services. Education of patients and their families about the implications of the disease is extremely important. Genetic, psychological, and social counseling is regularly required, and lay organizations specifically designed to help families with Huntington's disease often assist greatly in these tasks.

Medical treatment is symptomatic. Drugs that block postsynaptic dopamine receptors (neuroleptics) or deplete presynaptic dopamine terminals (reserpine, tetrabenazine, and α-methylparatyrosine) are the most useful in reducing chorea. It is not known exactly why antidopaminergic drugs decrease the chorea. They can also help with the emotional outbursts, paranoia, psychosis, and irritability sometimes seen in Huntington's disease. With respect to the movement disorder, these medications should be reserved for disabling dyskinesias because of the high incidence of serious side effects. In younger patients, concern about the superimposition of tardive dyskinesia on the underlying choreic disorder encourages the use of dopamine-depleting agents rather than neuroleptics. In elderly patients one might turn to neuroleptics more readily, as tetrabenazine is not generally available, reserpine may cause problematic hypotension, and there may be less concern regarding long-term side effects. Despite the ability of dopamine antagonists to strikingly reduce chorea, motor disability may not be altered given other deficits, such as bradykinesia and apraxia, that may be worsened by these drugs. Depression may be treated with conventional antidepressant agents. Akinetic-rigid patients occasionally benefit from antiparkinsonian medications; however, increasing chorea and psychiatric disturbances may ensue. Benzodiazepines are often helpful with anxiety. (See Chapter 29 for dis-

cussion of psychopharmacological agents in geriatric neuropsychiatric disorders.)

Other Choreas

Spontaneous orofacial dyskinesia.   Spontaneous abnormal movements in the lingual-facial-buccal region occur in a variety of populations and are not exclusive to patients treated with neuroleptics. The prevalence of this disorder in otherwise healthy individuals increases from 0.8% between the ages of 50 and 59, to 7.8% between the ages of 70 and 79 (Klawans and Barr 1982). Spontaneous orodyskinesia may be more likely to develop in the context of underlying brain dysfunction such as in patients with schizophrenia or Down's syndrome (Dinan and Golden 1990; Waddington and Youssef 1990). Often it is difficult to completely exclude a brief exposure to neuroleptics in these patients. Many patients described as having spontaneous orofacial dyskinesia actually have cranial dystonia or Meige's syndrome (discussed below) (Table 21–3.).

"Edentulous orodyskinesia" in elderly patients.   Elderly patients may develop orofacial dyskinesias following tooth extraction (Koller 1983b). This occurs in about 16% of patients, but only after a long period of edentulousness (average of 12 years). The movements are similar to those seen in tardive dyskinesia with stereotyped smacking and pursing of the lips and lateral deviation of the tongue or jaw. However, the absence of vermicular movements of the tongue when inside the mouth and the lack of involuntary movements of the limbs or trunk help distinguish "edentulous orodyskinesia" from tardive dyskinesia. Most often, patients are unaware of these movements, and they never cause disability. Wearing dentures often diminishes or dampens the movements.

"Senile chorea."   This uncommon condition is best considered a "syndrome" of late-onset generalized chorea (beginning after age 65) for which no underlying cause can be determined. There is no cognitive deterioration nor is there a family history of psychiatric disturbance or chorea. Few cases with pathological documentation are available. The findings are not uniform, but may resemble less severe degrees of the changes seen in Huntington's disease with degeneration of the caudate and putamen (Alcock 1936) or putamen alone (Friedman and Ambler 1990). Senile chorea probably represents a heterogeneous group of disorders, which may inadvertently include late-onset Huntington's disease as discussed above.

Vascular chorea.   An important consideration when assessing chorea presenting in elderly patients is the potential role of multiple infarctions involving the basal ganglia particularly caudate, putamen, and subthalamic nucleus (Sethi et al. 1987). This syndrome usually occurs in the setting of lacunar disease as a result of chronic hypertension. A wide range of other causes of cerebral infarction must also be considered. Although chorea due to systemic lupus erythematosus is usually a disorder of the young, it may also occur in older individuals, as may chorea due to the primary anticardiolipin syndrome (Lang et al. 1991). Here, the chorea is probably the result of vascular or immunologic processes.

Polycythemia rubra vera has been known to cause generalized chorea of acute, subacute, or gradual onset. The chorea may be the presenting complaint leading to the diagnosis of polycythemia rubra vera. Haloperidol may diminish the chorea; however, the abnormal movements often improve after venesection or treatment with phosphorous-32.

Hemiballismus

The term *hemiballismus* describes involuntary, proximal, large amplitude, flailing, or throwing movements that can be violent and potentially dangerous in severe cases. Hemiballismus is often classified as one extreme in the spectrum of chorea due to the clinical and pathological overlap between the two conditions. Many patients with hemiballismus have concomitant distal choreic movements. As patients with hemiballismus improve, they often go through a hemichoreic phase.

Most patients with hemiballismus have a lesion in the contralateral subthalamic nucleus, although lesions of the caudate, putamen, thalamus, and possibly even the cortex are able to induce similar movements (Shannon 1990). Most hemiballism is secondary to vascular insult in the form of either lacunar infarction or hemorrhage, typically presenting with sudden onset of the involuntary movements. Given the common causes, hemiballism is most often a disorder of elderly individuals, particularly those with predisposing factors such as hypertension and diabetes. The diagnostic study of choice is brain MRI. Other possible causes include metastatic tumor, basilar meningitis, infections (e.g., toxoplasmosis), drugs, and metabolic derange-

ment (e.g., hyperglycemic nonketotic states).

Injury to the STN results in disinhibition of thalamocortical efferents (Figure 21–1), leading to excessive involuntary movements. Vascular hemiballism usually resolves spontaneously after weeks or months, but may occasionally be persistent. Given the severe disability caused by the pronounced abnormal movements, most patients require treatment with either neuroleptics or dopamine-depleting agents. Drug-resistant or persistent hemiballism sometimes requires stereotactic thalamotomy.

Tardive Dyskinesia

Tardive dyskinesia refers to a variety of persistent, involuntary movements caused by drugs that are dopamine receptor blocking agents (DRBAs). Antipsychotic drugs, with the exception of clozapine, are the most common responsible agents. Medications less commonly recognized as DRBAs such as metoclopramide, promethazine, amoxapine, and perphenazine-amitriptyline (Etrafon) can also cause tardive dyskinesia. Other drugs such as antidepressants, antihistamines, and phenytoin may induce movements similar to those seen in tardive dyskinesia, however such movements are not, by definition, classified as tardive dyskinesia. Dopamine-depleting drugs such as reserpine, tetrabenazine, and α-methylparatyrosine have not been shown to cause tardive dyskinesia.

Tardive dyskinesia usually begins insidiously after several years of therapy with a DRBA but can occur after only 3 months of exposure. Tardive dyskinesia also commonly appears after a decrease in dose or drug withdrawal. There is no definite period of time between stopping a DRBA and onset of involuntary movements that excludes a diagnosis of tardive dyskinesia. However, it is widely accepted that the movement disorder must begin within 3 months of stopping the DRBA (Fahn 1992) for a diagnosis of tardive dyskinesia to be applied. In contrast to other neuroleptic-induced movement disorders, such as acute dystonic reactions, secondary parkinsonism, and acute akathisia, the movements of tardive dyskinesia usually worsen when the offending agent is withdrawn and improve when the dose of the DRBA is increased.

Tardive dyskinesia is now considered a syndrome that includes several categories of abnormal involuntary movements (Table 21–4). The typical movements of tardive dyskinesia are choreic in speed and amplitude, but their stereotypic and almost rhythmic pattern distinguish them from the classical random, flowing choreic movements seen in Huntington's disease. Occasionally, a more typical choreic picture is seen. The involuntary movements usually reach maximal severity quickly after onset and then tend to stabilize.

The oral-buccal-lingual muscles tend to be involved earliest and most frequently in tardive dyskinesia. One early sign is a fine, vermicular movement of the tongue when inside the mouth. This may progress to horizontal tongue movements and later to rolling, twisting, or curling with pressing of the tongue against the cheek ("bon bon sign"). There may be brief or prolonged involuntary tongue protrusion ("fly-catcher's tongue"). Jaw movements include chewing, biting, teeth clenching, and lateral side-to-side movements. There may be pouting, pursing, smacking, or sucking movements of the lips, which sometimes have an audible component. The corners of the mouth may retract ("bridling"), or the cheeks may puff out intermittently. Despite these movements, speech and eating are often unaffected, as volitional activity of the affected muscles often dampens or alleviates the dyskinesia. The hands, feet, neck, and trunk may also be affected. Movements of the fingers may have a "piano-playing" appearance. There may be tapping motions of the feet, side-to-side oscillations of the foot at the ankle, or marching in place without the report of restlessness. Respiratory dyskinesia due to diaphragm and intercostal muscle involvement may produce an irregular respiratory pattern, periodic tachypnea, or grunting. The term *copulatory dyskinesia* colorfully describes a rocking, undulating movement of the pelvis sometimes encountered as a tardive manifestation. Surprisingly the gait is usually little affected.

Many patients seem unaware of even pronounced involuntary movements. However, a significant minority of patients are embarrassed and/or disabled by the dyskinesias because of interference with speech and swallowing, oral ulceration, or life-threatening respiratory involvement. Schizophrenic patients with tardive dyskinesia may have twice the mortality rate of schizo-

phrenic patients without it, but the reasons for this are uncertain (Yagi et al. 1989).

The movements described above refer to "classical tardive dyskinesia," which should be distinguished from other subtypes of tardive dyskinesia such as tardive dystonia, tardive akathisia, and the withdrawal-emergent syndrome.

Unlike classical tardive dyskinesia, which occurs more frequently in elderly individuals, tardive dystonia is seen equally in all age groups. The prevalence of this condition among chronic psychiatric patients is approximately 2% (Yassa et al. 1986). Younger patients tend to have more generalized involvement, whereas older patients usually have a focal or segmental distribution. Retrocollis may be especially common in tardive dystonia with more severe forms demonstrating opisthotonic posturing, often with the arms extended and pronated. A history of exposure to DRBAs, early facial and neck involvement, and concomitant signs of other tardive syndromes (e.g., classical tardive dyskinesia and tardive akathisia) can support a diagnosis of tardive dystonia. Tardive dystonia is usually more disabling and more difficult to treat than classical tardive dyskinesia.

Patients taking neuroleptics often complain of inner restlessness or akathisia. Most often this is an early, dose-related complication referred to as *acute akathisia,* which resolves when the offending drug is stopped. In contrast, tardive akathisia is a persistent problem, resulting from chronic exposure to DRBAs. Patients demonstrate a variety of "akathitic" movements including rubbing the scalp, marching in place, crossing and uncrossing the legs, or rocking of the trunk. Moaning and shouting may also occur. As is true of the other tardive syndromes, tardive akathisia usually worsens on withdrawal of the DRBA and improves if the dose is increased. Like tardive dystonia, tardive akathisia can result in profound disability.

The withdrawal-emergent syndrome involves involuntary movements (usually choreic) that typically appear in children following the abrupt discontinuation of DRBAs. This is a self-limited disorder that usually disappears within 6–12 weeks of onset. Other tardive syndromes include myoclonus, tics, and possibly tremor, but they are much less common than those described above.

Differential diagnosis. The differential diagnosis of tardive dyskinesia is extensive, given the spectrum of movements seen in this condition (Table 21–5), and

---

Table 21–4. Tardive dyskinesia subtypes

"Classical tardive dyskinesia"
Tardive dystonia
Tardive akathisia
Withdrawal-emergent syndrome
Tardive myoclonus
Tardive tics

includes a variety of abnormal movements seen in elderly psychiatric populations. Manneristic movements such as rubbing, picking, or grimacing may also improve with neuroleptics and may be mistaken for tardive dyskinesia. Patients with Huntington's disease who have been on chronic neuroleptic therapy may develop superimposed tardive dyskinesia. Clinical points of distinction between Huntington's disease and tardive dyskinesia are listed in Table 21–3.

Epidemiology.   The prevalence of tardive dyskinesia among patients on chronic neuroleptic therapy has been estimated to be 20% (Kane and Smith 1982). Proven risk factors for the development of tardive dyskinesia include age, sex, and duration of treatment. The incidence of tardive dyskinesia in elderly patients may be four times higher than that in young adults. Tardive dyskinesia is probably more common in women. The longer a patient is exposed to neuroleptics, the greater is the chance of his or her developing tardive dyskinesia. The cumulative incidence is estimated to be 5% after 1 year, 10% after 2 years, and 19% after 4 years (Khot et al. 1992). Other proposed but controversial risk factors include preexisting "organic brain dysfunction," "negative features of schizophrenia," and affective disturbance (said to be a greater risk than schizophrenia).

Pathophysiology.   Although tardive dyskinesia has been recognized for over 30 years, its pathogenesis remains poorly understood. The most commonly proposed mechanism is supersensitivity of postsynaptic striatal dopamine receptors as a consequence of chemical denervation caused by chronic use of DRBAs. Supersensitive striatal neurons may then respond abnormally to the presence of dopamine and produce the movements of tardive dyskinesia. The discontinuation of DRBAs would be expected to facilitate more interaction between dopamine and supersensitive receptors, leading to worsening of symptoms. Increasing the dose of the offending drug would increase receptor blockade and improve (or mask) symptoms. The appearance of tardive dyskinesia during ongoing neuroleptic therapy suggests that competitive receptor blockade can sometimes be overcome by endogenous dopamine; the latter may be increased through enhanced activity of presynaptic nigrostriatal neurons responding to blockade of the postsynaptic receptors. Most neuroleptics are antagonists of the D_2 receptor. New classes of neuroleptics, such as clozapine, bind

other subclasses of dopamine receptors, which may explain why they do not cause tardive dyskinesia (Baldessarini and Frankenburg 1991). Recent animal studies have suggested that tardive dyskinesia may result not only from alterations in the D_2 receptor but possibly from complex interactions between D_1 and D_2 receptors (Rosengarten et al. 1991).

There are a number of inconsistencies with the dopamine receptor supersensitivity hypothesis of tardive dyskinesia (Fibiger and Lloyd 1984). Other proposed mechanisms include changes in GABAergic and glutamatergic neuronal function. The potential for neuroleptics to induce free-radical–mediated neuronal damage has been proposed (Cadet et al. 1986; Lohr et al. 1990). The ability of acetylcholine and noradrenaline agonists to reduce the movements of tardive dyskinesia suggests that these neurotransmitters also may be involved in its pathogenesis. The prominent and consistent involvement of the orofacial structures suggests changes in specific somatotopic basal ganglia regions. The pathophysiology of facial and limb dyskinesias may differ given certain clinical and epidemiological differences between them (Burke 1984).

Prevention.   Considering the iatrogenic nature of tardive dyskinesia, prevention should be emphasized. The indications for long-term antipsychotic medication should be clearly delineated and regularly reevaluated. Patients requiring chronic neuroleptic therapy should be maintained on the minimal dose needed for a therapeutic effect. Patients should be regularly evaluated for signs of tardive dyskinesia. Neuroleptics should be avoided in psychiatric conditions for which other categories of drugs may be effective. Metoclo-

---

Table 21–5.   Differential diagnosis of tardive dyskinesia in elderly patients

Schizophrenic stereotyped movements

Spontaneous orofacial dyskinesia

"Edentulous orodyskinesia"

Infarcts of the basal ganglia

Huntington's disease or other choreiform disorders (see Table 21–2)

Dyskinesias induced by other drugs (see Table 21–2)

Idiopathic dystonias: Meige's syndrome or oromandibular dystonia (see Table 21–3)

Hemifacial spasm

Mouthing movements said to be associated with cerebellar vermis lesions

pramide should not be given chronically unless other drugs have failed. The use of anticholinergic agents in addition to neuroleptics should be minimized, as they are known to aggravate movements of tardive dyskinesia and may actually increase the likelihood of the developing tardive dyskinesia, although this remains to be proven. It is common practice to use intermittent neuroleptic therapy, or "drug holidays," in hopes of determining whether early tardive dyskinesia has developed but is being masked by ongoing treatment. However, there is preliminary evidence that "drug holidays" may be associated with an increased risk of tardive dyskinesia (Jeste et al. 1979). Based on the free radical hypothesis there have been claims that free radical scavengers such as vitamin E may prevent the development of tardive dyskinesia. The results of well-designed placebo-controlled studies of antioxidant therapies in neuroleptic-treated patients are awaited with interest.

Treatment. Once the diagnosis of tardive dyskinesia is established, the offending agent should be gradually withdrawn if the psychiatric state allows (Figure 21–3). Anticholinergic and other antiparkinsonian medications should be discontinued. In patients who must continue on neuroleptic therapy, the movements of tardive dyskinesia usually remain static or gradually improve (Casey et al. 1986; Koshino et al. 1991). During the drug-withdrawal phase, involuntary movements will often transiently worsen over weeks, and it may be necessary to add a benzodiazepine such as diazepam or clonazepam or phenobarbital to ease the patient's discomfort and anxiety. Between one-quarter and one-half of patients will improve within 1 year of drug withdrawal, but others may require up to 5 years (Klawans et al. 1984). Sometimes tardive dyskinesia may be permanent. The severity of the movements does not predict outcome after drug withdrawal. Elderly patients have less chance for spontaneous remission once drugs are discontinued.

Patients requiring chronic neuroleptic treatment should be considered for conversion to lower-potency or atypical agents (e.g., loxapine, molindone, or thioridazine), though the efficacy of this strategy is unproven. Clozapine may suppress tardive dyskinesia and may someday become the drug of choice for psychotic patients with tardive dyskinesia (Khot et al. 1992).

For patients with disabling "classical" tardive dyskinesia, dopamine antagonists offer the most effective therapy for suppressing abnormal movements. Treat-

ment with DRBAs, however, significantly decreases the chance of remission. Presynaptic depletors such as reserpine and tetrabenazine may be very effective in suppressing tardive dyskinesia, but these may not be well tolerated because of secondary parkinsonism, akathisia, and depression. Therapeutic trials of GABA agonists (clonazepam, valproic acid, diazepam, and baclofen), noradrenergic antagonists (propranolol and clonidine), and cholinergic agonists (lecithin and choline chloride) may also be helpful, but are rarely as effective as treatment with dopamine antagonist drugs. Second-line agents include vitamin E, buspirone, and calcium channel blockers.

Whereas younger patients with tardive dystonia may benefit from anticholinergic agents such as trihexyphenidyl and ethopropazine, older patients are more likely to develop memory loss and confusion with these drugs, and they are relatively contraindicated in elderly patients. Dopamine antagonists, especially dopamine-depleting drugs, but sometimes even DRBAs, have the greatest likelihood of therapeutic success in disabling tardive dystonia. Dopamine depletors alone or in combination with other agents are helpful in over 50% of patients (Kang et al. 1986). Botulinum toxin injection may be extremely effective in selected patients with prominent focal involvement of cranial and cervical musculature.

In contrast to acute akathisia, tardive akathisia usually does not respond to beta-blockers, antiparkinsonian agents (e.g., anticholinergics and amantadine), or benzodiazepines. Management of this disabling tardive variant is difficult and usually involves dopamine depletors or receptor blockers. Electroconvulsive therapy may be effective in recalcitrant cases.

Dystonia

Dystonia is characterized by abnormal involuntary twisting movements that tend to be sustained and can result in abnormal postures. Some dystonic movements are slow and writhing and, when they occur distally, may be referred to as *athetosis*. Dystonic movements also may be quite rapid and resemble the lightening-like jerks of myoclonus. There may be superimposed rhythmic movements that are especially prominent when the patient tries to actively resist the dystonia (sometimes referred to as *dystonic tremor*). Dystonic movements frequently occur only during specific actions (e.g., writer's cramp). The movements are

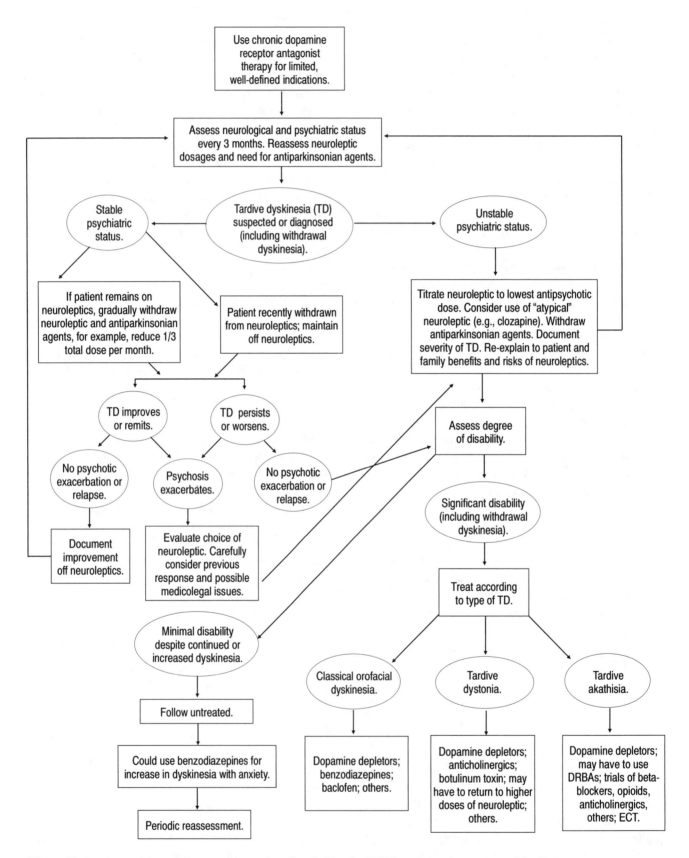

Figure 21–3. Approach to the management of tardive dyskinesia. DRBAs = dopamine receptor blocking agents; ECT = electroconvulsive therapy.
Source. Adapted from Weiner and Lang 1989.

often increased by stress and improve with relaxation. Patients often use a variety of tricks or antagonistic gestures to decrease the severity of the movements. Spontaneous remissions may occur in some forms of idiopathic dystonia, especially torticollis. Failure to recognize these unusual features has commonly resulted in dystonia being misdiagnosed as hysteria.

Dystonia is often classified by distribution, age at onset, and etiology. When a single body part is affected it is called *focal dystonia*. Involvement of two or more contiguous parts is called *segmental dystonia*, whereas it is called *multifocal dystonia* when distribution is not contiguous. The term *generalized dystonia* indicates involvement of one or both legs, the trunk, and some other body part. *Hemidystonia* is the involvement of one side of the body.

Dystonia beginning in adulthood typically affects the neck, face, or arm. Involuntary movements tend to remain limited to one or a small number of contiguous regions (i.e., face and neck). This is unlike dystonia of childhood onset in which signs usually begin in the legs and frequently generalize.

With respect to etiology, dystonia may be idiopathic or secondary to other disorders (Table 21–6). The age at onset and the distribution of the dystonia are often helpful in determining the cause. For example, in adulthood, generalized involvement or onset in the legs suggests that the dystonia is secondary to some underlying condition, whereas isolated focal or segmental dystonia is usually idiopathic. Involvement of one side of the body (hemidystonia) is often associated with a contralateral basal ganglia lesion. The nature of the dystonic movements also may assist in diagnosis. For example, as mentioned above, early in the course of dystonia patients may exhibit the abnormal movements only when performing specific actions. This feature is particularly common in idiopathic dystonia. When a patient demonstrates constant abnormal posturing of a limb early in the disease (i.e., dystonia at rest), this is suggestive of secondary cause.

Idiopathic Dystonia

Idiopathic torsion dystonia typically begins in childhood and often leads to severe disability by the age of 20. Occasional members of families with idiopathic torsion dystonia have onset delayed until later adulthood. The inheritance of idiopathic torsion dystonia seen in Ashkenazi Jewish and non-Jewish populations is autosomal dominant with variable penetrance. Link-

age studies have localized the genes for idiopathic torsion dystonia in Jewish and some non-Jewish families to chromosome 9 (Ozelius et al. 1989).

Focal dystonias. Idiopathic adult-onset focal dystonia is much more common than idiopathic torsion dystonia. Marsden (1976) provided compelling arguments in favor of classifying these disorders as variants of idiopathic torsion dystonia. The validity of this association awaits future developments in our understanding of the molecular basis of dystonia.

The most common forms of idiopathic adult-onset focal dystonia are spasmodic torticollis (cervical dysto-

Table 21–6. Causes of late-onset dystonia

Idiopathic dystonia
Generalized dystonia (rare)
Segmental/multifocal dystonia
Focal dystonias
  Spasmodic torticollis
  Cranial dystonia
    Blepharospasm
    Oromandibular dystonia
    Spasmodic dysphonia
  Writer's cramp

Secondary dystonia
Drugs: including neuroleptics, dopamine agonists, anticonvulsants, and antimalarial drugs
Stroke: hemorrhage or infarction[a]
Other focal lesions: vascular malformation, tumor, abscess, and demyelination
Trauma: head injury or peripheral injury[a] and subdural hematoma
Encephalitis
Toxins: manganese, carbon monoxide poisoning, methanol, and carbon disulfide
Paraneoplastic
Hypoparathyroidism
Central pontine myelinolysis
Degenerative diseases
  Parkinson's disease
  Progressive supranuclear palsy
  Cortical-basal ganglionic degeneration
  Multiple system atrophy (Shy-Drager syndrome, olivopontocerebellar atrophy, and striatonigral degeneration)

Disorders that may simulate dystonia
Psychogenic dystonia
Orthopedic: atlantoaxial subluxation[b]
Neurological: seizures, posterior fossa tumor, and oculomotor disturbance

[a]Dystonia is often delayed.
[b]Typically a disorder of childhood.

nia), cranial dystonia including blepharospasm and oromandibular dystonia, spasmodic dysphonia (laryngeal dystonia), and dystonia of the upper limb most often manifested as "writer's cramp."

Spasmodic torticollis is the most common type of adult-onset focal dystonia. It usually begins in the fourth or fifth decade and is more common in women. Involuntary activity of neck muscles causes abnormal postures and movements of the head. The movements may be sustained or may appear as twisting, shaking, or turning of the head. Commonly the head is turned to one side (torticollis), or tilted with the ear toward the shoulder (laterocollis). Less often there is excessive head flexion (anterocollis) or extension (retrocollis). The continuous muscle contraction may lead to muscle hypertrophy, frequently evident in the sternocleidomastoid muscle, and there may be associated shoulder elevation. Neck discomfort and pain are common. Although many patients initially report an involuntary pulling of the head in one direction, some are unaware of the abnormal head posture until a family member draws it to their attention. Up to 50% of patients will have additional dystonic features usually in the face or arm. Associated postural tremor of the hands is common.

Many patients use sensory tricks (*geste antagoniste*) to decrease the severity of the dystonic movements. Resting the head against a high-back chair, holding the back of the neck, or lightly touching the cheek may return the head to the normal position. Activities such as walking, writing, and combing the hair often aggravate the symptoms.

Symptoms usually increase during the first 5 years. Partial or full remission occurs in up to one-fifth of patients, but this is almost always transient (Jahanshahi et al. 1990). Symptoms may be mild, but most patients experience some degree of disability related to pain, abnormal head posture, and embarrassment. Patients with longstanding symptoms occasionally develop cervical root or cord compression. This complication may be more likely in elderly patients, who have a higher incidence of underlying cervical spondylosis.

Focal or segmental dystonia involving cranial muscles is called *cranial dystonia* (Meige's syndrome). The usual age at onset is the sixth decade, and women are more commonly affected than are men. The most common component of cranial dystonia is blepharospasm, characterized by involuntary, forced eye closure caused by excessive contraction of the orbicularis oculi muscles. The disorder usually begins with an increase in blink rate, which gradually progresses to more forceful closure of both eyelids. Aggravating factors include talking, watching television, reading, and exposure to bright lights. Tricks such as rubbing or lightly touching the eye, yawning or opening the mouth, or extending the neck may interrupt the eyelid closure. Blepharospasm may eventually result in functional blindness despite normal visual acuity.

Another component of cranial dystonia is oromandibular dystonia, featuring involuntary spasms of lower cranial muscles that cause mouth opening, jaw clenching, platysma contraction, tongue muscle contractions and protrusion, and contractions of the soft palate. There may be associated grunting, throat clearing, and inspiratory noises. This type of dystonia is usually seen in combination with blepharospasm or spasmodic dysphonia (see below), but it may occur in isolation. In contrast to classical tardive dyskinesia (for which oromandibular dystonia is commonly mistaken), the movements of oromandibular dystonia are typically brought out or aggravated by use of the involved muscles, such as in talking or chewing (Table 21–3). Injuries of the tongue, lips, and teeth are common. Touching the finger to the lips or teeth may lessen the spasms.

Involvement of laryngeal muscles is known as *spasmodic dysphonia*. Most patients have a voice disturbance due to hyperadduction of the vocal cords (adductor spasmodic dysphonia). The voice is strained, tight, hoarse, and often tremulous. The less common hyperabduction variety (abductor spasmodic dysphonia) results in breathy phonation and sudden drops in pitch.

Writer's cramp is the most common form of task-specific focal limb dystonia. Typically, the fingers and wrist flex excessively, causing the hand to tightly grasp the pen and press unnecessarily hard on the paper. Alternatively, the fingers may involuntarily extend or splay, making it difficult to hold the pen. Tremor or myoclonic jerks also may occur while writing. Initially, only writing may be affected (simple writer's cramp). Later, other manual tasks also may be impaired (dystonic writer's cramp). There are a wide variety of other "occupational palsies" or task-specific dystonias. As in the case of writer's cramp, these typically begin in mid-adult life and subsequently persist or progress. Like all other forms of dystonia, these disorders are commonly misdiagnosed as due to anxiety or "nerves." Both the chronic disability caused by the focal dystonia and the frequent mislabeling as a psychological disorder often result in emotional upset and reactive depression.

Pathophysiology. Little is known of the etiology or pathophysiology of idiopathic dystonia. Electrophysiological studies suggest disturbances of inhibitory mechanisms in the brain stem and spinal cord (Marsden and Quinn 1990). These changes may be secondary to aberrant suprasegmental influences, for example, originating from the basal ganglia. Routine histopathology studies have failed to demonstrate consistent abnormalities. Preliminary biochemical analyses suggest a disturbance of noradrenergic pathways (Hornykiewicz et al. 1986). Study of secondary dystonias may provide further clues to the origin and nature of the abnormalities in idiopathic dystonia.

Secondary Dystonia

Drug-induced dystonia. Levodopa-induced dystonia in Parkinson's disease is probably the most common form of drug-induced dystonia. Other important agents that can cause dystonia include DRBAs and, less commonly, anticonvulsants and antimalarial drugs (Lang 1992b). With respect to neuroleptics (antipsychotics and antiemetics such as prochlorperazine and metoclopramide), these drugs may cause short-lived dystonia very early in their course (acute dystonic reactions) or prolonged dystonia usually after long-term use (tardive dystonia). Unlike tardive dystonia, which has no age preference, and tardive dyskinesia and drug-induced parkinsonism, which are more common in elderly patients, neuroleptic-induced acute dystonia is more common in younger patients and indeed rarely develops in elderly patients. It may be more common in men and is more likely to occur with higher-potency neuroleptics. Of note is that clozapine has not been shown to cause acute dystonia. Dystonic reactions usually develop within the first 5 days of starting a neuroleptic, most often occurring on day 2 (Casey 1992). Patients may develop a sensation of thickness of the tongue, involuntary opening or closing of the mouth, facial grimacing, tongue protrusion, tightness in the throat, torticollis, retrocollis, oculogyric crisis (rolling of the eyes upward or off to the side), or laryngopharyngeal spasms. Limb or truncal spasm may result in bizarre posturing.

The pathophysiology of acute dystonia probably involves an increase in cholinergic activity with some alterations in dopaminergic pathways. It is still not known whether dopamine transmission at the time of the acute dystonic reaction is decreased or increased. Treatment consists of parenteral administration of an-

ticholinergic or antihistaminic agents followed by oral anticholinergics for 1–2 days.

Miscellaneous secondary dystonias. In childhood a wide variety of storage diseases and neurometabolic disorders can cause dystonia. All children presenting with dystonia require a trial of levodopa to exclude the diagnosis of dopa-responsive dystonia. Adults presenting with this disorder typically demonstrate features of Parkinson's disease rather than dystonia. Wilson's disease is an extremely important consideration; however, it rarely, if ever, presents de novo after the age of 45.

Dystonia can be seen after various acute brain insults such as stroke or head trauma. The dystonia secondary to stroke usually occurs weeks or even years after the initial insult. The involuntary movements often develop as a hemiparesis resolves. Lesions resulting in hemidystonia occur most often in the contralateral putamen, thalamus, caudate nucleus, and globus pallidus (Marsden et al. 1985). Occasionally, blepharospasm has been associated with lesions in the brain stem, thalamus, or basal ganglia (Jankovic 1986).

Many of the secondary dystonias due to environmental causes, such as encephalitis and exposure to toxins, have stabilization of symptoms once the destructive process is completed. However, for reasons that are not clearly known, the symptoms of a static encephalopathy, including dystonia, choreoathetosis, myoclonus, and even pyramidal tract deficits, may progress in later adult life.

There is increasing evidence that peripheral trauma may be associated with various forms of dystonia. In some instances there may be a genetic predisposition to idiopathic dystonia. Sometimes a seemingly inconsequential injury can result in severe, fixed dystonic postures with features of reflex sympathetic dystrophy.

Dystonia is a feature of a variety of neurodegenerative diseases. It is common in Parkinson's disease both as a manifestation of the disorder and as a complication of therapy with dopamine agonists (e.g., levodopa and bromocriptine). Patients often develop transient dystonia as their medications are "wearing off," in the fully developed "off" period, first thing in the morning, or as a peak-of-dose effect. Patients with progressive supranuclear palsy usually have pronounced neck and trunk rigidity, sometimes with nuchal extension, which has been referred to as *axial dystonia*. There may be associated dystonic posturing of the limbs, sometimes in a hemidystonic pattern. Cortical-basal ganglionic degeneration causes an akinetic-rigid syndrome with apraxia, cortical sensory deficit, action tremor, and frequent limb dystonia. Multiple system atrophy, which includes striatonigral degeneration, Shy-Drager syndrome, and olivopontocerebellar atrophy, may also manifest various forms of dystonia including excessive neck flexion (or anterocollis). An occasional feature of multiple system atrophy is laryngeal stridor, possibly secondary to vocal cord paralysis (Williams et al. 1979) or even laryngeal dystonia (Marion et al. 1992).

Psychogenic dystonia is uncommon, but when it does occur it can be severe enough to cause permanent contractures. Clinical clues that suggest psychogenic dystonia include "giving way" weakness, nondermatomal sensory loss, multiple somatizations, and especially inconsistency and incongruity of the abnormal movements (Fahn 1990).

Treatment

Dystonia has traditionally been one of the most difficult movement disorders to manage. Drug therapy is often unrewarding. The most effective drugs have a high incidence of side effects, especially in elderly patients. High doses of anticholinergic drugs (e.g., trihexyphenidyl, ethopropazine, and benztropine) may be at least partially effective in up to 50% of patients. Adults frequently experience intolerable side effects secondary to both peripheral and central anticholinergic effects. Peripheral side effects such as blurred vision and constipation may be lessened by the use of concomitant pilocarpine eye drops and oral bethanechol or pyridostigmine. However, central side effects including memory loss and confusion remain a major limiting factor especially in older patients. Tricyclic antidepressants, benzodiazepines, carbamazepine, dopamine antagonists, and baclofen may also be helpful.

Botulinum toxin injection has revolutionized the therapy of focal dystonia, particularly blepharospasm, spasmodic torticollis, spasmodic dysphonia, and oromandibular dystonia (Jankovic and Brin 1991). The toxin acts presynaptically at nerve terminals to decrease the amount of acetylcholine released into the neuromuscular junction. Chemical denervation of the muscle results in weakness and wasting. The duration of benefit is usually 3–4 months. Side effects mainly relate to excessive weakness of injected muscles and to spread of the toxin locally to other areas (e.g., causing dysphagia in patients treated for cervical dystonia).

Myoclonus

Myoclonus refers to sudden, brief, shock-like involuntary movements that are usually caused by active muscle contraction (positive myoclonus), but can also be caused by inhibition of ongoing muscle activity (negative myoclonus, including asterixis). Myoclonus may be focal, multifocal, segmental (involving two or more contiguous regions), or generalized. There is a wide clinical spectrum of myoclonic movements. They may be single, rare jerks or constant repetitive contractions. The amplitude may vary from a mild twitch that fails to move a joint to a gross jerk that moves the entire body. The pattern is usually irregular but sometimes may be rhythmic, giving a superficial appearance of tremor. Myoclonus may occur spontaneously at rest or on attempting movement (action myoclonus). Myoclonus is frequently triggered (stimulus sensitive) by a variety of stimuli such as sudden noise, light, visual threat, soft touch, pinprick, or muscle stretch.

Myoclonus can originate from a variety of locations in the central nervous system. Electrophysiological studies including back-average recording of electroencephalographic (EEG) potentials, evoked potentials, long-latency reflex recordings, and multichannel electromyographic (EMG) assessment are capable of separating myoclonus of cortical and subcortical (reticular) origin. Less often myoclonus originates at a segmental (brain stem or spinal) level, in which case the movements are often rhythmical. Rarely, myoclonic movements are due to lesions in the peripheral nervous system. Clinically, it is sometimes difficult to distinguish myoclonus from tics. Unlike tics, myoclonus cannot be willfully controlled nor is it associated with a conscious urge to move or with relief once the movement has been completed. Myoclonic movements are usually of shorter duration and less patterned than tics and are typically increased rather than diminished when the patient performs a motor act.

Causes of myoclonus in the elderly may include idiopathic disorders such as physiological myoclonus, nocturnal myoclonus, essential myoclonus, and startle syndromes. More commonly, however, myoclonus in elderly patients is secondary to metabolic disorders, infections, drugs, hypoxia, and degenerative diseases (Table 21–7). In earlier life, myoclonus is a common feature of idiopathic seizure disorders (epileptic myoclonus), and it may be a feature of progressive encephalopathies associated with seizures such as Lafora's disease (i.e., progressive myoclonic epilepsies).

Idiopathic Myoclonus

Physiological myoclonus. Physiological myoclonus occurs in healthy individuals and is often worsened by fatigue or stress. Hiccups and the jerking that most people experience on falling asleep (sleep starts or hypnic jerks) are other forms of myoclonus seen in healthy individuals.

Nocturnal myoclonus. Periodic movements in sleep are stereotyped, repetitive movements of the legs that appear during stages 1 and 2 of sleep. Typically, there is myoclonic jerking of one or both legs followed by tonic flexion at the knee and hip, dorsiflexion at the ankle, and extension of the big toe. The duration of the movements may be as long as 5 seconds, implying that they are not truly myoclonic in nature; they occur at regular intervals, usually every 20–40 seconds. The prevalence of periodic movements in sleep appears to increase with age, being present in 29% of patients over age 50 (Lugaresi et al. 1986).

Restless legs syndrome consists of nighttime unpleasant paresthesia and restlessness of the legs. These symptoms are relieved or lessened by activity, and patients may demonstrate a variety of secondary purposeful movements such as stretching, rubbing the legs, wiggling the ankles, or arising and pacing. Some patients also have myoclonic or dystonic involuntary movements in the legs while awake, and periodic movements in sleep are almost universal (Walters and Hening 1987). The symptoms interfere with sleep and, in fact, restless legs syndrome is the fourth leading cause of insomnia after psychiatric disorders, drug abuse, and sleep apneas (Coleman 1982). Restless legs syndrome can develop at any age but symptoms may become more severe in old age. Most cases are idiopathic, although strong associations exist with iron deficiency anemia, rheumatoid arthritis, and uremia. When no cause is apparent, restless legs syndrome may be inherited as an autosomal dominant trait. Neuroleptic treatment can exacerbate the symptoms of restless legs syndrome. Peripheral neuropathies may cause similar symptoms. Both periodic movements in sleep and restless legs syndrome respond to benzodiazepines including clonazepam and nitrazepam, dopamine agonists such as levodopa and bromocriptine, or μ-receptor opiate agonists such as codeine or propoxyphene.

Essential myoclonus. Essential myoclonus is an idiopathic disorder that is often inherited in an autosomal dominant pattern. Symptoms typically begin in childhood or early adult years and persist with a variable course over the remainder of the patient's life. Disability may be pronounced. Some patients also demonstrate a postural tremor, and others have features of

Table 21–7. Causes of myoclonus in elderly patients

Physiological myoclonus
Hiccup
Sleep starts
Exercise induced
Anxiety induced

Essential myoclonus

Secondary myoclonus
Metabolic causes
  Hepatic failure
  Renal failure
  Dialysis syndrome
  Hyponatremia
  Hypoglycemia
  Nonketotic hyperglycemia
Viral encephalopathies
  Herpes simplex encephalitis
  Arbovirus encephalitis
  Encephalitis lethargica
  Postinfectious encephalomyelitis
Drugs and toxins
  Bismuth
  Heavy metal poisons
  Methyl bromide, DDT
  Drugs: tricyclic antidepressants, levodopa, monoamine oxidase inhibitors, antibiotics, and lithium
Physical encephalopathies
  Postanoxic (Lance-Adams syndrome)
  Posttraumatic
  Heat stroke
  Electric shock
  Decompression injury
Dementing and degenerative diseases
  Creutzfeldt-Jakob disease
  Alzheimer's disease
  Cortical-basal ganglionic degeneration
  Parkinson's disease
  Huntington's disease
  Multiple system atrophy
  Pallidal degenerations
Focal central nervous system damage
  Poststroke
  Olivodentate lesions (palatal myoclonus)
  Spinal cord lesions (segmental/spinal myoclonus)
  Tumor
  Trauma
  Following thalamotomy (often unilateral asterixis)

Source. Adapted from Fahn et al. 1986.

focal or segmental dystonia. Whether these features are all manifestations of the same genotype or whether "essential myoclonus" represents several different genetic diseases remains to be determined (Bressman and Fahn 1986). Some patients experience a pronounced beneficial response with alcohol, and this has lead to problematic alcohol abuse (Quinn and Marsden 1984).

Startle syndromes. The startle syndromes represent exaggerations of the normal human alerting reaction (startle). There is excessive motor response to unexpected auditory or visual stimuli. Typically, this consists of a blink, contortion of the face, and flexion of the neck, trunk, and arms. Sometimes the condition is inherited in autosomal dominant fashion (hyperekplexia), but in rare cases it may result from acquired brain stem pathology such as anoxia, hemorrhage, or sarcoidosis (Brown et al. 1991a). Clonazepam is currently the treatment of choice.

Secondary Myoclonus

Myoclonus secondary to metabolic disturbances.
Myoclonus may result from a wide range of metabolic disturbances including severe hepatic failure, hyponatremia, hypoglycemia, and nonketotic hyperglycemia. The myoclonus commonly seen in uremia involves the face and upper extremities and is often aggravated by auditory or tactile stimuli. A significant number of patients with metabolic derangements will demonstrate asterixis. These brief lapses in postural tone (negative myoclonus) can be demonstrated by attempting to hold the wrist actively extended or the foot dorsiflexed. Toxic levels of anticonvulsants, especially phenytoin, may cause asterixis, as well as typical myoclonus. Unilateral asterixis may be caused by focal central nervous system lesions, which often involve the thalamus (Young and Shahani 1986).

Myoclonus secondary to infections or tumors. Multifocal or generalized myoclonus may be seen in patients with systemic infections, acute encephalitides, or postinfectious encephalomyelitis. Myoclonus may be accompanied by opsoclonus (dancing eye movements) in brain stem encephalitis, which is usually inflammatory or paraneoplastic in etiology.

Myoclonus secondary to drugs. There are a wide variety of medications that can cause myoclonus. Most often this occurs in the context of an acute toxic encephalopathy. For example, antibiotics, especially the penicillins and cephalosporins, can cause isolated myoclonus or more severe toxic encephalopathy with seizures, especially if given to patients with compromised renal function. A number of other drugs may cause myoclonus even in the absence of other features of toxicity: these include tricyclic antidepressants, levodopa, dopamine agonists, monoamine oxidase inhibitors, and lithium. In psychiatric practice, myoclonus occurs in up to 40% of patients taking tricyclic antidepressants (Garvey and Tollefson 1987).

Postanoxic myoclonus. Postanoxic myoclonus usually results from cardiac arrest, respiratory failure, or an anesthetic accident. Pronounced myoclonus in a patient with one of these conditions usually indicates a severe anoxic encephalopathy with poor prognosis. A unique syndrome of action myoclonus (the Lance-Adams syndrome) occurs in a minority of patients surviving severe cerebral anoxia. As the patient awakens from coma, action-induced myoclonic jerks emerge, as do lapses in posture (negative myoclonus), which frequently result in falling. In the more severely affected individuals, myoclonus interferes with all voluntary movement, including speech and swallowing. Additional cognitive and behavioral disturbances may accompany the myoclonus depending on the extent of anoxic cerebral damage.

The pathophysiology of postanoxic action myoclonus is strongly associated with dysfunction of brain stem serotonin pathways. The major metabolite of serotonin, 5-hydroxyindoleacetic acid (5-HIAA), is typically reduced in the cerebrospinal fluid of these patients. Agents that increase serotonin activity such as the serotonin precursor L-5-hydroxytryptophan (5-HTP) given with carbidopa are often markedly effective in reducing myoclonus. However, 5-HTP may cause a variety of side effects and is not readily available. For these reasons, the treatments of choice are valproic acid and/or clonazepam, agents that can also result in a striking reduction in the severity of the myoclonus.

Myoclonus related to dementing and neurodegenerative diseases. Myoclonus is a prominent feature of Creutzfeldt-Jakob disease, a disorder that causes subacute onset of dementia and personality change. Myoclonus may begin in the face or limbs, but later becomes more generalized as the disease progresses. Although present at rest, the myoclonus can often be triggered by loud noise. The EEG often shows periodic sharp discharges, occurring approximately once per second. The myoclonic jerks are sometimes time locked to these abnormal EEG discharges.

Myoclonus is present in 10% or more of patients with Alzheimer's disease. It can occur at any time in the course of the illness, but is often a late manifestation (Hauser et al. 1986). Focal, stimulus-sensitive myoclonus is a common feature of cortical-basal ganglionic degeneration (CBGD) and multiple system atrophy including striatonigral degeneration, Shy-Drager syndrome, and olivopontocerebellar degeneration. In Parkinson's disease, myoclonus rarely occurs as an early feature. Most often it develops as a late-stage side effect of levodopa especially in patients with psychiatric complications and concomitant dementia.

Segmental Myoclonus

Palatal myoclonus is characterized by unilateral or bilateral 1.5- to 3-Hz rhythmic (thus the more appropriate designation as a "tremor") movements of the soft palate. Synchronous movements of adjacent muscles of the face and neck frequently accompany the palatal activity. In most patients, a definitive cause can be identified, and these patients are said to have symptomatic palatal tremor. The most common etiology of symptomatic palatal tremor is stroke affecting the brain stem and cerebellum (Deuschl et al. 1990). The palatal tremor usually develops after a delay of up to 10 months following the initial stroke and persists as a permanent sequela.

Patients do not typically complain of the involuntary palatal movements, but rather they are more bothered by limb, gait, and oculomotor disturbances from the underlying infarction. MRI results often show hyperintense signal in the inferior olive (Pierot et al. 1992). Pathological examination shows vacuolar hypertrophic transsynaptic degeneration of the inferior olive with a lesion involving the connection between the cerebellar dentate nucleus (via the superior cerebellar peduncle) and the central tegmental tract to the contralateral inferior olive. When the lesion is unilateral, the olivary hypertrophy is on the side opposite the myoclonus.

One-quarter of patients with palatal tremor (myoclonus) have no underlying cause identified (Deuschl et al. 1990). These patients are considered to have essential palatal tremor, which typically occurs in young adulthood and presents with a clicking sound in the ear that can often also be heard by the examiner. The cause of the ear click is probably the sudden opening and closing of the eustachian tube as a result of intermittent contraction of the tensor veli palatini muscle.

Palatal myoclonus is typically resistant to pharmacological therapy, although occasional patients will respond to drugs such as clonazepam or anticholinergics. Bothersome ear click may be reduced by focal injections of botulinum toxin into the tensor veli palatini muscle (Deuschl et al. 1991).

Spinal myoclonus is also usually slow and rhythmic, involving the muscles of several spinal segments and resulting in movements of one or more limbs and/or trunk. Lesions in the spinal cord that may give rise to myoclonus include infection, demyelination, tumor, degenerative disease, and cervical myelopathy (Jankovic and Pardo 1986). Another rare form of spinal myoclonus is thought to originate in slowly conducting propriospinal pathways. Propriospinal myoclonus includes spontaneous and stimulus-sensitive nonrhythmic axial jerks causing symmetric flexion of the neck, trunk, hips, and knees (Brown et al. 1991b).

Hemifacial Spasm

Hemifacial spasm typically begins in adulthood and is more common in women. It begins as brief twitches around the eye that gradually increase in severity and may evolve to sustained contractions lasting many seconds to minutes. The movements may remain isolated to the orbicularis oculi or may spread to other ipsilateral facial muscles. The movements cannot be voluntarily suppressed and tend to persist in sleep. In most instances it is thought that hemifacial spasm is caused by mechanical compression of the facial nerve at the nerve root exit zone by an aberrant blood vessel (less commonly by a tumor, aneurysm, or other compressive lesions). Although surgical decompression of the facial nerve can be curative (Jannetta et al. 1977), botulinum toxin injection is extremely effective in reducing the involuntary movements and is the treatment of choice (Jankovic and Brin 1991).

Tics

Tics are intermittent, repetitive, stereotyped abnormal movements (motor tics) or sounds (vocal tics) that vary in intensity and are repeated at irregular intervals. Tics encompass an extremely broad range of movements and sounds. Although most tics are abrupt and brief, some tics may be slower in onset and prolonged (dystonic tics). Motor and vocal tics may be further classified as simple or complex. Simple motor tics involve one group of muscles and include eyeblinking, shoulder shrugging, or facial grimacing. Complex motor tics are coordinated sequences of movement such as touching, hitting, jumping, or copropraxia (obscene gestures). Simple vocal tics are inarticulate noises or sounds including throat clearing, sniffing, and grunting. Complex phonic tics involve saying words and include echolalia (repetition of others), palilalia (repetition of self), and coprolalia (swearing). Patients usually experience an inner urge to perform the movement, which is temporarily relieved by the execution of the movement. More than most other movement disorders, tics can be suppressed for prolonged periods of time and are decreased by distraction or concentration on complex mental or motor tasks.

Tics are most commonly idiopathic, but may result from a variety of other conditions such as encephalitis, head injury, stroke, and drugs (Table 21–8). Tics usually begin in childhood either as a simple transient motor tic or as part of the spectrum of manifestations of Gilles de la Tourette syndrome (Tourette syndrome). There is even evidence that a simple transient tic of childhood occasionally is the sole manifestation of the Tourette syndrome gene (Kurlan et al. 1988). Many patients with Tourette syndrome remit in adolescence, but for the remainder the syndrome is a lifelong disorder.

Table 21–8.   Causes of tics in elderly patients

Idiopathic
  Persistent childhood-onset tic disorder
  Simple tic
    Multiple motor tics
    Multiple motor and vocal tics (Tourette syndrome)
  Adult-onset tic disorder
Secondary
  Postencephalitic
  Head injury
  Carbon monoxide poisoning
  Poststroke
  Drugs: stimulants, levodopa, neuroleptics ("tardive Tourette"), carbamazepine, phenytoin, and phenobarbital
  Mental retardation syndromes: including chromosomal abnormalities
  Postrheumatic chorea (probably not seen in the elderly)

Unfortunately, there is limited information regarding the course of Tourette syndrome as patients reach the geriatric age period. Interestingly, the first well-described patient with Tourette syndrome reported by Itard in 1825 (included in Gilles de la Tourette's first paper) was 85 years old (Bruun 1988). The results of studies including elderly patients with Tourette syndrome indicate that most patients improve with maturity (except for occasional worsening in the fourth decade) and that when symptoms persist over the age of 50 they are typically mild (Bruun 1988; Burd et al. 1986). On the other hand, we have seen one patient with lifelong multiple simple motor tics who at the age of 72 developed the complex vocal tic of shouting the names of friends and 2 years later developed echolalia and coprolalia (Lang et al. 1983). Additional studies are required to understand the effects of aging on the course of tics. Further complicating this issue is the rare occurrence of idiopathic adult-onset tics. Epidemiological and clinical aspects of tics beginning in mid- to late-adult life have yet to be formally studied. The relationship between adult-onset tics and the more common childhood-onset tics, including Tourette syndrome, is unknown at present.

Summary

The hyperkinetic movement disorders include tremor, chorea, dystonia, myoclonus, and tics. A wide variety of these dyskinesias begin in late life, or their course is affected in some manner by the aging process. The idiopathic focal dystonias, including spasmodic torticollis, cranial dystonia, and writer's cramp, begin in mid to late life and can result in significant disability. Neurodegenerative disorders such as multiple system atrophy, progressive supranuclear palsy, CBGD, Alzheimer's disease, and Creutzfeldt-Jakob disease all may be associated with variable degrees of dystonia, myoclonus, or tremor. Parkinson patients who have been on long-term levodopa therapy often develop prominent choreiform and dystonic movements.

Increasing age is associated with a higher risk of cerebrovascular disease which can sometimes result in "cerebellar outflow tremor," chorea (including hemiballismus), delayed dystonia, palatal myoclonus, and occasionally asterixis. Elderly patients have a greater chance of developing tardive dyskinesia when exposed to neuroleptics and appear to have less potential for improvement after discontinuation of these drugs compared with that of younger patients. The incidence of periodic movements in sleep and "spontaneous orofacial dyskinesia" also increases with advancing age. Some disorders, such as essential tremor, may worsen with age. Conversely, there are examples in which advanced age appears to be an attenuating factor in the expression of hyperkinetic disorders. Patients with onset of Huntington's disease after age 50 have slower motor deterioration and milder cognitive dysfunction compared with those who develop symptoms in early adult life. The incidence of neuroleptic-induced acute dystonic reactions decreases with age, and these rarely occur in the elderly. Tics appear to lessen in severity after the third decade.

Treatment of hyperkinetic movements in older patients is often limited by medical contraindications or poor drug tolerance. An informed trial-and-error sequential use of several different medications may be necessary in disabled patients. Botulinum toxin has revolutionized the treatment of dystonia. Neuroleptics might be used more readily in elderly patients for the management of choreiform disorders, as there is less concern about long-term sequelae such as tardive dyskinesia; however, this possibility should remain a concern as should the greater risk of disabling drug-induced parkinsonism.

In summary, an elderly patient with a movement disorder may pose a diagnostic and therapeutic challenge for the clinician. The important first step is the classification of the dyskinesia, which then focuses the diagnostic considerations and guides the approach to treatment.

References

Alcock NS: A note on the pathology of senile chorea (non-hereditary). Brain 59:376–387, 1936

Alexander GE, Crutcher MD: Functional architecture of basal ganglia circuits: neural substrates of parallel processing. Trends Neurosci 13:266–271, 1990

Baldessarini RJ, Frankenburg FR: Clozapine: a novel antipsychotic agent. N Engl J Med 324:746–754, 1991

Bamford KA, Caine ED, Kido DK, et al: Clinical-pathologic correlation in Huntington's disease: a neuropsychological and computed tomography study. Neurology 39:796–801, 1989

Bateman D, Boughey AM, Scaravilli F, et al: A follow-up study of isolated cases of suspected Huntington's disease. Ann Neurol 31:293–298, 1992

Brandt J, Butters N: The neuropsychology of Huntington's disease. Trends Neurosci 9:118–120, 1986

Bressman S, Fahn S: Essential myoclonus, in Myoclonus (Advances in Neurology Series, Vol 43). Edited by Fahn S, Marsden CD, Van Woert M. New York, Raven, 1986, pp 287–294

Brown P, Rothwell JC, Thompson PD, et al: The hyperekplexias and their relationship to the normal startle reflex. Brain 114:1903–1928, 1991a

Brown P, Thompson PD, Rothwell JC, et al: Axial myoclonus of propriospinal origin. Brain 114:197–214, 1991b

Bruun RD: The natural history of Tourette's syndrome, in Tourette's Syndrome and Tic Disorders. Edited by Cohen DJ, Bruun RD, Leckman JF. New York, Wiley, 1988, pp 21–40

Burd L, Kerbeshian J, Wilkenheiser M, et al: Prevalence of Gilles de la Tourette's syndrome in North Dakota adults. Am J Psychiatry 143:787–788, 1986

Burke RE: Tardive dyskinesia: current clinical issues. Neurology 34:1348–1353, 1984

Cadet JL, Lohr JB, Jeste DV: Free radicals and tardive dyskinesia. Trends Neurosci 9:107–108, 1986

Caine ED, Hunt RD, Weingartner H, et al: Huntington's dementia. Arch Gen Psychiatry 35:377–384, 1978

Casey DE: Neuroleptic-induced acute dystonia, in Drug-Induced Movement Disorders. Edited by Lang AE, Weiner WJ. Mount Kisco, NY, Futura Publishing, 1992, pp 21–40

Casey DE, Povlsen UJ, Meidahl B, et al: Neuroleptic-induced tardive dyskinesia and parkinsonism: changes during several years of continuing treatment. Psychopharmacol Bull 22:250–253, 1986

Coleman RM: Periodic movements in sleep (nocturnal myoclonus) and restless legs syndrome, in Sleeping and Waking Disorders: Indications and Techniques. Edited by Guilleminault C. Palo Alto, CA, Addison-Wesley, 1982, pp 265–295

DeLong MR: Primate models of movement disorders of basal ganglia origin. Trends Neurosci 13:281–285, 1990

Deuschl G, Mischke G, Schenck E, et al: Symptomatic and essential rhythmic palatal myoclonus. Brain 113:1645–1672, 1990

Deuschl G, Lohle E, Heinen F, et al: Ear click in palatal tremor: its origin and treatment with botulinum toxin. Neurology 41:1677–1679, 1991

Dinan TG, Golden T: Orofacial dyskinesia in Down's syndrome. Br J Psychiatry 157:131–132, 1990

Fahn S: Recent concepts in the diagnosis and treatment of dystonias, in Movement Disorders. Edited by Chokroverty S. Costa Mesa, CA, PMA Publishing, 237–258, 1990

Fahn S: The tardive syndromes: phenomenology, concepts on pathophysiology, and treatment. Mov Disord 7 (suppl 1):7, 1992

Fahn S, Marsden CD, Van Woert MH: Definition and classification of myoclonus; in Myoclonus (Advances in Neurology Series, Vol 43). Edited by Fahn S, Marsden CD, Van Woert M. New York, Raven, 1986, pp 1–5

Farrer LA: Suicide and attempted suicide in Huntington disease: implications for preclinical testing of persons at risk. Am J Med Genet 24:305–311, 1986

Fibiger HC, Lloyd KG: Neurobiological substrates of tardive dyskinesia: the GABA hypothesis. Trends Neurosci 7:462–464, 1984

Friedman JH, Ambler M: A case of senile chorea. Mov Disord 5:251–253, 1990

Garvey MJ, Tollefson GD: Occurrence of myoclonus in patients treated with cyclic antidepressants. Arch Gen Psychiatry 44:269–272, 1987

Gusella JF, Wexler NS, Conneally PM, et al: A polymorphic DNA marker genetically linked to Huntington's disease. Nature 306:234–238, 1983

Gusella JF, MacDonald ME, Ambrose CM, et al: Molecular genetics of Huntington's disease. Arch Neurol 50:1157–1163, 1993

Harper PS: The epidemiology of Huntington's disease, in Huntington's Disease. Edited by Harper PS. London, WB Saunders, 1991, pp 251–280

Hauser WA, Morris ML, Heston LL, et al: Seizures and myoclonus in patients with Alzheimer's disease. Neurology 36:1226–1230, 1986

Hayden MR, Martin WRW, Stoessl AJ, et al: Positron emission tomography in the early diagnosis of Huntington's disease. Neurology 36:888–894, 1986

Hornykiewicz O, Kish SJ, Becker LE, et al: Brain neurotransmitters in dystonia musculorum deformans. N Engl J Med 315:347–353, 1986

Huggins M, Bloch M, Kanani S, et al: Ethical and legal dilemmas arising during predictive testing for adult-onset disease: the experience of Huntington disease. Am J Hum Genet 47:4–12, 1990

Jahanshahi M, Marion M-H, Marsden CD: Natural history of adult-onset idiopathic torticollis. Arch Neurol 47:548–552, 1990

Jankovic J: Blepharospasm with basal ganglia lesions. Arch Neurol 43:866–868, 1986

Jankovic J, Brin MF: Therapeutic uses of botulinum toxin. N Engl J Med 324:1186–1194, 1991

Jankovic J, Pardo R: Segmental myoclonus: clinical and pharmacologic study. Arch Neurol 43:1025–1031, 1986

Jannetta PJ, Abbasy M, Maroon JC, et al: Etiology and definitive microsurgical treatment of hemifacial spasm; operative techniques and results. J Neurosurg 47:321–328, 1977

Jeste DV, Potkin SG, Sinha S, et al: Tardive dyskinesia: reversible and persistent. Arch Gen Psychiatry 36:585–590, 1979

Kane JM, Smith JM: Tardive dyskinesia. Arch Gen Psychiatry 39:473–481, 1982

Kang UJ, Burke RE, Fahn S: Natural history and treatment of tardive dystonia. Mov Disord 1:193–208, 1986

Khot V, Egan MF, Hyde TM, et al: Neuroleptics and classic tardive dyskinesia, in Drug-Induced Movement Disorders. Edited by Lang AE, Weiner WJ. Mount Kisco, NY, Futura Publishing, 1992, pp 121–166

Klawans HL, Barr A: Prevalence of spontaneous lingual-facial-buccal dyskinesia in the elderly. Neurology 32:558–559, 1982

Klawans HL, Tanner CM, Barr A: The reversibility of "permanent" tardive dyskinesia. Clin Neuropharmacol 7:153–159, 1984

Koller WC: Alcoholism in essential tremor. Neurology 33:1074–1076, 1983a

Koller WC: Edentulous orodyskinesia. Ann Neurol 13:97–99, 1983b

Koller WC, Biary N, Cone S: Disability in essential tremor: effect of treatment. Neurology 36:1001–1004, 1986

Koshino Y, Wada Y, Isaki K, et al: A long-term outcome study of tardive dyskinesia in patients on antipsychotic medication. Clin Neuropharmacol 14:537–546, 1991

Kurlan R, Behr J, Medved L, et al: Transient tic disorder and the clinical spectrum of Tourette's syndrome. Arch Neurol 45:1200–1201, 1988

Kuwert T, Lange HW, Langen K-J, et al: Cortical and subcortical glucose consumption measured by PET in patients with Huntington's disease. Brain 113:1405–1423, 1990

Lang AE: Movement disorders: approach, definitions, and differential diagnosis, in Drug-Induced Movement Disorders. Edited by Lang AE, Weiner WJ. Mount Kisco, NY, Futura Publishing, 1992a, pp 1–20

Lang AE: Miscellaneous drug-induced movement disorders, in Drug-Induced Movement Disorders. Edited by Lang AE, Weiner WJ. Mount Kisco, NY, Futura Publishing, 1992b, pp 339–381

Lang AE, Moldofsky H, Awad AG: Long latency between the onset of motor and vocal tics in Tourette's syndrome. Ann Neurol 14:693–694, 1983

Lang AE, Sethi KD, Provias JP, et al: A severe and fatal systemic illness first presenting with a movement disorder. Mov Disord 4:362–370, 1991

Lohr JB, Kuczenski R, Bracha HS, et al: Increased indices of free radical activity in the cerebrospinal fluid of patients with tardive dyskinesia. Biol Psychiatry 28:535–539, 1990

Lugaresi E, Cirignotta F, Coccagna G, et al: Nocturnal myoclonus and restless legs syndrome, in Myoclonus (Advances in Neurology Series, Vol 43). Edited by Fahn S, Marsden CD, Van Woert MH. New York, Raven, 1986, pp 295–307

Marion M-H, Klap P, Perrin A, et al: Stridor and focal laryngeal dystonia. Lancet 339:457–458, 1992

Marsden CD: Dystonia: the spectrum of the disease, in The Basal Ganglia. Edited by Yahr MD. New York, Raven, 1976, pp 351–367

Marsden CD, Quinn NP: The dystonias. BMJ 300:139–144, 1990

Marsden CD, Obeso JA, Zarranz JJ, et al: The anatomical basis of symptomatic hemidystonia. Brain 108:463–483, 1985

Martin JB, Gusella JF: Huntington's disease: pathogenesis and management. N Engl J Med 315:1267–1276, 1986

Martin WRW, Clark C, Ammann W, et al: Cortical glucose metabolism in Huntington's disease. Neurology 42:223–229, 1992

Myers RH, Goldman D, Bird ED, et al: Maternal transmission in Huntington's disease. Lancet 1:208–210, 1983

Myers RH, Sax DS, Schoenfeld M, et al: Late onset of Huntington's disease. J Neurol Neurosurg Psychiatry 48:530–534, 1985

Nutt JG: Dyskinesia induced by levodopa and dopamine agonists in patients with Parkinson's disease, in Drug-Induced Movement Disorders. Edited by Lang AE, Weiner WJ. Mount Kisco, NY, Futura Publishing, 1992, pp 281–314

Ozelius L, Kramer PL, Moskowitz CB, et al: Human gene for torsion dystonia location on chromosome 9q34-q34. Neuron 2:1427–1434, 1989

Peyser CE, Folstein SE: Huntington's disease as a model for mood disorders: clues from neuropathology and neurochemistry. Mol Chem Neuropathol 12(2):99–119, 1990

Pierot L, Cervera-Pierot P, Delattre J-Y, et al: Palatal myoclonus and inferior olivary lesions: MRI-pathologic correlation. J Comput Assist Tomogr 16:160–163, 1992

Quinn NP, Marsden CD: Dominantly inherited myoclonic dystonia with dramatic response to alcohol. Neurology 34 (suppl 1):236–237, 1984

Reiner A, Albin RL, Anderson KD, et al: Differential loss of striatal projection neurons in Huntington disease. Proc Natl Acad Sci U S A 85:5733–5737, 1988

Rosengarten H, Schweitzer JW, Friedhoff AJ: Animal Models in Tardive Dyskinesia; in Neuromethods: Animal Models in Psychiatry, I. Edited by Boulton A, Baker G, Martin-Iverson M. Clifton, NJ, Humana Press, 1991, pp 245–266

Sethi KD, Nichols FT, Yaghmai F: Generalized chorea due to basal ganglia lacunar infarcts. Mov Disord 2:61–66, 1987

Shannon KM: Hemiballismus. Clin Neuropharmacol 13:413–425, 1990

Sotrel A, Paskevich PA, Kiely DK, et al: Morphometric analysis of the prefrontal cortex in Huntington's disease. Neurology 41:1117–1123, 1991

Starkstein SE, Brandt J, Folstein S, et al: Neuropsychological and neuroradiological correlates in Huntington's disease. J Neurol Neurosurg Psychiatry 51:1259–1263, 1988

Waddington JL, Youssef HA: The lifetime outcome and involuntary movements of schizophrenia never treated with neuroleptic drugs. Br J Psychiatry 156:106–108, 1990

Walters AS, Hening W: Clinical presentation and neuropharmacology of restless legs syndrome. Clin Neuropharmacol 10:225–237, 1987

Weinberger DR, Berman KF, Iadarola M, et al: Prefrontal cortical blood flow and cognitive function in Huntington's disease. J Neurol Neurosurg Psychiatry 51:94–104, 1988

Weiner WJ, Lang AE: Movement Disorders: A Comprehensive Survey. Mount Kisco, NY, Futura Publishing, 1989

Williams A, Hanson D, Calne DB: Vocal cord paralysis in the Shy-Drager syndrome. J Neurol Neurosurg Psychiatry 42:151–153, 1979

Yagi G, Takamuja M, Kauba S, et al: Mortality rates of schizophrenic patients with tardive dyskinesia during 10 years: a controlled study. Keio J Med 38:70–72, 1989

Yassa R, Nair V, Dimitry R: Prevalence of tardive dystonia. Acta Psychiatr Scand 73:629–633, 1986

Young RR, Shahani BT: Asterixis: one type of negative myoclonus; in Myoclonus (Advances in Neurology Series, Vol 43). Edited by Fahn S, Marsden CD, Van Woert M. New York, Raven, 1986, pp 137–156

Young AB, Penney JB: Biochemical and functional organization of the basal ganglia, in Parkinson's Disease and Movement Disorders. Edited by Jankovic J, Tolosa E. Baltimore, MD, Urban & Schwarzenberg, 1988, pp 1–11

Young AB, Penney JB, Starosta-Rubinstein S, et al: PET scan investigations of Huntington's disease: cerebral metabolic correlates of neurological features and functional decline. Ann Neurol 20:296–303, 1986

Young AB, Greenamyre JT, Hollingsworth Z, et al: NMDA receptor losses in putamen from patients with Huntington's disease. Science 241:981–983, 1988

22

Parkinson's Disease and Parkinsonism

William C. Koller, M.D., Ph.D.
Bernard B. Megaffin, M.D.

Introduction

Alterations of mental function in Parkinson's disease have been recognized since the late 1800s (Charcot 1878) and are now universally accepted as an integral part of the disease process. These alterations may take the form of cognitive dysfunction, clinical psychiatric illness, sleep disturbance, or any combination thereof. They are commonly encountered by clinicians representing the multiple medical specialties (e.g., family medicine, internal medicine, geriatrics, neurology, psychiatry, and neuropsychology) who manage this illness or provide general medical care. Unfortunately no uniform criteria for the diagnosis of the various manifestations of mental dysfunction in Parkinson's disease have yet been formulated. The establishment of specific diagnostic guidelines would facilitate recognition of, and reinforce the cause-and-effect relationship between, these abnormalities of mental function and Parkinson's disease.

In this chapter, our goal is to provide a description of the various changes of the mental state encountered in patients with Parkinson's disease. In doing so, we emphasize the clinical features and discuss the proposed pathogenetic mechanisms and the treatment options currently available.

Clinical Features

The four cardinal signs of parkinsonism are tremor, bradykinesia, rigidity, and postural abnormalities (including disturbance of balance, which may appear as the disease progresses). However, the clinical onset may be heralded by more nonspecific symptoms such as generalized fatigue; muscle tightness, aching, or cramping; focal dystonias; decreased manual dexterity; restlessness; sensory symptoms (e.g., extremity pain or paresthesias); and psychiatric complaints (e.g., anxiety and/or depression). Complaints may also be related to autonomic nervous system dysfunction such as postural hypotension, constipation, and/or paroxysmal sweating.

Epidemiology

The first comprehensive effort to estimate the community prevalence and annual incidence of Parkinson's disease was by Kurland (1958) in Rochester, Minnesota. This community-based study recognized persons receiving medical attention for Parkinson's disease and found a 187/100,000 prevalence and a 20/100,000 annual incidence. Prevalences found by community-based studies worldwide have varied from 31.4 to 347 per 100,000 (see Table 22–1).

A number of risk factors for the development of Parkinson's disease have been investigated. Toxins are known to cause parkinsonism, the most striking example of which is 1-methyl-4-phenyl-1,2,3,6-tetrahydropyridine (MPTP) (Langston et al. 1983). Other central nervous system toxins cause more widespread injury resulting in parkinsonism and a constellation of other clinical findings (Goetz 1985). MPTP produces clinical and anatomic findings identical to those seen in Parkinson's disease. Prevalence data suggest the development of Parkinson's disease may be related to resi-

Table 22–1. Estimated prevalence of Parkinson's disease in community-based studies

Study	Location	Patient acquisition setting	Prevalence per 100,000
Kurland 1958	Rochester, MN	Clinical	187
Gudmundsson 1967	Iceland	Clinical	162
Kessler 1972	Baltimore, MD	Clinical	128
Marttila and Rinne 1967	Finland	Clinical	120
Li et al. 1982	China	Door-to-door	44
Schoenberg et al. 1985	Copian County, MS	Door-to-door	347
Mutch et al. 1986	Scotland	Clinical	164
Ashok et al. 1986	Libya	Clinical	31
Schoenberg et al. 1988	Nigeria	Door-to-door	59
Okada et al. 1990	Japan	Clinical	82
Rocca and Morgante 1990	Sicily, Italy	Door-to-door	243

dence in industrialized nations (Aquilonius and Hartvig 1986), or in rural areas with exposure to well water, herbicides, or pesticides (Koller et al. 1990; Tanner et al. 1987, 1989). Presumably this is due, at least in part, to a toxicant exposure.

Golbe et al. (1990a) reported a large Italian kindred with apparent autosomal-dominant inherited, typical Parkinson's disease. Unfortunately an indeterminant degree of intermarriage in preceding generations may have resulted in a pattern of inheritance that only resembles autosomal-dominant transmission. For the most part, genetic factors do not appear to play a primary role in the pathogenesis of Parkinson's disease (Maraganore et al. 1991). However, they may provide a predisposition to Parkinson's disease (e.g., there is a greater prevalence of Parkinson's disease in white populations compared with other ethnic groups) and, in conjunction with an environmental exposure (e.g., toxic or viral), may lead to the appearance of the clinical syndrome (Barbeau and Pourcher 1982).

Increasing age uniformly increases the risk for the development of Parkinson's disease. The onset of Parkinson's disease before the fourth decade is rare (Rajput et al. 1987). A number of studies (e.g., Burch 1981; Kahn 1966) have found a lower prevalence of Parkinson's disease in cigarette smokers versus nonsmokers. However, a subsequent study conducted in China (Li et al. 1982) found no such effect. This suggests alternatively that the premorbid Parkinson's disease personality may be less prone to nicotine addiction. In addition, it has been proposed that the ingestion of foods rich in antioxidant vitamins (i.e., presuming that oxidative mechanisms are involved in the pathogenesis of Parkinson's disease [Jenner et al. 1992]) may be protective for its development (Golbe et al. 1990b; Li et al. 1982).

Differential Diagnosis

The differential diagnosis includes any disorder manifesting parkinsonism (Table 22–2), a syndrome that

Table 22–2. Classification of parkinsonism

Infectious and postinfectious causes of parkinsonism
Encephalitis lethargica
Encephalitides
Syphilis

Toxic causes of parkinsonism
Manganese
Carbon monoxide
Carbon disulfide
Cyanide
Methanol
1-methyl-4-phenyl-1,2,3,6-tetrahydropyridine (MPTP)

Pharmacological causes of parkinsonism
Neuroleptics
  Phenothiazines
  Butyrophenones (e.g., haloperidol)
  Thioxanthenes (e.g., thiothixene)
  Benzamides (e.g., metoclopramide)
Reserpine, tetrabenazine
Miscellaneous agents
  α-Methyldopa
  Lithium

Multiple system atrophies with parkinsonian features
Striatonigral degeneration
Progressive supranuclear palsy
Olivopontocerebellar degeneration
Shy-Drager syndrome

Other degenerative diseases of the nervous system with parkinsonian features
Primary pallidal atrophy

Idiopathic dystonia-parkinsonism
Corticobasal ganglionic degeneration
Hemiatrophy-hemiparkinsonism
Parkinsonism-ALS (amyotrophic lateral sclerosis)-dementia complex of Guam
"Atherosclerotic" or "senile" parkinsonism
Alzheimer's and Pick's diseases
Creutzfeldt-Jakob disease
Gerstmann-Straüssler-Schneider disease
Rett's disease

Central nervous system disorders that may cause parkinsonism
Normal pressure hydrocephalus
Stroke
Tumor
Trauma
Subdural hematoma
Syringomesencephalia

Metabolic causes of parkinsonism
Hypoparathyroidism and basal ganglia calcification
Chronic hepatocerebral degeneration

Hereditary diseases of the nervous system associated with parkinsonism
Wilson's disease
Huntington's disease
Disorder with diffuse pathology
Spinocerebellonigral degeneration
Parkinsonism with ataxia and neuropathy
Parkinsonism with alveolar hypoventilation

may result from a variety of etiologies. The group of disorders designated *multiple system degenerations* (also known as *parkinsonism-plus syndromes*) share parkinsonian features with Parkinson's disease, but manifest additional findings (e.g., supranuclear ophthalmoplegia in progressive supranuclear palsy and dysautonomia in Shy-Drager syndrome). Early in their courses, these disorders may be difficult to distinguish from Parkinson's disease. One useful characteristic in this regard is their poor responsiveness to levodopa or dopamine agonists.

Treatment

Treatment goals should be individualized for each patient. Patient education and reassurance are important in the newly diagnosed, mild Parkinson's disease patient. Each should be encouraged to contact a local Parkinson's disease support group or a national Parkinson's disease organization.

Since the discovery of its markedly reduced concentration in the striatum of Parkinson's disease patients, levodopa has been the mainstay of drug therapy for the motor manifestations of the disease. Its absorption is highly variable in the proximal small intestine, with competition for transport from amino acid components of ingested protein (Riley and Lang 1988; Wade and Katzman 1975). It is decarboxylated to dopamine in the gut and liver and, after crossing the blood-brain barrier, in the brain by the surviving dopaminergic neurons and by decarboxylase-containing serotonergic and adrenergic neurons (Melamed et al. 1980).

The initiation of levodopa therapy, most often at a time when Parkinson's disease has begun to interfere with the activities of daily living, usually results in dramatic improvement in motor symptoms. The absence of a therapeutic effect at high doses necessitates reappraisal of the diagnosis. Bradykinesia and rigidity respond best, there may be some degree of improvement of tremor, but usually there is no improvement in postural stability, changes of the mental state, or autonomic nervous system dysfunction.

Levodopa is combined with a peripheral dopa decarboxylase inhibitor (carbidopa in the United States, benserazide in Europe) to counteract the adverse effects of peripherally produced dopamine (e.g., nausea, vomiting, and postural hypotension). Most patients are started at a dose of one tablet of Sinemet 25/100 (25

mg carbidopa and 100 mg levodopa) tid, 30 minutes before or 1 hour after meals. The subsequent dosage is adjusted to obtain an optimal motor response.

A long-acting preparation, Sinemet CR (controlled-release) 50/200, is a slowly eroding tablet that is absorbed over a more protracted period of time. Its onset of effect is slower than that of standard Sinemet, but it has been shown to decrease "off" time (return of symptoms due to subtherapeutic drug effects), early morning dystonia, and nocturnal disturbances. Standard Sinemet and Sinemet CR may be given separately or in combination based on the desired clinical effect. Although not yet approved by the Food and Drug Administration at the time of this writing, it is anticipated that generic carbidopa-levodopa preparations will eventually be marketed in the United States.

In addition to those mentioned, dyskinesias are prominent among the adverse effects caused by levodopa. Choreic movements are most common, and dyskinesias may interfere with speech, swallowing, respiration, and balance (Tanner 1986). They are dose-related and may improve by lowering the dose, although this may exacerbate the parkinsonism. In addition, motor fluctuations (e.g., early morning akinesia) and "wearing-off" and "on-off" phenomena are more severe in patients treated with levodopa. Smaller and multiple doses may improve this end-of-dose deterioration. The psychic complications of levodopa therapy are discussed below.

The natural history of Parkinson's disease includes gradual deterioration of speech and posture and gait abnormalities. Levodopa does little to affect progression to disability in this regard. However, its efficacy may continue for rigidity, bradykinesia, tremor, and micrographia after many years of levodopa therapy (Klawans 1986), and levodopa has reduced premature mortality in Parkinson patients (Curtis et al. 1984).

Selegiline (l-deprenyl, Eldepryl), a monoamine oxidase–B inhibitor, has been shown to delay the requirement for symptomatic therapy in early disease (Parkinson Study Group 1989) and has been demonstrated effective as initial therapy in some mildly affected Parkinson's disease patients (Myllyla et al. 1989). There is general agreement that all Parkinson's disease patients, if tolerant, should be started on selegiline. This indication is due in part to the demonstration that pretreatment with the drug before the administration of a known toxin to nigral neurons, MPTP, prevented their destruction (Heikkila et al. 1984) and to the uncontrolled observations that patients receiving selegiline and levodopa lived longer than those receiving only levodopa (Birkmayer et al. 1985). The mechanism by which selegiline may protect nigral neurons is unknown.

Anticholinergic drugs (e.g., benztropine and trihexyphenidyl) and amantadine (Symmetrel) may be beneficial when tremor is a major problem. Because of their adverse effects (especially mental status changes), they are best avoided in those patients over age 70. The dopamine agonists bromocriptine (Parlodel) and pergolide (Permax) may be used effectively in combination with levodopa and should be started in small, once-daily (bedtime) doses to minimize the occurrence of orthostatic hypotension. The dosage may be gradually increased until the desired therapeutic benefit is realized.

Unilateral surgical thalamotomy is effective for severe tremor, especially if there is an action component. Chronic thalamic stimulation, achieved by the stereotactic placement of an electrode in the ventralis intermediate nucleus of the thalamus, has been demonstrated to be well tolerated and effective in controlling tremor and reducing dyskinesias (Caparros-Lefebvre et al. 1993). Ventroposterior medial globus pallidotomy has been demonstrated, in small numbers of patients, to cause significant improvement in parkinsonian symptoms, with alleviation of contralateral, medication-induced dyskinesias (Fazzini et al. 1993).

The intrastriatal implantation of autologous adrenal medullary tissue has resulted in modest improvement in motor function in some Parkinson's disease patients (Goetz et al. 1989). More recently, small numbers of patients have undergone intrastriatal grafting of fetal tissue. Early results (5 months postgraft) have revealed improvement in objective measures of parkinsonism, and positron-emission tomography (PET) scan evidence of increased uptake of fluorine-18-labelled dopa ([^{18}F]dopa) on the grafted side (Defer et al. 1993). Although the results of ablative and implantation procedures justify further research, at present they remain investigational.

Parkinson's Disease Dementia

Overview

The occurrence of a primary degenerative dementia in Parkinson's disease is no longer disputed. Indeed, the dementia of Parkinson's disease and the dementia of Alzheimer's disease are clinically and pathologically similar. The dementia of Parkinson's disease is a major obstacle to successful symptomatic pharmacotherapy.

Despite Charcot's 1861 observation that, "in general, psychic faculties are definitely impaired" (Charcot and Vulpian 1862), researchers in the late 19th and early 20th centuries found no association between Parkinson's disease and dementia (Konig 1912; Oppenheim 1911; Wollenberg 1899). Charcot's conclusion, based on astute clinical observation, was made before the invention of comprehensive neuropsychological testing. It was not until 1949 that a Swedish study documented a 3.2% incidence of "senile psychosis" (i.e., senile dementia) in 194 Parkinson's disease patients (Mjones 1949). At that time, dementia in the Swedish general population had a prevalence of less than 1%. In 1966, before the widespread use of levodopa, a study that distinguished idiopathic Parkinson's disease from other forms of parkinsonism found the prevalence of dementia in Parkinson's disease patients to be 8% (Pollack and Hornabrook 1966).

A genetic predisposition to the dementia of Parkinson's disease has been proposed. The risk of dementia among the first-degree relatives of Parkinson's disease patients with dementia is sixfold greater than that in relatives of Parkinson's disease patients without dementia (Marder et al. 1990). However, the risk factors most often associated with Alzheimer's disease are not found in Parkinson's disease patients with dementia. A familial association between Parkinson's disease and Alzheimer's disease has been reported; first-degree relatives with Alzheimer's disease had a threefold risk of Parkinson's disease, suggesting a common genetic etiology (Hofman et al. 1989).

The technical aspects of epidemiological studies to determine the prevalence of dementia in Parkinson's disease warrant consideration. Studies of the prevalence of dementia to date have been either community based (i.e., population based: the number of cases of Parkinson's disease within a population defined by political or geographic boundaries) or case controlled (comparison of patients with a disease to similar persons not yet afflicted).

A community-based study acquires patients from a clinic or hospital setting (i.e., clinic- or hospital-based study) and is composed of symptomatic individuals seeking medical treatment. This may not provide a true representation of the population from which the subjects are drawn, introducing a greater likelihood for selection bias. Another type of community-based study, conducted door-to-door, offers the best opportunity for the detection of mild cases of Parkinson's disease (i.e., greatest sensitivity) not yet receiving medical attention and, if present, the mildest degrees of cognitive decline. Unfortunately it is often impossible to distinguish whether early signs of parkinsonism are due to Parkinson's disease or one of the variant syndromes (i.e., a parkinsonism-plus syndrome).

Some early studies suggested prevalences of dementia up to 90%, but these are probably not valid because of their failure to base the diagnosis on specific criteria (Mayeux 1992). In all likelihood, age is an important factor in predisposing to the appearance of dementia, although few studies have assessed this. Mayeux et al. (1988b) found an age-specific prevalence of 21% in patients whose motor manifestations did not begin until after age 70.

Studies completed before the widespread use of levodopa found a prevalence of dementia of less than 10% in Parkinson's disease patients (Mjones 1949; Pollock and Hornabrook 1966). More recent studies have estimated the prevalence to be two to three times as great (Mayeux 1992). The best explanation is that subsequent studies have included more comprehensive neuropsychological testing, but the effects of pharmacological therapies are also a consideration.

Marttila and Rinne (1976) divided a large population of Parkinson's disease patients in Finland into idiopathic and postencephalitic forms and reported a dementia prevalence rate of 29%. Several subsequent studies have confirmed a similar rate of prevalence (Huber et al. 1989; Mindham et al. 1982; Rajput and Rozdilsky 1975), although other studies indicated rates as low as 12% (Mayeux et al. 1988b). The consensus of published studies indicates a rate of prevalence of dementia in Parkinson's disease of approximately 30%. The use of standardized criteria for the diagnosis would allow more meaningful comparison between groups studied.

Incidence rates in the study of chronic diseases of long duration such as Parkinson's disease estimate, within a given population, the probability for the development of a symptom or disorder. Mindham et al. (1982) reported that 3 years after initial evaluation, Parkinson's disease patients were four times as likely as control subjects to satisfy DSM-III-R (American Psychiatric Association 1987) criteria for dementia. Rajput et al. (1987) reported a similar finding at a magnitude of 3.8 times that of control subjects at 5 years. From a follow-up study of nearly 5 years (Mayeux et al. 1990), the incidence rate of dementia was estimated to be 69/1,000 population per years of follow-up. Consequent with increasing age was an increased risk of dementia, reaching 65% by age 85.

An analysis of the Mindham study (Mindham et al. 1982) illustrates the importance of considering incidence rates. Four of their 16 patients died during the study interval, with zero mortality for the age-matched patients and control subjects. The mortality lowered the dementia prevalence within the study group, without affecting incidence. Controlling for age, significantly greater mortality has been reported in Parkinson's disease patients with dementia versus those without dementia (Marder et al. 1990). Taking these considerations into account, the risk for developing dementia appears to be significantly higher than indicated by prevalence studies.

Definition

Diagnostic criteria for dementia have been defined by the American Psychiatric Association (Table 22–3). The diagnosis of dementia in the Parkinson's disease patient is complicated by the likelihood of intellectual dysfunction before the satisfaction of the requirements specific for a diagnosis of dementia (Huber et al. 1989). The various disorders of cognition that compose the syndrome of dementia are discussed below.

Modifications of these criteria have been proposed by some due to the requirement for interference in so-

---

Table 22–3.   Diagnostic criteria for dementia

A. The development of multiple cognitive deficits manifested by both
   1. Memory impairment (impaired ability to learn new information or to recall previously learned information)
   2. One (or more) of the following cognitive disturbances:
      a. Aphasia (language disturbance)
      b. Apraxia (impaired ability to carry out motor activities despite intact motor function)
      c. Agnosia (failure to recognize or identify objects despite intact sensory function)
      d. Disturbance in executive functioning (i.e., planning, organizing, sequencing, abstracting)
B. The cognitive deficits in criteria A1 and A2 each cause significant impairment in social or occupational functioning and represent a significant decline from a previous level of functioning.

Source. Adapted from American Psychiatric Association 1994.

cial and occupational capabilities (Brown and Marsden 1984; McCarthy et al. 1985). The issue of functional impairment in the Parkinson's disease patient may be related to the motor disability and not necessarily to intellectual decline. It has also been suggested that because of performance expectations, especially in the workplace, dementia in men may be recognized sooner than in the homebound, female homemaker (Rajput et al. 1990).

To facilitate the future study of dementia in Parkinson's disease, criteria for the diagnosis should be standardized. A revision of the DSM-IV criteria (American Psychiatric Association 1994) specific for the Parkinson's disease patient (i.e., taking into account the physical disability and its social and occupational consequences) would be welcome.

Pathology

Parkinson's disease is characterized by the loss of pigmented neurons from the pars compacta of the substantia nigra and by the appearance of Lewy bodies in the substantia nigra, locus coeruleus, ventral tegmental area, nucleus basalis of Meynert, thalamus, dorsal raphe nuclei, cerebral cortex, and entire autonomic nervous system. Lewy bodies contain cytoskeletal elements, and the mechanism of their formation is unknown.

The typical dementia syndrome (discussed in the next section) of Parkinson's disease has been termed *subcortical*, in contrast to the *cortical* dementia typical of Alzheimer's disease (Cummings and Benson 1984). However, there is considerable overlap of pathological findings (i.e., subcortical versus cortical) in patients with clinical findings diagnostic of Parkinson's disease versus Alzheimer's disease.

The evidence relating the dementia of Parkinson's disease and Alzheimer-type pathology (neuritic plaques, neurofibrillary tangles, and granulovacular degeneration) is contradictory. Several studies (e.g., Boller et al. 1980; Gaspar and Gray 1984) have shown a high incidence of Alzheimer-type pathology in Parkinson's disease patients with dementia, whereas others (e.g, Ball 1984; Perry et al. 1983) have reported an infrequent association. Another (Jellinger 1987) found a relationship only in the age at death of Parkinson's disease patients and Alzheimer-type pathology, with a twofold increase in coincidence over age 70.

Dementia has been present in patients with pathology restricted to the brain stem pigmented nuclei, in the absence of Alzheimer-type pathology. The amount of cell loss from the substantia nigra is highly variable in Parkinson's disease and has not been shown to be predictive of the presence or severity of dementia (Gaspar and Gray 1984). Although dementia can occur with intact basal nuclei, neuronal loss in the nucleus basalis of Parkinson's disease patients with dementia is usually more severe than in those without dementia (Whitehouse et al. 1983). However, dementia in Parkinson's disease may occur in the absence of both Alzheimer-type changes and atrophy of the nucleus basalis (Helig et al. 1985).

In 1980, Kosaka et al. described a new clinico-pathological entity characterized by Lewy bodies present not only in brain stem neurons but distributed throughout the cerebral cortex. Variously labeled *diffuse Lewy body disease* (DLBD) or the *Lewy body variant of Alzheimer's disease,* the clinical characteristics were more recently reviewed (Kosaka 1990). Dementia was the presenting syndrome in more than half the cases, with cortical findings (e.g., aphasia and apraxia) commonly present. Extrapyramidal signs gradually appeared, but were often mild. In one-third of the cases, Alzheimer's disease was the clinical, antemortem diagnosis, and in one-fourth it was Parkinson's disease. The clinicopathological spectrum of DLBD is varied (de Bruin et al. 1992). Lewy body predominance in the brain stem and diencephalic nuclei is more likely to present clinically as akinetic parkinsonism (Mark et al. 1992).

The typical clinical findings of the subcortical dementia of Parkinson's disease (i.e., affective disturbance and bradyphrenia) and the cortical dementia of Alzheimer's disease (e.g., aphasia and apraxia) are usually, but not invariably, confirmed at autopsy. Thus it is apparent that the dementia associated with Parkinson's disease has a diverse pathological basis. Additional studies of selected populations with control subjects, using standardized histopathological criteria, are required to better define the anatomic relationship between Parkinson's disease and Alzheimer's disease.

Clinical Features

Dementia is an acquired clinical syndrome, not a single entity or outcome. It may result from a number of etiologies and present in various forms depending on which facets of intellect are most affected. Cummings and Benson (1983) defined dementia as loss of function in at least three of five areas: 1) memory; 2) language; 3) visuospatial function; 4) complex cognition, that is, executive function (e.g., abstraction, calculation, and judgment); or 5) affect, that is, mood or personality. Neuropsychological deficits have not been found to develop in a uniform manner during the progression of Parkinson's disease (Huber et al. 1989). Patients with major depression have shown significantly greater cognitive decline, deterioration of the activities of daily living, and motor dysfunctions than those with minor or no depression (Starkstein et al. 1992).

Cortical versus subcortical findings. Dementia syndromes have been subdivided, on the basis of neuropsychological deficits, into two categories: cortical and subcortical (Cummings 1986). The prototypical cortical dementia is senile dementia of the Alzheimer type (SDAT). Examples of subcortical dementia occur in Parkinson's disease, Huntington's disease, and progressive supranuclear palsy. A comparison of the features of these categories of dementia is presented in Table 22–4.

Memory. The memory deficits of Parkinson's disease are not as pervasive as those in SDAT, with better delayed recall and recognition. Studies have suggested

that Parkinson's disease patients are better able to store information for delayed recall, but that retrieval of stored information is impaired (Flowers et al. 1984; Heikala et al. 1988). Verbal cues are effective in improving word retrieval in Parkinson's disease dementia, but not in SDAT. These findings have been found reproducible for verbal and nonverbal (geometric designs) information (Sullivan et al. 1989). Immediate recall is impaired in both Parkinson's disease and SDAT.

Language. The language disturbance that characterizes SDAT is aphasia, a distinguishing feature from Parkinson's disease. Abnormal language capabilities are present early in the course of SDAT. Circumlocutions result from word-finding difficulties, resulting in frequent, meaningless phrases. As the disease progresses, a transcortical sensory aphasia (dysnomia, paraphasias, impaired written and auditory comprehension, and aphasic dysgraphia) appears. Speech remains fluent, with intact repetition and ability to read aloud (Cummings and Benson 1983).

Language difficulties in Parkinson's disease are related to hypophonia and dysarthria, with rare paraphasic errors. Mild impairments of word generation and

Table 22–4. Comparison of cortical and subcortical types of dementia

Feature	Cortical dementia	Subcortical dementia
Language	Aphasia	Relatively preserved
Memory Functions		
Recall	Impaired	Impaired
Recognition cues	Ineffective	Effective
Encoding	Ineffective	Effective
Priming	Absent	Present
Procedural	Intact	Impaired
Visuoperception	Severe impairment	Mild impairment
Calculation	Acalculia	Relatively preserved
Executive/frontal systems function	Proportionate to overall intellectual impairment	Affected greater than overall impairment
Speed of information processing	Normal	Slowed
Personality and mood	No insight; unconcerned; depression infrequent	Insight; apathetic; depression frequent
Motor functions		
Speech	Normal articulation until late	Dysarthria early
Motor speed	Normal until late	Slowed
Posture	Normal until late	Stooped, rigid
Gait	Normal until late	Abnormal
Coordination	Normal until late	Abnormal
Adventitious movements	Absent except for myoclonus late in course	Chorea, tremor, dystonia, and tics

Source. Adapted from Ross et al. 1992.

retrieval are felt to be consistent with frontal lobe dysfunction (Matison et al. 1982). This form of anomia has been termed the *tip-of-the-tongue phenomenon*, and may be overcome by providing a phonemic cue. Visual naming, comprehension skills, and writing ability are preserved.

Visuospatial function. Impaired visuospatial and visuoconstructive abilities are characteristic of SDAT. Similar deficits have been found consistently in Parkinson's disease, even when tasks have been designed to eliminate the contribution of the motor disability. The results of studies comparing the abilities of both groups are not conclusive. Huber et al. (1986) found that SDAT patients outperformed Parkinson's disease patients with dementia on Raven's Progressive Matrices (a test of spatial reasoning). Their Parkinson's disease patients performed better at block design than did the SDAT group, suggesting more severe involvement of frontal systems in Parkinson's disease and more severe posterior hemispheric changes in Alzheimer's disease.

Visuospatial impairments do not improve with dopamine replacement and do not vary during "on" and "off" periods. If the dopamine deficit plays a role in these abnormalities, it must be in conjunction with other neurochemical or pathological processes (Pillon and Dubois 1989).

Complex cognition. Executive functions of the brain depend largely on frontal lobe integrity and are influenced greatly by subcortical connections. Frontal lobe dysfunction in Parkinson's disease most likely results from the deficit of dopamine within the basal ganglia. This is supported by the fact that there is greater preservation of dopamine in the caudate than in the putamen, resulting in the retention of complex cognition in the occurrence of early Parkinson's disease with motor disability (Taylor et al. 1990).

The disturbance of cortical-subcortical pathways has been suggested to be responsible for poor performance of tasks that require coordination of mental and motor functions (e.g., resulting in frequent falling or poor operation of an automobile). The loss of these abilities may be conditioned by visuospatial deficits leading to the defective planning and execution of strategies to accomplish a task (e.g., turning a corner while walking or driving) (Marsden 1982). This gives rise to the hypothesis that the basal ganglia serve as a subcognitive, internal navigational system that places

limits on the options available to efficiently solve a problem (Robertson and Flowers 1990; Sullivan et al. 1989). Demands placed by a new situation could then rely only on conscious control.

Affect. Disorders of mood are more extensively discussed below. In contrast to SDAT, depression is much more frequently seen in Parkinson's disease dementia. It is considered an important feature that distinguishes subcortial from cortical syndromes.

Neuroimaging

Brain imaging studies often accompany the workup of the patient manifesting a dementia syndrome. They are most useful in eliminating the possibility of dementia secondary to a structural brain abnormality, such as a space-occupying lesion (tumor or vascular malformation) or hydrocephalus. The contribution of these studies to the evaluation of dementia secondary to other types of organic brain disease is less clear.

Cerebral atrophy is the most frequent finding of brain-imaging studies in neurodegenerative disorders. Computed tomography (CT) studies attempting to relate nonspecific measures of atrophy (i.e., ventricular enlargement or size of the sulci) with the severity of dementia, determined by less than rigorous neuropsychological criteria, have yielded conflicting results (deLeon et al. 1980; Wilson et al. 1982). Even when it was demonstrated that greater atrophy was present in dementia patients, there was significant overlap with the control groups.

Subsequently, studies were conducted relating specific neuropsychological test results to measures of structural brain changes (from CT) in Parkinson's disease patients (Inzelberg et al. 1987; Lichter et al. 1988). Measures of general cerebral cortical atrophy were not found to be predictive of dementia in these studies. However, findings suggesting subcortical atrophy (e.g., increase in intercaudate distance or ventricular enlargement) or frontal atrophy (e.g., increased width of the anterior interhemispheric fissure) were associated with the presence of cognitive dysfunction (Starkstein and Leiguarda 1993).

Magnetic resonance imaging (MRI) provides more precise visualization of brain abnormalities including cerebral cortical loss, ventricular enlargement, and changes in the periventricular white matter. Despite this enhanced sensitivity, the correlation of MRI abnormalities and dementia in Parkinson's disease patients parallels that of the CT studies. Cerebral cortical atrophy correlates poorly with dementia. Findings consistent with subcortical atrophy (e.g., ventricular enlargement and increase in intercaudate width) were associated with cognitive impairment (Inzelberg et al. 1987; Korczyn et al. 1986; Lichter et al. 1988).

PET provides images that measure the binding of positron-emitting radio-pharmaceuticals, [^{18}F]6-fluorodopa, to specific neurochemical receptors. Studies using this compound have demonstrated asymmetry in striatal dopaminergic storage in patients with hemiparkinsonism (Garnett et al. 1984), and significantly impaired striatal dopamine metabolism in advanced Parkinson's disease patients compared with patients with mild disease (Leenders et al. 1986). PET has been shown to detect asymptomatic dopaminergic lesions that may be a preclinical indicator for the development of Parkinson's disease (Karbe et al. 1992)

Estimates of metabolic activity and regional cerebral blood flow via the utilization of oxygen-15 or [^{18}F]fluorodeoxyglucose are measurable by PET. It has been demonstrated that cerebral metabolism in Parkinson's disease patients (without dementia) is decreased globally (especially in the frontal lobes) (Brooks and Frackowaik 1989). These findings would be consistent with the current concept that subcortical dementia is most likely symptomatic of frontal lobe dysfunction (e.g., slowing of cognitive function and affective disorders). To date, no PET studies have been conducted to specifically correlate changes in neurotransmission or cerebral metabolism and dementia.

Treatment

The drugs piracetam and phosphatidylserine have been the subjects of controlled clinical trials in the treatment of the dementia of Parkinson's disease. Neither resulted in improvement of cognition (Funfgeld et al. 1989; Sano et al. 1990).

Bradyphrenia

Bradyphrenia has been defined as the psychic equivalent of akinesia (Birkmayer et al. 1983). It was first described by the French neurologist, Naville (1922), in victims of the epidemic of encephalitis lethargica. Bradyphrenia encompasses not only slowing of mental function, but also inattention, apathy, and the inability to sustain effort for completion of the task at hand.

This description also characterizes the syndrome of subcortical dementia. However, the Parkinson's disease patient manifesting bradyphrenia without dementia would exhibit a persistent impairment of attention and vigilance, in the absence of depression and impairment of consciousness, memory, and/or executive function (Mayeux 1992).

Pillon and associates studied cognitive processing after withdrawal of levodopa, followed by reinstitution of the medication. They found no benefit from levodopa therapy (Sullivan et al. 1989). This would suggest that the cognitive slowing is related to a non-dopaminergic neurotransmitter system. Additional studies have suggested a failure of noradrenergic transmission based on changes in metabolite concentrations in the cerebrospinal fluid (CSF) during mental exercise (Mayeux et al. 1987).

An alternative hypothesis involves the documented degeneration of the locus ceruleus (the site in the brain stem of norepinephrine production) in Parkinson's disease (Gaspar and Gray 1984). Pathways from the locus ceruleus to the cortex are felt to be important in the maintenance of attention and vigilance (Mason and Fibiger 1979).

Psychiatric Conditions

The psychiatric manifestations of Parkinson's disease may be as or more disabling than the motor dysfunction. They may occur as a complication of pharmacotherapy for the motor symptoms or result from the disease itself. The specific syndromes are discussed below, and various ranges of prevalence are presented in Table 22–5.

Table 22–5. Prevalence of psychiatric conditions in Parkinson's disease

Condition	Prevalence
Generalized anxiety	35%–40%
Psychosis	< 1%
Depression	40%–50%
Drug-related	
Hallucinations	5%–35%
Delusions	3%–30%
Confusion and delirium	4%–33%
Mania	1%–5%

Source. Adapted from Huber and Bornstein 1992.

Depression

General considerations. Parkinson's original description characterized his patients as manifesting "melancholy" and appearing "dejected." Subsequent studies found a high prevalence of depression in Parkinson's disease. Approximately 50% of patients become depressed at some time during the disease (Dooneief et al. 1992; Mayeux 1982), and depression is present in up to one-third of patients at the time of their diagnosis (Santamaria et al. 1986). In addition, it is important to distinguish dementia from depression (i.e., pseudodementia) and examine the relationship, if any, between the two.

Any chronic, disabling disease state may produce depression. Some investigators (e.g., Gotham et al. 1986) have suggested that the depression of Parkinson's disease is a reactive process, secondary to the development of motor dysfunction. Factors favoring the reactive etiology include the finding that patients with rheumatoid arthritis with a similar degree of physical disability as Parkinson's disease patients have depression at approximately the same prevalence (Gotham et al. 1986). No increased prevalence of depression has been found among unaffected family members of Parkinson's disease patients, discouraging the likelihood of a genetic predisposition (Winokur et al. 1978), except in the event that depression antedated the onset of Parkinson's disease (Santamaria et al. 1986).

On the other hand, Mayeux et al. (1981) found that 43% of Parkinson's disease patients were depressed prior to the appearance of motor signs, suggesting endogenous depression. In addition, the depressed patients tended to be younger and with lesser degrees of physical impairment. Some investigators (Gotham et al. 1986; Mayeux et al. 1981) have found a relationship between the severity of disability (both motor and cognitive) and the incidence of depression. However, others (Kostic et al. 1987; Santamaria et al. 1986) have failed to confirm this relationship, arguing against the hypothesis that the depression of Parkinson's disease is a form of "adjustment disorder," a diagnosis rarely seen in this population.

Pathophysiology. Studies of the CSF of patients with depression have shown decreased concentrations of the serotonin metabolite 5-hydroxyindoleacetic acid (5-HIAA) (Van Praag and de Haan 1979). Similar results have been reported in Parkinson's disease patients with depression (Kostic et al. 1987; Mayeux et al.

1984). An improvement in the depression of Parkinson's disease patients has been demonstrated following the administration of L-5-hydroxytryptophan (5-HTP), the precursor of serotonin, in addition to concomitant increases in CSF 5-HIAA (Mayeux et al. 1988a; McCance-Katz et al. 1992).

It has been shown that the brain content of serotonin at autopsy in Parkinson's disease patients is reduced; the raphe nuclei, which produce serotonin, have a reduced ability to decarboxylate amino acids in Parkinson's disease. Using PET, Mayberg et al. (1990) demonstrated caudate and inferior frontal lobe hypometabolism in Parkinson's disease patients, which has implications for both the dopaminergic and serotonergic pathways therein. Dysfunction of the latter pathway may be involved in the pathogenesis of the disturbance of mood in Parkinson's disease.

Clinical features. The most frequent manifestations of depression in Parkinson's disease conform to the DSM-IV criteria for major depression or dysthymic disorder (Tables 22–6 and 22–7). The two differ in that the former is characterized by periods of depression separated by intervals with normal affect; the latter is a chronic condition with more mild mood changes.

The depression is usually mild to moderate; very infrequently is it severe. Suicide is rare in Parkinson's disease patients. Two studies have found a greater likelihood for depression in Parkinson's disease with a younger age at onset (Mayeux et al. 1981; Santamaria et al. 1986), but others have found no difference when compared with an age at onset from 55 to 70 (Jankovic et al. 1990).

Methodological differences between longitudinal studies make it difficult to determine the effect of treatment on the course of the affective illness. Recent-onset levodopa therapy has been found to transiently improve mood, but this effect is rarely sustained (Shaw et al. 1980). Virtually all studies of depression in Parkinson's disease include patients receiving chronic levodopa therapy.

Treatment: pharmacotherapy. Prior to discussing specific drug therapy for depression in Parkinson's disease, it is important to consider the effects of antiparkinsonian medication on mood. Levodopa may produce symptoms of psychosis (discussed below). In addition, because of its effects on serotonin metabolism, it may predispose to depression (Anderson and Aabro 1980). Bromocriptine (Sitland-Marken et al.

Table 22–6. Diagnostic criteria for major depressive syndrome

A. Five (or more) of the following symptoms have been present during the same 2-week period and represent a change from previous functioning; at least one of the symptoms is either 1) depressed mood or 2) loss of interest or pleasure.

Note: Do not include symptoms that are clearly due to a general medical condition, or mood-incongruent delusions or hallucinations.

1. Depressed mood most of the day, nearly every day, as indicated by either subjective report (e.g., feels sad or empty) or observation made by others (e.g., appears tearful).

2. Markedly diminished interest or pleasure in all, or almost all, activities most of the day, nearly every day (as indicated by either subjective account or observation made by others)

3. Significant weight loss when not dieting or weight gain (e.g., a change of more than 5% of body weight in a month), or decrease or increase in appetite nearly every day.

4. Insomnia or hypersomnia nearly every day

5. Psychomotor agitation or retardation nearly every day (observable by others, not merely subjective feelings of restlessness or being slowed down)

6. Fatigue or loss of energy nearly every day

7. Feelings of worthlessness or excessive or inappropriate guilt (which may be delusional) nearly every day (not merely self-reproach or guilt about being sick)

8. Diminished ability to think or concentrate, or indecisiveness, nearly every day (either by subjective account or as observed by others)

9. Recurrent thoughts of death (not just fear of dying), recurrent suicidal ideation without a specific plan, or a suicide attempt or a specific plan for committing suicide

B. The symptoms do not meet criteria for a mixed episode.

C. The symptoms cause clinically significant distress or impairment in social, occupational, or other important areas of functioning.

D. The symptoms are not due to the direct physiological effects of a substance (e.g., a drug of abuse, a medication) or a general medical condition (e.g., hypothyroidism).

E. The symptoms are not better accounted for by bereavement (i.e., after the loss of a loved one, the symptoms persist for longer than 2 months or are characterized by marked functional impairment, morbid preoccupation with worthlessness, suicidal ideation, psychotic symptoms, or psychomotor retardation).

Source. Adapted from American Psychiatric Association 1994.

1990), anticholinergic drugs (e.g., trihexyphenidyl) (Kaspar et al. 1981), amantadine (Bavazzano and Guarducci 1980), and deprenyl (Eisler et al. 1981; Parkinson Study Group 1989) have been shown to have beneficial effects on mood in some studies. Should levodopa exacerbate the symptoms of depression, either lowering the dosage or combining it with one of the above agents may be effective in treating the motor and depressive symptoms of Parkinson's disease (Silver and Yudofsky 1992).

Table 22–7. Diagnostic criteria for dysthymia

A. Depressed mood for most of the day, for more days than not, as indicated either by subjective account or observation by others, for at least 2 years.

B. Presence, while depressed, of two (or more) of the following:
   1. Poor appetite or overeating
   2. Insomnia or hypersomnia
   3. Low energy or fatigue
   4. Low self-esteem
   5. Poor concentration or difficulty making decisions
   6. Feelings of hopelessness

C. During the 2-year period of the disturbance, the person has never been without the symptoms in criteria A and B for more than 2 months at a time.

D. No major depressive episode has been present during the first 2 years of the disturbance (i.e., the disturbance is not better accounted for by chronic major depressive disorder, or major depressive disorder, in partial remission).

Note: There may have been a previous major depressive episode provided there was a full remission (no significant signs or symptoms for 2 months) before development of the dysthymic disorder. In addition, after the initial 2 years of dysthymic disorder, there may be superimposed episodes of major depressive disorder, in which case both diagnoses may be given when the criteria are met for a major depressive episode.

E. There has never been a manic episode, a mixed episode, or a hypomanic episode, and criteria have never been met for cyclothymic disorder.

F. The disturbance does not occur exclusively during the course of a chronic psychotic disorder, such as schizophrenia or delusional disorder.

G. The symptoms are not due to the direct physiological effects of a substance (e.g., a drug of abuse or a medication) or a general medical condition (e.g., hypothyroidism).

H. The symptoms cause clinically significant distress or impairment in social, occupational, or other important areas of functioning.

Source. Adapted from American Psychiatric Association 1994.

For the purpose of directing the most appropriate intervention, Silver and Yudofsky (1992) proposed subtypes of Parkinson's disease and depression (see Table 22–8). The specific subtype results from an assessment of the current clinical status of the Parkinson's disease and the type of depressive syndrome manifested (i.e., *partial* versus *full*) (Table 22–9). A listing of commonly used antidepressant medications appears in Table 22–10, with the relative pharmacological properties of some of these agents detailed in Table 22–11. Table 22–12 provides guidelines for pharmacological intervention in the management of the depression of Parkinson's disease (Silver and Yudofsky 1988). The guidelines are effected on the determination of the subtype from Table 22–8. A detailed discussion of the pharmacological properties of these drugs is beyond the scope of this chapter and may be found elsewhere (Baldessarini 1985; Bernstein 1991; Cassem 1991; Silver and Yudofsky 1988; see also Chapter 29, this volume).

Table 22–8.   Subtypes of depression in Parkinson's disease

Subtype	Treatment	Result	Depressive syndrome
I	Treated	Controlled	Partial
II	Treated	Uncontrolled	Partial
III	Treated	Controlled	Full
IV	Treated	Uncontrolled	Full
V	Not treated	Mild	Full

Source. Adapted from Silver and Yudofsky 1992.

Table 22–9.   Symptoms of full versus partial depressive syndrome

Symptom	Full syndrome	Partial syndrome
Depressed mood	Present	Present
Lack of reactivity	Present	Absent
Diminished interest	Present	Can be motivated
Loss of appetite	Present	Absent
Sleep disorder	Present	Present
Fatigue	Present	Present, but patient can become involved
Guilt	Present	Absent
Decreased concentration	Present	Short-term memory intact
Suicidal thoughts	Present	Absent

Source. Adapted from Silver and Yudofsky 1992.

Table 22–10.   Selected antidepressant drugs and their usual daily dosages

Generic name (by class)	Trade name(s)	Oral dose (mg)
Tertiary amine tricyclic		
Imipramine	Tofranil; Tofranil PM SK-Pramine; Janimine	300
Amitriptyline	Elavil; Endep	300
Doxepin	Adapin; Sinequan	300
Trimipramine	Surmontil	200
Secondary amine tricyclic		
Desipramine	Norpramin; Pertofrane	300
Nortriptyline	Aventyl; Pamelor	150
Protriptyline	Vivactil	60
Tetracyclic		
Maprotiline	Ludiomil	200
Dibenzoxazepine		
Amoxapine	Asendin	400
Triazolopyridine		
Trazodone	Desyrel	600
Bicyclic		
Fluoxetine	Prozac	60
Naphthylamine		
Sertraline	Zoloft	100
Unicyclic		
Bupropion	Wellbutrin	450

Source. Adapted from Silver and Yudofsky 1992.

The side effects of these medications require caution in their administration. Patients with Parkinson's disease are particularly sensitive to certain of these effects. Many experience orthostatic hypotension that may be exacerbated by drugs, resulting in syncope with injury (e.g., fractures and lacerations). Nortriptyline is less likely to cause postural hypotension than is imipramine (Roose and Glassman 1981).

The anticholinergic effects inherent to some of these agents may cause confusion and worsen preexisting cognitive problems. Among the heterocyclic antidepressants, desipramine and nortriptyline are less likely than amitriptyline to cause these effects. Trazodone and fluoxetine have no anticholinergic effects.

Several antidepressant agents, via different actions, are known to cause parkinsonian symptoms.

These include amoxapine (which is metabolized to loxapine) (Thornton and Stahl 1984), fluoxetine (Bouchard et al. 1989), and phenelzine (Gillman and Sandy 1986; Waldmeier and Delini-Stula 1979).

Fluoxetine, a serotonin-reuptake inhibitor, has a known dopamine-antagonistic activity (Brod 1989). Steur (1993) reported a transient, but significant, increase in parkinsonian signs and symptoms in 4 Parkinson's disease patients taking fluoxetine for depression. These patients were receiving fluoxetine 20 mg/day. On the other hand, Caley and Friedman (1982) reported no exacerbation of parkinsonian symptoms in 20 depressed Parkinson's disease patients receiving up to 40 mg/day of fluoxetine. An additional 3 patients experienced mild worsening of symptoms. This antidepressant should be administered with cau-

Table 22–11. Selected antidepressant drugs and their pharmacological properties

Antidepressant	Postural hypotension	Anticholinergic effect	Sedative effect	Reuptake inhibition	
				NE	5-HT
Amitriptyline	++++	+++++	+++++	+	++++
Imipramine	+++	++++	+++	++	+++
Doxepin	+++	+++	++++	++	+++
Desipramine	++	+	+	+++++	0
Nortriptyline	++	+++	++	+++	++
Trazodone	+++	++	+++++	0	+++++
Fluoxetine	0/+	+	+	0	+++++
Bupropion	0/+	+	+	0	0
Amoxapine	++	++	++	++++	+

Note. NE = norepinephrine; 5-HT = 5-hydroxytryptamine (serotonin); 0 = not present; 0/+ = very mild; + = mild; ++ = mild to moderate; +++ = moderate; ++++ = moderate to severe; +++++ = severe.
Source. Adapted from Bernstein 1991.

Table 22–12. Guidelines for use of antidepressants in Parkinson's disease

1. Reevaluate antiparkinsonian medications.
2. Categorize subtype of Parkinson's disease based on severity and response of symptoms to treatment, and presence of full or partial depressive syndrome (see Table 22–8).
3. For subtypes I and II (and III and IV if depression is not severe), consider lowering the dosage of levodopa-carbidopa (Sinemet) and using other dopaminergic agents.
4. For subtypes III and IV, use antidepressant medications with low anticholinergic effects and low incidence of orthostatic hypotension; preferred tricyclic antidepressants are nortriptyline and desipramine. If

bupropion is used, watch for increased dopaminergic function; if fluoxetine is used, watch for increased symptoms; and if trazodone is used, watch for orthostatic hypotension.
5. For subtype V, consider the tricyclic antidepressants nortriptyline and desipramine, bupropion, and deprenyl.
6. Start at relatively low dosages (i.e., nortriptyline 10 mg bid) and increase slowly (i.e., by 10 mg every third day). The usual full therapeutic dosage ultimately may be required. Monitor plasma levels when appropriate.
7. Maintain the patient on antidepressants for at least 6 months after full therapeutic effect has been obtained.

Source. Adapted from Silver and Yudofsky 1988.

tion to patients who have Parkinson's disease.

Bupropion is mildly dopaminergic and may induce dyskinesias or hallucinations. Lithium alone may produce extrapyramidal symptoms (Tyrer et al. 1980) and, when given with levodopa, may produce signs of dopaminergic excess (Coffey et al. 1984).

Drugs that may offer specific advantages include deprenyl, which, when given at dosages selective for monoamine oxidase–B receptor activity, may improve mood and postpone the requirement for levodopa early in the course of the disease (Parkinson Study Group 1989). Trazodone and fluoxetine, by virtue of negligible anticholinergic properties, have little adverse effect on cognition. As does fluoxetine, sertraline (recently approved in the United States for the treatment of depression) inhibits serotonin reuptake. Its efficacy in Parkinson's disease has not been reported.

There have been no long-term studies of antidepressant therapy in Parkinson's disease patients. Therefore, general principles of antidepressant drug therapy are applicable. An adequate trial should last at least 6 weeks. The drug should be titrated to the dose necessary (within the recommended guidelines) to achieve a satisfactory antidepressant effect, in the absence of intolerable side effects.

Plasma levels are not required for the management of patients receiving antidepressant therapy. Guidelines were developed by the American Psychiatric Association Task Force on the Use of Laboratory Tests in Psychiatry (1985) to determine optimal plasma levels in patients with major depression (excluding patients with neurodegenerative disorders, such as Parkinson's disease). An optimal trial of the medication is assumed when plasma levels fall within the guidelines. It is not known if the results of these determinations are applicable to more complicated clinical settings (i.e., in the setting of a documented brain disorder). Levels of imipramine and its desmethyl metabolite, desipramine, should be greater than 200–250 ng/ml, levels of desipramine greater than 125 ng/ml, and a level of nortriptyline between 50 and 150 ng/ml. Levels should be drawn 10–14 hours after the last dose.

Treatment: electroconvulsive therapy. Electroconvulsive therapy (ECT) has been shown to be effective in the treatment of psychiatric disorders, especially depression (Brandon et al. 1984; Faber and Trimble 1991; Gregory et al. 1985; see Chapter 30). In controlled comparison studies with antidepressant medications, it has been demonstrated to be superior

(Abrams 1988). Dating back to the 1950s (Lebensohn and Jenkins 1975; Savitsky and Karliner 1953; Shapiro and Goldberg 1957), ECT has also been observed to benefit the tremor and motor symptoms of Parkinson's disease patients undergoing the procedure for depression, as well as to improve parkinsonism secondary to neuroleptic medications (Goswami et al. 1989).

A number of recent series (Andersen et al. 1987; Douyon et al. 1986; Zervas and Fink 1991) have reported ECT to be effective in relieving motor symptoms of Parkinson's disease in patients undergoing the procedure for depression. The primary indication for ECT in Parkinson's disease is in the treatment of depression, especially when antidepressant medications are ineffective or when side effects make them intolerable. The latter may include impairment of cognition, glaucoma, ileus, heart conduction block, or urinary retention. In addition, ECT may be preferable in life-threatening situations requiring a more rapid response (e.g., suicidal depression or malnutrition secondary to apathy and psychomotor retardation).

Other psychiatric uses of ECT include the treatment of mania (Small and Millstein 1986), uncommon in Parkinson's disease patients, and psychoses, including psychotic depression, schizophrenia, and psychoses secondary to neurological disease or toxicity from medications. Roth et al. (1988) reported improvement in both motor and affective signs in a manic Parkinson's disease patient treated with ECT. ECT has been used effectively in the treatment of psychosis induced by dopaminergic therapy (see section on "Drug-Related Conditions" below).

In Parkinson's disease patients without psychiatric disease, Balldin and associates (Balldin and Eden 1980; Balldin and Granerus 1981) and Andersen et al. (1987) found improvement in motor symptoms, especially those exhibiting motor fluctuations (i.e., "on-off phenomenon," end-of-dose deterioration, and so on). The latter study included a group of control subjects who received no benefit from sham ECT, but several of whom improved after crossover to ECT. In contrast, no motor benefit was reported by Ward and Stern (1980) in five of six Parkinson's disease patients who were not clinically depressed and underwent ECT. One patient improved transiently.

The mechanism by which ECT results in improvement of parkinsonism is not known. Experimental evidence indicates a dopamine-enhancing effect that may occur due to changes in autoreceptors (Clark and White 1987), postsynaptic receptors (White and Barrett 1981), postreceptor events (Heal and Green 1978), and/or neurotransmitters (Green et al. 1978).

Included with the risks of ECT are those attendant with the induction of and recovery from anesthesia. Psychotropic drugs are discontinued prior to ECT, and levodopa dosage should be reduced. The latter is required to minimize the occurrence of dyskinesias and posttreatment delirium, which may result from increased dopamine sensitivity. The cardiovascular risks of ECT are small (Kramer 1985), with a mortality of one death per 50,000 treatments. Neither permanent electroencephalographic (EEG) changes nor subsequent spontaneous seizures follow ECT. Postictal confusion is common for up to 30 minutes after the procedure. Figiel et al. (1991) reported prolonged interictal delirium in each of seven depressed Parkinson patients, suggesting that pathological changes in the basal ganglia may play a role in the pathogenesis of this mental status abnormality. Bilateral electrode placement results in some degree of memory impairment for at least 6 months (Weiner et al. 1986). However, unilateral electrode placement with brief pulse stimulation produces a memory disturbance no greater in ECT-treated patients than in antidepressant-treated control subjects (Weiner et al. 1986).

ECT is safe and effective in dementia patients (Tsuang et al. 1979). The distinction between the dementia and depression is problematic in some patients because of the occurrence of apathy and psychomotor retardation in both disorders (McAllister and Price 1976). Depression itself, and the antidepressant medications required for its treatment, may exacerbate cognitive impairment. Improvement in depression, cognition, and extrapyramidal symptoms has been reported in an ECT-treated Parkinson's disease patient (Jaeckle and Dilsaver 1986). The cost of ECT is considerable, ranging from $10,000 to $15,000 for the initial year, and from $5,000 to $10,000 in subsequent years. Additional costs (e.g., medication and office visits) may also be expected. However, the cost of ECT may be considerably less, with fewer other attendant risks and more promising beneficial effects, than investigative neurosurgical procedures (e.g., autologous adrenal medullary or fetal tissue transplant) (Goetz et al. 1989) for progressive, poorly controlled disease.

Mania

Manic behavior secondary to bipolar illness is rare among Parkinson patients, but has been associated with levodopa therapy (Celesia and Barr 1970) and Parkinson's disease dementia. Hyperactivity may occur as a manifestation of a schizophrenic-like disorder that has been described rarely in Parkinson's disease (Crow et al. 1976). Management is difficult because of the likelihood of the exacerbation of manic symptoms by levodopa and the risk of increasing extrapyramidal symptoms (e.g., tardive dyskinesia) by lithium.

Anxiety Disorders

Generalized anxiety disorder.   Generalized anxiety is a frequent finding in patients with Parkinson's disease. Stein et al. (1990) found the disorder in 38% of Parkinson's disease patients and with no relationship to their degree of motor disability or treatment with levodopa. Symptoms of anxiety or panic may also coexist with depression (i.e., atypical depression) (Henderson et al. 1992; Schiffer et al. 1988).

Benzodiazepines are effective in the treatment of anxiety. In addition, they may be used in conjunction with antidepressants and are effective in counteracting the not-infrequent occurrence of stimulant effects by small, initial doses of antidepressants (e.g., in the treatment of panic disorder). Buspirone, a nonbenzodiazepine with both anxiolytic and antidepressant properties, may be administered in conjunction with antidepressant drugs to treat coexistent anxiety (Fabre 1990). However, in a double-blind placebo-controlled crossover study of 16 Parkinson patients, buspirone in doses of 10 mg/day to 100 mg/day had no effect on anxiety, depression scales, or extrapyramidal symptoms (Ludwig et al. 1986). Panic disorder may be effectively treated with the heterocyclic antidepressants nortriptyline, desipramine, and imipramine and the non-heterocylic fluoxetine (Silver and Yudofsky 1988).

Phobic disorder.   Phobic disorders are characterized by irrational fear (fully defined by DSM-IV), such as fear of crowded places. Initially fear manifested by Parkinson's disease patients may be justified (e.g., fear of falling because of impaired postural reflexes), but later it may be exaggerated to include situations in which it is not reasonable. This disorder rarely begins before the onset of Parkinson's disease.

Obsessive-Compulsive Disorder

Obsessive-compulsive symptomatology (OCS) has been linked to dysfunction of the basal ganglia. It is sometimes present in disorders involving the basal ganglia (e.g., Gilles de la Tourette syndrome, Huntington's disease, and Sydenham's chorea) and has been observed in postencephalitic parkinsonism patients. It has also been associated with lateralized brain abnormalities in both left and right hemispheres.

Tomer et al. (1993), using the Leyton Obessional Inventory (Cooper 1970), studied the relationship between OCS and the lateralization of motor symptoms in 30 patients with idiopathic Parkinson's disease. The severity of left-sided motor dysfunction was found to be a reliable predictor of the overall severity of OCS. The variables that most significantly correlated with left-sided motor impairment were overconscientiousness, repetition, disturbing thoughts, and obsessions with cleanliness. This may reflect a relatively greater deficiency of dopamine in the right basal ganglia of Parkinson's disease patients manifesting OCS.

Psychosis

No convincing association has been found between Parkinson's disease and psychosis (i.e., schizophrenia). Psychotic depression is an extreme manifestation of depressive illness and is also rare in Parkinson's disease. Symptoms that may be shared (e.g., hallucinations or delusions) are more closely related to drug toxicity in the treatment of Parkinson's disease (discussed below) or occur in the setting of dementia.

Drug-Related Conditions

Virtually every drug used in the treatment of Parkinson's disease, because of their various effects on brain neurochemistry, can produce clinically significant psychiatric symptoms. Included are the anticholinergics, amantadine, deprenyl, levodopa, and dopamine receptor agonists. These adverse effects significantly limit the efficacy of antiparkinsonian medication in some patients. Data reported in some studies regarding the incidence of certain effects (e.g., hallucinations, delusions, and delirium) may be inaccurate (i.e., most likely an underestimation) because of imprecise psychiatric interviewing techniques, the reluctance of patients and families to relate these disturbing events, and failure to distinguish the exact nature of the adverse effect.

Hallucinations. Visual hallucinations are the most common medication-induced side effect (tactile and auditory hallucinations are rare) and may occur with the use of any antiparkinsonian. The overall incidence is estimated to be about 20% and is greatest with the use of dopaminergic agents (Goetz et al. 1982). It is thought that bromocriptine has a greater potential to cause psychiatric side effects than levodopa.

The hallucinations most frequently occur in the absence of delirium, at night, and most often they involve seeing formed objects (e.g., people or animals). Sleep disturbances may also be present. Increasing age, a history of multiple-drug therapy, a premorbid history of psychiatric illness, and the use of anticholinergic medications have been found to be predictors for the occurrence of hallucinations (Glantz et al. 1986; Tanner et al. 1983).

Hallucinatory syndromes differ depending on the offending agent. Anticholinergic drugs are more likely to produce hallucinations that are threatening, be combined with tactile or auditory components, and accompanied by delirium (Goetz et al. 1982). They usually respond to decreasing the dosage of the causative agent(s). (Additional treatment options are discussed below.) A few Parkinson's disease patients experience "benign hallucinations": vivid, nonthreatening visual hallucinations in the absence of delirium or other cognitive impairment, with insight remaining intact. Dosage reduction, if possible, is usually effective in lessening or eliminating hallucinations.

Delusions. As in the occurrence of hallucinations, delusions (false beliefs based on faulty inference, held despite evidence to the contrary, and ordinarily not accepted by members of a person's culture or subculture) have been reported with all types of antiparkinsonian medication. The reported incidence range is from 3% to 30% (but may be higher if more scrupulously sought), and it is greater at higher doses.

If caused by levodopa, delusions may often be predicted by the occurrence of dreams and/or visual hallucinations (Klawans 1978). Delusions may occur in the setting of a clear or clouded sensorium (Moskovitz et al. 1978). They may be self-persecutory. Older patients with dementia are particularly susceptible (Fischer et al. 1990), and delusions are rarely associated with a schizophrenic-like thought disorder (Beardsley and Puletti 1971).

Management of delusions includes withdrawal of anticholinergic agents and amantadine and reduction of the dosage of levodopa or other dopaminergic drugs. Toxic (i.e., drug-induced) psychoses resulting from antiparkinsonian medications have been successfully treated using neuroleptic medications. They are limited by their tendencies to produce extrapyramidal symptoms and, thus, worsen the parkinsonism. Low dosages of molindone, thioridazine, perphenazine, and haloperidol may be administered with caution to alleviate symptoms (Hale and Bellizzi 1980). However, in our experience, a successful result is rarely achieved because of exacerbation of the parkinsonian features with these drugs. In addition, L-tryptophan has been reported to reduce paranoid delusions in a few patients (Miller and Nieburg 1974).

Clozapine, an atypical antipsychotic that produces fewer parkinsonian side effects, has been used successfully in the treatment of drug-induced psychosis. Van Tol et al. (1991) hypothesized that clozapine may bind to a specific dopamine receptor (i.e., the dopamine, subtype 4 [D_4], receptor) that has a greater affinity for this compound than the D_1, D_2, or D_3 receptors. Factor and Brown (1992) reported a study of eight patients being treated with clozapine whose psychiatric disorders were improved significantly by the use of every-other-day dosing (which prevented the recurrence of psychosis during intervals of significant dosage increases of levodopa and the addition of other antiparkinsonian medications). They also reported improvement in motor disability with these medication adjustments. Clozapine may cause bone marrow suppression, and hematologic monitoring (i.e., weekly complete blood counts) is required.

In our experience, the administration of low dosages of clozapine (25–50 mg at night) is very helpful in reducing or eliminating levodopa-induced hallucinations. These are smaller doses than those used to treat drug-resistant schizophrenia. Parkinson's disease patients with dementia are less tolerant of clozapine. In patients whose psychiatric symptoms (i.e., adverse drug effects) would have otherwise precluded increasing levodopa dosages to better control motor symptoms, the use of clozapine makes it possible. We have also noticed an antitremor effect of clozapine in some patients. Others have reported improvement in insomnia (especially early morning awakening) when the medication is taken at bedtime. ECT is an additional alternative in the treatment of levodopa-induced psychosis (Hurwitz et al. 1988).

Confusion/delirium. The terms *confusion* and *delirium* are often used interchangeably and refer to a syndrome consisting of an altered state of consciousness,

incoherent speech, altered psychomotor activity, memory impairment, and sudden onset and rapid fluctuation (Table 22–13). Mild forms may be unrecognized. This syndrome has been noted to complicate all forms of antiparkinsonian therapy with a prevalence of 5%–25% and seems to be more frequent among higher-potency ergot derivatives (e.g., bromocriptine and pergolide).

Depression. Despite its mood-elevating effects in some Parkinson's disease patients, levodopa has also been implicated as a depression-causing agent. Huber et al. (1988) found that depressed Parkinson's disease patients had taken the drug for longer periods and were receiving significantly higher dosages than were nondepressed patients. However, the prevalence range of depressive symptoms in Parkinson's disease patients treated with levodopa compared with those untreated is approximately the same, ranging from 2% to 50%. Levodopa may in some way effect the appearance of depressive symptoms, but has not been found to make them more prevalent. Treatment of depression in the setting of levodopa therapy is by the conventional use of antidepressants and ECT.

Mania. Levodopa has the capability of mood elevation along a spectrum from a simple feeling of well-being to full blown episodes of mania (e.g., elation, grandiosity, pressured speech, racing thoughts, hyperactivity, reduced requirement for sleep, increased libido, and risk-taking behavior) (Celesia and Barr 1970; Ryback and Schwab 1971). Pergolide has also been reported to cause mania (Lang and Quinn 1982). In

---

Table 22–13. Diagnostic criteria for delirium

A. Disturbance of consciousness (i.e., reduced clarity of awareness of the environment) with reduced ability to focus, sustain, or shift attention.

B. A change in cognition (such as memory deficit, disorientation, language disturbance) or the development of a perceptual disturbance that is not better accounted for by a preexisting, established, or evolving dementia.

C. The disturbance develops over a short period of time (usually hours to days) and tends to fluctuate during the course of the day.

D. There is evidence from the history, physical examination, or laboratory findings that the disturbance is caused by the direct physiological consequences of a general medical condition.

Source. Adapted from American Psychiatric Association 1994.

Parkinson's disease patients with a premordid history of mania, hypomania has resulted from levodopa and bromocriptine therapy (Goodwin 1971; Jouvent et al. 1983). It usually subsides with dosage reduction.

Anxiety. Symptoms of anxiety and panic (e.g., apprehension, irritability, nervousness, feelings of impending doom, palpitations, and hyperventilation) have been attributed to levodopa therapy, especially when occurring in patients not so predisposed before the onset of Parkinson's disease (Celesia and Barr 1970). Those with similar prior symptomatology have reported worsening of their anxiety syndromes (Rondot et al. 1984). Pergolide and deprenyl (in combination with levodopa) therapies have also been associated with a significant incidence of anxiety (Lang and Quinn 1982; Yahr et al. 1983). It occurs in approximately two-thirds of patients with motor fluctuations, especially in the "off" state (Nissenbaum 1987). Treatment is by adjustment (usually reduction) of the agent and use of anxiolytic agents (e.g., benzodiazepines).

Altered sexual behavior. Increased libido, resulting from antiparkinsonian therapy, may occur in conjunction with or in the absence of a manic syndrome. Its expression may range from a renewed sexual interest with increased potency to a pathological state (i.e., hypersexuality). Increases in libido in case series reports range from 1% to 10%, but may be more frequent. The hypersexuality may be manifested by increased masturbation, marked increase in marital intercourse, and extramarital affairs to attain gratification. Males are predominantly affected, and levodopa is the most common causative agent (Harvey 1988; Vogel and Schifter 1983). The behavior has also been reported with pergolide (Quinn et al. 1984). Paraphiliac (i.e., sexually deviant) behavior has been reported in Parkinson's disease patients both with and without a prior history, but is more likely in those with a predisposition. Paraphiliac disorders that have been reported include sexual masochism, pedophilia, voyeurism, sadomasochistic fantasies, and exhibitionism.

Sleep disturbances. Sleep disturbances are more likely in Parkinson's disease patients with drug-related psychiatric conditions. Hallucinosis and confusional episodes are significantly more common in patients with sleep complaints than in those without (Nausieda and Weiner 1982). Vivid dreams and nightmares complicate both levodopa and pergolide treatment (Lang

and Quinn 1982). Sleep disturbances are also more common in Parkinson's disease patients with major depression (Starkstein et al. 1991). Sleep studies in Parkinson patients have found diminished stage III and IV sleep, with multiple arousals and awakenings (Emser et al. 1988). Symptomatic treatment with hypnotic agents (e.g., chloral hydrate or benzodiazepines) have been effective anecdotally, and antidepressants may be effective if secondary to depression.

Summary

Cognitive and psychiatric disorders are important aspects of the clinical syndrome resulting from Parkinson's disease. Although the motor symptoms often receive the majority of attention, deterioration of the mental state is not uncommon and virtually inevitable if the disease is longstanding. Behavioral disturbances may result from the disease itself and from the medications used to improve motor function.

Following recognition of changes in the mental state, it is necessary to distinguish those that may be more likely to respond to treatment (e.g., depression and drug-induced psychosis) from those that will not (e.g., dementia and bradyphrenia). This determination will be facilitated when specific diagnostic guidelines are formulated that take into account both the behavioral and the motor manifestations of Parkinson's disease. For the neuropsychiatric manifestations, effective therapies (e.g., drug and ECT) are available and may significantly improve the quality of life of the Parkinson's disease patient.

References

Abrams R: Electroconvulsive Therapy. New York, Oxford, 1988

American Psychiatric Association: Diagnostic and Statistical Manual of Mental Disorders, 3rd Edition, Revised. Washington, DC, American Psychiatric Association, 1987

American Psychiatric Association: Diagnostic and Statistical Manual of Mental Disorders, 4th Edition. Washington, DC, American Psychiatric Association, 1994

American Psychiatric Association Task Force on the Use of Laboratory Tests in Psychiatry: Blood level measurements and clinical outcome: an APA Task Force report. Am J Psychiatry 142:155–162, 1985

Andersen K, Balldin J, Gottfries CG, et al: A double-blind evaluation of electroconvulsive therapy in Parkinson's disease with "on-off" phenomena. Acta Neurol Scand 76:191–199, 1987

Anderson J, Aabro E: Antidepressant treatment in Parkinson's disease: a controlled trial of the effect of nortriptyline in patients with Parkinson's disease treated with L-dopa. Acta Neurol Scand 62:210–219, 1980

Aquilonius SM, Hartvig P: A Swedish country with unexpected high utilization of antiparkinsonian drugs. Acta Neurol Scand 74:379–382, 1986

Ashok PP, Radhakrishan K, Sridharan R, et al: Parkinsonism in Benghazi, East Libya. Clin Neurol Neurosurg 88:109–113, 1986

Baldessarini RJ: Chemotherapy in Psychiatry: Principles and Practice. Boston, MA, Harvard University Press, 1985

Ball M: The morphological basis of dementia in Parkinson's disease. Can J Neurol Sci 11:180–184, 1984

Balldin J, Eden S: Electroconvulsive therapy in Parkinson's syndrome with "on-off" phenomenon. Journal of Neural Transmission 47:11–21, 1980

Balldin J, Granerus A: Predictors for improvement after electroconvulsive therapy in parkinsonian patients with on-off symptoms. Journal of Neural Transmission 52:199–211, 1981

Barbeau A, Pourcher E: New data on the genetics of Parkinson's disease. Can J Neurol Sci 9:53–60, 1982

Bavazzano A, Guarducci R: Clinical trial with amantidine and hydergine in elderly patients. J Clin Exp Neuropsychol 2:289–299, 1980

Beardsley JV, Puletti F: Personality (MMPI) and cognitive (WAIS) changes after levodopa treatment. Arch Neurol 25:145–150, 1971

Bernstein JG: Psychotropic drug prescribing: antidepressant drugs, in Massachusetts General Hospital Handbook of General Hospital Psychiatry. Edited by Cassem NH. St. Louis, MO, Mosby Year Book, 1991, pp 245–255

Birkmayer W, Danielczyk W, Riederer P: Symptoms and side effects in the course of Parkinson's disease. J Neural Transm [Suppl] 19:185–199, 1983

Birkmayer W, Knoll J, Riederer P, et al: Increased life expectancy resulting from addition of L-deprenyl to Madopar treatment in Parkinson's disease: a long-term study. Journal of Neural Transmission 64:113–127, 1985

Boller F, Mizutani R, Roessmann U, et al: Parkinson's disease, dementia and Alzheimer's disease: clinicopathologic correlations. Ann Neurol 7:329–335, 1980

Bouchard RH, Bourcher E, Vincent P: Fluoxetine and extrapyramidal side effects. Am J Psychiatry 146:1352–1353, 1989

Brandon S, Cowley P, McDonald C, et al: Electroconvulsive therapy: results in depressive illness from the Leicestershire trial. BMJ 288:22–25, 1984

Brod TM: Fluoxetine and extrapyramidal side effects. Am J Psychiatry 146:1352–1353, 1989

Brooks DJ, Frackowaik R: PET and movement disorder. J Neurol Neurosurg Psychiatry (suppl) 52:68–77, 1989

Brown RG, Marsden CD: How common is dementia in Parkinson's disease? Lancet 2:1262–1265, 1984

Burch PRJ: Cigarette smoking and Parkinson's disease. Neurology 31:500–503, 1981

Caley CF, Friedman JH: Does fluoxetine exacerbate Parkinson's disease? J Clin Psychiatry 53:278–282, 1982

Caparros-Lefebvre D, Blond S, Vermersch P, et al: Chronic thalamic stimulation improves tremor and levodopa induced dyskinesias in Parkinson's disease. J Neurol Neurosurg Psychiatry 56:268–273, 1993

Cassem NH: Depression: choice of antidepressant treatment, in Massachusetts General Hospital Handbook of General Hospital Psychiatry. Edited by Cassem NH. St. Louis, MO, Mosby Year Book, 1991, pp 209–225

Celesia GG, Barr AN: Psychosis and other psychiatric manifestations of levodopa therapy. Arch Neurol 23:193–200, 1970

Charcot JM: Lectures on Diseases of the Nervous System, Vol 1. English translation by Sigerson G. London, New London Society, 1878

Charcot JM, Vulpian A: De la paralysie agitante. Gaz Hebdomadaire Med Chir 9:54–59, 1862

Clark D, White FJ: Review D_1 dopamine receptors: the search for a function: a critical evaluation of the D_1/D_2 dopamine receptor classification and its functional implications. Synapse 1:347–388, 1987

Coffey CE, Ross ER, Massey EW, et al: Dyskinesias associated with lithium therapy in parkinsonism. Clin Neuropharmacol 7:223–229, 1984

Cooper J: The Leyton Obsessional Inventory. Psychol Med 1:48–64, 1970

Crow TJ, Johnstone EC, McClelland HA: The coincidence of schizophrenia and parkinsonism: some neurochemical implications. Psychol Med 6:227–233, 1976

Cummings JL: Subcortical dementia: neuropsychology, neuropsychiatry and pathophysiology. Br J Psychiatry 149:682–687, 1986

Cummings JL, Benson DF: Dementia: a clinical approach. Boston, MA, Butterworths, 1983

Cummings JL, Benson DF: Subcortical dementia: review of an emerging concept. Arch Neurol 41:874–879, 1984

Curtis L, Lees AJ, Stern GM, et al: Effect of L-dopa on the course of Parkinson's disease. Lancet 2:211–212, 1984

de Bruin VMS, Lees AJ, Daniel SE: Diffuse Lewy body disease presenting with supranuclear gaze palsy, parkinsonism and dementia: a case report. Mov Disord 4:355–358, 1992

Defer G, Cesaro P, Nguyen JP, et al: Fetal grafting in Parkinson's disease: results for the first three patients (abstract). Neurology 43 (suppl):A222, 1993

deLeon MJ, Ferris SH: Computed tomography evaluation of brain-behavior relationships in senile dementia of the Alzheimer's type. Neurobiol Aging 1:59–79, 1980

Dooneief G, Mirabello E, Bell K, et al: An estimate of the incidence of depression in idiopathic Parkinson's disease. Arch Neurol 49:305–307, 1992

Douyon R, Selby M, Klutchko B, et al: ECT and Parkinson's disease revisited: a "naturalistic" study. Am J Psychiatry 37:819–825, 1986

Eisler T, Teravaiinen H, Nelson R, et al: Deprenyl in Parkinson's disease. Neurology 31:19–23, 1981

Emser W, Brenner M, Stober T, et al: Changes in nocturnal sleep in Huntington's and Parkinson's diseases. J Neurol 235:177–179, 1988

Faber R, Trimble MR: Electroconvulsive therapy in Parkinson's disease and other movement disorders. Mov Disord 6:293–303, 1991

Fabre LF: Buspirone in the management of major depression: a placebo-controlled comparison. J Clin Psychiatry 51 (suppl):55–61, 1990

Factor SA, Brown D: Clozapine prevents recurrence of psychosis in Parkinson's disease. Mov Disord 7:125–131, 1992

Fazzini E, Dogali M, Eidelberg D, et al: Long-term follow-up on patients with Parkinson's disease receiving unilateral ventroposterior medial pallidotomy (abstract). Neurology 43 (suppl):A222, 1993

Figiel GS, Hassen MA, Zorumski C, et al: ECT-induced delirium in depressed patients with Parkinson's disease. J Neuropsychiatry Clin Neurosci 3:405–411, 1991

Fischer P, Danielczyk W, Simyani M, et al: Dopaminergic psychosis in advanced Parkinson's disease, in Parkinson's Disease: Anatomy, Pathology & Therapy (Advances in Neurology Series, Vol 53). Edited by Streifler MB, Korczyn AD, Melamed E, et al. New York, Raven, 1990, pp 391–397

Flowers KA, Pearce I, Pearce JMS: Recognition memory in Parkinson's disease. J Neurol Neurosurg Psychiatry 47:1174–1181, 1984

Funfgeld EW, Baggen M, Nedwidek P, et al: Double-blind study with phosphatidylserine in parkinsonian patients with senile dementia of the Alzheimer's type. Prog Clin Biol Res 317:1235–1246, 1989

Garnett ES, Nahmais C, Firnau G: Central dopaminergic pathways in hemiparkinsonism examined by positron emission tomography. Can J Neurol Sci 11:174–179, 1984

Gaspar P, Gray F: Dementia in idiopathic Parkinson's disease. Acta Neuropathol 64:43–52, 1984

Gillman MA, Sandy KR: Parkinsonism induced by a monoamine oxidase inhibitor. Postgrad Med J 62:235–236, 1986

Glantz RH, Bielauskaus L, Paleogos N: Behavioral indicators of hallucinosis in levodopa-treated Parkinson's disease, in Parkinson's Disease (Advances in Neurology Series, Vol 45). Edited by Yahr MD, Bergmann KJ. New York, Raven, 1986, pp 417–420

Goetz CG: Neurotoxins in Clinical Practice. New York, SP Medical & Scientific Books, 1985

Goetz CG, Tanner CM, Klawans HL: Pharmacology of hallucinations induced by long-term drug therapy. Am J Psychiatry 139:494–497, 1982

Goetz CG, Olanow C, Koller W, et al: Multicenter study of autologous adrenal medullary transplantation to the corpus striatum in patients with advanced Parkinson's disease. N Engl J Med 320:337–341, 1989

Golbe LI, DiIorio G, Bonavita V, et al: A large kindred with autosomal dominant Parkinson's disease. Ann Neurol 27:276–282, 1990a

Golbe LI, Farrell TM, Davis PH: Follow-up study of early life protective and risk factors in Parkinson's disease. Mov Disord 5:66–70, 1990b

Goodwin FK: Psychiatric side effects of levodopa in man. JAMA 218:1915–1920, 1971

Goswami U, Dutta S, Kuruvilla K, et al: Electroconvulsive therapy in neuroleptic-induced parkinsonism. Biol Psychiatry 26:234–238, 1989

Gotham A-M, Brown RG, Marsden CD: Depression in Parkinson's disease: a quantitative and qualitative analysis. J Neurol Neurosurg Psychiatry 49:381–389, 1986

Green AR, Peralta E, Hong JS, et al: Alteration in GABA metabolism and metenkephalin content in rat brain following repeated electroconvulsive shocks. J Neurochem 31:607–611, 1978

Gregory S, Schawcross CR, Gill D: The Nottingham ECT study: a double-blind comparison of bilateral, unilateral and simulated ECT in depressive illness. Br J Psychiatry 146:520–524, 1985

Gudmundsson KR: A clinical survey of parkinsonism in Iceland. Acta Neurol Scand 33:9–61, 1967

Hale MS, Bellizzi J: Low-dose perphenazine and levodopa/carbidopa therapy in a patient with parkinsonism and a psychotic illness. J Nerv Ment Dis 168:312–314, 1980

Harvey NS: Serial cognitive profiles in levodopa-induced hypersexuality. Br J Psychiatry 153:833–836, 1988

Heal DJ, Green AR: Repeated electroconvulsive shock increases the behavioural responses of rats to injection of both dopamine and dibutyryl cyclic AMP into the nucleus acumbens. Neuropharmacology 17:1085–1087, 1978

Heikala E-V, Laulumaa V, Soininen H, et al: Recall and recognition memory in patients with Alzheimer's and Parkinson's diseases. Ann Neurol 24:214–217, 1988

Heikkila RE, Manzino L, Cabbat FS: Protection against the dopaminergic neurotoxicity of 1-methyl-4-phenyl-1,2,4,6-tetrahydropyridine by monoamine oxidase inhibitors. Nature 311:467–469, 1984

Helig CW, Knopman DS, Mastri AR, et al: Dementia without Alzheimer pathology. Neurology 35:762–765, 1985

Henderson R, Kurlan R, Kersun JM, et al: Preliminary examination of the comorbidity of anxiety and depression in Parkinson's disease. J Neuropsychiatry Clin Neurosci 4:257–264, 1992

Hofman A, Schulte W, Tanja TA, et al: History of dementia and Parkinson's disease in first-degree relative of patients with Alzheimer's disease. Neurology 39:1589–1592, 1989

Huber ST, Bornstein RA: Neuropsychological evaluations of Parkinson's disease, in Parkinson's Disease: Neurobehavioral Aspects. Edited by Huber SJ, Cummings JL. New York, Oxford University Press, 1992, pp 32–45

Huber SJ, Shuttleworth EC, Paulson GW: Dementia in Parkinson's disease. Arch Neurol 43:987–990, 1986

Huber SJ, Paulson GW, Shuttleworth EC: Depression in Parkinson's disease. Neuropsychiatry, Neuropsychology, and Behavioral Neurology 1:47–51, 1988

Huber SJ, Freidenberg DL, Shuttleworth EC, et al: Neuropsychological impairments associated with the severity of Parkinson's disease. J Neuropsychiatry Clin Neurosci 1:154–158, 1989

Hurwitz TA, Calne DB, Waterman K: Treatment of dopaminomimetic psychosis in Parkinson's disease with electroconvulsive therapy. Can J Neurol Sci 15:32–34, 1988

Inzelberg R, Treves T, Reider I, et al: Computed tomography brain changes in Parkinson's disease. Neuroradiology 29:535–539, 1987

Jaeckle RS, Dilsaver SC: Covariation of depressive symptoms, parkinsonism and post-dexamethasone plasma cortisone in a bipolar patient: simultaneous response to ECT and lithium carbonate. Acta Psychiatr Scand 74:68–72, 1986

Jankovic J, McDermott M, Carter J, et al: Variable expression of Parkinson's disease: a baseline analysis of the DATATOP cohort. Neurology 40:1529–1534, 1990

Jellinger LK: Pathological correlations of dementia in Parkinson's disease. Arch Neurol 44:690–691, 1987

Jenner P, Schapira AHV, Marsden CD: New insights into the cause of Parkinson's disease. Neurology 42:2241–2250, 1992

Jouvent R, Abensour P, Bonnet AM, et al: Antiparkinsonian and antidepressant effects of high doses of bromcriptine. J Affect Disord 5:141–145, 1983

Kahn HA: The Dorn study of smoking among United States veterans, in National Cancer Institute: Epidemiologic Approaches to the Study of Cancer and Other Diseases (Monograph 19). Washington DC, US Government Printing Office, 1966, pp 1–125

Karbe N, Holthoff V, Rudolf J, et al: Positron emission tomography in degenerative disorders of the dopaminergic system. J Neural Transm Park Dis Dement Sect 4:121–130, 1992

Kaspar S, Moises HW, Beckman H: The anticholinergic biperiden in depressive disorders. Pharmacopsychiatry 14:195–198, 1981

Kessler II: Epidemiologic studies of Parkinson's disease, III: a community-based survey. Am J Epidemiol 96:242–254, 1972

Klawans HL: Levodopa-induced psychosis. Am J Psychiatry 8:447–451, 1978

Klawans HL: Individual manifestations of Parkinson's disease after ten or more years of levodopa. Mov Disord 1:187–192, 1986

Koller WC, Vetere-Overfield B, Gray C, et al: Environmental risk factors in Parkinson's disease. Neurology 40:1218–1221, 1990

Konig H: Zur Psychopathogie der paralysis Agitans. Archiv für Psychiatrie und Nervenkrankheiten 50:285–305, 1912

Korczyn AD, Inzelberg R, Treves T, et al: Dementia of Parkinson's disease. in Parkinson's Disease (Advances in Neurology Series, Vol 45). Edited by Yahr MD, Bergmann KJ. New York, Raven, 1986, pp 399–403

Kosaka K: Diffuse Lewy body disease in Japan. J Neurol 237:197–204, 1990

Kosaka K, Matsushita M, Oyanagi S, et al: A clinicopathological study of the "Lewy body disease." Seishin Shinkeigaku Zasshi (Psychiatria et Neurolica Japonica) 82:292–311, 1980

Kostic VS, Djuricic BM, Covickovic-Sternic N, et al: Depression and Parkinson's disease: possible role of serotonergic mechanisms. J Neurol 12:94–96, 1987

Kramer BA: The use of ECT in California, 1977–1983. Am J Psychiatry 142:1190–1192, 1985

Kurland LT: Epidemiology: incidence, geographic distribution and genetic consideration, in Pathogenesis and Treatment of Parkinsonism. Edited by Field W. Springfield, IL, Charles C Thomas, 1958, pp 5–43

Lang AF, Quinn N: Pergolide in late-stage Parkinson's disease. Ann Neurol 12:243–247, 1982

Langston JW, Ballard PA, Tetrud JW, et al: Chronic parkinsonism in humans due to a product of meperidine-analog synthesis. Science 219:979–980, 1983

Lebensohn ZM, Jenkins RB: Improvement of parkinsonism in depressed patients treated with ECT. Am J Psychiatry 132:283–285, 1975

Leenders KL, Wolfson L, Gibbs TM, et al: The effect of L-dopa on regional cerebral blood flow and oxygen metabolism in patients with Parkinson's disease. J Neurol Neurosurg Psychiatry 49:853–860, 1986

Li SC, Schoenberg BS, Wang CC, et al: A prevalence study of Parkinson's disease and other movement disorders in the People's Republic of China. Arch Neurol 42:655–657, 1982

Lichter DG, Corbett AJ, Fitzgibbon GM, et al: Cognitive and motor dysfunction in Parkinson's disease. Arch Neurol 45:854–860, 1988

Ludwig CL, Weinberger DR, Bruno G, et al: Buspirone, Parkinson's disease and the locus ceruleus. Clin Neuropharmacol 9:373–378, 1986

Maraganore DM, Harding AE, Marsden CD: A clinical and genetic study of familial Parkinson's disease. Mov Disord 3:205–211, 1991

Marder K, Mirabello E, Chen J, et al: Death rates among demented and nondemented patients with Parkinson's disease (abstract). Ann Neurol 28:295, 1990

Mark MH, Sage JI, Dickson DW, et al: Levodopa non-responsive Lewy body parkinsonism: clinicopathologic study of two cases. Neurology 42:1323–1327, 1992

Marsden R: The mysterious motor function of the basal ganglia: the Robert Wartenberg lecture. Neurology 32:514–539, 1982

Marttila RJ, Rinne UK: Epidemiology of Parkinson's disease in Finland. Acta Neurol Scand 43 (suppl 33):9–61, 1967

Marttila RJ, Rinne UK: Dementia in Parkinson's disease. Acta Neurol Scand 54:431–441, 1976

Mason ST, Fibiger HC: Noradrenaline and selective attention. Life Sci 25:1949–1956, 1979

Matison R, Mayeux R, Rosen J, et al: "Tip-of-the-tongue" phenomenon in Parkinson's disease. Neurology 32:567–570, 1982

Mayberg NS, Starkstein SE, Sadzot B, et al: Selective hypometabolism in the inferior frontal lobe of depressed patients with Parkinson's disease. Ann Neurol 26:57–64, 1990

Mayeux R: Depression and dementia in Parkinson's disease, in Movement Disorders. Edited by Marsden CO, Fahn S. London, Butterworth, 1982, pp 75–95

Mayeux R: The mental state in Parkinson's disease, in The Handbook of Parkinson's Disease, 2nd Edition. Edited by Koller WC. New York, Marcel Dekker, 1992, pp 159–184

Mayeux R, Stern Y, Rosen J, et al: Depression, intellectual impairment and Parkinson's disease. Neurology 31:645–650, 1981

Mayeux R, Stern Y, Cote L, et al: Altered serotonin metabolism in depressed patients with Parkinson's disease. Neurology 34:642–646, 1984

Mayeux R, Stern Y, Sano M, et al: Clinical and biochemical correlates of bradyphrenia in Parkinson's disease. Neurology 37:1130–1134, 1987

Mayeux R, Stern Y, Sano M, et al: The relationship of serotonin to depression in Parkinson's disease. Mov Disord 3:237–244, 1988a

Mayeux R, Stern Y, Rosenstein R, et al: An estimate of the prevalence of dementia in Parkinson's disease. Arch Neurol 45:260–262, 1988b

Mayeux R, Chen J, Mirabello E, et al: An estimate of the incidence and prevalence of dementia in idiopathic Parkinson's disease. Neurology 40:1513–1516, 1990

McAllister TW, Price TRP: Severe depressive pseudodementia with and without dementia. Am J Psychiatry 139:626–629, 1976

McCance-Katz EF, Marek KL, Price LH: Serotonergic dysfunction in depression associated with Parkinson's disease. Neurology 42:1813–1814, 1992

McCarthy R, Gresty M, Findley LJ: Parkinson's disease and dementia. Lancet 1:407–408, 1985

Melamed E, Hefti F, Wurtman RJ: Nonaminergic striatal neurons convert exogenous L-dopa to dopamine in parkinsonism. Ann Neurol 8:558–563, 1980

Miller EM, Nieburg HA: L-tryptophan in the treatment of levodopa-induced psychiatric disorders. Diseases of the Nervous System 35:20–23, 1974

Mindham RHS, Ahmed SWA, Clough CG: A controlled study of dementia in Parkinson's disease. J Neurol Neurosurg Psychiatry 45:969–974, 1982

Mjones H: Paralysis agitans: clinical and genetic study. Acta Psychiatrica et Neurologica 54 (suppl):1–195, 1949

Moskovitz C, Moses H III, Klawans HL: Levodopa-induced psychosis: a kindling phenomenon. Am J Psychiatry 135:669–675, 1978

Mutch WJ, Dingwall-Fordyce I, Downie AW, et al: Parkinson's disease in a Scottish city. BMJ 292:534–536, 1986

Myllyla VV, Sotaniemi KA, Tuominen J: Selegeline as primary treatment in early phase Parkinson's disease: an interim report. Acta Neurol Scand 126:177–182, 1989

Nausieda PA, Weiner WJ: Sleep disruption in the course of chronic levodopa therapy: an early feature of levodopa psychosis. Clin Neuropharmacol 5:183–194, 1982

Naville F: Les complications et les sequelles mentales de l'encephalite epidemique. Encephale (Paris) 17:369–375, 423–436, 1922

Nissenbaum H, Quinn NP, Brown RG, et al: Mood swings associated with the "on-off" phenomenon in Parkinson's disease. Psychol Med 17:899–904, 1987

Okada K, Kobayashi S, Tsunematso T: Prevalence of Parkinson's disease in Izumo City, Japan. Gerontology 36:340–344, 1990

Oppenheim H: Textbook of Nervous Diseases. Edinburgh, Otto Schulze, 1911

Parkinson Study Group: Effect of deprenyl on the progression of disability in early Parkinson's disease. N Engl J Med 321:1364–1371, 1989

Perry RH, Tomlinson BE, Candy JM, et al: Cholinergic deficit in mentally impaired parkinsonian patients. Lancet 2:789–790, 1983

Pillon B, Dubois B: Cognitive slowing in Parkinson's disease fails to respond to levodopa treatment: the 15-objects test. Neurology 39:762–768, 1989

Pollock M, Hornabrook RW: The prevalence, natural history and dementia of Parkinson's disease. Brain 89:429–448, 1966

Quinn NP, Lang AE, Thompson C, et al:. Pergolide in the treatment of Parkinson's disease, in Parkinson-Specific Motor and Mental Disorders (Advances in Neurology Series, Vol 40). Edited by Hassler RG, Christ JF. New York, Raven, 1984, pp 509–513

Rajput AH, Rozdilsky B: Parkinsonism and dementia: effects of levodopa (letter). Lancet 1:1084, 1975

Rajput AH, Offord KP, Beard CM, et al: A case-control study of smoking habits, dementia and other illnesses in idiopathic Parkinson's disease patients. Neurology 37:226–232, 1987

Rajput, AH, Rozdilsky B, Rajput A: Alzheimer's disease with idiopathic Parkinson's disease: clinical, pharmacological and pathological observations (abstract). Neurology 40:339, 1990

Riley D, Lang AE: Practical application of a low-protein diet for Parkinson's disease. Neurology 38:1026–1031, 1988

Robertson C, Flowers KA: Motor set in Parkinson's disease. J Neurol Neurosurg Psychiatry 59:583–592, 1990

Rocca WA, Morgante M: Prevalence of Parkinson's disease and other parkinsonisms: a door-to-door survey in two Sicilian communities. Neurology 40 (suppl 1):422, 1990

Rondot P, de Recondo J, Coignet A, et al: Mental disorders in Parkinson's disease after treatment with L-dopa, in Parkinson-Specific Motor and Mental Disorders (Advances in Neurology Series, Vol 40). Edited by Hassler RG, Christ JF. New York, Raven, 1984, pp 259–269

Roose SP, Glassman AH: Comparison of imipramine- and nortriptyline-induced orthostatic hypotension: a meaningful difference. J Clin Psychopharmacol 1:316–319, 1981

Ross GW, Mahler ME, Cummings JL: The dementia syndromes of Parkinson's disease: cortical and subcortical features, in Parkinson's Disease: Neurobehavioral Aspects. Edited by Huber SJ, Cummings JL. New York, Oxford University Press, 1992, pp 132–148

Roth SD, Mukherjee S, Sackeim HA: Electroconvulsive therapy in a patient with mania, parkinsonism and tardive dyskinesia. Convulsive Therapy 4:92–97, 1988

Ryback RS, Schwab RS: Manic response to levodopa therapy: report of a case. N Engl J Med 285:788–789, 1971

Sano M, Stern Y, Marder K, et al: A controlled trial of piracetam in intellectually impaired patients with Parkinson's disease. Mov Disord 5:230–234, 1990

Santamaria J, Tolosa E, Valles A: Parkinson's disease with depression: a possible subgroup of idiopathic parkinsonism. Neurology 36:1130–1133, 1986

Savitsky N, Karliner W: Electroshock in the presence of organic disease of the central nervous system. Journal of the Hillside Hospital 2:3–22, 1953

Schiffer RB, Kurlan R, Rubin A, et al: Evidence for atypical depression in Parkinson's disease. Am J Psychiatry 145:1020–1022, 1988

Schoenberg BS, Anderson DW, Haerer AF, et al: Prevalence of Parkinson's disease in the biracial population of Copiah County, Mississippi. Neurology 35:841–845, 1985

Schoenberg BS, Osuntokun BO, Adeuja AO, et al: Comparison of the prevalence of Parkinson's disease in black populations in the rural US and Nigeria: door-to-door community studies. Neurology 38:645–646, 1988

Shapiro MF, Goldberg HH: Electroconvulsive therapy in patients with structural disease of the nervous system. Am J Med Sci 233:186–195, 1957

Shaw KM, Lees AJ, Stern GM: The impact of treatment with levodopa on Parkinson's disease. Q J Med 49:283–293, 1980

Silver JM, Yudofsky SC: Psychopharmacology and electroconvulsive therapy, in The American Psychiatric Press Textbook of Psychiatry. Edited by Talbott JA, Hales RE, Yudofsky SC. Washington, DC, American Psychiatric Press, 1988, pp 767–853

Silver JM, Yudofsky SC: Drug treatment of depression in Parkinson's disease, in Parkinson's Disease: Neurobehavioral Aspects. Edited by Huber SJ, Cummings JL. New York, Oxford University Press, 1992, pp 240–254

Sitland-Marken PA, Wells BG, Froemming JH, et al: Psychiatric applications of bromocriptine therapy. J Clin Psychiatry 51:68–82, 1990

Small JG, Millstein V: Electroconvulsive therapy in the treatment of manic episodes, in Electroconvulsive Therapy: Clinical and Basic Research Issues. Edited by Malitz S, Sackeim HA. New York, New York Academy of Sciences, 1986, pp 37–49

Starkstein SE, Leiguarda R: Neuropsychological correlates of brain atrophy in Parkinson's disease: a CT-scan study. Mov Disord 1:51–55, 1993

Starkstein SE, Preziosi TJ, Robinson RG: Sleep disorders, pain and depression in Parkinson's disease. Eur Neurol 31:352–355, 1991

Starkstein SE, Maybert NS, Leiguarda R, et al: A longitudinal prospective study of depression, cognitive decline and physical impairments in patients with Parkinson's disease. J Neurol Neurosurg Psychiatry 55:377–382, 1992

Stein MB, Heuser IJ, Juncos JL, et al: Anxiety disorders in patients with Parkinson's disease. Am J Psychiatry 147:217–220, 1990

Steur ENHJ: Increase of Parkinson disability after fluoxetine medication. Neurology 43:211–213, 1993

Sullivan EV, Sagar HJ, Gabrieli JD, et al: Different cognitive profiles on standard behavioral tests in Parkinson's disease and Alzheimer's disease. J Clin Exp Neuropsychol 11:799–820, 1989

Tanner CM: Drug-induced movement disorders, in Extrapyramidal Disorders: Handbook of Clinical Neurology, Vol. 5. Edited by Vinken PJ, Bruyn GW, Klawans HL. Amsterdam, Elsevier Science, 1986, pp 185–204

Tanner CM, Vogel C, Goetz CG, et al: Hallucinations in Parkinson's disease: a population study (abstract). Ann Neurol 14:136, 1983

Tanner CM, Chen B, Wang WZ, et al: Environmental factors in the etiology of Parkinson's disease. Can J Neurol Sci 14:419–423, 1987

Tanner CM, Chen B, Wang W, et al: Environmental factors and Parkinson's disease: a case-control study in China. Neurology 39:660–664, 1989

Taylor AE, Saint-Cyr JA, Lang AE: Frontal lobe dysfunction in early Parkinson's disease: evidence for a "frontal lobe syndrome." Alzheimer Dis Assoc Disord 4:150–160, 1990

Thornton JE, Stahl SM: Case report of tardive dyskinesia associated with amoxapine therapy. Am J Psychiatry 141:704–705, 1984

Tomer R, Levin BE, Weiner WJ: Obsessive-compulsive symptoms and motor asymmetries in Parkinson's disease. Neuropsychiatry, Neuropsychology, and Behavioral Neurology 6:26–30, 1993

Tsuang MT, Tidball JS, Geller D: ECT in a depressed patient with shunt in place for normal pressure hydrocephalus. Am J Psychiatry 136:1205–1206, 1979

Tyrer P, Alexander MS, Regan A, et al: An extrapyramidal syndrome after lithium therapy. Br J Psychiatry 136:191–194, 1980

Van Tol HHM, Bunzow JR, Guan HC, et al: Cloning of the gene for a human D_4 receptor with high affinity for the antipsychotic clozapine. Nature 350:610–614, 1991

Van Praag HM, de Haan S: Central serotonin metabolism and frequency of depression. Psychiatr Res 1:219–224, 1979

Vogel HP, Schifter R: Hypersexuality: a complication of dopaminergic therapy in Parkinson's disease. Pharmacopsychiatry 16:107–110, 1983

Wade LA, Katzman R: Synthetic amino acids and the nature of L-dopa transport at the blood-brain barrier. J Neurochem 25:837–842, 1975

Waldmeier PC, Delini-Stula AA: Serotonin-dopamine interactions in the nigrostriatal system. Eur J Pharmacol 55:363–373, 1979

Ward C, Stern G: Electroconvulsive therapy in parkinsonian patients with the "on-off" syndrome. Journal of Neural Transmission 49:133–135, 1980

Weiner RD, Rogers HJ, Davidson JR, et al: Effects of stimulus parameters on cognitive side effects, in Electroconvulsive Therapy: Clinical and Basic Research Issues. Edited by Malitz S, Sackeim HA. New York, New York Academy of Sciences, 1986, pp 315–325

White DK, Barrett RJ: The effects of electroconvulsive shock on the discriminative stimulus properties of d-amphetamine and apomorphine: evidence for dopamine receptor alteration subsequent to ECS. Psychopharmacology 73:211–214, 1981

Whitehouse PJ, Hedreen JC, White CL III, et al: Basal forebrain neurons in the dementia of Parkinson's disease. Ann Neurol 13:243–248, 1983

Wilson RS, Fox JH, Huckman MS, et al: Computed tomography in dementia. Neurology 32:1054–1057, 1982

Winokur A, Dugan J, Mendels J, et al: Psychiatric illness in relatives of patients with Parkinson's disease: an expanded survey. Am J Psychiatry 135:854–855, 1978

Wollenberg R: Paralysis agitans, in Specielle Pathologie und Therapie. Edited by Nothnagel H. Vienna, Austria, Alfred Holder, 1899

Yahr MD, Mendoza MR, Moros D, et al: Treatment of Parkinson's disease in early and late phases: use of pharmacological agents with special reference to deprenyl (Selegeline). Acta Neurol Scand 95 (suppl):95–102, 1983

Zervas IM, Fink M: ECT for refractory Parkinson's disease (letter). Convulsive Therapy 7:222–223, 1991

23

Neuropsychiatric Aspects of Stroke

Sergio E. Starkstein, M.D., Ph.D.
Robert G. Robinson, M.D.

Introduction

Cerebrovascular disease is one of the most common life-threatening problems among the elderly population in the United States, and it ranks as the third leading cause of death (behind only heart disease and cancer) in patients over 50 years old. The prevalence of stroke increases steadily with age, rising from 10/100,000 for those under age 35 to 5,970/100,000 for those over age 75 (Wolf et al. 1984). The National Survey of Stroke estimated there will be 500,000 new cases of stroke each year (Walker et al. 1981). During the past 10 years, however, there has been a steady decline in the incidence of stroke, which most investigators have attributed to the improved control of hypertension (Hachinski and Norris 1985; Wolf et al. 1984). Nevertheless, 75% of stroke survivors are left with physical or intellectual impairments of sufficient severity to limit their vocational capacity (Hachinski and Norris 1985).

The psychiatric complications of stroke lesions, although recognized for more than 100 years (Kraepelin 1921), have never received the attention that has been devoted to poststroke motor deficits, language problems, or intellectual disturbances. This relative neglect of emotional impairments following stroke is difficult to understand for several reasons. First, psychiatric complications of stroke, such as depression or apathy, have a high prevalence (Robinson et al. 1983; Starkstein et al. 1993a). Second, these behavioral disorders have been shown to significantly impair the physical recovery (Parikh et al. 1990) and to increase the long-term mortality (Morris et al. 1993) of stroke patients. Third, clinical-pathological correlations derived from the study of stroke lesions may constitute a valuable model for illuminating the mechanisms of psychiatric disorders in patients without known neuropathological disorders (i.e., functional disorders).

In this chapter, we briefly review the classification and nature of cerebrovascular disease and then discuss the most frequent emotional-behavioral sequela of stroke lesions. Some of these psychiatric complications of stroke, such as depression, have been the focus of intense research, whereas other complications, such as anxiety or emotional lability, have not been characterized as well.

Cerebrovascular Disease

Classification

One obvious way of classifying cerebrovascular disease is based on the cause of the anatomic-pathological process within the blood vessels that perfuse the central nervous system. Such a classification would include infectious, connective tissue, neoplastic, hematologic, pharmacological, and traumatic causes. Alternatively, the classification of cerebrovascular disease may be based on the mechanisms of these different pathological processes, such as the interactive effects of systemic hypertension and atherosclerosis on the resilience of large arteries, integrity of vessel lumens, and production of end-organ ischemia; developmental abnormalities leading to the formation of aneurysmal dilations or weakness of the arterial wall; or the effect of cardiac arrhythmias on the propagation of emboli.

The most pragmatic way of classifying cerebrovascular disease, however, is categorizing disorders based on the way in which parenchymal changes in the brain do or do not occur (Starkstein and Robinson 1992). The first of these, ischemia, may occur with or without parenchymal infarction. Ischemic disorders include transient ischemic attacks, which do not produce parenchymal changes, and infarctions, which do produce parenchymal lesions. The causes of infarctions include atherosclerotic thrombosis, cerebral embolism, lacunae, and others, such as arteritis and fibromuscular dysplasia. The other cause of parenchymal changes is hemorrhage. Hemorrhages may cause direct parenchymal damage by extravasation of blood into the surrounding brain tissue, as in intracerebral hematoma, or indirect parenchymal damage by hemorrhage into the ventricles, subarachnoid space, extradural space, or subdural regions.

There are five major categories of cerebrovascular disease that produce focal parenchymal lesions: atherosclerotic thrombosis, cerebral embolism, lacunae, intracranial hemorrhage, and vascular malformations, such as aneurysms and arteriovenous malformations. Ischemic infarcts constitute the most prevalent type of stroke and the ratio of infarcts to hemorrhages is about 5:1; atherosclerotic thrombosis and cerebral embolism

This work was supported by the following National Institute of Mental Health Grants RSA MH00163 (to RGR), MH40355, and a grant from the Instituto DiTella (to SES).

account for about one-third of all strokes (Caplan and Stein 1986).

Atherosclerotic Thrombosis

Atherosclerotic thrombosis is often a result of a dynamic interaction between hypertension and atherosclerotic deposition of hyaline-lipid material in the walls of peripheral, coronary, and cerebral arteries. Hypertension is the most important risk factor for thrombotic stroke and other factors such as hyperlipidemia, diabetes mellitus, smoking, and obesity are of less importance. Atheromatous plaques tend to propagate at the bifurcation of the internal carotid artery or the carotid sinus, the "top" of the basilar artery, the posterior cerebral arteries at the midbrain level, and the anterior cerebral arteries as they curve over the corpus callosum. These plaques may lead to stenosis of one or more of these cerebral arteries or to complete occlusion.

Transient ischemic attacks, defined as periods of transient focal ischemia associated with reversible neurological deficits within a few hours, are usually produced by a thrombotic process. Most commonly, transient ischemic attacks have a duration of 2–15 minutes, with a range from a few seconds to up to 12–24 hours. Whereas the neurological examination between episodes of transient ischemic attacks is entirely normal, permanent neurological deficits (i.e., more than 24 hours) indicate that infarction has occurred.

Cerebral Embolism

Cerebral embolism, which accounts for approximately one-third of all strokes, is usually caused by a fragment breaking way from a thrombus within the heart and traveling up the carotid artery. The source of the embolism may also be from an atheromatous plaque within the lumen of the carotid sinus or from the distal end of a thrombus within the internal carotid artery, or less frequently it may represent a fat, tumor, or air embolus within the internal carotid artery. The causes of thrombus formation within the heart include cardiac arrhythmias, congenital heart disease, infectious processes, valve prostheses, postsurgical complications, and myocardial infarction with mural thrombus. Of all strokes, those caused by cerebral embolism develop most rapidly. A large embolus may occlude the internal carotid artery or the stem of the middle cerebral artery producing a severe hemiplegia. More often,

however, the embolus is smaller and passes into one of the branches of the middle cerebral artery, producing infarction distal to the site of the arterial occlusion. This is characterized by a pattern of neurological deficits consistent with that specific vascular distribution, which may be transient if the embolus fragments and travels into more distal arteries.

Lacunae

Lacunae, accounting for nearly one-fifth of strokes, are the result of occlusion of small penetrating cerebral arteries. These are small infarcts that may produce no recognizable deficits, or, depending on their location, they may be associated with pure motor or sensory deficits. There is a strong association between lacunae and both atherosclerosis and hypertension, suggesting that lacunar infarction is the result of the effect of arteriosclerosis on small-diameter vessels.

Intracranial Hemorrhage

Intracranial hemorrhage is the fourth most frequent cause of stroke. The main causes of intracranial hemorrhage are hypertension, rupture of saccular aneurysms or arteriovenous malformations, hemorrhagic disorder, and trauma. Primary (hypertensive) intracranial hemorrhage occurs in deep parenchymal brain areas. The extravasation of blood forms a roughly circular or oval-shaped mass that disrupts and displaces the parenchyma. Adjacent tissue is compressed and seepage into the ventricular system may occur. Intracranial hemorrhages can range in size from massive bleeds of several centimeters in diameter to petechial hemorrhages of a millimeter or less. They most commonly occur within the putamen and the adjacent internal capsule, thalamus, cerebellum, lobar white matter, and brain stem. Severe headache is a common accompaniment of intracranial hemorrhage and occurs in about 50% of cases. The prognosis is grave, with 70%–75% of patients dying within 1–30 days (Adams and Victor 1985).

Aneurysms and Arteriovenous Malformations

Ruptured aneurysms and arteriovenous malformations are the most common type of cerebrovascular disease after thrombosis, embolism, lacunae, and intracranial hemorrhage. Aneurysms are usually located at arterial bifurcations and are presumed to result from developmental defects in the formation of the arterial wall; rupture occurs when the intima bulges outward and eventually breaks through the adventitia. Arteriovenous malformations consist of a tangle of dilated vessels that form an abnormal communication between arterial and venous systems. They are developmental abnormalities consisting of persistent embryonic blood vessels. Hemorrhage from aneurysms or arteriovenous malformations may occur within the subarachnoid space or the brain parenchyma.

Neuropsychiatric Syndromes

Poststroke Depression

Frequency.   Depression is one of the most common psychiatric sequela to occur after a cerebrovascular lesion. Cross-sectional studies have demonstrated that 20%–50% of consecutive samples of stroke patients have depression, regardless of whether these patients are in specialized stroke units, general clinical units, rehabilitation hospitals, or the community (Eastwood et al. 1989; Robinson et al. 1983; Wade et al. 1987). In our studies of patients admitted to the hospital with an acute stroke, 25% met DSM-III (American Psychiatric Association 1980) criteria for major depression, whereas another 20% met criteria for dysthymic (minor) depression (Robinson et al. 1983). This high prevalence of poststroke depression was observed in both acute and chronic stroke patients (Morris et al. 1990; Robinson et al. 1987).

Phenomenology of poststroke depression.   We have identified two types of poststroke depressive disorders: the diagnosis of major depression is based on DSM-III criteria for major depression (excluding the time constraint), and the diagnosis of minor (dysthymic) depression is based on patients meeting DSM-III criteria for dysthymic disorder (also excluding the time constraint) (Table 23–1). Lipsey et al. (1986) compared the frequency and type of depressive symptoms in a group of 43 patients with major poststroke depression and a group of 43 age-matched patients with "functional" major depression. Both groups showed the same frequency and types of depressive symptoms (Figure 23–1). The only exception was that the major poststroke depression group had a greater frequency of "slowness" than did the other group. This study, however, demonstrated that major poststroke depression is

not an atypical form of depression and that these patients present with symptoms identical to elderly patients with major depression. Several studies have validated the distinction between major and minor poststroke depression and have demonstrated these two types of depression to have different courses of longitudinal evolution (Morris et al. 1990; Robinson et al. 1987), biological markers (Barry and Dinan 1990; Lipsey et al. 1985), effects on cognitive function (Robinson et al. 1986), and correlation with brain location (Robinson et al. 1984; Starkstein et al. 1988b).

Clinical correlates.   Poststroke depression has a significant influence on both the recovery in activities of daily living (ADLs) and the intellectual impairment of stroke patients. In a recent study, we (Parikh et al. 1990) compared the 2-year recovery from impairments in ADLs between 25 patients with poststroke depres-

---

Table 23–1.   Criteria for major depression and dysthymia

Major depression
  A. Dysphoric mood
  B. At least four of the following symptoms:
     1. Poor appetite or significant weight loss.
     2. Insomnia
     3. Loss of interest or pleasure in usual activities, or decrease in sexual drive
     4. Feelings of worthlessness, self-reproach, or excessive or inappropriate guilt
     5. Complaints or evidence of diminished ability to think or concentrate, such as slowed thinking, or indecisiveness
     6. Recurrent thoughts of death, suicidal tendencies, wishes to be dead, or suicide attempt

Dysthymia
  A. Dysphoric mood
  B. Presence of at least three of the following symptoms:
     1. Insomnia
     2. Feelings of inadequacy, loss of self-esteem, or self-depreciation
     3. Decreased effectiveness or productivity
     4. Decreased attention, concentration, or ability to think clearly
     5. Social withdrawal
     6. Loss of interest in or enjoyment of pleasurable activities
     7. Inability to respond with apparent pleasure to praise or rewards
     8. Pessimistic attitude toward the future, brooding about past events, or feeling sorry for self
     9. Tearfulness or crying
     10. Recurrent thoughts of death or suicide

Source. Adapted from American Psychiatric Association 1980.

sion (either major or minor depression) and 38 stroke patients with no mood disorders who were matched for their in-hospital severity of ADL impairments. After controlling for all the variables that have been shown to influence stroke outcome (e.g., acute treatment on a stroke unit, size, nature and location of brain injury, age, education, and duration of rehabilitation services), we found that patients with in-hospital poststroke depression had a significantly poorer recovery than did nondepressed stroke patients even after their depressions had subsided (Figure 23–2).

In another study, we (Robinson et al. 1986) compared patients with major poststroke depression and nondepressed stroke patients for the presence of cognitive impairments. We found that patients with major poststroke depression after left-hemisphere lesions had significantly more cognitive deficits than did non-

depressed patients with a similar size and location of brain lesion. These deficits were observed in a wide range of cognitive tasks including orientation, language, visuoconstructional ability, executive motor functions, and frontal lobe tasks (Figure 23–3) (Bolla-Wilson et al. 1989). In contrast, among patients with right-hemisphere lesions, patients with major depression did not differ from nondepressed patients on any of the measures of cognitive impairment. This finding suggests that left-hemisphere lesions that lead to major depression may produce a different kind of depression than do right-hemisphere lesions. Left-hemisphere lesions can produce a dementia of depression, which does not occur with major depressions following right-hemisphere lesions. It remains to be determined whether these dementias of depression will improve with treatment of depression.

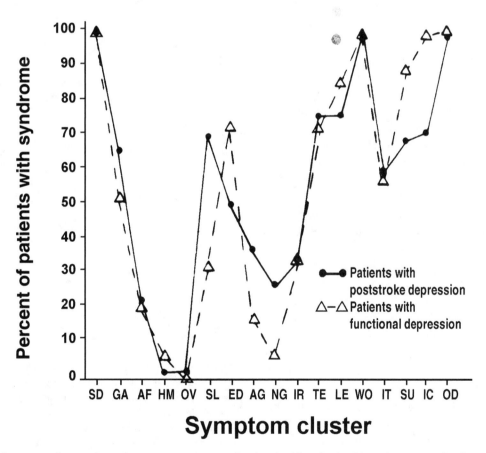

Figure 23–1. Symptom clusters from the present state examination in 43 patients with major poststroke depression and 43 patients with functional depression. SD = simple depression; GA = general anxiety; AF = affective flattening; HM = hypomania; OV = overactivity; SL = slowness; ED = special features of depression; AG = agitation; NG = self-neglect; IR = ideas of reference; TE = tension; LE = lack of energy; WO = worrying; IT = irritability; SU = social unease; IC = loss of interest and concentration; and OD = other symptoms of depression.

Source. Reprinted from Lipsey JR, Spencer WC, Rabins PV, et al: "Phenomenological Comparison of Functional and Post-stroke Depression." *American Journal of Psychiatry* 143:527–529, 1986. Used with permission.

Clinical-pathological correlates and mechanism. In several prospective studies using different samples of stroke patients, we have consistently found a significant association between poststroke depression and lesion location: patients with major poststroke depression showed a significantly higher frequency of lesions in anterior areas of the left hemisphere, namely the left frontal dorsolateral cortex and the head of the caudate (Robinson et al. 1984; Starkstein et al. 1987). Among patients with right-hemisphere stroke lesions, those with frontal or parietal damage showed the highest frequency of depression (Starkstein et al. 1989). Although some, but not all, of these findings have been replicated by other investigators (Eastwood et al. 1989; House et al. 1991; Morris et al. 1992), a consensus has emerged that there is a significant correlation between proximity of the lesion to the frontal pole and severity of depression.

In 1981, we first reported that in a group of 29 patients with left-hemisphere lesions produced by trauma or stroke there was an inverse correlation between severity of depression and distance of the anterior border of the lesion from the frontal pole ($r = -.76$, $P < .001$) (Figure 23–4) (Robinson and Szetela 1981). Since then, using computed tomography (CT) imaging, we found the same phenomenon in another group of 10 right-handed patients with single stroke lesions of the anterior left hemisphere ($r = -.92$, $P < .001$) (Robinson et al. 1984). When patients with left-posterior-hemisphere lesions were added ($n = 18$), the correlation decreased ($r = -.54$, $P < .05$) (Table 23–2). This inverse correlation was also found in other groups of patients with purely cortical lesions of the left hemisphere ($n = 16$; $r = -.52$, $P < .05$) (Starkstein et al. 1987), purely left-sided subcortical lesions ($n = 13$) ($r = -.68$, $P < .01$) (Starkstein et al. 1987), and single left-hemisphere lesions in left-handed patients ($n = 13$; $r = -.78$, $P < .01$) (Robinson et al. 1985). This phenomenon has now been replicated by four different groups of investigators using patients from Canada, England, and Australia (Table 23–2).

Some investigators have found a correlation between severity of depression and proximity of the lesion to the frontal pole in combined right- and left-hemisphere lesion groups, whereas others found it only with left-sided lesions (Table 23–2). Although there is some difference in the strength of this correlation (and, therefore, the amount of variance in severity of depression explained by lesion location), this phenomenon has emerged as one of the most consistent

and robust clinical-pathological correlations ever described in neuropsychiatry. Future experiments aimed at elucidating the mechanism of poststroke depression must provide an explanation for this remarkably consistent phenomenon.

The mechanism by which left anterior lesions produce depression is not known. One possibility is that both the frontal dorsolateral cortex and the dorsal cau-

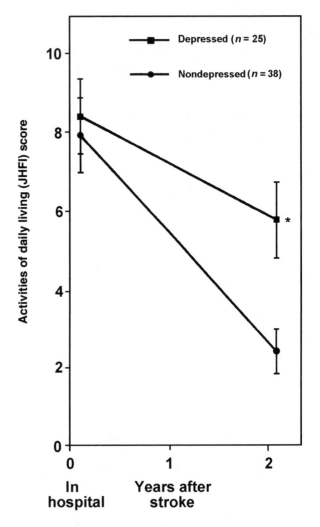

Figure 23–2. Johns Hopkins Functioning Inventory (JHFI) scores in the hospital and at 2-year follow-up in patients who were depressed or nondepressed. Higher scores on the JHFI indicate greater impairment in activities of daily living. There was a significant group-by-time interaction, with the nondepressed patients having significantly lower (i.e., less impaired) scores than the depressed patients at 2-year follow-up. * = $P < .05$.
Source. Reprinted from Parikh RM, Robinson RG, Lipsey JR, et al: "The Impact of Post-Stroke Depression on Recovery in Activities of Daily Living Over Two-Year Follow-Up." *Archives of Neurology* 47:785–789, 1990. Used with permission.

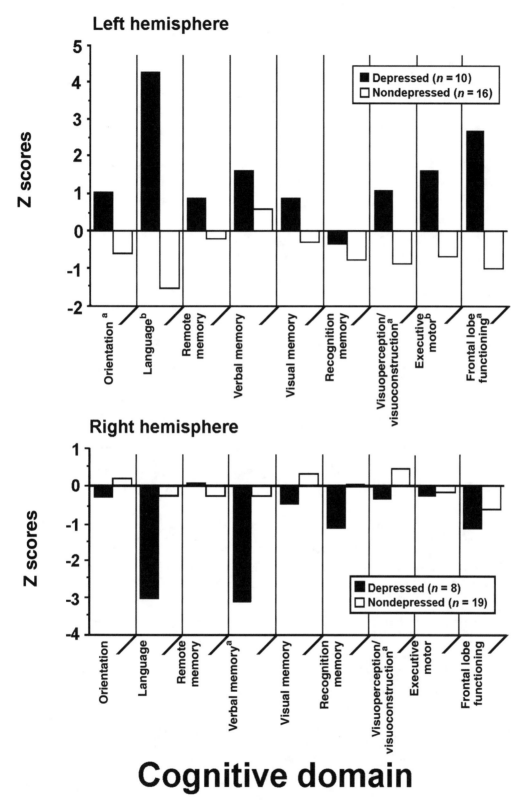

Figure 23–3. Performance on the nine cognitive domains by depressed and nondepressed patients with left- or right-hemisphere stroke.

[a]P < .05 comparing depressed and nondepressed groups using one-way analysis of variance (ANOVA).

[b]P < .01 comparing depressed and nondepressed groups using one-way ANOVA.

Source. Reprinted from Bolla-Wilson K, Robinson RG, Starkstein SE, et al: "Lateralization of Dementia of Depression in Stroke Patients." *American Journal of Psychiatry* 146:627–634, 1989. Used with permission.

date play an important role in mediating locomotor, intellectual, and instinctive behavior through their connection with the supplementary motor area, temporoparietal association cortex, and limbic system. A lesion of these anterior brain areas may result in low activation of locomotor, sensory, or limbic areas and produce the autonomic and affective symptoms of depression. We (Robinson et al. 1984) have suggested that biogenic amines may also play an important role in poststroke depression. The anatomy of these path-

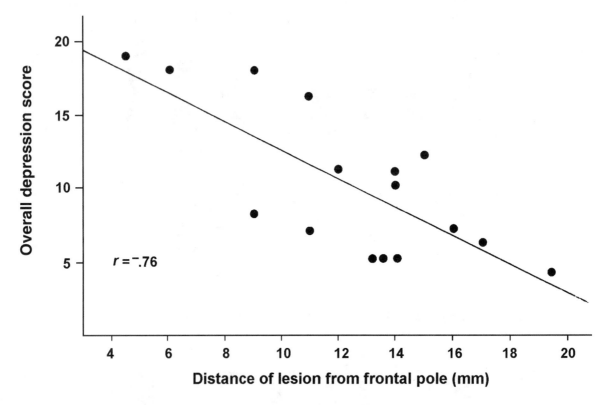

Figure 23–4. Relationship between severity of depression as measured by overall depression score and mean distance of the lesion from the frontal pole for patients with lesions that extended into the frontal lobe. The closer the lesion was to the frontal pole, the greater the depression was ($r = -.76$, $P < .001$).
Source. Reprinted from Robinson RG, Szetela B: "Mood Change Following Left Hemispheric Brain Injury." *Annals of Neurology* 9:447–453, 1981. Used with permission.

Table 23–2. Depression severity and proximity of lesion to frontal pole

Study	N patients	Patient population	Lesion hemisphere	Correlation	P<
Robinson and Szetela 1981	29	Stroke or trauma	Left	− .76	.001
Robinson et al. 1984	10	Single stroke, right handed	Left anterior	− .92	.001
	18		Left anterior and posterior	− .54	.05
Lipsey et al. 1983	15	Bilateral stroke lesions	Left only	− .65	.01
Robinson et al. 1985	13	Left handed, single stroke	Left	− .78	.01
Starkstein et al. 1987	16	Cortical lesions only	Left	− .52	.05
	13	Subcortical lesion only	Left	− .68	.01
Sinyor et al. 1986	27	Single stroke	Left and right	− .47	.05
Eastwood et al. 1989	11	Single stroke	Left	− .74	.01
House et al. 1991	63	Single stroke	Left and right	− .28	.01
	33	6 months	Left	− .38	.05
Morris et al. 1992	14	Single stroke remove prior depression	Left	− .87	.001

ways (i.e., they begin in brain stem nuclei and ascend through subcortical regions, around the corpus callosum to posterior cortex) may explain the correlations with lesion location, as anterior lesions close to the frontal pole would interrupt more "downstream" pathways than posterior lesions (Robinson et al. 1984).

Treatment. In a randomized, double-blind, and placebo-controlled study of the efficacy of treatment of poststroke depression, we demonstrated the utility of the tricyclic antidepressant nortriptyline in the treatment of poststroke depression (Lipsey et al. 1984). Patients received 25 mg for 1 week, 50 mg for 2 weeks, 75 mg for 1 week, and 100 mg for 2 weeks. The group on active drug (11 completed the study) showed a significant decrease in depression scores compared with the placebo group (15 completed) (Figure 23–5). Side effects were observed in 6 of 17 patients: 3 developed delirium, 1 had syncope, 1 complained of oversedation, and 1 complained of dizziness.

One other controlled study demonstrated the usefulness of another antidepressant drug (trazodone) for poststroke depression (Reding et al. 1986). Depressed patients taking trazodone were found to have greater improvements in ADL scores than were patients treated with placebo. This trend became statistically significant when the treatment groups were restricted

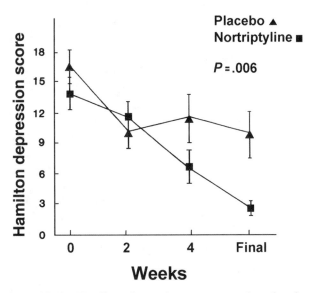

Figure 23–5. Hamilton depression scores over 6 weeks of treatment for poststroke depression.
Source. Reprinted from Lipsey JR, Robinson RG, Pearlson GD, et al: "Nortriptyline Treatment of Post-Stroke Depression: A Double-Blind Treatment Trial." *Lancet* 1:297–300, 1984. Used with permission.

to patients with abnormal dexamethasone tests. Although antidepressants are effective in the treatment of poststroke depression, the high rate of complications such as delirium dictate that tricyclic drugs should be used cautiously in elderly stroke patients.

Poststroke Anxiety

Although anxiety is one of the most frequent complaints in the general population, it has rarely been the focus of empirical research among stroke patients.

Phenomenology and frequency. In a recent study on the prevalence of anxiety disorders in stroke patients, we examined 309 patients admitted to the hospital with acute stroke using DSM-III criteria for generalized anxiety disorders (Castillo et al. 1993). We found that 78 patients (26.9%) met criteria for generalized anxiety disorder. However, the presence of the disorder was strongly associated with the presence of depression, as 58 out of 78 stroke patients meeting criteria for generalized anxiety disorder were also depressed. Thus although generalized anxiety disorder is a common finding among stroke patients, it frequently coexists with depression.

Clinical correlates and mechanism. We examined the clinical and lesion correlates of anxiety and depression in the study of 309 acute stroke patients (Castillo et al. 1993). The anxious and nonanxious groups were not significantly different in their demographic backgrounds or neurological findings. The nondepressed anxious patients, however, had a significantly higher frequency of alcoholism compared with the nonanxious patients (26% generalized anxiety disorder versus 8% nonanxious, $P < .05$). When patients with both generalized anxiety disorder and depression were compared to patients with depression only, patients with anxious-depression had a significantly higher frequency of cortical lesions (mainly left frontal), whereas the patients with depression only had a significantly higher frequency of subcortical lesions (mainly left basal ganglia) (Starkstein et al. 1990a). Among the anxious patients without depression, 67% had right-hemisphere lesions compared to 43% of the anxious depressed patients ($P = .04$) (Castillo et al. 1993). Finally, among patients with right-hemisphere lesions, the anxious patients had lesions that were significantly more posterior than those of the nonanxious patients ($P = .038$) (Castillo et al. 1993).

Although the mechanism of anxiety is still unknown, several studies have reported a significant decrease in cortical metabolic activity with increased anxiety, as well as a lack of correlation between the severity of anxiety and subcortical metabolic rate (Bartlett et al. 1988; Gur et al. 1987). This is in agreement with our finding of significantly more severe anxiety after cortical as compared with subcortical lesions and suggests a critical role for cortical-subcortical interaction in the modulation of anxious states.

Poststroke Apathy

Apathy is the absence or lack of feeling, emotion, interest, or concern and has been reported frequently among stroke patients. We recently examined a consecutive series of 80 patients with single stroke lesions and no significant impairment in comprehension using the Apathy Scale (Table 23–3). We demonstrated both validity and reliability of this scale in the assessment of apathy in patients with cerebrovascular lesions (Starkstein et al. 1993a). A score of 14 on this scale separated apathetic from nonapathetic patients with high sensitivity and specificity.

Prevalence and clinical correlates. In this study of poststroke apathy (Starkstein et al. 1993a), we found that 9 of 80 patients (11%) showed apathy as their only

psychiatric disorder, whereas another 11% had both apathy and depression. The only demographic correlate of apathy was age, as apathetic patients (with or without depression) were significantly older than were nonapathetic patients. Also, apathetic patients showed significantly more severe deficits in ADLs, and there was a significant interaction between depression and apathy (i.e., Johns Hopkins Functioning Inventory [JHFI] scores were 4.8 ± 4.0 for patients with no disorder, 6.21 ± 3.9 for depressed patients, 7.6 ± 5.8 apathetic patients, and 13.7 ± 5.5 for depressed and apathetic patients; effect of apathy $P < .001$, effect of depression $P < .002$, and interaction $P = .05$).

Clinical-pathological correlates and mechanism of poststroke apathy.
Patients with apathy (without depression) showed a significantly higher frequency of lesions involving the posterior limb of the internal capsule as compared with patients with no apathy (Starkstein et al. 1993a). Lesions in the internal globus pallidus and the posterior limb of the internal capsule have been reported to produce important behavioral changes, such as motor neglect, psychic akinesia, and akinetic mutism (Helgason et al. 1988). The ansa lenticularis is one of the main internal pallidal outputs, and it ends in the pedunculopontine nucleus after going through the posterior limb of the internal capsule (Nauta 1989). In rodents, this pathway has a prom-

Table 23–3. Apathy Scale

Questions	Not at all	Slightly	Some	A lot
1. Are you interested in learning new things?				
2. Does anything interest you?				
3. Are you concerned about your condition?				
4. Do you put much effort into things?				
5. Are you always looking for something to do?				
6. Do you have plans and goals for the future?				
7. Do you have motivation?				
8. Do you have the energy for daily activities?				
9. Does someone have to tell you what to do each day?				
10. Are you indifferent to things?				
11. Are you unconcerned with many things?				
12. Do you need a push to get started on things?				
13. Are you neither happy nor sad, just in between?				
14. Would you consider yourself apathetic?				

Note. For questions 1–8, the scoring system is the following: *Not at all* = 3 points; *Slightly* = 2 points; *Some* = 1 point; *A lot* = 0 points.
For questions 9–14, the scoring system is the following: *Not at all* = 0 points; *Slightly* = 1 point; *Some* = 2 points; *A lot* = 3 points.

inent role in goal-oriented behavior (Bechara and van der Kooy 1989), and dysfunction of this system may explain the presence of apathy in stroke patients.

Poststroke Psychosis

The phenomenon of hallucinations and delusions in stroke patients has been called *agitated delirium, acute atypical psychosis, peduncular hallucinosis, release hallucinations,* or *acute organic psychosis.* We consider *secondary hallucinations* to be sensory perceptions in the absence of appropriate stimuli, with the important qualification that first the patient believes the (nonexistent) sensory perception is real and second this disorder started after a lesion. We use the term *secondary hallucinosis* to refer to a perception without a stimulus, where the patient does not believe the (nonexistent) sensory perception is real and the disorder occurs after a stroke lesion. Finally, we use the term *secondary psychosis* to refer to patients who develop either secondary hallucinations or secondary hallucinosis after stroke lesion. Patients with secondary psychosis, hallucination type, are delusional (i.e., they do not recognize the perception as false), whereas those with secondary psychosis, hallucinosis type, are usually not delusional, unless there is some other independent delusional idea.

Prevalence and clinical-pathological correlates. In a recent study of secondary psychosis after stroke lesions, we (Rabins et al. 1991) found a very low prevalence of this phenomenon among stroke patients (only 5 in more than 300 consecutive admissions). All 5 patients had right-hemisphere lesions, primarily involving frontoparietal regions. When compared with 5 age-matched patients with cerebrovascular lesions in similar locations but no psychosis, patients with secondary psychosis had significantly greater subcortical atrophy, as manifested by significantly larger areas of both the frontal horn of the lateral ventricle and the body of the lateral ventricle (measured on the side contralateral to the brain lesion). Several other investigators have reported a high frequency of seizures among patients with secondary psychosis (e.g., Levine and Finklestein 1982). These seizures usually started after the brain lesion but before the onset of psychosis. We also found seizures in 3 of our 5 patients with poststroke psychosis, as compared to none of the 5 poststroke nonpsychiatric control subjects.

Mechanism. We conclude from these observations that three factors may be important in the mechanism of secondary psychosis, hallucination type, namely a right-hemisphere lesion involving the temporoparietal cortex, seizures, and/or subcortical brain atrophy. The mechanism of secondary hallucinosis is even less clear than secondary hallucinations. Although most patients with secondary hallucinosis in the literature had peduncular lesions, patients with lesions in other brain areas, such as the diencephalon, also showed the phenomenon (Cascino and Adams 1986; Geller and Bellur 1987). These lesions have frequently been found to involve primary sensory pathways, mainly visual and auditory. Thus secondary hallucinosis may be a "release phenomenon" secondary to damage to reticular activating brain stem pathways, and the presence of primary sensory deficits in these patients may be a necessary predisposing factor.

In conclusion, secondary psychosis is a rare finding in stroke patients. We believe that there are at least two types of secondary psychosis. The first is the hallucination type, which is characterized by hallucinations perceived by the patient as real and may result from right temporoparietal lesions in the presence of preexisting subcortical brain atrophy and poststroke seizures. The second is the hallucinosis type, which is characterized by hallucinations perceived by the patient as unreal and may be secondary to lesions in primary sensory or reticular activating pathways.

Anosognosia

Anosognosia is a term coined by Babinski (1914) to describe the lack of unawareness of hemiplegia, but was later used to refer to the unawareness of other poststroke deficits, such as cortical blindness, hemianopia, and amnesia (Heilman 1991).

Prevalence and clinical correlates. In a recent study, we examined the prevalence of anosognosia in a consecutive series of 80 patients with single acute stroke lesions (Starkstein et al. 1992). We developed an Anosognosia Questionnaire (Table 23–4), which we used to definite the existence of anosognosia. To rate the severity of this phenomenon, we also developed the Denial of Illness Scale (DIS) (Table 23–5), which allows the classification of patients into those with mild, moderate, or severe anosognosia. Patients with aphasia were included only if they had intact verbal comprehension as measured by their ability to complete part one of the Token Test (De Renzi and Vignolo 1962). The assessment of anosognosia, however, only examined motor, sensory, and visual field disturbances and did not evaluate anosognosia for aphasia.

The first important finding from this study was that about one-third of this consecutive series of patients had anosognosia (19% mild, 11% moderate, and 13% severe anosognosia) (Starkstein et al. 1992). We also examined potential correlates of anosognosia and found this phenomenon to be significantly associated with the presence of a neglect syndrome (i.e., failure to respond to or orient to stimuli contralateral to the lesion), as well as deficits in recognizing facial emotions and the emotional content of speech (prosody). There also was a significant association between anosognosia and right-hemisphere lesions involving the temporal and parietal lobes, thalamus, and basal ganglia.

Two important negative findings should also be noted. First, the frequency of depression was similar among patients with and without anosognosia. Thus the existence of anosognosia does not preclude stroke patients from experiencing or reporting depressive

---

Table 23–4.   Anosognosia Questionnaire

1. Why are you here?
2. What is the matter with you?
3. Is there anything wrong with your arm or leg?
4. Is there anything wrong with your eyesight?
5. Is your arm or leg weak, paralyzed, or numb?
6. How does your arm or leg feel?

If denial is elicited ask the following:

   a. (*pick up the patient's arm*) What is this?
   b. Can you lift it?
   c. Do you have some problem with this?
   d. (*ask the patient to lift both arms*) Can you see that your two arms are not at the same level?
   e. (*ask the patient to identify finger movements in and out of the abnormal visual field*) Can't you see that you have a problem with your eyesight?

Scoring

0 = The disorder is spontaneously reported or mentioned following a general question about the patient's complaints.

1 = The disorder is reported only after a specific question about the strength of the patient's limb, or visual problems.

2 = The disorder is acknowledged only after its demonstration through routine techniques of neurological examination.

3 = The disorder is not acknowledged.

Table 23–5.   Denial of Illness Scale

Questions	Scoring		
1. Patient minimizes present symptoms (at interview).	0 (no)	1 (once or twice)	2 (more than twice)
2. Patient alludes to there being nothing really wrong with her or him and that she or he is ready to go home.	0 (no)	1 (once or twice)	2 (more than twice)
3. Patient (past or present) displaces source of symptoms to organs other than brain or complains of symptoms unrelated to the central nervous system.	0 (no)	1 (once or twice)	2 (more than twice)
4. Did the patient at any time admit to fear of death?	0 (yes)	1 (no)	
5. Did the patient at any time admit to fear of invalidism?	0 (yes)	1 (no)	
6. Patient verbally denies being in the hospital.	0 (not at all)	1 (sometimes)	2 (every time)
7. Patient displays, at least on the surface, a carefree, cheerful, jovial approach to life.	0 (no)	1 (once or twice)	2 (more than twice)
8. Patient's behavior during interview is characterized by nonchalance, coolness, imperturbability.	0 (no)	1 (once or twice)	2 (more than twice)
9. Patient displaces fear for his or her own illness to family, older patients, weaker patients, and so on.	0 (no)	1 (at least 1 time during the interview)	
10. Patient projects illness or weakness to family, spouse, and so on.	0 (no)	1 (at least 1 time during the interview)	

feelings. Second, anosognosic patients did not show more severe sensory deficits than did nonanosognosic patients (i.e., anosognosia is not related to the presence of sensory deficits) (Starkstein et al. 1992).

Mechanism.   In our study (Starkstein et al. 1992), we also found that brain atrophy, probably preexisting the brain lesion, may have been an important predisposing factor for anosognosia, as anosognosic patients had significantly more frontal subcortical and diencephalic atrophy (but no cortical atrophy) than did patients with no anosognosia. Moreover, patients with anosognosia had significantly more deficits in frontal-lobe–related cognitive tasks than did patients with no anosognosia, but lesions in similar brain areas.

These findings suggest that lesions in specific cortical and subcortical areas of the right hemisphere, although necessary, may not be sufficient to produce anosognosia; concomitant frontal lobe dysfunction (as expressed by frontal subcortical atrophy and deficits in frontal-lobe–related cognitive tasks) may be necessary to produce the syndrome.

Heilman (1991) proposed that anosognosia may result from a dysfunction of a system that monitors the intention to move, as well as the actual performance of movements. This mismatch between the intention to move and the (lack of) movement may convey the impression that the movement was actually performed and that the limb is normal. The systems monitoring single sensory and motor modalities may be located in the right parietal lobe, whereas the frontal lobe may constitute a supramodal monitoring structure.

In conclusion, anosognosia is present in one-third of acute stroke patients and is significantly associated with right-hemisphere lesions in the temporoparietal cortex, basal ganglia, or thalamus. The presence of neglect and frontal lobe dysfunction may constitute important predisposing factors.

Catastrophic Reaction

Catastrophic reaction is a term coined by Goldstein (1939) to describe the "inability of the organism to cope when faced with physical or cognitive deficits," and is expressed by anxiety, tears, aggressive behavior, swearing, displacement, refusal, renouncement, and, sometimes, compensatory boasting.

Prevalence and clinical correlates.   The catastrophic reaction has been reported to be a frequent finding among aphasic patients (Gainotti 1972) and has been given the status of a separate neuropsychiatric syndrome. There are no empirical studies regarding the construct validity of the catastrophic reaction, however, and it is possible that the catastrophic reaction may represent a symptom of a major depressive syndrome or anxiety disorder in stroke patients. To empirically examine this issue, we assessed a consecutive series of 62 patients with a Catastrophic Reaction Scale (CRS), which we developed to assess the existence and severity of the catastrophic reaction (Table 23–6). We have demonstrated the CRS to be a reliable instrument in the measurement of catastrophic reaction symptoms (Starkstein et al. 1993b).

We identified the catastrophic reaction in 12 of 62 consecutive patients (19%) with acute stroke lesions (Starkstein et al. 1993b). Three major findings

---

Table 23–6.   Catastrophic Reaction Scale

1. Patient appeared to be anxious (i.e., patient showed an apprehensive attitude or expressed fears).

2. Patient complained of feeling anxious or afraid (i.e., patient referred to feeling tense or having psychological concomitants of anxiety).

3. Patient became tearful (i.e., patient cried at some point during the evaluation).

4. Patient complained of feeling sad or depressed (i.e., patient spontaneously reported sad feelings during the evaluation).

5. Patient behaved in angry manner (i.e., patient shouted, contradicted the examiner, or performed tasks in a careless way).

6. Patient complained of feeling angry (i.e., patient reported being upset with the evaluation and/or the examiner).

7. Patient swore (i.e., patient swore at some point during the evaluation).

8. Patient expressed displaced anger (i.e., patient complained about the hospital, doctors, and fellow patients).

9. Patient refused to do something (i.e., patient stopped doing a task or refused to answer some questions).

10. Patient described a feeling of suddenly becoming depressed or hopeless (i.e., patient reported feeling worthless and sad and had a lack of confidence).

11. Patient boasted about self (i.e., patient reported being able to perform the tasks flawlessly; he or she explained failures as due to lack of concentration and tiredness).

Note.   Scoring key: 0 = None; 1 = Slight (once during the interview); 2 = Moderate (several times during the interview); 3 = Extreme (most of the interview).

emerged from this study. First, patients with catastrophic reaction were found to have a significantly higher frequency of familial and personal history of psychiatric disorders (mostly depression) than were patients without the catastrophic reaction. Second, catastrophic reaction was not significantly more frequent among aphasic (33%) compared with nonaphasic patients (66%), which does not support the suggestion that catastrophic reaction is more frequent among "frustrated" aphasic patients (Gainotti 1972). Third, 9 (75%) of the 12 patients with catastrophic reaction also had major depression, 2 (17%) had minor depression, and only 1 (8%) was not depressed. On the other hand, among patients without catastrophic reaction (i.e., 50 patients), 7 (14%) had major depression, 6 (12%) had minor depression, and 37 (74%) were not depressed. Thus catastrophic reaction was significantly associated with major depression ($\chi^2 = 20.9$, df = 2, $P = .0001$). Moreover, patients with a catastrophic reaction had significantly higher scores on the Hamilton Anxiety and Depression Scales compared with patients with no catastrophic reaction.

Mechanism.   Patients with a catastrophic reaction had a significantly higher frequency of lesions involving the basal ganglia (Starkstein et al. 1993b). When 10 depressed patients with a catastrophic reaction were compared to 10 depressed patients without a catastrophic reaction, the catastrophic reaction group showed significantly more anterior lesions, which were mostly located in subcortical regions (8 of 9 depressed patients with catastrophic reaction had subcortical lesions; 3 of 9 depressed patients without catastrophic reaction had subcortical lesions) ($\chi^2 = 5.84$, df = 1, $P = .01$).

We may conclude from the above evidence that the catastrophic reaction is not just a behavioral response of patients confronted with their limitations, as patients with and without a catastrophic reaction showed a similar frequency of aphasia and physical impairments. On the contrary, the catastrophic reaction seems to characterize a specific type of poststroke major depression (i.e., major depressions associated with anterior subcortical lesions). Anterior brain lesions (both cortical and subcortical) have been consistently associated with poststroke depression. Subcortical damage, however, has usually been hypothesized to underlie the "release" of emotional display by removing inhibitory input to the limbic areas of the cortex (Ross and Stewart 1987).

In conclusion, the catastrophic reaction occurs in about 20% of stroke patients (Starkstein et al. 1993b), mainly among those with a positive familial or personal history of psychiatric disorders. The catastrophic reaction is significantly associated with major depression and may be mediated by a release of emotional display produced by anterior subcortical lesions. Thus the catastrophic reaction may not represent an independent clinical syndrome, but may be a behavioral and emotional expression of depressed patients with anterior subcortical damage.

Emotional Lability

Emotional lability is a common complication of stroke lesions. It is characterized by sudden, easily provoked episodes of crying, which, although occurring frequently, generally occur in appropriate situations and are accompanied by a congruent mood change. Pathological laughing and crying is a more severe form of emotional lability and is characterized by episodes of laughing and/or crying that are not appropriate to the context. They may appear spontaneously or may be elicited by nonemotional events and do not correspond to underlying emotional feelings. Other terms for these disorders have been *emotional incontinence* or *pseudobulbar affect*.

Prevalence and clinical correlates.   We examined the clinical correlates and treatment of emotional lability (including pathological laughter and crying) in 28 patients with either acute or chronic stroke (Robinson et al. 1993). We developed a Pathological Laughter and Crying Scale (PLACS) (Appendix 1) to assess the existence and severity of emotional lability. We demonstrated in 18 treatment patients and 54 acute stroke patients the reliability and validity of this instrument in the assessment of emotional lability (Robinson et al. 1993). We also found that PLACS scores did not correlate with either Hamilton Depression Scale scores, MMSE scores, ADL scores, or Social Ties scores, indicating that the PLACS was assessing a factor other than the ones being measured by these instruments.

A double-blind drug trial of nortriptyline was conducted in 31 patients with emotional lability (Robinson et al. 1993). After randomization, patients were given active drug or placebo in a single bedtime dose. Patients were started on 25 mg of nortriptyline for 1 week, 50 mg for 2 weeks, 70 mg for 1 week, and 100 mg for the last 2 weeks of the study. One patient dropped out during the study, and 2 patients withdrew before initiation of the study; there were 28 who completed the 6-week protocol. Patients on nortriptyline showed significant improvements in PLACS scores compared with the placebo-treated patients; these differences became statistically significant at weeks 4 and 6 (Figure 23–6). Although a significant improvement in depression scores was also observed, improvements in PLACS scores were significant for both depressed and nondepressed patients with pathological laughing and crying, indicating that treatment response was not simply related to an improvement in depression.

Mechanism. Pseudobulbar affect has classically been explained as secondary to the bilateral interruption of neocortical upper motor neuron innervation of bulbar motor nuclei (Poeck 1969). The finding that emotional lability can be successfully treated with tricyclic drugs suggests that biogenic amine systems may also play a role in the pathogenesis of this disorder.

In conclusion, our study (Robinson et al. 1993) suggests that poststroke depression and emotional lability are independent phenomena, although they may coexist. Moreover, we also found that both depressed

and nondepressed patients with emotional lability showed significant improvements in the severity of their emotional lability after nortriptyline treatment.

Mania

Prevalence and clinical correlates.   Mania, or disinhibited behavior, is a relatively rare consequence of acute stroke lesions. Using DSM-III criteria for affective disorder, manic type, we found only 3 cases of secondary mania among a consecutive series of 309 acute stroke patients in an unpublished study. On the other hand, secondary mania is more frequent among patients with traumatic brain injury. In a recent study of 66 patients with acute traumatic brain injury (Jorge et al. 1993), we found 6 cases (9%) of secondary mania. Patients with traumatic brain injury frequently sustain damage to orbitofrontal and basotemporal cortical areas, which may be related to the mechanism of mania. These brain areas are rarely damaged in stroke patients, and this difference in the frequency of frontal and temporal cortical injury between traumatic and ischemic brain injury may explain the different prevalence of mania in these two populations. Cummings and Mendez (1984) found right thalamic stroke lesions in two cases of secondary mania.

In a series of 17 patients with post–brain-injury mania, we (Robinson et al. 1988) reported a high frequency of lesions involving the basal and polar areas of the right temporal lobe and subcortical areas of the right hemisphere, such as the head of the caudate and right thalamus. In a study using positron-emission tomography (PET) with [18F]fluorodeoxyglucose, we (Starkstein et al. 1990b) examined metabolic abnormalities in 3 patients with mania following right basal ganglia strokes. The patients had focal hypometabolic deficits in the right basotemporal cortex. This finding suggested that lesions leading to secondary mania may do so through their distant effects on the right basotemporal cortex. This phenomenon of lesions producing distant effects is a well-recognized consequence of some brain lesions and has been termed *diaschesis*.

Because not every patient with a right orbitofrontal or basotemporal lesion develops a manic syndrome, we have also looked for potential predisposing factors for secondary mania (Robinson et al. 1988; Starkstein et al. 1987). In these studies, we found that patients with secondary mania had a significantly higher frequency of familial history of psychiatric disorders, as well as significantly more subcortical brain atrophy (as

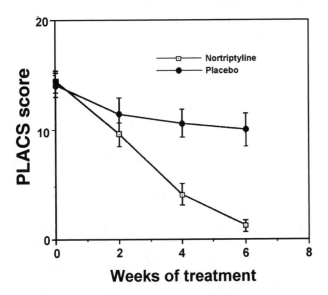

Figure 23–6. Mean Pathological Laughter and Crying Scale (PLACS) scores during 6 weeks of double-blind treatment. The nortriptyline-treated group had significantly lower (more improved) PLACS scores at 4 ($t = 3.9$, df = 26, $P = .0005$) and 6 ($t = 5.1$, df = 26, $P = .0001$) weeks of treatment compared with the placebo-treated group.
Source. Adapted from Robinson et al. 1993. Used with permission.

determined by increased ventricular-to-brain ratios), than did patients with similar brain lesions but no mania. Interestingly, those patients without a genetic predisposition had significantly more subcortical atrophy than did secondary mania patients with a genetic burden, suggesting that subcortical atrophy and genetic predisposition may be independent risk factors for mania following brain injury.

Mechanism.   To postulate a mechanism for secondary mania, two clinical-pathological correlations need to be explained. First, most lesions associated with secondary mania involve, directly or indirectly, limbic or limbic-related areas of the brain. Second, virtually all of these lesions are localized to the right hemisphere.

The basotemporal cortex appears to be a crucial area in the production of mania. This paralimbic area receives projections from secondary sensory and multimodal association regions (e.g., the frontal, temporal, and parietal association area), limbic regions, and paralimbic areas (e.g., the insula and the parahippocampal gyrus) (Moran et al. 1987). The basotemporal cortex is strongly connected to the orbitofrontal cortex through the uncinate fasciculus, and both may exert a tonic inhibitory control over limbic and dorsal cortical regions. Thus lesions or dysfunction of these areas may result in motor disinhibition (i.e., hyperactivity and pressured speech), intellectual disinhibition (i.e., flight of ideas and grandiose delusions), and instinctive disinhibition (i.e., hyperphagia and hypersexuality).

The second finding, which needs to be incorporated into any explanation of poststroke mania, is that the manias almost always occur following right hemisphere lesions. In our laboratory studies of the neurochemical and behavioral effects of brain lesions in rats (Robinson 1979), we found that small suction lesions in the right (but not left) frontal cortex of rats produced a significant increase in locomotor activity. Similar abnormal behavior was also found after electrolytic lesions of the right (but not left) nucleus accumbens (which is considered part of the ventral striatum) (Kubos et al. 1987). Moreover, right frontocortical suction lesions also produced a significant increment in dopaminergic turnover in the nucleus accumbens that was not seen with left-hemisphere lesions (Starkstein et al. 1988a). Thus it is possible that, in the presence of predisposing factors such as a genetic burden or subcortical atrophy, significant increments in biogenic amine turnover in the nucleus accumbens produced by specific right-hemisphere lesions may be part of the

mechanism that results in a manic syndrome.

In conclusion, secondary mania is a rare complication of stroke lesions. We have identified two risk factors: a genetic burden for psychiatric disorders and increased subcortical atrophy. Most patients with secondary mania have right-hemisphere lesions, which involve the orbitofrontal or basotemporal cortex, or subcortical structures, such as the thalamus or head of the caudate. Secondary mania may result from disinhibition of dorsal cortical and limbic areas and/or dysfunction of asymmetric biogenic amine pathways.

Conclusions

We have discussed several of the emotional and behavioral disorders that occur following cerebrovascular lesions (Table 23–7). Depression occurs in about 40% of stroke patients with approximately equal distributions of major depression and minor depression. Patients with poststroke depression often have a greater degree of cognitive impairment (i.e., dementia of depression) and significantly less recovery in ADLs than do patients who never develop depression. Poststroke depression is significantly associated with left frontal and left basal ganglia lesions and may be successfully treated with tricyclic antidepressants. Anxiety, which is present in about 27% of stroke patients, is associated with depression in the vast majority of cases. Among the few patients with poststroke anxiety and no depression, there was a high frequency of alcoholism and lesions of the right hemisphere. Apathy is present in about 20% of stroke patients. It is associated with older age, more severe deficits in ADLs, and a significantly higher frequency of lesions involving the posterior limb of the internal capsule.

Hallucinations and hallucinosis are rare complications of stroke lesions. Poststroke hallucinations are associated with right-hemisphere temporoparietal lesions, subcortical brain atrophy, and seizures. Poststroke hallucinosis is associated with damage to reticular activating and primary sensory pathways. Anosognosia is present in about 30% of patients with acute stroke lesions. It is associated with right-hemisphere temporoparietal, basal ganglia, and thalamic lesions; neglect; and subcortical brain atrophy.

Catastrophic reactions occur in about 20% of stroke patients; they are not related to the severity of impairment or the presence of aphasia but may represent a defining symptom for one clinical type of post-

Table 23–7. Poststroke neuropsychiatric syndromes

Neuropsychiatric syndrome	Prevalence	Neuropathological correlates
Depression		
Major	10.25%	Left frontal cortex and basal ganglia; enlarged ventricles
Minor	10%–40%	Not established
Generalized anxiety		
With depression	20%	Left frontal cortex
Without depression	7%	Right parietal cortex
Apathy		
With depression	11%	Left frontal cortex and basal ganglia
Without depression	11%	Posterior internal capsule
Psychosis	Unknown, rare	Right parietal-temporal-occipital junction
Anosognosia	24%–43%	Right hemisphere and enlarged ventricles; frontal dysfunction
Catastrophic reaction	19%	Anterior cortical lesion
Emotional lability	20%	Bilateral injury
Mania	Unknown, rare	Right hemisphere, or bifrontal, basotemporal, basal ganglia, and thalamus

stroke major depression. Catastrophic reactions are associated with anterior subcortical lesions and may result from a "release" of emotional display in depressed patients. Emotional lability is another common complication of stroke lesions that sometimes coexists with depression and may be successfully treated with tricyclic antidepressants. Finally, mania is a rare complication of stroke lesions. It is strongly associated with right-hemisphere damage involving the orbitofrontal cortex, basal temporal cortex, thalamus, or basal ganglia. Risk factors for mania include a familial history of psychiatric disorders and subcortical atrophy.

References

Adams RD, Victor M: Principles of Neurology. New York, McGraw-Hill, 1985

American Psychiatric Association: Diagnostic and Statistical Manual of Mental Disorders, 3rd Edition. Washington, DC, American Psychiatric Association, 1980

Babinski J: Contribution a l'etude des troubles mentaux dans l'hemiplegie organique cerebrale (anosognosie). Rev Neurol (Paris) 27:845–848, 1914

Barry S, Dinan TG: Alpha-2 adrenergic receptor function in post-stroke depression. Psychol Med 10:305–309, 1990

Bartlett EJ, Brodie JD, Wolf AP, et al: Reproducibility of cerebral glucose metabolic measurements in resting human subjects. J Cereb Blood Flow Metab 8:502–512, 1988

Bechara A, van der Kooy D: The tegmental pedunculopontine nucleus: a brainstem output of the limbic system critical for the conditioned place preferences produced by morphine and amphetamine. J Neurosci 9:3400–3409, 1989

Bolla-Wilson K, Robinson RG, Starkstein SE, et al: Lateralization of dementia of depression in stroke patients. Am J Psychiatry 146:627–634, 1989

Caplan LR, Stein RW: Stroke: A Clinical Approach. Boston, MA, Butterworths, 1986

Cascino GD, Adams RD: Brainstem auditory hallucinosis. Neurology 36:1042–1047, 1986

Castillo CS, Starkstein SE, Fedoroff JP, et al: Generalized anxiety disorder following stroke. J Nerv Ment Dis 181:100–106, 1993

Cummings JL, Mendez MF: Secondary mania with focal cerebrovascular lesions. Am J Psychiatry 141:1084–1087, 1984

De Renzi E, Vignolo LA: The Token Test: a sensitive test to detect disturbances in aphasics. Brain 85:665–678, 1962

Eastwood MR, Rifat SL, Nobbs H, et al: Mood disorder following cerebrovascular accident. Br J Psychiatry 154:195–200, 1989

Gainotti G: Emotional behavior and hemispheric side of the brain. Cortex 8:41–55, 1972

Geller TJ, Bellur SW: Peduncular hallucinosis: magnetic confirmation of mesencephalic infarction during life. Ann Neurol 21:602–604, 1987

Goldstein K: The Organism: A Holistic Approach to Biology Derived From Pathological Data in Man. New York, American Books, 1939

Gur RC, Gur RE, Resnick SM, et al: The effect of anxiety on cortical cerebral blood flow and metabolism. J Cereb Blood Flow Metab 7:173–177, 1987

Hachinski V, Norris JW: The Acute Stroke. Philadelphia, PA, FA Davis, 1985

Heilman KM: Anosognosia: possible neuropsychological mechanisms, in Awareness of Deficit After Brain Injury. Edited by Prigatano GP, Schacter DL. New York, Oxford University Press, 1991, pp 53–62

Helgason C, Wilbur A, Weiss A, et al: Acute pseuobulbar mutism due to discrete bilateral capsular infarction in the territory of the anterior choroidal artery. Brain 111:507–519, 1988

House A, Dennis M, Mogridge L, et al: Mood disorders in the year after stroke. Br J Psychiatry 158:83–92, 1991

Jorge RE, Robinson RG, Starkstein SE, et al: Secondary mania following traumatic brain injury. Am J Psychiatry 150:916–921, 1993

Kraepelin E: Manic Depressive Insanity and Paranoia. Edinburgh, Livingstone, 1921

Kubos KL, Moran TH, Robinson RG: Mania after brain injury: a controlled study of etiological factors. Arch Neurol 44:1069–1073, 1987

Levine DN, Finklestein S: Delayed psychosis after right temporoparietal stroke or trauma: relation to epilepsy. Neurology 32:267–273, 1982

Lipsey JR, Robinson RG, Peralson GD, et al: Mood change following bilateral hemisphere brain injury. Br J Psychiatry 143:266–273, 1983

Lipsey JR, Robinson RG, Pearlson GD, et al: Nortriptyline treatment of post-stroke depression: a double-blind treatment trial. Lancet 1:297–300, 1984

Lipsey JR, Robinson RG, Pearlson GD, et al: Dexamethasone suppression test and mood following stroke. Am J Psychiatry 142:318–323, 1985

Lipsey JR, Spencer WC, Rabins PV, et al: Phenomenological comparison of functional and post-stroke depression. Am J Psychiatry 143:527–529, 1986

Moran MA, Mufson EJ, Mesulam MM: Neural imputs into the temporopolar cortex of the rhesus monkey. J Comp Neurol 256:88–103, 1987

Morris PLP, Robinson RG, Ralphael B: Prevalence and course of depressive disorders in hospitalized stroke patients. Int J Psychiatry Med 20:349–364, 1990

Morris PLP, Robinson RG, Ralphael B: Lesion location and depression in hospitalized stroke patients: evidence supporting a specific relationship in the left hemisphere. Neuropsychiatry, Neuropsychology and Behavioral Neurology 3:75–82, 1992

Morris PLP, Robinson RG, Andrezejewski P, et al: Association of depression with 10-year post-stroke mortality. Am J Psychiatry 150:124–129, 1993

Nauta WJH: Reciprocal links of the corpus striatum with the cerebral cortex and the limbic system: a common substrate for movement and thought? in Neurology and Psychiatry: A Meeting of Minds. Edited by Muller J. Basel, Karger, 1989, pp 43–63

Parikh RM, Robinson RG, Lipsey JR, et al: The impact of post-stroke depression on recovery in activities of daily living over two-year follow-up. Arch Neurol 47:785–789, 1990

Poeck K: Pathophysiology of emotional disorders associated with brain damage, in Handbook of Clinical Neurology. Edited by Vinken PJ, Bruyn GW. Amsterdam, North-Holland, 1969

Rabins PV, Starkstein SE, Robinson RG: Risk factors for developing atypical (schizophreniform) psychosis following stroke. J Neuropsychiatry Clin Neurosci 3:6–9, 1991

Reding MJ, Orto LA, Winter SW, et al: Antidepressant therapy after stroke: a double-blind trial. Arch Neurol 43:763–765, 1986

Robinson RG: Differential behavioral and biochemical effects of right and left hemispheric cerebral infarction in the rat. Science 105:707–710, 1979

Robinson RG, Szetela B: Mood change following left hemispheric brain injury. Ann Neurol 9:447–453, 1981

Robinson RG, Starr LB, Kubos KL, et al: A two-year longitudinal study of post-stroke mood disorders: findings during the initial evaluation. Stroke 14:736–744, 1983

Robinson RG, Kubos KL, Starr LB, et al: Mood disorders in stroke patients: importance of location of lesion. Brain 107:81–93, 1984

Robinson RG, Lipsey JR, Bolla-Wilson K, et al: Mood disorders in left-handed stroke patients. Am J Psychiatry 142:1424–1429, 1985

Robinson RG, Bolla-Wilson K, Kaplan E, et al: Depression influences intellectual impairment in stroke patients. Br J Psychiatry 148:541–547, 1986

Robinson RG, Bolduc P, Price TR: A two-year longitudinal study of post-stroke depression: diagnosis and outcome at one- and two-year follow-up. Stroke 18:837–843, 1987

Robinson RG, Boston JD, Starkstein SE, et al: Comparison of mania with depression following brain injury: causal factors. Am J Psychiatry 145:172–178, 1988

Robinson RG, Parikh RM, Lipsey JR, et al: Pathological laughing and crying following stroke: validation of measurement scale and double blind treatment study. Am J Psychiatry 150:286–293, 1993

Ross ED, Stewart RS: Pathological display of affect in patients with depression and right frontal brain damage. J Nerv Ment Dis 175:165–172, 1987

Sinyor D, Jacques P, Kaloupek DG, et al: Post-stroke depression and lesion location: an attempted replication. Brain 109:537–546, 1986

Starkstein SE, Robinson RG: Neuropsychiatric aspects of cerebral vascular disorders, in The American Psychiatric Press Textbook of Neuropsychiatry, 2nd Edition. Edited by Yudofsky SC, Hales RE. Washington DC, American Psychiatric Press, 1992, pp 449–472

Starkstein SE, Pearlson GD, Robinson RG: Mania after brain injury: a controlled study of etiological factors. Arch Neurol 44:1069–1073, 1987

Starkstein SE, Moran TH, Bowersox JA, et al: Behavioral abnormalities induced by frontal cortical and nucleus accumens lesions. Brain Res 473:74–80, 1988a

Starkstein SE, Robinson RG, Berthier ML, et al: Differential mood changes following basal ganglia versus thalamic lesions. Arch Neurol 45:725–730, 1988b

Starkstein SE, Robinson RG, Honig MA, et al: Mood changes after right hemisphere lesion. Br J Psychiatry 155:79–85, 1989

Starkstein SE, Cohen BS, Fedoroff P, et al: Relationship between anxiety disorders and depressive disorders in patients with cerebrovascular injury. Arch Gen Psychiatry 47:246–251, 1990a

Starkstein SE, Mayberg HS, Berthier ML, et al: Mania after brain injury: neuroradiological and metabolic findings. Ann Neurol 27:652–659, 1990b

Starkstein SE, Fedoroff JP, Price TR, et al: Anosognosia in patients with cerebrovascular lesions: a study of causative factors. Stroke 23:1446–1453, 1992

Starkstein SE, Fedoroff JP, Price TR, et al: Apathy following cerebrovascular lesions. J Neurol Neurosurg Psychiatry 24:1625–1630, 1993a

Starkstein SE, Fedoroff JP, Price TR, et al: Catastrophic reaction after cerebrovascular lesions: frequency, correlates, and validation of a scale. J Neuropsychiatry Clin Neurosci 5:189–194, 1993b

Wade DT, Legh-Smith J, Hewer RA: Depressed mood after stroke: a community study of its frequency. Br J Psychiatry 151:200–205, 1987

Walker AE, Robins M, Weinfeld FD: Clinical findings in the National Survey of Stroke. Stroke 12 (suppl 1):I13–I31, 1981

Wolf PA, Kannel WB, Verter J: Cerebrovascular disease in the elderly: epidemiology, in Clinical Neurology of Aging. Edited by Albert ML. New York, Oxford University Press, 1984, pp 458–477

Appendix 23–1   Pathological Laughter and Crying Scale (PLACS)

Ratings are based on clinical assessment. Initial probe questions are given for each item. However, further questions may be used for clarification. Write the number in the spaces provided that most accurately reflects clinical symptoms.

Part I: Patient Interview

1. Have you recently experienced sudden episodes of laughter?
    ___ Rate the frequency of the episodes during the past two weeks.
    0. Rarely or not at all
    1. Occasionally
    2. Quite often
    3. Frequently

2. Have you recently experienced sudden episodes of crying?
    ___ Rate the frequency of the episodes during the past two weeks.
    0. Rarely or not at all
    1. Occasionally
    2. Quite often
    3. Frequently

If you have experienced sudden **episodes of laughter,** *please answer the following (questions 3–10), otherwise skip to question 11.*

3. Have these episodes occurred without any cause in your surroundings?
    ___ Rate the frequency with which the episodes have occurred without external stimuli in the past 2 weeks.
    0. Rarely or not at all
    1. Occasionally
    2. Quite often
    3. Frequently

4. Have these episodes lasted for a long period of time?
    ___ Rate the average duration of the episodes during the past two weeks.
    0. Very brief
    1. Few seconds
    2. Moderate (less than 30 seconds)
    3. Prolonged (more than 30 seconds)

5. Have these episodes been uncontrollable by you?
    ___ Rate the ability to control the episodes during the past two weeks.
    0. Rarely or not at all
    1. Occasionally
    2. Quite often
    3. Frequently

6. Have these episodes occurred as a result of feelings of happiness?
    ___ Rate the frequency with which the episodes have occurred as a result of happiness in the past two weeks.
    0. Rarely or not at all
    1. Occasionally
    2. Quite often
    3. Frequently

7. Have these episodes occurred in excess of feelings of happiness?
    ___ Rate the frequency with which the episodes have been disproportionate to the emotional state in the past two weeks.
    0. Rarely or not at all
    1. Occasionally
    2. Quite often
    3. Frequently

8. Have these episodes of laughter occurred with feelings of sadness?
    ___ Rate the frequency of association between the episode and the paradoxical emotion in the past two weeks. The sadness must precede or accompany the episode and not be a reaction to it.
    0. Rarely or not at all
    1. Occasionally
    2. Quite often
    3. Frequently

9. Have these episodes occurred with any emotions other than happiness or sadness, such as, nervousness, anger, fear, etc.?
    ___ Rate the frequency of association between the episodes and emotions in the past two weeks. The emotions must precede or accompany the episode and not be a reaction to it.
    0. Rarely or not at all
    1. Occasionally
    2. Quite often
    3. Frequently

Appendix 23–1   Pathological Laughter and Crying Scale (PLACS)

10. Have these episodes caused you any distress or social embarrassment?

   ___ Rate the degree of distress or embarrassment caused by the episodes in the past two weeks.

   0. Rarely or not at all

   1. Occasionally

   2. Quite often

   3. Frequently

If you have experienced sudden **episodes of crying,** *please answer the following (questions 11–18).*

11. Have these episodes occurred without any cause in your surroundings?

   ___ Rate the frequency with which the episodes have occurred without an external stimuli in the past two weeks.

   0. Rarely or not at all

   1. Occasionally

   2. Quite often

   3. Frequently

12. Have these episodes lasted for a long period of time?

   ___ Rate the average duration of the episodes during the past two weeks.

   0. Very brief

   1. Short (few seconds)

   2. Moderate (less than 30 seconds)

   3. Prolonged (more than 30 seconds)

13. Have these episodes been uncontrollable by you?

   ___ Rate the ability to control the episodes during the past two weeks.

   0. Rarely or not at all

   1. Occasionally

   2. Quite often

   3. Frequently

14. Have these episodes occurred as a result of feelings of sadness?

   ___ Rate the frequency with which the episodes have occurred as a result of sadness in the past two weeks. The sadness must proceed or accompany the crying and not be a reaction to it.

   0. Rarely or not at all

   1. Occasionally

   2. Quite often

   3. Frequently

15. Have these episodes occurred in excess of feelings of sadness?

   ___ Rate the frequency with which the episodes have been disproportionate to the emotional state in the past two weeks.

   0. Rarely or not at all

   1. Occasionally

   2. Quite often

   3. Frequently

16. Have these episodes of crying occurred with feelings of happiness?

   ___ Rate the frequency of association between the episode and the paradoxical emotion in the past two weeks. The happiness must precede or accompany the crying.

   0. Rarely or not at all

   1. Occasionally

   2. Quite often

   3. Frequently

17. Have these episodes occurred with any emotions other than sadness or happiness, such as nervousness, anger, fear, etc.?

   ___ Rate the frequency of association between the episodes and emotions in the past two weeks. The emotions must precede or accompany the episode and not be a reaction to it.

   0. Rarely or not at all

   1. Occasionally

   2. Quite often

   3. Frequently

18. Have these episodes caused you any distress or social embarrassment?

   ___ Rate the degree of distress or embarrassment caused by the episodes in the past two weeks.

   0. Rarely or not at all

   1. Occasionally

   2. Quite often

   3. Frequently

24

Traumatic Brain Injury

Robert B. Fields, Ph.D.
C. Edward Coffey, M.D.

Introduction

The topic of traumatic brain injury in the elderly represents a paradox in neuropsychiatry. Among young adults, traumatic brain injury is the leading cause of organically based neurobehavioral disturbances, and, among patients with neuropsychiatric disorders in general, advancing age is a leading risk factor. Yet despite these well-established findings, research regarding the overlap of these two topics (i.e., the neuropsychiatric impact of a traumatic brain injury on an older person and on an older brain) has been limited.

Comprehensive reviews of the literature on traumatic brain injury can be found elsewhere (Bigler 1990b; Finger et al. 1988; Levin et al. 1982; Parker 1990; Richardson 1990; Wood 1990). In this chapter, we discuss studies relevant to the potential differential vulnerability of elderly patients. To support an age-based "differential vulnerability" hypothesis about outcome after brain injury, several points must be established. First, there must be evidence that traumatic brain injury in the elderly is sufficiently common to warrant attention. Second, outcome after such injuries must be sufficiently different among the elderly to suggest that they constitute a population "at risk." Third, and of particular relevance to this volume, is the question of whether the pattern of postinjury neuropsychiatric symptoms among the elderly distinguishes this group from younger adults. Finally, if the elderly are in fact at greater risk for negative outcome, we should be able to identify markers of that vulnerability and to specify age-specific treatment strategies.

We begin this chapter with an overview of the methodology used to study traumatic brain injury. In subsequent sections, we review the pathophysiology and epidemiology of brain injury, general and neurobehavioral outcome following traumatic brain injury, and the diagnosis and treatment of the consequences of traumatic brain injury. Finally, we discuss conceptual models and future directions, including possible markers of vulnerability. Each section includes a general review of the traumatic brain injury literature followed by a discussion of what is known about older adults who sustain such injuries.

Methodological Issues

Our purpose in this section is to review terminology and assessment strategies in order to provide a context for discussing research relevant to traumatic brain injury in elderly patients.

Terminology

The use of general terms such as *head injury, brain injury,* and *traumatic brain injury* can be both informative and problematic. The utility of these terms stems from the implied causal connection between an acquired lesion and abnormal behavior. Among patients who have sustained a traumatic brain injury, there is an assumption that subsequent alterations in thinking, mood, and behavior are due to the specific neurological damage associated with the traumatic event. However, the use of these terms can also be misleading. Among younger adults, for example, the term *brain injury* typically connotes a traumatic injury, whereas among older adults, the term *brain injury* is often used to describe a variety of etiologies (e.g., stroke, aneurysm, and tumor, as well as traumatic injury). These terms also imply a misleading homogeneity of patients across studies. Just as strokes of different types, sizes, and locations can produce a wide range of neurological and neurobehavioral dysfunction, so too can traumatic brain injuries of different types and severities cause different symptoms. Comparing studies of outcome following "brain injury," therefore, will likely produce different conclusions if this anatomic heterogeneity is not taken into account. A third problem with these terms is the risk of assuming a direct correspondence between the brain injury and subsequent behavior and of minimizing other factors that have been shown to contribute to outcome. These factors include, but are not limited to, premorbid personality, previous brain injury or dysfunction, substance abuse, vocational history, social support network, involvement in treatment, and the experience of being in a traumatic event (Parker 1990; Richardson 1990; Wood 1990).

Classification

Classification by mechanism or cause of injury. An injury to brain tissue may be the result of an internal (e.g., stroke or surgery) or external (e.g., gunshot wound, toxic exposure, or motor vehicle accident) event. Externally produced head injuries can be further categorized as being either "open" or "closed" depending on whether or not the skull has been penetrated. As might be expected, the manner in which an injury is sustained has important implications for the neuroanatomical, neurochemical, metabolic, and neurobehavioral disruption that follows. Missile wounds, for example, usually produce neuroanatomical damage and behavioral disturbances that are different from the effects of closed head injuries and that are dependent on factors such as the path of the bullet, tissue disruption by associated force waves, the spread of bone chips, and the development of cerebral edema (Bigler 1991; Kirkpatrick and DiMaio 1978). The well-known case of Phineas Gage in the 1860s is an example of an open head injury (i.e., penetration by a railroad spike through the left frontal lobe) that produced specific and dramatic changes in personality and social comportment with no other apparent gross neurological dysfunction (Harlow 1868). In contrast, closed head injuries sustained during high-velocity motor vehicle accidents are likely to produce a multitude of deficits as a result of a rapid acceleration and deceleration of the brain within the cranial vault.

Classification by severity of injury. Severity is an important dimension of a brain injury. Traditionally, most classification systems of severity have focused on an assessment of a patient's neurological status immediately following the injury and the duration of neurological and neuropsychological dysfunction over time. The categories "mild," "moderate," and "severe" are typically used to differentiate brain injuries based on criteria such as degree of initial neurological dysfunction, length of period of unconsciousness, and duration of posttraumatic amnesia.

Patients classified as having "mild" traumatic brain injuries usually have only transient loss of, or changes in, consciousness; brief periods of amnesia; and short or no hospitalizations (Barth et al. 1983; Bigler 1990a, 1991; Bohnen and Jolles 1992; Rimel et al. 1981). Patients with "moderate" brain injuries often demonstrate impaired consciousness or disorientation an hour or so after the injury and may have posttraumatic amnesia for approximately 1 to 24 hours (Bigler 1991; Rimel et al. 1982). Patients whose injuries are considered to be "severe" generally display more pronounced and longstanding deficits in consciousness and posttraumatic amnesia for longer than 24 hours (Bigler 1991; Russell 1971). The terms *very severe* or *profound brain injury* are reserved for patients who display persistent coma and who, if they survive, may either be in a vegetative state, permanently neurologically impaired, or have posttraumatic amnesia that usually lasts longer than 7 days (Bigler 1991).

Assessment of the severity of neurological impairment following a traumatic brain injury is most often accomplished with the Glasgow Coma Scale (GCS; Teasdale and Jennett 1974). The GCS is a global measure of level of consciousness that assesses functions in three domains (eye opening, verbal response, and motor response) and yields a score ranging from 3 to 15 (Table 24–1). GCS scores are generally interpreted as follows: 13–15 = mild, 9–12 = moderate, 3–8 = severe. The GCS predicts outcome well, with more impaired patients having poorer prognoses (Alexandre et al. 1983; Jennett 1979; Levin et al. 1990).

However, the utility of the GCS is limited in selected populations (e.g., children, patients with chronic disabilities, and patients whose injuries affect the eyes and mouth) (Sorenson and Kraus 1991). As a result, other scales of injury severity have been developed that take into account the fact that brain injuries often co-occur with other injuries. The Abbreviated Injury Scale (AIS; American Association for Automotive Medicine 1985), for example, was designed to rate overall injury severity based on several sources of information (e.g., loss of consciousness, duration of period of unconsciousness, and brain imaging). The AIS includes the Injury Severity Scale (ISS; Baker et al. 1976), which measures cumulative damage across six body regions, including the head. The total score is computed based on the three areas that are most impaired.

Other means of classifying severity also exist. One recent classification system (Marshall et al. 1991) used

Table 24–1.   Glasgow Coma Scale

Eye opening response	Spontaneous	4
	To voice	3
	To pain	2
	None	1
Best verbal response	Oriented	5
	Confused	4
	Inappropriate words	3
	Incomprehensive sounds	2
	None	1
Best motor response	Obeys	6
	Localizes pain	5
	Withdraws (pain)	4
	Flexion (pain)	3
	Extension (pain)	2
	None	1

Source.   Reprinted from Teasdale G, Jennett B: "Assessment of Coma and Impaired Consciousness: A Practical Scale." *Lancet* 2:81–84, 1974. Used with permission.

quantitative and qualitative analyses of the initial brain computed tomography (CT) scans of brain injury patients to assess severity. By determining the status of the mesencephalic cisterns, the degree of midline shift, and the presence or absence of surgical masses, four levels of severity were obtained (i.e., "diffuse injury" I through IV). Using this classification system, along with an assessment of type of intracranial hemorrhage, there was improved prediction of gross outcome measures such as mortality and level of disability over the traditional method of categorizing lesions as either focal or diffuse. Of interest, when patients with similar injury severity scores were separated by age (40 or younger [$n = 153$] versus older than 40 [$n = 24$]), older patients had significantly poorer outcomes than did their younger counterparts.

Classification by stages of recovery and outcome.
Patients who have sustained mild traumatic brain injuries may exhibit transient disruptions in cognitive processing, as well as in physical and neurobehavioral functioning ("postconcussion syndrome") (Alexander 1992; Binder 1986; Bohnen and Jolles 1992; Levin et al. 1987c). Because some of these symptoms are nonspecific, however, the process of identifying stages of recovery and determining differential diagnosis following mild traumatic brain injury is difficult.

Among patients whose traumatic brain injuries can be classified as severe, the early stages of recovery are more easily defined. Although it is dependent on factors such as the focality and overall severity of the injury, the initial recovery phase can be characterized by the three stages of coma, unresponsive vigilance, and mute responsiveness (Alexander 1982). The next phase of recovery is usually referred to as the *posttraumatic amnesia state* (Alexander 1982; Stuss and Buckle 1992). The term *posttraumatic amnesia* emphasizes a hallmark feature of this phase (i.e., the inability of a patient to recall recent events). This term may be somewhat misleading, however, because disturbances in arousal, attention, mood, and personality or behavior may also occur (Alexander 1982). This term is used clinically to describe the postacute injury period and should be differentiated from the more permanent syndromes of posttraumatic amnestic disorder and posttraumatic dementia. In general, the duration of posttraumatic amnesia can be predicted from the duration of coma. However, among elderly patients, relatively longer periods of amnesia may follow relatively shorter periods of coma (Richardson 1990; Von

Wowern 1966). The association between posttraumatic amnesia and eventual outcome appears to be stronger among older adults than among younger adults (Richardson 1990; Russell and Smith 1961).

There have been several approaches to describing the long-term recovery process following severe traumatic brain injuries (Alexander 1982; Stuss and Buckle 1992). During the first year or so after the injury, intellectual and social competencies typically improve and dependence on caregivers decreases (Alexander 1982; Stuss and Buckle 1992). Neurobehavioral progress beyond the first year has been characterized by slower and more heterogeneous neuropsychological improvement, additional personality and psychosocial or familial difficulties, continued disturbances in areas such as self-monitoring and self-awareness, and variability in behavior and vocational or test performance (Stuss and Buckle 1992).

Assessment of global progress through the initial stages of recovery is often accomplished with the Rancho Los Amigos Scale (Hagen et al. 1972), and specific improvement in cognitive functioning may be monitored via serial administrations of cognitive screening tests such as the Galveston Orientation and Amnesia Test (GOAT; Levin et al. 1979b). Global outcome during the later stages of recovery is most often assessed via the 5-point Glasgow Outcome Scale (GOS; Jennett and Bond 1975): 1) good recovery, 2) moderate disability, 3) severe disability, 4) vegetative state, and 5) dead. Quantification of neuropsychiatric functioning has been accomplished primarily via neuropsychological testing, symptom checklists, and clinician's rating scales such as the Neurobehavioral Rating Scale (Levin et al. 1987b). Following mild brain injury, global outcome is frequently assessed by criteria such as capacity to return to work. The determination of more subtle or specific neurobehavioral deficits generally requires comprehensive neuropsychiatric assessment and neuropsychological testing.

In conclusion, several studies have reported that outcome is worse for older adults following traumatic brain injury, but many of such studies fail to control for other factors that also contribute to outcome such as total injury severity. Similarly, studies may assume increased vulnerability where there is none if they fail to take into account age differences in performance among "normal" adults on the neuropsychological tests or symptom checklists they use to assess outcome. Finally, the validity of traditional psychiatric assessment tools for assessing the impact of traumatic brain injuries on patients in different age groups remains to be determined.

Pathophysiology and Sequelae of Traumatic Brain Injury

Initial or primary effects of the injury are typically distinguished from the subsequent processes or secondary injuries that follow (Jennett and Teasdale 1981; Katz 1992; Pang 1989; Parker 1990; Richardson 1990). Although somewhat arbitrary, this distinction is useful for descriptive purposes.

Primary Brain Injury

Several destructive processes take place when a traumatic brain injury occurs. Among patients who experience closed head injuries, the two most important processes are contact and acceleration-rotation (Katz 1992). Consequences of contact include distorted or fractured skulls and contusions or lacerations of the brain. Contrecoup injuries are also common, although the term *contrecoup* may be somewhat misleading because the location of these injuries may not be exactly opposite the point of initial impact (Richardson 1990).

In addition to contact with an external object, many traumatic brain injuries also involve linear acceleration or rotational movements of the brain within the skull. In severe cases, dramatic rotation of the brain around the brain stem may lead to coma (Parker 1990). In other cases, the accelerating and decelerating or twisting movements of the brain produce lacerations or contusions when the moving brain comes into contact with the more stationary bony protuberances of the base of the skull. Within the cranial vault, the orbital, frontal, and temporal areas are most vulnerable to this type of injury (Adams et al. 1977; Bigler 1990a, 1991; Ommaya et al. 1971; Richardson 1990). An important byproduct of these movements is diffuse axonal injury (Adams 1988; Adams et al. 1982). Straining, shearing, and rupture of axonal fibers are common following traumatic brain injury of all severities and are generally associated with more significant neuropsychiatric disorders (Jennett and Teasdale 1981; Parker 1990; Richardson 1990).

Secondary Brain Injury

Damage to the structure and function of the brain often continues following the initial trauma (Jennett and Teasdale 1981). As a result, it may be more appropriate to consider a severe traumatic brain injury as a "process" rather than an "event" (Parker 1990). Intracranial hematomas and brain swelling are considered to be two of the most frequent types of acute secondary brain injury (Richardson 1990). In his review of this literature, Richardson (1990) reported that intracranial hemorrhage occurs in approximately 50% of patients with severe injuries and often is responsible for the development of delayed coma or other types of neurological deterioration. The presence of a skull fracture dramatically increases the risk of intracranial hematomas (Jennett and Teasdale 1981). Diffuse brain swelling develops in approximately 10% of patients who have sustained severe brain injuries (Adams et al. 1989; Richardson 1990). Brain edema may lead to herniation or to occlusion of intracranial vessels with secondary strokes (e.g., subfalcial herniation may occlude the anterior cerebral artery, and transtentorial herniation may occlude the posterior cerebral artery). The occurrence of subdural hematomas secondary to the tearing of veins is particularly problematic in elderly patients in whom brain atrophy increases the distance from the brain surface to the venous sinuses, thus increasing the vulnerability of bridging veins to rupture with even minor trauma (Cummings and Benson 1992).

Other types of secondary consequences may also occur following severe injuries. Experimentally induced traumatic brain injuries in animals produce widespread depolarization of neurons (Katayama et al. 1990) and release of excitatory neurotransmitters (Gorman et al. 1989; Katayama et al. 1990). An example of the consequences of this "neurotoxic cascade" is the release of free radicals and excitotoxic neurotransmitters (e.g., glutamate) (Becker et al. 1988; Faden et al. 1989; Silver et al. 1992). Such alterations in neurochemistry may affect basic vascular and metabolic functioning and may cause changes in intracranial pressure, heart rate, blood pressure, and nutritional state (Bigler 1991; Parker 1990).

The postinjury course may also be complicated by sequelae such as ischemia, infection, ventricular enlargement, or posttraumatic epilepsy (Bachman 1992; Katz 1992; Parker 1990; Richardson 1990). Ventricular enlargement, for example, is common following moderate to severe traumatic brain injury (Levin et al. 1981) and has been associated with greater neuropsychological impairment (Cullum and Bigler 1986) and worse prognosis (Gudeman et al. 1981; Kishore et al. 1978). Changes in ventricular size may not be fully apparent (via CT scan analysis) until 1–3 months after the injury (Cope et al. 1988; Gudeman et al. 1981).

Posttraumatic epilepsy is another delayed consequence of brain injury that can affect eventual outcome. Approximately 5% of patients develop seizures within the first week after a traumatic brain injury. Risk factors for "early" posttraumatic epilepsy include prolonged posttraumatic amnesia, depressed skull fracture, intracranial hematoma, and childhood (Bachman 1992; Hendrick and Harris 1968; Jennett and Teasdale 1981). "Late" seizures (i.e., beyond the first week) have also been reported in approximately 5% of patients following traumatic brain injury, but may not develop until more than a year after the injury. Risk factors for late epilepsy include severity of injury, early epilepsy, and depressed skull fracture (Annegers et al. 1980a; Bachman 1992; Jennett and Teasdale 1981). Mathematical models exist to predict the likelihood of seizures for individual patients (Feeney and Walker 1990). Among patients who have already had one late seizure, 75% continue to have seizures (Bachman 1992). The use of prophylactic anticonvulsant medication following brain injury reduces the risk of early seizures, but not late seizures (Temkin et al. 1990). Because anticonvulsants often produce sedation, their use among elderly patients may be problematic (e.g., increased risk of subsequent head injuries due to falls). (The diagnosis and management of seizures in the elderly is reviewed in Chapter 25.)

Special consideration for geriatric populations. Age may contribute to an elderly individual's vulnerability to particular injuries in several ways. For example, changes in bone structure are thought to predispose elderly individuals to fractures during traumatic injuries (Dries and Gamelli 1992). However, in one large study of patients with traumatic brain injuries (Pentland et al. 1986), no age differences were found in the frequency of skull fracture, and, in another study (Vollmer et al. 1991), only a slight increase with age was found. It is not known whether the aging brain is more vulnerable to axonal shearing injuries after trauma-induced accelerational and rotational movements. It has been suggested that the older brain is more vulnerable to damage from excitotoxic neurotransmitters following traumatic brain injury (Hamm et al. 1991, Hamm et al. 1992), although the extent to which this occurs is not known. Posttraumatic epilepsy and brain swelling do not appear to occur more commonly in

older adults than in younger adults following brain injury (Richardson 1990).

Older adults are, however, more vulnerable to the development of posttraumatic infections, subdural hematomas, and intracranial hemorrhages (Dries and Gamelli 1992; Fogel and Duffy 1994; Miller and Pentland 1989). For example, Pentland et al. (1986) reported a threefold increase in intracranial hematomas among their older sample (older than 65 [n = 449]) compared with their younger sample (younger than 65 [n = 1,571]) following traumatic brain injury. This age discrepancy was particularly noteworthy for patients who had experienced mild to moderate injuries. Among patients whose injuries were severe, the frequency of intracranial hematomas was high in both age groups and not significantly different. In contrast, the frequency of intracranial hematoma among patients who sustained mild to moderate brain injuries was six times greater in the older sample. In another study (Vollmer et al. 1991), both intracerebral and extracerebral hemorrhages were significantly more common in older (56 or older [n = 74]) than younger (age 16–55 [n = 580]) patients following moderate to severe traumatic brain injuries. In this study, it was also noted that the size of these lesions (particularly those that were extracerebral) increased with age, as did the frequency of subarachnoid hemorrhage and the likelihood of shift of midline structures on CT.

A complicating factor in elderly patients is that intra- and extracerebral hemorrhages may go unrecognized in the presence of other injuries, or they may develop in a delayed fashion over time (Fogel and Duffy 1994). In one study, 10% of older patients who were admitted to a hospital because of a fractured bone were found to have a subdural hematoma as well (Oster 1977). The presence of psychiatric disorders can also complicate the diagnostic process. The patient described in Figure 24–1, for example, was referred for a course of electroconvulsive therapy to treat his recurrent depression. Because increased cognitive deficits were observed during treatment (relative to his previous baselines), an additional evaluation was conducted, which revealed the presence of a subacute subdural hematoma sustained during a prior mild brain injury (i.e., fall with no loss of consciousness).

Although the finding of increased posttraumatic intracerebral hematomas in elderly patients is consistent with a differential vulnerability hypothesis, two points are worth noting. First, intracranial hematomas are more common following falls than other types of brain injuries (Gennarelli et al. 1982), and, as discussed below, falls are more common among elderly individuals (Sorenson and Kraus 1991). Second, the incidence of nontraumatic intracerebral hemorrhage in the general population increases exponentially with age and at a much greater rate than other types of hemorrhage (e.g., subarachnoid) (Broderick et al. 1993). As a result, it has not yet been firmly established whether the increased risk of posttraumatic intracerebral hematomas found among older patients reflects

an age difference in response to injury or age differences in the type of injury sustained and general vulnerability to intracerebral hemorrhage.

Epidemiology

Studies of the epidemiology of traumatic brain injury have generally considered three major questions. First, how common are these injuries among a specific population? Second, are there demographic differences in the occurrence of brain injuries? And third, are there differences in the types of injuries sustained by different groups? Among the general population, the annual rate of traumatic brain injury in the United States is approximately 150–200 per 100,000 people (Kraus et al. 1984; Naugle 1990; Sorenson and Kraus 1991). These injuries do not, however, occur randomly. Traumatic brain injuries are most common among young adult males (ages 16–25) and typically are the result of a motor vehicle accident. Children are also at risk for head injuries (Goldstein and Levin 1990; Rosenthal et al. 1990). What is less well appreciated is that older adults are also a high-risk group.

Figure 24–2 presents epidemiological data regarding the occurrence of head injuries from San Diego County (Kraus et al. 1984). These data are generally consistent with surveys from other locations (Sorenson and Kraus 1991), and reveal that following a period of relative low risk in middle adulthood, adults are at increased risk for a traumatic brain injury when they reach age 65 or 70. In addition, the large sex difference in incidence rate that exists in young adults is not present in elderly adults.

Differences also exist across age groups in how injuries are sustained. Among the general population, motor vehicle accidents are the leading cause of head injury, and falls are the second leading cause. Among the elderly, this order is reversed (Parker 1990; Sorenson and Kraus 1991). In a study of head injury in Rhode Island for example, Fife et al. (1986) reported that among teenagers, young adults, and middle aged adults a motor vehicle accident was the most likely cause of head injury, whereas among children and those over age 65, the injury was most likely due to a fall. Although geographic differences exist (e.g., more assaults with firearms in larger cities), the basic findings of increased falls and pedestrian accidents among elderly subjects, as well as a corresponding decrease in motor vehicle accidents, hold up across studies (Soren-

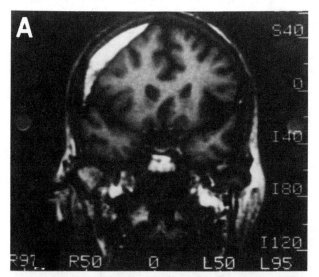

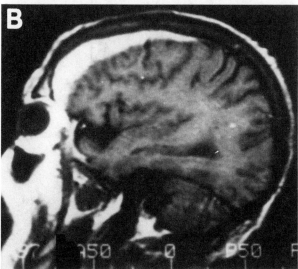

Figure 24–1. T1-weighted (TR = 500 milliseconds, TE = 20 milliseconds) magnetic resonance image (MRI) in the coronal (*panel A*) and parasagittal (*panel B*) planes demonstrating fluid collection with increased signal consistent with subacute subdural hematoma. This subdural hematoma was discovered in a 69-year-old man who had previously had a mild head injury (i.e., fall with no loss of consciousness).

son and Kraus 1991) including our own (Fields 1991) (Figure 24–3).

Regarding the severity of these injuries (as determined by GCS), "mild" head injuries are the most common for all age groups and account for approximately 80% of all traumatic brain injuries (Sorenson and Kraus 1991). Compared with younger patients, the percentage of "severe" injuries may be greater in elderly patients, and (as noted above) these injuries are more likely to result in cerebral hemorrhages (Sorenson and Kraus 1991). Several factors increase the risk of having a traumatic brain injury including previous head injury and alcohol use (Naugle 1990; Sparadeo et al. 1990). Among the elderly population, the risk of accidental traumatic brain injuries is also increased by factors that may impair perception, reaction time, coordination, or judgment; these include chronic illness, sensory loss, medication, and cognitive decline (Dries and Gamelli 1992).

Outcome

For patients and families of patients who experience traumatic brain injuries, the most pressing injury-related issues pertain to survival and quality of life in the postinjury period.

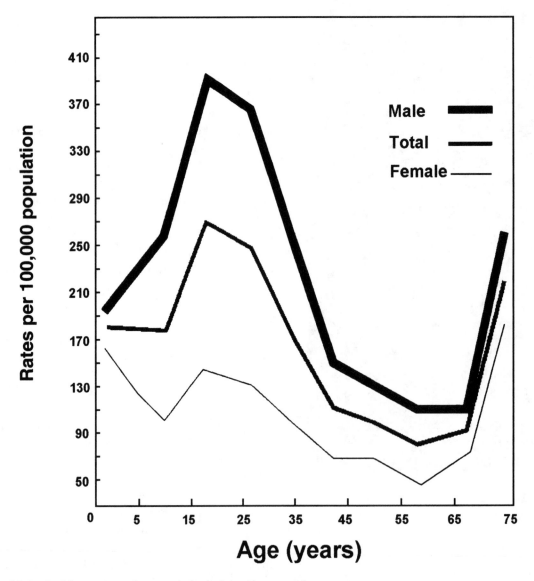

Figure 24–2. Incidence rates of traumatic brain injury by age and sex.
Source. Adapted from Kraus et al. (1984). Used with permission.

Global Outcome

Initial outcome.   The best predictor of outcome during the first few weeks after a traumatic brain injury is the severity of the initial injury (as measured by scales such as the GCS). Patients whose injuries are more severe are at greater risk for death, longer hospital stays, and placement in supervised care settings following hospitalization (Jennett and Teasdale 1981; Marshall et al. 1983; Richardson 1990; Russell and Smith 1961). In one sample of adults (ages 25–54 [$n = 1,487$]) hospitalized for traumatic brain injury (Fields 1991), the rate of in-hospital mortality following a severe injury (GCS score = 3–8 [$n = 363$]) was 32.8%, whereas, mortality following a mild injury (GCS = 13–15 [$n = 1,124$]) was 1.4%. Similar differences were found in length of hospital stay (severe = 50% were discharged in 19 days; mild = 50% were discharged in 5 days) and likelihood of placement in a rehabilitation facility or nursing home (severe = 55.8%; mild = 5.8%).

Longer-term outcome.   Severity of injury is also the most important predictor of longer-term outcome. Se-

vere injuries are associated with greater generalized impairment than are mild injuries. In one representative study, for example, Vollmer et al. (1991) found the following outcome statistics (based on GOS) for a sample of adults (ages 26–55 [$n = 279$]) 6 months after a severe brain injury: good recovery = 22%, moderate to severe disability = 35%, vegetative survival or death = 43%. Return to work is infrequent among patients who survive severe traumatic brain injuries (Ben Yishay et al. 1987). Kreutzer et al. (1988), for example reported a 70% unemployment rate in their sample 7 years postinjury.

Following mild brain injuries, brief periods of amnesia, as well as symptoms of headache, vertigo, and poor memory, are common initial sequelae (Bohnen and Jolles 1992; Levin et al. 1987c; Rutherford 1989). Although return to normal functioning usually occurs within 2–4 weeks, a subset of patients continue to report these difficulties, which interfere with cognitive, physical, interpersonal, and vocational functioning (Bohnen et al. 1992). Inability to return to work after mild traumatic brain injury is relatively rare among executives, business managers, and other professionals

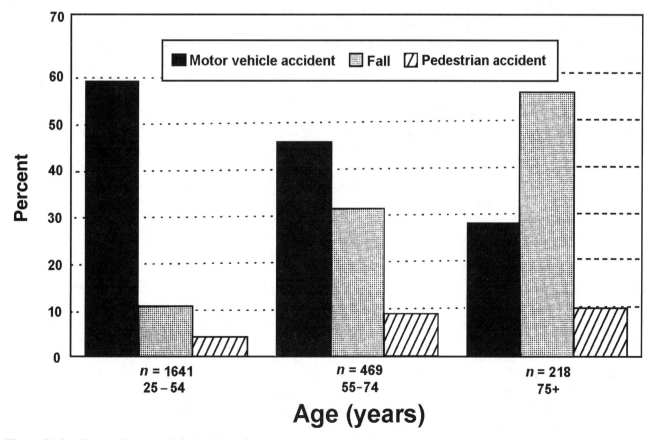

Figure 24–3.   Causes of traumatic brain injury by age.

(Rimel et al. 1981), but considerably more common among patients with lower IQ or those whose jobs require motor speed, safety, and efficiency (Adamovich et al. 1985; Dikmen et al. 1989; Rimel et al. 1981).

Outcome in the elderly.   Older adults are usually thought to have less favorable outcomes than are younger adults following traumatic brain injury. In 1932, for example, Russell reported an increase in mortality associated with traumatic brain injury beginning in the fifth decade of life. In their influential work, Jennett and Teasdale (1981) described a "continuous" and essentially linear relationship between age and negative outcome across the life span. Other studies have also documented increased mortality rates, increased length of hospital stay, increased likelihood of nursing home placement, increased long-term disability, and other signs of poor prognosis among older adults following brain injury (e.g., Annegers et al. 1980b; Carlsson et al. 1968; Cartlidge and Shaw 1981; Edna 1983; Fife et al. 1986; Jennett and Teasdale 1981; Kotwica and Jakubowski 1992; Luerssen et al. 1988; Marshall et al. 1991; Pentland et al. 1986; Vollmer et al. 1991). In addition, the literature on general trauma in humans (Dries and Gamelli 1992) and the limited experimental literature on brain injury in animals (Hamm et al. 1991) also suggest that advanced age is a risk factor for adverse outcome.

Although the weight of the evidence is impressive, studies comparing the effects of traumatic brain injury on older versus younger adult humans have been problematic for a number of reasons. First is the influence of preexisting conditions on subsequent outcome. The relationship between preexisting neurological impairment and a brain injury in elderly patients may affect the cause of injury (e.g., a dementia patient who falls), initial presentation (e.g., inaccurate history or delay in seeking treatment), postinjury course (e.g., exaggeration of injury-related neuropsychological deficits), and diagnosis (e.g., attribution of dementia-related cognitive impairment to the brain injury).

Whether a traumatic brain injury is the cause or the result of brain dysfunction is more likely to be a question among older adults in whom degenerative changes, medication sensitivity, and so on are more common than in younger adults. In a study of brain injury among the "old old" (ages 80–96) for example, a factor that contributed to the injury (e.g., previous stroke, postural dizziness, and medication) could be identified for 75% of the patients whose injury was the result of a fall (Amacher and Bybee 1987). Assessing outcome in this sample, therefore, might underestimate the potential recovery of "normal" elderly individuals who fall for other reasons.

A second problem has been controlling for severity of brain injury, as well as for total body injuries, when comparing samples of different age groups. If older adults have more severe injuries (as Sorenson and Kraus [1991] contended), increased negative outcome among the elderly may be simply a reflection of severity of injury rather than of age. A third problem is that, even when severity of injury is controlled, comparisons of different age groups generally do not control for differences in the type of injury sustained. Finally, the definition of "age" varies considerably from study to study. Many reports of change in outcome with "age" involve a comparison between young adults (usually ages 20–40) and middle-aged adults (ages 40–65), with very little representation of geriatric patients.

A few studies have addressed these issues. For example, Vollmer et al. (1991) investigated more than 600 patients age 15 and older whose nonpenetrating head injuries resulted in traumatic coma. Consistent with other studies, the types of injuries sustained in their sample differed by age. However, no differences in GCS score or presence of multiple injuries were found among the elderly patients suggesting that findings of increased negative outcome could not be attributed to group differences in severity of brain injury or severity of global injuries. With these factors controlled, mortality was significantly more likely and good recovery significantly less likely among those age 56 and older. Furthermore, when a higher-order regression analysis was performed to determine the combined effect of multiple variables on outcome, age remained an independent predictor.

In a study of traumatic brain injury in the United Kingdom, Pentland et al. (1986) included a large sample of younger (under 65 [n = 1,571]) and older (65 or older [n = 449]) patients who were heterogeneous in terms of severity of injury. Using the GOS, age was related to outcome following moderate and severe brain injuries. For example, among patients whose injuries were severe (GCS score less than 8), the mortality rate for the older group was 77% compared to a rate of 39% for younger patients. Among patients whose injuries were moderate (i.e., GCS scores 8–12), severe disability or death was also significantly more likely in the older group (55%) than the younger group (15%). Among patients whose injuries were mild (GCS scores 13–14),

GOS scores did not differ, but, length of hospital stay was longer in the older group.

These findings are supported by another study of severely injured patients based on data collected for the multicenter Trauma Coma Data Bank (Ruff et al. 1990). This study was designed to assess the effects of alcohol on outcome following traumatic brain injury and used age as an independent variable. Their data documented the increased likelihood of negative outcome (based on GOS) among older adults (50 or older [n = 55]) versus younger adults (15–49 [n = 352]) independent of level of alcohol consumption. Finally, Katz et al. (1990) reported from their study of 192 brain injury patients (age 8–88) that, although older patients (over 60) did not have longer periods of coma, they did demonstrate longer confusional states, slower recovery, and worse overall recovery compared with younger patients with equivalent injury severity (as measured by GOS).

Studies at our institution (e.g., Fields 1991) have also included samples of traumatic brain injury patients who are older and more heterogeneous in terms of severity of injury. Our studies were designed to include a large sample of older adults and to control for the variables of severity of head injury, severity of total body injury, and type of injury. Data from our large urban trauma center were accumulated over a 5-year period (1985–1990), with a primary goal of determining the extent to which age contributed to outcome during hospitalization for traumatic brain injury. As can be seen in Table 24–2 our sample included a large population of younger (25–64 [n = 1,867]) and older (65–95 [n = 461]) adults whose injuries spanned the continuum of severity (mild = 67%, moderate = 10%, severe = 23%). In keeping with other studies, age dif-ferences were found for type of injury, but not for severity of head injury (based on GCS) or severity of global injury (based on ISS).

We examined three outcome measures: in hospital mortality, length of hospital stay, and discharge destination. For the sample as a whole (i.e., all ages, all types of injuries, and all levels of severity of injury), a marked age-related increase in risk of death was found, beginning at age 55. In contrast to the finding of Jennett and Teasdale (1981), the in-hospital mortality rates for patients in the three groups between ages 25 and 54 were all stable and approximately 9% overall. The mortality rate, however, was approximately 18% in the subjects 55–64, 23% in those 65–84, and 35% in those 85 and older (Figure 24–4).

Dividing the sample according to whether the injury was mild or severe revealed a relationship between increased age and increased mortality at both levels of severity. As expected, in-hospital mortality for all age groups was greater following severe injuries. However, as can be seen in Figure 24–5, older patients were at greater risk for death following either mild or severe injuries. The mortality rate following "mild" traumatic brain injury (GCS score 13–15) was almost 12% for patients age 75 and older, whereas the corresponding rate for patients 25–54 was only 1.4%.

Age differences were also noted in average length of hospital stay and discharge destination, with older adults more likely to remain hospitalized longer and to return home less often. Although these findings seem to imply that older adults take longer to recover from a traumatic brain injury, the data are not entirely clear. As can be seen in Table 24–3, the mean length of hospital stay for patients returning home and for those who were placed in a nursing home did not differ by

Table 24–2.   Demographics of traumatic brain injury patient sample by age

Variable	Age						
	25–34	**35–44**	**45–54**	**55–64**	**65–74**	**75–84**	**85+**
n patients	907	462	272	226	243	166	52
Sex (%)							
Men	78.4	74.9	69.1	66.8	62.1	48.8	55.8
Women	21.6	25.1	30.9	33.2	37.9	51.2	44.2
Race (%)							
White	90.0	90.5	95.2	94.7	96.7	97.0	90.4
Black	8.5	9.0	3.7	4.4	1.6	1.2	1.9
Other	1.5	0.5	1.1	0.9	1.7	1.8	7.7
Glasgow Coma Scale mean ± SD	12.0 ± 4.7	12.3 ± 4.4	12.2 ± 4.4	11.7 ± 4.3	11.9 ± 4.5	11.9 ± 4.5	11.5 ± 4.6
Injury Severity Scale mean ± SD	18.4 ± 12.7	18.2 ± 12.4	19.0 ± 10.7	20.2 ± 12.0	20.0 ± 12.9	18.2 ± 10.0	19.6 ± 10.4

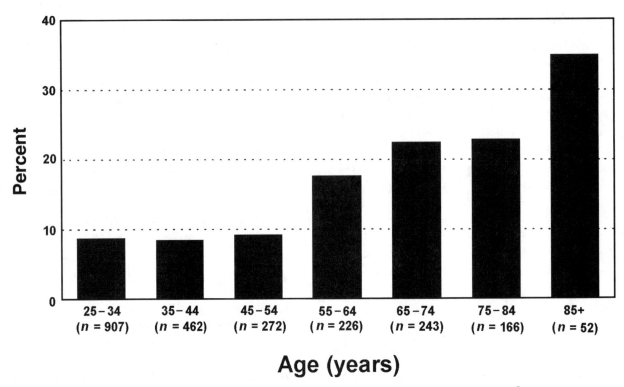

Figure 24–4. Age differences in mortality rate following traumatic brain injury—all levels of severity ($\chi^2 = 87.8$, df = 7, $P < .001$.

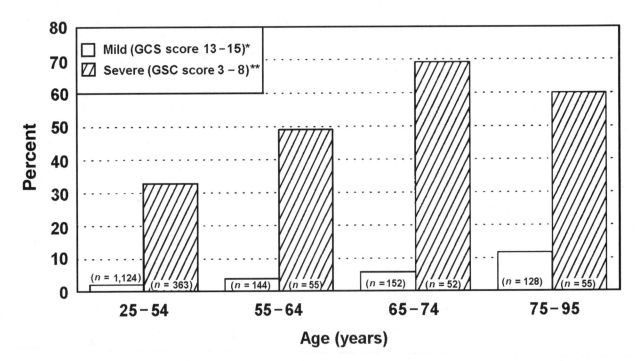

Figure 24–5. Age differences in mortality rate following traumatic brain injury—mild versus severe injuries. GCS = Glasgow Coma Scale (Teasdale and Jennett 1974).
$^*\chi^2 = 50.3$, df = 3, $P < .001$; $^{**}\chi^2 = 36.9$, df = 3, $P < .001$.

age. What did differ was the likelihood of being discharged to different destinations. The average length of stay for elderly brain injury patients was increased relative to those of the younger groups because patients of any age who are discharged to a nursing home stay in hospital longer than do patients who return home and because elderly patients are discharged to nursing homes more often than are younger adults.

Finally, our large sample size allowed a comparison of younger and older adults who sustained injuries of similar type (i.e., motor vehicle accidents and falls) and severity (i.e., mild and severe). In general, the overall pattern of increased risk for negative outcome with age was found in this analysis as well. Equating for type and severity of injury did, however, suggest that these factors need to be taken into account when assessing the influence of age (see Table 24–4). Thus, for example, although mortality rates were higher in the older sample for both types of injuries, the older adult (age 55 and older) mortality rate following a mild head injury due to a motor vehicle accident was 9.4% (versus 1.1% for those 25–54), whereas the mortality rate after a mild head injury due to a fall was 4.1% (versus 2.4% for those 25–54) (Fields 1991).

Neurobehavioral Outcome

Animal studies. One strategy for understanding the factors that contribute to general and neurobehavioral outcome following traumatic brain injury is to use animal models. Most of the experimental literature has focused on the neuropathological changes that are associated with traumatic brain injuries and the course of progression or resolution of these injuries over time. Two paradigms that have gained acceptance in the an-

imal literature are the angular acceleration model and the fluid percussion model (Povlishock and Coburn 1989). These paradigms have been helpful in elucidating the type and extent of axonal injuries that occur following traumatic brain injuries at different levels of severity. Studies have demonstrated that the greater plasticity of an immature central nervous system enhances the ability of very young animals to recover from experimental brain injuries (Finger 1978). To date, however, the effect of advanced age on head injury in animals has received only limited attention (Hamm et al. 1992).

In one study, Hamm et al. (1991) reported that the mortality rate for older rats (20 months) was approximately three times greater than that for younger rats (3 months) following experimentally produced (fluid percussion) "mild" brain injury. Following a more severe fluid percussion brain injury (i.e., "moderate injury") mortality was five times greater among the older rats. Using a similar model, Hamm et al. (1992) also found age-related motoric and cognitive deficits following a lower level (i.e., "mild") fluid percussion brain injury. In this study, weight was used as an index of general health, balance beam performance as an index of motor skill, and the Morris Water Maze Task as an index of cognitive capacity. Older rats (20 months) suffered no general health changes following the injury but did demonstrate significant motoric and cognitive deficits. In contrast, the younger rats (3 months) did not display any postinjury motor deficits and had less severe cognitive deficits than did the older rats.

Behavioral outcome in humans. A number of studies have sought to investigate the presence of specific neurobehavioral symptoms following traumatic brain

Table 24–3. Percentage of survivors discharged to various destinations and length of hospital stay based on discharge destination (by age)

	Age			
	25–54 (*n* = 1,497)	55–64 (*n* = 186)	65–74 (*n* = 188)	75+ (*n* = 161)
Discharge destination for survivors of traumatic brain injury (%)				
Home	78.3	66.6	63.4	57.5
Rehabilitation facility	15.6	25.5	25.3	26.0
Skilled nursing facility	0.9	7.8	11.3	16.4
Length of stay (in days) for patients discharged to:				
Home	8.3	10.5	10.5	10.9
Rehabilitation facility	28.8	33.4	32.8	31.5
Skilled nursing facility	36.1	37.8	37.5	34.8

injuries. In the cognitive domain, mild traumatic brain injuries are generally associated with observable, but time-limited, neuropsychological deficits, particularly in the areas of attention and information processing. For the first week after a single uncomplicated mild brain injury, deficits in selected areas of attention, memory, and higher cognitive processing can be expected (Gentilini et al. 1989; Gronwall 1989b; Ruff et al. 1989b). Most of these deficits resolve within 1 month of the injury, although for some patients recovery of cognitive capacities may take several months and may be related to other neurobehavioral deficits (Bohnen et al. 1992; Ruff et al. 1989b). For example, in a recent 6-month follow-up study of patients who experienced mild traumatic brain injuries, Bohnen et al. (1992) found that patients with postconcussive symptoms performed less well on tests of divided and selective attention than did patients without postconcussive symptoms or healthy control subjects.

Following severe traumatic brain injuries, the presence of cognitive dysfunction is more long lasting (Parker 1990). Persistent deficits in intellectual functioning have been found in most patients following severe traumatic brain injury (Levin et al. 1979a) although the pattern of impairment is not always uniform. For example, Levin et al. (1990) found that although basic language and visuospatial skills had returned to normal 1 year after a severe traumatic brain injury, young adult patients continued to demonstrate memory impairment and slowed information processing.

In general, the pattern of neuropsychological impairment and the potential for recovery following moderate to severe brain injury is dependent on a number of factors including the type, severity, and location of the injury, as well as the individual's premorbid history and postinjury course. With regard to specific cognitive domains, attentional and memory deficits are common sequelae of severe traumatic brain injury. Impairment in speeded and sustained attention is seen most often, but, hemi-inattention, distractibility, and diminished arousal may also be postinjury consequences (Cullum et al. 1990; Gronwall 1987). A reduction in the ability to learn and remember new information is likely following severe traumatic brain injuries, although global amnesias have also been reported (Cullum et al. 1990; Levin et al. 1982). Other neuropsychological deficits that may result from severe diffuse, or focal, brain injuries include psychomotor slowing, language impairment (e.g., word retrieval problems and paraphasic errors), speech impairment

(e.g., dysarthria), nonverbal intellectual processing, and novel problem solving (Cullum et al. 1990; Marquardt et al. 1990).

With regard to affective symptoms, there is a lack of consistent findings in the literature. This inconsistency is probably due to the considerable variability in methodologies used to assess affective changes (e.g., regarding severity of injury, time since injury, definition of symptom, and approach to assessment). For example, studies of depressive symptoms following mild brain injury have found prevalence rates varying from 6% to 39%, and following severe brain injury from 10% to 77% (Silver et al. 1991, 1992). Depressive symptoms are apparently not related to factors such as length of unconsciousness, length of posttraumatic amnesia, or presence of skull fracture (Silver et al. 1992), but may be related to neuropsychological status (Bornstein et al. 1989) and lesion location (Federoff et al. 1992).

Other causes of mood or behavioral change following traumatic brain injury include psychologically based grief or other adjustment-related reactive mood disturbances and neurologically based changes such as apathy, amotivation, slowed cognitive processing, and affective lability (Silver et al. 1991). In addition, whether depressive symptoms predated or caused the head injury (e.g., suicidal car crash) must be taken into account when assessing the role of brain injury in "causing" depression (Silver et al. 1991).

The use of comprehensive assessment procedures and an agreed-on classification system to diagnose mood disturbance (and other neuropsychiatric disor-

Table 24–4. Mortality rates following mild head injury (by age and cause of injury)

Cause of injury	Age		
	35–50	55–70	75–90
Falls			
n subjects	64	79	71
Mean GCS score	14.7	14.7	14.7
Mean ISS score	14.6	14.6	14.3
% died in hospital	3.1	3.8	2.8
Motor vehicle accidents			
n	293	136	50
Mean GCS score	14.8	14.8	14.8
Mean ISS score	14.0	18.9	17.5
% died in hospital	0.3	5.9	10.0

Note. GCS = Glasgow Coma Scale (Teasdale and Jennett 1974); ISS = Injury Severity Scale (Baker et al. 1976).

ders) following traumatic brain injury has been rare (Taylor and Price, in press). Even when structured interviews and specific diagnostic criteria are used, reported prevalence rates vary and depend, in part, on the point at which patients are assessed. For example, in a sample of patients who were assessed during the first year after a traumatic brain injury (Jorge et al. 1993b), the frequency of major depression based on DSM-III (American Psychiatric Association 1980) criteria was 42%, whereas the frequency of major depression among a sample assessed 2–8 years after their injury was 77% (Varney et al. 1987). In both studies, a substantial portion of these patients reported that their depressive symptoms developed at least 3–6 months after the injury (i.e., 39% in the Jorge et al. study and 46% in the Varney et al. study).

Recently, a series of studies took an important step toward clarifying the causes and course of depressive symptoms following traumatic brain injury (Federoff et al. 1992; Jorge et al. 1993a, 1993b). The presence of neurobehavioral disturbance was assessed among 66 young adults on an inpatient trauma service with a structured psychiatric interview (i.e., modified Present State Exam) and scales of depression, cognitive capacity, activities of daily living, and social functioning. Patients were initially evaluated during the acute postinjury period and then reassessed 3, 6, and 12 months later. During the 1-year follow-up period, 42.4% of the patients met DSM-III criteria for major depression (25.7% during the acute period and 16.7% during one of the follow-up examinations). Both the "acute-" and "delayed-" onset depression patients had a higher frequency of previous psychiatric problems and impaired social functioning than did the nondepressed patients, but these groups also differed on a number of other dimensions. Lesions in the left frontal region (particularly left dorsolateral frontal and/or left basal ganglia) were associated with major depression among the acute-onset depression patients only. In contrast, patients with delayed-onset depression had significantly poorer social functioning, but less severe depression and less impairment in activities of daily living than did the acute-onset group. Based on these findings, Jorge et al. (1993b) suggested that acute-onset depression may be more related to biological changes in an injured brain, whereas delayed-onset depression may be more psychologically based.

Regarding other symptoms of mood disturbance, manic symptoms occur less frequently than do depressive symptoms following traumatic brain injury (Silver

et al. 1992) and have been associated with right-hemisphere lesions (Starkstein et al. 1988, 1990). Reports of the frequency of postinjury anxiety symptoms have varied considerably, apparently depending on severity of injury and source of information (Silver et al. 1992). Family members of patients who experience severe brain injuries reported that 60% of these patients displayed increased anxiety (McKinlay et al. 1981), whereas two studies (Dikmen et al. 1986; Schoenhuber and Gentilini 1988) found no increased self-report of anxiety symptoms among patients following a mild brain injury. Anxiety symptoms may also occur solely as a result of the experience of being involved in a traumatic event. Patients who sustain mild traumatic brain injuries may be more vulnerable to the development of symptoms of posttraumatic stress disorder. They are, for example, better able to recall the events surrounding the injury than are patients whose injuries are severe and, as a result, may be at greater risk for intrusive distressing recollections.

Jennett and Teasdale (1981) found personality changes in approximately two-thirds of patients who sustained severe brain injuries. Changes that are commonly associated with traumatic brain injury include impulsivity, irritability, diminished drive, altered frustration tolerance, agitation, aggression, and impaired social judgment (Bigler 1991; Jennett and Teasdale 1981; Silver et al. 1987). In general, neurobehavioral symptoms differ based on injury severity. Following severe traumatic brain injuries, long-term changes in personality and behavior, as well as mood, are common (Bigler 1991; Parker 1990; Prigatano 1992; Richardson 1990). Frequently, some of these problems occur, or become exacerbated, several months after the injury when rehabilitation ends, attempts to return to work fail, and family members become stressed or frustrated by the continuing disruption in their lives. Behavioral and personality changes (rather than cognitive deficits) are typically the most distressing to family members (Oddy et al. 1978).

Neurobehavioral sequelae, including postconcussive symptoms, are also common following mild traumatic brain injuries (Binder 1986; Bohnen and Jolles 1992). These symptoms however, may not be as short lived as the neuropsychological deficits (Middelboe et al. 1992) and may develop some time after the injury. For example, Rutherford (1989) described early (e.g., headache, dizziness, vomiting, nausea, drowsiness, and blurred vision) and late (e.g., headache, dizziness, irritability, anxiety, depression, concentration/memory deficits, sleep disturbance, and fatigue) postconcussive symptomatology following mild traumatic brain injury. Although the development of postconcussive symptoms occurs independent of litigation status, (Merskey and Woodforde 1972; Steadman and Graham 1970), several factors including pending litigation, preinjury personality, length of posttraumatic amnesia, alcohol use, fault for injury, and social network, all must be evaluated when assessing the relationship between a traumatic brain injury and late postconcussive symptomatology (Alexander 1992; Rutherford 1989). In addition, age appears to be a contributing factor, as increased postconcussive symptoms have been reported by older patients 6 weeks (Rutherford et al. 1977) and 1 year (Rutherford et al. 1979) after a brain injury. Finally, psychotic symptoms have also been reported to be more common following severe traumatic brain injuries than in the general population (Achté et al. 1991; Thomsen 1984).

Anatomic correlates of behavioral disorders.   Both location and severity of brain injury affect the ensuing constellation of symptoms. Left-hemisphere damage has been associated with generalized cognitive dysfunction, whereas right-hemisphere damage has been linked to more specific visuospatial deficits (Bigler et al. 1981). Bifrontal injuries are associated with deficits in attention, memory, and "executive" functions, as well as with changes in personality and behavior (Levin et al. 1991). Lesions in the orbitofrontal area have been linked to a behavioral dyscontrol syndrome that includes disinhibition, impulsivity, emotional lability, hyperactivity, and diminished awareness or concern for the implications of one's behavior (Cummings 1985; Gualtieri 1991; Mattson and Levin 1990). Lesions in other areas of the frontal lobes have been associated with perseveration, apathy, indifference, amotivation, and abulia (Lewis et al. 1992; Taylor and Price, in press). Temporal lobe injuries have been associated with memory deficits, emotional lability, mania, and delusions (Gualtieri 1991). Finally, as noted above, there is recent evidence that depression during the acute postinjury phase may be more common following injuries that cause left anterior brain damage (Jorge et al. 1993a).

Neurobehavioral outcome in the elderly.   The assessment of neurobehavioral outcome following traumatic brain injury in older adults presents special problems. Normal aging results in changes in many of the speeded attentional and memory capacities that are assessed in postinjury neuropsychological test batteries. As Gronwall (1989a) pointed out, comparing the performances of younger and older brain injury patients will be misleading if only "raw" scores are used. A more appropriate strategy would be to use measures of the departure from age norms as an index of impairment. Age-appropriate control groups should also be used when comparing symptom checklists, as apparent age differences in symptomatology may also simply be a reflection of base rate differences in older patients.

The few studies of brain injury that have reported age-related differences in outcome variables such as depression (Cartlidge and Shaw 1981) have generally not addressed these methodological issues. In addition, conclusions have frequently been drawn from relatively small samples of older subjects. For example, return to work has been reported to be slower in "older" brain injury patients since the 1930s (Russell 1934), yet, not all studies have supported this conclusion (e.g., Uzell et al. 1987), and this variable is obviously of limited validity in a retirement-age group. Similarly, Rutherford (1989) reported a trend toward increased postconcussive symptoms in a group of brain injury patients above age 40, even though the pattern of results was actually curvilinear: both the 20 or younger group and the 40 or older group reported more symptoms (13% and 24%, respectively) than did the 20–39 group (6%) 1 year after a mild brain injury.

Neuropsychological test performance may be differentially affected in older patients following head injury. Gronwall (1989b) compared the performance of patients in their 40s with patients in their 20s on a test of speeded attentional processing at 1, 4, and 8 weeks after a mild traumatic brain injury. One week after the injury, no age differences were found. Although both groups demonstrated improvement over time, by 8 weeks the performance of the younger group was significantly better than that of the older group. Whether this difference represents a differential rate of recovery or a return to an age-appropriate baseline was not reported. In another recent study, Goldstein et al. (1993) compared the performance of patients above age 50 who had sustained mild to moderate injuries with age-matched control subjects. Patients demonstrated significantly poorer performance on tests of effortful processing under timed conditions, recall of visual and verbal material, and inferences of similarities.

In a preliminary attempt to assess the natural history of posttraumatic brain injury complaints among geriatric patients, Fields et al. (1993) compared younger (18–45 [$n = 139$]) and older (50–95 [$n = 49$]) patients 1 and 4 months after mild to moderate traumatic brain injury (i.e., GCS score 9–15). The Posttraumatic Neurobehavioral Screening Inventory (PTNSI), a questionnaire that assesses symptoms commonly reported following traumatic brain injury, was used in this study (see Appendix 24–1).[1] One hundred eighty-eight patients completed the PTNSI during their first outpatient trauma clinic visit, which took place approximately 1 month after their injury. Approximately 3 months later, 79 (42%) of these patients (ages 18–45 [$n = 54$]; 50–95 [$n = 25$]) could be reached by telephone, at which time the PTNSI was readministered.

The two age groups were found not to differ in terms of severity of head injury (based on GCS scores) or total body injury (based on ISS scores). One month after the injury, neurobehavioral complaints were common among both younger and older patients. The symptom profiles for the two age groups were generally similar, although the younger patients endorsed significantly more symptoms of posttraumatic stress disorder, whereas the older patients reported more fatigue. When reevaluated 4 months after their brain injury, however, more age-related differences were present (Table 24–5). The older patients endorsed more fatigue, difficulty processing information, dysphoric mood, dizziness, and sensitivity to noise than did the younger patients. Most striking was the apparent age-by-time interaction noted for the posttraumatic stress disorder, cognitive, and behavioral subscales. The older sample reported greater distress in these areas at 4 months than they had at 1 month, whereas the younger sample reported decreased distress on all of the subscales across the same time period. Although preliminary, these findings suggest that the course of neurobehavioral recovery following traumatic brain injury in elderly patients may be different, and worse, than in younger patients.

To summarize, severity of injury is the best predictor of general outcome following traumatic brain injury. With regard to the differential vulnerability hypothesis, recent studies lend support to the long-standing belief that the variable of age plays a role in mediating outcome. Although important, age accounts for much less variance than do other variables when predicting outcome. Factors that determine increased individual risk within the elderly population have not been identified.

Diagnosis and Management of Posttraumatic Neurobehavioral Sequelae

The neurobehavioral assessment and treatment of patients who sustain traumatic brain injuries will be more straightforward once diagnosis becomes more accurate, double-blind medication trials for specific syndromes have been completed, and the role of factors, such as age, in mediating response to treatment is understood. Until then, the literature suggests a number of potential principles that may provide guides for developing assessment and treatment strategies.

Diagnosis

The diagnosis of a psychiatric disturbance in patients with brain dysfunction is often problematic (Coffey 1987; Ross and Rush 1981). For example, valid and reliable historical information may be difficult to obtain in patients with language deficits (e.g., aphasia) or neglect syndromes (e.g., unawareness or denial or ill-

Table 24–5. Age differences in symptom report at 1 month and 4 months following traumatic brain injury using the Posttraumatic Neurobehavioral Screening Inventory (PTNSI)

Symptom	Percentage of sample endorsing symptom		
	Age 18–45	Age 50–95	P
1 month	($n = 139$)	($n = 49$)	
Fatigue	48.6	66.0	< .05
4 months	($n = 54$)	($n = 25$)	
Fatigue	30.9	72.0	< .001
Difficulty processing information	12.0	44.0	< .005
Dysphoric mood	20.1	45.8	< .05
Dizziness	5.4	24.0	< .05
Sensitivity to noise	5.4	20.0	< .05

---

[1] The PTNSI was developed at our institute to screen a large trauma patient population for neuropsychiatric symptoms. It assesses six symptom domains: cognitive, mood, behavior, psychosis, postconcussive symptoms, and symptoms of posttraumatic stress disorder.

ness). In addition, brain disorders may distort the signs and symptoms of psychiatric disturbances (e.g., complaints of hopelessness and helplessness secondary to depression may appear unconvincing in a patient with aprosody). Behavioral disturbances that result from traumatic brain injury may be misdiagnosed as a psychiatric disorder, or, conversely, the behavioral disturbances that often accompany psychiatric illness may be mistakenly attributed to a brain disorder (e.g., psychomotor retardation of depression attributed to posttraumatic parkinsonism). These difficulties in recognizing psychiatric illness in patients with traumatic brain injury impede efforts to determine the neuroanatomical correlates of behavior and may lead to inappropriate diagnosis and treatment.

Diagnostic process and tools. Accurate diagnosis requires an understanding of the neurobehavioral sequelae and the course of recovery of traumatic injuries of different types, locations, and severities (Taylor and Price, in press). In addition, because there are multiple possible causes of neurobehavioral symptoms, the evaluation of the patient with a traumatic brain injury needs to include a review of prior head trauma, developmental and academic history, occupational history, and social history, as well as a comprehensive psychiatric, medical, neurological, and substance abuse assessment (Taylor and Price, in press). Because discrepancies between the reports of patients and families are common following traumatic brain injury (Oddy et al. 1985), the importance of collateral history from relatives and hospital records is also critical.

With these general guidelines in mind, the assessment of specific disorders may require flexible strategies. Regarding the assessment of depression, for example, Ross and Rush (1981) suggested that in addition to obtaining history from the patient and a reliable informant, clinical cues such as a complicated recovery from the brain injury, multiple "vegetative signs" of depression, atypical emotional outbursts, aprosody, and an abrupt deterioration in the patient's neurological status can be used to make a diagnosis. Among elderly patients, additional factors that must be considered include the presence of systemic medical conditions, preexisting neurodegenerative disorders, and possible developmental changes in the phenomenology of depressive symptoms related to aging (Caine et al. 1993).

The labor intensive process of comprehensive assessment is further complicated by the lack of assessment tools and an inadequate classification system. Although current psychiatric diagnostic systems provide a useful starting point for studying patients with traumatic brain injuries, it is quite possible that neuropsychiatric symptomatology following such injuries may be better classified by other approaches. For example, the "bottom up" approach of the Schedules for Clinical Assessment in Neuropsychiatry (SCAN; World Health Organization 1992) is promising in that it assesses the presence and severity of a comprehensive list of symptoms rather than (or in addition to) the traditional method of establishing a specific diagnosis. This approach allows for the generation of clusters of symptoms that may have clinical significance but that do not meet diagnostic criteria.

A related issue pertains to the limits of the current diagnostic classification system for patients with neuropsychiatric disorders. Following traumatic brain injuries, patients may have an identifiable pattern of symptoms, but may not meet criteria for a DSM-IV disorder (American Psychiatric Association 1994). Furthermore, even when diagnostic criteria are met, it may be difficult to determine whether the brain disease is causal of the neuropsychiatric symptoms. Such etiologic judgments may at times be unreliable and invalid, and it has been suggested that Axis I diagnoses such as major depression be kept purely phenomenological, with relevant causal or contributory organic factors identified on Axis III (Fogel 1991).

Imaging. An improved diagnostic classification system for patients with traumatic brain injuries will ultimately depend on the sensitivity of neuropsychiatric and neuropsychological assessment instruments and the correlation between these measures and neuroradiological indices of brain structure and function. Brain imaging is critical for the assessment of most patients who sustain traumatic brain injury. CT scanning remains the most widely used technology and is the modality of choice for assessing the presence of skull fractures and hemorrhage in the acute (1–3 days) posttrauma period (Chakares and Bryan 1986; Taylor and Price, in press; Yoshino and Seeger 1989).

Brain magnetic resonance imaging (MRI) is more sensitive than CT for the assessment of parenchymal damage, including the diffuse axonal "shear" lesions (Alavi 1989; Levin et al. 1985; Levin et al. 1987a; Taylor and Price, in press). MRI also provides a better view of brain tissue adjacent to the skull (e.g., inferior frontal regions and temporal lobes), because, unlike CT, it is not subject to beam-hardening artifact. However, because MRI does not image bone, it is not helpful in assessing possible fractures, nor can MRI be used in patients attached to metal respirators or in those who have metal fragments (e.g., bullets or shrapnel) in their heads. Increased sensitivity of MRI to the presence of brain lesions is particularly apparent among patients with mild to moderate traumatic brain injuries (Levin et al. 1992) and follow-up MRI studies have been shown to be more predictive of eventual outcome than are acute studies for some patients (Wilson et al. 1988). Of course, structural brain imaging studies of elderly patients must be interpreted within the context of changes that occur with normal aging (see Chapter 9, this volume).

Metabolic brain imaging studies (e.g., regional cerebral blood flow [rCBF], single photon emission computerized tomography [SPECT], and positron-emission tomography [PET]) have not yet found a role in the routine assessment of patients with traumatic brain injury. Cerebral blood flow and metabolism are reduced acutely after brain injury, and the degree of metabolic suppression may be related to the severity of injury (Fieschi et al. 1974; Obrist et al. 1979). Metabolic imaging techniques appear to be more sensitive than either CT or MRI in detecting areas of brain abnormalities after traumatic brain injury (Alavi 1989; Alavi et al. 1986; Langfitt et al. 1986; Ruff et al. 1989a), and such abnormalities correlate more closely with neuropsychological performance postinjury than do the structural changes seen on CT or MRI (Ruff et al. 1989a). The clinical use of these metabolic imaging techniques and their particular characteristics in elderly patients must await further research.

Management

Early considerations.   Based on age-related differences in the occurrence, pathophysiology, and sequelae of traumatic brain injury in elderly individuals, Fogel and Duffy (1994) recommended guidelines for the acute and subacute assessment and treatment of older adults. In the acute postinjury phase, these recommendations include increased vigilance regarding possible early or delayed vascular complications (e.g., subdural hematoma and intracranial hemorrhage); identification and management of neuropsychiatric comorbidities (e.g., preexisting cognitive impairment, depression, and alcoholism); and ongoing monitoring of neuropsychiatric status if other medical problems

predominate (e.g., serial assessment of mental status or functional capacity during treatment for orthopedic injuries). In the postacute phase, neuropsychiatric input is recommended for determining capacity to benefit from formal rehabilitation (e.g., based on degree of cognitive impairment, as well as physical deficits); assessing and managing functional deficits (e.g., capacity to take medication, live independently, or drive); and treating the neurobehavioral and psychosocial consequences of the traumatic brain injury (Fogel and Duffy 1994).

Pharmacological strategies.   Despite an absence of double-blind placebo-controlled medication trials for neuropsychiatric sequelae of traumatic brain injury, a number of studies offer suggestions for treatment, as well as avenues for further research. Two recent reviews of the literature (Dubovsky 1992; Silver et al. 1992) make several general points regarding the pharmacological treatment of younger and older adults with neuropsychiatric symptoms. First, until therapeutic interventions are able to limit the initial brain damage from the traumatic injury, a primary role for medication will be to control certain target symptoms such as depression, anergia, mania, mood lability, agitation, anxiety, psychosis, and aggression (Silver et al. 1992). Control of such symptoms will have the additional beneficial effect of increasing the patient's capacity to participate in other ongoing therapies, including psychotherapy and cognitive rehabilitation (Silver et al. 1992).

Second, patients who have experienced traumatic brain injuries and patients who are elderly may be more sensitive to the therapeutic effects of many psychotropic medications including heterocyclic antidepressants, monoamine oxidase inhibitors, lithium, antianxiety agents, and neuroleptics (Dubovsky 1992; Silver et al. 1992). As a result, starting with lower doses, titrating medications in smaller increments, and ultimately using lower maintenance doses have been recommended (Dubovsky 1992; Silver et al. 1992).

Third, a similar increase in sensitivity to side effects can be expected among patients who have acquired brain lesions or who are elderly. Sedative and anticholinergic side effects are of particular concern (Dubovsky 1992; Silver et al. 1992). Other side effects include the risk of lowering seizure threshold among patients with traumatic brain injury (Silver et al. 1992) and the risk of cardiovascular changes among elderly patients (Dubovsky 1992). To date, the extent to which the interaction between a traumatic brain injury and an older brain alters sensitivity to medication is not known.

One example of the process of balancing efficacy with the possible complications associated with pharmacotherapy after brain injury concerns the treatment of depressive and anergic-abulic states. As noted above, one important limiting factor in this type of treatment is the risk of lowering seizure threshold in patients who are already at greater risk for seizures because of their brain injury (Silver et al. 1991; Silver et al. 1992). Tricyclic antidepressants, for example, have been reported to increase the likelihood of seizures after severe brain injuries (Wroblewski et al. 1990), whereas methylphenidate apparently does not (Wroblewski et al. 1992). Therefore, methylphenidate may be a superior agent in retarded depressive and apathetic states following brain injury.

Although modest improvement in depressive symptoms has been reported among patients with traumatic brain injuries following trials of tricyclic antidepressants, carbamazepine (Varney et al. 1987), and fluoxetine (Cassidy 1989), other studies have had less optimistic results. Dinan and Mobayed (1992), for example, reported improvement in depressive symptoms in only 4 of 13 patients who met DSM-III criteria for depression and who were treated with amitriptyline after a mild traumatic brain injury. In contrast, 11 of the 13 patients with "functional" DSM-III depression in this study improved with the same treatment. Similarly, Saran (1985) found no significant improvement in mood in a sample of patients with mild brain injuries who were treated with phenelzine or amitriptyline. These studies are consistent with the hypothesis that traumatic brain injuries may alter the responsiveness of the brain to traditional methods of pharmacotherapy (Dinan and Mobayed 1992).

Variability in responsiveness to treatment for depression across studies may be due to several factors including differences in degree of structural brain changes (Coffey et al. 1989) and differences in diagnostic criteria (Silver et al. 1991). It is also possible that different subtypes of depression exist among this population. For example, Silver et al. (1991) hypothesized that depressive symptoms related to strokelike focal disruption of neurotransmitter receptors may be more responsive to reuptake inhibitors than those symptoms that may be caused by the release of neurotoxins during more diffuse and severe injuries. Similarly, as discussed above, Jorge et al. (1993b) proposed subtypes of

depression based, in part, on the point at which symptoms develop (i.e., early-onset depression was associated with lesion location and delayed-onset depression with social factors). Until issues relating to diagnostic subtypes have been resolved and effective treatment strategies have been established, the focus of pharmacotherapy for posttraumatic neuropsychiatric disorders among elderly patients will remain the application of conventional treatment strategies for symptom management. (This topic is reviewed in Chapter 29 in this volume and by Fogel and Duffy [1994].)

Psychotherapeutic strategies.   For most of this century, a brain injury was considered to be an exclusionary criterion for psychotherapy. However, a number of authors have now argued convincingly for the role of psychotherapy following traumatic brain injury (Cicerone 1991; Lewis 1991; Lewis et al. 1992; Prigatano 1991a; Prigatano and Klonoff 1990). As with pharmacological strategies, this literature has focused on younger patients and lacks well-controlled studies.

In a review of the literature, Starratt and Fields (1991) suggested that two major themes are consistently emphasized by those conducting psychotherapy with brain injured patients: 1) maintenance of self-identity and self-esteem in the face of loss and 2) the management of anxiety and affect. Attempts to adjust to the emotional dysregulation and to the cognitive, physical, vocational, and interpersonal losses that often accompany traumatic brain injury are complicated by factors such as embarrassment, guilt, and premorbid attitudes and beliefs about persons with disabilities. The process of therapy, therefore, includes efforts to help patients understand their changed experience of the world, to facilitate the process of mourning over personal and other losses, and to promote adaptation to different types of existence (Lewis et al. 1992).

Although psychotherapeutic strategies for brain injury patients range from psychoanalytic to social learning and behavioral, a common denominator has been the need to depart from traditional approaches (Forrest 1992). The importance of this point cannot be overstated as the demands and process of traditional psychotherapy can clearly make some patients more distressed. Prigatano et al. (1988), for example, warned of increased paranoia among delusional patients with brain injury in "insight-oriented" groups and of behavior modification programs that may be perceived by patients as overly intrusive or controlling.

Based on the degree to which brain injury patients

are able to tolerate individual therapy sessions, the length, frequency, and location of these sessions may need to be modified. Barth and Boll (1981) suggested a number of such modifications. First, the behavior of brain injury patients should not necessarily be equated with that of other therapy patients. For example, failure to keep an appointment may reflect a cognitive deficit rather than "avoidance."

Second, the type(s) of therapy will differ based on the nature and the severity of the injury. Some patients with significant cognitive and memory deficits may have limited awareness of their deficits (Prigatano 1991b) and may become increasingly distressed when confronted with their impairments (e.g., patients with frontal lobe lesions who demonstrate "catastrophic" reactions during challenging neuropsychological testing). Others may be able to identify their deficits, but may not have the executive functioning capacities necessary to deal with them in an insight-oriented manner and, as a result, may become overwhelmed by this approach. Psychoeducational approaches are often helpful in providing the context for promoting postinjury adjustment, but all approaches should be tailored to the needs and resources of the individual patient. Insight-oriented, interpersonal, supportive, and cognitive approaches may be useful with patients whose relatively mild injuries have resulted in narcissistic injuries, survival guilt, and adjustment disorders. In contrast, behavioral approaches may be more applicable for patients with significant cognitive impairment who display more severe behavioral disruption.

Third, the timing of the intervention is important. Early in the postinjury period, patients may deny or may be unaware of the existence of neurobehavioral problems and may resist treatment. Fourth, the pace of therapy may need to be slower with more frequent sessions. Finally, establishing goals for therapy may be different with brain injury patients. Rather than seeking a complete resolution of conflicts, more appropriate goals such as increasing tolerance for frustration, improving acceptance of deficits, and establishing contingency plans for daily stressors may be necessary (Starratt and Fields 1991).

Psychotherapy with older adults who have sustained traumatic brain injuries is similar to psychotherapy with older adults who have experienced other types of physical or cognitive losses. Like patients with traumatic brain injuries, some patients who have had strokes or signs of early dementia are distressed by their losses, whereas others have limited awareness of these changes in functioning. Dealing with issues such as loss, mortality, financial concerns, environment change, and unresolved personal and family matters are common among older adults in distress. Among those patients who are less distressed, the focus of intervention is typically on the caregiver who may experience both the burden of caregiving and the loss of emotional support from the injured patient. A number of "barriers" exist that limit the use of mental health services by elderly individuals (Gatz et al. 1985). These barriers include those related to the patients themselves (e.g., lack of psychological sophistication and importance of self-reliance), their therapists (e.g., ageist stereotypes, countertransference issues, and economic considerations), and their environments (e.g., travel and accessibility of buildings).

Rehabilitation and family considerations. Because traumatic brain injuries often result in neurological dysfunction, involvement in rehabilitation (i.e., physical therapy, occupational therapy, and speech therapy) is frequently an essential component of the postinjury treatment process. Deficits in physical functioning (e.g., hemiparesis), perception (e.g., hemianopsia), motor planning (e.g., apraxia), and communication (e.g., dysarthria and aphasia) may occur after brain injury and may impact on a patient's capacity to function independently and to benefit from traditional psychotherapeutic techniques. Similarly, postinjury changes in mood (e.g., depression), behavior (e.g., impulse control), or cognitive processing (e.g., attention and memory) can reduce participation in rehabilitation. Thus as noted above, neuropsychiatric consultation for patients in rehabilitation settings is often required, and progress in rehabilitation may be an important marker of psychiatric improvement.

The treatment of patients with traumatic brain injuries must also take into account the resources of the patient's social support network. Involvement with the family may need to include psychoeducational approaches, stress management, and episodic or prolonged grief therapy. Such involvement also needs to take into account the specific neurobehavioral deficits of the patient. For example, patients whose frontotemporal injuries affect their capacity to tolerate frustration, learn new information, and deal with ambiguity may do better if families provide them with highly structured, predictable, and low-stress environments. In contrast, patients with frontal or right-hemisphere lesions who are anergic and may not perceive, or who misperceive, subtle nuances of verbal and nonverbal communication may do better when family members exaggerate facial expression and voice quality to increase the likelihood that they are understood accurately. Among elderly patients, intervention strategies such as these become problematic when social support systems are limited in size or capacity (e.g., spouse with dementia).

Future Directions

The supposition that an older brain is more vulnerable to the effects to a traumatic injury is a reasonable one and fits with common notions of changes that occur with age. However, the literature discussed above suggests that there is not a simple linear relationship between age and negative outcome. Future studies in this area will need to delineate the factors that increase the risk of specific groups of elderly patients to negative outcome after traumatic brain injury.

Two lines of research may be helpful in this regard. First, the study of aging among healthy elderly individuals (e.g., Coffey et al. 1992) may provide information about the factors that increase risks or, alternatively, provide "protection" from negative consequences after traumatic brain injury. For example, several chapters in this volume present data on neurobiological changes that occur across the normal lifespan. The observations that structural changes become most noteworthy after age 55 and that the mortality rate following traumatic brain injury also dramatically increases after age 55 suggests a potential relationship that is worthy of additional research (see below). In addition, studies suggesting age-related changes in catecholamine and excitatory amino acid neurotransmitter function may be helpful in explaining age differences in outcome after traumatic brain injury (Fogel and Duffy 1994).

Second, a number of investigators have proposed models to explain increased vulnerability based on presumed brain capacity. Constructs such as "cognitive reserve capacity" (Baltes et al. 1992), "brain reserve capacity," and "threshold for functional impairment" (Satz 1991) have been used to account for differential outcome among elderly or brain injury patients. In his review of this literature, Satz (1991) suggested a threshold theory in which vulnerability factors (e.g., prior brain injury or aggregate brain lesions) and protective factors (e.g., higher level of general intelligence and

education) determine the threshold at which functional impairment occurs following a brain injury. Severe injuries will produce impairment regardless of brain reserve capacity; milder insults, however, will produce functional impairment based on the threshold for a specific individual. In one empirical test of this theory, we (Fields and Coffey, in press) found a significant relationship between ventricular enlargement (on CT) and functional capacity at the time of discharge in a sample of older adults (55–90 [$n = 36$]) who were hospitalized after a mild head injury. Although preliminary, this work suggests that measures of presumed premorbid brain integrity (e.g., CT and MRI) may have a role as possible markers of vulnerability or negative outcome among older patients after a traumatic brain injury.

Summary

Epidemiological studies consistently document age-related differences in the pattern of occurrence of traumatic brain injury. These injuries are a relatively common phenomenon among elderly patients and are most often the result of a fall. In addition, it appears that in comparison to younger adults, traumatic brain injury in elderly individuals is associated with fewer gender differences and more severe injuries. Research in the area of global outcome after brain injury also supports the long-held belief that elderly patients are at greater risk for negative outcome and that age plays an independent role in mediating outcome. In terms of in-hospital mortality, hospital length of stay, discharge destination, and other measures of long-term outcome, older adults generally fare worse than younger adults even after controlling for injury severity. However, not all elderly patients do worse, and the factors that contribute to the increased risk for any particular older adult have not been identified.

Very little is known about the neuropsychiatric sequelae of traumatic brain injury and their treatment in elderly patients. There is preliminary evidence that the course of neurobehavioral recovery may be worse among older adults. However, studies have rarely taken into account age differences in neuropsychological test performance and symptom reporting. Similarly, the treatment of older patients who sustain traumatic brain injuries is in its infancy. Principles such as 1) increased sensitivity to side effects, 2) altered responsiveness to treatment, 3) reduced seizure threshold, and 4) consideration of nontraditional pharmacological and psychotherapeutic strategies may all be useful guides. Finally, a number of areas of research (including the neurology of normal aging and studies of diminished brain reserved capacity) are under way that may increase our understanding of the neuropsychiatry of traumatic brain injury in elderly patients and may help to identify which elderly patients are at risk for negative outcome.

References

Achté K, Jarho L, Kyykka T, et al: Paranoid disorders following war brain damage: preliminary report. Psychopathology 24:309–315, 1991

Adamovich BB, Henderson JA, Averbach S: Cognitive Rehabilitation of Closed Head Injured Patients. San Diego, CA, College Hill Press, 1985

Adams JH: The autopsy in fatal non-missile head injuries, in Neuropathology (Current Topics in Pathology, Vol 76). Edited by Berry CL. Berlin, Springer-Verlag, 1988, pp 1–22

Adams JH, Mitchell DE, Graham DI, et al: Diffuse brain damage of immediate impact type. Brain 100:489–502, 1977

Adams JH, Graham DI, Murray LS, et al: Diffuse axonal injury due to nonmissile head injury in humans: an analysis of 45 cases. Ann Neurol 12:557–563, 1982

Adams JH, Doyle D, Ford I, et al: Diffuse axonal injury in head injury: definition, diagnosis and grading. Histopathology 15:49–59, 1989

Alavi A: Functional and anatomic studies of head injury. J Neuropsychiatry Clin Neurosci 1 (suppl):S45–S50, 1989

Alavi A, Langfitt T, Fazekas F, et al: Correlation studies of head trauma with PET, MRI, and XCT. J Nucl Med 27:919–920, 1986

Alexander MP: Traumatic brain injury, in Psychiatric Aspects of Neurologic Disease, Vol II. Edited by Benson DF, Blumer D. New York, Grune & Stratton, 1982, pp 219–249

Alexander MP: Neuropsychiatric correlates of persistent postconcussive syndrome. Journal of Head Trauma Rehabilitation 7:60–69, 1992

Alexandre A, Colombo F, Nertempi P, et al: Cognitive outcome and early indices of severity of head injury. J Neurosurg 59:751–761, 1983

Amacher AL, Bybee DE: Toleration of head injury by the elderly. Neurosurgery 20:954–958, 1987

American Association for Automotive Medicine: Abbreviated Injury Scale (AIS), 1985 Revision. Arlington Heights, IL, American Association for Automotive Medicine, 1985

American Psychiatric Association: Diagnostic and Statistical Manual of Mental Disorders, 3rd Edition. Washington, DC, American Psychiatric Association, 1980

American Psychiatric Association: Diagnostic and Statistical Manual of Mental Disorders, 4th Edition. Washington, DC, American Psychiatric Association, 1994

Annegers JF, Grabow JD, Groover RV, et al: Seizures after head trauma: a population study. Neurology 30:683–689, 1980a

Annegers JF, Grabow JD, Kurland LT, et al: The incidence, causes, and secular trend of head trauma in Olmsted County, Minnesota, 1935–1974. Neurology 30:912–919, 1980b

Bachman DL: The diagnosis and management of common neurologic sequelae of closed head injury. Journal of Head Trauma Rehabilitation 7:50–59, 1992

Baker SP, O'Neil B, Haddon WJ, et al: The injury severity score: a method of describing patients with multiple injuries and evaluating emergency care. J Trauma 14:187–196, 1976

Baltes MM, Kuhl KP, Sowarka D: Testing for limits of cognitive reserve capacity: a promising strategy for early diagnosis of dementia? J Gerontol 47(3):P165–P167, 1992

Barth JT, Boll TJ: Rehabilitation and treatment of central nervous system dysfunction: a behavioral medicine perspective, in Medical Psychology: Contributions to Behavioral Medicine. Edited by Prokop CP, Bradley LA. New York, Academic Press, 1981, pp 241–266

Barth JT, Macciocchi SN, Giordani B, et al: Neuropsychological sequelae of minor head injury. Neurosurgery 13:529–533, 1983

Becker DP, Verity MA, Povlishock J, et al: Brain cellular injury and recovery: horizons for improving medical therapies in stroke and trauma. West J Med 148:670–684, 1988

Ben Yishay Y, Silver SM, Piasetsky E, et al: Relationship between employability and vocational outcome after intensive holistic cognitive rehabilitation. Journal of Head Trauma Rehabilitation 2:35–48, 1987

Bigler ED: Neuropathology of traumatic brain injury, in Traumatic Brain Injury. Edited by Bigler ED. Austin, TX, Pro-Ed, 1990a, pp 13–49

Bigler ED: Traumatic Brain Injury. Austin, TX, Pro-Ed, 1990b

Bigler ED: Diagnostic Clinical Neuropsychology. Austin, TX, University of Texas Press, 1991

Bigler ED, Steinman DS, Newton JS: Clinical assessment of cognitive deficit in neurologic disorder, II: cerebral trauma. Clinical Neuropsychology 3:13–18, 1981

Binder LM: Persisting symptoms after mild head injury: a review of the postconcussive syndrome. J Clin Exp Neuropsychol 8:323–346, 1986

Bohnen N, Jolles J: Neurobehavioral aspects of postconcussive symptoms after mild head injury. J Nerv Ment Dis 180:683–692, 1992

Bohnen N, Jolles J, Twijnstra A: Neuropsychological deficits in patients with persistent symptoms six months after mild head injury. Neurosurgery 30:692–696, 1992

Bornstein RA, Miller HB, Van Schoor JT: Neuropsychological deficit and emotional disturbance in head-injured patients. J Neurosurg 70:509–513, 1989

Broderick JP, Brott T, Tomsick T, et al: Intracerebral hemorrhage more than twice as common as subarachnoid hemorrhage. J Neurosurg 78:188–191, 1993

Caine ED, Lyness JM, King DA: Reconsidering depression in the elderly. Am J Geriatr Psychiatry 1:4–20, 1993

Carlsson CA, vonEssen C, Lofgren J: Factors affecting the clinical course of patients with severe head injuries. J Neurosurg 29:242–251, 1968

Cartlidge NEF, Shaw DA: Head Injury. London, WB Saunders, 1981

Cassidy JW: Fluoxetine: a new serotonergically active antidepressant. Journal of Head Trauma Rehabilitation 4:67–69, 1989

Chakares DW, Bryan RN: Acute subarachnoid hemorrhage: in vitro comparison of MRI and CT. American Journal of Neuroradiology 7:223–228, 1986

Cicerone KD: Psychotherapy after mild traumatic brain injury: relation to the nature and severity of subjective complaints. Journal of Head Trauma Rehabilitation 6(4):30–43, 1991

Coffey CE: Cerebral laterality and emotion: the neurology of depression. Compr Psychiatry 28:197–219, 1987

Coffey CE, Figiel GS, Djang WT, et al: Subcortical white matter hyperintensity on magnetic resonance imaging: clinical and neuroanatomic correlates. J Neuropsychiatry Clin Neurosci 1:135–144, 1989

Coffey CE, Wilkinson WE, Parashos IA, et al: Quantative cerebral anatomy of the aging human brain: a cross-sectional study using magnetic resonance imaging. Neurology 42:527–536, 1992

Cope DN, Date ES, Mar EY: Serial computerized tomographic evaluations in traumatic head injury. Arch Phys Med Rehabil 69:483–486, 1988

Cullum CM, Bigler ED: Ventricle size, cortical atrophy and the relationship with neuropsychological status in closed head injury: A quantitative analysis. J Clin Exp Neuropsychol 8:437–452, 1986

Cullum CM, Kuck J, Ruff RM: Neuropsychological assessment of traumatic brain injury in adults, in Traumatic Brain Injury. Edited by Bigler ED. Austin, TX, Pro-Ed, 1990, pp 129–163

Cummings JL: Clinical Neuropsychiatry. Orlando, FL, Grune & Stratton, 1985

Cummings JL, Benson DF: Dementia: A Clinical Approach, 2nd Edition. Boston, MA, Butterworths, 1992

Dikmen S, McLean A, Temkin N: Neuropsychological and psychosocial consequences of minor head injury. J Neurol Neurosurg Psychiatry 49:1227–1232, 1986

Dikmen SS, Temkin N, Armsden G: Neuropsychological recovery: relationship to psychosocial functioning and postconcussional complaints, in Mild Head Injury. Edited by Levin HS, Eisenberg HM, Benton AL. New York, Oxford University Press, 1989, pp 229–241

Dinan TG, Mobayed M: Treatment resistance of depression after head injury: a preliminary study of amitriptyline response. Acta Psychiatr Scand 85:292–294, 1992

Dries DJ, Gamelli RL: Issues in geriatric trauma, in Trauma 2000: Strategies for the Millennium. Edited by Gamelli RL, Dries DJ. Austin, TX, RG Landes, 1992, pp 191–197

Dubovsky SL: Psychopharmacological treatment in neuropsychiatry, in American Psychiatric Press Textbook of Neuropsychiatry, 2nd Edition Edited by Yudofsky SC, Hales RE. Washington, DC, American Psychiatric Press, 1992, pp 663–701

Edna TH: Risk factors in traumatic head injury. Acta Neurochir 69:15–21, 1983

Faden AI, Demediuk P, Panter SS, et al: The role of excitatory amino acids and NMDA receptors in traumatic brain injury. Science 244:798–800, 1989

Federoff JP, Starkstein SE, Forrester AW, et al: Depression in patients with acute traumatic brain injury. Am J Psychiatry 149:918–923, 1992

Feeney DM, Walker AE: The prediction of posttraumatic epilepsy: a mathematical approach. Arch Neurol 36: 8–12, 1990

Fields RB: The effects of head injuries on older adults (abstract). Clinical Neuropsychologist 5:252, 1991

Fields RB, Coffey CE: CT scan predictors of outcome following geriatric head injury (abstract). Archives of Clinical Neuropsychology (in press)

Fields RB, Taylor C, Starratt GK: Neuropsychiatric complaints following geriatric head injury (abstract). Arch Clin Neuropsychol 8:223–224, 1993

Fieschi C, Battistini N, Beduschi A, et al: Regional cerebral blood flow and intraventricular pressure in acute head injuries. J Neurol Neurosurg Psychiatry 37:1378–1388, 1974

Fife D, Faich G, Hollinshead WI, et al: Incidence and outcome of hospital-treated head injury in Rhode Island. Am J Public Health 76:773–778, 1986

Finger S: Recovery From Brain Damage. New York, Plenum, 1978

Finger S, Levere TE, Almli CR, et al: Brain Injury and Recovery. New York, Plenum, 1988

Fogel BS: Major depression versus organic mood disorder: A questionable distinction. J Clin Psychiatry 51:53–56, 1991

Fogel BS, Duffy J: Elderly patients, in Neuropsychiatry of Traumatic Brain Injury. Edited by Silver JM, Yudofsky SC, Hales RE. Washington, DC, American Psychiatric Press, 1994, pp 412–441

Forrest DV: Psychotherapy of patients with neuropsychiatric disorders, in American Psychiatric Press Textbook of Neuropsychiatry, 2nd Edition. Edited by Yudofsky SC, Hales RE. Washington, DC, American Psychiatric Press, 1992, pp 703–739

Gatz M, Popkin SJ, Pino CD, et al: Psychological interventions with older adults, in Handbook of the Psychology of Aging. Edited by Birren JE, Schaie KW. New York, Van Nostrand Reinhold, 1985, pp 755–785

Gennarelli TA, Spielman GM, Langfitt TW, et al: Influence of the type of intracranial lesion on outcome from severe head injury. J Neurosurg 56:26–32, 1982

Gentilini M, Nichelli P, Schoenhuber R: Assessment of attention in mild head injury, in Mild Head Injury, Edited by Levin HS, Eisenberg HM, Benton AL. New York, Oxford University Press, 1989, pp 163–175

Goldstein FC, Levin HS: Epidemiology of traumatic brain injury: incidence, clinical characteristics, and risk factors, in Traumatic Brain Injury. Edited by Bigler ED. Austin, TX, Pro-Ed, 1990, pp 51–67

Goldstein FC, Levin HS, Presley RM, et al: Neurobehavioral consequences of closed-head injury in older adults (abstract). J Clin Exp Neuropsychol 15:59, 1993

Gorman LK, Fu K, Hovda DA, et al: Analysis of acetylcholine release following concussive brain injury in the rat (abstract). J Neurotrauma 6:203, 1989

Gronwall D: Advances in the assessment of attention and information processing after head injury, in Neurobehavioral Recovery from Head Injury. Edited by Levin HS, Grafman J, Eisenberg HM. New York, Oxford University Press, 1987, pp 355–371

Gronwall D: Behavioral assessment during the acute stages of traumatic brain injury, in Assessment of the Behavioral Consequences of Head Trauma. Edited by Lezak MD. New York, Alan R Liss, 1989a, pp 19–36

Gronwall D: Cumulative and persisting effects of concussion on attention and cognition, in Mild Head Injury. Edited by Levin HS, Eisenberg HM, Benton AL. New York, Oxford University Press, 1989b, pp 153–162

Gualtieri CT: Neuropsychiatry and Behavioral Pharmacology. Springer-Verlag, New York, 1991

Gudeman SK, Kishore PR, Becker DP, et al: Computerized tomography in the evaluation of incidence and significance of post-traumatic hydrocephalus. Radiology 141:397–402, 1981

Hagen C, Malkmus D, Durham P: Levels of Cognitive Functioning. Downey, CA, Rancho Los Amigos Hospital, 1972

Hamm RJ, Jenkins LW, Lyeth BG, et al: The effect of age on outcome following traumatic brain injury in rats. J Neurosurg 75:916–921, 1991

Hamm RJ, White-Gbadebo DM, Lyeth BG, et al: The effect of age on motor and cognitive deficits after traumatic brain injury in rats. Neurosurgery 31:1072–1078, 1992

Harlow JM: Recovery from the passage of an iron bar through the head. Publications of the Massachusetts Medical Society 2:327–347, 1868

Hendrick EB, Harris L: Post-traumatic epilepsy in children. J Trauma 8:547–556, 1968

Jennett B: Predictors of recovery in evaluation of patients in coma. Adv Neurol 22:129–135, 1979

Jennett B, Bond MR: Assessment of outcome after severe brain injury: a practical scale. Lancet 1:480–484, 1975

Jennett B, Teasdale G: Management of Head Injuries. Philadelphia, PA, FA Davis, 1981

Jorge RE, Robinson RG, Arndt S: Are there symptoms that are specific for depressed mood in patients with traumatic brain injury. J Nerv Ment Dis 181(2):91–99, 1993a

Jorge RE, Robinson RG, Arndt S, et al: Comparison between acute- and delayed-onset depression following traumatic brain injury. J Neuropsychiatry Clin Neurosci 5:43–49, 1993b

Katayama Y, Becker DP, Tamura T, et al: Massive increases in extracellular potassium and the indiscriminate release of glutamate following concussive brain injury. J Neurosurg 73:889–900, 1990

Katz DI: Neuropathology and neurobehavioral recovery from closed head injury. Journal of Head Trauma Rehabilitation 7:1–15, 1992

Katz DI, Kehs GJ, Alexander MP: Prognosis and recovery from traumatic head injury: the influence of advancing age (abstract). Neurology 40 (suppl):276, 1990

Kirkpatrick JB, DiMaio V: Civilian gunshot wounds of the brain. J Neurosurg 49:185–198, 1978

Kishore PR, Lipper MH, Miller JD, et al: Post-traumatic hydrocephalus in patients with severe head injuries. Neuroradiology 16:261–265, 1978

Kotwica Z, Jakubowski JK: Acute head injuries in the elderly: an analysis of 136 patients. Acta Neurochir 118:98–102, 1992

Kraus JF, Black MA, Hessol N, et al: The incidence of acute brain injury and serious impairment in a defined population. Am J Epidemiol 119:186–201, 1984

Kreutzer JS, Wehman P, Morton MV, et al: Supported employment and compensatory strategies for enhancing vocational outcome strategies. Brain Inj 2:205–233, 1988

Langfitt TW, Obrist WD, Alavi A, et al: Computerized tomography, magnetic resonance imaging and positron emission tomography in the study of brain trauma. J Neurosurg 64:760–767, 1986

Levin HS, Grossman RG, Rose JE, et al: Long-term neuropsychological outcome of closed head injury. J Neurosurg 50:412–422, 1979a

Levin HS, O'Donnell VM, Grossman RG: The Galveston Orientation and Amnesia Test: a practical scale to assess cognition after head injury. J Nerv Ment Dis 167:675–684, 1979b

Levin HS, Meyers CA, Grossman RG, et al: Ventricular enlargement after closed head injury. Arch Neurol 38:623–629, 1981

Levin HS, Benton Al, Grossman RG: Neurobehavioral Consequences of Closed Head Injury. New York, Oxford University Press, 1982

Levin HS, Handel SF, Goldman AM, et al: Magnetic resonance imaging after "diffuse" nonmissile head injury: a neurobehavioral study. Arch Neurol 42:963–968, 1985

Levin HS, Amparo E, Eisenberg HM, et al: Magnetic resonance imaging and computerized tomography in relation to the neurobehavioral sequelae of mild and moderate head injuries. J Neurosurg 66:706–713, 1987a

Levin HS, High WM, Goethe KE, et al: The neurobehavioral rating scale: assessment of the behavioral sequelae of head injury by the clinician. J Neurol Neurosurg Psychiatry 50:183–193, 1987b

Levin HS, Mattis S, Ruff RM, et al: Neurobehavioral outcome following minor head injury: a three-center study. J Neurosurg 66:234–243, 1987c

Levin HS, Gary HE, Eisenberg HM, et al: Neurobehavioral outcome 1 year after severe head injury. J Neurosurg 73:699–709, 1990

Levin HS, Eisenberg HM, Benton AL: Frontal Lobe Function and Dysfunction. New York, Oxford University Press, 1991

Levin HS, Williams DH, Eisenberg HM, et al: Serial MRI and neurobehavioral findings after mild to moderate closed head injury. J Neurol Neurosurg Psychiatry 55:255–262, 1992

Lewis L: A framework for developing a psychotherapy treatment plan with brain-injured patients. Journal of Head Trauma Rehabilitation 6:22–29, 1991

Lewis L, Athey GI, Eyman J, et al: Psychological treatment of adult psychiatric patients with traumatic frontal lobe injury. J Neuropsychiatry Clin Neurosci 4:323–330, 1992

Luerssen TG, Klauber MR, Marshall LF: Outcome from head injury related to patient's age: a longitudinal prospective study of adult and pediatric head injury. J Neurosurg 68:409–416, 1988

Marshall LF, Becker DP, Bowers SA, et al: The national traumatic coma data bank, I: design, purpose, goals, and results. J Neurosurg 59:276–84, 1983

Marshall LF, Marshall SB, Klauber MR, et al: A new classification of head injury based on computerized tomography. J Neurosurg 75 (suppl):S14–S20, 1991

Marquardt TP, Stoll J, Sussman H: Disorders of communication in traumatic brain injury, in Traumatic Brain Injury. Edited by Bigler Ed. Austin, TX, Pro-Ed, 1990, pp 181–205

Mattson AJ, Levin HS: Frontal lobe dysfunction following closed head injury. J Nerv Ment Dis 178:282–291, 1990

McKinlay WW, Brooks DN, Bond MR, et al: The short-term outcome of severe blunt head injury as reported by the relatives of the injured person. J Neurol Neurosurg Psychiatry 44:527–533, 1981

Merskey H, Woodforde JM: Psychiatric sequelae of minor head injury. Brain 95:521–528, 1972

Middelboe T, Andersen HS, Birket-Smith M, et al: Minor head injury: impact on general health after 1 year: a prospective follow-up study. Acta Neurol Scand 85:5–9, 1992

Miller JD, Pentland B: The factors of age, alcohol, and multiple injury in patients with mild and moderate head injury, in Mild to Moderate Head Injury. Edited by Hoff JT, Anderson TE, Cole TM. Boston, MA, Blackwell Scientific, 1989, pp 125–133

Naugle RI: Epidemiology of traumatic brain injury in adults, in Traumatic Brain Injury. Edited by Bigler Ed. Austin, TX, Pro-Ed, 1990, pp 69–103

Obrist WD, Gennarelli TA, Segawa H, et al: Relation of cerebral blood flow to neurological status and outcome in head-injury patients. J Neurosurg 51:292–300, 1979

Oddy M, Humphrey M, Uttley D: Stresses upon the relatives of head-injured patients. Br J Psychiatry 133:507–513, 1978

Oddy M, Coughlan T, Tyerman A, et al: Social adjustment after closed head injury: a further follow-up seven years after injury. J Neurol Neurosurg Psychiatry 48:564–568, 1985

Ommaya AK, Grubb RL Jr, Naumann RA: Coup and contrecoup injury: Observations on the mechanics of visible brain injuries in the rhesus monkey. J Neurosurg 35:503–516, 1971

Oster C: Signs of sensory deprivation versus cerebral injury in post-hip fracture patients. J Am Geriatr Soc 25:368–370, 1977

Pang D: Physics and pathophysiology of closed head injury, in Assessment of the Behavioral Consequences of Head Trauma. Edited by Lezak MD. New York, Alan R Liss, 1989, pp 1–18

Parker RS: Traumatic Brain Injury and Neuropsychological Impairment. New York, Springer-Verlag, 1990

Pentland B, Jones PA, Roy CW, et al: Head injury in the elderly. Age Aging 15:193–202, 1986

Povlishock JT, Coburn TH: Morphopathological change associated with mild head injury, in Mild Head Injury. Edited by Levin HS, Eisenberg HM, Benton AL. New York, Oxford University Press, 1989, pp 37–53

Prigatano GP: Disordered mind, wounded soul: the emerging role of psychotherapy in rehabilitation after brain injury. Journal of Head Trauma Rehabilitation 6(4):1–10, 1991a

Prigatano GP: Disturbances of self-awareness of deficit after traumatic brain injury, in Awareness of Deficit After Brain Injury. Edited by Prigatano GP, Schacter DL. New York, Oxford University Press, 1991b, pp 111–126

Prigatano GP: Personality disturbances associated with traumatic brain injury. J Consult Clin Psychol 60:360–368, 1992

Prigatano GP, Klonoff PS: Psychotherapy and neuropsychological assessment after brain injury, in Traumatic Brain Injury. Edited by Bigler ED. Austin, TX, Pro-Ed, 1990, pp 313–330

Prigatano GP, O'Brien KP, Klonoff PS: The clinical management of paranoid delusions in postacute traumatic brain injured patients. Journal of Head Trauma Rehabilitation 3(3):23–32, 1988

Richardson JTE: Clinical and Neuropsychological Aspects of Closed Head Injury. London, Taylor & Francis, 1990

Rimel RW, Giordani B, Barth JT, et al: Disability caused by minor head injury. Neurosurgery 9:221–228, 1981

Rimel RW, Giordani B, Barth JT, et al: Moderate head injury: completing the clinical spectrum of brain trauma. Neurosurgery 11:344–351, 1982

Rosenthal M, Bond MR, Griffith ER, et al: Rehabilitation of the Adult and Child With Traumatic Brain Injury. Philadelphia, PA, FA Davis, 1990

Ross ED, Rush MD: Diagnosis and neuroanatomical correlates of depression in brain-damaged patients. Arch Gen Psychiatry 38:1344–1354, 1981

Ruff RM, Buchsbaum MS, Troster AI, et al: Computerized tomography, neuropsychology, and positron emission tomography in the evaluation of head injury. Neuropsychiatry, Neuropsychology, and Behavioral Neurology 2:103–123, 1989a

Ruff RM, Levin HS, Mattis S, et al: Recovery of memory after mild head injury: a three center study, in Mild Head Injury. Edited by Levin HS, Eisenberg HM, Benton AL. New York, Oxford University Press, 1989b, pp 176–188

Ruff RM, Marshall LF, Klauber MR, et al: Alcohol abuse and neurological outcome of the severely head injured. Journal of Head Trauma Rehabilitation 5(3):21–31, 1990

Russell WR: Cerebral involvement in head injury: a study based on the examination of two hundred cases. Brain 55:549–603, 1932

Russell WR: The after-effects of head injury. Edinburgh Medical Journal 41:129–44, 1934

Russell WR: The Traumatic Amnesias. London, Oxford University Press, 1971

Russell WR, Smith A: Post-traumatic amnesia in closed head injury. Arch Neurol 5:4–17, 1961

Rutherford WH: Post-concussion symptoms: relationship to acute neurological indices, individual differences, and circumstances of injury in Mild Head Injury. Edited by Levin HS, Eisenberg HM, Benton AL. New York, Oxford University Press, 1989, pp 217–228

Rutherford WH, Merrett JD, McDonald JR: Sequelae of concussion caused by minor head injuries. Lancet 1:1–4, 1977

Rutherford WH, Merrett JD, McDonald JR: Symptoms at one year following concussion from minor head injuries. Injury 10:225–230, 1979

Saran AS: Depression after minor closed head injury: role of dexamethasone suppression test and antidepressants. J Clin Psychiatry 46:335–338, 1985

Satz P: Threshold theory: brain reserve capacity on symptom onset after brain injury: a formulation and review of evidence. Paper presented at the annual meeting of the American Psychological Association, San Francisco, CA, August 1991

Schoenhuber R, Gentilini M: Anxiety and depression after mild head injury: a case control study. J Neurol Neurosurg Psychiatry 51:722–724, 1988

Silver JM, Yudofsky SC, Hales RE: Neuropsychiatric aspects of traumatic brain injury, in American Psychiatric Press Textbook of Neuropsychiatry. Edited by Hales RE, Yudofsky SC. Washington, DC, American Psychiatric Press, 1987, pp 179–190

Silver JM, Yudofsky SC, Hales RE: Depression in traumatic brain injury. Neuropsychiatry, Neuropsychology, and Behavioral Neurology 4:12–23, 1991

Silver JM, Hales RE, Yudofsky SC: Neuropsychiatric aspects of traumatic brain injury, in American Psychiatric Press Textbook of Neuropsychiatry, 2nd Edition. Edited by Yudofsky SC, Hales RE. Washington, DC, American Psychiatric Press, 1992, pp 363–395

Sorenson SB, Kraus JF: Occurrence, severity, and outcomes of brain injury. Journal of Head Trauma Rehabilitation 6(2):1–10, 1991

Sparadeo FR, Strauss D, Barth JT: The incidence, impact, and treatment of substance abuse in head trauma rehabilitation. Journal of Head Trauma Rehabilitation 5(3):1–8, 1990

Starkstein SE, Boston JD, Robinson RG: Mechanisms of mania after brain injury 12 case reports and review of the literature. J Nerv Ment Dis 176(2):87–100, 1988

Starkstein SE, Mayberg HS, Berthier ML, et al: Mania after brain injury: neuroradiological and metabolic findings. Ann Neurol 27:652–659, 1990

Starratt C, Fields R: Psychotherapy following brain injury. Allegheny General Hospital Neuroscience Journal 2(3):32–36, 1991

Steadman J, Graham J: Rehabilitation of the brain injured. Proceedings of the Royal Society of Medicine 63: 23–27, 1970

Stuss DT, Buckle L: Traumatic brain injury: neuropsychological deficits and evaluation at different stages of recovery and in different pathologic subtypes. Journal of Head Trauma Rehabilitation 7(2):40–49, 1992

Taylor CT, Price TRP: Neuropsychiatric assessment, in Neuropsychiatry of Traumatic Brain Injury. Edited by Silver JM, Yudofsky SC, Hales RE. Washington, DC, American Psychiatric Press (in press)

Teasdale G, Jennett B: Assessment of coma and impaired consciousness: a practical scale. Lancet 2:81–84, 1974

Temkin NR, Dikmen SS, Wilensky AJ, et al: A randomized, double-blind study of phenytoin for the prevention of post-traumatic seizures. N Engl J Med 323:497–502, 1990

Thomsen IV: Late outcome of very severe blunt head trauma: a 10–15 year second follow-up. J Neurol Neurosurg Psychiatry 47:260–268, 1984

Uzell BP, Langfitt TW, Dolinskas CA: Influence of injury severity on quality of survival after head injury. Surg Neurol 27:419–429, 1987

Varney NR, Martzke JS, Roberts RJ: Major depression in patients with closed head injury. Neuropsychology 1:7–9, 1987

Vollmer DG, Torner JC, Jane JA, et al: Age and outcome following traumatic coma: why do older patients fare worse. J Neurosurg 75 (suppl):S37–S49, 1991

Von Wowern F: Post-traumatic amnesia and confusion as an index of severity in head injury. Acta Neurol Scand 42:373–378, 1966

Wilson JTL, Wiedman KD, Hadley DM, et al: Early and late magnetic resonance imaging and neuropsychological outcome after head injury. J Neurol Neurosurg Psychiatry 51:391–396, 1988

Wood RL: Neurobehavioral Sequelae of Traumatic Brain Injury. New York, Taylor & Francis, 1990

World Health Organization: Schedules for Clinical Assessment in Neuropsychiatry. Geneva, World Health Organization, 1992

Wroblewski BA, McColgan K, Smith K, et al: The incidence of seizures during tricyclic antidepressant drug treatment in a brain-injured population. J Clin Psychopharmacol 10:124–128, 1990

Wroblewski BA, Leary JM, Phelan AM, et al: Methylphenidate and seizure frequency in brain injured patients with seizure disorders. J Clin Psychiatry 53(3):86–89, 1992

Yoshino MT, Seeger JF: CT still exam of choice in closed head trauma. Diagnostic Imaging 11:88–92, 1989

Appendix 24–1 Posttraumatic Neurobehavioral Screening Inventory

Instructions

The following questions will help us find out if you have noticed differences in yourself following your injury. Each question will ask about a specific problem area. If you have noticed a definite change in this area, circle "2." If you have not noticed a change, circle "0." If you have noticed only a little change, circle "1." If you really don't know, circle "9." Please ask staff if you have any questions, but please fill this out yourself without help from family or friends, if possible.

Question	No	A little	Yes	Don't know
1. Are you having more trouble concentrating than before your injury (as in reading a newspaper, following conversations, paying attention to television, or carrying out tasks at work)?	0	1	2	9
2. Are you more forgetful than you were before your injury?	0	1	2	9
3. Do you have trouble handling as much information as well or as quickly as you did before your injury?	0	1	2	9
4. Are you more easily angered than you were before your injury?	0	1	2	9
5. Do you yell or strike out more than you did before your injury?	0	1	2	9
6. Do you act without thinking more often than you did before your injury?	0	1	2	9
7. Do you think or act in ways now that you would not have before your injury?	0	1	2	9
8. Are you more mistrustful of others than before your injury?	0	1	2	9
9. Have you had any of the following experiences since your injury?				
a. Hearing voices when no one is around	0	1	2	9
b. Seeing things that others do not see	0	1	2	9
c. Smelling odors that others do not smell	0	1	2	9
10. Do you feel more sad, blue, or hopeless than you did before the injury?	0	1	2	9
11. Do you feel more nervous, restless, or panicky than you did before your injury?	0	1	2	9
12. Does your mood fluctuate more than it did before your injury (easy tearfulness or sudden changes in feelings)?	0	1	2	9
13. Do you have more energy and require less sleep than you did before your injury?	0	1	2	9

14. Are you bothered by the following problems more now than
before your injury?

a. Headaches	0	1	2	9
b. Fatigue	0	1	2	9
c. Dizziness	0	1	2	9
d. Blurred vision	0	1	2	9
e. Sensitivity to noise	0	1	2	9
f. Sensitivity to light	0	1	2	9
g. Trouble sleeping	0	1	2	9
h. Irritability	0	1	2	9

15. Have you had any of the following problems since your injury?

a. Nightmares or bad dreams about the injury	0	1	2	9
b. Recurring distressing thoughts or memories of the injury	0	1	2	9
c. Feelings that the injury is happening again	0	1	2	9
d. Avoiding things or places that are associated with the injury	0	1	2	9
e. Feelings of being upset when thinking about the injury	0	1	2	9
f. Being more easily startled by noises or people	0	1	2	9

Craig Taylor, M.D., and Robert B. Fields, Ph.D.; Allegheny Neuropsychiatric Institute, Oakdale, Pennsylvania.

25

Neuropsychiatric Aspects of Epilepsy

Mario F. Mendez, M.D., Ph.D.

Introduction

Epilepsy is associated with a variety of behavioral conditions that may be especially severe in elderly patients (Table 25–1). Seizure disorders can have psychosocial consequences, neuropsychological effects, and seizure-related behavioral manifestations. Moreover, throughout much of recorded history, epileptic patients have been prone to psychopathology during their seizure-free periods (Kraepelin 1923). In modern times, the belief in a universal epileptic predisposition to psychopathology has declined in favor of a specific predisposition of temporal lobe epilepsy (TLE) to psychosis, depression, and other psychopathology (Gibbs et al. 1948). Although not systematically studied in the elderly population, this psychopathology can persist in later years. In this chapter, I explore the behavioral aspects of epilepsy that might affect elderly patients and conclude with a discussion of management issues.

Demography and Definitions

Epileptic seizures result from abnormal neuronal discharges in the brain. They are sudden, involuntary behavioral events caused by excessive or hypersynchronous electrical discharges, often from hyperexcitable neurons. Epileptic seizures can be primary, secondary to a brain lesion, or symptomatic from acute, situational conditions such as sleep deprivation or drug withdrawal. The term *epilepsy* refers specifically to recurrent unprovoked seizures and includes primary and secondary epileptic seizures, but excludes symptomatic ones. The International Classification of Epileptic Seizures (Commission on Classification and Terminology of the International League Against Epilepsy 1981) further divides seizures into generalized (characterized by an initial widespread bihemispheric involvement) and partial (characterized by an initial focal onset in part of one hemisphere) (Table 25–2).

Epilepsy is a common neurological disorder. It affects up to 50 million people worldwide, has a prevalence of at least 0.63% and has an overall annual incidence of about 50/100,000 (Hauser and Kurland 1986). The incidence of new-onset epilepsy is highest in the first year, drops to a minimum in individuals in their 30s and 40s, and increases again in those over age 60 to an annual incidence of 77–92/100,000 (Hauser 1992; Luhdorf et al. 1986a). Although two-thirds of ep-

ilepsy in young adults is idiopathic, more than half of elderly epilepsy patients have a known cause (Hauser 1992). In those over age 65, about one-third have a cerebrovascular etiology for their seizures, approximately 10%–15% have brain tumors, and up to 23% have infections, trauma, or other secondary lesions (Luhdorf et al. 1986b; Sanders and Murray 1991). Furthermore, in a study of elderly people with unexplained seizures, small vascular changes occurred more commonly in those with epilepsy than in nonepileptic control subjects (Shorvon et al. 1984).

Clinical Aspects of Epilepsy

In adults, the three most common types of seizures are 1) generalized tonic-clonic seizures (GTCSs), with convulsions (also known as *grand mal seizures*); 2) complex partial seizures (CPSs), with an alteration of consciousness; and 3) simple partial seizures (SPSs), with isolated motor, somatosensory, autonomic, or psychic

---

Table 25–1. Behavioral disorders in epilepsy

Psychosocial
  Low self-esteem, dependency, and helplessness
  Fear of loss of control
  Stigmatization
  Loss of independence
  Associated marital, job, transportation, and related
    problems
Neuropsychological
  From seizures
  From underlying lesions and/or disease
  From antiepileptic drugs (AEDs)
Ictally related
  Prodromal symptoms: dysphoria, apprehension, and
    so on
  Ictal automatisms and psychic symptoms
  Nonconvulsive status: simple partial seizures, complex
    partial seizures, absence, and periodic lateralizing
    epileptiform discharges
  Postictal confusion and other postictal behaviors
  Ictal or postictal intermixed behaviors: "twilight states"
    and so on
  Psychotic episodes related to the ictus
Interictal
  Chronic schizophrenic psychosis
  Depression
  Suicide
  "Heightened significance" and other personality changes
  Miscellaneous: hyposexuality, aggression, dissociative
    states, and so on

symptoms (Table 25–2). SPSs that evolve to CPSs are considered "auras," and CPSs that evolve to GTCSs are "secondarily generalized." Although about one-third of all epileptic patients have CPSs, about one-half of elderly epileptic patients have CPSs, reflecting the increased specific focal causes of their epilepsy (Hauser 1992). On electroencephalography (EEG), these seizure disorders may have interictal spikes and other markers of abnormal electrical activity, most commonly emanating from a temporal lobe. In addition, variants of childhood absence (petit mal) seizures, which result in brief lapses of consciousness, occur occasionally in elderly patients.

The evaluation of new-onset seizures in the elderly includes the identification of cerebrovascular, neoplastic, and other acquired neuropathology; the exclusion of acute, symptomatic seizures; and the characterization of any epileptiform discharges. These patients need neuroimaging of the brain, preferably magnetic resonance imaging with its superior resolution for most parenchymal lesions. Routine X-ray and laboratory studies help exclude the presence of symptomatic seizures. In addition, a lumbar puncture is indicated in the presence of a persistent alteration of consciousness, especially if accompanied by fever and meningeal signs. EEGs are more likely to define the type of epilep-

tiform changes if the patient attains drowsiness or sleep during the tracing. However, computerized EEG techniques, which may help in mapping a structural lesion, are not very useful for evaluating these discharges.

Epileptic seizures must be differentiated from syncope and from nonepileptic seizures. Patients with brief lapses of consciousness but without typical ictal features or postictal confusion usually have syncope from a cardiovascular, toxic-metabolic, or cerebrovascular cause; however, these lapses could be atypical seizures, particularly if they are of frontal lobe origin. Some elderly patients may have syncope-like ictal events such as brief periods of amnesia or falling episodes (Godfrey 1989). Nonepileptic seizures, or pseudoseizures, are the most frequent conversion reaction among seizure patients. Patients with nonepileptic seizures are most commonly young women with psychological stressors and poor coping skills, but nonepileptic seizures have occurred in elderly patients (Gates et al. 1985; Meierkord et al. 1991). Nonepileptic seizures are characterized by a sudden collapse or by motor activity that does not fit a typical CPS or GTCS, ictal durations of two or more minutes, occurrence in the presence of a witness, possible induction with injections or suggestion, poor responsiveness to antiepilepsy drugs (AEDs), and lack of a seizure-induced rise in serum prolactin levels (Gates et al. 1985; Meierkord et al. 1991).

The neuropsychiatric aspects of epilepsy include four categories: psychosocial, neuropsychological, ictally related behavioral alterations, and interictal psychopathology (Table 25–1). Psychosocial aspects are those directly due to the stress of having a seizure disorder, and neuropsychological aspects refer to persistent disturbances in cognitive abilities. Temporary behavior changes also occur either before, during, or after a seizure as a direct result of ictal or seizure discharges. A final group of behaviors manifest as sustained psychopathology during the interictal or seizure-free period. Although these categories overlap and some behaviors may change groups as underlying mechanisms are identified, these categories are useful for discussing the neuropsychiatric aspects of epilepsy (Smith et al. 1991).

Table 25–2. The International Classification of Epileptic Seizures

I. Partial (focal, local) seizures
  A. Simple partial seizures (SPSs)
    Motor, somatosensory, autonomic, or psychic symptoms
  B. Complex partial seizures (CPSs)
    1. Begin with symptoms of simple partial seizure but progress to impairment of consciousness
    2. Begin with impairment of consciousness
  C. Partial seizures with secondary generalization
    1. Begin with simple partial seizure
    2. Begin with complex partial seizure (including those with symptoms of simple partial seizures at onset)

II. Generalized seizures (convulsive or nonconvulsive)
  A. Absence (typical and atypical)
  B. Myoclonus
  C. Clonic
  D. Tonic
  E. Tonic-clonic (GTCSs)
  F. Atonic/akinetic

III. Unclassified

Source. From Commission on Classification and Terminology of the International League Against Epilepsy 1981.

Psychosocial Impact of Seizures

The presence of a seizure disorder in later life has important psychosocial implications (Table 25–1). First, patients with epilepsy are subject to low self-esteem, particularly arising from the greater dependency that the disorder engenders (Dodrill et al. 1984). Self-esteem problems can be greater in elderly individuals, who may already be heavily reliant on family and others. Second, the possibility of having a seizure at any time results in feelings of loss of control (Hermann and Wyler 1989). Elderly subjects tend to be cautious and conservative, and the potential for public loss of control can be particularly distressing. In addition to an overall increased sense of vulnerability, there is a very real fear of falling and sustaining incapacitating hip fractures or other trauma. Third, there is continued stigmatization from the disorder, and people often misunderstand and fear those with epilepsy (Dodrill et al. 1984). This can lead to housing problems; some nursing homes do not accept elderly patients with seizures. Fourth, the independence of elderly patients may already be impaired or tenuous, and epilepsy further narrows their ability to function independently (Luhdorf et al. 1986b). Seizures may critically compromise the function of the elderly individuals who are still able to keep a job, provide their own transportation, maintain their economic status, and perform other independent activities. Although seizures by themselves rarely result in institutionalization, in an already impaired elder, seizures may be the final condition that terminates independent living. In addition, given the higher frequency of secondary epilepsy in the elderly, older patients are often already disabled from underlying neurological disorders such as stroke or dementia.

Neuropsychological Impact of Seizures

Neuropsychological functions are vulnerable to the effects of seizures. Prolonged seizures can result in metabolic and direct electrical injury to the brain. By age 70, there has been significant loss of neuronal tissue and a decline in cognitive efficiency, particularly on time-dependent tasks and in memory retrieval (Botwinick 1981). With this decreased neuronal reserve, elderly patients have a greater neuropsychological decline from neuronal damage due to ongoing seizure activity than do younger patients. For this reason alone, seizure duration and rate of recurrence of seizures are important clinical variables in the elderly.

In older patients with secondary epilepsy, seizures are often associated with disorders that impair cogni-

tion. Seizures can temporarily exacerbate stroke or tumor deficits such as aphasias (Godfrey 1989). Furthermore, seizures occur in dementing disorders including Alzheimer's disease, multi-infarct dementia, Pick's disease, and other neurodegenerative disorders (McAreavey et al. 1992). Alzheimer's disease, the most prevalent dementia, may have seizures (usually GTCSs) in 10% or more of patients, particularly late in the course (Hauser et al. 1986; Romanelli et al. 1990).

Although most seizures can be controlled with AEDs, these medications have potential neuropsychological side effects. Elderly patients have a slowed elimination of these drugs, require lower doses, are often on multiple interacting medications, and are, therefore, more likely to experience AED toxicity (Leppik 1992). With the already significant susceptibility to confusional states of the aged brain, the addition of AEDs greatly adds to the possibility of drug-induced delirium. Even at therapeutic levels, some drugs can cause specific problems. For example, barbiturates may need discontinuation because of drug-induced depression, suicidal ideation, sedation, psychomotor slowing, and paradoxical hyperactivity (Brent et al. 1990). The added susceptibility for AED-induced toxicity in elderly patients indicates the need for closer monitoring, especially of free phenytoin levels, carbamazepine epoxide levels, renal and liver function tests, and AED-induced hyponatremia.

Ictally Related Behavioral Alterations

Ictally related behavioral alterations occur before, during, and after seizures (Table 25–1). First, a prodrome of dysphoria, insomnia, anxiety, or build-up of tension may precede seizures or be relieved by them. Second, ictal discharges can produce both reactive automatisms involving semipurposeful activity and psychic manifestations producing affective, cognitive, language, memory, and perceptual changes. Examples of automatisms include ictal laughter from left-hemisphere discharges and ictal crying from right-hemisphere discharges (Sackeim et al. 1982). Examples of psychic manifestations include affective changes such as ictal fear and depression and cognitive changes such as forced thinking, derealization, and depersonalization. Moreover, prolonged alterations of responsiveness may result from nonconvulsive status epilepticus or from recurrent electrical discharges with EEG complexes known as *periodic lateralizing epileptiform discharges* (PLEDs) (Engel et al. 1978). Third, the postictal period includes a confusional state lasting minutes to hours or, occasionally, days. The postictal period can be particularly prolonged in elderly patients, who may take longer to recover from the disruption of seizures (Godfrey 1989). Rarer postictal changes include depression after left-hemisphere seizures and hypomania after right-hemisphere seizures (Hurwitz et al. 1985). Although semidirected, ictally related aggression is extremely rare, nondirected destructive behavior frequently occurs during the postictal confusional state as a response to attempts at restraint (Treiman 1991). Finally, occasional, protracted periods with intermixed ictal and postictal changes can produce "twilight states," compulsive wandering or "poriomania," an agitated state, and "depressive delirium" (Betts 1981a).

One final ictally related behavioral manifestation is brief psychotic episodes, which are precipitated or relieved by or alternate with seizures (Dongier 1959/60; Ervin et al. 1955). These episodes involve days to weeks of agitated, hallucinatory, paranoid, and impulsive behaviors often with sudden mood swings and suicide attempts. Some patients develop their psychotic episodes concomitant with an increase in seizure frequency or AED withdrawal and, on control of the seizures, have resolution of the psychotic symptoms (Wells 1975). Others develop psychotic episodes 12–48 hours after a flurry of seizures and may occasionally continue to display psychotic symptoms for an extended period of time (Logsdail and Toone 1988). A third group develop psychotic episodes after seizures are controlled, and this "alternating psychosis" promptly resolves once the seizures recur (Pakalnis et al. 1987). *Forced* (or *paradoxical*) *normalization* refers to this subgroup with an antagonism between psychotic episodes and the seizures or EEG discharges (Landolt 1958).

Interictal Psychopathology

Epileptic patients are susceptible to psychopathology during the seizure-free periods (Table 25–1). These behavioral disorders usually occur in patients with long-standing, incompletely controlled seizures, and, although not specifically studied in the elderly, these disorders can occur in older patients. Community epidemiological studies have shown a high prevalence of interictal psychiatric problems among epileptic patients (Gudmundsson 1966; Pond and Bidwell

1959/60). The percentage of epileptic patients in psychiatric hospitals has ranged from 5% to 10%, significantly higher than the prevalence of epilepsy in the general population (Betts 1981b; Mendez et al. 1986). Furthermore, of patients attending epilepsy clinics, about 30% have had a prior psychiatric hospitalization (Stevens 1975), and about 18% were on at least one psychotropic drug (Wilensky et al. 1981). Recent studies report more psychopathology among epileptic patients than among other neurological control subjects (Mendez et al. 1993a, 1993c). In summary, although most epileptic patients do not have psychiatric disease, about one-quarter of epileptic patients, particularly those with long-standing CPSs, have interictal psychosis, depression, suicidality, hyposexuality, and other psychopathology.

Interictal Psychosis

The best known psychiatric disorder in epilepsy is the chronic "schizophreniform" psychosis. The influential study by Slater and Beard (1963) reported 69 patients with both epilepsy and an interictal schizophrenic disorder and concluded that these two disorders occurred together more frequently than expected by chance. Although some investigators have interpreted this association as reflecting selective sampling (Stevens 1991), most subsequent studies indicate that 7%–12% of epileptic patients develop a psychotic disorder, usually a chronic, interictal schizophrenic illness (Trimble 1991). For example, in a recent controlled investigation of 1,611 epileptic outpatients, interictal schizophrenic disorders were 9–10 times more common among epilepsy patients than among other neurological control subjects (Mendez et al. 1993c).

Other studies found psychosis in 12% of 1,675 patients with CPSs of TLE origin, especially those with left-sided foci, compared to less than 1% of 6,671 generalized epilepsy patients (Gibbs 1951), and a psychotic illness occurred in 9 (10%) of 87 children with TLE epilepsy followed for up to 30 years (Lindsay et al. 1979). Moreover, on the Minnesota Multiphasic Personality Inventory (MMPI) patients with epilepsy had more elevated schizophrenia and paranoia scale scores than did patients with other neurological disabilities (Dikmen et al. 1983). In conclusion, epileptic patients have a severalfold greater risk for a chronic schizophrenic illness than does the general population, and the risk is particularly high for CPS patients, regardless of age.

Unlike ictally related psychotic episodes, chronic interictal schizophrenic disorder has no direct relationship to individual seizures (Mendez et al. 1993c; Trimble 1991). However, there is often an 11–15 year history of poorly controlled seizures (Slater and Beard 1963), and, compared with nonpsychotic epilepsy patients, schizophrenic epilepsy patients may have a later age at onset (Mendez et al. 1993c). Furthermore, the schizophrenic symptoms commonly emerge with increased CPS activity or with AED withdrawal (Mendez et al. 1993c) and may less frequently emerge with successful seizure treatment or disappearance of EEG discharges (Figure 25–1). Although removal of the seizure focus does not prevent the development of psychosis (Falconer 1973), left temporal mediobasal lesions are associated with this psychotic disorder (Sherwin et al. 1982).

The schizophrenic disorder resembles an episodic schizoaffective psychosis with prominent paranoia, positive symptoms, relatively preserved affect, and normal premorbid personality (Perez and Trimble 1980; Slater and Beard 1963; Trimble 1991). Compared with process schizophrenia, there may be more hallucinations and religiosity and less social withdrawal, system-

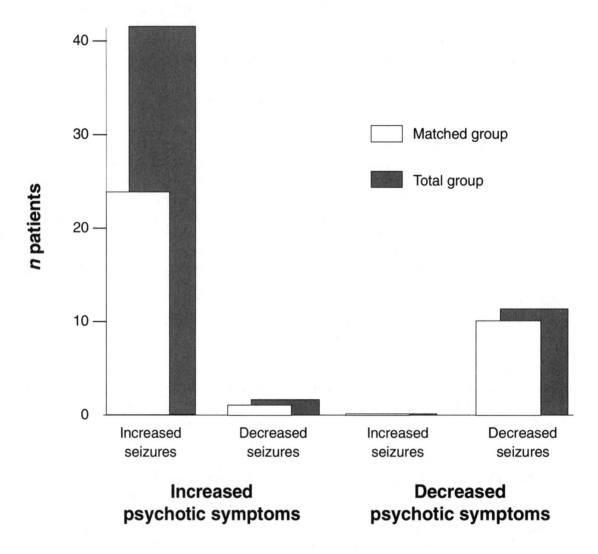

Figure 25–1. The correspondence of psychotic symptoms to seizure frequency. *Increased psychotic symptoms:* Total schizophrenic epilepsy group ($n = 149$): increased seizures in 42 and decreased seizures in 2 ($\chi^2 = 40.56$, df = 1, $P < .001$). Matched schizophrenic epilepsy group ($n = 62$): increased seizures in 24 and decreased seizures in 1 ($\chi^2 = 24.25$, df = 1, $P < .001$). *Decreased psychotic symptoms:* Total group: increased seizures in 9 and decreased seizures in 0 ($\chi^2 = 7.33$, df = 1, $P < .007$). Matched group: increased seizures in 8 and decreased seizures in 0 ($\chi^2 = 6.55$, df = 1, $P < .011$).
Source. Reprinted from Mendez MF, Grau R, Doss RC, et al: "Schizophrenia in Epilepsy: Seizure and Psychosis Variables." *Neurology* 43:1073–1077, 1993c. Used with permission.

atized delusions, Schneiderian first-rank symptoms, and family history of schizophrenia. However, these features are not clearly atypical or unique psychotic symptoms, and most schizophrenic syndromes in epilepsy can correspond to typical schizophrenic disorder categories (Mendez et al. 1993c).

Depression

Less well-known than the interictal psychosis is the problem of depression in epilepsy. The elderly are particularly prone to this disorder, and depression is undoubtedly a frequent neuropsychiatric disturbance in older seizure patients. Depression occurs in up to 75% of patients in mixed epilepsy groups (Standage and Fenton 1975), and there are elevations in depressive traits in epileptic patients compared with control subjects (Robertson 1991). Depression is also the main reason for the psychiatric hospitalization of epileptic patients (Betts 1981b; Mendez et al. 1986). Furthermore, despite contrary studies (Dodrill and Batzel 1986), most investigations report a twofold greater frequency of interictal depression among seizure patients than among comparably disabled individuals (Kogeorgos et al. 1982; Mendez et al. 1986; Rodin and Schmaltz 1984; Standage and Fenton 1975). The percentages of depressed patients specifically among those with CPSs ranges from 19% to 65% (Currie et al. 1971; Dongier 1959/60; Roy 1979), including more depression in those with CPSs compared with other seizure patients (Dongier 1959/60; Roy 1979).

Depressed epileptic patients most commonly have a chronic interictal depression or dysthymia that is distinct from ictal depression (Devinsky and Bear 1991; Weil 1955), post-ictal depression (Hurwitz et al. 1985), "depressive delirium" (Betts 1981a), or depression induced by barbiturates (Brent et al. 1990). The interictal depression frequently has endogenous features, paranoia, and other symptoms suggesting a continuum with schizoaffective disorder (Mendez et al. 1986). According to most investigators, seizures relieve depression in epilepsy patients (similar to the effects of electroconvulsive therapy [ECT]), whereas better seizure control or decreased secondarily generalized seizures make it worse (Betts 1981a; Mendez et al. 1993a; Robertson 1991). A few investigators have also reported depression with increased seizure activity or no relationship (Dodrill and Batzel 1986; Roy 1979). Depression is specifically associated with CPSs from left-sided temporal foci, suggesting an organic mood

disorder rather than a nonspecific psychosocial reaction to a chronic disability (Altshuler et al. 1990; Mendez et al. 1986; Perini and Mendius 1984). Conversely, studies have not established the proposed association of right-hemisphere foci with the much rarer cases of mania found in epilepsy (Flor-Henry 1969).

Suicide

Elderly individuals with epilepsy are at greater risk for suicide than those without epilepsy. Among all epileptic patients, the estimated risk of death by suicide is 3%–22% or 4–5 times higher than that for the general population (Mathews and Barabas 1981). Among those with CPSs of TLE origin, the risk of suicide is as much as 25 times greater (Barraclough 1981). Furthermore, as many as one-third of all epileptic patients have attempted suicide at some point in time. A comparison of suicide attempts among epileptic patients and comparably impaired nonepileptic control subjects revealed suicide attempts in 30% of the epileptic subjects compared to only 7% of the control subjects (Mendez et al. 1986), and this increased risk of suicide continued even long after temporal lobectomy and successful control of seizures (Jensen 1975).

Epileptic patients are likely to attempt suicide not only from psychosocial stress, but also because of the increased interictal psychopathology such as depression, psychosis, and borderline personality characteristics (Mendez et al. 1989). They are most likely to complete suicide when they have psychosis with paranoid hallucinations, agitated compunction to kill themselves, and occasional ictal command hallucinations to commit suicide (Mendez and Doss 1992). Ictal depression has also resulted in successful suicide attempts (Mendez and Doss 1992). One important contributing factor to the suicide risk among epileptic patients is the ease of overdose from ready access to AEDs (MacKay 1979).

Personality Characteristics

Although there is no general epileptic personality, specific personality traits have occurred in a subset of patients with CPSs regardless of age. Because most studies with the MMPI proved insensitive to the personality traits attributed to epilepsy, the Bear-Fedio Inventory was developed to assess the "TLE personality" (Bear and Fedio 1977). Bear and Fedio found that patients with CPSs of TLE origin had a personality characterized by a sense of "heightened significance" indicated by sobriety and humorlessness, tenaciousness or "viscosity" in interpersonal encounters, a deepened affect, a pronounced sense of personal destiny, and an intense interest in religious, moral, and philosophical issues. Such patients are circumstantial and may spend a long time getting to the point, give detailed background information, and write copiously about their thoughts and feelings (Geschwind 1983). In addition, patients with left-sided temporal foci tended to maximize their problems, whereas those with right-sided foci minimized them (Bear and Fedio 1977).

In contrast, other patients with CPSs of TLE origin are explosive and dyscontrolled with emotional lability and poor impulse control (Blumer 1991). Other applications of the Bear-Fedio Inventory found the same "TLE personality" characteristics in nonepileptic patients with psychiatric disorders or with comparable physical disabilities (Rodin and Schmaltz 1984). Rather than specific personality traits of patients with CPSs of TLE origin, the Bear-Fedio Inventory may reflect the presence of psychosis, depression, and an increased frequency of the common personality disorders, such as borderline, dependent, antisocial, explosive, and others (Mendez et al. 1993b).

Hyposexuality and Other Behavioral Disorders

The association of epilepsy with other conditions is less certain. Surveys suggest that incompletely treated epileptic patients tend to experience hyposexuality (Toone 1987), a problem that can still affect elderly patients. Epileptic patients appear to lack libido and may experience impotence or frigidity, and this hyposexuality improves after seizures are controlled (Toone 1987). Other sexual disorders are probably rare and must be distinguished from ictal sexual behaviors manifested by libidinous or erotic feelings, orgasm, masturbation, or even promiscuity after sensory seizures in the genital region.

Most directed aggression in epilepsy correlates less with seizures than with psychosis, "episodic dyscontrol" (intermittent explosive disorder with ictal-like features), subnormal intelligence, lower socioeconomic status, prior head injuries, and possible orbital frontal damage (Elliott 1982; Herzberg and Fenwick 1988; Rodin 1973; Whitman et al. 1984). There are case reports of dissociative states in epilepsy (i.e., multiple personality disorder, possession and fugue states, and

psychogenic amnesia); however, the relationship with epilepsy is not clear.

Etiology and Pathology

Although the mechanisms of psychopathology are not established, current theories of the psychopathology of epilepsy emphasize an organic disturbance in the temporal limbic system rather than psychodynamic processes. As previously described, psychosis, depression, personality disorders, and hyposexuality are 2–3 times more common in patients with CPSs (most of whom have a temporal focus) compared with GTCS patients. The most common pathological findings in epileptic patients are mediobasal temporal lobe lesions involving limbic structures. Stimulation and ablation studies in animals and man link these temporal limbic structures to emotional behavior. Psychotic-like behavior in animal subjects has followed repeated application of epileptic agents to "kindle" limbic structures (Adamec 1990; Stevens and Livermore 1978), schizophrenic patients have had limbic discharges on depth electrode monitoring (Heath 1982), and disinhibition of the mesolimbic dopamine system has resulted from kindling in the limbic system (Stevens and Livermore 1978).

There are several specific organic mechanisms potentially responsible for psychiatric disturbances in epilepsy (Table 25–3). First, the underlying brain lesions could be the source of both seizures and behavioral changes. Psychosis may be more common with left temporal lobe pathology such as hamartomas or gangliogliomas (Taylor 1972), and depression is associated with strokes and other hypoactive lesions in the left hemisphere (Robinson and Szetela 1981). Second, ictal discharges could kindle behavioral changes by facilitating limbic-sensory associations and other neuronal connections. The schizophrenic psychosis is associated with increased frequencies of CPSs, and personality disorders may occur in those with auras (Mendez et al. 1993b). Third, decreased function, such as the focal interictal hypometabolism observed on positron-emission tomography (PET) (Bromfield et al. 1992), may lead to interictal behavioral changes. Depression often follows seizure control sufficient to inhibit secondary generalization to GTCS (i.e., the surrounding hypometabolism may result in depression by preventing the spread of temporal limbic epileptic foci). Fourth, seizures may result in neuroendocrine or neurotransmitter changes including increased dopaminergic or inhibitory transmitters, decreased prolactin, increased testosterone, and increased endogenous opioids. These changes probably explain, at least in part, the hyposexuality found in some epileptic patients. Finally, organic factors may be potentiated by psychodynamic factors. For example, a proposed role for auras in personality disorders or psychosis may relate to their impact on reality testing (Mendez et al. 1993b).

Table 25–3. Proposed relationships of psychiatric disturbances to epilepsy

Common neuropathology, genetics, or developmental disturbance

Ictal or subictal discharges potentiate abnormal behavior

Kindling or facilitation of a distributed neuronal matrix

Changes in spike frequency or inhibitory-excitatory balance

Altered receptor sensitivity (e.g., dopamine receptors)

Secondary epileptogenesis

Absence of function at the seizure focus

Inhibition and hypometabolism surrounding the focus

Release or abnormal activity of remaining neurons

Dysfunction or downregulation of associated areas

Neurochemical alterations
  Dopamine and other neurotransmitters
  Endorphins

Gonadotrophins and other neuroendocrinologic changes

Psychodynamic influences

Dependence, learned helplessness, and low self-esteem

Disruption of reality testing

Weakening of defense mechanisms

Organic and psychodynamic factors potentiating each other

Sleep disturbance

Drug-induced neurophysiological changes

Treatment

Most epileptic seizures respond to AEDs. Phenytoin, carbamazepine, and valproate are effective drugs for partial seizures and GTCS, the main seizures of adulthood (Table 25–4). Side effects and elimination half-lives are other important considerations in choosing between AEDs. Monitoring of blood levels helps avoid dose-dependent side effects, but clinical monitoring of patients for idiosyncratic side effects is also necessary. Moreover, the more sedative AEDs are considered secondary drugs in the management of seizures.

Another important property of AEDs is the time it takes for their serum concentrations to be reduced by half. For example, one may choose to use phenytoin over carbamazepine because it has a consistently longer half-life and can be potentially given once per day. The use of multiple AEDs affects efficacy, side effects, and half-lives; therefore, it is preferable to treat seizures with one AED rather than with several. For those patients who do not respond to the common AEDs, several newer drugs are available or are awaiting approval by the Food and Drug Administration (FDA). Ultimately, when drug therapy fails to control seizures, patients may be considered for epilepsy surgery.

Table 25–4. Antiepileptic drugs (AEDs)

AEDs (brand names)	Indications	Half-life (hours)	Level (µg/ml)	Dose (mg/kg body weight)
Primary drugs				
Phenytoin (Dilantin)	GTCS, CPS, SPS	10–34	10–20	4–6
Carbamazepine (Tegretol, Epitol)	GTCS, CPS, SPS	11–32	4–12	15
Valproic acid (Depakene, Depakote)	GTCS, CPS, SPS, absence, atonic, myoclonic	5–20	40–150	15–30
Ethosuximide (Zarontin)	Absence	30–60	40–100	10–30
Secondary drugs				
Phenobarbital (various)	GTCS, CPS, SPS	46–140	15–40	1–3
Primidone (Mysoline)	GTCS, CPS, SPS	5–18	5–12	10–20
Clonazepam (Klonopin)	Absence, atonic, myoclonic	20–40	.005–.07	.01–.3

Note. GTCS = generalized tonic-clonic seizure; CPS = complex partial seizure; SPS = simple partial seizure.

In managing the neuropsychiatric aspects of epilepsy in elderly patients, a first consideration is the role of AEDs. These medications may relieve some behavioral symptoms either through direct psychotropic properties or through their effects on seizure control (Post et al. 1985). The psychotropic properties of AEDs are particularly important in the management of depression (Robertson and Trimble 1985). If possible, discontinue phenobarbital and other barbiturates, which may promote depression in elderly patients, and use carbamazepine or valproate, which stabilize mood and provide prophylaxis against recurrent depressive episodes. In addition, carbamazepine may be helpful for rapid cycling, dysphoria, personality features, and dyscontrolled, aggressive behavior (Dalby 1971). Clonazepam, in addition to its anxiolytic properties, can serve as a supplement to other antimanic therapies. The alleviation of seizures with any AED has improved libido, often resulting in the dramatic return of sexual functioning (Blumer 1991), but may worsen or precipitate depression (Mendez et al. 1993a). Successful seizure control less frequently affects the emergence of psychosis, suicide, or personality characteristics.

Another therapeutic consideration is the seizure-threshold–lowering effect of psychotropic medications (Itil and Soldatos 1980; Luchins et al. 1984; Oliver et al. 1982) (Table 25–5). This is usually not a problem but can occasionally reach clinical significance. Psychotropic drugs are most convulsive with rapid introduction of the drug and in high doses. Clozapine and bupropion, particularly in combination, may be especially convulsant. When initiating psychotropic therapy, it is best to start low and go slow while monitoring AED levels and EEGs.

There is a potential for interaction of anticonvulsant and psychotropic medications (Table 25–6). Attention to drug interactions is particularly important in elderly patients, who are often on multiple medications. In addition to increasing the metabolism of other AEDs, the addition of an AED most commonly increases the metabolism of a psychotropic drug with a consequent decrease in its therapeutic efficiency (Linnoila et al. 1980). Withdrawal of AEDs can precipitate rebound elevations in psychotropic levels. Alternatively, the initiation of a psychotropic may result in competitive inhibition of anticonvulsant metabolism with elevations of AED levels to toxicity (Vincent 1980).

Other therapeutic considerations that can affect the neuropsychiatric aspects of epilepsy include epilepsy surgery, ECT, and allowing patients to experience occasional partial or generalized seizures. Although epilepsy surgeries such as temporal lobectomy or corpus callosotomy are rarely performed in elderly patients, the removal of a secondary epileptogenic lesion

Table 25–5. Seizure threshold effect of psychotropic medications

Potential	Antipsychotic	Antidepressant	Other psychotropic
Proconvulsant			
High	Clozapine	Bupropion	
	Chlorpromazine	Imipramine	
		Maprotiline	
		Amitriptyline	
		Amoxapine	
		Nortriptyline	
Moderate	Most piperazines	Protriptyline	Lithium
	Thiothixene	Clomipramine	
Low	Fluphenazine	Doxepin	Ethchlorvynol
	Haloperidol	Desipramine	Glutethimide
	Loxapine	Fluoxetine	Hydroxyzine
	Molindone	Trazodone	Meprobamate
	Pimozide	Trimipramine	Methaqualone
	Thioridazine		
Anticonvulsant			
Low		Monoamine oxidase inhibitors	Oral benzodiazepine
	Methylphenidate		
	Dextroamphetamine		
High		Barbiturates	

Table 25–6. Anticonvulsant-psychotropic drug effects on blood levels

Anticonvulsant	Indication	Psychotropic[a] effects on anticonvulsant	Anticonvulsant effect on psychotropic[a]
Carbamazepine	SPS, CPS, GTCS	Potentially decreased	Decreased
Phenytoin	SPS, CPS, GTCS	Potentially decreased or increased, rarely toxic levels	Decreased
Phenobarbital and primidone	SPS, CPS, GTCS	Potentially decreased	Significantly decreased
Valproic acid	CPS, GTCS, absence	Potentially increased, rarely toxic levels	Potentially decreased
Ethosuximide	Absence	None known	None known
Clonazepam	Myoclonic	Potentially decreased	Potentially decreased

[a]Antipsychotic and antidepressant drugs; lithium and the minor tranquilizers have few drug interactions with anticonvulsants.
Note. GTCS = generalized tonic-clonic seizures; CPS = complex partial seizures; SPS = simple partial seizures.

such as a tumor may ameliorate associated behavioral disturbances. Unfortunately, most epileptic patients continue to develop psychosis, personality changes, and suicidal behavior even long after primary epilepsy surgery (Falconer 1973; Jensen 1975; Koch-Weser et al. 1988). In addition to the occasional behavior alleviated by strict seizure control, allowing seizures under carefully controlled conditions, much like ECT, can relieve interictal depression, some cases of ictally related psychotic episodes, episodic dyscontrol, and, less frequently, other behaviors.

Summary

The neuropsychiatric aspects of epilepsy include a broad range of behavioral changes that can occur in elderly patients. The incidence of seizure disorders in those over age 65 is higher than at any time since infancy; consequently, there is benefit in understanding the particular psychosocial impact of seizures on older people. In later life, there are increased neuropsychological effects from seizures, from the causative brain lesions, and from anticonvulsant medications. There may be an increased severity of ictally related behavioral disturbances such as prolonged periods of postictal confusion. Moreover, epileptic patients have an increased frequency of interictal psychiatric disturbances, such as depression, psychosis, suicide, personality disorders, hyposexuality, and others. Management of these behavioral disorders requires attention to the behavioral effects of anticonvulsant medications, the convulsant effects of psychotropic medications, and the interactions between them.

References

Adamec RE: Does kindling model anything clinically relevant? Biol Psychiatry 27:249–279, 1990

Altshuler LL, Devinsky O, Post RM, et al: Depression, anxiety, and temporal lobe epilepsy: laterality of focus and symptoms. Arch Neurol 47:284–288, 1990

Barraclough B: Suicide and epilepsy, in Epilepsy and Psychiatry. Edited by Reynolds E, Trimble MR. New York, Churchill Livingstone, 1981, pp 72–76

Bear D, Fedio P: Quantitative analysis of interictal behavior in temporal lobe epilepsy. Arch Neurol 34:454–467, 1977

Betts TA: Depression, anxiety and epilepsy, in Epilepsy and Psychiatry. Edited by Reynolds E, Trimble MR. New York, Churchill Livingstone, 1981a, pp 60–71

Betts TA: Epilepsy and the mental hospital, in Epilepsy and Psychiatry. Edited by Reynolds E, Trimble MR. New York, Churchill Livingstone, 1981b, pp 175–184

Blumer D: Personality in epilepsy. Semin Neurol 11:155–166, 1991

Botwinick J: Neuropsychology of aging, in The Handbook of Clinical Neuropsychology. Edited by Fiskov SB, Boll TJ. New York, Wiley, 1981, pp 135–171

Brent DA, Crumrine PK, Varma R, et al: Phenobarbital treatment and major depressive disorder in children with epilepsy: a naturalistic follow-up. Pediatrics 85:1086–1091, 1990

Bromfield EB, Altshuler L, Leiderman BD, et al: Cerebral metabolism and depression in patients with complex partial seizures. Arch Neurol 49:617–623, 1992

Commission on Classification and Terminology of the International League Against Epilepsy: Proposal for revised clinical and electroencephalographic classification of epileptic seizures. Epilepsia 22:489–501, 1981

Currie S, Heathfield KWG, Henson RA, et al: Clinical course and prognosis of temporal lobe epilepsy: a survey of 666 patients. Brain 92:173–190, 1971

Dalby MA: Antiepileptic and psychotropic effect of carbamazepine (Tegretol) in the treatment of psychomotor epilepsy. Epilepsia 12:325–334, 1971

Devinsky O, Bear DM: Varieties of depression in epilepsy. Neuropsychiatry Neuropsychology and Behavioral Neurology 4:49–61, 1991

Dikmen S, Hermann BP, Wilensky AJ, et al: Validity of the Minnesota Multiphasic Personality Inventory (MMPI) to psychopathology in patients with epilepsy. J Nerv Ment Dis 171:114–122, 1983

Dodrill CB, Batzel LW: Interictal behavioral features of patients with epilepsy. Epilepsia 27 (suppl 2):S64–S76, 1986

Dodrill CB, Breyer DN, Diamond MB, et al: Psychosocial problems among adults with epilepsy. Epilepsia 25:168–175, 1984

Dongier S: Statistical study of clinical and electroencephalographic manifestations of 536 psychotic episodes occurring in 516 epileptics between clinical seizures. Epilepsia 1:117–142, 1959/60

Elliott FA: Neurological findings in adult minimal brain dysfunction and the dyscontrol syndrome. J Nerv Ment Dis 170:680–687, 1982

Engel J, Ludwig B, Fetell M: Prolonged partial complex status epilepticus: EEG and behavioral observations. Neurology 28:863–866, 1978

Ervin F, Epstein RW, King HE: Behavior of epileptic and nonepileptic patients with "temporal spikes." Arch Neurol Psychiatry 74:488–497, 1955

Falconer MA: Reversibility by temporal-lobe resection of the behavioral abnormalities of temporal-lobe epilepsy. N Engl J Med 289:451–455, 1973

Flor-Henry P: Depressive-like reactions and affective psychosis associated with temporal lobe epilepsy: etiologic factors. Am J Psychiatry 126:400–403, 1969

Gates JR, Ramani V, Whalen S, et al: Ictal characteristics of pseudoseizures. Arch Neurol 42:1183–1187, 1985

Geschwind N: Pathogenesis of behavior change in temporal lobe epilepsy, in Epilepsy. Edited by Ward AA Jr, Penry JK, Purpura E. New York, Raven, 1983, pp 355–370

Gibbs FA: Ictal and non-ictal psychiatric disorders in temporal lobe epilepsy. J Nerv Ment Dis 113:522–528, 1951

Gibbs FA, Gibbs EL, Fuster B: Psychomotor epilepsy. Arch Neurol Psychiatry 60:331–339, 1948

Godfrey JBW: Misleading presentation of epilepsy in elderly people. Age Ageing 18:17–20, 1989

Gudmundsson G: Epilepsy in Iceland: a clinical and epidemiological investigation. Acta Neurol Scand (suppl 25): 1–124, 1966

Hauser WA: Seizure disorders: the changes with age. Epilepsia 33 (suppl 4):S6–S14, 1992

Hauser WA, Kurland LT: The epidemiology of epilepsy in Rochester, Minnesota, 1935 through 1967. Epilepsia 27:135–141, 1986

Hauser WA, Morris ML, Heston LL, et al: Seizures and myoclonus in patients with Alzheimer's disease. Neurology 36:1226–1260, 1986

Heath RG: Psychosis and epilepsy: similarities and differences in the anatomic-physiologic substrate. Advances in Biological Psychiatry 8:106–116, 1982

Hermann BP, Wyler AR: Depression, loss of control, and the effects of epilepsy surgery. Epilepsia 30:332–338, 1989

Herzberg JL, Fenwick PB: The aetiology of aggression in temporal lobe epilepsy. Br J Psychiatry 153:50–55, 1988

Hurwitz TA, Wada JA, Kosaka BD, et al: Cerebral organization of affect suggested by temporal lobe seizures. Neurology 35:1335–1337, 1985

Itil TM, Soldatos C: Epileptogenic side effects of psychotropic drugs. JAMA 244:1460–1463, 1980

Jensen I: Temporal lobe epilepsy: late mortality in patients treated with unilateral temporal lobe resections. Acta Neurol Scand 52:374–380, 1975

Koch-Weser M, Garron DC, Gilley DW, et al: Prevalence of psychological disorders after surgical treatment of seizures. Arch Neurol 45:1308–1313, 1988

Kogeorgos J, Fonagy P, Scott DF: Psychiatric symptom patterns of chronic epileptics attending a neurological clinic: a controlled investigation. Br J Psychiatry 140:236–243, 1982

Kraepelin E: Psychiatrie, 8th Edition. Leipzig, Germany, Johann Ambrosius Barltz, 1923

Landolt H: Serial electroencephalographic investigations during psychotic episodes in epileptic patients and during schizophrenic attacks, in Lectures on Epilepsy. Edited by L de Haas. New York, Elsevier Science, 1958, pp 91–133

Leppik IE: Metabolism of antiepileptic medication: newborn to elderly. Epilepsia 33 (suppl 4):S32–S40, 1992

Lindsay J, Ounsted C, Richards P: Long-term outcome in children with temporal lobe seizures, III: psychiatric aspects in childhood and adult life. Dev Med Child Neurol 21:630–636, 1979

Linnoila M, Viukari M, Vaisanen K, et al: Effect of anticonvulsants on plasma haloperidol and thioridazine levels. Am J Psychiatry 137:819–821, 1980

Logsdail SJ, Toone BK: Post-ictal psychosis, a clinical and phenomenological description. Br J Psychiatry 152:246–252, 1988

Luchins DH, Oliver AP, Wyatt RJ: Seizures with antidepressants: an in vitro technique to assess relative risk. Epilepsia 25:25–32, 1984

Luhdorf K, Jensen LK, Plesner AM: Epilepsy in the elderly: incidence, social function and disability. Epilepsia 27:135–141, 1986a

Luhdorf K, Jensen LK, Plesner AM: Etiology of seizures in the elderly. Epilepsia 27:458–463, 1986b

MacKay A: Self-poisoning: a complication of epilepsy. Br J Psychiatry 134:277–282, 1979

Mathews WS, Barabas G: Suicide and epilepsy: a review of the literature. Psychosomatics 22:515–524, 1981

McAreavey MJ, Ballinger BR, Fenton GW: Epileptic seizures in elderly patients with dementia. Epilepsia 33:657–660, 1992

Meierkord H, Will B, Fish D, et al: The clinical features and prognosis of pseudoseizures diagnosed using video-EEG telemetry. Neurology 41;1643–1646, 1991

Mendez MF, Doss RC: Ictal and psychiatric aspects of suicide among epileptics. Int J Psychiatry Med 22:231–237, 1992

Mendez MF, Cummings JL, Benson DF: Depression in epilepsy, significance and phenomenology. Arch Neurol 43:766–770, 1986

Mendez MF, Lanska DJ, Manon-Espaillet R, et al: Causative factors for suicide attempts by overdose in epileptics. Arch Neurol 46:1065–1068, 1989

Mendez MF, Doss RC, Taylor JL, et al: Interictal depression in epilepsy: relationship to seizure variables. J Nerv Ment Dis 181:444–447, 1993a

Mendez MF, Doss RC, Taylor JL, et al: Relationship of seizure variables to personality disorders in epilepsy. J Neuropsychiatry Clin Neurosci 5:283–286, 1993b

Mendez MF, Grau R, Doss RC, et al: Schizophrenia in epilepsy: seizure and psychosis variables. Neurology 43:1073–1077, 1993c

Oliver AP, Luchins DH, Wyatt RJ: Neuroleptic-induced seizures. Arch Gen Psychiatry 39:206–209, 1982

Pakalnis A, Drake ME, John K, et al: Normalizations: acute psychosis after seizure control in seven patients. Arch Neurol 44:289–292, 1987

Perez MM, Trimble MR: Epileptic psychosis-diagnostic comparison with process schizophrenia. Br J Psychiatry 37:245–249, 1980

Perini G, Mendius R: Depression and anxiety in complex partial seizures. J Nerv Ment Dis 172:287–290, 1984

Pond DA, Bidwell BH: A survey of epilepsy in 14 general practices, II: social and psychological aspects. Epilepsia 1:285–299, 1959/60

Post RM, Uhde TW, Joffe RT: Anticonvulsant drugs in psychiatric illness: new treatment alternatives and theoretical implications, in The Psychopharmacology of Epilepsy. Edited by Trimble MR. New York, Wiley, 1985, pp 141–171

Robertson MM: Depression in patients with epilepsy: an overview. Semin Neurol 11:182–189, 1991

Robertson MM, Trimble MR: The treatment of depression in patients with epilepsy: a double blind trial. J Affective Dis 9:127–136, 1985

Robinson RG, Szetela B: Mood change following left hemisphere brain injury. Ann Neurol 9:447–453, 1981

Rodin EA: Psychomotor epilepsy and aggressive behavior. Arch Gen Psychiatry 28:210–213, 1973

Rodin E, Schmaltz S: The Bear-Fedio personality inventory and temporal lobe epilepsy. Neurology 34:591–596, 1984

Romanelli M, Morris JC, Ashkin K, et al: Advanced Alzheimer's disease is a risk factor for late-onset seizures. Arch Neurol 47:847–850, 1990

Roy A: Some determinants of affective symptoms in epileptics. Can J Psychiatry 24:554–556, 1979

Sackeim HA, Greenberg MS, Weiman AL, et al: Hemispheric asymmetry in the expression of positive and negative emotions: neurologic evidence. Arch Neurol 39:210–218, 1982

Sanders KM, Murray GB: Geriatric epilepsy: a review. J Geriatr Psychiatry Neurol 4:98–105, 1991

Sherwin I, Peron-Magnon P, Bancaud J, et al: Prevalence of psychosis in epilepsy as a function of laterality of the epileptogenic lesion. Arch Neurol 39:621–625, 1982

Shorvon SD, Gilliatt RW, Cox TCS, et al: Evidence of vascular disease from CT scanning in late onset epilepsy. J Neurol Neurosurg Psychiatry 47:225–230, 1984

Slater E, Beard A: The schizophrenia-like psychosis of epilepsy: psychiatric aspects. Br J Psychiatry 109:95–150, 1963

Smith DB, Treiman DM, Trimble MR: Neurobehavioral Problems in Epilepsy. New York, Raven Press, 1991

Standage KF, Fenton GW: Psychiatric symptom profiles of patients with epilepsy: a controlled investigation. Psychol Med 5:152–160, 1975

Stevens JR: Interictal clinical manifestations of complex partial seizures. Adv Neurol 2:85–112, 1975

Stevens JR: Psychosis and the temporal lobe, in Neurobehavioral Problems in Epilepsy. Edited by Smith DB, Treiman DM, Trimble MR. New York, Raven, 1991, pp 79–96

Stevens JR, Livermore A: Kindling of the mesolimbic dopamine system: animal model of psychosis. Neurology 28:36–46, 1978

Taylor D: Mental state and temporal lobe epilepsy: a correlative account of 100 patients treated surgically. Epilepsia 13:727–765, 1972

Toone B: Sexual disorders in epilepsy, in Recent Advances in Epilepsy, 3rd Edition. Edited by Pedley TA, Meldrum BS. New York, Churchill Livingstone, 1987 pp 233–259

Treiman DM: Psychobiology of ictal aggression, in Neurobehavioral Problems in Epilepsy. Edited by Smith DB, Treiman DM, Trimble MR. New York, Raven, 1991, pp 341–356

Trimble MR: The Psychosis of Epilepsy. New York, Raven, New York, 1991

Vincent FM: Phenothiazine-induced phenytoin intoxication. Ann Intern Med 93:56–57, 1980

Weil AA: Depressive reactions associated with temporal lobe-uncinate seizures. J Nerv Ment Dis 121:505–510, 1955

Wells CE: Transient ictal psychosis. Arch Gen Psychiatry 32:1201–1203, 1975

Whitman S, Coleman TE, Patmon C, et al: Epilepsy in prison: elevated prevalence and no relationship to violence. Neurology 34:775–782, 1984

Wilensky AJ, Leal KW, Dudley DL, et al: Characteristics of psychotropic drug use in an epilepsy center population (abstract). Epilepsia 22:247, 1981

26

Neuropsychiatric Aspects of Neoplastic, Demyelinating, Infectious, and Inflammatory Brain Disorders

Douglas W. Scharre, M.D.

Introduction

Acquired diseases of the brain are common in the elderly population. Neuropsychiatric disorders are frequent complications of these conditions and may be the sole manifestations of the brain dysfunction. In this chapter, I discuss the neuropsychiatric manifestations of the major neoplastic, demyelinating, infectious, and inflammatory diseases of the brain.

Neoplastic Disorders

Demography

Primary and metastatic neoplasms of the central nervous system (CNS) are common in the geriatric population. The overall incidence of CNS tumors is 15/100,000 per year, and the age-specific incidence peaks between 60 to 80 years. Eighty-five percent of all primary neoplasms occur intracranially; the rest are intraspinal. In clinical series, 45% of intracranial tumors are gliomas, 15% are meningiomas, 7% are pituitary adenomas, and 6% are metastatic (Tyler and Byrne 1992). However, many tumors go unrecognized during life, and in autopsy series meningiomas account for up to 40% and metastatic tumors for up to 18% of all intracranial neoplasms (Kurtzke and Kurland 1983). The most common cancers to metastasize to the brain are lung, breast, kidney, colon, testis, melanoma, and lymphoma (Alvord and Shaw 1991).

Physiology

There are multiple ways for CNS neoplasms to alter brain function. Direct invasion and compression will produce focal neurological deficits such as aphasia, hemiparesis, amnesia, or visual field deficits. Vasogenic brain edema is produced in many neoplasms secondary to capillary leakage across a defective blood-brain barrier (Adams and Victor 1985). This edema in conjunction with the mass effect of the tumor often leads to increased intracranial pressure. The typical signs and symptoms of increased intracranial pressure are headache, nausea, vomiting, papilledema, sixth cranial nerve palsy, and mental status changes. These mental status changes include diminished arousal, impaired attention, irritability, emotional lability, impaired cognition, and psychomotor retardation. Eventually, with continued increased intracranial pressure, bradycardia, hypertension, and herniation syndromes develop.

Tumors located near the ventricular system often cause obstructive hydrocephalus. Headache, cognitive decline, and gait disturbances are frequent sequela. Tumors may also cause vascular obstruction, particularly of the venous system, resulting in ischemic infarctions, hemorrhages, and increased intracranial pressure. Finally, 30% of tumors will produce focal or generalized seizures.

Pathology

Intracranial neoplasms consist of rapidly growing tumor cells, tumor-related blood vessels, and necrotic tissue. Astrocytomas are classified as low grade, intermediate grade, or high grade (glioblastoma multiforme) according to the degree of nuclear atypism, mitosis, endothelial proliferation, and necrosis exhibited. Elderly individuals tend to have higher-grade astrocytomas. Oligodendrogliomas frequently contain calcifications and may bleed. Meningiomas are derived from cells of the arachnoid, pia mater, and dura mater and do not invade the brain parenchyma. Pituitary adenomas arise from one of several cell types in the anterior lobe of the pituitary. Most of the adenomas in the geriatric age range are nonfunctional chromophobe types (Alvord and Shaw 1991).

Laboratory Evaluations

Lumbar puncture is generally avoided because of the risk of precipitating a herniation syndrome when there is a mass lesion in the brain. When cerebrospinal fluid (CSF) is collected, it typically reveals a mild pleocytosis, elevated protein, and normal glucose (Cummings and Benson 1992). CSF cytology is helpful in cases of meningeal carcinomatosis.

Electroencephalography (EEG) in patients with brain tumors is usually abnormal revealing either focal or generalized slowing, sharp waves and spikes, or frank epileptiform activity. Angiography demonstrates the amount of tumor vascularity, which, in gliomas, is often correlated to tumor growth rate. Angiography of

This chapter is from a project supported by a National Institute on Aging training grant.

meningiomas often show a meningeal blood supply and a distinct vascular blush (Tyler and Byrne 1992).

Magnetic resonance imaging (MRI) and computed tomography (CT) reveal evidence of mass processes, edema, midline shifts, hydrocephalus, and hemorrhage. Contrast enhancement greatly improves tumor detection. MRI is more sensitive than CT in the detection of small tumors, but CT can demonstrate calcifications and bony erosions better. Unfortunately, neither CT nor MRI can accurately define intraparenchymal tumor boundaries. For most intracranial tumors, MRI shows increased signal on T2-weighted and gadolinium-enhanced T1-weighted images. Meningiomas exhibit an extra-axial location, dural base, and marked enhancement with contrast agents. MRIs of a glioblastoma multiforme and a meningioma are shown in Figures 26–1 and 26–2, respectively. Cerebral metastases often appear as multiple ring-enhancing nodular masses (Tyler and Byrne 1992).

Magnetic resonance angiography (MRA), single photon emission tomography (SPECT), and positron-emission tomography (PET) can now provide information on tumor blood flow, grade, recurrence, and response to treatment (Tyler and Byrne 1992).

Treatment and Prognosis

The location and type of CNS neoplasms determines the approach to treatment. Surgical removal or debulking, chemotherapy, or radiation therapy are often used in some combination. Chemotherapy agents depend on the breakdown of the blood-brain barrier at the tumor site for selective drug delivery. The complications of radiation therapy include hypothalamic-pituitary dysfunction with resultant hypothyroidism, hypogonadism, or panhypopituitarism (Constine et al. 1993). Postradiation and chemotherapy leukoencephalopathy complications are discussed in the demyelinating disorders section below.

Corticosteroids are useful in reducing cerebral edema secondary to CNS neoplasms and thereby also aid in reduction of any associated increased intracranial pressure. Anticonvulsants are given to prevent seizures. Psychosis is treated with very low dose haloperidol (0.5 to 1 mg/day) and increased slowly until an adequate response is achieved. Depression is treated with antidepressants or methylphenidate. Mania is treated with carbamazepine, valproate, or a benzodiazepine; lithium is usually avoided because of its po-

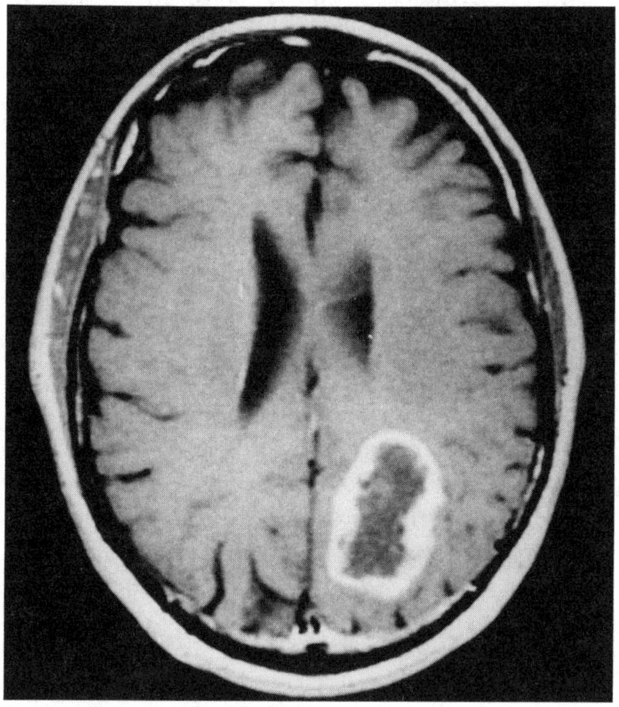

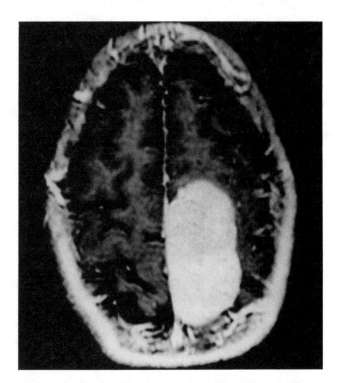

Figure 26–1. Gadolinium-enhanced, T1-weighted magnetic resonance image (MRI) of a 56-year-old man with a left parieto-occipital glioblastoma multiforme. The MRI reveals a ring-enhancing mass with a necrotic center.

Figure 26–2. T1-weighted magnetic resonance image (MRI) of a 56-year-old woman with a left-sided posterior falx meningioma. A large, dural-based, extra-axial mass homogeneously enhances with gadolinium.

tential for exacerbating seizures (T. R. P. Price et al. 1992).

Astrocytomas and oligodendrogliomas are treated with surgery, radiation therapy, and chemotherapy depending on their degree of malignancy. Meningiomas can be completely removed surgically in approximately 90% of cases but have a high rate of recurrence. Pituitary microadenomas are removed through a transphenoidal approach or treated with chemotherapy. Macroadenomas with extensive extraglandular extension often require craniotomies for removal and postsurgical hormonal replacement is often required. Thirty percent of metastases are solitary and are candidates for surgical removal (Alvord and Shaw 1991). The 5-year survival rate for meningiomas is 60%, for gliomas is 20%, and the median survival for glioblastoma multiforme is about 1 year (Kurtzke and Kurland 1983).

Neuropsychiatric Manifestations of Neoplastic Disorders

Frontal lobe tumors.   Frontal lobe tumors produce mental status and personality changes in 90% of cases and frank dementia in 70% of cases, but few focal neurological findings (Cummings and Benson 1992). Apathy, disinhibition, or impulsivity are the hallmarks of frontal involvement. Euphoria or depression, irritability, lack of concern, poor judgment, disorientation, and poor attention are additional frequent early findings. Patients with right frontal tumors may display more euphoria, whereas those with left frontal tumors may display more depression and abulia (Belyi 1987). Psychosis with paranoia, delusions, and hallucinations can also be observed. Impaired word list generation and aphasia with dominant hemisphere tumors, decreased design fluency with nondominant hemisphere tumors, constructional deficits, motor programming deficits, perseveration, forgetfulness, poor abstraction, and psychomotor retardation characterize the dementia. Large subfrontal meningiomas, gliomas spreading to both frontal lobes, and metastatic tumors frequently result in severe dementia. Fifty percent of patients with frontal lobe tumors develop seizures, usually focal motor (Jacksonian) type, and a few develop hydrocephalus due to obstruction of the interventricular foramen. Tumors located in the posterofrontal region produce hemiparesis, olfactory groove meningiomas produce anosmia, sphenoid ridge meningiomas produce unilateral exophthalmos and cranial nerve palsies, prefrontal tumors often produce a grasp reflex, and involvement of the frontal eye fields produces a conjugate deviation of the eyes to the side of the tumor.

Temporal lobe tumors.   Temporal lobe tumors cause personality changes, irritability, euphoria, depression, anxiousness, psychosis, hallucinations (auditory, formed visual, and simple olfactory or gustatory), and cognitive impairment early in their course. Dominant hemisphere tumors produce aphasia and verbal memory deficits (amnesia), whereas nondominant hemisphere tumors produce nonverbal memory deficits. Hydrocephalus may result from obstruction of the third ventricle or compression of the midbrain with obstruction of the cerebral aqueduct. Partial complex seizures are frequent and manifest with staring, blinking, complex motor activity, déjà vu phenomena, visual distortions, hallucinations, and other psychomotor disturbances.

Parietal lobe tumors.   Tumors that are located in the anterior parietal area produce somatosensory disturbances including deficits in two-point discrimination; identification of finger writing (agraphesthesia); identification of objects by their shape, size, texture, or weight (astereognosis); simultaneously identifying bilateral stimulation (inattention); and localization of tactile stimuli (atopognosia). Parietal lobe tumors may cause a contralateral lower-quadrant field cut due to disruption of the superior optic radiations. Difficulties in drawing, apraxia, and focal sensory seizures may also occur with parietal lobe lesions.

Tumors involving the nondominant parietal lobe are most likely to cause a neglect syndrome of the contralateral body and extrapersonal space (inattention). In this condition, patients will not see, dress, shave, or groom the neglected side of the body and do not respond to stimuli in the neglected hemispace. They may deny a contralateral hemiparesis (anosognosia). Dominant parietal lobe tumors in the angular gyrus region cause Gerstmann's syndrome including difficulties with writing (dysgraphia), finger identification, calculations (acalculia), and distinguishing right from left. Often, aphasia and constructional disturbances are also present.

Occipital lobe tumors.   Occipital lobe tumors commonly produce contralateral homonymous visual field deficits, simple visual seizures with generalization, and visual hallucinations consisting of unformed images such as flashes, streaks, or simple geometric patterns. Bilateral medial occipitotemporal tumors may cause a disturbance in visual recognition of objects (visual agnosia), identification of familiar faces (prosopagnosia), or recognition of familiar environments (environmental agnosia). Occasionally right-sided lesions alone may produce some of these syndromes.

Deep midline tumors.   Deep midline tumors often cause bihemispheric dysfunction due to invasion or brain compression by surrounding edema. Tumors within or near the third ventricle can obstruct the interventricular foramen or the cerebral aqueduct and cause hydrocephalus. Tumors within the ventricle can cause intermittent obstruction resulting in severe headaches and vomiting that are position dependent.

Pituitary and hypothalamic area tumors often cause bitemporal hemianopsia, optic atrophy, endocrine disturbances, diabetes insipidus, somnolence, personality changes, and cognitive decline. Excessive somnolence, rage attacks, and hyperphagia are occasionally seen with direct hypothalamic involvement.

Thalamic tumors produce memory loss, confusional states, emotional lability, hemiparesis, and hemihypesthesia with hemianesthesia (Dejerine-Roussy syndrome). Basal ganglia tumors result in impaired attention, memory loss, personality changes, depression, and movement disorders including chorea, dystonia, or rigidity.

Pineal tumors compress the superior colliculus, producing aqueduct occlusion, hydrocephalus, and Parinaud's syndrome with paralysis of upward gaze and ptosis. Brain stem tumors produce cranial nerve deficits, long tract signs, cerebellar symptoms, and hydrocephalus. Personality changes, lethargy, disorientation, memory impairment, and mutism may also occur (Cummings and Benson 1992).

Posterior fossa tumors.   Tumors in this area can obstruct the fourth ventricle or the outflow into the basal cisterns resulting in hydrocephalus. Prominent signs and symptoms include headache, vomiting, mental status changes, cranial nerve palsies, nystagmus, ataxia, dysmetria, hypotonia, and intention tremor.

Paraneoplastic Syndromes

The remote effects of carcinoma are poorly understood. The symptoms usually develop rapidly over a few weeks; they may occur before the discovery of the neoplasm. An autoantibody mechanism is the most likely etiology (Posner 1992).

Limbic encephalitis has been seen with small-cell lung carcinoma, as well as carcinoma of the breast, uterus, ovary, prostate, and kidney; multiple myeloma; lymphosarcoma; reticulum cell sarcoma; and acute leukemia. The age at onset is typically 50–80 years, and men are more commonly affected. The condition may last several years. The syndrome is characterized by an amnestic memory disturbance, cognitive decline, depression, anxiety, personality changes, paranoia, hallucinations, and diminished alertness. Often a severe sensory neuropathy is present. Occasionally seizures, cerebellar deficits, brain stem signs, myelopathy, and autonomic failure are observed.

Neuronal loss and perivascular inflammatory infiltrates particularly in the medial temporal areas are found at autopsy (Newman et al. 1990). Sometimes the cerebellum, brain stem, spinal cord, dorsal root ganglia, and autonomic ganglia are involved. Neuroimaging is typically unrevealing. Rarely, MRI demonstrates increased signal on T2-weighted images in the frontal and temporal lobes. CSF examination usually shows mild lymphocytic pleocytosis, elevated protein, and increased immunoglobulin G (IgG). Anti-Hu antibodies are seen in many cases and found in the nuclei of neurons. No treatment is currently available (Dalmau et al. 1992; Kodama et al. 1991; Posner and Furneaux 1990).

Demyelinating Disorders

Although demyelinating conditions are more common in young individuals, there are many examples of these disorders with late survival or presentation in the elderly population. A comprehensive list of common and rare white matter disorders is presented in Table 26–1. Primary demyelination involves the loss of the myelin sheath leaving the axon intact but denuded. Dysmyelinating conditions reflect impairment in the formation or development of the myelin sheath. These two types of myelin disease give similar clinical and neuropsychiatric features.

Multiple Sclerosis

Multiple sclerosis (MS) is the most common demyelinating disorder of the CNS. Typically it presents in young adults, but 0.6% of the patients do not have their first symptom until age 60 or later (Hooge and

Redekop 1992). The prevalence at age 70 is about 50/100,000 (Kurtzke and Kurland 1983). It is rare in the tropics, but its frequency increases in more northern latitudes. Women are affected more often than men by a ratio of 2 to 1.

Clinical features. The clinical course of MS has three forms: exacerbating-remitting, acute progressive, and chronic progressive. Exacerbating-remitting type is characterized by symptoms that may evolve over a few days and then partially or totally resolve over weeks. Rarely there is an acute rapidly progressive course to death over a few weeks or months. The most common

---

Table 26–1. Causes of demyelinating disorders in elderly patients

Autoimmune
Multiple sclerosis (MS)
Behcet's syndrome
Systemic lupus erythematosus (SLE)
Sjögren's syndrome
Acute disseminated encephalomyelitis
Vogt-Koyanagi-Harada syndrome
Postinfectious encephalomyelitis

Vascular
Binswanger's disease (subcortical arteriosclerotic encephalopathy)

Metabolic-toxic
Marchiafava-Bignami disease
Central pontine myelinolysis
Subacute combined degeneration (vitamin B_{12} deficiency)
Thiamine deficiency (vitamin B_1)
Vitamin B_6 deficiency
Vitamin E deficiency
Postanoxic/posthypoxic state
Postradiation leukoencephalopathy
Chemotherapy-related leukoencephalopathy

Hereditary-metabolic
Metachromatic leukodystrophy (MLD)
Adrenoleukodystrophy (ALD)
Adrenomyeloneuropathy
Cerebrotendinous xanthomatosis
Membranous lipodystrophy
Hereditary adult-onset leukodystrophy
Globoid cell leukodystrophy, late onset

Infectious
Human immunodeficiency virus–type 1 (HIV-1)–associated cognitive/motor complex
Progressive multifocal leukoencephalopathy (PML)
Lyme disease

Neoplastic
Lymphoma of the central nervous system
Paraneoplastic syndromes

---

pattern, particularly in those with onset over age 40, is a chronic, slowly progressive course.

Neurological signs and symptoms include optic neuritis, diplopia, internuclear ophthalmoplegia, spastic weakness, myelopathy, acute transverse myelitis, gait imbalance, appendicular and truncal ataxia, intention tremor, dysmetria, bladder dysfunction, urinary frequency and urgency, urinary incontinence, constipation, autonomic dysfunction, sensory disturbances, paresthesias, loss of vibratory and position sense, pain syndromes particularly of the back and lower extremities, bilateral trigeminal neuralgia, vertigo, paroxysmal disorders, and neuropsychiatric syndromes. Most patients with the onset of symptoms after age 50 or 60 have a slowly progressive myelopathy with spastic paraparesis, gait imbalance, and bladder impairment (Hooge and Redekop 1992; Noseworthy et al. 1983).

Neuropsychiatric aspects. Neuropsychiatric symptoms may be the presenting complaint and like other MS symptoms may exacerbate and remit or may be continuously present after onset. Treatment with steroids or other medications can contribute to these symptoms. Table 26–2 lists the principal neuropsychiatric manifestations of MS and their approximate frequencies. It is important to distinguish between how the patient subjectively feels (mood) and the outward expression of his emotion (affect). About 11% of MS patients have difficulties regulating their emotional expression, resulting in rapid mood swings or inappropriate emotional responses (Minden and Schiffer 1990). Many patients have depressed moods in spite of a euphoric affect.

Table 26–2. Frequency of neuropsychiatric manifestations in multiple sclerosis

Neuropsychiatric manifestation	Frequency
Emotional lability	11%
Depression	50%
Euphoria	25%
Mania	13%
Psychosis	1%–3%
Personality changes	40%
Fatigue	75%
Sexual dysfunction	50% (in women) 75% (in men)
Hypersexuality	4%
Cognitive dysfunction	30%–50%

Compared with patients with other chronic neurological diseases, MS patients have significantly more depression. About half of all MS patients experience at least one major depression during their illness. No association has been found between their depression and a family history of depression, duration of illness, age, gender, or socioeconomic status (Minden et al. 1987). Depression is associated with recent exacerbations of MS symptoms requiring steroid therapy, but not with severity of disability or cognitive impairment in most studies (Good et al. 1992; Schiffer and Caine 1991).

Euphoria—a cheerful affect inappropriate to the situation—occurs in about 25% of MS patients (Rabins 1990). It is not associated with steroid use and does not have other features of hypomania. In fact, many euphoric patients have a depressed mood. Euphoria appears to be produced by bilateral subfrontal demyelination (Minden and Schiffer 1990) and patients with euphoria have more neurological and cognitive deficits than those who do not (Rabins 1990).

Mania occurs in up to 13% of MS patients (Joffe et al. 1987), and MS patients have twice the risk of developing bipolar disorder as the general population.

Human leukocyte antigen (HLA) analysis and family history studies suggest a genetic predisposition for bipolar disorder in MS patients who manifest manic behavior (Schiffer et al. 1988).

Psychosis in MS—including auditory or visual hallucinations, delusions, or paranoia—is seen in about 1%–3% of patients, and it occurs at a later age than in idiopathic schizophrenia (Feinstein et al. 1992; Ron and Logsdail 1989). It can occur without steroid use and without a family history of schizophrenia. Psychosis in MS is associated with increased temporal and temporoparietal lobe abnormalities on MRI (Feinstein et al. 1992; Honer et al. 1987; Ron and Logsdail 1989).

Apathy, irritability, poor judgment, and slowed mental processing are personality changes observed in as many as 40% of MS patients (Mahler 1992). Fatigue—a sense of tiredness or lack of energy that is greater than expected for the effort required for a task or the degree of disability evidenced by the patient (The Canadian MS Research Group 1987)—occurs in about 75% of MS patients, often preventing normal activities (Murray 1985). It must be differentiated from symptoms of depression, weakness, lack of rest, or excessive exercise. Fatigue in MS patients is exacerbated by heat and improves with cooler temperatures (Krupp et al. 1988).

About 75% of men and 50% of women with MS report sexual dysfunction (Stenager et al. 1992). In men, two-thirds have erectile dysfunction and one-third report decreased libido. In women, painful genital dysesthesias, inability to achieve orgasm, and decreased libido are common. Nearly 90% of the men have neurogenic causes for their erectile dysfunction (Kirkeby et al. 1988). Hypersexuality has been noted in as high as 4% of MS patients (Mahler 1992).

Cognitive dysfunction occurs in 30%–50% of MS patients (Fennell and Smith 1990; Rao et al. 1991), with most investigators emphasizing memory impairment. About 20%–30% of MS patients meet criteria for a dementia with defects primarily involving poor retrieval memory, impaired conceptual reasoning, visuospatial abnormalities, and slowed information processing: a pattern suggestive of a subcortical dementia syndrome (Huber et al. 1987; Rao 1986). Corpus callosal atrophy on MRI and increased plaque volume correlate with the severity of cognitive impairment (Huber et al. 1992b; Swirsky-Sacchetti et al. 1992). The cognitive changes do not correlate with duration of disease or depression, but may be more severe in the chronic progressive type of MS typical of elderly patients (Minden et al. 1990; Rao et al. 1991). The cognitive changes weakly correlate with physical disability in some studies (Rao et al. 1991), but not in others (Maurelli et al. 1992).

Both verbal and nonverbal memory are impaired, with spatial memory being more severely affected in most studies (Beatty et al. 1988; Grafman et al. 1990). The memory deficit is a retrieval abnormality and not a true amnesia (Rao 1986). Remote memory is usually spared (Rao et al. 1991). Verbal IQ is generally better preserved than performance IQ (Rao 1986). However, word list generation, also called *verbal fluency* (the number of words beginning with a certain letter produced in 1 minute or the number of animals named per minute), is often decreased (Beatty et al. 1988; Rao et al. 1991). Rarely aphasic syndromes have been described (Achiron et al. 1992). Executive functions including planning, abstraction, concept formation, set shifting, sustained attention, and organization skills are affected in MS (Fennell and Smith 1990) and suggest frontal lobe dysfunction (Beatty et al. 1989). Left frontal lesions on MRI correlate with these disturbances (Huber et al. 1992a). Signs of corpus callosal disconnection have been identified with dichotic listening tasks (Rubens et al. 1985), with tachistoscopic object-naming tasks (Rao et al. 1989), and from the clinical examination demonstrating left-hand apraxia, agraphia, and astereognosis (Schnider et al. 1993). Corpus callosal atrophy on MRI has been demonstrated in these patients.

Pathophysiology and diagnosis.   MS is believed to be caused by an immune-mediated response triggered by exposure to an unknown environmental agent in the genetically predisposed individual. This response results in multifocal discrete inflammatory demyelinated areas scattered throughout the white matter, including the arcuate U-fiber regions. MRI shows these plaques in the white matter as areas of high signal on T2-weighted images (Figure 26–3) and gadolinium contrast can distinguish active from inactive plaques (Bastianello et al. 1990). Diagnosis is aided by finding increased immunoglobulin production in the CSF and prolonged latencies on evoked potential testing (Poser et al. 1983).

Treatment.   Prednisone, methylprednisolone, and adrenocorticotropic hormone (ACTH) appear to speed the recovery of an acute exacerbation. Immunotherapies may decrease the rate of disease progression. Many experimental therapies that are aimed at treating the underlying disease process are currently under investigation.

Management of specific symptoms may contribute to improved patient functioning. Spasticity is treated with a combination of physical therapy, baclofen, benzodiazepines, botulinum toxin, or dantrolene. Paroxysmal disorders respond to anticonvulsants. Bladder disorders and urinary tract infections are reduced by anticholinergics, self-catheterization, and prophylactic antibiotics.

Treatments for the neuropsychiatric manifestations are also available. Pathological laughing or crying can be treated with low-dose amitriptyline (Schiffer et al. 1985) or fluoxetine (Seliger et al. 1992). Depression is treated with tricyclic antidepressants and bipolar disorder with lithium (Schiffer 1990). Anticholinergic agents may impair cognition but aid bladder symptoms; the choice of treatment in any single individual will depend on the relative anticholinergic effect desired. Fatigue may be ameliorated by amantadine (Murray 1985; The Canadian MS Research Group 1987) or pemoline (Weinshenker et al. 1992) or with steroids if associated with an acute exacerbation. Pharmacotherapy reassessment is essential to eliminate agents no longer needed.

Support groups and psychotherapy are useful for information exchange, social interaction, stress reduction, and emotional support (Minden and Moes 1990). The use of memory aids, lists, routinization of daily activities, and other cognitive retraining techniques may improve function but more investigation is needed to establish their utility (LaRocca 1990).

Acute Disseminated Encephalomyelitis

Acute necrotizing hemorrhagic, postinfectious, and postvaccinal encephalomyelitis are forms of acute disseminated encephalomyelitis, an immune-mediated-condition resulting in CNS demyelination. It can occur at any age. It is a monophasic illness presenting with fever, headache, and altered consciousness and typically preceded days or weeks earlier by either a viral illness or vaccination (Geerts et al. 1991). The hemorrhagic form is usually, but not always, rapidly fatal (Huang et al. 1988). If the individual survives the acute condition, gradual recovery over days to weeks ensues. Hemiparesis, sensory deficits, seizures, dysarthria, or dysphasia may be present initially (Geerts et al. 1991). The neuropsychiatric residua vary depending on the degree of injury and extent of recovery. A subcortical dementia syndrome similar to that seen in multiple sclerosis is typical. Inflammation, demyelination, and variable hemorrhage occurs in the white matter and spares the cortex. Imaging studies show either multifocal abnormalities or a focal mass process (Huang et al. 1988). CSF cultures are negative. A brain biopsy may be required to rule out infection or tumor. Treatment is supportive and may require reduction of increased intracranial pressure. Surgical decompression has been recommended for the hemorrhagic form (Huang et al. 1988). Immunosuppression has been used with some success (Seales and Greer 1991).

Binswanger's Disease

Binswanger's disease, also called *subcortical arteriosclerotic encephalopathy,* is a vascular dementia involving the small penetrating vessels supplying the deep white matter of the cerebral hemispheres. It occurs in elderly individuals with a history of chronic hypertension. A gradually progressive course with dementia and personality change is typical. Neuropsychiatric findings include memory impairment, poor judgment, lack of spontaneity, perseveration, pseudobulbar palsy, and at times euphoria, elation, and aggressiveness (Babikian and Ropper 1987). Weakness, ataxia, rigidity, dysarthria, and urinary incontinence are frequent neurological abnormalities. White matter demyelination is seen pathologically, and MRI reveals hyperintensities on T2-weighted images in the periventricular and deep white matter regions. Binswanger's disease and lacunar state commonly co-occur. (This condition is discussed in more detail in Chapter 20.)

Marchiafava-Bignami Disease

Marchiafava-Bignami disease is characterized by demyelination of the corpus callosum and adjacent white matter. It is rare and occurs mostly in middle- to late-adult men with chronic alcoholism. Many individuals exhibit a chronic dementia syndrome that progresses over months to years. Remissions are possible. Patients with severe cases present in stupor or coma and die rapidly.

The neuropsychiatric features vary widely from case to case. Dementia, limb apraxia, seizures, and personality changes are common. Violence, apathy, and

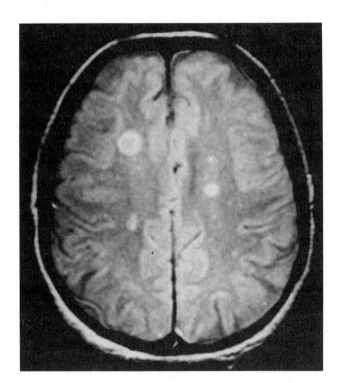

Figure 26–3. Magnetic resonance image (MRI) of a 65-year-old woman with chronic progressive multiple sclerosis. MRI shows multiple areas of increased signal on the proton-density–weighted image in the right and left centrum semiovale regions.

sexual deviations have been reported. The neurological manifestations include dysarthria, incontinence, aphasia, hemiparesis, apraxic gait, and frontal release signs (Victor 1986). Signs of corpus callosum interhemispheric disconnection are evident with left-sided apraxia and left-handed anomia and agraphia (Lechevalier et al. 1977).

Demyelination of the corpus callosum with relative sparing of the splenium and absence of inflammatory changes is the characteristic pathology. Less often, the anterior or posterior commissures, centrum semiovale, superior cerebellar peduncles, or the white matter of the pons are involved. CT or MRI scans help identity the demyelination (Chang et al. 1992).

Subacute Combined Degeneration

Subacute combined degeneration is caused by vitamin B_{12} (or rarely folate) deficiency, which produces demyelination in the spinal cord and brain. This condition can occur at any age and may be secondary to pernicious anemia, malabsorption syndromes, a total gastrectomy, or, rarely, a dietary B_{12} deficiency. Pernicious anemia is a disease with onset usually between ages 35 and 60. Clinical features of subacute combined degeneration include myelopathy, peripheral neuropathy, megaloblastic anemia, and dementia.

Confusion, memory impairment, slow reaction time, and depression are common neuropsychiatric manifestations (Cummings and Benson 1992). The dementia may occasionally precede other systemic manifestations of the vitamin deficiency (Karnaze and Carmel 1990). Paranoia, agitation, delusions, and hallucinations also occur (Lindenbaum et al. 1988). Numbness, tingling, lower-extremity weakness, and gait disturbance may progress to flaccid paralysis and incontinence.

The dorsal and lateral columns of the spinal cord and the white matter in the brain show areas of spongiform degenerative demyelination. EEG reveals generalized slowing in those with dementia. A low serum B_{12} level is usually diagnostic, and malabsorption is demonstrated by performing a Schilling test. Administration of vitamin B_{12} may reverse or stop the progression of the neurological findings and the dementia.

Postanoxic/Posthypoxic States

Elderly individuals are particularly prone to anoxia/hypoxia from cardiopulmonary failure or sleep apnea.

Chronic hypoxia results in a slowly progressive dementia syndrome, whereas acute anoxia can lead to profound neuronal injury and death. Rarely, patients may develop extensive white matter demyelination a few weeks after apparent recovery from an acute anoxic insult. The delayed symptoms include slowed responses, somnolence, irritability, depression, inattentiveness, disorientation, forgetfulness, pseudobulbar palsy, mutism, incontinence, gait disturbances, and spasticity (Plum et al. 1962). Death often occurs but moderate recovery has been observed. Postanoxic demyelination is seen diffusely over both cerebral hemispheres on MRI.

Postradiation and Chemotherapy-Related Leukoencephalopathy

Neoplastic conditions are very common in the geriatric population and both radiation therapy and chemotherapy are often used either alone or in combination to treat the tumors. These therapies can be used either to reduce the tumor burden or as a prophylactic to reduce the likelihood of potential brain or spinal cord metastases. However, both may also lead to a delayed demyelination of the CNS occurring from 3 months to 5 years after the treatment. The neurological complications of cranial irradiation include memory loss, cognitive decline, abulia, gait disturbance, ataxia, long tract signs, and tremors. Patients may become severely disabled with dementia and paresis (B. E. Johnson et al. 1985).

Chemotherapeutic agents cause a delayed demyelination thought to be secondary to oligodendrocyte neurotoxicity. The neurological findings are similar to the delayed effects of radiation treatment. Methotrexate is the most notable example of such an agent, especially when given intrathecally (Ojeda 1982). Cyclosporine (de Groen et al. 1987), cytosine arabinoside (AraC) (Lee et al. 1986), and 5-fluorouracil combined with levamisole (C. C. Hook et al. 1992) have all been reported to cause demyelination. The combination of radiation therapy and chemotherapy, particularly when using methotrexate, cisplatin, lomustine (CCNU]) or amphotericin B, appears to enhance the neurotoxicity (So et al. 1987; Walker and Rosenblum 1992).

Demyelination with necrosis is the pathological finding seen with the delayed effects of radiation on the CNS. Demyelination with or without necrosis has also been reported with the use of chemotherapeutic agents (C. C. Hook et al. 1992; Ojeda 1982). Diffuse symmetric white matter low attenuation, cerebral atrophy, ventricular dilatation, and occasionally mass effect are seen with CT scanning of the head (So et al. 1987). MRI reveals increased signal on the T2-weighted images in the periventricular white matter in a diffuse, symmetric, and confluent pattern. Scattered focal lesions that enhance with gadolinium are also common (C. C. Hook et al. 1992; So et al. 1987).

Metachromatic Leukodystrophy

Metachromatic leukodystrophy (MLD) is a dysmyelinating disorder with infantile, juvenile, and adult forms. The adult form may present from ages 16 to 40 and will usually last from 5 to 20 years, but occasionally as long as 40 years. The enzyme deficient in this autosomal recessive inheritable disorder is arylsulfatase A. Personality changes and cognitive decline mark the insidious onset of the adult form (Baumann et al. 1991). Disinhibition, poor judgment, dishevelment, inappropriate affect, emotional lability, looseness of associations, diminished attention span, memory deficits, abstraction and calculation difficulties, spatial disorientation, and constructional problems are seen (Merriam et al. 1990). This progresses to psychosis (present in more than 50% of cases), occasionally mania, and dementia (Hyde et al. 1992). Spasticity, ataxia, and seizures are often present. Resting and postural tremors and choreoathetosis have occasionally been described (Merriam et al. 1990). Peripheral neuropathy, in the adult form, may not be clinically evident though present electrophysiologically. Sulfatide deposits are present around both central and peripheral nerves and in viscera. Demyelination sparing the arcuate fibers (U-fibers) is present in the cerebral hemispheres and evident on neuroimaging. Motor and sensory nerve conduction velocities are mildly slowed, and increased CSF protein is occasionally found. Diagnosis is made by measuring the enzyme deficiency in leukocytes or measuring the amount of sulfatide in urine (Baumann et al. 1991). Genetic counseling is indicated.

Adrenoleukodystrophy

Adrenoleukodystrophy (ALD) is an X-linked dysmyelinating disorder featuring a deficiency of a peroxisomal enzyme that results in the excessive storage of very long chain fatty acids (VLCFAs) (Naidu and Moser 1990). There are neonatal, juvenile, adolescent, and adult cerebral forms as well as an X-linked adrenomyeloneuropathy (AMN) form. The adult cerebral form, representing about 3% of all cases, may present from ages 18 to 57 (Weller et al. 1992). The AMN form, found in 21% of all cases, typically has its onset between ages 20 and 35 and rarely occurs in later adult life. About 10%–15% of the female ALD carriers develop neurological deficits resembling AMN with onset between age 15 and 76 (Naidu and Moser 1990).

The initial finding in the adult cerebral form of ALD is usually dementia. Other neurological findings include upper motor neuron signs, paresis, ataxia, gait apraxia, dysarthria, homonymous hemianopsia, impaired visual acuity leading to cortical blindness, ocular movement disorders, and hearing loss. Seizures are a late finding. Psychiatric features are seen in nearly 40% of patients, often occur early in the course, and include hypomania, emotional lability, depression, hyperactivity, physical and sexual aggression, and psychosis (Kitchin et al. 1987). Adrenal insufficiency and a bronze discoloration of the skin typically become evident after the neurological symptoms begin. The AMN form begins with a progressive spastic paraparesis and a mild peripheral neuropathy, with 20% eventually developing dementia. Emotional lability and depression have also been observed (Naidu and Moser 1990). In ALD, there is demyelination of cerebral white matter sparing the arcuate fibers. Increased signal on T2-weighted images is present in the periventricular white matter on MRI scanning, typically starting occipitally and progressing anteriorly. CSF protein is increased. Diagnosis is made by assaying VLCFAs in plasma or skin fibroblasts. A low cortisol level or a reduced adrenal response to stimulation indicates adrenal insufficiency. Treatment includes a low-VLCFA diet with erucic and oleic acid; adrenal steroids are used for the adrenal dysfunction.

Cerebrotendinous Xanthomatosis

Cerebrotendinous xanthomatosis is an autosomal recessive disorder resulting in impaired hepatic synthesis of bile salts, leading to markedly increased levels of cholestanol. Age at onset ranges from infancy to the seventh decade. The clinical features include cataracts, tuberous and tendon xanthomas, dementia, ataxia, pyramidal tract signs, spasticity, dysarthria, seizures, depression, and a demyelinating neuropathy. Early atherosclerosis with coronary artery disease is also common. The tendon xanthomas often begin between ages 20 and 40. Cognitive decline can appear in childhood or be delayed well past middle age. Spasticity and ataxia progress, and, in the terminal stage, incontinence and pseudobulbar palsy are present. Pathology shows extensor tendon xanthomas and brain deposition of high-density lipoprotein. CSF examination demonstrates a mildly elevated protein. CT and MRI scanning reveal atrophy, focal tuberous xanthomas, and demyelination in the cerebellum and cerebrum (Hokezu et al. 1992). Diagnosis is confirmed by finding elevated levels of cholestanol in plasma or bile. Early treatment with chenodeoxycholic acid to reduce the formation of cholestanol may reverse and prevent the clinical findings (Bjorkhem and Skrede 1990).

Infectious Disorders

Infectious conditions producing neuropsychiatric signs and symptoms are common at all ages. In the elderly population, diagnosis is more difficult as certain systemic signs such as fever may not be present whereas other nonspecific symptoms such as confusion, headache, malaise, generalized weakness, and diminished appetite may be more prominent. Progression to an acute confusional state or delirium with hallucinations, delusions, paranoia, impaired attention, disorientation, cognitive deficits, sleep disturbance, and tremors may occur rapidly. Consideration of infectious etiologies at an early stage enables prompt diagnosis and treatment. Neuroimaging with MRI or CT followed by lumbar puncture and, potentially, brain biopsy are often necessary to determine the specific pathogen. Common CNS infections of the geriatric age group are listed in Table 26–3.

Prion Infections

Prions are *pro*teinaceous *in*fectious particles consisting of protein with little or no nucleic acid and causing transmissible diseases (Hsiao and Prusiner 1990; Prusiner 1991). The gene responsible for the prion protein is located on the short arm of chromosome 20. Aberrant prion protein isoforms, produced by a posttranslational process, are hypothesized to lead to disease (Meiner et al. 1992). Additionally, point mutations in the prion protein gene are associated with the familial forms of prion disease (Prusiner 1991).

Three of the human neurodegenerative diseases—Gerstmann-Straüssler-Scheinker syndrome (GSS),

Creutzfeldt-Jakob disease (CJD), and kuru—are caused by prions and are transmissible to laboratory animals (Prusiner 1991). GSS is an autosomal dominant disorder with onset between ages 40 and 60. It is characterized by a mild dementia with pyramidal, extrapyramidal, and cerebellar signs (Farlow et al. 1989). Kuru is seen in certain New Guinea tribes who practice ritualistic cannibalism. Two additional rare neurodegenerative diseases, fatal familial insomnia and a familial form of thalamic dementia, which do not appear to be transmissible, have both been linked to a mutation at codon 178 of the prion protein (Medori et al. 1992; Petersen et al. 1992), suggesting that they are the same prion disorder. These conditions have courses and presentations similar to those of CJD with the addition of progressive insomnia and dysautonomia.

CJD has a worldwide incidence of approximately 1/1,000,000. About 90% of CJD cases arise sporadically without evidence of any infectious source, and 5%–15% are familial with an autosomal dominant inheritance (Hsiao and Prusiner 1990). The only transmitted cases in humans have occurred iatrogenically with corneal transplants, depth electrodes, neurosurgical instruments, a cadaveric dura matter graft, and when giving human growth hormone that was extracted from human cadaveric pituitaries (Rappaport 1987).

The usual age at onset is between 50 and 70, with a range from 20 to 79 (Cummings and Benson 1992). The clinical course is typically very rapid, with death usually within several months to 1 year. Occasionally, individuals have survived for several years. The familial forms have an earlier age at onset and a longer duration of illness (Brown et al. 1992).

Initially, the patient has complaints of generalized fatigue, anxiety, sleep disturbance, appetite change, depression, impaired concentration, and forgetfulness. After a few weeks, a progressive dementia ensues with aphasia, amnesia, apraxia, agnosia, and severe cognitive deficits. Other neurological features appear with the dementia and include myoclonus, chorea, tremor, ataxia, cerebellar signs, pyramidal signs, spasticity, rigidity, and seizures. Hallucinations and delusions are also seen. Mutism, incontinence, decerebrate rigidity, and akinesis occur in the final phases (Brown et al. 1986; Cummings and Benson 1992).

Pathology shows a spongiform state in the cortical and subcortical gray matter with loss of neurons and gliosis (Masters et al. 1981). The spongiform changes reflect the occurrence of intracellular vacuoles. Occasionally, white matter gliosis and demyelination are also seen. Some CJD patients have amyloid plaques in the cerebellum and cerebrum similar to those found in kuru. An abnormal isoform of the prion protein accumulates in the brain and in the amyloid plaques (Serban et al. 1990). MRI results may be normal or reveal mild atrophy and areas of increased signal on T2-weighted images corresponding to the pathological regions (Milton et al. 1991). PET shows multiple diffuse areas of hypometabolism in both cortical and subcortical regions (Holthoff et al. 1990) (Figure 26–4). Lumbar puncture is abnormal in only 20% of patients, showing mild lymphocytosis and elevations in protein and IgG (Table 26–4). The EEG shows background slowing and a very characteristic periodic polyspike discharge (Chiofalo et al. 1980); this EEG pattern may be absent in the familial forms of CJD (Brown et al. 1992). Diagnosis can be made by the clinical features and EEG changes and is confirmed by brain biopsy if the features are atypical. Treatment is not available except for supportive care.

Table 26–3. Causes of central nervous system infections in elderly patients

Prions
   Creutzfeldt-Jakob disease (CJD)
   Gerstmann-Sträussler-Scheinker syndrome (GSS)
   Fatal familial insomnia
   Thalamic dementia
Virus
   Acute viral encephalitis
      Herpes simplex encephalitis
      Other meningoencephalitides
   Slow viral encephalitis
      Human immunodeficiency virus–type 1 (HIV-1)
      Progressive multifocal leukoencephalopathy (PML)
Bacteria
   Acute bacterial meningitis
   Brain abscess
   Subdural empyema
   Epidural abscess
   Tuberculosis (meningitis)
   Whipple's disease
Fungus
   Chronic meningitis
Spirochetes
   Syphilis
   Lyme disease
Parasites
   Toxoplasma
   Cysticercosis
   Amoeba

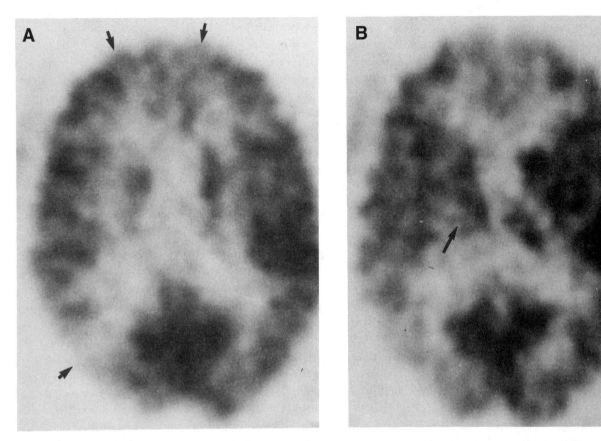

Figure 26–4. Positron-emission tomography (PET) image of a 63-year-old man with autopsy-proven Creutzfeldt-Jakob disease. *Panel A:* PET shows multifocal areas of cortical hypometabolism involving the right parieto-occipital region and the bilateral frontal areas (*arrows*). *Panel B:* A slightly caudal PET slice revealing the relative hypometabolism seen in the right basal ganglia region (*arrow*).

Table 26–4.   Cerebrospinal fluid profiles of infections

Infection	White cells	Protein (mg/dl)	Glucose (mg/dl)	Miscellaneous
Creutzfeldt-Jakob disease	0–15 lymphocytosis	Normal, 50–120	Normal	Occasional IgG increase
Herpes simplex encephalitis	50–1000 lymphocytosis	50–400	Normal	Culture, serology
Aseptic meningoencephalitis	5–1000 lymphocytosis	45–80	20–40, normal	Culture
HIV-1 dementia complex	0–8 lymphocytosis	< 80	Occasional decrease	IgG increase, culture
PML	0–8 lymphocytosis	< 80	Normal	
Acute bacterial meningitis	100–60,000 PMN	100–1000	5–40	Culture, serology
Brain abscess	0–500 PMN, lymphocytes	40–100	Occasional decrease	
Fungal meningitis	5–800 lymphocytosis	45–500	10–40, normal	Culture, cryptococcal antigen
Neurosyphilis	5–1000 lymphocytosis	50–100	< 40, normal	VDRL test, IgG increase
Neuroborreliosis (Lyme disease)	0–150 lymphocytosis	40–100	Normal	IgG increase, serology

Note. IgG = immunoglobulin G; HIV-1 = human immunodeficiency virus–type 1; PML = progressive multifocal leukoencephalopathy; PMN = polymorphonuclear cells; VDRL = venereal disease research laboratory.
Sources.   From Bale 1991; Fishman 1992; Halperin et al. 1991; Kirschbaum 1968; Levy et al. 1985; Marshall et al. 1988; Navia et al. 1986b; Schmidt 1989.

Viral Infections

Viral infections can be classified as either acute with a rapid onset of symptoms or slow with a chronic course over months to years (Table 26–3). The clinical features of the infection relate to the selective vulnerability of certain cell types to the particular virus (R. T. Johnson 1982).

Herpes simplex encephalitis.   This acute infection is a very common cause of encephalitis in elderly patients and it is often treatable, but mortality is high. Incidence is about 1/400,000 per year, with half of all cases occurring in those over age 50 (Whitley 1991).

Initial clinical features include headache, fever, stiff neck, and photophobia. This progresses over a few days to produce lethargy, mental status changes, memory impairment, aphasia, focal neurological deficits such as hemiparesis and visual field deficits, seizures, and eventually coma (Whitley 1991). Behavioral changes and hallucinations may be prominent (Bale 1991). Recovery may be complete or partial. The most common residual cognitive deficit is an amnesia due to frequent medial temporal lobe damage. The Klüver-Bucy syndrome—with hyperoral behavior, dietary changes, hypersexuality, placidity, visual agnosia, and hypermetamorphosis (excessive tactile exploration of the environment)—can be seen with bilateral temporal damage. An aphasia or a dementia syndrome may also be permanent sequela (Cummings and Benson 1992).

Hemorrhagic necrosis and petechial hemorrhages are seen in the brain pathologically. The medial temporal, insular, cingulate, and orbitotemporal regions are the areas most commonly involved (Okazaki 1983). Periodic lateralized epileptiform discharges (PLEDs) are the usual focal EEG abnormality, seen in 80% of patients (Bale 1991). MRI scan often shows focal areas of increased signal on T2-weighted images in the temporal-insular regions, and CT demonstrates hypodensity in those same areas (Schroth et al. 1987). An imaging study is often necessary before the lumbar puncture to rule out a mass lesion. The lumbar puncture usually suggests a viral infection (Table 26–4). Serology and viral cultures may be helpful. Brain biopsy is diagnostic but is not always accurate, and it has an acute morbidity of at least 3% (Whitley 1991). Therapy with acyclovir (30 mg/kg body weight per day in three divided doses for 10 days) is started empirically and immediately; the toxic effects of this drug are minimal, and its use reduces mortality from 70% to 19% (Whitley 1991).

Other meningoencephalitides.   The arboviruses are frequent causes of meningoencephalitis in the elderly population (Ho and Hirsch 1985). All are mosquito borne, and all have seasonal and geographic preferences. St. Louis encephalitis is the most common type in the United States. In a study of eastern equine encephalitis, 40% of all cases occurred in patients over age 50 (Przelomski et al. 1988). Western equine encephalitis is common particularly in young children and the elderly. Rubella, mumps, measles, Coxsackie viruses, polio, and adenoviruses typically occur in younger age groups (Bale 1991).

The acute prodrome of the viral meningoencephalitides are all similar to that described for herpes simplex encephalitis above. The specific neurological deficits depend on the extent and distribution of the infection. Lethargy, mental status changes, focal neurological deficits, seizures, and coma may occur. The syndrome of inappropriate antidiuretic hormone (SIADH) secretion is common with St. Louis encephalitis (Ho and Hirsch 1985). Permanent postencephalitic intellectual deficits have been observed with several arbovirus infections including western equine, eastern equine, Japanese, and St. Louis encephalitis (Cummings and Benson 1992).

Human immunodeficiency virus–type 1.   Human immunodeficiency virus–type 1 (HIV-1) is a retrovirus that preferentially infects helper T cells (Pantaleo et al. 1993). Gradually over years, the number of helper T cells declines, causing an immunodeficiency disorder called *acquired immunodeficiency syndrome* (AIDS) and making the individual susceptible to numerous opportunistic infections. The virus is constantly mutating and certain virus types are able to enter the CNS easily and early in the course of the infection, making neurological symptoms common. High-risk groups include homosexual men, intravenous drug users, individuals who receive contaminated blood products, heterosexual partners of HIV-1–infected individuals, and children of HIV-1–infected mothers (Rosenblum et al. 1988). Although this disease is most prevalent among men between ages 25 and 44, undoubtedly an increasing number of cases will be identified in the geriatric population.

It was estimated that in 1991 15 million people in the United States and 30 million worldwide would be infected with HIV-1 (Rosenblum et al. 1988). Nearly everyone infected is expected to eventually develop AIDS. In 1991 there were more than 45,000 new cases of AIDS reported in the United States alone (Centers for Disease Control 1992a). The median period of time between the initial infection and the development of AIDS is 10 years. Elderly individuals, however, have a more rapid course.

The most common signs and symptoms of HIV-1 infection include lymphadenopathy, diarrhea, fever, night sweats, weight loss, and lethargy (Bale 1991). Opportunistic infections account for many additional clinical syndromes.

Neurological and neuropsychiatric manifestations in HIV-1 infection are frequent and include those conditions associated with direct HIV-1 infection and those secondary to the immunodeficiency syndrome (Table 26–5). In AIDS, neurological complications occur in 40%–60% of patients, whereas autopsy studies indicate neurological damage in 70%–90% (Kieburtz and Schiffer 1989). The HIV-1–associated dementia complex (subacute encephalopathy, HIV encephalopathy, or AIDS dementia complex) is the initial manifestation of AIDS in 7% of all AIDS patients, but in those over age 74 it is the initial manifestation in 19% (Janssen et al. 1992). It is characterized by progression over weeks to months of a subcortical dementia syndrome with mental slowness, impaired concentration, forgetfulness, cognitive abnormalities, apathy, social withdrawal, slowed motor skills, ataxia, and weakness potentially resulting in severe global cognitive dysfunction, paraplegia, mutism, and incontinence (American Academy of Neurology AIDS Task Force 1991; R. W. Price et al. 1988; Van Gorp et al. 1989). Agitation, delusions, and hallucinations occur in a few patients (Cummings and Benson 1992). The HIV-1–associated vacuolar myelopathy presents as a progressive paraparesis (American Academy of Neurology AIDS Task Force 1991). Opportunistic infections and neoplasms involving the CNS are listed in Table 26–5 (Bale 1991; Kieburtz and Schiffer 1989; Levy and Bredesen 1988). Intracerebral hemorrhages, embolic infarctions from nonbacterial thrombotic endocarditis, strokes due to vasculitis, and medication effects also contribute to the neurological deficits (Engstrom et al. 1989; Ochitill and Dilley 1988) (Table 26–5).

Although most neurological complications seen in HIV-1–infected individuals occur in AIDS patients, there are HIV-1 antibody seropositive patients who do not fit the criteria for AIDS (Centers for Disease Control 1992b) but who have HIV-1–related neurological and neuropsychiatric syndromes. At the time of seroconversion some individuals develop a primary HIV-1 meningitis consisting of fever, headache, meningismus, and CSF pleocytosis (Cooper et al. 1985). Asymptomatic HIV-1 individuals have either mild (Bornstein et al. 1992) or no (McArthur et al. 1989) abnormalities on neuropsychological testing. However, once systemic findings appear (lymphadenopathy

Table 26–5. Neurological disorders in human immunodeficiency virus–type 1 (HIV-1) infection

Primary HIV-1 infection
  Aseptic meningitis
  HIV-1–associated minor cognitive/motor disorder
  HIV-1–associated dementia complex
  HIV-1–associated myelopathy
  HIV-1–associated acute inflammatory demyelinating polyradiculoneuropathy (HIV-1 associated Guillain-Barré syndrome)
  Chronic inflammatory demyelinating polyneuropathy
  HIV-1–associated predominantly sensory polyneuropathy
  Mononeuritis multiplex
  HIV-1–associated myopathy
  Vasculitis (stroke)
Opportunistic infections
  Viral
    Cytomegalovirus (meningoencephalitis, retinitis, myelitis)
    Papovavirus (progressive multifocal leukoencephalopathy)
    Herpes simplex virus (myelitis, encephalitis)
    Varicella zoster virus (myelitis, encephalitis)
  Nonviral
    Toxoplasma gondii (meningoencephalitis)
    Mycobacteria (meningitis)
    Cryptococcus neoformans (meningitis, brain abscess)
    Aspergillus fumigatus (meningitis, brain abscess)
    Histoplasma capsulatum (meningitis, brain abscess)
    Candida albicans (meningitis, brain abscess)
    Coccidioides immitis (meningitis, brain abscess)
    Nocardia asteroides (brain abscess)
    Mucormycosis (brain abscess)
    Listeria monocytogenes (meningitis)
    Escherichia coli (meningitis)
    Syphilis (meningovascular)
    Amoebic infections (brain abscess)
Opportunistic neoplasms
  Primary central nervous system lymphoma
  Metastatic systemic lymphoma
  Metastatic Kaposi's sarcoma
Other conditions
  Stroke (endocarditis, tumor hemorrhage)
  Drug intoxication or withdrawal

syndrome or AIDS-related complex [ARC]), 50% of these individuals have neurological signs or symptoms, and 50% have abnormalities on neuropsychological testing (Janssen et al. 1988). Mental and motoric slowness (Kieburtz and Schiffer 1989) referred to as the *HIV-1–associated minor cognitive/motor disorder* is the most common abnormality (American Academy of Neurology AIDS Task Force 1991).

The pathology of the HIV-1–associated dementia complex consists of white matter pallor, reactive gliosis, multinucleated giant cells, and microglial nodules, especially in the subcortical white and gray matter (Masliah et al. 1992; Navia et al. 1986a). CT and MRI scans show cerebral atrophy and periventricular white matter abnormalities (Ekholm and Simon 1988; Navia et al. 1986b). EEG results are either normal or show moderate diffuse slowing (Koppel et al. 1985). CSF examination shows mild pleocytosis, an elevation of protein, occasional low glucose, and an increased IgG index (Marshall et al. 1988; Navia et al. 1986b) (Table 26–4). For the various opportunistic conditions, MRI scanning, CSF results, and, occasionally, brain biopsy aid in diagnosis (Bale 1991) (Figure 26–5). Diagnosis of HIV-1 infection itself is made by detecting serum antibodies to HIV-1 proteins using western blot analysis (Steckelberg and Cockerill 1988). Treatment with zidovudine slows the progression of HIV-1–associated dementia complex and lowers the frequency and mortality of opportunistic infections (Schmitt et al. 1988). Specific treatments are also available for many of the opportunistic infections and neoplasms (Bale 1991).

Progressive multifocal leukoencephalopathy.   Progressive multifocal leukoencephalopathy is a demyelinative condition caused by the JC virus, a papovavirus, which typically occurs in patients with deficits in cell-mediated immunity, particularly in association with AIDS or lymphoproliferative diseases, or in those receiving immunosuppressive therapy (Holman et al. 1991). Onset is usually between ages 30 and 70, but can range from ages 6 to 84 (Stoner et al. 1988). The disease typically progresses to death in less than 1 year, but occasional patients have survived several years (Bale 1991).

The neurological manifestations are multifocal. Impaired concentration, visuospatial deficits, memory impairment, speech disturbance, aphasia, calculation deficits, cognitive decline, hemianopsia, slowing of motor speed, paresis, sensory deficits, incoordination, or ataxia are common (Berger et al. 1987; Cummings

and Benson 1992). Depression and agitation have been reported (Stagno et al. 1990). Fever or other systemic signs are not present.

Foci of demyelination are seen in the subcortical white matter. In these subcortical regions, axons are spared, but the oligodendrocytes and myelin are destroyed. Circling the demyelinative foci, enlarged oligodendrocytes with intranuclear inclusions consisting of papovavirus are present (R. T. Johnson 1982). MRI reveals multifocal white matter regions with increased signal on T2-weighted images consistent with demyelination (Berger et al. 1987), and PET studies show diminished metabolism in the same areas (Kiyosawa et al. 1988). CSF test results are usually normal, but may show a mild increase in protein or rarely a lymphocytic pleocytosis (Table 26–4). Diagnosis is made by brain biopsy and treatment is supportive.

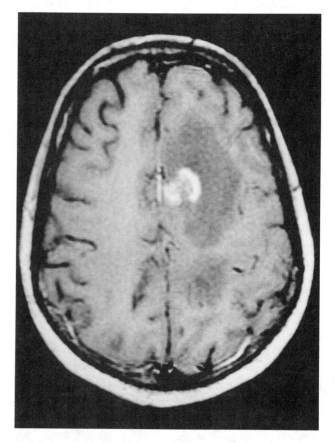

Figure 26–5.   Gadolinium-enhanced T1-weighted magnetic resonance image (MRI) of an individual with acquired immunodeficiency syndrome (AIDS) and a cerebral abscess due to toxoplasmosis. MRI reveals a mass lesion in the left medial frontal region with surrounding edema.

Bacterial Infections

Acute bacterial meningitis. The incidence of bacterial meningitis is 5/100,000 per year. Mortality can be as high as 35% in those over age 65 (Behrman et al. 1989). Common organisms causing acute bacterial meningitis in the elderly population are *Streptococcus pneumoniae, Neisseria meningitidis, Listeria monocytogenes, Hemophilus influenzae* type B, and other gram-negative bacilli (Behrman et al. 1989; Durand et al. 1993; Stacy and Roeltgen 1991). Predisposing conditions such as diabetes, cancer, recent craniotomy, or immunosuppressive therapy are present in about 35% of cases, and concurrent infections occur in approximately 40% of cases (Behrman et al. 1989).

Typical features of a bacterial meningitis include fever, headache, stiff neck, photophobia, agitation, lethargy, and often, especially in the elderly, an acute confusional state. Mental status changes are more common than meningismus or headache (Behrman et al. 1989). Focal neurological deficits can occur, including hemiparesis, visual field defects, aphasia, or cranial nerve palsies, and are usually due to acute obstructive hydrocephalus or stroke (Durand et al. 1993). Long-term sequelae include dementia, hydrocephalus, seizures, and persistent focal neurological deficits. Purulent meningitis and brain edema are seen at autopsy. CT or MRI may show evidence of hydrocephalus or edema. CSF examination shows polymorphonuclear pleocytosis, elevated protein, hypoglycorrhachia, and positive cultures and serology (Table 26–4). Diagnosis is made by CSF analysis, and antibiotics are required for treatment.

Brain abscess and epidural abscess. Abscesses consist of collections of purulent material that may be present in brain parenchyma, subdural space, or epidural space. The incidence of brain abscess is 4/1,000,000 per year. Fifteen percent of all brain abscesses and 25% of all spinal epidural abscesses occur in patients over age 60. Typical organisms for brain abscesses include aerobic and anaerobic streptococci, bacteroides, fusobacteria, and clostridium species. In immunocompromised individuals, various fungal species, cysticercosis, and toxoplasmosis are prevalent. *Staphylococcus aureus* and gram-negative organism infections are frequently seen in epidural abscesses, which often represent an extension of a frontal sinusitis or middle ear infection (Stacy and Roeltgen 1991). In brain abscesses, headache, fever, mental status changes, and focal neurolog-

ical signs are common (Behrman et al. 1989). Seizures and increased intracranial pressure may occur. Long-term sequela include late seizures and persistent focal neurological deficits. Enhanced MRI is very helpful in diagnosing brain abscesses (Sze and Zimmerman 1988), and EEG usually shows focal delta activity. Lumbar puncture may precipitate a herniation syndrome and is contraindicated in brain abscesses (Table 26–4). Treatments for brain abscesses include broad coverage antibiotics and occasionally surgical drainage (Stacy and Roeltgen 1991).

Fungal Infections

Half of all chronic fungal meningitis infections occur in individuals with depressed immune systems or chronic debilitation (Cummings and Benson 1992), making these infections frequent among the geriatric population. Cryptococcal meningitis is the most common of these infections. Other causative organisms include coccidioidomycosis, histoplasmosis, candida species, blastomycosis, and aspergillus. The disease begins insidiously and progresses slowly over weeks to months. Headache, fever, and stiff neck are common, but may not always be present. Mental status changes occur more frequently and include lethargy, apathy, disorientation, poor concentration, memory deficits, and aphasia. Focal neurological deficits, cranial nerve dysfunction, gait imbalance, dementia, or hydrocephalus may also occur (Cummings and Benson 1992). CSF examination reveals lymphocytic pleocytosis, increased protein, and hypoglycorrhachia (Table 26–4) (Fishman 1992). Cryptococcal antigen in the CSF is specific for cryptococcal meningitis. Cultures or titers are necessary for diagnosis of other infections. Intravenous or intrathecal antibiotics are the mainstays of treatment.

Spirochete Infections

Syphilis. Syphilis is caused by the spirochete *Treponema pallidum* and is spread by intimate contact. Prior to penicillin treatment, general paresis accounted for up to 30% of all admissions to mental hospitals. Syphilis is again increasing in frequency, and it is most commonly seen in HIV-1 patients (E. W. Hook 1989). The annual incidence of syphilis of all types was 20/100,000 in the United States in 1990 (E. W. Hook and Marra 1992); for neurosyphilis it is estimated to be 2/100,000 (Simon 1985). Primary syphilis presents as a chancre that heals in several weeks and is followed by a diffuse skin rash indicative of the bacteremia of secondary syphilis. Meningeal neurosyphilis may be seen at this early stage. Tertiary syphilis occurs 2–20 years after the primary infection and occurs in various forms including cardiovascular (aortitis), meningovascular, paretic, and tabetic. Because of the long incubation times, neurosyphilis frequently begins between ages 30 and 60 (Cummings and Benson 1992).

General paresis results from syphilitic invasion into the brain parenchyma, and its neuropsychiatric features include inattention, memory deficits, cognitive impairment, anomia, dementia, tremulous speech, impaired judgment, irritability, pseudobulbar palsy, paralysis, tremor, ataxia, incontinence, optic atrophy, and Argyll Robertson pupils. Mania is seen in 20%–40% of patients, depression in 6%, and peculiar deportment, grandiose delusions, paranoia, and hallucinations in 3%–6% (Cummings and Benson 1992).

The pathology of syphilis is varied and includes meningitis, vasculitis, stroke, gummas, neuronal loss, and gliosis. General paresis features predominant involvement of the frontal lobes. Screening for neurosyphilis should be done with the fluorescent treponemal antibody absorption (FTA-ABS) test; other screening tests may be nonreactive in tertiary syphilis (Simon 1985). False positives can occur with systemic lupus erythematosus and some infectious conditions (E. W. Hook and Marra 1992). If the FTA-ABS is positive, a lumbar puncture is indicated. CSF examination in neurosyphilis shows lymphocytic pleocytosis, elevated protein, positive venereal disease research laboratory (VDRL) test, occasional hypoglycorrhachia, and increased IgGs (Table 26–4). Penicillin is the treatment of choice for all forms of syphilis with the intravenous route and longer duration of treatments required for patients with neurosyphilis and for patients with syphilis associated with HIV-1 (E. W. Hook and Marra 1992). Desensitization is recommended for those with penicillin allergies (Centers for Disease Control 1989).

Lyme disease. Lyme disease is caused by the tickborne spirochete *Borrelia burgdorferi.* Age at onset ranges from 7 to 86 (Halperin et al. 1991). The acute localized infection consists of an erythema chronicum migrans rash and a viral-like syndrome. Dissemination occurs after a few weeks to months and is followed by a multifocal erythema chronicum migrans rash, acute arthritis, cardiac conduction block, myocarditis, myositis, hepatitis, or meningoradiculoneuritis. Some individuals develop a chronic course leading to chronic arthritis, radiculoneuritis, or, after invasion of the brain parenchyma, an encephalitis.

Early neurological manifestations occur in 10% of patients and may include bilateral seventh nerve palsies, oculomotor disturbances, other cranial neuropathies, radiculopathies, mononeuritis multiplex, myopathy, or an acute lymphocytic meningitis with headache, photophobia, and meningismus (Finkel and Halperin 1992). Chronic neurological features are frequent and typically include memory loss, anomia, cognitive deficits, mild dementia, depression, and irritability. Rarely, patients develop focal CNS deficits including paresis, ataxia, seizures, or a severe dementia with CSF evidence of an encephalitis (Halperin et al. 1991).

Neuropsychiatric manifestations include psychosis with paranoia and hallucinations, anorexia nervosa, fatigue, depression ranging from mild to severe, emotional lability, irritability, and violent outbursts (Fallon et al. 1992). Pathologically, peripheral neuritis, vasculitis, focal demyelination, and, in the late stages, signs of brain parenchyma infection are observed. MRI reveals multifocal regions of increased signal in the white matter consistent with demyelination (Halperin et al. 1991). CSF examination shows a lymphocytic pleocytosis, elevated protein, increased IgG, and positive serology (Table 26–4). Diagnosis is made with a positive serology in the setting of appropriate clinical findings. Antibiotics can prevent or halt the neurological complications and may lead to significant improvement.

Inflammatory Disorders

The inflammatory disorders include the vasculitides and the collagen vascular diseases. Most of these conditions can present at any age, but some are particularly prevalent in elderly individuals. Common causes of inflammatory disorders involving the CNS in the geriatric age group are listed in Table 26–6.

Vasculitides

Temporal arteritis. Temporal arteritis is a systemic vasculitis seen predominantly in the geriatric population. Nearly all patients are over age 50, and women are affected twice as often as are men. The incidence is as high as 7/100,000 per year (Boesen and Sorensen 1987), and it rises dramatically with increasing age to over 25/100,000 per year over age 80. Systemic symptoms are rarely absent and include fever, weight loss, anorexia, and malaise. Pain and stiffness in the muscles of the neck, shoulders, and pelvis, which represent the classic features of polymyalgia rheumatica, are seen in 50% of those with temporal arteritis. Scalp necrosis, muscular wasting, and angina occur infrequently.

Neurological manifestations classically include a new-onset headache characterized by a stabbing or throbbing pain, which is centered over the temple and radiates over the scalp and face. Jaw claudication, scalp tenderness, and tenderness and nodularity of the superior temporal artery are common (Berlit 1992; Chmelewski et al. 1992). Less frequently depression, facial neuralgia, blurred vision, vertigo, amaurosis fugax, diplopia, neuropathy, dementia, and cerebral or brain stem stroke occur (Nadeau and Watson 1990). Blindness occurs in about 10%, usually without warning (Caselli et al. 1988).

Pathology shows a patchy giant cell arteritis frequently involving the branches of the external carotid and ophthalmic arteries. The large and medium-sized arteries throughout the body are also involved but are rarely symptomatic. Involvement of the intracranial arteries is uncommon. Multinucleated giant cells with destruction of the internal elastic lamina are seen. Anemia is common, and an elevated Westergren sedi-

Table 26–6. Causes of inflammatory disorders involving the central nervous system in elderly patients

Vasculitides
Temporal arteritis
Polyarteritis nodosa
Allergic granulomatosis
Granulomatous angiitis
Wegener's granulomatosis
Takayasu's arteritis
Lymphomatoid granulomatosis
Eales' disease (idiopathic retinal vasculitis)

Collagen vascular diseases
Systemic lupus erythematosus (SLE)
Antiphospholipid antibody syndrome
Behcet's syndrome
Scleroderma
Rheumatoid arthritis
Sjögren's syndrome
Dermatomyositis
Cogan's syndrome
Mixed connective tissue disease

Other
Vogt-Koyanagi-Harada syndrome
Paraneoplastic disorders

mentation rate (over 50 mm/hour and often over 100 mm/hour) is almost always found. A superior temporal artery biopsy is positive in about 70% of cases and should be done in all suspected cases (Nadeau and Watson 1990). Negative biopsies should not dissuade treatment in those with the typical clinical features. Prednisone, typically in doses of 40–60 mg/day, is an effective treatment and should be initiated without waiting for biopsy confirmation (Berlit 1992).

Polyarteritis nodosa. Polyarteritis nodosa characterizes a group of acute systemic necrotizing vasculitides that includes allergic granulomatosis. Immune complex deposition in polyarteritis nodosa causes a relapsing and remitting vasculitis that eventually leads to infarction or hemorrhage in multiple organs. The incidence of polyarteritis nodosa is about 0.2/100,000 per year, with males affected twice as often as females. Age at onset ranges from 6 to 80, with a mean of about 45. Common systemic findings include fever, weight loss, anorexia, asthma, dyspnea, proteinuria, arthralgias, skin rash, congestive heart failure, gastrointestinal pain, and hypertension.

Neurological manifestations occur in up to 80% of cases, with mononeuritis multiplex being the most common finding. Myopathy, polyneuropathy, cranial neuropathy, headache, dementia, encephalopathy, seizures, and strokes are also common. Mental status changes occur in about 20% of patients and include disorientation, attentional deficits, visual hallucinations, mania, paranoia, memory impairment, cognitive deterioration, and hypoarousal progressing to coma. Hemiparesis, homonymous hemianopia, and ataxia occur secondary to the strokes. A necrotizing vasculitis of the small and medium muscular arteries is seen on pathological examination. Elevated sedimentation rate, anemia, leukocytosis, and thrombocytosis are common. Angiography reveals aneurysms and arteriopathy. MRI and CT may reveal evidence of infarction. CSF examination shows increased pressure, elevated protein, lymphocytic pleocytosis, and occasionally subarachnoid bleeding. Diagnosis is made clinically and confirmed by tissue biopsy (muscle, skin, sural nerve, or kidney) and angiography. Corticosteroids and immunosuppressive agents are the treatments of choice and often lead to remissions or recovery (Nadeau and Watson 1990).

Granulomatous angiitis. This rare vasculitis of unknown etiology, also known as *isolated CNS vasculitis,* is confined to the CNS. It occurs at any age, age at onset ranging from 3 to 96. Fever and weight loss are noted in 25% of cases. Lymphoma, sarcoidosis, and herpes zoster conditions have occasionally been associated with this vasculitis. A subacute presentation with headache, encephalopathy, strokes, and focal neurological deficits progressing to a vascular dementia syndrome is typical.

Other common manifestations include seizures, supranuclear cranial nerve palsies, aphasia, cerebellar signs, and myelopathy. Increased intracranial pressure may occur leading to papilledema and potentially coma and brain stem herniation. A segmental vasculitis with fibrinoid necrosis and giant cells is found in the medium and small arteries, capillaries, and veins of the CNS. The sedimentation rate is increased in 60% of the patients but only to a mean of about 35 mm/hour. CT results may be normal or may reveal masses or infarctions. Angiography may show vasculopathy but is often normal. CSF findings include an elevated protein, lymphocytic pleocytosis, and often increased pressure. Diagnosis is made clinically and confirmed by brain biopsy. Treatment with prednisone and immunosuppressive agents is often ineffective, and there is an 87% mortality rate, with deaths occurring a mean of 6 months after onset of symptoms (Younger et al. 1988).

Collagen Vascular Diseases

Systemic lupus erythematosus. Systemic lupus erythematosus (SLE) is a multisystem immunological disorder of uncertain etiology. It has the highest incidence of neuropsychiatric manifestations of any of the collagen vascular disorders, and these manifestations are often the first symptoms of the illness. The incidence of SLE is about 5/100,000 per year, and the prevalence is about 45/100,000 (Nadeau and Watson 1990). Women are much more often affected. Although SLE is a disease primarily of young to middle-aged adults it can occur in the very old. Systemic manifestations may include fever, anorexia, rash, lymphadenopathy, arthralgias, pericarditis, valvular disease, pleuritis, Raynaud's phenomenon, alopecia, vasculitis, renal insufficiency, nephrotic syndrome, and hypertension (Nadeau and Watson 1990).

Neuropsychiatric manifestations are seen in 40%–75% of cases and often occur early in the disease course. Over 60% of cases develop memory and cognitive deficits (Carbotte et al. 1986), whereas 35%–60% have symptoms of impaired attention, an acute confu-

sional state or delirium, psychosis with hallucinations and delusions, depression, hypomania, or anxiety. Seizures, strokes, supranuclear cranial nerve deficits, and focal paresis are present in 10%–35% of cases (McCune and Golbus 1988). Also reported are visual disturbances, optic neuritis, ptosis, ophthalmoplegia, transverse myelitis, tremor, chorea, and myositis (Nadeau and Watson 1990).

An antiphospholipid antibody syndrome consisting of the presence of antiphospholipid antibodies (particularly lupus anticoagulant and anticardiolipin antibodies) and evidence of venous or arterial thrombotic strokes or ischemia, recurrent abortions, or thrombocytopenia are not uncommon in SLE (Lockshin 1992; Rosove and Brewer 1992). The antibodies are present in up to 50% of SLE patients. Myelopathy, deep vein thrombosis, Guillain-Barré syndrome, migraine, chorea, and seizures have also been associated with this syndrome (Levine and Welch 1987).

The main pathological feature of SLE is a vasculopathy with fibrinoid degeneration and endothelial proliferation of the small vessels resulting in microinfarcts and microhemorrhages. Less commonly, a true vasculitis is seen. MRI is useful in localizing strokes (McCune et al. 1988). Angiography usually is unable to identify the microangiopathy of SLE. CSF findings are abnormal in one-third of patients, with evidence of a lymphocytic pleocytosis, elevated protein, and increased IgG. Diagnosis of SLE is based on clinical features, a positive antinuclear antibody test, and other specific antibody tests (Tan et al. 1982). Treatments include nonsteroidal anti-inflammatory agents, steroids, and immunosuppressive agents. Oral anticoagulants or antiplatelet agents may prevent the recurrent thrombotic events seen with antiphospholipid antibodies. Neuroleptics are used for psychosis and anticonvulsants for seizures.

Behcet's syndrome. Behcet's syndrome is an inflammatory disorder of uncertain etiology characterized by oral and genital ulcers and uveitis. Up to 40% have neurological features. Prevalence is uncertain, with reports ranging from 4 to 100 per 100,000. Cases have been reported from ages 6 to 72. Systemic features include arthritis, vasculitis, thrombophlebitis, and gastrointestinal disturbances (Nadeau and Watson 1990). A relapsing focal meningoencephalitis affecting the brain stem with headache, cranial nerve deficits, dysarthria, long tract signs, and bulbar and pseudobulbar palsies is the most common neurological manifestation. A dementia syndrome with memory deficits, cognitive impairment, and emotional disturbance can occur. Seizures, aphasia, intracranial hypertension, and peripheral neuropathy have also been reported (Serdaroglu et al. 1989). A chronic inflammatory vasculopathy is seen pathologically with retinal and cutaneous vasculitis commonly found. Ischemic foci with chronic inflammation are noted in the CNS especially in the brain stem, spinal cord, globus pallidus, and hypothalamus (Totsuka et al. 1985). Meningeal inflammation is also common. MRI scanning reveals increased signal on T2-weighted images in the deep subcortical and brain stem regions (Al Kawi et al. 1991). CSF shows a lymphocytic pleocytosis and elevated protein. Diagnosis is based on clinical features. Treatment for Behcet's syndrome includes high-dose steroids and azathioprine.

Summary

Most acquired brain disorders occur in the geriatric population. Some conditions have their onset in late life, whereas other conditions have chronic courses and persist into advanced age. Diagnosis and treatment of these disorders in the elderly patient is influenced by the frequent co-occurrence of other chronic medical conditions, multiple medication regimens, and the normal physiological changes that accompany aging.

Neoplastic disorders involving the CNS occur frequently in elderly individuals, and they present as primary tumors, metastatic tumors, or paraneoplastic syndromes. MS often begins in early adulthood, but many patients survive well past 70. Its neuropsychiatric features include depression, psychosis, and mania. Toxic and metabolic causes of demyelination may begin in elderly patients. Both common and rare infectious disorders affecting the CNS have characteristic presentations in the elderly population, and most are treatable. Temporal arteritis occurs almost exclusively in patients over age 50. Finally, SLE is a common disorder with frequent late survival and significant CNS manifestations.

References

Achiron A, Ziv I, Djaldetti R, et al: Aphasia in multiple sclerosis: Clinical and radiologic correlations. Neurology 42:2195–2197, 1992

Adams RD, Victor M: Principles of Neurology, 3rd Edition. New York, McGraw-Hill, 1985

Al Kawi MZ, Bohlega S, Banna M: MRI findings in neuro-Behcet's disease. Neurology 41:405–408, 1991

Alvord EC Jr, Shaw C-M: Neoplasms affecting the nervous system of the elderly, in The Pathology of the Aging Human Nervous System. Edited by Duckett S. Philadelphia, PA, Lea & Febiger, 1991, pp 210–286

American Academy of Neurology AIDS Task Force: Nomenclature and research case definitions for neurologic manifestations of human immunodeficiency virus-type 1 (HIV-1) infection. Neurology 41:778–785, 1991

Babikian V, Ropper AH: Binswanger's disease: a review. Stroke 18:2–12, 1987

Bale JF Jr: Encephalitis and other virus-induced neurologic disorders, in Clinical Neurology. Edited by Baker AB, Joynt RJ. New York, Harper & Row, 1991, chapter 26, pp 1–86

Bastianello S, Pozzilli C, Bernardi S, et al: Serial study of gadolinium-DPTA MRI enhancement in multiple sclerosis. Neurology 40:591–595, 1990

Baumann N, Masson M, Carreau V, et al: Adult forms of metachromatic leukodystrophy: clinical and biochemical approach. Dev Neurosci 13:211–215, 1991

Beatty WW, Goodkin DE, Monson N, et al: Anterograde and retrograde amnesia in patients with chronic progressive multiple sclerosis. Arch Neurol 45:611–619, 1988

Beatty WW, Goodkin DE, Beatty PA, et al: Frontal lobe dysfunction and memory impairment in patients with chronic progressive multiple sclerosis. Brain Cogn 11:73–86, 1989

Behrman RE, Myers BR, Mendelson MH, et al: Central nervous system infections in the elderly. Arch Intern Med 149:1596–1599, 1989

Belyi BI: Mental impairment in unilateral frontal tumors: role of the laterality of the lesion. Int J Neurosci 32:799–810, 1987

Berger JR, Kaszovitz B, Post JD, et al: Progressive multifocal leukoencephalopathy associated with human immunodeficiency virus infection. Ann Intern Med 107:78–87, 1987

Berlit P: Clinical and laboratory findings with giant cell arteritis. J Neurol Sci 111:1–12, 1992

Bjorkhem I, Skrede S: Familial diseases with storage of sterols other than cholesterol: cerebrotendinous xanthomatosis and phytosterolemia, in The Metabolic Basis of Inherited Disease, 6th Edition. Edited by Scriver CR, Beaudet AL, Sly WS, et al. New York, McGraw-Hill, 1990, pp 1283–1293

Boesen P, Sorensen SF: Giant cell arteritis, temporal arteritis, and polymyalgia rheumatica in a Danish county: a prospective investigation, 1982–1985. Arthritis Rheum 30:294–299, 1987

Bornstein RA, Nasrallah HA, Para MF, et al: Neuropsychological performance in asymptomatic HIV infection. J Neuropsychiatry Clin Neurosci 4:386–394, 1992

Brown P, Cathala F, Castaigne P, et al: Creutzfeldt-Jakob disease: clinical analysis of a consecutive series of 230 neuropathologically verified cases. Ann Neurol 20:597–602, 1986

Brown P, Goldfarb LG, Kovanen J, et al: Phenotypic characteristics of familial Creutzfeldt-Jakob disease associated with the codon 178Asn PRNP mutation. Ann Neurol 31:282–285, 1992

Carbotte RM, Denburg SD, Denburg JA: Prevalence of cognitive impairment in systemic lupus erythematosus. J Nerv Ment Dis 174:357–364, 1986

Caselli RJ, Hunder GG, Whisnant JP: Neurologic disease in biopsy-proven giant cell (temporal) arteritis. Neurology 38:352–359, 1988

Centers for Disease Control: Sexually transmitted diseases treatment guidelines. MMWR 38 (S-8):5–15, 1989

Centers for Disease Control: Update: acquired immunodeficiency syndrome—United States, 1991. MMWR 41:463–468, 1992a

Centers for Disease Control: 1993 revised classification system for HIV infection and expanded surveillance case definition for AIDS among adolescents and adults. MMWR 41 (RR-17):1–19, 1992b

Chang KH, Cha SH, Han MH, et al: Marchiafava-Bignami disease: serial changes in corpus callosum on MRI. Neuroradiology 34:480–482, 1992

Chiofalo N, Fuentes A, Galvez S: Serial EEG findings in 27 cases of Creutzfeldt-Jakob disease. Arch Neurol 37:143–145, 1980

Chmelewski WL, McKnight KM, Agudelo CA, et al: Presenting features and outcomes in patients undergoing temporal artery biopsy: a review of 98 patients. Arch Intern Med 152:1690–1695, 1992

Constine LS, Woolf PD, Cann D, et al: Hypothalamic-pituitary dysfunction after radiation for brain tumors. N Engl J Med 328:87–94, 1993

Cooper DA, Gold J, MacLean P, et al: Acute AIDS retrovirus infection. Lancet 1:537–540, 1985

Cummings JL, Benson DF: Dementia: A Clinical Approach, 2nd Edition. Stoneham, MA, Butterworth, 1992

Dalmau J, Graus F, Rosenblum MK, et al: Anti-Hu-associated paraneoplastic encephalomyelitis/sensory neuronopathy: a clinical study of 71 patients. Medicine 71:59–72, 1992

de Groen PC, Aksamit AJ, Rakela J, et al: Central nervous system toxicity after liver transplantation: the role of cyclosporine and cholesterol. N Engl J Med 317:861–866, 1987

Durand ML, Calderwood SB, Weber DJ, et al: Acute bacterial meningitis in adults: a review of 493 episodes. N Engl J Med 328:21–28, 1993

Ekholm S, Simon JH: Magnetic resonance imaging and the acquired immunodeficiency syndrome dementia complex. Acta Radiol 29:227–230, 1988

Engstrom JW, Lowenstein DH, Bredesen DE: Cerebral infarctions and transient neurologic deficits associated with acquired immunodeficiency syndrome. Am J Med 86:528–532, 1989

Fallon BA, Nields JA, Burrascano JJ, et al: The neuropsychiatric manifestations of Lyme borreliosis. Psychiatr Q 63:95–117, 1992

Farlow MR, Yee RD, Dlouhy SR, et al: Gerstmann-Sträussler-Scheinker disease, I: extending the clinical spectrum. Neurology 39:1446–1452, 1989

Feinstein A, du Boulay G, Ron MA: Psychotic illness in multiple sclerosis. A clinical and magnetic resonance imaging study. Br J Psychiatry 161:680–685, 1992

Fennell EB, Smith MC: Neuropsychological assessment, in Neurobehavioral Aspects of Multiple Sclerosis. Edited by Rao SM. New York, Oxford University Press, 1990, pp 63–81

Finkel MJ, Halperin JJ: Nervous system Lyme borreliosis-revisited. Arch Neurol 49:102–107, 1992

Fishman RA: Cerebrospinal Fluid in Diseases of the Nervous System, 2nd Edition. Philadelphia, PA, WB Saunders, 1992

Geerts Y, Dehaene I, Lammens M: Acute hemorrhagic leucoencephalitis. Acta Neurol Belg 91:201–211, 1991

Good K, Clark CM, Oger J, et al: Cognitive impairment and depression in mild multiple sclerosis. J Nerv Ment Dis 180:730–732, 1992

Grafman J, Rao SM, Litvan I: Disorders of memory, in Neurobehavioral Aspects of Multiple Sclerosis. Edited by Rao SM. New York, Oxford University Press, 1990, pp 102–117

Halperin JJ, Volkman DJ, Wu P: Central nervous system abnormalities in Lyme neuroborreliosis. Neurology 41:1571–1582, 1991

Ho DD, Hirsch MS: Acute viral encephalitis. Med Clin North Am 69:415–429, 1985

Hokezu Y, Kuriyama M, Kubota R, et al: Cerebrotendinous xanthomatosis: cranial CT and MRI studies in eight patients. Neuroradiology 34:308–312, 1992

Holman RC, Janssen RS, Buehler JW, et al: Epidemiology of progressive multifocal leukoencephalopathy in the United States: analysis of national mortality and AIDS surveillance data. Neurology 41:1733–1736, 1991

Holthoff VA, Sandmann J, Pawlik G, et al: Positron emission tomography in Creutzfeldt-Jakob disease. Arch Neurol 47:1035–1038, 1990

Honer WG, Hurwitz T, Li DKB, et al: Temporal lobe involvement in multiple sclerosis patients with psychiatric disorders. Arch Neurol 44:187–190, 1987

Hooge JP, Redekop WK: Multiple sclerosis with very late onset. Neurology 42:1907–1910, 1992

Hook CC, Kimmel DW, Kvols LK, et al: Multifocal inflammatory leukoencephalopathy with 5-fluorouracil and levamisole. Ann Neurol 31:262–267, 1992

Hook EW III: Syphilis and HIV infection. J Infect Dis 160:530–534, 1989

Hook EW III, Marra CM: Acquired syphilis in adults. N Engl J Med 326:1060–1069, 1992

Hsiao K, Prusiner SB: Inherited human prion diseases. Neurology 40:1820–1827, 1990

Hsiao K, Baker HF, Crow TJ, et al: Linkage of a prion protein missense variant to Gerstmann-Sträussler syndrome. Nature 338:342–345, 1989

Huang C-C, Chu N-S, Chen T-J, et al: Acute haemorrhagic leucoencephalitis with a prolonged clinical course. J Neurol Neurosurg Psychiatry 51:870–874, 1988

Huber SJ, Paulson GW, Shuttleworth EC, et al: Magnetic imaging correlates of dementia in multiple sclerosis. Arch Neurol 44:732–736, 1987

Huber SJ, Bornstein RA, Rammohan KW, et al: Magnetic resonance imaging correlates of executive function impairments in multiple sclerosis. Neuropsychiatry, Neuropsychology, and Behavioral Neurology 5:33–36, 1992a

Huber SJ, Bornstein RA, Rammohan KW, et al: Magnetic resonance imaging correlates of neuropsychological impairment in multiple sclerosis. J Neuropsychiatry Clin Neurosci 4:152–158, 1992b

Hyde TM, Ziegler JC, Weinberger DR: Psychiatric disturbances in metachromatic leukodystrophy: insights into the neurobiology of psychosis. Arch Neurol 49:401–406, 1992

Janssen RS, Saykin AJ, Kaplan JE, et al: Neurological complication of human immunodeficiency virus infection in patients with lymphadenopathy syndrome. Ann Neurol 23:49–55, 1988

Janssen RS, Nwanyanwu OC, Selik RM, et al: Epidemiology of human immunodeficiency virus encephalopathy in the United States. Neurology 42:1472–1476, 1992

Joffe RT, Lippert GP, Gray TA, et al: Mood disorder and multiple sclerosis. Arch Neurol 44:376–378, 1987

Johnson BE, Becker B, Goff WB II, et al: Neurologic, neuropsychologic and computed cranial tomography scan abnormalities in 2- to 10-year survivors of small-cell lung cancer. J Clin Oncol 3:1659–1667, 1985

Johnson RT: Viruses and chronic neurologic diseases. Johns Hopkins Medical Journal 150:132–140, 1982

Karnaze DS, Carmel R: Neurologic and evoked potential abnormalities in subtle cobalamin deficiency states, including deficiency without anemia and with normal absorption of free cobalamin. Arch Neurol 47:1008–1012, 1990

Kieburtz K, Schiffer RB: Neurologic manifestations of human immunodeficiency virus infections. Neurol Clin 7:447–468, 1989

Kirkeby HJ, Poulsen EU, Petersen T, et al: Erectile dysfunction in multiple sclerosis. Neurology 38:1366–1371, 1988

Kirschbaum WR: Jakob-Creutzfeldt Disease. New York, American Elsevier, 1968, p 132

Kitchin W, Cohen-Cole SA, Mickel SF: Adrenoleukodystrophy: frequency of presentation as a psychiatric disorder. Biol Psychiatry 22:1375–1387, 1987

Kiyosawa M, Bosley TM, Alavi A, et al: Positron emission tomography in a patient with progressive multifocal leukoencephalopathy. Neurology 38:1864–1867, 1988

Kodama T, Numaguchi Y, Gellad FE, et al: Magnetic resonance imaging of limbic encephalitis. Neuroradiology 33:520–523, 1991

Koppel BS, Wormser GP, Tuchman AJ, et al: Central nervous system involvement in patients with acquired immune deficiency syndrome (AIDS). Acta Neurol Scand 71:337–353, 1985

Krupp LB, Alvarez LA, LaRocca NG, et al: Fatigue in multiple sclerosis. Arch Neurol 45:435–437, 1988

Kurtzke JF, Kurland LT: The epidemiology of neurologic disease, in Clinical Neurology. Edited by Baker AB, Joynt RJ. New York, Harper & Row, 1983, chapter 66, pp 1–143

LaRocca NG: A rehabilitation perspective, in Neurobehavioral Aspects of Multiple Sclerosis. Edited by Rao SM. New York, Oxford University Press, 1990, pp 215–229

Lechevalier B, Andersson JC, Morin P: Hemispheric disconnection syndrome with a "crossed avoiding" reaction in a case of Marchiafava-Bignami disease. J Neurol Neurosurg Psychiatry 40:483–497, 1977

Lee Y-Y, Nauert C, Glass JP: Treatment-related white matter changes in cancer patients. Cancer 57:1473–1482, 1986

Levine SR, Welch KMA: The spectrum of neurologic disease associated with antiphospholipid antibodies: lupus anticoagulants and anticardiolipin antibodies. Arch Neurol 44:876–883, 1987

Levy RM, Bredesen DE: Central nervous system dysfunction in acquired immunodeficiency syndrome, in AIDS and the Nervous System. Edited by Rosenblum ML, Levy RM, Bredesen DE. New York, Raven, 1988, pp 29–63

Levy RM, Bredesen DE, Rosenblum ML: Neurological manifestations of the acquired immunodeficiency syndrome (AIDS): experience at UCSF and review of the literature. J Neurosurg 62:475–495, 1985

Lindenbaum J, Healton EB, Savage DG, et al: Neuropsychiatric disorders caused by cobalamin deficiency in the absence of anemia or macrocytosis. N Engl J Med 318:1720–1728, 1988

Lockshin MD: Antiphospholipid antibody syndrome. JAMA 268:1451–1453, 1992

Mahler ME: Behavioral manifestations associated with multiple sclerosis. Psychiatr Clin North Am 15:427–438, 1992

Marshall DW, Brey RL, Cahill WT, et al: Spectrum of cerebrospinal fluid findings in various stages of human immunodeficiency virus infection. Arch Neurol 45:954–958, 1988

Masliah E, Achim CL, Ge N, et al: Spectrum of human immunodeficiency virus-associated neocortical damage. Ann Neurol 32:321–329, 1992

Masters CL, Gajdusek DC, Gibbs CJ Jr: Creutzfeldt-Jakob disease virus isolation from the Gerstmann-Sträussler syndrome with an analysis of the various forms of amyloid plaque deposition in the virus-induced spongiform encephalopathies. Brain 104:559–588, 1981

Maurelli M, Marchioni E, Cerretano R, et al: Neuropsychological assessment in MS: clinical, neurophysiological and neuroradiological relationships. Acta Neurol Scand 86:124–128, 1992

McArthur JC, Cohen BA, Selnes OA, et al: Low prevalence of neurological and neuropsychological abnormalities in otherwise healthy HIV-1-infected individuals: results from the multicenter AIDS cohort study. Ann Neurol 26:601–611, 1989

McCune WJ, Golbus J: Neuropsychiatric lupus. Rheum Dis Clin North Am 14:149–167, 1988

McCune WJ, MacGuire A, Aisen A, et al: Identification of brain lesions in neuropsychiatric systemic lupus erythematosus by magnetic resonance scanning. Arthritis Rheum 31:159–166, 1988

Medori R, Tritschler H-J, LeBlanc A, et al: Fatal familial insomnia: a prion disease with a mutation at codon 178 of the prion protein gene. N Engl J Med 326:444–449, 1992

Meiner Z, Halimi M, Polakiewicz RD, et al: Presence of prion protein in peripheral tissues of Libyan Jews with Creutzfeldt-Jakob disease. Neurology 42:1355–1360, 1992

Merriam AE, Hegarty AM, Miller A: The mental disabilities of metachromatic leukodystrophy: implications concerning the differentiation of cortical, subcortical gray, and white matter dementias. Neuropsychiatry, Neuropsychology, and Behavioral Neurology 3:217–225, 1990

Milton WJ, Atlas SW, Lavi E, et al: Magnetic resonance imaging of Creutzfeldt-Jakob disease. Ann Neurol 29:438–440, 1991

Minden SL, Moes E: A psychiatric perspective, in Neurobehavioral Aspects of Multiple Sclerosis. Edited by Rao SM. New York, Oxford University Press, 1990, pp 230–250

Minden SL, Schiffer RB: Affective disorders in multiple sclerosis: review and recommendations for clinical research. Arch Neurol 47:98–104, 1990

Minden SL, Orav J, Reich P: Depression in multiple sclerosis. Gen Hosp Psychiatry 9:426–434, 1987

Minden SL, Moes EJ, Orav J, et al: Memory impairment in multiple sclerosis. J Clin Exp Neuropsychol 12:566–586, 1990

Murray TJ: Amantadine therapy for fatigue in multiple sclerosis. Can J Neurol Sci 12:251–254, 1985

Nadeau SE, Watson RT: Neurologic manifestations of vasculitis and collagen vascular syndromes, in Clinical Neurology. Edited by Baker AB, Joynt RJ. New York, Harper & Row, 1990, chapter 59, 1–166

Naidu S, Moser HW: Peroxisomal disorders. Neurol Clin 8:507–519, 1990

Navia BA, Cho E-S, Petito CK, et al: The AIDS dementia complex, II: neuropathology. Ann Neurol 19:525–535, 1986a

Navia BA, Jordan BD, Price RW: The AIDS dementia complex, I: clinical features. Ann Neurol 19:517–524, 1986b

Newman NJ, Bell IR, McKee AC: Paraneoplastic limbic encephalitis: neuropsychiatric presentation. Biol Psychiatry 27:529–542, 1990

Noseworthy J, Paty D, Wonnacott T, et al: Multiple sclerosis after age 50. Neurology 33:1537–1544, 1983

Ochitill HN, Dilley JW: Neuropsychiatric aspects of acquired immunodeficiency syndrome, in AIDS and the Nervous System. Edited by Rosenblum ML, Levy RM, Bredesen DE. New York, Raven, 1988, pp 315–325

Ojeda VJ: Necrotising leucoencephalopathy associated with intrathecal/intraventricular methotrexate therapy. Med J Aust 2:289–293, 1982

Okazaki H: Fundamentals of Neuropathology, 1st Edition. New York, Igaku-Shoin, 1983, pp 134–136

Pantaleo G, Graziosi C, Fauci AS: The immunopathogenesis of human immunodeficiency virus infection. N Engl J Med 328:327–335, 1993

Petersen RB, Tabaton M, Berg L, et al: Analysis of the prion protein gene in thalamic dementia. Neurology 42:1859–1863, 1992

Plum F, Posner JB, Hain RF: Delayed neurologic deterioration after anoxia. Arch Intern Med 110:18–25, 1962

Poser CM, Paty DW, Scheinberg L, et al: New diagnostic criteria for multiple sclerosis: guidelines for research protocols. Ann Neurol 13:227–231, 1983

Posner JB: Pathogenesis of central nervous system paraneoplastic syndromes. Rev Neurol (Paris) 148:502–512, 1992

Posner JB, Furneaux HM: Paraneoplastic syndromes, in Immunologic Mechanisms in Neurologic and Psychiatric Disease. Edited by Waksman BH. New York, Raven, 1990, pp 187–219

Price RW, Sidtis JJ, Navia BA, et al: The AIDS dementia complex, in AIDS and the Nervous System. Edited by Rosenblum ML, Levy RM, Bredesen DE. New York, Raven, 1988, pp 203–219

Price TRP, Goetz KL, Lovell MR: Neuropsychiatric aspects of brain tumors, in The American Psychiatric Press Textbook of Neuropsychiatry, 2nd Edition. Edited by Yudofsky SC, Hales RE. Washington, DC, American Psychiatric Press, 1992, pp 493–494

Prusiner SB: Molecular biology of prion diseases. Science 252:1515–1522, 1991

Przelomski MM, O'Rourke E, Grady GF, et al: Eastern equine encephalitis in Massachusetts: a report of 16 cases, 1970–1984. Neurology 38:736–739, 1988

Rabins PV: Euphoria in multiple sclerosis, in Neurobehavioral Aspects of Multiple Sclerosis. Edited by Rao SM. New York, Oxford University Press, 1990, pp 180–185

Rao SM: Neuropsychology of multiple sclerosis: a critical review. J Clin Exp Neuropsychol 8:503–542, 1986

Rao SM, Bernardin L, Leo GJ, et al: Cerebral disconnection in multiple sclerosis: relationship to atrophy of the corpus callosum. Arch Neurol 46:918–920, 1989

Rao SM, Leo GJ, Bernardin L, et al: Cognitive dysfunction in multiple sclerosis, I: frequency, patterns, and prediction. Neurology 41:685–691, 1991

Ron MA, Logsdail SJ: Psychiatric morbidity in multiple sclerosis: a clinical and MRI study. Psychol Med 19:887–895, 1989

Rosenblum ML, Levy RM, Bredesen DE: Overview of AIDS and the nervous system, in AIDS and the Nervous System. Edited by Rosenblum ML, Levy RM, Bredesen DE. New York, Raven, 1988, pp 1–12

Rosove MH, Brewer PMC: Antiphospholipid thrombosis: clinical course after the first thrombotic event in 70 patients. Ann Intern Med 117:303–308, 1992

Rappaport EB: Iatrogenic Creutzfeldt-Jakob disease. Neurology 37:1520–1522, 1987

Rubens AB, Froehling B, Slater G, et al: Left ear suppression on verbal dichotic tests in patients with multiple sclerosis. Ann Neurol 18:459–463, 1985

Schiffer RB: Disturbances of affect, in Neurobehavioral Aspects of Multiple Sclerosis. Edited by Rao SM. New York, Oxford University Press, 1990, pp 186–195

Schiffer RB, Caine ED: The interaction between depressive affective disorder and neuropsychological test performance in multiple sclerosis patients. J Neuropsychiatry Clin Neurosci 3:28–32, 1991

Schiffer RB, Herndon RM, Rudick RA: Treatment of pathologic laughing and weeping with amitriptyline. N Engl J Med 312:1480–1482, 1985

Schiffer RB, Weitkamp LR, Wineman NM, et al: Multiple sclerosis and affective disorder: family history, sex, and HLA-DR antigens. Arch Neurol 45:1345–1348, 1988

Schmidt RP: Neurosyphilis, in Clinical Neurology. Edited by Baker AB, Joynt RJ. New York, Harper & Row, 1989, chapter 28, pp 1–23

Schmitt FA, Bigley JW, McKinnis R, et al (and the AZT Collaborative Working Group): Neuropsychological outcome of zidovudine (AZT) treatment of patients with AIDS and AIDS-related complex. N Engl J Med 319:1573–1578, 1988

Schnider A, Benson DF, Rosner LJ: Callosal disconnection in multiple sclerosis. Neurology 43:1243–1245, 1993

Schroth G, Gawehn J, Thron A, et al: Early diagnosis of herpes simplex encephalitis by MRI. Neurology 37:179–183, 1987

Seales D, Greer M: Acute hemorrhagic leukoencephalitis. A successful recovery. Arch Neurol 48:1086–1088, 1991

Seliger GM, Hornstein A, Flax J, et al: Fluoxetine improves emotional incontinence. Brain Inj 6:267–270, 1992

Serban D, Taraboulos A, DeArmond SJ, et al: Rapid detection of Creutzfeldt-Jakob disease and scrapie prion proteins. Neurology 40:110–117, 1990

Serdaroglu P, Yazici H, Ozdemir C, et al: Neurologic involvement in Behcet's syndrome: a prospective study. Arch Neurol 46:265–269, 1989

Simon RP: Neurosyphilis. Arch Neurol 42:606–613, 1985

So NK, O'Neill BP, Frytak S, et al: Delayed leukoencephalopathy in survivors with small cell lung cancer. Neurology 37:1198–1201, 1987

Stacy M, Roeltgen D: Infection of the central nervous system in the elderly, in The Pathology of the Aging Human Nervous System. Edited by Duckett S. Philadelphia, PA, Lea & Febiger, 1991, pp 374–392

Stagno SJ, Naugle RI, Roca C, et al: Progressive multifocal leukoencephalopathy appearing as language disturbance. Neuropsychiatry, Neuropsychology, and Behavioral Neurology 3:283–289, 1990

Steckelberg JM, Cockerill FR: Serologic testing for human immunodeficiency virus antibodies. Mayo Clin Proc 63:373–380, 1988

Stenager E, Stenager EN, Jensen K: Sexual aspects of multiple sclerosis. Semin Neurol 12:120–124, 1992

Stoner GL, Walker DL, Webster HdF: Age distribution of progressive multifocal leukoencephalopathy. Acta Neurol Scand 78:307–312, 1988

Swirsky-Sacchetti T, Mitchell DR, Seward J, et al: Neuropsychological and structural brain lesions in multiple sclerosis: a regional analysis. Neurology 42:1291–1295, 1992

Sze G, Zimmerman RD: The magnetic resonance imaging of infections and inflammatory diseases. Radiol Clin North Am 26:839–859, 1988

Tan EM, Cohen AS, Fries JF, et al: The 1982 revised criteria for the classification of systemic lupus erythematosus. Arthritis Rheum 25:1271–1277, 1982

The Canadian MS Research Group: A randomized controlled trial of amantadine in fatigue associated with multiple sclerosis. Can J Neurol Sci 14:273–278, 1987

Totsuka S, Hattori T, Yazaki M, et al: Clinicopathologic studies on neuro-Behcet's disease. Folia Psychiatrica et Neurologica Japonica 39:155–166, 1985

Tyler JL, Byrne TN: Neoplastic disorders, in Clinical Brain Imaging: Principles and Applications. Edited by Mazziotta JC, Gilman S. Philadelphia, PA, FA Davis, 1992, pp 166–216

Van Gorp WG, Mitrushina M, Cummings JL, et al: Normal aging and the subcortical encephalopathy of AIDS: a neuropsychological comparison. Neuropsychiatry, Neuropsychology, and Behavioral Neurology 2:5–20, 1989

Victor M: Neurologic disorders due to alcoholism and malnutrition, in Clinical Neurology. Edited by Baker AB, Joynt RJ. New York, Harper & Row, 1986, chapter 61, pp 1–94

Walker RW, Rosenblum MK: Amphotericin B-associated leukoencephalopathy. Neurology 42:2005–2010, 1992

Weinshenker BG, Penman M, Bass B, et al: A double-blind, randomized, crossover trial of pemoline in fatigue associated with multiple sclerosis. Neurology 42:1468–1471, 1992

Weller M, Liedtke W, Petersen D, et al: Very-late-onset adrenoleukodystrophy: possible precipitation of demyelination by cerebral contusion. Neurology 42:367–370, 1992

Whitley RJ: Herpes simplex virus infections of the central nervous system: encephalitis and neonatal herpes. Drugs 42:406–427, 1991

Younger DS, Hays AP, Brust JCM, et al: Granulomatous angiitis of the brain: an inflammatory reaction of diverse etiology. Arch Neurol 45:514–518, 1988

27

Neuropsychiatric Aspects of Medical Therapies

Harry McConnell, M.D., F.R.C.P.C.
James Duffy, M.D.

Introduction

Although medications are vital and effective for the treatment or control of disease in elderly patients, they frequently produce significant adverse side effects. In particular, the behavioral consequences of prescription medications are frequently devastating. Unfortunately, physicians often fail to recognize the drug-related etiology of these behavioral changes and often prescribe further psychotropic medications in an attempt to control symptoms. This results in a pattern of escalating medications with further side effects and drug interactions.

Although the elderly (defined as those over age 65) represent 12% of the population in the United States, they consume almost one-third of all prescriptions (Baum et al. 1987). Furthermore, although data vary widely among people taking medications, the elderly are two to three times more likely to experience adverse reactions compared with younger patients (Vestal and Cusack 1990). The significance and severity of adverse drug reactions in elderly patients is exemplified by the observation that as many as 10% of geriatric psychiatric admissions may be attributed to adverse drug reactions (Nelson and O'Malley 1988).

The frequency of prescription and "over-the-counter" (OTC) drug use increases with age, with 83% of community-dwelling elderly individuals consuming at least one medication (Ostrom et al. 1985). The quantity of prescription medications consumed is alarming, with an average of 3.1 prescription drugs per elderly community dweller (Ouslander 1981). Not unexpectedly, this figure is even higher in the nursing home population in which the average resident receives 7 prescribed medications (H. D. Bergman 1975), and it reaches astounding proportions in hospitalized elderly patients who receive an average of 10 medications (Ouslander 1981). Table 27–1 lists the ten most frequently prescribed medications in elderly patients.

When considering drug use in the elderly population, it is important to remember that elderly patients frequently self-prescribe OTC drugs such as nonsteroidal anti-inflammatory drugs (NSAIDs), antihistamines, analgesics, and psychostimulants including caffeine or phenylpropanolamine. Each of these agents may have significant behavioral side effects that may not be recognized if a full history of OTC drug usage is not obtained (Chaiton et al. 1976).

There is considerable overlap in the ten most frequently prescribed drugs in the elderly (Table 27–1) and the ten most frequent drugs associated with psychiatric adverse reactions. The Boston Collaborative Drug Surveillance Program (1971) looked at 90,000 drug exposures occurring during 10,600 admissions and found the following drugs to be most frequently associated with behavioral side effects: prednisone, isoniazid, methyldopa, insulin, diazepam, furosemide, phenobarbital, chlordiazepoxide, and aminophylline. In this chapter, we review the neuropsychiatric effects of prescribed and OTC medications in elderly patients and summarize how these agents may interfere with different aspects of neurobehavioral function including cognition, mood, arousal, sleep, ambulation, and sexual function.

Special Considerations in Geriatric Medical Therapy

Elderly patients are particularly susceptible to the neuropsychiatric complications of medical therapies because of the influence of aging on drug-taking behavior (compliance), central nervous system (CNS) vulnerability (pharmacodynamics), and the body's ability to absorb, distribute, metabolize, and excrete drugs (pharmacokinetics). The high prevalence of concomitant physical illness and the use of multiple drugs (polypharmacy), as well as environmental factors and the underrecognition of drug abuse in the elderly population, may also contribute to the development of neuropsychiatric complications of medical therapy. Rational medical treatment depends on an understanding of the interrelationships between these factors.

Table 27–1. Ten most frequently prescribed drugs in elderly patients

1. Diuretics
2. Antihypertensives
3. Coronary artery vasodilators
4. Digitalis preparations
5. Psychotropics
6. Alpha- and beta-blockers
7. Antiarthritics
8. Narcotic analgesics
9. Corticosteroids
10. Bronchodilators

Source. Adapted from Lamy et al. 1992.

Compliance

Noncompliance with medical therapy may predispose the patient to neuropsychiatric (as well as other) complications in three ways. First, underutilization of the prescribed drug can cause a recurrence or exacerbation of the illness being treated (e.g., refractory seizures due to noncompliance with anticonvulsants). Second, underutilization of one prescribed medication can result in increased toxicity of another. For example, Brook et al. (1971) found the compliance rates of digoxin, hydrochlorothiazide, and potassium chloride were 92%, 83%, and 60%, respectively, in patients followed up after hospitalization. The resultant hypokalemia resulting from potassium chloride noncompliance may present with delirium or may contribute to digoxin toxicity with delirium or psychosis (Hussar 1975). Finally, overutilization of the prescribed drug can place the patient at an increased risk of adverse reactions (e.g., the patient who forgets a dose and doubles up on the next dose or the patient who feels that if one tablet is good, two must be better) (Swinyard 1987).

Although estimates for noncompliance in elderly patients are generally similar to those for patients in other age groups, the data vary considerably (see Vestal and Cusack 1990). Certain elderly populations may require particularly careful monitoring, including patients seeking medications from several physicians or sharing medications with a spouse, those with even mild cognitive impairment (Kennedy 1992), and those on multiple medications (U. Bergman and Wilholm 1981).

As many as 75% of the elderly individuals living at home are likely to be noncompliant with their medications. The likelihood of noncompliance rises with the number of prescribed drugs and the disability of the patient (Ostrom et al. 1985). Confusion over exactly what patients are consuming (as opposed to what they are prescribed) is further compounded by the fact that elderly patients frequently take medication prescribed previously or prescribed for someone else (Jackson et al. 1989). In addition, as many as one-third of geriatric patients will provide different drug histories to independent examiners (Jackson et al. 1989). Because elderly patients may "shop around" for different physicians or consult more than one specialist, the likelihood of adverse events is often increased by their failure to identify a single physician responsible for orchestrating care.

Pharmacodynamics: CNS Vulnerability

The normal aging process is associated with predictable physiological alterations that influence the elderly person's response to medications. Although there is substantial inter- and intraindividual variability in the extent and type of change associated with the aging process, certain characteristic cognitive, neurochemical, and hemodynamic changes have been well documented. An understanding of these changes enables the clinician to predict and avoid adverse drug reactions in elderly patients.

Sunderland (1992) outlined four factors that contribute to the increased sensitivity of the elderly person to medications:

1. Age-related alterations in neuronal cell numbers and neurotransmitter production and breakdown
2. Selective alteration in the number of pre- and postsynaptic receptors with age
3. Age-related alterations in the receptor binding site–second messenger system.
4. An increase in the CNS concentration of drugs in elderly patients secondary to altered pharmacokinetics

Although some of the data remain contradictory, certain characteristic alterations in neurotransmitters have been ascribed to the aging process. These changes have significant implications for the effect of neuroactive drugs in elderly patients. A decrease in both serotonin production (Shih and Young 1978) and serotonin receptor number and sensitivity (Lawlor et al. 1989) has been linked to the alterations in appetite and sleep seen in elderly patients and may explain their apparently reduced response to serotonergic drugs (Sunderland 1992). A reduction in the number of cholinergic neurons in the nucleus basalis of Meynert (Mesulam et al. 1987), as well as decreased muscarinic and nicotinic receptors (Flynn and Mash 1986), accounts for increased sensitivity to anticholinergics among the elderly. A reversal in the normal superior ratio of dopamine, subtype 2 (D_2), to subtype 1 (D_1) receptors together with a decrease in dopamine production (Robinson et al. 1977) explains the increased incidence of neuroleptic-induced extrapyramidal side effects in elderly patients (Jeste and Wyatt 1987). The increased sensitivity of the elderly to benzodiazepines may be explained by an age-associated increase in γ-aminobutyric acid (GABA) receptor numbers and receptor sensitivity (Hare et al. 1982).

In addition to alterations in the specific neurotransmitters described, other age-related physiological changes may have significant implications for drug effects. These changes render the older person more susceptible to the adverse side effects of many medications and include 1) decreased cerebral circulation and metabolism (Fazekas et al. 1952; Sokoloff 1966); 2) neurodegenerative changes in the autonomic nervous system (predisposing to orthostatic hypotension and thermal dysregulation) (Brocklehurst 1974; Caird et al. 1987; Nemeroff 1989); and 3) a loss in neurons, particularly in the prefrontal cortex and substantia nigra (Nemeroff 1989).

The elderly patient with an identified neuropathological process is in even greater peril of developing adverse drug effects. The characteristic changes associated with neurodegenerative processes such as Alzheimer's disease, Parkinson's disease, subcortical atherosclerotic encephalopathy, and multi-infarct dementia produce a predictable vulnerability to drugs. An understanding of these changes allows the physician to avoid many adverse drug effects in such elderly patients.

Senile dementia of the Alzheimer type (SDAT) is characterized by a dramatic degradation of cholinergic systems. Anticholinergic drugs are likely to have a deleterious effect on the already compromised memory of these patients; many patients are also liable to develop an acute confusional state with even low doses of anticholinergics. In addition to changes in the cholinergic system, persons with SDAT exhibit alterations in adrenergic and serotonergic systems. The impact of these changes on drug response remains to be determined.

The reduction in dopaminergic receptors associated with SDAT implies that these patients will be more susceptible to the extrapyramidal effects of the neuroleptics they are often prescribed for control of their agitated behavior (Cross et al. 1984). The profound dopamine depletion (and subsequent neuroleptic supersensitivity) associated with primary or secondary Parkinsonism often poses a therapeutic dilemma because these patients frequently develop delusional disorders and/or hallucinations as a consequence of dopamine agonist treatment (Cummings 1991). The selective dopamine, subtype 4 (D_4), receptor blocking agent clozapine provides a viable therapeutic option in such situations (Rosenthal et al. 1992). Patients with Parkinson's disease also demonstrate an increased sensitivity to anticholinergic agents; one study found the development of an acute confusional state in 93% of Parkinson's disease patients taking anticholinergic medications (De Smet et al. 1982). Patients with cortical or subcortical vascular disease are likely to be sensitive to a wide range of psychoactive drugs. The degree and nature of these changes is somewhat idiosyncratic and dependent on the nature and site of the vascular pathology.

Although these age-related physiological and pathological changes make the elderly more sensitive to the CNS effects of medical therapies, older patients may actually be less sensitive to the peripheral effects of some drugs (e.g., the chronotropic effects of isoproterenol, β-adrenergic blockage by propranolol, PR prolongation by verapamil and diltiazem, and the hypoglycemic effect of tolbutamide (Vestal and Cusack 1990). The clinician must be aware of and carefully balance the altered central and peripheral pharmacodynamics in prescribing for elderly patients to avoid neuropsychiatric adverse reactions. The age-related changes in pharmacodynamics for some specific drugs are shown in Table 27–2.

Pharmacokinetics

The process of aging results in physiological and environmental changes, as well as in an increased incidence of certain disease states that alter the absorption, distribution and transport, metabolism, and excretion of drugs. These factors are summarized in Table 27–3.

Absorption.   Decreases in the number of absorptive cells, in some active transport processes, and in the gastric acidity, motility, and blood flow occurring with age might all be expected to affect drug absorption. However, the rate and extent of drug absorption is largely unaltered in elderly patients, and except for drugs with first-pass metabolism (e.g., prazosin, propranolol, and lidocaine), bioavailability tends to be the same in young and old subjects for most drugs (Vestal and Cusack 1990). These age-related physiological changes in the gastrointestinal tract may, however, have a direct effect on the bioavailability of the benzodiazepine clorazepate and of levodopa. The increased gastric pH may contribute to decreased steady-state concentrations of clorazepate, and the decreased dopa decarboxylase in the gastric mucosa can cause a threefold increase in the bioavailability of levodopa in elderly patients (P. Wood and Castleden 1991).

Distribution. The changes in body composition noted in Table 27–3 result in an increased apparent volume of distribution for lipophilic drugs (e.g., thiopental and benzodiazepines). Hydrophilic drugs that are distributed mainly in body fluids (e.g., alcohol and acetaminophen) will thus exhibit higher blood levels in elderly individuals due to a reduced volume of distribution (Erwin 1993). Drugs with a basic pH will exhibit an increased binding (and thus a decreased free fraction) to the elevated levels of α_1 acid glycoprotein in the elderly, whereas acidic drugs will demonstrate an increased free fraction as they bind predominantly to albumin. The latter is moderately decreased in elderly individuals (Vestal and Cusack 1990).

Metabolism and excretion. Decrease in hepatic mass and blood flow and increased prevalence of slow acetylator status in elderly individuals cause a decrease in the first-pass effect, with less drug removed after absorption into the portal vein as the drug passes through the liver to the systemic circulation, resulting in increased bioavailability for drugs typically metabolized by first-pass effects. Because the elimination half-life is dependent on clearance and volume of distribution,

Table 27–2. Pharmocodynamics and aging

Drug	Age change in dynamics	Method of measurement of effect
Antidepressants[a]	No change	Systolic time intervals
Chlormethiazole	Increase	Choice reaction time, flicker-fusion threshold, postural sway
Coumarins[b]	Increase	Prothrombin time
Deslanoside	No change	Systolic time intervals
Diazepam	Increase	Sedation for endoscopy
Diazepam	Increase	Sedation for cardioversion
Diazepam	Increase	Postural sway
Dichloralphenazone	Increase	Postural sway
Diltiazem	Increase	Acute antihypertensive effect
Diphenhydramine	No change	Psychomotor function
Enalapril	Increase	Acute antihypertensive effect
Furosemide	Decrease	Latency and size of peak diuretic response
Heparin	No change	Activated partial thromboplastin time
Isoproterenol	Decrease	Chronotropic effect
Isoproterenol	Decrease	Forearm blood flow, chronotropic effect, renin output response
Isoproterenol	Decrease	Chronotropic effect
Levodopa	?Increase	Dose limitation due to side effects
Morphine	Increase	Analgesic effect
Morphine	Increase	Extent and duration of pain relief
Nitrazepam	Increase	Psychomotor function, sedation
Pancuronium	No change	Depression of muscle twitch tension
Pentazocine	Increase	Analgesic effect
Propranolol	Decrease	Chronotropic effect
Temazepam	Increase	Postural sway, flicker-fusion threshold, choice reaction time, sedation
Tolbutamide	Decrease	Hypoglycemic effect
Verapamil	Increase	Acute peak antihypertensive effect
Warfarin	Increase	Thrombotest
Warfarin	Increase	Prothrombin time, clotting factor synthesis
Warfarin[c]	Increase	Prothrombin time

[a]Including amitriptyline, trimipramine, imipramine, maprotiline, and mianserin.
[b]Including warfarin, phenoprocoumarin, and dicumarol.
[c]Only in patients treated for thromboembolic disease and coronary artery disease and not in patients with peripheral vascular disease or valvular heart disease.
Source. Adapted from Cusack and Vestal 1986; Vestal and Cusack 1990.

those drugs with an increased volume of distribution and a decreased hepatic clearance (e.g., diazepam) will have a significantly prolonged half-life in elderly patients. Oxidation, reduction, and hydrolysis of drugs (phase I enzymatic reactions) are affected by aging far more than are the conjugation of drugs and metabolites (phase II enzymatic reactions). Drugs requiring oxidation for biotransformation will thus have a greatly prolonged half-life in elderly patients (Erwin 1993).

Renal functioning in those over age 65 is, on average, about 35% reduced compared with that of the young. The aging kidney is also at greater risk for nephrotoxicity, and, although there is significant individual variation in renal function in elderly individuals, these factors may be important for the excretion of water-soluble drugs and metabolites, diminishing plasma clearance of these substances in elderly patients with impaired renal function.

Concomitant Physical Illness

Elderly patients are at increased risk for a variety of disease states that may affect pharmacokinetics (Table 27–3). The effects of age-related pathology on pharmacodynamics was discussed above.

Polypharmacy

As discussed above, elderly patients are also at increased risk from neuropsychiatric complications of medical therapy by virtue of the effects of polypharmacy, which may affect compliance and cause drug-drug interactions. U. Bergman and Wilholm (1981) showed that in patients over 65 the rate of noncompliance doubles when more than three drugs are prescribed (32% versus 69%). Whereas in patients under 65, the rates are similar (28% versus 33%). Drug-drug interactions may cause neuropsychiatric adverse reactions by either direct CNS toxicity or through indirect effects on the periphery (e.g., by drug-induced hypoglycemia or electrolyte disturbances). The most significant drug-drug interactions leading to neuropsychiatric effects in elderly patients are shown in Table 27–4.

Environmental Factors

Environmental conditions in elderly patients that may affect medical therapy include 1) diet, with secondary effects on the pharmacokinetics of some drugs (Vestal and Cusack 1990); 2) the patient's living situation, which may affect compliance (Kennedy 1992); and

Table 27–3. Summary of factors affecting drug disposition in elderly patient

Pharmacokinetic parameter	Age-related physiological changes	Pathological conditions	Environmental factors
Absorption	Increased gastric pH Decreased absorptive surface Decreased splanchnic blood flow Decreased gastrointestinal motility	Achlorhydria Diarrhea Postgastrectomy state Malabsorption syndromes Pancreatitis	Antacids Anticholinergics Cholestyramine Drug interactions Food or meals
Distribution	Decreased cardiac output Decreased total body water Decreased lean body mass Decreased serum albumin Increased α_1-acid glycoprotein	Congestive heart failure Dehydration Edema or ascites Hepatic failure Malnutrition Renal failure	Drug interactions Protein-binding displacement
Metabolism	Decreased hepatic mass Decreased enzyme activity Decreased hepatic blood flow	Congestive heart failure Fever Hepatic insufficiency Malignancy Malnutrition Thyroid disease Viral infection or immunization	Dietary composition Drug interactions Insecticides Tobacco (smoking)
Excretion	Decreased renal blood flow Decreased glomerular filtration rate Decreased tubular secretion	Hypovolemia Renal insufficiency	Drug interactions

Source. From Vestal and Dawson 1985.

Table 27–4. Significant potential drug-drug interactions in psychogeriatrics

Drugs	Interacting drugs	Consequences
Salicylates	β-Adrenergic blockers	Decreased antihypertensive action
	Hypoglycemics (chlorpropamide)	Large acetylsalicylic acid doses may cause hypoglycemia
	Lithium	Possible lithium toxicity
	Valproate	Possible valproate toxicity
Nonsteroidal anti-inflammatory drugs	Beta-blockers	Decreased antihypertensive action
	Captopril	Indomethacin-decreased antihypertensive action
	Furosemide	Decreased diuretic action and antihypertensive effect
	Haloperidol	Possible severe sedation with indomethacin
	Potassium	Indomethacin-induced hyperkalemia
	Thiazide diuretics	Hyponatremia
Antidepressants: tricyclic	Clonidine	Decreased antihypertensive effect
	Disulfiram	Organic mental disorder
	Guanethidine	Decreased antihypertensive effect
	Hypoglycemics (chlorpropamide)	Doxepin-induced hypoglycemia
	Nitroglycerin (sublingual; tolazamide)	Nortriptyline-induced hypoglycemia
	Trimethoprim: sulfamethoxazole	Nitroglycerine may not dissolve; loss of antidepressant effect
Antidepressants: nontricyclic	Tricyclic antidepressants	Fluoxetine and maprotiline may inhibit metabolism of some tricyclic antidepressants
	Digoxin	Trazodone may increase risk of digoxin toxicity
	Phenothiazines	Trazodone combined may produce severe hypotension
Carbamazepine	Anticoagulants	Prothrombin time decreased
	Cimetidine	Carbamazepine levels increased
	Desipramine	Carbamazepine and desipramine levels increased
	Diltiazem	Neurotoxicity
	Metoclopramide	Neurotoxicity
	Theophylline	Theophylline concentration decreased
	Thiazide diuretics	Hyponatremia
	Verapamil	Carbamazepine levels increased
β-Adrenergic blockers	Alcohol	May block signs of delirium tremens
	Cimetidine	Decreased β-adrenergic blocker metabolism
	Clonidine	Paradoxical hypertension
	Diltiazem	Heart failure
	Haloperidol	Profound hypotension
	Sulfonylureas	Prolonged hypoglycemia with hypoglycemic overdose
	Insulin	Prolonged hypoglycemia with hypoglycemic overdose
	Maprotiline	Decreased maprotiline metabolism
	Methyldopa	Hypertensive reaction
	Nifedipine	Heart failure
	Chlorpromazine	Levels increased of both medications
	Thioridazine	Thioridazine levels increased
	Sympathomimetic bronchodilators	Decreased bronchodilation
	Theophyllines	Theophylline toxicity
	Thiazide diuretics	Cardiac arrhythmias
	Verapamil	Heart failure
Lithium	Methyldopa	Lithium toxicity
	Phenytoin	Lithium toxicity
	Verapamil	Neurotoxicity, bradycardia

Source. From Kennedy 1992.

3) their economic status and accessibility to medical care, which may affect their use or misuse of OTC medications (Atkinson et al. 1992).

The Underrecognition of Drug Abuse and Misuse

Substance abuse in elderly patients may lead to a variety of neuropsychiatric complications of medical therapy (Gambert 1992; Lawson 1989). Alcohol, prescription sedatives and analgesics, OTC medications, tobacco, and caffeine are the most frequent substances of abuse. Many patients will conceal their OTC drug use or may not consider them as drugs. Only one-sixth of patients will inform their physicians of their OTC use, and those with cognitive impairment are particularly vulnerable to OTC misuse (Atkinson et al. 1992).

The anticholinergic effects of diphenhydramine and other antihistamines found in most OTC sleep and cold remedies may cause significant cognitive effects, delirium, and psychosis in elderly patients, even in therapeutic doses. There is also an age-associated increased sensitivity to caffeine and other stimulants such as phenylpropanolamine, ephedrine, and pseudoephedrine found in OTC allergy and cold preparations. Patients on monoamine oxidase inhibitors (MAOIs) may unknowingly take OTC preparations with phenylpropanolamine, putting them at increased risk for hypertensive crisis. Elderly patients may also be at increased risk from the neuropsychiatric effects of NSAIDs in OTC preparations, including aseptic meningitis, psychosis, and cognitive dysfunction (Hoppmann et al. 1991). (The neuropsychiatric aspects of drug abuse and misuse in the elderly population are discussed further in Chapter 19.)

The clinician must thus take into account age-related compliance, as well as pharmacokinetic/dynamic, environmental, and behavioral factors in prescribing for elderly patients. Family members and caretakers should be included in discussions about treatment whenever possible and may help with the cognitively impaired patient in assuring the correct administration of medications. Elderly patients' visual deficits and hearing impairments may result in errors in the frequency and dose of their prescriptions, and tamper-resistant packaging of medications may also interfere with compliance. Attention to these simple factors may avoid tragic errors.

Drug-Induced Neuropsychiatric Syndromes

Appendix 27–1 summarizes the drugs associated with specific neuropsychiatric syndromes in elderly patients. These are further discussed below.

Delirium and Cognitive Impairment

The most common disorder of attention and cognition encountered in clinical practice is delirium (acute confusional state [ACS]). Identified factors predisposing to the development of a confusional state are 1) age greater than 60 years (Lipowski 1984; Liston 1982) and 2) brain dysfunction (Erkinjuntti et al. 1986; Lipowski 1990). A large multicenter trial found that as many as one-third of patients over age 65 were found to be in ACSs on admission to a general hospital. Drugs, particularly anticholinergic agents, represent the most common cause of confusional states across all age groups (Hodkinson 1973). (Delirium is also discussed further in Chapter 19, and dementia in Chapters 20 and 21.)

Many of the same drugs that produce ACSs may also cause chronic cognitive impairment in elderly patients. Katzman et al. (1988) reviewed nine published series and found drug-induced states to be the most common of the reversible causes of dementia, accounting for 2.7% of all cases. Larson et al. (1987) implicated drugs as either a primary or contributing cause in 35 of their 300 patients evaluated for dementia. The incidence of adverse drug reactions increased from 2.7% for those taking two to three prescription drugs to 9.3% for those taking four to five and to 13.7% for those taking six or more. Sedative-hypnotic agents, especially long-acting benzodiazepines, were the drugs most commonly associated with cognitive impairment. Appendix 27–1 indicates the various medical therapies reported to be associated with the development of delirium and dementia. The most important agents causing cognitive impairment are discussed below.

Anticholinergics.   Narcotic analgesics, antidepressants, antiparkinsonian drugs, neuroleptics, antispasmodics, and OTC cold and sleep preparations containing antihistamines all have significant anticholinergic effects. Anticholinergic agents are particularly likely to induce ACS and are postulated to induce an imbalance in the cholinergic and adrenergic pathways of the reticular activating system and thalamocortical projections, thereby disrupting the attentional matrix (Itil and Fink 1966).

As discussed above, the elderly brain is likely to be more sensitive to the anticholinergic effects of drugs, particularly if there is associated neurodegenerative disease. Indeed, the neurologically compromised elderly patient may develop an ACS even after receiving 1% scopolamine eye drops or transdermal patches (Danielson et al. 1981; MacEwan et al. 1985). The increased neurological sensitivity of the elderly is further aggravated by the pharmacokinetic changes associated with aging (discussed above). The extent of the hazard faced by elderly patients is highlighted by the finding that 60% of nursing home residents and 23% of elderly community dwellers are receiving at least one anticholinergic drug at any one time (Blazer et al. 1983). P. S. Miller et. al. (1988) evaluated the effects of low-dose scopolamine (.005 mg/kg body weight) versus placebo in presurgical elderly patients and found the degree of impairment on the Saskatoon Delirium Symptom Checklist and performance on the Rey Auditory-Verbal Learning test to relate to both serum and cerebrospinal fluid anticholinergic levels. Katz et al. (1988) suggested that background EEG slowing combined with cognitive tests may help identify patients with cognitive impairment caused by anticholinergic toxicity.

Antidepressants.   Elderly patients are frequently prescribed antidepressants, and, prior to the advent of "novel" antidepressants, these were almost exclusively tricyclic agents. The risk of tricyclic-induced anticholinergic toxicity rises with age (Livingston et al. 1983), and as many as 5% of elderly patients are reported to develop a confusional state—even at therapeutic levels (Cole et al. 1983). It is important to recognize that elderly patients may experience the central muscarinic toxicity that produces a confusional state or a dementia-like syndrome without necessarily manifesting the characteristic autonomic (nicotinic) changes of urinary retention, tachycardia, piloerection, or pupillary dilatation (Crawshaw and Mullen 1984). The incidence of delirium with the serotonin selective reuptake inhibitors such as sertraline, fluoxetine, and fluvoxamine remains to be determined. The minimal anticholinergic effects of these agents is likely to present a significant clinical advantage over the tricyclic agents. Bupropion (Branconnier et al. 1983) and trazodone (Burns et. al. 1986) appear to have less toxicity in elderly patients on formal testing than do the tricyclic antidepressants.

Cardiovascular medications.   Several antihypertensives have been reported to produce an ACS. Beta-blockers in particular have been implicated in producing not only an ACS (Kuhr 1979) but also hallucinosis, sleep disruption, and chronic fatigue (McGahan et al. 1984). The association between beta-blockers and the development of a major depressive disorder is inconclusive (Bartels et al. 1988). Similar to the topical anticholinergics, the topical beta-blocker timolol, used to treat glaucoma, may also produce an ACS (Shore et al. 1987). Other antihypertensives implicated in the production of an ACS include calcium channel blockers, clonidine, and methyldopa (Adler 1981; Hoffman and Ladogana 1981; Jacobson et al. 1987). Methyldopa, propranolol, hydrochlorothiazide, and reserpine may also produce significant global cognitive impairment in the elderly (Larson et al. 1987).

An ACS may occur with therapeutic blood levels (Eisendrath and Sweeney 1987) of digoxin and herald the onset of potentially fatal cardiac arrhythmias (Sagel and Matisonn 1975). In addition to alterations in attention, digoxin may produce hallucinosis, sleep disruption, dysphoria, and irritability (Eisendrath and Sweeney 1987). The muscarinic-blocking properties of the antiarrhythmics quinidine and disopyramide may also result in cognitive impairment in elderly patients.

NSAIDs.   Any of the NSAIDs may produce ACS and cognitive impairment in elderly patients (Allison and Shantz 1987; J. S. Goodwin and Regan 1982; Thornton 1980). Although the opiate analgesics are less likely to produce an ACS, the anticholinergic effects of normeperidine (a metabolite of meperidine) may result in a syndrome characterized by agitation, hallucinosis, and confusion (Eisendrath et al. 1987). Elderly individuals are particularly susceptible to acute or chronic salicylate toxicity that may occur at "therapeutic levels" and frequently presents with an ACS (Cupit 1982).

Histamine, subtype 2 (H2) receptor antagonists. The H2 receptor blockers cimetidine and ranitidine are widely prescribed in elderly patients and are usually considered to have a benign side effect profile. These agents (particularly cimetidine) have, however, been reported to produce an ACS in as many as 17% of elderly patients with renal or hepatic insufficiency (Schentag et al. 1979). The observation that physostigmine can reverse cimetidine-induced delirium (Jenike and Levy 1983) suggests that there may be indirect cholinergic involvement.

Antiparkinsonian medications. Although the frequency remains uncertain, there is no doubt that Parkinson's disease patients receiving levodopa are at risk for developing an ACS. Parkinson's disease patients with significant cortical atrophy appear to be at most risk for developing not only an ACS but also other behavioral side effects such as hallucinosis (Celesia and Barr 1970; Fennelly 1987). Not surprisingly, the anticholinergics often prescribed to treat Parkinson's disease also frequently produce confusion and cognitive impairment. The dopamine agonists bromocriptine and amantadine have also been reported to produce delirium in as many as 20% of patients (Cummings 1991; Lieberman et al. 1979; Postma and Vantilburg 1975).

Anesthesia. A postoperative ACS is not uncommon in elderly patients. Several possible etiologies should be considered including anticholinergic preoperative preparations, hypoxia, metabolic disturbances, infection, fat embolism, hemodynamic disturbances, meperidine intoxication, pulmonary embolism, and sedative-hypnotic withdrawal (Lipowski 1990).

Other drugs causing delirium and cognitive impairment. The anticholinergic effects of neuroleptics, particularly the lower-potency phenothiazines, may cause both ACS and cognitive impairment in elderly patients, even at therapeutic doses. Low doses of benzodiazepines can also cause significant cognitive impairment in elderly patients, relating to the plasma concentration (Pomara et al. 1984). The long-acting benzodiazepines may pose a greater problem with increased accumulation and persistence of side effects. The Veterans Affairs cooperative study studied the cognitive effects of anticonvulsants in 622 epileptic patients, finding patients on phenobarbital, primidone, and phenytoin to exhibit significant cognitive impairment, whereas those on carbamazepine exhibited stable performance on cognitive tasks (Smith et al. 1987). Carbamazepine and sodium valproate have shown less tendency to induce cognitive impairment in most studies, although the latter has been implicated as causing a dementia-like syndrome associated with reversible cerebral atrophy (McLachlan 1987). Other drugs reported to cause cognitive impairment include lithium, corticosteroids, various antibiotics, radiocontrast agents, interferon, alcohol, heavy metals, organic solvents, carbon monoxide, organophosphates, cyclosporine, various antineoplastic agents, metaclo-

pramide, phenylpropanolamine, and caffeine. (For an excellent review, see Morrison and Katz 1989.)

Anxiety

Anxiety may be caused by a variety of pharmacological agents (see Appendix 27–1). There is an increased sensitivity to stimulants with aging, and the elderly may be particularly susceptible to caffeinism even without a history of excessive intake (Williams and Caranasos 1992). Caffeine may also be taken unknowingly in various OTC cold and allergy preparations. Sympathomimetic amines, which may also be present in such OTC preparations, are also common causes of secondary anxiety in elderly patients (Lader 1982). Elderly individuals are susceptible to paradoxical excitement manifested by anxiety and agitation due to alcohol, benzodiazepines, barbiturates, and other sedative-hypnotics, as well as some antidepressants. Tricyclic antidepressants, bupropion, and fluoxetine have all been reported to produce restlessness, anxiety, and insomnia (Williams and Caranasos 1992).

The withdrawal effects of narcotics, alcohol, benzodiazepines, and other sedative-hypnotics are also frequent causes of anxiety. Erratic use of sedative-hypnotics may cause withdrawal insomnia and daytime anxiety. Other drugs implicated as causing anxiety include thyroxine, antiparkinsonian drugs (particularly levodopa and bromocriptine), various cardiac drugs (disopyramide and nifedipine), cycloserine, anticonvulsants, antihistamines, anticholinergics, theophylline, and various respiratory drugs. Ten percent to 15% of patients treated with dopaminergic agents will develop anxiety symptoms (Cummings 1991).

Depression, Mania, and Psychosis

Drugs implicated in causing affective and psychotic disorders are shown in Appendix 27–1. Here we discuss the most important of these as they pertain to elderly patients.

Cardiac medications. Cardiac glycosides, antiarrhythmics, and antihypertensives have all been associated with the development of psychotic and affective symptoms. The catecholamine-depleting effects of reserpine account for the frequent association of depression with the use of this antihypertensive, occurring in 20% of patients on average and generally resolving with discontinuation of treatment (F. K. Goodwin and

Bunney 1971). α-Methyldopa is an antihypertensive agent also associated with depressive symptoms, acting primarily via its metabolite α-methyl norepinephrine, a potent α_2-adrenergic agonist. Paykel et al. (1982) have reviewed 65 clinical trials with 2,320 patients, finding 83 cases (3.6%) of depression reported, of which 25 cases warranted discontinuing the drug. In their extensive review of the literature, they also found an incidence of depression of 1.5% for clonidine, another α_2-adrenergic agonist; 1.1% for the β-adrenoreceptor blocker propranolol; and 1.9% for guanethidine. Propranolol has also been reported to cause visual hallucinations and psychosis (Fleminger 1978; Fraser and Carr 1976). Fleminger (1978) found 17.5% of 115 patients had visual hallucinations and/or illusions with propranolol. Although the incidence of depression with propranolol is probably much less than originally thought, atenolol, being less lipophilic than propranolol and thus crossing the blood-brain barrier less easily, is probably the preferable beta-blocker to use in those susceptible to the development of depression.

Digitalis has a very narrow therapeutic index and toxic levels may produce delirium, aphasia, and hallucinations (Levenson 1979). Depression may occur as a side effect at therapeutic levels, particularly in elderly patients (Pascualy and Veith 1989). The psychiatric side effects of digoxin are associated with elevated serum levels, and the susceptibility of elderly patients is probably related to decreased clearance of the drug.

The antiarrhythmics quinidine, procainamide, and disopyramide have all been associated with the development of hallucinations and psychosis. This may relate to their anticholinergic effects, although their psychiatric side effects are frequently associated with polypharmacy (K. A. Wood et. al. 1988).

Corticosteroids. The Boston Collaborative Drug Surveillance Program study (1971) found prednisone to be the most frequent cause of moderate or severe psychiatric side effects, occurring in 2.6% of patients. Lewis and Smith (1983), in an extensive review of the literature, found a 5% incidence of serious psychiatric symptoms in patients on corticosteroids. Depression, mania, euphoria, and psychosis have all frequently been reported and appear to be dose-related and/or related to withdrawal. Female sex, systemic lupus erythematosus, and high doses of prednisone are risk factors, and decreasing the steroid dose, neuroleptics, and ECT are generally effective treatments. Tricyclic antidepressants do not appear to be as effective.

NSAIDs. Hoppmann et al. (1991) have recently reviewed the neuropsychiatric reports of side effects of NSAIDs. Elderly patients are particularly susceptible, especially with NSAIDs that are mostly protein bound. Psychosis has been reported as a side effect of both indomethacin and sulindac, agents that are structurally related. The mechanism of inducing psychosis could relate to the indolic moiety of indomethacin, similar to serotonin. Ibuprofen, naproxen, salicylates, and other NSAIDs have also been associated with depression and cognitive impairment, particularly in elderly patients.

Antiparkinsonian drugs. Cummings (1991) reviewed the neuropsychiatric complications of the treatment of Parkinson's disease. He found that 30% of patients treated with dopaminergic agents develop visual hallucinations, 10% have delusional syndromes, 10% euphoria, 1% mania, and 10%–15% anxiety symptoms. Elderly patients and dementia patients appear more susceptible to these complications. Clozapine may be effective in treating psychotic symptoms if they do not resolve with dosage reduction (Friedman and Lannon 1989; Rosenthal et al. 1992). Anticholinergics used in Parkinson's disease are more frequently associated with delirium but may also present with delusions and/or hallucinations.

H_2 blockers. The H_2 blockers cimetidine and, less frequently, ranitidine have been reported to cause depression, mania, and psychosis (Billings and Stein 1986; Billings et al. 1981; Hubain et al. 1982; Russell and Lopez 1980). As the role of histamine as a central neurotransmitter is still unclear, the mechanism of action of these effects is also not certain. Cimetidine interacts significantly with a number of other medications (see Table 27–3), and thus care must be taken in patients taking numerous drugs. As cimetidine and ranitidine are both excreted primarily by the kidney, the clinician should be particularly cautious in prescribing H_2 blockers in elderly patients with diminished renal function.

Psychotropics. Reports of benzodiazepine-induced depression and psychosis are difficult to evaluate because the patients often had preexisting psychiatric illness and/or concomitant therapies. In a retrospective review, Greenblatt et al. (1976) reported that 3% of more than 2,000 patients on flurazepam manifested depression, although almost half of these were on other drug therapy as well. The psychiatric effects of benzodiazepines are most likely secondary to inhibition via the neurotransmitter GABA. Confusion, hallucinations, and seizures may also occur with benzodiazepine withdrawal. There has been considerable debate over the depression-inducing effects of neuroleptics. Hogarty and Munetz (1984) found no difference in depressive symptoms in their control subjects compared with their neuroleptic subjects in a double-blind study. There have also been a number of cases of mania reported with antidepressant therapy and withdrawal, as well as with stimulants and sympathomimetics (Sultzer and Cummings 1989). (The neuropsychiatric aspects of psychotropic medication are discussed further in Chapter 30.)

Disorders of Gait and Mobility

Disorders of gait, particularly those that result in a fall, represent a significant source of hazard and subsequent disability in elderly people. As many as 15% of people over age 65 have a gait disorder (Newman et. al 1960); the incidence rises to 25% after age 79 (Lungren-Lindquist et al. 1983). Medications are important contributors to these statistics and profoundly influence the ability of elderly patients to ambulate safely and efficiently. The magnitude of the problem is highlighted by the finding that more than one-third of community-dwelling people over age 75 fall each year (Tinetti 1977) and as many as 10% of these falls result in serious (sometimes fatal) injury (Smallegan 1983). The psychological and physical repercussions of these falls frequently necessitate placement in a nursing home (Kellogg International 1987). The problem in nursing homes reaches catastrophic proportions where the annual incidence of falls is 1,600 per 1,000 residents (Sudarsky 1990).

Normal changes in ambulation associated with aging include 1) shorter, broader strides; 2) decreased speed; 3) diminished pelvic rotation; and 4) a decreased capacity for adjusting posture in response to environmental demands (MacDonald and MacDonald 1977). In addition to these expected changes, the elderly person may also develop gait abnormalities as a consequence of some other identifiable pathology such as musculoskeletal changes, Parkinson's disease, myelopathies (e.g., cervical spondylosis), cerebellar degeneration, normal pressure hydrocephalus, and subcortical atherosclerotic disease (Sudarsky 1990). Medications may aggravate these pathological processes or may produce gait abnormalities independently. The risk of falls in an elderly person rises proportionally to the number of medications he or she is taking. Medications that have been conclusively demonstrated to increase the risk of falling include barbiturates, tricyclic antidepressants, neuroleptics (particularly phenothiazines), antihypertensives, levodopa, benzodiazepines, and diuretics (Davie et al. 1981; MacDonald 1983; MacDonald and MacDonald 1977; Prudnam and Evans 1981; Ray et. al. 1989; Wild et al. 1981). In particular, combinations of medications that have additive side-effects (e.g., antihypertensives in combination with sedative-hypnotics) appear to be most hazardous (MacDonald 1983).

Sleep Disorders Produced by Medical Therapies

The predictable alterations in sleep architecture associated with aging are reviewed in Chapter 17. The incidence of insomnia increases as a function of age and physical status (Gillin and Byerly 1990). Many elderly persons therefore complain of poor sleep and/or unacceptable daytime drowsiness and frequently seek treatment—either from their physician or via OTC medications. In the context of neurodegenerative disorders, sleep problems frequently exhaust relatives and precipitate the family's decision to seek institutionalization of a loved one (Berry and Webb 1985). Medications may play a significant role in producing sleep disturbances in the elderly. In addition, the particular vulnerabilities of the aging brain demand the judicious selection of appropriate treatment strategies for sleep disorders—failure to do so may result in escalating sleep and behavioral problems.

The use of benzodiazepines, which are frequently prescribed in elderly patients, presents particular hazards (Closser 1991). The elderly are more sensitive to benzodiazepines secondary to their altered pharmacokinetics and enhanced postsynaptic receptor sensitivity (Swift 1986). Benzodiazepines are frequently administered to elderly patients who complain of insomnia. The extent of benzodiazepine use is highlighted by one study that reported that half of all elderly medical admissions were receiving benzodiazepines (Foy et al. 1986).

Ironically, although benzodiazepines are usually initially prescribed to treat insomnia, they are a frequent cause of deteriorating sleep quality (Schneider-Heimert 1988). Sustained use results in diminished slow-wave and rapid-eye-movement (REM) sleep, with no alteration in total sleep time (Schneider-Heimert 1988). The problem may be further compounded when the elderly person develops rebound insomnia after missing even a single dose of a short-acting preparation, often resulting in escalating hypnotic use (Gillin et al. 1989). Patients receiving ultra-short acting benzodiazepines such as triazolam may experience this rebound phenomenon within a few hours of their last dose and may require more than one dose per evening to maintain sleep and avoid becoming agitated or confused. In addition, the ultra-short acting benzodiazepines have been reported to produce a myriad of behavioral changes in susceptible individuals including anterograde amnesia, delirium, anxiety, and dysphoria (Patterson 1987; Reynolds et al. 1985).

The long half-life benzodiazepines (e.g., flurazepam and clonazepam) should be avoided in elderly patients, as they are likely to produce prolonged daytime drowsiness, cognitive disturbances, and potentially hazardous ataxia (Carskadon et al. 1982). Sleep apnea increases with age and may be significantly aggravated by the use of sedative-hypnotics, thereby creating a potentially serious risk (Ancoli-Israel et al. 1985). Overall, the use of benzodiazepines for insomnia in elderly patients remains controversial. Their administration should probably be limited to the brief use of the intermediate benzodiazepines in stressful situations.

Several cardiovascular drugs have been reported to exert a powerful influence on sleep architecture. Beta-blockers (particularly lipophilic agents such as propranolol, metoprolol, and pindolol) and reserpine have been associated with nightmares, hallucinations, fatigue, and diminished sleep quality (Henningsen and Mattiason 1979). Clonidine causes REM suppression with decreased time in deep sleep and more awakenings (i.e., decreased quality of sleep) (Spiegel and Devos 1980). Several antiarrhythmics including amiodarone, lorcainide, and quinidine have been reported to produce insomnia (Greene et al. 1983; Guillemenault and Silvestri 1982; Karacan et al. 1976).

Methylxanthines, found in theophylline, theobromine, and caffeine, are common causes of insomnia. Caffeine, available in beverages such as tea or coffee and frequently found in OTC preparations, produces difficulty initiating sleep and delays the onset of REM sleep to the latter part of the night (Karacan et. al. 1976). Psychostimulants such as methylphenidate that are sometimes used to treat depression in the elderly produce a significant reduction in slow-wave and REM sleep (Kay et al. 1976).

Finally, nonspecific causes of diminished sleep quality should be considered. These include prolonged confinement to bed, physical discomfort caused by medical illness (e.g., arthritis, Parkinson's disease, and orthopnea), and the alteration in sleep cycle characteristic of confusional states.

Sexual Disorders

Sexuality in older people is a subject of considerable misunderstanding. Older people do experience some age-associated alterations in sexual function, but these do not preclude an active and satisfying sex life. Sexual activity between marital partners continues well into later life. A recent national survey reported that more than half of married persons between ages 66 and 70 report having sex at least four times per month. More than one-quarter of married people over age 76 report an active sex life, with an average frequency of sex of more than twice per month (Marsiglio and Donnelly 1991). It is important to note that, unless physical disability intervenes, the sexual behavior of older people tends to remain consistent over time (George and Weiler 1981). These statistics highlight the importance of obtaining a sexual history in all older patients. Any change from their premorbid baseline may herald recent physical or psychosocial stressors.

Although growing older does not mandate an abandonment of sexuality, predictable age-related physiological changes do affect the elderly person's sexual functioning (Grenshaw 1985). The older male is likely to experience some decrease in libido and a slowing of sexual arousal that may delay ejaculation. The postmenopausal woman is likely to experience a number of physiological changes that may reduce the pleasure of sexual intercourse. These changes include decreased vaginal lubrication, atrophic changes in the mucosal lining of the vaginal wall, and decreased turgidity of the vaginal outlet. In addition, physical disability is likely to exert a powerful negative influence on the older person's sexual activity (Marsiglio and Donnelly 1991). As a consequence, elderly people are likely to be more vulnerable to the drug-induced disorders in sexual functioning outlined in Table 27–5.

Movement Disorders

The age-related changes in CNS vulnerability in elderly patients discussed above may predispose them to drug-induced movement disorders. (The problems of hyperkinetic movement disorders are discussed further in Chapter 22 and tardive dyskinesia is discussed in Chapter 30.) Neuroleptics are the most common cause of drug-induced movement disorders, but dopamine agonists also frequently produce dyskinesias, and a variety of other medical therapies have been associated with movement abnormalities (Table 27–6). Elderly patients are at an increased risk particularly for drug-induced parkinsonism from antiemetic and antipsychotic medications, related, perhaps, to the diminished number of nigral dopaminergic neurons associated with aging (Friedman 1992). This may be a significant cause of immobility, gait disturbance, falls, and mortality in elderly patients (Wilson and MacLennen 1989). (For excellent reviews, see L. G. Miller and Jankovic 1992 and Lang and Weiner 1992.)

Summary

Four percent to 10% of geriatric psychiatric admissions may be attributed to adverse drug reactions, and

Table 27–5. Effects of commonly prescribed drugs on sexual function

Drugs	Effects on sexual function		
	Libido	Arousal or erection	Orgasm or ejaculation
Psychotropic agents			
Amphetamines and cocaine	Enhanced with low doses; decreased with high doses	Decreased with chronic use	Increased with low doses; diminished with high doses
Monoamine oxidase–inhibiting antidepressants	—	—	Impaired
Tricyclic antidepressants	May be impaired	May be impaired	May be impaired; may cause spontaneous seminal emission
Bupropion	Increased	—	—
Trazodone	Increased	May cause priapism	—
Fluoxetine	Increased	—	—
Lithium carbonate	Impaired	Impaired	—
Neuroleptic agents	May be decreased	Impaired (rare priapism)	Retrograde ejaculation rarely
Sedative-hypnotics[a]	Reduced	Reduced	—
Benzodiazepines	—	Impaired with chronic usage	—
Buspirone	Increase	—	—
Narcotics	Impaired in high doses	Impaired in high doses	Impaired in high doses
Antihypertensive agents			
Reserpine, α-methyldopa	Decreased	Decreased (common)	May be impaired
Diuretics	—	May be impaired	—
Clonidine	—	—	May block emission in males
Propranolol	May be decreased	May be decreased	—
Anticholinergic agents	—	May be impaired	—
Sympathomimetics			
Phendimetrazine	Increased	—	—
Fenfluramine	Increased	—	—
Hormonal agents			
Androgens	Increased	Increased (men)	Increased (men)
Estrogens	Decreased (men); Variable (women)	May cause impotence in men	Delayed
Thyroxine	Increased	—	—
Adrenal steroids	Decreased in high doses	—	—
Miscellaneous			
Levodopa	May be increased	—	—
Cholestyramine	Increased	—	—
Disulfiram	—	Occasional impotence	Delayed

[a]Alcohol, barbiturates, etc.
Source. Adapted from Cummings 1985a. Used with permission.

Table 27–6. Drug-induced movement disorders

Movement disorders	Drugs
Accentuated physiological tremor	Epinephrine, isoproterenol, caffeine, theophylline, lithium, tricyclic antidepressants, thyroid hormone, hypoglycemic agents, sodium valproate, nicotinic acid, cyclosporine
Cerebellar ataxia and tremor	Phenytoin, barbiturate, lithium, 5-fluorouracil, cimetidine-triazolam interaction
Chorea-dyskinesia	Neuroleptics, levodopa, bromocriptine, phenytoin, ethosuximide, carbamazepine, oral contraceptives, chloroquine, antidepressants, metoclopramide, lithium, antidepressants, benzodiazepines, antihistamines, calcium channel blockers, cocaine, methyldopa, cimetidine
Dystonia	Neuroleptics, levodopa, bromocriptine, lithium, metoclopramide, carbamazepine, cimetidine, chlorzoxazone, calcium channel blockers
Myoclonus and tics	Neuroleptics, amphetamines, methylphenidate, fenfluramine, levodopa, bromocriptine, antidepressants, pemoline, cocaine
Parkinsonism	Neuroleptics, reserpine, tetrabenazine, methyldopa, α-methyltyrosine, lithium, diazoxide, physostigmine, metoclopramide, trazodone, meperidine, etretinate, cimetidine, cinnarizine, flunarizine
Akathisia	Neuroleptics, reserpine, tetrabenazine, metoclopramide, antidepressants, calcium channel blockers, buspirone, methysergide, cimetidine

the increased susceptibility of the elderly to the neuropsychiatric side effects of medical therapies should always be considered in treating older patients. Medical therapies may cause depression, mania, psychosis, sexual disorders, movement disorders, delirium, dementia, anxiety, and sleep and gait disturbances. To minimize the risk of these adverse effects, one must consider the following factors in prescribing medications to elderly patients:

1. Understand alterations in cognition, pharmacokinetics, and neurochemistry associated with "normal" aging.
2. Identify the presence of any neurodegenerative process and understand the possible ramifications of these diseases for drug effects and sensitivity.
3. Identify social determinants of medication (non-) compliance (e.g., living alone and financial circumstances).
4. Always consider the possible involvement of OTC medications.
5. Always consider the possibility that the patient has consumed medications other than those prescribed (e.g., drugs from more than one physician or taking a friend's or spouse's prescriptions).
6. Always consider drug toxicity when the patient exhibits an alteration in attention or cognition or any behavioral change.
7. Always consider the physical barriers to medication compliance (e.g., hearing and visual loss).
8. Always determine the lowest effective dose for the elderly patient.
9. Follow the elderly patient's mental status carefully. Subtle changes in attention may be the first manifestation of impending serious drug toxicity.
10. Avoid the prolonged use of sedative-hypnotics and anticholinergics in elderly patients.

References

Adler S: Methyldopa-induced decrease in mental activity. JAMA 230:1428–1429, 1981

Allison N, Shantz I: Delirium due to tiaprofenic acid. Can Med Assoc J 137:1022–1023, 1987

Ancoli-Israel S, Kripke DF, Mason W, et al: Sleep apnea and periodic movements in an aging sample. J Gerontol 40:419–425, 1985

Atkinson RM, Ganzini L, Bernstein MJ: Alcohol and substance-use disorders in the elderly, in Handbook of Mental Health and Aging. Edited by Birren JE, Sloane R, Cohen GD. San Diego, CA, Academic Press, 1992, pp 515–555

Bartels D, Glasser M, Wang A, et al: Association between depression and propranolol use in ambulatory patients. Clin Pharm 7:2:146–150, 1988

Baum C, Kennedy DL, Knapp DE, et al: Drug Utilization in the U.S.—1986: Eighth Annual. Springfield, VA, National Technical Information Service, Office of Epidemiology and Biostatistics, Center for Drug Evaluation and Research, 1987

Bergman HD: Prescribing drugs in a nursing home. Drug Intelligence and Clinical Pharmacy 9:365, 1975

Bergman U, Wilholm BE: Patient medication on admission to a medical clinic. Eur J Clin Pharmacol 20:185–191, 1981

Berry DTR, Webb WB: Sleep and cognitive functions in normal older adults. J Gerontol 40:331–335, 1985

Billings R, Stein M: Depression associated with ranitidine. Am J Psychiatry 143:915–916, 1986

Billings R, Tang SW, Rafkoff VM: Depression associated with cimetidine. Can J Psychiatry 26:260–261, 1981

Blazer DG, Fedrespiel CF, Ray WA, et al: The risk of anticholinergic toxicity in the elderly: a study of prescribing practices in two populations. J Gerontol 38:31–35, 1983

Boston Collaborative Drug Surveillance Program: Psychiatric side effects of nonpsychiatric drugs. Seminars in Psychiatry 3:4:406–420, 1971

Branconnier RJ, Cole JO, Ghazvinian S, et al: Clinical pharmacology of bupropion and imipramine in elderly depressives. J Clin Psychiatry 44 (5 [sec. 2]):130–133, 1983

Brocklehurst JC: Aging in the autonomic nervous system. Aging 4 (suppl):7, 1974

Brook RH, Appel FA, Avery C, et al: Effectiveness of inpatient follow-up care. N Engl J Med 285:1509–1514, 1971

Burns M, Moskowitz H, Jaffe J: A comparison of the affects of trazadone and amitriptyline on skills performance by geriatric subjects. J Clin Psychiatry 47:252–254, 1986

Caird FI, Andrews GR, Kennedy RD: Effect of posture on blood pressure in the elderly. Br Heart J 35:448, 1987

Callahan CM: Psychiatric syndromes in elderly patients due to medications. Annual Review of Gerontology and Geriatrics 12:41–75, 1992

Carskadon MA, Seidel WF, Greenblatt DJ, et al: Daytime carryover of triazolam and flurazepam, elderly insomniacs. Sleep 5:361–371, 1982

Celesia GG, Barr AN: Psychosis and other psychiatric manifestations of levodopa therapy. Arch Neurol 23:193–200, 1970

Chaiton A, Spitzer WO, Roberts RS, et al: Patterns of medical drug use: a community focus. Can Med Assoc J 114:33–37, 1976

Closser MH: Benzodiazepines and the elderly. J Subst Abuse Treat 8:35–41, 1991

Cole JO, Branconnier R, Salomon M, et al: Tricyclic use in the cognitively impaired elderly. J Clin Psychiatry 44:14–19, 1983

Crawshaw JA, Mullen PEW: A study of benhexol abuse. Br J Psychiatry 145:300–303, 1984

Cross AJ, Crow TJ, Johnson JA, et al: Studies on neurotransmitter receptor systems in neocortex and hippocampus in senile dementia of the Alzheimer type. J Neurol Sci 64:109–117, 1984

Cummings JL: Disturbances of sleep, appetite, and sexual behavior, in Clinical Neuropsychiatry. Edited by Cummings JL. New York, Grune & Stratton, 1985a, pp 234–250

Cummings JL: Clinical Neuropsychiatry. New York, Grune & Stratton, 1985b

Cummings JL: Organic psychoses: delusional disorders and secondary mania. Psychiatr Clin North Am 9:2:293–311, 1986

Cummings JL: Behavioral complications of drug treatment of Parkinson's disease. J Am Geriatr Soc 39:708–716, 1991

Cupit GC: The use of non-prescription analgesics in an older population. J Am Geriatr Soc 30 (suppl):76–80, 1982

Cusack BJ, Vestal RE: Clinical pharmacology: special consideration in the elderly, in Practice of Geriatric Medicine. Edited by Calkins E, Davis PJ, Ford AB. Philadelphia, PA, WB Saunders, 1986, pp 115–134

Danielson DA, Porter JB, Lawson DH, et al: Drug induced psychiatric disturbances in medical inpatients. Psychopharmacology 74:105–108, 1981

Davie JW, Blumenthal MD, Robinson-Hawkins S: A model of risk of falling for psychogeriatric patients. Arch Gen Psychiatry 38:463–467, 1981

De Smet Y, Ruberg M, Serdaru M, et al: Confusion, dementia and anticholinergics in Parkinson's disease. J Neurol Neurosurg Psychiatry 45:1161–1164, 1982

Eisendrath SJ, Sweeney MA: Toxic neuropsychiatric effects of digoxin at therapeutic serum concentrations. Am J Psychiatry 144:506–507, 1987

Eisendrath SJ, Goldman B, Douglas J, et al: Meperidine-induced delirium. Am J Psychiatry 144:1062–1065, 1987

Erkinjuntti T, Wikstrom J, Palo J: Dementia among medical inpatients. Arch Intern Med 146:1923–1926, 1986

Erwin WG: Geriatrics, in Pharmacotherapy: A Pathophysiologic Approach. Edited by Kepiro JT, Talbert RL, Hayes PE, et al. Norwalk, CT, Appleton & Lange, 1993, pp 64–70

Estroff TW, Gold MS: Medication-induced and toxin-induced psychiatric disorders, in Medical Mimics of Psychiatric Disorders. Edited by Extein I, Gold MS. Washington, DC, American Psychiatric Press, 1986, pp 163–198

Fazekas JF, Alivan RW, Bessman AN: Cerebral physiology of the aged. Am J Med Sci 223:245, 1952

Fennelly ME: Ranitidine-induced mental confusion. Crit Care Med 15:1165–1166, 1987

Fleminger R: Visual hallucinations and illusions with propanolol. BMJ 1:1182, 1978

Flynn DD, Mash DC: Characterization of L-H3 nicotine binding in human cerebral cortex: comparison between Alzheimer's disease and normals. J Neurochem 47:1948–1954, 1986

Foy A, Drinkwater V, March S: Confusion after admission to hospital in elderly patients using benzodiazepines. BMJ 293:1072, 1986

Fraser HS, Carr AC: Propanolol psychosis. Br J Psychiatry 129:508–509, 1976

Friedman JH: Drug-induced parkinsonism, in Drug-Induced Movement Disorders. Edited by Lang AE, Weiner WJ. Mount Kisco, NY, Futura Publishing, 1992, pp 41–84

Friedman JH, Lannon MC: Clozapine in the treatment of psychosis in Parkinson's disease. Neurology 39:1219–1221, 1989

Gambert SR: Substance abuse in the elderly, in Substance Abuse: A Comprehensive Textbook, 2nd Edition. Edited by Lawison JH, Ruit P, Millman RB, et al. Baltimore, MD, Williams & Wilkins, 1992, pp 213–234

George LK, Weiler SJ: Sexuality in middle and late life. Arch Gen Psychiatry 38:912–992, 1981

Gillin JC, Byerly WF: The diagnosis and management of insomnia. N Engl J Med 322:239–248, 1990

Gillin JC, Spinweber CL, Johnson LC: Rebound insomnia: a critical review. J Clin Psychopharmacol 9:161–172, 1989

Goodwin FK, Bunney WE: Depressions following reserpine: a reevaluation. Seminars in Psychiatry 3(4):435–448, 1971

Goodwin JS, Regan M: Cognitive dysfunction associated with naproxen and ibuprofen in the elderly. Arthritis Rheum 25:1013–1015, 1982

Greenblatt D, Allen M, Shader R: Toxicity of high dose flurazepam in the elderly. Clin Pharmacol Ther 21:355, 1976

Greene HL, Graham EL, Werner JA, et al: Toxic and therapeutic effects of amiodorone in the treatment of cardiac arrythmias. J Am Coll Cardiol 2:1114–1128, 1983

Grenshaw TL: Age-related changes in sexual function. Geriatric Consultant 3(5):26–29, 1985

Guillemenault C, Silvestri R: Aging, drugs and sleep. Neurobiol Aging 3:379–386, 1982

Hall RC, Stickney SK, Garner ER: Behavioral toxicity of neuropsychiatric drugs, in Psychiatric Presentations of Mental Illness. Edited by Hall CW. New York, Spectrum Publication, 1980, pp 337–349

Hare TA, Wood JH, Manyam BV, et al: Central nervous system gamma-aminobutyric acid activity in man: relationship to age and sex as reflected in CSF. Arch Neurol 39:247–249, 1982

Henningsen NC, Mattiason I: Long-term clinical experience with atenolol—a new selective beta-1-blocker with few side-effects from the central nervous system. Acta Medica Scandinavica 205:61–66, 1979

Hodkinson HM: Mental impairment in the elderly. J R Coll Physicians Lond 7:305–317, 1973

Hoffman WF, Ladogana L: Delirium secondary to clonidine therapy. N Y State J Med 81:382–383, 1981

Hogarty GI, Munetz MR: Pharmacogenic depression among outpatient schizophrenic patients: a failure to substantiate. J Clin Psychopharmacol 4:17–24, 1984

Hoppmann RA, Peden JG, Ober K: Central nervous system side effects of nonsteroidal anti-inflammatory drugs: aseptic meningitis, psychosis, and cognitive dysfunction. Arch Intern Med 151:1309–1313, 1991

Hubain P, Sobolski J, Mendlewicz J: Cimetidine-induced mania. Neuropsychobiology 8:223–224, 1982

Hussar DA: Patient noncompliance. Journal of the American Pharmaceutical Association 15:183–190, 201, 1975

Itil T, Fink M: Anticholinergic drug-induced delirium: experimental modification, quantitative EEG and behavioral correlations. J Nerv Ment Dis 143:492–507, 1966

Jackson JE, Ramsdell JW, Renvall M, et al: Reliability of drug histories in a specialized geriatric outpatient clinic. J Gen Intern Med 4:39–43, 1989

Jacobsen FM, Sack DA, James SP: Delirium induced by verapamil (letter). Am J Psychiatry 144:248, 1987

Jenike MA, Levy JC: Physostigmine reversal of cimetidine-induced delirium and agitation. J Clin Psychopharmacol 3:43–44, 1983

Jeste DV, Wyatt RJ: Aging and tardive dyskinesia, in Schizophrenia and Aging. Edited by Miller NE, Cohen GD. New York, Guilford, 1987, pp 275–286

Karacan I, Thornby JI, Anch AM, et al: Dose related sleep disturbance produced by coffee and caffeine. Clin Pharmacol Ther 20:682–689, 1976

Katz IR, Stoff D, Muhly C, et al: Identifying persistent adverse effects of anticholinergic medications in the elderly. J Geriatr Psychiatry Neurol 1:212–217, 1988

Katzman R, Lasker B, Bernstein N: Advances in the diagnosis of dementia accuracy of diagnosis and consequences of misdiagnosis of disorders causing dementia. Aging and the Brain 32:17–62, 1988

Kay DC, Blackburn AB, Buckingham JA: Human pharmacology of sleep, in Pharmacology of Sleep. Edited by Williams RL, Karacan I. New York, Wiley, 1976, pp 83–210

Kellogg International Work Group on the Prevention of Falls by the Elderly: The prevention of falls in later life. Dan Med Bull 34 (suppl 4):1–24, 1987

Kennedy JS: Adverse drug effects in the older adult, in Drug-Induced Dysfunction in Psychiatry. Edited by Kesharen MS, Kennedy JS. New York, Hemisphere, 1992, pp 93–101

Kuhr BM: Prolonged delirium with propanolol. J Clin Psychiatry 40:194–195, 1979

Lader M: Differential diagnosis of anxiety in the elderly. J Clin Psychiatry 43 (9 [sec 2]):4–7, 1982

Lamy PP, Salzman C, Nevis-Olesen J: Drug prescribing patterns, risks, and compliance guidelines, in Clinical Geriatric Psychopharmacology, 2nd Edition. Edited by Salzman S. Baltimore, MD, Williams & Wilkins, 1992, pp 15–37

Lang AE, Weiner WJ: Drug-Induced Movement Disorder. Mount Kisco, NY, Futura Publishing, 1992

Larson EB, Kukull WA, Buchner D, et al: Adverse drug reactions associated with global cognitive impairment in elderly persons. Ann Intern Med 107:169–173, 1987

Lawlor BA, Sunderland T, Mellow AM, et al: A preliminary study of the effects of intravenous m-chlorphenylpiperazine, a serotonin, in elderly subjects. Biol Psychiatry 25:679–686, 1989

Lawson AW: Substance abuse problems of the elderly: considerations for treatment and prevention, in Alcoholism and Substance Abuse in Special Populations. Edited by Lawson GW, Lawson AW. Rockville, MD, Aspen, 1989, pp 95–133

Levenson JJ: Neuropsychiatric Side Effects of Drugs in the Elderly. New York, Raven, 1979

Lewis DA, Smith RE: Steroid-induced psychiatric syndromes. J Affect Disord 5:319–332, 1983

Lieberman AN, Kupersmith M, Gopinathan G, et al: Bromocriptine in Parkinson's disease: further studies. Neurology 29:363–369, 1979

Lipowski ZJ: Acute confusional states in the elderly, in Clinical Neurology of Aging. Edited by Albert ML. New York, Oxford University Press, 1984, pp 277–297

Lipowski ZJ: Delirium: Acute Confusional States. New York, Oxford University Press, 1990

Liston EH: Delirium in the aged. Psychiatr Clin North Am 5:49–66, 1982

Livingston RL, Zucker DK, Isenberg K, et al: Tricyclic antidepressants and delirium. J Clin Psychiatry 44:173–176, 1983

Lundgren-Lindquist B, Aniansson A, Rundgren A: Functional studies in 79 year olds, III: walking performance and climbing capacity. Scand J Rehabil Med 15:125–131, 1983

MacDonald JB: The role of drugs in falls in the elderly. Clin Geriatr Med 1:3:621–636, 1983

MacDonald JB, MacDonald ET: Nocturnal femoral fracture and continuing widespread use of barbiturate hypnotics. BMJ 2:483–485, 1977

MacEwan GW, Remick RA, Noone JA: Psychosis due to transdermally administered scopolamine. Can Med Assoc J 133:431–432, 1985

Marsiglio W, Donnelly D: Sexual relations in later life: a national study of married persons. J Gerontology 46 (suppl 6):338–344, 1991

McGahan DJ, Wojslaw A, Prasad V, et al: Propanolol-induced psychosis. Drug Intelligence and Clinical Pharmacy 18:601–603, 1984

McLachlan RS: Pseudoatrophy of the brain with valproic acid monotherapy. Can J Neurol Sci 14:294–296, 1987

Mesulam M-M, Mufson EJ, Rogers J: Age-related shrinkage of cortically projecting cholinergic neurons: a selective effect. Ann Neurol 22:31–36, 1987

Miller LG, Jankovic J: Drug-induced movement disorders: an overview, in Movement Disorders in Neurology and Neuropsychiatry. Edited by Joseph AB, Young RR. Oxford, England, Blackwell, 1992, pp 5–32

Miller PS, Richardson S, Jyu CA, et al: Association of low serum anticholinergic levels and cognitive impairment in elderly presurgical patients. Am J Psychiatry 145:342–345, 1988

Morrison RL, Katz IR: Drug-related cognitive impairment: current progress and recurrent problems, in Annual Review Gerontology and Geriatrics, Vol 9. Edited by Lawton MP. New York, Springer, 1989, pp 232–279

Nelson L, O'Malley K: Prescribing for the elderly, II: prescribing patterns: differences due to age. J Am Geriatr Soc 36:245–254, 1988

Nemeroff CB: Chemical messengers of the brain, in Geriatric Psychiatry. Edited by Busse E, Blazer DG. Washington DC, American Psychiatric Press, 1989, pp 97–134

Newman G, Dovenmuehle RH, Busse EW: Alterations in neurological status with age. J Am Geriatr Soc 8:915–917, 1960

Ostrom JR, Hammarlund ER, Christensen DB, et al: Medication use in the elderly population. Med Care 23:157–164, 1985

Ouslander J: Drug therapy in the elderly. Ann Intern Med 95:711–722, 1981

Pascualy M, Veith RC: Depression as an adverse drug reaction, in Aging and Clinical Practice: Depression and Coexisting Disease. Edited by Robinson RG, Rabins PV. New York, Igaku-Shoin, 1989, pp 132–151

Patterson JF: Triazolam syndrome in the elderly. South Med J 80:1425–1426, 1987

Paykel ES, Flemingero RF, Watson JP: Psychiatric side effects of antihypertensives other than reserpine. J Clin Psychopharmacol 2:14–39, 1982

Pomara N, Stanley B, Block R, et al: Adverse effects of single therapeutic doses of diazepam on performance in normal geriatric subjects: relationship to plasma concentration. Psychopharmacology 84:342–346, 1984

Postma JU, Vantilburg W: Visual hallucinations and delirium during treatment with amantadine. J Am Geriatr Soc 23:212–215, 1975

Prudnam D, Evans JG: Factors associated with falls in the elderly: a community study. Age Aging 10:141–146, 1981

Ray WA, Griffin MR, Downey W: Benzodiazepines of long and short half-life and the risk of hip fracture. JAMA 262:3303–3307, 1989

Reynolds CF, Kupfer DJ, Hoch CC, et al: Sleeping pills in the elderly: are they ever justified? J Clin Psychiatry 46:9–12, 1985

Robinson DS, Sourkes TL, Nies A, et al: Monoamine metabolism in human brain. Arch Gen Psychiatry 34:89–92, 1977

Rosenthal SH, Fenton ML, Harnett DS: Clozapine for the treatment of levodopa-induced psychosis in Parkinson's disease. Gen Hosp Psychiatry 14:285–286, 1992

Russell WL, Lopez LM: Cimetidine-induced mental status changes: case report and literature review. Am J Hosp Pharm 37:1667–1671, 1980

Sagel J, Matisonn R: Neuropsychiatric disturbance as the initial manifestation of digitalis toxicity. S Afr Med J 46:512–521, 1975

Schentag J, Cerra F, Calleri G, et al: Pharmacokinetics and clinical studies in patients with cimetidine-associated confusion. Lancet 1:117–181, 1979

Schneider-Heimert D: Why low-dose-benzodiazepine dependent insomniacs can't escape their sleeping pills. Acta Psychiatr Scand 78:706–711, 1988

Shih JC, Young H: The alteration of serotonin binding sites in aging human brain. Life Sci 23:1441–1448, 1978

Shore JH, Fraunfelder FT, Meyer SM: Psychiatric side effects from topical ocular timolol, a beta-adrenergic blocker. J Clin Psychopharmacol 7:264–267, 1987

Smallegan M: How families decide on nursing home admission. Geriatric Consultant 1:21–24, 1983

Smith DB, Mattson RH, Cramer JA, et al: Results of a nationwide VA cooperative study comparing the efficacy and toxicity of carbamazepine, phenobarbitol phenytoin and primidone. Epilepsia 28 (suppl 3):S50–S58, 1987

Sokoloff L: Cerebral circulatory and metabolic changes associated with aging. Res Publ Assoc Nerv Ment Dis 41:237–254, 1966

Spiegel R, Devos JE: Central effects of guanfacine and clonidine during wakefulness and sleep in healthy subjects. British Journal of Clinical Psychopharmacology 10 (suppl):165–168, 1980

Sudarsky L: Geriatrics: gait disorders in the elderly. N Engl J Med 20:1441–1445, 1990

Sultzer DL, Cummings JL: Drug-induced mania: causative agents, clinical characteristics and management: a retrospective analysis of the literature. Medical Toxicology and Adverse Drug Experience 4:127–143, 1989

Sunderland T: Neurotransmission in the aging central nervous system, in Clinical Geriatric Psychopharmacology, 2nd Edition. Edited by Salzman S. Baltimore, MD, Williams & Wilkins, 1992, pp 41–60

Swift CG: Special problems relating to the use of hypnotics in the elderly. Acta Psychiatr Scand Suppl 73:92–98, 1986

Swinyard EA: Principles of prescription order writing and patient compliance instruction, in Goodman and Gilman's Pharmacological Basis of Therapeutics. Edited by Gilman AG, Goodman LS, Rall TW, et al. New York, Macmillan, 1987, pp 1651–1662

Thornton TL: Delirium associated with suindac. JAMA 243:1630–1631, 1980

Tinetti ME: Factors associated with serious injury during falls in an elderly population, I: incidence and morbidity. Age Aging 6:210–210, 1977

Vestal RE, Cusack BJ: Pharmacology and Aging, in Handbook of the Biology of Aging. Edited by Schneider EL, Roew JW. San Diego, CA, Academic Press, 1990, pp 349–383

Vestal RE, Dawson GW: Pharmacology and aging, in Handbook of the Biology of Aging, 2nd Edition. Edited by Finch CE, Sneider EL. New York, Van Nostrand Reinhold, 1985, pp 744–819

Wild D, Nayak US, Isaacs B: How dangerous are falls in old people at home? BMJ 282:2166–268, 1981

Williams L, Caranasos GJ: Neuropsychiatric effects of drugs in the elderly. J Fla Med Assoc 79:6:371–375, 1992

Wilson JA, MacLennen WJ: Review: drug-induced parkinsonism in elderly patients. Age Aging 18:208–210, 1989

Wood KA, Harris MJ, Morreale A, et al: Drug-induced psychosis and depression in the elderly. Psychiatr Clin North Am 11:167–189, 1988

Wood P, Castleden CM: Psychopharmacology in the elderly, in Psychiatry in the Elderly. Edited by Jacob R, Oppenheimer C. Oxford, England, Oxford University Press, 1991, pp 339–372, 1991

Appendix 27–1 Drug- and toxin-induced neuropsychiatric disorders

	Depression	Mania	Anxiety or agitation	Delirium	Psychosis	Visual hallucinations	Dementia-like syndrome
Antihypertensive drugs							
Clonidine	✔	✔	✔	✔			✔
Oxyprenolol	✔						
Propranolol	✔	✔		✔	✔	✔	
Reserpine	✔						
Methyldopa	✔			✔	✔		
Guanethidine	✔						
Hydralazine	✔			✔			
Bethanidine	✔						
Captopril		✔	✔				
Nifedipine	✔						
Prazosin	✔						
Cardiac glycosides	✔	✔		✔	✔	✔	✔
Antiarrhythmics							
Procainamide	✔	✔		✔	✔		
Lidocaine	✔			✔	✔		
Quinidine				✔			
Disopyramide				✔	✔		
Antiparkinsonian drugs							
Amantadine	✔		✔	✔	✔	✔	
Bromocriptine	✔	✔	✔	✔	✔	✔	
Levodopa	✔	✔	✔	✔	✔	✔	✔
Pergolide					✔		
Lisuride		✔			✔		
Piribedil		✔					
Trihexyphenidyl				✔		✔	
Procyclidine				✔		✔	
Biperidine				✔		✔	
Analgesics							
NSAIDs	✔			✔	✔		
Salicylates			✔	✔	✔		
Narcotics	✔		✔	✔		✔	
Ibuprofen					✔		
Phenacetin	✔				✔		
Naproxen					✔		
Indomethacin	✔	✔			✔	✔	

	Depression	Mania	Anxiety or agitation	Delirium	Psychosis	Visual hallucinations	Dementia-like syndrome
Anticonvulsants							
Carbamazepine	✔	✔		✔	✔		
Valproate				✔			✔
Phenytoin	✔			✔	✔	✔	✔
Barbiturates	✔		✔	✔			✔
Ethosuximide	✔		✔		✔	✔	
Clonazepam					✔		✔
Phenacemide					✔		
Sedative-hypnotics							
Benzodiazepines	✔	✔	✔	✔	✔		✔
Chloral Hydrate	✔			✔			✔
Ethanol	✔			✔			✔
Clomethiazole	✔			✔			✔
Chlorazepate	✔			✔			✔
Meprobamate				✔	✔		✔
Anticholinergics/ antispasmodics							
Atropine				✔	✔	✔	✔
Benztropine				✔	✔	✔	✔
Propantheline				✔	✔	✔	✔
Scopolamine				✔	✔	✔	✔
Dicyclomine				✔	✔	✔	✔
Hyoscyamine				✔	✔	✔	✔
Lithium		✔		✔			✔
Antidepressants							
TCAs		✔	✔	✔	✔	✔	✔
MAOIs		✔			✔		
Bupropion			✔				
Trazodone		✔			✔		
Fluoxetine		✔	✔	✔			
Sertraline		✔					
Maprotiline						✔	
Neuroleptics							
Butyrophenones	✔			✔			✔
Phenothiazines	✔			✔	✔		✔
Clozapine				✔			
Thiothixene				✔			

Appendix 27–1   Drug- and toxin-induced neuropsychiatric disorders *(continued)*

	Depression	Mania	Anxiety or agitation	Delirium	Psychosis	Visual hallucinations	Dementia-like syndrome
Neuroleptics *(continued)*							
Molindone				✔			
Antidiarrheals							
Diphenoxylate/ atropine				✔			
Loperamide				✔			
Antimicrobial agents							
Podophyllin					✔		
Penicillins	✔		✔			✔	
Sulfamethoxazole	✔			✔			
Clotrimazole	✔						
Cycloserine	✔		✔	✔	✔		
Dapsone	✔	✔	✔				
Ethionamide	✔						
Tetracycline	✔					✔	
Griseofulvin	✔						
Metronidazole	✔						
Streptomycin	✔						
Nitrofurantoin	✔						
Nalidixic acid	✔						
Antimalarials					✔	✔	
Sulfonamides	✔		✔			✔	
Procaine penicillin	✔		✔	✔	✔		
Thiocarbanilide	✔						
Acyclovir	✔			✔			
Isoniazid	✔	✔	✔		✔	✔	
Mefloquine				✔			
Iproniazid		✔			✔	✔	
Cephalosporins				✔	✔		
Ciprofloxacin				✔			
Amphotericin B				✔			
Antihistamines (H$_1$ blocking agents)							
Diphenhydramine				✔			
Chlorpheniramine				✔			
H$_2$ blockers							
Cimetidine	✔	✔		✔	✔	✔	

	Depression	Mania	Anxiety or agitation	Delirium	Psychosis	Visual hallucinations	Dementia-like syndrome
H₂ blockers *(continued)*							
Ranitidine	✔			✔			
Drugs for urinary incontinence							
Oxybutynin				✔			
Flavoxate				✔			
Hyoscyamine				✔			
Withdrawal syndromes							
Barbiturates			✔	✔		✔	
Alcohol	✔		✔	✔	✔	✔	
Benzodiazepines			✔	✔	✔	✔	
Amphetamines	✔	✔	✔	✔	✔		
Chloral hydrate			✔	✔		✔	
Corticosteroids	✔		✔	✔			
Propranolol		✔	✔				
Reserpine		✔	✔				
MAOIs		✔	✔				
TCAs		✔	✔				
Caffeine			✔				
Meprobamate			✔			✔	
Opiates			✔		✔	✔	
Hallucinogens							
Phencyclidine		✔			✔	✔	
Indole hallucinogens	✔	✔			✔	✔	
Cannabinols			✔		✔	✔	
Ketamine						✔	
Nitrous oxide						✔	
Antineoplastic drugs							
Azathioprine	✔						✔
C-Asparaginase	✔			✔	✔		
Plicamycin (mithramycin)	✔						
Vincristine	✔						
6-Azauridine	✔						
Bleomycin	✔						
Trimethoprim	✔						
Interferon	✔		✔	✔			

Appendix 27–1 Drug- and toxin-induced neuropsychiatric disorders *(continued)*

	Depression	Mania	Anxiety or agitation	Delirium	Psychosis	Visual hallucinations	Dementia-like syndrome
Endocrine agents							
Corticosteroids	✔	✔		✔	✔	✔	
ACTH		✔					
Oral contraceptives	✔						
Thyroid hormones		✔	✔		✔	✔	
Triamcinolone	✔						
Norethisterone	✔						
Danazol	✔						
Clomiphene citrate					✔		
Central nervous system stimulants							
Cocaine		✔	✔				
Sympathomimetics		✔	✔		✔	✔	
Amphetamine	✔	✔	✔		✔		
Fenfluramine	✔		✔				
Diethylpropion	✔		✔		✔		
Phenmetrazine	✔		✔				
Caffeine			✔	✔			
Methylphenidate		✔	✔		✔		
Pseudoephedrine		✔	✔		✔		
Pemoline		✔	✔				
Isoetharine		✔	✔				
Phenypropanolamine		✔	✔		✔		
Ephedrine		✔	✔		✔		
Phenylephrine		✔	✔		✔		
Epinephrine			✔				
Isoproterenol			✔				
Miscellaneous drugs							
Acetazolamide	✔						
Albuterol					✔		
Anticholinesterase	✔		✔	✔			
Aprindine					✔		
Arsenic			✔		✔	✔	✔
Aspartame		✔					
Baclofen	✔	✔			✔		

	Depression	Mania	Anxiety or agitation	Delirium	Psychosis	Visual hallucinations	Dementia-like syndrome
Miscellaneous drugs *(continued)*							
Benzene			✔				
Bromide		✔			✔	✔	✔
Calcium		✔					
Carbon disulfide			✔		✔		✔
Carbon monoxide					✔		✔
Choline	✔						
Cocaine		✔	✔		✔		
Cyclobenzaprine		✔		✔			
Cyclosporin A		✔					
Cyproheptadine	✔	✔					
Diethyl-m-toluamide		✔					
Diltiazem	✔	✔					
Diphenoxylate	✔						
Disulfiram	✔	✔		✔	✔	✔	✔
Flutamide		✔					
Halothane	✔						
Heavy metals			✔		✔	✔	✔
Isosafrole					✔		
L-Glutamine		✔					
Manganese					✔		✔
Mebeverine	✔						
Meclizine	✔						
Mepacrine		✔					
Mercury			✔		✔		✔
Methoserpidine	✔						
Methysergide	✔						
Metoclopramide	✔	✔		✔			
Metrizamide		✔			✔	✔	
Organophosophates			✔				✔
Oxandrolone		✔					
Oxymetholone		✔					
Pentazocine					✔		
Phenindione	✔						
Phosphorous			✔				

Appendix 27–1   Drug- and toxin-induced neuropsychiatric disorders *(continued)*

	Depression	Mania	Anxiety or agitation	Delirium	Psychosis	Visual hallucinations	Dementia-like syndrome
Miscellaneous drugs *(continued)*							
Pizotifen	✔						
Procaine	✔			✔			
Procarbazine		✔					
Procyclidine		✔					
Propafenone		✔					
Salbutamol	✔						
Tetrabenazine	✔						
Thallium					✔		✔
Theophylline		✔	✔				
Tryptophan		✔					
Veratrum	✔						
Yohimbine		✔	✔				
Zidovudine (AZT)		✔					

Note. NSAIDs = nonsteroidal anti-inflammatory drugs; TCAs = tricyclic antidepressants; MAOIs = monoamine oxidase inhibitors; H_1 = histamine, subtype 1, receptor; H_2 = histamine, subtype 2, receptor; ACTH = adrenocorticotropic hormone.
Source. From Callahan (1992); Cummings (1985b, 1986); Estroff and Gold (1986); Hall et al. (1980); Levinson (1979); Morrison and Katz (1989); Pascualy and Veith (1989); Sultzer and Cummings (1989); Williams and Caranasos (1992); K. A. Wood et al. (1988).

Principles of Neuropsychiatric Treatment of the Elderly

Section Editor
C. Edward Coffey, M.D.

chapter 28

Pharmacological and Neuroendocrine Probes in
Neuropsychiatric Illness

chapter 29

Geriatric Neuropsychopharmacology

chapter 30

Electroconvulsive Therapy in Geriatric Neuropsychiatry

chapter 31

Psychosocial Therapies

chapter 32

Neuropsychiatry in Nursing Homes

28

Pharmacological and Neuroendocrine Probes in Neuropsychiatric Illness

Marc Cantillon, M.D.
Susan E. Molchan, M.D.
John Little, M.D.
Trey Sunderland, M.D.

Introduction

Because alterations in brain neurotransmitter and neurohormone function are thought to be involved in the etiology and physiology of neuropsychiatric illness, it has long been assumed that pharmacological studies of neuroendocrine abnormalities will give clues about neurochemical alterations in the brain. As a result, a veritable cottage industry of pharmacological and neuroendocrine challenge tests have been developed over the past decade in which drugs and hormones are used as probes of human physiology and behavior. The implicit promise in these challenge approaches is that individual patient subgroups may have specific and characteristic responses that allow for better diagnostic or prognostic accuracy during subsequent clinical treatment. Furthermore, some pharmacological and neuroendocrine probes have been tested as challenge or modeling agents for individual illnesses to further the understanding of their pathophysiology. Unfortunately, clinicians have thus far derived little direct benefit, because the challenges have still not established absolute specificity and validity, even in controlled research samples. There is also a paucity of studies in elderly neuropsychiatric patients, as well as a lack of clear understanding of how the aging process itself modifies responses to various challenges. Nonetheless, the hope that the challenge test model will provide direct clinical benefits still runs high within research circles. For the purposes of this chapter, therefore, we review the plethora of currently available challenge paradigms in neuropsychiatry with a special emphasis on those most pertinent to the elderly populations.

For orientation purposes, we have included several tables in this chapter. Table 28–1 is a summary of challenge approaches with clinical symptoms as the focal point. Although this table does not cover all the pharmacological challenges available, it does offer an overview of the field from a clinical perspective. The latter tables are targeted toward specific neurotransmitter systems and are more complete archives of challenges or probes within that selected area. Each table is divided into adult studies and aging studies to focus attention on the general imbalance of our knowledge in the aging field. Many more pharmacological and neuroendocrine challenges need to be completed; these tables set an outline of which areas have been explored and which still need to be tested.

Table 28–1.   Summary of target behaviors and currently available pharmacological challenge agents

Precipitating symptoms as dependent variables	Challenge agents	Representative studies
Attention/anxiety	Lactate (not altered by naloxone)	Pitts and Allen 1979; Uhde et al. 1985
	Caffeine	Charney et al. 1985
	Yohimbine	Davis et al. 1979; Coupland et al. 1992
	CO_2	Elam et al. 1981
	Inverse agonists (i.e., β CCE or FG71)	Paul et al. 1986
	Naloxone (increases symptoms in obsessive-compulsive disorder but not panic attacks)	Liebowitz et al. 1984
	Benzodiazepine antagonist (RO 15–1788)	Duka 1988; Duka et al. 1992
	Cholecystokinin (CCK4), idazoxan	Jackson et al. 1992; Bourin and Bradwejn 1991
Amnesia	Scopolamine	Sunderland et al. 1992
	Benzodiazepines	Duka et al. 1992; Block et al. 1985
	Tricyclic antidepressants	Curran et al. 1988
Memory/cognition	Glucose	Manning et al. 1990
	Nicotine	Newhouse et al. 1988a, 1992
	Arecoline	Raffaele et al. 1991
	Physostigmine, Lecithin	Peters and Levin 1979
	Benzodiazepine antagonist (ZK 93426)	Duka et al. 1992
Depression	Naloxone	Gerner et al. 1980; Tariot et al. 1988
	Physostigmine	Molchan et al. 1991c
	Oxotremorine	Davis et al. 1987
Psychosis	Phencyclidine (PCP)	Allen and Young 1978; Snyder et al. 1981
	Amphetamine	Antelman and Chiodo 1981

Pharmacological Probes of the Central Nervous System

Cholinergic System

One of the best-studied neurotransmitter systems in the elderly population is the acetylcholine system. Because of the links of cholinergic transmission with sleep, mood, and memory, there have been multiple pharmacological challenges established in this area in both young and older subjects (Table 28–2). For example, there are precursor loading tests with lecithin, postsynaptic agonist challenges with arecoline and nicotine, cholinesterase inhibition with physostigmine, and anticholinergic blockade with scopolamine, just to name a few (Corkin 1981; Sunderland et al. 1987; Warburton 1992).

Table 28–2 illustrates the increasing diversity of pharmacological probes for the cholinergic system. However, these approaches are lagging behind our knowledge of the receptor subtyping, because the development of specific pharmacological probes is still in its infancy (Bonner 1989). In all neurotransmission systems, our agonist and antagonist probes have limited selectivity (e.g., between various nicotinic and muscarinic subtypes). Each functional subtype study could be unique because of each subtype's separate effector pathways or ion channels.

Before accepting the conclusions of these cholinergic studies, however, three basic concepts regarding pharmacological challenges should be reviewed. Although these points are focused on the cholinergic model, they are applicable to each of the subsequent systems we review as well.

1. *Drug specificity:* In addition to the traditional distinction between muscarinic and nicotinic receptors within the cholinergic system, we now have the molecular biological techniques to characterize muscarinic receptor subtypes. However, our pharmacological challenges, as mentioned above, are still relatively nonspecific, and we must approach each challenge with the thought of utilizing a mixed agonist and/or antagonist across a host of receptor subtypes.

2. *Choice of dependent variables:* Neuroendocrine and

Table 28–2. Selected cholinergic challenge studies in adult and aging populations

Challenge agent	Adult studies	References	Aging studies	References
Scopolamine	Impaired serial learning	Russell et al. 1986; Beatty et al. 1986	Increased behavioral and cognitive sensitivity in Alzheimer's disease (AD)	Sunderland et al. 1988; Wesnes and Revell 1984
	Increased sensitivity in affective disorder	Caine 1981; Janowsky and Risch 1987	Increased cognitive sensitivity Major depressive disorder less cognitively affected than AD	Molchan et al. 1992; Curran et al. 1988; Newhouse et al. 1988b
Arecoline	? Improved serial learning	Hollander et al. 1986	No improvement in AD	Bruno et al. 1986; Tariot et al. 1988
Choline	Improved serial learning	Sitaram et al. 1984	No significant benefit in AD	Corkin 1981
Lecithin	No cognitive improvement	Bartus et al. 1982	No significant benefit in AD	Thal et al. 1990
Physostigmine	Increased depression and cognition, blood pressure, growth hormone, prolactin, cortisol, and β-endorphin	Risch et al. 1983; Davis et al. 1987	? Memory enhancement in AD	Davis et al. 1979; Stern et al. 1987; Raskind et al. 1989b
Nicotine	Increased cognition	Warburton 1992	? Memory enhancement in AD	Newhouse et al. 1990
	Blockade caused decreased cognition, even in nonsmokers	Newhouse et al. 1992	Increased ability to withhold inappropriate responses	Warburton 1992
Mecamylamine	Increased learning of passive avoidance	Elrod and Buccafusco 1991	rCBF changes as in AD	Gitelman and Prohovnik 1992

Note: rCBF = regional cerebral blood flow.

even behavioral measures can easily be con-founded by noncholinergic effects. For example, unwanted side effects usually occur long before any beneficial effect of a procholinergic drug is re-alized (Davis et al. 1987). In addition, the behav-ioral and physical side effects cannot always be predicted by the in vitro binding of a cholinergic compound. As a result, the dependent variables for any cholinergic study must be carefully planned and studied in pilot form before being used in drug trials.

3. *Underlying age and medical condition of the subject:* Al-though this point may seem obvious, it is clear in any study of cholinergic function in humans that age, medical condition, and severity of illness may greatly influence the outcome, especially in a geri-atric population. Scrupulous attention to detail to this point may subsequently lead to less variance in the data analysis later.

The abundance of cholinergic challenge tests in elderly subjects (Table 28–2) is impressive. Because Alzheimer's dementia has long been considered a nat-urally occurring cholinergic deficit state (Bartus et al. 1982; Gottfries 1985; Whitehouse and Kellar 1987), subjects with Alzheimer's disease were obvious choices for cholinergic challenge studies. Comparisons of stud-ies across the age spectrum suggest a strong effect of age, especially with the antagonist compounds (Mol-chan et al. 1992).

For example, increased sensitivity was found fol-lowing scopolamine challenge in patients with Alzheimer's disease compared with control subjects, as measured by behavioral and cognitive, but not physio-logical, parameters, suggesting a possible centrally me-diated "functional hypersensitivity" in Alzheimer subjects (Sunderland et al. 1987). Similar increases in sensitivity have also been noted in other elderly neuro-psychiatric populations including patients with Parkinson's disease or Korsakoff's syndrome (Sunder-land et al. 1990), but not elderly depression patients (Newhouse et al. 1988b). Of the muscarinic receptors, subtype 1 (M_1) and subtype 2 (M_2) have been most studied. There is as yet no clear agreement on subtype alteration in Alzheimer's disease, partly because of the lack of selective ligands. Some studies have found that M_2 receptor binding is substantially decreased, and M_1 binding appears to be unchanged in Alzheimer's dis-ease (Mash et al. 1985). To date at least five distinct muscarinic receptor genes (m1 through m5) have

been cloned and sequenced (Bonner 1989), but only the M_1 and M_2 receptor subtypes have been associated with their respective genes.

The cognitive effects of nicotinic blockade with mecamylamine are less well studied in the elderly pop-ulation, but then there is the intriguing finding of Gitelman and colleagues (see Gitelman and Prohovnik 1992) that mecamylamine and scopolamine together in control subjects mimic the cerebral blood flow pat-tern of dementia. Further study in this area is certainly warranted. Nicotine subtyped ligands are also needed. From another perspective, subjects with Alzheimer's disease seem less responsive than do control subjects to challenges with the cholinesterase inhibitor physostig-mine, as measured by increases in plasma arginine vasopressin, β-endorphin, and epinephrine levels (Janowsky and Risch 1987; Raskind et al. 1989b). These data would suggest that Alzheimer's disease results in decreased responsiveness of neuroendocrine systems regulated by central cholinergic systems.

In conclusion, further study is needed with other cholinergic agents, particularly once more receptor-subtype–selective agonist and antagonists become available. Cholinergic system deficits in Alzheimer's disease remain the most substantiated neurotransmit-ter change, so it appears that challenges in this area will continue to be important in the future, both for possi-ble prognostic and diagnostic purposes.

Adrenergic System

Peripheral measures of catecholamine function in-crease with age, both at rest and under the physiologi-cal stress of standing (Halbreich et al. 1987; Ziegler et al. 1976). Centrally, abnormalities of the adrenergic system have been noted in aging, major depression, and Alzheimer's disease (Davis et al. 1979; Raskind et al. 1989a). At autopsy, decreases in numbers of neu-rons in the locus coeruleus and other adrenergic changes have been seen in both elderly control sub-jects and patients with Alzheimer's disease (Mann et al. 1982; McGeer 1981; Vijayashankar and Brody 1979). In some cases, the adrenergic deficits of pa-tients with Alzheimer's disease have been correlated with behavioral changes before death (Zubenko 1992).

Although multiple pharmacological probes of the noradrenergic system have been developed and used in the younger adult population, there has been rela-tively little study thus far in the field of aging (Table

28–3). What is known is that older men show an increased cerebrospinal fluid (CSF) norepinephrine response to challenge with clonidine but that there is no obvious cognitive benefit to older control subjects with clonidine (Raskind et al. 1988).

Adrenergic challenge agents have most often been used in the study of anxiety and depression, and it is now generally accepted that the midbrain locus coeruleus, containing almost half the brain's norepinephrine neurons, is a fundamental mediator of the "fight or flight" response (Aston-Jones and Bloom 1981; Simson and Weiss 1988). Consequently, researchers have used peripheral measures of adrenergic function to determine the degree of adrenergic dysregulation in anxious patients. However, data from studies of anxious young adults do not always correspond to studies in elderly subjects. Villacres et al. (1987) found normal norepinephrine but increased epinephrine levels at rest in young adults with panic disorder. This finding contrasts with the discovery of increased plasma norepinephrine but normal plasma levels of epinephrine in older male control subjects, using an

oral clonidine challenge 5 µg/kg body weight (Raskind et al. 1988). Halbreich et al. (1987) also reported that the norepinephrine metabolite, 3-methoxy-4-hydroxyphenylglycol (MHPG), increases with age.

In aging studies, α-adrenergic responsiveness has been shown to be either decreased or normal (Scarpace 1986; Supiano et al. 1987). Although Brown et al. (1988) showed decreased numbers of α_3-adrenergic sites on peripheral lymphocytes in younger adult panic disorder patients, several studies in elderly subjects revealed a normal number of α_3-adrenergic sites but a decreased affinity or responsiveness of these sites to normal stimulation (Feldman et al. 1984; Heinsimer and Kefowitz 1985; Vestal et al. 1979). In a study of young versus older controls, Raskind et al. (1988) reported that clonidine caused decreased CSF norepinephrine levels in younger but not older subjects, suggesting a possible decreased responsivity with age.

Because the adrenergic projection to the forebrain has been implicated in motor, emotional, and cognitive functions, it is possible that locus coeruleus loss of neurons (McGeer and McGeer 1976) may underlie

Table 28–3. Selected adrenergic challenge studies in adult and aging populations

Challenge tests	Adult studies	References	Aging studies	References
Clonidine	Decreased growth hormone response in panic disorder and major depressive disorder	Amsterdam et al. 1989; Uhde et al. 1992; Glue et al. 1991	Increased cerebrospinal fluid norepinephrine (NE) in older men	Raskind et al. 1988
	Increased drop in blood pressure (BP) and MHPG	Charney et al. 1984	Decreased NE response in Alzheimer's disease and aging	Kalaria and Andorn 1991
Yohimbine	Increased BP, MHPG, and cortisol in panic attacks	Charney et al. 1990	—	—
	No change in growth hormone in panic attacks	Gurguis and Uhde 1990	—	—
Amphetamine	Increased growth hormone in major depressive disorder; no change in cognition in control subjects	Mewaldt and Ghoneim 1979; Rapoport et al. 1980	Minimal reversal of scopolamine-induced impairment	Martinez et al. 1990
Desipramine	Decreased growth hormone response in major depressive disorder	Rudorfer et al. 1991	—	—
Idazoxan	Increased BP, arousal, and NE	Glue et al. 1991		
Orthostatic tests	NE increased in major depressive disorder	Rudorfer et al. 1985	Increased NE in Alzheimer's disease	Vitiello 1993
	NE greatly increased in major depressive disorder with desipramine	Coupland et al. 1992	Decreased responsiveness (α-adrenergic receptors)	Scarpace 1986; Supiano et al. 1987

Note. MHPG = 3-methoxy-4-hydroxyphenylglycol.

some of the observed deficits in locomotion, anxiety threshold, and cognition in elderly patients. Recent findings of increased behavioral problems in patients with Alzheimer's disease and marked loss of locus coeruleus neurons suggest this hypothesis, but further study with specific adrenergic challenges in elderly subjects are needed (Chan-Palay and Asan 1989; Zweig et al. 1988).

Serotonergic System

Brain levels of the neurotransmitter serotonin (5-hydroxytryptamine [5-HT]) and its synthetic enzyme, tryptophan hydroxylase, have been documented to decline with age in animal studies (Meek et al. 1977). In older human subjects, CSF levels of the 5-HT metabolite 5-hydroxyindoleacetic acid (5-HIAA) have been reported to be increased compared with those in younger subjects (Gottfries et al. 1971), which is thought to reflect increased turnover secondary to 5-HT receptor loss that has been reported to occur with aging (Middlemiss et al. 1986; Sparks et al. 1988). The functional significance of changes in the serotonergic system that occur with aging is unknown, but it may be related to symptoms such as insomnia, decreased appetite, and poor memory, which not uncommonly appear with aging. Further, the increased rate of suicide in elderly people may be related to serotonergic system alterations (Rifai et al. 1992).

The 5-HT agonist m-chlorophenylpiperazine (m-CPP) has been used as a pharmacological probe of the serotonergic system in studies in elderly subjects (Lawlor et al. 1989b). Healthy elderly subjects showed decreased behavioral, but not neuroendocrine, responses (plasma levels of cortisol and prolactin) to intravenous m-CPP when compared with young subjects (Table 28–4).

This m-CPP study used the National Institute of Mental Health Self-Rating Scale (Murphy et al. 1982). The measures in which decreases were documented included "anxiety," "depression," and "altered self-reality." These decreased behavioral responses were taken to indicate a functionally less responsive 5-HT subsystem in the older subjects, which, it was hypothesized, may be related to the low incidence of new-onset anxiety disorders reported in elderly patients (Lawlor et al. 1989a). Further, as m-CPP is thought to be a relatively more selective 5-HT, subtype 1 (5-HT$_1$), receptor agonist, the decrease in responsivity may be related to the documented loss of 5-HT$_1$ brain receptors that occurs with age (Middlemiss et al. 1986).

The lack of a difference in neuroendocrine response between the two age groups may be contrasted with results from earlier studies using the indirect 5-HT agonist fenfluramine and the 5-HT precursor L-tryptophan. These studies showed a decreased prolactin response to these agents in older subjects (DeMeo et al. 1988; Heninger et al. 1984). The apparent discrepancy

Table 28–4.   Selected serotonergic challenges in adult and aging populations

Challenge agent	Adult studies	References	Aging studies	References
Tryptophan (iv)	Normal prolactin (PRL) response in Parkinson's disease; and increased prolactin in obsessive-compulsive disorder	Charney et al. 1985; Murphy et al. 1989	Decreased PRL response in older women	Heninger et al. 1984; DeMeo et al. 1988
m-CPP (po)	Increased behavioral and cortisol response in control subjects	Kahn et al. 1988	Increased behavioral and cognitive sensitivity	Lawlor et al. 1989b; Mueller et al. 1986
	Partial attenuation with metergoline	Pigott et al. 1992	Decreased behavioral but not neuroendocrine sensitivity with age	Lawlor et al. 1989a
Fenfluramine (po)	? Decreased PRL in major depressive disorder	Mitchell and Smythe 1990	Decreased PRL response with age	McBride et al. 1990
Ondansetron	No change in cognition in control subjects	Hall and Ceuppens 1991; Broocks et al. 1992	No improvement in Scopolamine-induced impairment	Little et al. 1993
	Partial anxiolysis after m-chlorophenylpiperazine (m-CPP)			

between these findings and those of Lawlor et al. (1989a) has been hypothesized to be due to the fact that fenfluramine and L-tryptophan are thought to act presynaptically and indirectly by increasing 5-HT production or release, and m-CPP is thought to act on prolactin release by directly affecting postsynaptic 5-HT receptors (Lawlor et al. 1989a). It is possible that presynaptic and not postsynaptic mechanisms mediate this neuroendocrine response decline with age (Lawlor et al. 1989a).

Patients with Alzheimer's disease were shown by Lawlor et al. (1998b) (Table 28–4) to have increased behavioral responsivity and cognitive sensitivity to m-CPP compared with that of elderly control subjects. Patients with Alzheimer's disease became anxious, restless, and experienced psychomotor activation and perceptual abnormalities after intravenous infusion of the drug. Cognitive effects of m-CPP were minimal, though the patients had a greater performance decrement on some measures of recent and knowledge memory as compared with controls. Neuroendocrine responses did not differ between the two groups (Lawlor et al. 1989b).

These findings were postulated to be related to damaged brain 5-HT neurons or other neuronal systems that interact with 5-HT neurons in Alzheimer's disease. Such damage to 5-HT systems has been documented in postmortem studies (Cross 1990). 5-HT, subtype 2 (5-HT$_2$), receptors especially have been shown to be decreased in Alzheimer's disease brain in some (Cross 1990), though not all, studies (Dewar et al. 1990); they have been shown to have an inhibitory effect on 5-HT$_1$ receptors. The increased behavioral sensitivity to m-CPP in Alzheimer's disease has been hypothesized to be secondary to decreased inhibition from 5-HT$_2$ receptors, or possibly from decreased inhibition from damaged cholinergic neurons on 5-HT systems (Lawlor et al. 1989a). This hyperresponsiveness has been postulated to reflect a contribution of 5-HT systems to some of the behavioral disturbances (e.g., anxiety, depression, agitation, and sleeplessness) that occur in Alzheimer's disease. The increased memory impairment produced in the patients with Alzheimer's disease after m-CPP is consistent with animal data showing that 5-HT agonists impair and antagonists enhance memory function, possibly through interactions with the cholinergic system (Lawlor et al. 1989b).

Although the results from these studies appear complicated and at times contradictory, they do suggest a complex interrelationship between the serotonergic system and other neurotransmitter systems. Furthermore, it is clear that the serotonergic system changes considerably with aging and in neuropsychiatric illnesses. As a consequence, further pharmacological and neuroendocrine probing of this system in the elderly population will be of great importance in coming years.

GABA-ergic System

The inhibitory neurotransmitter γ-aminobutyric acid (GABA) has been shown to be altered in Huntington's disease, Parkinson's disease, and tardive dyskinesia (Zorumski and Isenberg 1991). Markers of GABA neurotransmission have also been reported to be decreased in aging and include decreased synthetic enzymes for GABA, decreased GABA levels in CSF, and decreased receptor numbers (Komiskey et al. 1988). These findings may relate to the increased sensitivity to benzodiazepines observed to occur with aging (Pomara et al. 1991; Swift et al. 1985). The benzodiazepine class of drugs interacts with the benzodiazepine-GABA receptor complex to enhance GABA activity, which is thought to lead to their anxiolytic action (Zorumski and Isenberg 1991). Studies of anxiety disorders in the elderly are few (see Chapter 14, this volume), as are studies that have used pharmacological probes of the GABA-benzodiazepine receptor complex in elderly subjects (Table 28–5).

The increased sensitivity of elderly patients to the cognitive, psychomotor, and sedative effects of benzodiazepines is not explained or is only partly explained by alterations in pharmacokinetics and plasma concentrations (Greenblatt et al. 1989). Increased central nervous system depression from benzodiazepines has been confirmed in older versus younger animals, despite similar brain concentrations of drug. Because alterations in receptor concentrations or binding sites have not been reported to occur consistently with age, it has been hypothesized that the increased sensitivity may be due to alterations in coupling between receptors and their effector mechanisms, such as second messenger systems (Greenblatt et al. 1989).

In a recent study (Pomara et al. 1991), older volunteer control subjects were shown to have decreased plasma cortisol after receiving a single dose of the benzodiazepine diazepam; younger subjects had no significant decrease in cortisol. No correlations were found between cortisol levels and performance on tasks of memory, attention, and reaction time. In a follow-up study, Pomara et al. (1992) found that single doses of diazepam decreased plasma cortisol in both elderly control subjects and elderly subjects with generalized anxiety disorder. Plasma cortisol was also measured in these subjects after chronic treatment with diazepam and acute diazepam rechallenge; no significant response was found, indicating the development of tolerance. Although the functional implications of these deficits in the GABA system are not clear, the very ubiquity of GABA neurons suggests that changes may relate to decline in global neurological functioning.

Many studies in young subjects have shown that the cognitive effects of benzodiazepines resemble cognitive changes that occur in organic amnestic syndromes (Wolkowitz et al. 1987). In one study of elderly subjects (Sunderland et al. 1989), cognitive and behavioral effects of the benzodiazepine lorazepam were compared between patients with Alzheimer's disease and elderly control subjects. Drug-induced cognitive impairments in the patients with Alzheimer's disease were found to be predominantly attentional; in the control subjects,

errors were indicative of disinhibition. It was hypothesized that one possible reason for the difference between the groups was altered benzodiazepine sensitivity in the patients with Alzheimer's disease, secondary, for example, to decreased benzodiazepine receptor numbers, as has been reported in that group (Greenamyre et al. 1987).

It would be difficult to summarize the results of GABA-ergic studies in the elderly population because there is still relatively little information available. However, earlier studies with GABA-ergic active agents in young adults make it clear that this system must be studied in much greater detail, especially in relation to the effects of benzodiazepines on memory in elderly patients.

Dopaminergic System

A number of studies have reported alterations in dopaminergic markers with age, including decreased levels of synthetic enzymes (McGeer 1981), decreased

Table 28–5. Selected GABA-ergic challenges in adult and aging populations

Challenge agent	Adult studies	References	Aging studies	References
Benzodiazepine	Anterograde amnesia Amnesia not reversed by physostigmine	Wolkowitz et al. 1987; Duka 1988	Increased central nervous system sedation, sensitivity Decreased cortisol in control subjects and generalized anxiety disorder *Low dose:* decreased attention in Alzheimer's disease and increased disinhibition in control subjects *High dose:* recognition decreased in Alzheimer's disease and control subjects; increased sensitivity with advancing age	Greenblatt et al. 1989 Pomara et al. 1991, 1992; Sunderland et al. 1989 Block et al. 1985
Benzodiazepine antagonists:				
RO15-1788	Reverses the anterograde amnesia	O'Boyle et al. 1983		
β-carboline (βZK93 426)	? Reverses scopolamine-induced amnesia Less amnesia than with benzodiazepine	Duka et al. 1992; Sarter et al. 1988a Roache et al. 1993	? Increased cognition in Alzheimer's disease	Sarter et al. 1988b; Sarter et al. 1988c
Baclofen	Decreased growth hormone in schizophrenia	Montelesone et al. 1988	Increased growth hormone secretion in Parkinson's disease	Volpi et al. 1991

Note. GABA = γ-aminobutyric acid.

numbers of neurons (Morgan et al. 1987), decreased receptors (at least the subtype 2 [D2] receptors) (Morgan et al. 1987; Wolkowitz et al. 1987), and increased monoamine oxidase, a primary enzyme involved in the degradation of dopamine (Gottfries et al. 1971; Sunderland et al. 1992) (Table 28–6). These changes with aging may contribute to the development of Parkinson's disease, a neurodegenerative disease predominantly of the nigrostriatal dopaminergic system, and to the increased sensitivity of elderly patients to the extrapyramidal side effects of neuroleptic drugs, including tardive dyskinesia (American Psychiatric Association 1980).

Drugs, such as neuroleptics, that have prominent effects on the dopaminergic system also affect other neurotransmitter systems to a significant degree. Few studies have therefore been done using specifically dopaminergic system probes, especially in nonpsychiatric samples (Table 28–6). There are age-related changes in the dopaminergic tuberoinfundibular tract, as reflected in changes in pituitary hormone secretion (Greenspan et al. 1991). Dopamine has strong modulatory effects on a number of these hormones,

suppressing, for example, thyroid-stimulating hormone (TSH [or thyrotropin]) secretion and stimulating gonadotropin secretion. Studies using the dopamine antagonist metoclopramide and levodopa showed some differences in older compared with younger volunteer control subjects in the dopaminergic modulation of TSH and gonadotropins, but not of prolactin or growth hormone (Cusimano et al. 1991; Greenspan et al. 1991).

A number of studies using dopamine agonists have been done in patients with Parkinson's disease. Results of one study (Cusimano et al. 1991) indicated that patients who showed a therapeutic response to bromocriptine had a lower prolactin and TSH response to acute bromocriptine followed by thyrotropin-releasing hormone (TRH), and to TRH alone. When challenged with bromocriptine followed by TRH, patients with Parkinson's disease showed a greater decrease in plasma prolactin than did control subjects. As dopamine is known to be inhibitory to prolactin release, the decreased response was interpreted to indicate hypersensitivity of dopamine receptors secondary to a chronic decrease in dopamine release by the hypothal-

Table 28–6. Selected dopaminergic system challenges

Challenge agent	Adult studies	References	Aging studies	References
Levodopa	Growth hormone increased in control subjects; ? in bipolar depression	Sachar et al. 1975	Preserved thyrotropin pulsatile secretion	Greenspan et al. 1991
			No change in growth hormone, prolactin, or thyrotropin with age	Franceschi et al. 1988
			Decreased enkephalins after levodopa in Parkinson's disease	Baronti et al. 1991
Amantadine or trihexyphenidyl	Cognitive improvement as increased visual attention	Andersson 1992	No memory impairment	McEvoy et al. 1987
Apomorphine	Decreased prolactin in control subjects ?	Lal et al. 1980	—	—
	? Growth hormone blunting in major depressive disorder	Insel et al. 1982		
Bromocriptine	—	—	Growth hormone release in Parkinson's disease	Urakami et al. 1990; Cusimano et al. 1991
			Decreased prolactin-thyrotropin response to thyrotropin-releasing hormone alone in Parkinson's disease	Cusimano et al. 1991
Methylphenidate	—	—	Increased mood in Parkinson's disease	Cantello et al. 1989

amus. Cusimano et al. (1991) also found that the growth hormone response to the stimuli was increased. As dopamine has a facilitatory effect on growth hormone release, these data are also consistent with a hypersensitivity phenomenon in the Parkinson's patients. The authors also pointed out that growth hormone response has not been as consistent among reports as has that of the other hormones discussed.

In another study (Gancher et al. 1990), improvement on motor tasks was measured as a clinical response to acute infusion of the dopamine agonist apomorphine. The response was shown to lag behind peak plasma concentrations of the drug and to persist beyond the time the plasma concentration fell below what had been established as response threshold levels. Gancher et al. (1990) interpreted these results to indicate that the drug effects outlasted the period of agonist receptor occupancy and that information from such studies may provide clues on how to control the fluctuating response to levodopa therapy. Another recent study (Baronti et al. 1991) investigated CSF levels of opioid peptides in patients with Parkinson's disease and control subjects after infusion of levodopa. These peptides have neuromodulatory effects on dopamine and are important in striatal output. CSF levels of a proenkephalin derivative were lower in the patients with Parkinson's disease than in the control subjects. Studies of this type may provide insights into interactions between various neurotransmitter systems.

Behavioral symptoms are common in patients with neuropsychiatric illnesses such as Alzheimer's disease and Parkinson's disease, and it is speculated that these symptoms are related to neurotransmitter alterations caused by the illnesses (Baronti et al. 1991; Insel et al. 1984). A study that evaluated mood response to the stimulant methylphenidate, which enhances catecholamines including dopamine, showed that Parkinson's patients with major depression lacked an euphoriant response compared with patients with major depression without Parkinson's disease and with control subjects (Cantello et al. 1989). The dopaminergic neurons in the ventral tegmental area of the mesencephalon (i.e., the mesolimbic dopaminergic system) have been shown to be important in reward effects in animals, and stimulant-mediated euphoria has been shown to be blocked by dopamine receptor blockers in humans (Cantello et al. 1989). The authors interpreted the above results to indicate that the depressed patients with Parkinson's disease had a deficiency in the mesolimbic dopaminergic system. They also noted

that, consistent with prior studies, some motoric symptoms, specifically rigidity and akinesia, were relieved by methylphenidate (Cantello et al. 1989). Further studies using drugs that affect dopamine and pituitary hormones may provide clues to the alterations in neuroendocrine function that occur with age and to the age-related pathology of neuropsychiatric and endocrine system illnesses.

Neuroendocrine Probes of the Central Nervous System

Dexamethasone Suppression Test

The dexamethasone suppression test (DST) has received unique evaluation among biological tests for clinical use in neuropsychiatry. The DST has also been extensively studied in the elderly population. Some researchers have found that healthy elderly individuals have no significant increase in dexamethasone nonsuppression or in postdexamethasone cortisol levels (Balldin et al. 1983; Tourigny-Rivard et al. 1981). However, a review of the literature (Greden et al. 1986) indicated that a moderate loss of the specificity of the 1-mg DST occurs in healthy elderly populations, whereas in major depression this was further complicated by variables such as illness severity and chronicity, in addition to comorbid medical conditions. The DST has also been widely studied in populations with Alzheimer's disease but without major depression. Here the consensus has been that a nonsuppression rate in nondepressed patients with Alzheimer's disease or multi-infarct dementia can be indistinguishable from primary melancholia (Carroll and Mendels 1976; Georgotas et al. 1984; Molchan et al. 1990; Skare et al. 1990). In fact, the DST does not appear to be useful in distinguishing dementia from depression, though conflicting evidence exists for its use as a severity measure of depression (Molchan et al. 1990; Skare et al. 1990).

Multiple explanations have been posited regarding the cause of dexamethasone nonsuppression, in young and older patients alike. For the sake of review, we summarize below the five most prominent theories:

1. *Increased endogenous corticotropin-releasing hormone (CRH) production.* Following a CRH stimulation test, patients with depression or Alzheimer's disease have been found to have a blunted adrenocorticotropic hormone (ACTH) response, consistent

with hypersecretion of CRH (Holsboer et al. 1984; Kathol et al. 1989; Lesch et al. 1990; Nemeroff et al. 1984). This finding implies a pathological process at the level of the hypothalamus or above.

2. *Glucocorticoid receptor alterations.* Resistance of cortisol to suppression by dexamethasone has been shown to increase with age in both Alzheimer's disease (Greenwald et al. 1986) and major depression (Georgotas et al. 1984). The hippocampus is involved in the neuropathology of Alzheimer's disease, and it has the greatest number of glucocorticoid receptors in the brain. It has been postulated that age itself is of etiologic significance in the observed hypothalamus-pituitary-adrenal (HPA) axis abnormalities in these diseases and that chronically higher baseline cortisol levels could account in part for some of the neuropathology associated with aging (Sapolsky et al. 1986).

3. *Monoamine transmitter alterations.* Hypersecretion of glucocorticoids may change monoamine neurotransmission (Lesch et al. 1990) and affect psychobiological functioning such as the HPA axis abnormalities in Alzheimer's disease and major depression (McEwen 1987).

4. *Adrenal hyperresponsivity.* Hyperresponsivity of the adrenal gland to ACTH has been demonstrated in patients with depression (Kathol et al. 1989). This abnormality has been postulated to be secondary to adrenal hypertrophy that has occurred due to chronic stimulation with ACTH.

5. *Cholinergic abnormality.* Endogenous acetylcholine and drugs that enhance cholinergic transmission have been shown in most studies to have a stimulatory effect on the HPA axis (Davous et al. 1988; Mohs et al. 1985). Overactivation of the muscarinic cholinergic system is seen in major depression (Janowsky and Risch 1987), whereas cholinergic depletion is a disease hallmark in patients with Alzheimer's disease. Because both diseases are associated with abnormal DSTs, a simple cholinergic explanation is unlikely. Future studies may examine the specific role of nicotinic versus muscarinic receptors in the HPA axis.

In summary, continued study of the HPA axis alterations that occur in Alzheimer's disease and major depression should help elucidate whether these endocrine responses are an adaptational response to other changes or whether the HPA system has a primary etiologic role in these illnesses.

Thyrotropin-Releasing Hormone (TRH) Stimulation Test

Many studies have reported associations between thyroid dysfunction and psychiatric symptoms, especially depressed mood (Franceschi et al. 1988; Loosen 1987; Molchan et al. 1991b). A number of studies have reported decreased TSH response to TRH with age, especially in men (Targum et al. 1989; Tsuboyama et al. 1992; Warner et al. 1990). One recent study (Targum et al. 1989) found that responses to TRH in elderly subjects, both control subjects and patients with major depression, were highly variable. Findings included a decreased TSH response in men versus women, but no difference in response between control subjects and depressed subjects. In a large study by Molchan et al. (1991b), elderly depression patients had lower stimulated TSH levels and a higher rate of blunted responses than did patients with Alzheimer's disease or age-matched control subjects. Depressed patients with a blunted response had lower basal TSH levels, consistent with prior studies in younger patients (Loosen 1987). The depressed patients also had higher thyroxine and free thyroxine levels than did the patients with Alzheimer's disease or the control subjects.

Clinically, patients with Alzheimer's disease and major depression often have overlapping clinical syndromes, but studies of the TRH stimulation test in Alzheimer patients have shown mixed results (Lampe et al. 1989; Molchan et al. 1990; Sunderland et al. 1986; Tsuboyama et al. 1992; Warner et al. 1990). Most studies have found no correlations between degree of dementia severity or depression and TSH response (Franceschi et al. 1988). Prolactin, growth hormone, and cortisol responses to TRH have been quite variable in patients with Alzheimer's disease (Tsuboyama et al. 1992). Reasons for discrepancies among studies may include the heterogeneity of patients with Alzheimer's disease, the study of patients at different stages of the illness, the small number of subjects in some studies, and the inclusion of patients with slight baseline thyroid function test abnormalities. Further research in this area is still needed.

Peptide Probes of the Central Nervous System

More than 40 neuropeptides, acting as another class of chemical messenger, have been identified in the central nervous system neurons. Because endogenous peptides in the systemic circulation do not cross the blood-brain barrier, they have been limited as probes in clinical challenge studies (Mazurek et al. 1986; Peabody et al. 1985). Oxytocin and vasopressin improved visual memory in young control subjects, though results have been mixed in patients with Alzheimer's disease (Peabody et al. 1986). Pentagastrin, angiotensin, and cholecystokinin (CCK4) are being studied in young adults to ascertain hypothalamic control of neuroendocrine secretion and autonomic function (Becker et al. 1992).

The levels of several neuropeptides are decreased in the Alzheimer's disease cortex, including somatostatin, corticotropin-releasing factor (CRF), neuropeptide Y, and substance P (Allen et al. 1983; Bareggi et al. 1985; Beal and Mazurek 1987; Beal et al. 1986; Cugini et al. 1992; Lesch et al. 1990). Patients with Alzheimer's disease and major depression have been consistently shown to have decreased concentrations of CSF somatostatin-like immunoreactivity (SLI) (Bissette et al. 1985; Cantillon et al. 1993; Molchan et al. 1991a) and substance P–like immunoreactivity (Bouras et al. 1990). Like many other neuropeptides, somatostatin would be an obvious choice for challenge studies if it were available in a form that could cross the blood-brain barrier. Unfortunately, until smaller peptides, lipophilic peptide analogs, or lipophilic carriers are made available, this challenge approach will have limited success.

Summary and Future Directions

Our purpose in this chapter has been to focus attention on the pharmacological and neuroendocrine probes of brain neurochemistry in the elderly population. For the well-known neurotransmitter systems such as the cholinergic, noradrenergic, and serotonergic, there are already multiple probes available. And although there is an obvious paucity of studies focusing specifically on elderly subjects, at least the tools needed for such studies are currently available (Table 28–1). The job for the future will be to characterize and contrast the responses of elderly subjects, using ill patients and control subjects alike, with those of younger populations. Furthermore, it will be a future goal to improve the pharmacological specificity of the challenge agents to come more in line with the rapidly advancing knowledge of receptor subtypes provided by modern molecular biology techniques. Similarly, we

must advance our knowledge surrounding the neuroendocrine challenges by tracking these approaches with specific biological processes.

Using drugs as tools, we will continue to update our theories on neurotransmitter physiology (Nutt and Cowen 1987). For example, certain aspects of amnesia can be mimicked by benzodiazepines in control subjects, and centrally acting anticholinergics can be used to briefly recreate in healthy elderly subjects some of the patterns of memory loss of Alzheimer's disease. Furthermore, these effects can perhaps be blocked or attenuated with peptides like TRH or other neurotransmitter specific agents such as serotonin reuptake inhibitors. These modeling approaches may eventually lead us to more rational pharmacological treatments. Prior to these pharmacological challenges, central nervous system research placed much reliance on neuropsychological testing or animal brain lesion experiments and single case trauma studies. As our measurement techniques become more sophisticated, we may also link these pharmacological and neuroendocrine challenge tests with studies of second messenger function and dynamic central nervous system imaging. In any case, better understanding and treatment of neuropsychiatric illnesses in the elderly population will be our central focus.

References

Allen RM, Young SF: Phencyclidine-induced psychosis. Am J Psychiatry 133:1081–1084, 1978

Allen SJ, Benton JS, Goodhardt MJ, et al: Biochemical evidence of selective nerve cell changes in the normal aging human and rat brain. J Neurochem 41:256–265, 1983

American Psychiatric Association: Task Force Report: Tardive Dyskinesia. Washington, DC, American Psychiatric Association, 1980

Amsterdam JD, Maislin G, Skolnick B, et al: Multiple hormone responses to clonidine administration in depressed patients and healthy volunteers. Biol Psychiatry 26:265–278, 1989

Andersson S, Berstad J, Finset A, et al: Amantadine in cognitive failure in patients with traumatic head injuries. Tidsskr Nor Laegeforen 112:2070–2072, 1992

Antelman SM, Chiodo LA: Dopamine autoreceptor subsensitivity: a mechanism common to the treatment of depression and the induction of amphetamine psychosis. Biol Psychiatry 16:717–727, 1981

Aston-Jones G, Bloom EE: Norepinephrine-containing locus coeruleus neurons in behaving rats exhibit pronounced response to non-noxious environmental stimuli. J Neurosci 1:887–900, 1981

Balldin J, Gottfries C-G, Karlsson I, et al: Dexamethasone suppression test and serum prolactin in dementia disorders. Br J Psychiatry 143:277–281, 1983

Bareggi SR, Franceschi M, Smirne S: Neurochemical findings in cerebrospinal fluid in Alzheimer's disease, in Normal Aging, Alzheimer's Disease, and Senile Dementia: Aspects on Etiology, Pathogenesis, Diagnosis, and Treatment. Edited by Gottfries CG. Brussels, Editions de l'Universite de Bruxelles, 1985, pp 203–212

Baronti F, Conant KE, Giuffra M, et al: Opioid peptides in Parkinson's disease: effects of dopamine repletion. Brain Res 560:92–96, 1991

Bartus RT, Dean RL, Beer B, et al: The cholinergic hypothesis of geriatric memory dysfunction. Science 217:408–417, 1982

Beal MF, Mazurek MF: Substance P-like immunoreactivity is reduced in Alzheimer's disease. Neurology 37:1205–1209, 1987

Beal MF, Growdon JH, Mazurek MF: CSF somatostatin-like immunoreactivity in dementia. Neurology 36:294–297, 1986

Beatty WW, Butters N, Janowsky DS: Patterns of memory failure after scopolamine treatment: implications for cholinergic hypotheses of dementia. Behav Neural Biol 45:196–211, 1986

Becker JB, Breedlove SM, Crews D (eds): Behavioral Endocrinology. Cambridge, MA, MIT Press, 1992

Bissette G, Reynolds GP, Kilts CH, et al: Corticotrophin-releasing factor-like immunoreactivity in senile dementia of the Alzheimer type. JAMA 254:3067–3069, 1985

Block RI, DeVoe M, Stanley B, et al: Memory performance in individuals with primary degenerative dementia: its similarity to diazepam-induced impairments. Exp Aging Res 11:151–155, 1985

Bonner TI: New subtypes of muscarinic acetylcholine receptors. Trends Pharmacol Sci 10:11–15, 1989

Bouras C, Vallet PG, Hof PR, et al: Substance P immunoreactivity in Alzheimer's disease: a study in cases presenting symmetric or asymmetric cortical atrophy. Alzheimer Dis Assoc Disord 4:24–34, 1990

Bourin M, Bradwejn J: Les antagonistes de la cholecystokinine: anxiolytiques de demain? Pathol Biol 40:215–217, 1991

Broocks A, Pigott TA, Canter S, et al:. Acute administration of ondansetron and m-CPP patients with obsessive-compulsive disorder (OCI and controls: behavioral and biological results. Biol Psychiatry 31:174A, 1992

Brown GM, Koslow SH, Reichlin S: Neuroendocrinology and Psychiatric Disorder. New York, Raven, 1988

Bruno G, Mohr E, Gillespie M, et al: Muscarinic agonist therapy of Alzheimer's disease: a clinical trial of RS-86. Arch Neurol 43:659–661, 1986

Caine ED: Pseudodementia: current concepts and future directions. Arch Gen Psychiatry 38:1359–1364, 1981

Cantello R, Aguggia M, Gilli M, et al: Major depression in Parkinson's disease and the mood response to intravenous methylphenidate: possible role of the "hedonic" dopamine synapse. J Neurol Neurosurg Psychiatry 52:724–731, 1989

Cantillon M, Martinez R, Molchan S, et al: Somatostatin and cerebral atrophy in elderly neuropsychiatric subjects. Abstract presented at the biennial meeting of the International Psychogeriatric Association, Berlin, Germany, September 1993

Carroll BJ, Mendels J: Neuroendocrine regulation in affective disorders, in Hormones, Behavior, and Psychopathology. Edited by Sacher EJ. New York, Raven, 1976, pp 193–224

Chan-Palay V, Asan E: Alterations in catecholamine neurons of the locus coeruleus in senile dementia of the Alzheimer type and in Parkinson's disease with and without dementia and depression. J Comp Neurol 287:373–392, 1989

Charney DS, Heninger GR, Breier A: Noradrenergic function and panic anxiety effects of yohimbine in healthy subjects and patients with agoraphobia and panic disorder. Arch Gen Psychiatry 41:751–763, 1984

Charney DS, Heninger GR, Jatlow PI: Increased anxiogenic effects of caffeine in panic disorders. Arch Gen Psychiatry 42:233–243, 1985

Charney DS, Woods SW, Krystal JH, et al: Neurobiological mechanisms of human anxiety, in The Biological Basis of Psychiatric Treatment. Pohl P, Gershon S. Basel, Karger, 1990, pp 242–283

Corkin S: Acetylcholine, aging and Alzheimer's disease: implications for treatment. Trends Neurosci 4:287–290, 1981

Coupland N, Glue P, Nutt DJ: Challenge tests: assessment of the noradrenergic and GABA systems in depression and anxiety disorders. Mol Aspects Med 13:221–247, 1992

Cross AJ: Serotonin in Alzheimer-type dementia and other dementing illnesses. Ann N Y Acad Sci 600:405–415, 1990

Cugini P, Lucia P, DiPalma L, et al: The circadian rhythm of atrial natriuretic peptide, vasoactive intestinal peptide, β-endorphin and cortisol in healthy young and elderly subjects. Clin Auton Res 2(2):113–118, 1992

Curran HV, Sakulsriprong M, Lader M: Antidepressants and human memory: an investigation of four drugs with different sedative and anticholinergic profiles. Psychopharmacology 95:520–527, 1988

Cusimano G, Capriani C, Bonifati V, et al: Hypothalamo-pituitary function and dopamine dependence in untreated parkinsonian patients. Acta Neurol Scand 83(3):145–150, 1991

Davis KL, Mohs RC, Tinklenberg JR: Enhancement of memory by physostigmine (letter). N Engl J Med 301:946 1979

Davis KL, Hollander E, Davidson M, et al: Induction of depression with oxotremorine in patients with Alzheimer's disease. Am J Psychiatry 144:468–471, 1987

Davous P, Roudier M, Piketty ML, et al: Pharmacological modulation of cortisol secretion and dexamethasone suppression in Alzheimer's disease. Biol Psychiatry 23:13–24, 1988

DeMeo MD, McBride PA, Mann JJ, et al: Fenfluramine challenge in major depression. Abstract presented at the annual meeting of the American Psychiatric Association, Montreal, Canada, May 1988

Dewar D, Graham DL, McCulloch J: 5-HT$_2$ receptors in dementia of Alzheimer type: a quantitative autoreceptors in dementia of Alzheimer type: a quantitative autoradiographic study of frontal cortex and hippocampus. J Neural Transm Park Dis Dement Sect 2:129–137, 1990

Duka T: Benzodiazepine receptor ligands, memory, and information processing: psychometric, psychopharmacological, and clinical issues. Psychopharmacology 95:463–471, 1988

Duka T, Edelmann V, Schutt B, et al: Scopolamine-induced amnesia in humans: lack of effects of the benzodiazepine receptor antagonist β-carboline ZK 93426. J Psychopharmacol 6:382–388, 1992

Elam M, Yoat TP, Svensson TH: Hypercapnia and hyper-Chemo-receptor-mediated control of locus ceruleus neurons and splanchnic, sympathetic nerves. Brain Res 222:373–381, 1981

Elrod K, Buccafusco J: Correlation of the amnestic effects of nicotinic antagonists with inhibition of regional brain acetylcholine synthesis in rats. J Pharmacol Exp Ther 258:403–409, 1991

Feldman RD, Limbird LE, Nadeau J, et al: Alterations in leukocyte b-receptor affinity with aging. N Engl J Med 310:815–819, 1984

Franceschi M, Perego L, Ferini-Strambi L, et al: Neuroendocrinological function in Alzheimer's disease. Neuroendocrinology 48:367–370, 1988

Gancher ST, Woodward WR, Gliessman P, et al: The short-duration response to apomorphine: implications for the mechanism of dopaminergic effects in Parkinsonism. Ann Neurol 27:660–665, 1990

Georgotas A, Stokes P, Krakowski M, et al: Hypothalamic-pituitary-adrenocortical function in geriatric depression: diagnosis and treatment implications. Biol Psychiatry 19:685–689, 1984

Gerner RH, Catlin DH, Gorelick DA, et al: β-Endorphin: intravenous infusion causes behavioral change in psychiatric inpatients. Arch Gen Psychiatry 37:642–647, 1980

Gitelman DR, Prohovnik I: Muscarinic and nicotinic contributions to cognitive function and cortical blood flow. Neurobiol Aging 13:313–318, 1992

Glue P, Wilson S, Lawson C, et al: Acute and chronic idazoxan in normal volunteers: biochemical, physiological and psychological effects. J Psychopharmacol 5:396–403, 1991

Gottfries CG: Alzheimer's disease and senile dementia: biochemical characteristics and aspects of treatment. Psychopharmacology 86:245–252, 1985

Gottfries CG, Gottfries I, Johansson B, et al: Acid monoamine metabolites in human CSF and their relation to age and sex. Neuropharmacology 10:665–672, 1971

Greden JF, Flegel P, Haskett R, et al: Age effects in serial hypothalamic-pituitary-adrenal monitoring. Psychoneuroendocrinology 11:195–204, 1986

Greenamyre JT, Penny JB, D'Amato CJ, et al: Dementia of the Alzheimer's type: changes in hippocampal l-[3H]glutamate binding. J Neurochem 48:543–551, 1987

Greenblatt DJ, Shader RI, Harmatz JS: Implications of altered drug disposition in the elderly: studies of benzodiazepines. J Clin Pharmacol 29:866–872, 1989

Greenspan SL, Klibanski A, Rowe JW, et al: Age-related alterations in pulsatile secretion of TSH: role of dopaminergic regulation. Am J Physiol 260:E486–E491, 1991

Greenwald BS, Mathe AA, Mohs RC, et al: Cortisol and Alzheimer's disease, II: dexamethasone suppression, dementia severity, and affective symptoms. Am J Psychiatry 143:442–446, 1986

Gurguis GNM, Uhde TW: Plasma MHPG and growth hormone response to yohimbine in panic disorder patients and normal controls. Psychoneuroendocrinology 15:217–224, 1990

Halbreich U, Sharpless N, Asnis GM, et al: Afternoon continuous plasma levels of 3-methoxy-4-hydroxyphenylglycol and age. Arch Gen Psychiatry 44:804–812, 1987

Hall ST, Ceuppens PR: A study to evaluate the effect of ondansetron on psychomotor performance after repeated oral dosing in health subjects. Psychopharmacology 104:86–90, 1991

Heinsimer JA, Kefowitz RJ: The impact of aging on adrenergic receptor function: clinical and biochemical aspects. J Am Geriatr Soc 33:184–188, 1985

Heninger GR, Charney DS, Sternberg DE: Serotonergic function in depression: prolactin response to intravenous tryptophan in depressed patients and healthy subjects. Arch Gen Psychiatry 41:398–402, 1984

Hollander E, Mohs RC, Davis KL: Cholinergic approaches to the treatment of Alzheimer's disease. Br Med Bull 42:97–100, 1986

Holsboer F, Bardeleben U, Gerken A, et al: Blunted corticotropin and normal cortisol responses to human corticotropin-releasing factor in depression (letter). N Engl J Med 311:1127, 1984

Insel TR, Kalin NH, Guttmacher LB, et al: The dexamethasone suppression test in patients with primary obsessive-compulsive disorder. Psychiatry Res 6:153–160, 1982

Insel TR, Mueller EAI, Gillin JC: Biological markers in obsessive-compulsive and affective disorders. J Psychiatr Res 18:407–423, 1984

Jackson HC, Griffin IJ, Nutt DJ: Endogenous opioids may be involved in idazoxan-induced food intake. Neuropharmacology 31:771–776, 1992

Janowsky DS, Risch SC: Role of acetylcholine mechanisms in the affective disorders, in Psychopharmacology: The Third Generation of Progress. Edited by Meltzer HY. New York, Raven, 1987, pp 527–533

Kahn J-P, Rubinow DR, Davis CL, et al: Salivary cortisol: a practical method for evaluation of adrenal function. Biol Psychiatry 23:335–349, 1988

Kalaria RN, Andorn AC: Adrenergic receptors in aging and Alzheimer's disease: decreased alpha 2-receptors demonstrated by [^{3}H]p-aminoclonidine binding in prefrontal cortex. Neurobiol Aging 12:131–136, 1991

Kathol RG, Jaeckle RS, Lopez JF, et al: Pathophysiology of HPA axis abnormalities in patients with major depression: an update. Am J Psychiatry 146:311–317, 1989

Komiskey HL, Raemont LM, Mundinger KL: Aging: Modulation of GABA, binding sites by ethanol and diazepam. Brain Res 458:37–44, 1988

Lal S, Young SN, Cervantes P, et al: Effect of l-tryptophan on apomorphine-induced growth hormone secretion in normal subjects. Pharmakopsychiatrie Neuro-Psychopharmakologie 13:331–335, 1980

Lampe TH, Veith RC, Plymate SR, et al: Pressor, norepinephrine, and pituitary responses to two TRH doses in Alzheimer's disease and normal older men. Psychoneuroendocrinology 14:311–320, 1989

Lawlor BA, Sunderland T, Hill JL, et al: Evidence for a decline with age in behavioral responsivity to the serotonin agonist, m-chlorophenylpiperazine, in healthy human subjects. Psychiatry Res 29:1–10, 1989a

Lawlor BA, Sunderland T, Mellow AM, et al: Hyperresponsivity to the serotonin agonist m-chlorophenylpiperazine in Alzheimer's disease: a controlled study. Arch Gen Psychiatry 46:542–549, 1989b

Lesch KP, Ihl R, Frolich L, et al: Endocrine responses to growth hormone releasing hormone and corticotropin releasing hormone in early-onset Alzheimer's disease. Psychiatry Res 33:107–112, 1990

Liebowitz MR, Gorman JM, Fyer AJ, et al: Effects of naloxone on patients with panic attacks. Am J Psychiatry 141:995–997, 1984

Little JT, Broocks A, Martin A, et al: Serotonergic modulation of scopolamine in older normal volunteers. Abstract presented at the annual meeting of the Society of Biological Psychiatry, San Francisco, CA, May 1993

Loosen PT: The TRH stimulation test in psychiatric disorders: a review, in Handbook of Clinical Psychoneuroendocrinology. Edited by Nemeroff CB, Loosen PT. New York, Guilford, 1987, pp 336–360

Mann DM, Yates PO, Hawkes J: The noradrenergic system in Alzheimer and multi-infarct dementias. J Neurol Neurosurg Psychiatry 45:113–119, 1982

Manning CA, Hall JL, Gold PE: Glucose effects on memory and other neuropsychological tests in elderly humans. Psychological Science 1(5):307–311, 1990

Martinez R, Molchan S, Hill J, et al: Amphetamine effects on acute scopolamine in neuropsychiatric subjects. Abstract presented at the annual meeting of the Society of Biological Psychiatry, May 1990

Mash DC, Flynn DD, Potter LT: Loss of M_2 muscarine receptors in the cerebral cortex in Alzheimer's disease and experimental cholinergic denervation. Science 228:1115–1117, 1985

Mazurek MF, Growdon JH, Beal MF, et al: CSF vasopressin concentration is reduced in Alzheimer's disease. Neurology 36:1133–1137, 1986

McBride PA, Tierney H, DeMeo M, et al: Effects of age and gender on CNS serotonergic responsivity in normal adults. Biol Psychiatry 27:1143–1155, 1990

McEvoy JP, McCue M, Spring B, et al: Effects of amantadine and trihexyphenidyl on memory in elderly normal volunteers. Am J Psychiatry 144:573–577, 1987

McEwen BS: Glucocorticoid-biogenic amine interactions in relation to mood and behavior. Biochem Pharmacol 36:1755–1763, 1987

McGeer EG: Neurotransmitter systems in aging and senile dementia. Prog Neuropsychopharmacol 5:435–445, 1981

McGeer E, McGeer PL: Neurotransmitter metabolism in the aging brain, in Neurobiology of Aging. Edited by Terry RD, Gershon S. New York, Raven, 1976, pp 389–403

Meek JL, Bertilsson K, Cheney DL, et al: Age induced changes in acetylcholine and serotonin content of discrete brain nuclei. J Gerontol 32:129–131, 1977

Mewaldt SP, Ghoneim MM: The effects of interactions of scopolamine, physostigmine and methamphetamine on human memory. Pharmacol Biochem Behav 10:205–210, 1979

Middlemiss DM, Palmer AM, Edel N, et al: Binding of the novel serotonin agonist 8-hydroxy-2-(di-n-propylamino) tetralin in normal and Alzheimer brain. J Neurochem 46:993–996, 1986

Mitchell P, Smythe G: Hormonal responses to fenfluramine in depressed and control subjects. J Affect Disord 19:43–51, 1990

Mohs RC, Davis BN, Johns CA, et al: Oral physostigmine treatment of patients with Alzheimer's disease. Am J Psychiatry 142:28–33, 1985

Molchan SE, Hill JL, Mellow AM, et al: The dexamethasone suppression test in Alzheimer's disease and major depression: relationship to dementia severity, depression, and CSF monoamines. Int Psychogeriatr 2:99–122, 1990

Molchan SE, Lawlor BA, Hill JL, et al: CSF monoamine metabolites and somatostatin in Alzheimer's disease and major depression. Biol Psychiatry 29:1110–1118, 1991a

Molchan SE, Lawlor BA, Hill JL, et al: The TRH stimulation test in Alzheimer's disease and major depression: relationship to clinical and CSF measures. Biol Psychiatry 30:567–576, 1991b

Molchan SE, Vitiello B, Minichiello M, et al: Reciprocal changes in psychosis and mood after physostigmine in a patient with Alzheimer's disease. Arch Gen Psychiatry 48:1113–1114, 1991c

Molchan SE, Martinez RA, Hill JL, et al: Increased cognitive sensitivity to scopolamine with age and a perspective on the scopolamine model. Brain Research Review 17:215–226, 1992

Montelesone P, Maj M, Iovino M, et al: Baclofen-induced growth hormone secretion is blunted in chronic schizophrenics: neuroendocrine evidence for a GABA disturbance in schizophrenia. Psychiatry Res 26:1–9, 1988

Morgan DG, May PC, Finch CE: Dopamine and serotonin systems in human and rodent brain: Effects of age and neurogenerative disease. J Am Geriatr Soc 35:334–345, 1987

Mueller EA, Murphy DL, Sunderland T: Further studies of the putative serotonin agonist m-chlorophenylpiperazine: evidence for a serotonin receptor mediated mechanism of action in humans. Psychopharmacology 89:388–391, 1986

Murphy DL, Pickar D, Alterman IS: Methods for the quantitative assessment of depressive and manic behavior, in Quantitative Techniques for the Evaluation of the Behavior of Psychiatric Patients. Edited by Burdock EI, Sudilovsky A, Gershon S. New York, Marcel Dekker, 1982, pp 355–392

Murphy DL, Mueller, EA, Hill JL, et al: Comparative anxiogenic, neuroendocrine, and other physiologic effects of m-chlorophenylpiperazine given intravenously or orally to healthy volunteers. Psychopharmacology 98:275–282, 1989

Nemeroff CB, Widerlov E, Bissette G, et al: Elevated concentrations of CSF corticotropin-releasing factor-like immunoreactivity in depressed patients. Science 226:1342–1344, 1984

Newhouse P, Sunderland T, Tariot P, et al: Intravenous nicotine in Alzheimer's disease: A pilot study. Psychopharmacology 95:171–175, 1988a

Newhouse PA, Sunderland T, Tariot PN, et al: The effects of acute scopolamine in geriatric depression. Arch Gen Psychiatry 45:906–912, 1988b

Newhouse PA, Sunderland T, Narang PK, et al: Neuroendocrine, physiologic, and behavioral responses following intravenous nicotine in nonsmoking healthy volunteers and in patients with Alzheimer's disease. Psychoneuroendocrinology 15:471–484, 1990

Newhouse PA, Potter A, Corwin J, et al: Acute nicotinic blockade produces cognitive impairment in normal humans. Psychopharmacology 108:480–484, 1992

Nutt DJ, Cowen PJ: Monoamine function in anxiety and depression: Information from neuroendocrine challenge tests. Human Psychopharmacol 2:211–220, 1987

O'Boyle C, Lambe R, Darragh A, et al: RO-15-1788 antagonizes the effects of diazepam in man without affecting its bioavailability. Br J Anaesth 55:349–355, 1983

Paul SM, Crawley JN, Skilnick P: The neurobiology of anxiety and the role of the GABA/benzodiazepine receptor complex, in American Handbook of Psychiatry, 8. Edited by Berger PA, Brodie KH. New York, Basic Books, 1986, pp 581–596

Peabody CA, Thiemann S, Pigache R: Desglycinamide-9-arginine-8-vasopressin [DGAVP, Organon 5667] in patients with dementia. Neurobiol Aging 6:95–100, 1985

Peabody CA, Davies H, Berger PA, et al: Desamino-D-arginine-vasopressin (DDAVP) in Alzheimer's disease. Neurobiol Aging 7:301–303, 1986

Peters BH, Levin HS: Effects of physostigmine and lecithin on memory in Alzheimer's disease. Ann Neurol 6:219–221, 1979

Pigott TA, Grady TA, Bernstein SE, et al: A comparison of oral and IV m-CPP in patients with OCD (abstract). Biol Psychiatry 31:173A, 1992

Pitts FN, Allen RE: Biochemical induction of anxiety. New York, Spectrum, 1979

Pomara N, Deptula D, Singh R, et al: Increased cortisol response to diazepam in the aged (abstract). Biol Psychiatry 29:121A, 1991

Pomara N, Deptula D, Singh R, et al: The effects of diazepam on plasma cortisol levels in the elderly (abstract). Biol Psychiatry 31:61A, 1992

Raffaele KC, Berardi A, Morris PP, et al: Effects of acute infusion of the muscarinic cholinergic agonist arecoline on verbal memory and visuo-spatial function in dementia of the Alzheimer type. Prog Neuropsychopharmacol Biol Psychiatry 15:643–648, 1991

Rapoport JL, Buchsbaum MS, Weingartner H, et al: Dextroamphetamine. Arch Gen Psychiatry 37:933–943, 1980

Raskind MA, Peskind ER, Veith RC, et al: Increased plasma and cerebrospinal fluid norepinephrine in older men: differential suppression by clonidine. J Clin Endocrinol Metab 66:438–443, 1988

Raskind MA, Peskind ER, Veith RC, et al: Neuroendocrine responses to physostigmine in Alzheimer's disease. Arch Gen Psychiatry 46:535–540, 1989a

Raskind MA, Peskind ER, Veith RC, et al: Neuroendocrine responses to physostigmine in Alzheimer's disease. Arch Gen Psychiatry 46:535–540, 1989b

Rifai AH, Reynolds CF, Mann JJ: Biology of elderly suicide. Suicide Life Threat Behav 22:48–61, 1992

Risch SC, Klain NH, Janowsky DL, et al: Corelease of ACTH and β-endorphin immunoreactivity in human subjects in response to central cholinergic stimulation. Science 222:77, 1983

Roache JD, Cherek DR, Bennett RH, et al: Differential effects of triazolam and ethanol on awareness, memory, and psychomotor performance. J Clin Psychopharmacol 13:3–15, 1993

Rudorfer MV, Ross RJ, Linnoila M, et al: Exaggerated orthostatic responsivity of plasma norepinephrine in depression. Arch Gen Psychiatry 42:1186–1192, 1985

Rudorfer MV, Sherer MA, Lane EA, et al: Acute noradrenergic effects of desipramine in depression. J Clin Psychopharmacol 11:22–27, 1991

Russell RW, Ehlert FJ, Hwa JJ: Relation between behaviorally augmented tolerance and upregulation of muscarinic receptors in the CNS: effects of chronic administration of scopolamine. Psychopharmacology 88:33–39, 1986

Sachar EJ, Altman N, Gruen PH, et al: Human growth hormone response to levodopa. Arch Gen Psychiatry 32:502–503, 1975

Sapolsky RM, Krey LC, McEwen BS: The neuroendocrinology of stress and aging: the glucocorticoid cascade hypothesis. Endocr Rev 7:284–301, 1986

Sarter M, Bodewitz G, Stephens DN: Attenuation of scopolamine-induced impairment of spontaneous alterations behaviour by antagonist but not inverse agonist and agonist b-carbolines. Psychopharmacology 94:491–495, 1988a

Sarter M, Duka T, Stephens DN: Nootropic properties of antagonist 8-carbolines: a symptomatological treatment for early senile dementia? (abstract). Neuropsychopharmacology 5:25, 1988b

Sarter M, Schneider HH, Stephens DN: Treatment strategies for senile dementia: antagonist b-carbolines. Trends Neurosci 11:13–16, 1988c

Scarpace PJ: Decreased α-adrenergic responsiveness during senescence. Federal Proceedings 45:51–54, 1986

Simson PE, Weiss JM: Altered activity of locus coeruleus in an animal model of depression. Neuropsychopharmacology 1:287–295, 1988

Sitaram N, Gillin C, Bunney WE: Cholinergic and catecholaminergic receptor sensitivity in affective illness: strategy and theory, in Neurobiology of Mood Disorders. Edited by Post RM, Ballenger JC. Baltimore, MD, Williams & Wilkins, 1984, pp 629–651

Skare S, Pew B, Dysken M: The dexamethasone suppression test in dementia: a review of the literature. J Geriatr Psychiatry Neurol 3(3):124–138, 1990

Snyder EW, Schlehuber C, Dustman RE, et al: Phencyclidine-induced alterations of rat electrophysiology. Brain Res Bull 7:249–253, 1981

Sparks DL, DeKosky ST, Markelsbery WR: Alzheimer's disease: aminergic-cholinergic alterations in hypothalamus. Arch Neurol 45:994–999, 1988

Stern Y, Sano M, Mayeux R: Effects of oral physostigmine in Alzheimer's disease. Ann Neurol 22:306–310, 1987

Sunderland T, Mellow AM, Gross M, et al: Thyrotropin-releasing hormone and dementia (letter). Am J Psychiatry 143:1318, 1986

Sunderland T, Tariot PN, Cohen RM, et al: Anticholinergic sensitivity in patients with dementia of the Alzheimer type and age-matched controls: a dose-response study. Arch Gen Psychiatry 44:418–426, 1987

Sunderland T, Tariot PN, Newhouse PA: Differential responsivity of mood, behavior, and cognition to cholinergic agents in elderly neuropsychiatric populations. Brain Res Rev 13:371–389, 1988

Sunderland T, Weingartner H, Cohen RM, et al: Low-dose oral lorazepam administration in Alzheimer subjects and age-matched controls. Psychopharmacology 99:129–133, 1989

Sunderland T, Molchan SE, Martinez RA, et al: Drug challenge strategies in Alzheimer's disease: a focus on the scopolamine model, in Alzheimer's Disease: Current Research in Early Diagnosis. Edited by Becker RE, Giacobini E. New York, Taylor & Francis, 1990, pp 173–181

Sunderland T, Molchan S, Putnam KT, et al: CSF monoamine effects of long-term deprenyl and hydergine in Alzheimer patients. Paper presented at the annual meeting of the Society of Biological Psychiatry, Washington, DC, May 1992

Supiano MA, Linares OA, Halter JB, et al: Functional uncoupling of the platelet α_2-adrenergic receptor-adenylate cyclase complex in the elderly. Clin Endocrinol Metab 64:1160–1164, 1987

Swift CG, Ewen JM, Clarke P, et al: Responsiveness to oral diazepam in the elderly: relationship to total and free plasma concentrations. Br J Clin Pharmacacol 20:111–118, 1985

Targum SD, Marshall LE, Magac-Harris K, et al: TRH Tests in a healthy elderly population: demonstration of gender differences. J Am Geriatr Soc 37:533–536, 1989

Tariot PN, Gross M, Sunderland T, et al: High-dose naloxone in older normal subjects: implications for Alzheimer's disease. J Am Geriatr Soc 36:681–686, 1988

Thal LJ, Masur DM, Sharpless NS, et al: Acute and chronic effects of oral physostigmine and lecithin in Alzheimer's disease. Prog Neuropsychopharmacol Biol Psychiatry 33:107–112, 1990

Tourigny-Rivard MF, Raskind M, Rivard D: The dexamethasone suppression test in an elderly population. Biol Psychiatry 16:1177–1184, 1981

Tsuboyama GK, Gabriel SS, Davis BM, et al: Neuroendocrine dysfunction in Alzheimer's disease: results following TRH stimulation. Biol Psychiatry 32:195–198, 1992

Uhde TW, Roy-Byrne PP, Vittone BJ: Phenomenology and neurobiology of panic disorder, in Anxiety and the Anxiety Disorders. Edited by Tuma M. Hillsdale, NJ, Erlbaum, 1985, pp 557–576

Uhde TW, Tancer ME, Rubinow DR, et al: Evidence for hypothalamo-growth hormone dysfunction in panic disorder; profile of growth hormone (GH) responses to clonidine, yohimbine, caffeine, glucose, GRH and TRH in panic disorder patients versus healthy volunteers. Neuropsychopharmacology 6:101–118, 1992

Urakami K, Takahashi K, Matsushima E, et al: The threshold of pain and neurotransmitter's change on pain in Parkinson's disease. Jpn J Psychiatry Neurol 44(3):589–593, 1990

Vestal RE, Wood AJJ, Shand DG: Reduced b-adrenoceptor sensitivity in the elderly. Clin Pharmacol Ther 26:181–186, 1979

Vijayashankar N, Brody H: A quantitative study of the pigmented neurons in the nuclei locus coeruleus and subcoeruleus in man as related to aging. J Neuropathol Exp Neurol 38:490–497, 1979

Villacres EC, Hollifield M, Katon WJ, et al: Sympathetic nervous system activity in panic disorder. Psychiatry Res 21:313–321, 1987

Vitiello B, Veith RC, Molchan SE, et al: Autonomic dysfunction in patients with dementia of the Alzheimer type. Biol Psychiatry 34:428–433, 1993

Volpi R, Scaglioni A, Marcato A, et al: Failure of the gamma-aminobutyric acid (GABA) derivative, baclofen, to stimulate growth hormone secretion in Parkinson's disease. J Neural Transm 3:259–264, 1991

Warburton DM: Nicotine as a cognitive enhancer. Prog Neuropsychopharmacol Biol Psychiatry 16:181–191, 1992

Warner MD, Vinogradov S, Peabody CA, et al: TRH/LHRH Stimulation test and Alzheimer's disease. Biol Psychiatry 28:358–362, 1990

Wesnes K, Revell A: The separate and combined effects of scopolamine and nicotine on human information processing. Psychopharmacology 84:5–11, 1984

Whitehouse PJ, Kellar KH: Nicotinic and muscarinic cholinergic receptors in Alzheimer's disease and related disorders. J Neural Transm Suppl 24:175–182, 1987

Wolkowitz OW, Weingartner H, Thompson K, et al: Diazepam induced amnesia: a neuropharmacological model of an "organic amnestic syndrome." Am J Psychiatry 144:25–29, 1987

Ziegler MG, Lake CR, Kopin IJ: Plasma noradrenaline increases with age. Nature 261:333–335, 1976

Zorumski CF, Isenberg KE: Insights into the structure and function of GABA-benzodiazepine receptors: ion channels and psychiatry. Am J Psychiatry 148:162–173, 1991

Zubenko GS: Biological correlates of clinical heterogeneity in primary dementia. Neuropsychopharmacology 6:77–93, 1992

Zweig RM, Ross CA, Hedreen JC, et al: The neuropathology of aminergic nuclei in Alzheimer's disease. Ann Neurol 24:233–242, 1988

29

Geriatric Neuropsychopharmacology

Steven L. Dubovsky, M.D.

Introduction

Accounting for 11% of the population, elderly individuals take 20%–25% of all prescribed medications (Sargenti et al. 1988). The average nursing home patient takes 9.3 medications (Pollock et al. 1992), at least one of which is likely to be a psychotropic medication (Avorn et al. 1992). Patients may continue for many years to take medications that contribute to neurological morbidity. For example, in one study (Salzman 1992) 1.3% of patients over the age of 80 were found to have been taking meprobamate for more than 25 years.

A number of factors complicate the prescription of psychotropic medications for geriatric patients with neurological illnesses (Ahronheim 1992; Salzman 1992; Sargenti et al. 1988). Adding these drugs to medications the patient already is taking—including over-the-counter substances that may not be reported to the physician—not only increases the risk of interactions, but makes it difficult for patients with memory impairment to keep track of which pills must be taken when. Further, patients with tremor, arthritis, visual problems, or confusion find it difficult to open the child-proof containers that pharmacists are required by many states to dispense unless directed otherwise.

In this chapter, I review the pharmacological treatment of neuropsychiatric conditions in elderly patients. To facilitate an understanding of parameters that affect pharmacotherapy in older patients with neuropsychiatric disorders, I briefly review general principles of pharmacology and physiology applicable to geriatric neuropsychiatry. I then review the use of the major classes of psychotropic medications and the treatment of special problems such as delirium and agitated dementia. Medication doses and half-lives in elderly patients are provided in tables and in the text. (Electroconvulsive therapy [ECT] is considered in detail in Chapter 30.)

Changes in the Aging Nervous System Relevant to Psychopharmacology

Even in the absence of frank neurological disease, changes in brain structure and function as the nervous system ages make older patients more vulnerable to side effects of psychotropic medications (Ahronheim 1992; Rovner 1990; Salzman 1990; Sargenti et al. 1988). Loss of neurons in the cortex, locus coeruleus,

and hippocampus makes sedative and psychomotor side effects more pronounced. A gradual decline in central cholinergic transmission increases sensitivity to anticholinergic side effects such as confusion and amnesia, which are even more marked in the presence of dementia. Reduced sensitivity of baroreceptors in the carotid artery and of hypothalamic blood pressure regulatory centers, along with decreased numbers of α_1-noradrenergic receptors, make it difficult to maintain blood pressure in the face of the hypotensive effects of antidepressants and neuroleptics. A decline in neurons in the substantia nigra and of dopamine receptors in the corpus striatum increases sensitivity to extrapyramidal side effects, which is usually a limiting side effect in the presence of Parkinson's disease.

Although it is clearly established that elderly patients are more sensitive to side effects of psychotropic medications, especially sedation, psychomotor impairment, orthostatic hypotension, and anticholinergic side effects (Abernathy 1992), there is no empirical support in most cases for the common assertion that geriatric patients are also more sensitive to therapeutic actions at the same blood levels (versus doses) (Abernathy 1992; Young and Meyers 1991). Indeed, reduced sensitivity of beta (Ahronheim 1992; Rovner 1990), benzodiazepine (Young and Meyers 1991), and other receptors may make some drugs less efficient in elderly patients. This issue is considered in more detail in discussions of specific medications.

Formal research into psychotropic drug effects in elderly patients with neuropsychiatric illnesses has not been extensive. It is therefore necessary to extrapolate from anecdotal experience and from studies in the broader field of geropsychiatry to develop pharmacological principles for geriatric neuropsychiatry.

Psychopharmacological Principles

A few basic concepts help to predict medication actions in elderly neuropsychiatric patients (Ahronheim 1992; Abernathy 1992). *Pharmacokinetics,* or what the body does to a drug, refers to factors influencing drug disposition including absorption, distribution, metabolism, and excretion. *Pharmacodynamics,* the processes influencing the action of drugs at tissue sites, describes what the medication does to the body. The *volume of distribution* is the hypothetical volume in which a medication is in equilibrium, reflecting how widely a drug is distributed throughout the body.

The *elimination half-life* is the time required to eliminate half the amount of medication in the body. It takes four to five half-lives, which for many drugs administered to elderly patients is more than 2 weeks (Abernathy 1992), to eliminate about 90% of a drug. When the interval between doses is less than the elimination half-life, the medication accumulates until the amount entering the plasma equals the amount being cleared (Abernathy 1992). This is the *steady state concentration,* which is directly proportional to the dose and inversely proportional to the clearance (Young and Meyers 1991). It takes four to five half-lives to achieve about 90% of a steady state (Abernathy 1992).

Although gastrointestinal absorption is essentially unchanged in elderly patients (Abernathy 1992; Young and Meyers 1992), anticholinergic drugs and antacids frequently used by older neurological patients delay absorption of other medications (Abernathy 1992). Once a medication is absorbed, its metabolism is altered in aging in several ways (Abernathy 1992; Sargenti et al. 1988; Young and Meyers 1992). First-pass metabolism, which occurs when a drug is carried from the gut to the liver following absorption, is slowed because hepatic blood flow decreases with age. As a result, the blood level and, therefore, the effect of drugs with extensive first-pass metabolism (e.g., triazolam, midazolam, neuroleptics, and all antidepressants except trazodone) can be increased.

After return to the circulation following first-pass metabolism, medications undergo another series of metabolic transformations (Ahronheim 1992; Salzman 1990). Phase I (or oxidative) metabolism is mediated by the cytochrome P450 oxidase system and produces demethylated biologically active metabolites. For example, diazepam is metabolized to desmethyldiazepam, desmethyldiazepam is metabolized to oxazepam, amitriptyline is metabolized to nortriptyline, and nortriptyline is metabolized to 11-hydroxy-nortriptyline. Because phase I metabolism slows with aging, blood levels and half-lives of parent compounds of many tricyclic antidepressants (TCAs), benzodiazepines, neuroleptics, and anticonvulsants tend to increase, causing more toxic, as well as therapeutic, effects at the same dose. Phase II metabolism, which through glucuronidation, acetylation, or sulfation produces inactive water-soluble metabolites that are excreted by the kidney, is not altered by the aging process.

Slowed oxidative metabolism should result in a lower dose of most psychotropic medications being necessary to achieve the same blood level. However,

metabolic rates vary substantially from person to person, and the number of individuals with slow metabolism by the P450 system does not increase with age (Pollock et al. 1992). Some older patients therefore will continue to demonstrate rapid phase I metabolism throughout the life span and will need the same medication doses as younger patients to achieve a therapeutic level (Pollock et al. 1992).

The distribution of psychotropic drugs changes significantly with age. Because all psychotropics—with the exception of lithium—are lipid soluble, they distribute into fatty tissue, which increases as a percentage of total body weight from 19% at age 25 to 35% at age 70 (Young and Meyers 1991). As a result, psychotropic medications distribute more widely in peripheral tissues and remain in the body longer, and the proportion diffusing into the brain slows because of increased distribution elsewhere (Abernathy 1992). Because equilibration in the body takes longer, it takes more time to reach a steady state and the onset of therapeutic effect may be delayed. Side effects and drug accumulation may also begin later than anticipated (Abernathy 1992). The reverse effects occur with lithium, which, being hydrophilic, has a decreased volume of distribution in elderly patients (Abernathy 1992).

All psychotropic medications except lithium are extensively bound to plasma protein, and only the unbound fraction is available both for pharmacological action and for metabolism (Abernathy 1992; Young and Meyers 1991). Changes in protein binding do not produce noticeable changes in drug action in healthy elderly patients, but those with significant decreases in serum albumin concentration (e.g., because of inanition) may develop elevated levels of free benzodiazepines and anticonvulsants (Young and Meyers 1991). Acutely ill geriatric patients may have elevated levels of α_1-glycoprotein, which binds heterocyclic antidepressants (HCAs) and neuroleptics, leading to reduced therapeutic effects of these drugs at the same total blood level (Sargenti et al. 1988).

All psychotropic drugs are excreted by the kidneys, lithium directly and other medications after metabolic transformation in the liver to hydrophilic metabolites (Abernathy 1992; Young and Meyers 1991). As a result of reduced renal blood flow, creatinine clearance falls by up to 60% in elderly patients (Abernathy 1992; Young and Meyers 1991). Reduced renal lithium clearance, combined with its smaller volume of distribution, leads to higher lithium levels and a half-life increased by up to 50% (Abernathy 1992; Young and Meyers

1991). Diminished clearance of water-soluble metabolites of TCAs with cardiotoxic potential (e.g., 11-hydroxy-nortriptyline) can enhance cardiac and other toxic effects of these drugs.

Longer half-lives, longer times to reach a steady state, larger volumes of distribution of lipid-soluble drugs, and slower elimination, along with hypersensitivity of the central nervous system (CNS) to many toxic effects, necessitates changes in prescribing practices for elderly neuropsychiatric patients. Initial doses should be lower than those for younger patients, and more time should elapse between dosage increments. Some patients may achieve therapeutic levels at lower final doses, but others may ultimately require the same doses as younger patients. The appearance of toxicity, especially in the CNS, as well as therapeutic effects, may be delayed longer than in younger adults. Approaches to these problems are outlined in the following discussions of specific medication categories.

Heterocyclic Antidepressants (HCAs)

Depression, the most common psychiatric disorder in elderly patients, often is a neuropsychiatric condition in this population in that it is often associated with cognitive complaints (McMahon and DePaulo 1992), cortical and subcortical atrophy and basal ganglia lesions (Coffey et al. 1993; Rabins et al. 1991), and treatment resistance (Coffey et al. 1991; Rabins et al. 1991). Disruption of systems for affective expression caused by brain lesions can result in atypical presentations of depression that may include unusual course of the neurological illness, lack of initiative, pseudodementia, and toothache and other odd forms of pain (Ruegg et al. 1988; Salzman 1985).

Poststroke depression and depression associated with Parkinson's disease are the two best-studied forms of geriatric neuropsychiatric depression. Both raise principles that apply to the general use of antidepressants in geriatric neuropsychiatry. Poststroke depression (see Chapter 23) is more likely to occur in patients with left-sided and right posterior lesions; enlarged ventricles and poorer functioning on mental status examination are additional risk factors (Dagon 1990; Robinson et al. 1984). Further, poststroke depression may represent an interaction between premorbid risk factors such as previous depressive episodes, side of lesion, and location of lesion (frontal versus non frontal and dorsal versus ventral) (C. A. Ross 1992). No matter

what the pathophysiology, poststroke depression may respond to antidepressants (Lipsey et al. 1984; Robinson et al. 1984).

Depression is also a common complication of Parkinson's disease, and this syndrome also may respond to antidepressant therapy (Cummings 1992). As discussed below, some dementia patients who do not appear depressed because the full depressive syndrome is masked by the organic mental disorder may benefit from antidepressants (E. D. Ross and Rush 1981). Antidepressants are less useful for elderly patients with dysphoria not meeting criteria for major depression (Salzman 1990).

Antidepressants produce about a 60% remission rate in elderly patients, compared with a 13% remission rate with placebo (Georgotas et al. 1986). However, relapse is common (Georgotas et al. 1988; Zis and Goodwin 1979), especially in patients with an incomplete remission, chronic depression, and three or more previous depressive episodes (Georgotas et al. 1988). Continuation therapy for 8 months to 2 years has been found to decrease relapse rates significantly compared with placebo (Young and Meyers 1991).

Neurological Uses of HCAs

HCAs have been used as primary treatments for some neurological disorders, but such applications have not been studied formally in elderly neuropsychiatric patients, and older neuropsychiatric patients have not been compared with younger ones. Amitriptyline, imipramine, desipramine, doxepin, and trazodone have been found to reduce chronic pain in both usual antidepressant doses and lower doses (Hoogiverf 1985; Rosenblatt et al. 1984). Rectal doxepin in doses of 25–150 mg/day has been found to ameliorate chronic pain in terminally ill cancer patients who were too weak to take the medication orally (Storey and Trumble 1992). Even though many patients with chronic pain are depressed, the antinociceptive effect does not seem to be dependent on an antidepressant action in that one state may improve with an antidepressant but not the other. The finding that desipramine, but not fluoxetine, was as effective as amitriptyline for neuropathic pain suggests that a serotonergic mechanism may not be essential for pain relief by antidepressants, as is commonly assumed (Max et al. 1992).

In younger patients, amitriptyline is frequently used as a prophylactic agent for migraine headaches (Mathew 1981). Other TCAs are probably effective too, although propranolol may be a more reliable anti-migraine drug (Goodman and Charney 1985). Many patients find that migraine headaches become less frequent and severe with age, permitting a reduction in migraine prophylaxis. Highly serotonergic antidepressants such as fluoxetine and sertraline often make migraine headaches worse. Fluoxetine (Lauterbach and Schiveri 1991) and amitriptyline (Schiffer et al. 1985) have been noted to ameliorate pseudobulbar affect in some patients with cerebral disease.

Available Preparations

HCAs (Table 29–1) have different structures containing rings comprised of carbon, nitrogen, and/or oxygen with varying side chains. Tertiary amine TCAs such as amitriptyline and imipramine are used as reference antidepressants in many studies, but they are poorly tolerated by older patients with organic brain disease. Secondary amine congeners of these drugs such as nortriptyline and desipramine, which have the additional advantage of demonstrated correlations between blood level and clinical response, are better choices for older patients (Young and Meyers 1991).

Table 29–1. Heterocyclic antidepressants in use in the United States

Medication	Trade name	Starting dose (mg)[a]	Daily dose (mg)
Amitriptyline[b]	Elavil	10	25–100
Nortriptyline[b,c,d]	Pamelor, Aventyl	10	10–50[c]
Protriptyline[b]	Vivactil	5	5–20
Imipramine[b,d]	Tofranil	10	25–100[c]
Desipramine[b,c,d]	Norpramin, Pertofrane	10	25–100[c]
Trimipramine[b]	Surmontil	10	25–100
Clomipramine[b]	Anafranil	10	50–150
Doxepin[b]	Sinequan, Adapin	10	10–75
Amoxapine	Asendin	10	25–300
Maprotiline	Ludiomil	10	25–75
Trazodone	Desyrel	25	25–200
Fluoxetine	Prozac	5	5–20
Bupropion	Wellbutrin	75	75–450
Sertraline	Zoloft	50	50–150
Paroxetine	Paxil	10	20–40

[a]All doses are geriatric doses.
[b]Tricyclic antidepressant.
[c]Secondary amine.
[d]Dose adjusted according to blood level.

Newer antidepressants are no more effective than the TCAs for nonpsychotic depression and may be less effective for psychotic depression (Rockwell et al. 1988), but they have fewer sedative, anticholinergic, cardiotoxic, and psychomotor side effects (Gottfries and Hesse 1990; Roose et al. 1991).

HCA Metabolism and Dosing in the Elderly

Certain aspects of antidepressant metabolism that change with aging must be taken into consideration in prescribing these drugs to older neuropsychiatric patients (Abernathy 1992; Alexopoulos 1992; Rockwell et al. 1988; C. K. Cohen et al. 1990). Tertiary amine antidepressants are demethylated to secondary amines, and these and other antidepressants are hydrolyzed by the P450 system to water-soluble hydroxy metabolites that are cleared by the kidneys. Some of these metabolites (e.g., 10-hydroxy-nortriptyline, 2-hydroxy-desipramine) have been linked to cardiac conduction defects, and some (e.g., 2-hydroxy-desipramine) may have antidepressant properties.

Because the efficiency of demethylation diminishes with age, conversion of tertiary amines to secondary amine metabolites is slower, and the parent compounds, which have more adverse effects, tend to accumulate. In addition, reduced renal clearance of cardiotoxic hydroxy metabolites enhances cardiac side effects at therapeutic doses. Phase I clearance of newer antidepressants such as fluoxetine, sertraline, and bupropion is impaired by age, but less so than that of the TCAs. However, even in younger patients, the half-life of fluoxetine is 1–3 days and the half-life of its active metabolite norfluoxetine can increase from 9 days to 3 weeks with chronic use (Pato et al. 1991). Slower metabolism of antidepressants results in longer half-lives, more time to reach a steady state, and higher blood levels of the parent drug. These factors are not affected by brain disease.

Although therapeutic and toxic blood levels may be achieved with lower antidepressant doses in the elderly, the same blood levels and even the same doses as in younger patients may be necessary for an antidepressant effect in many elderly depressed patients. Young et al. (1985) found a mean dose of 75 mg/day of nortriptyline to be effective for the treatment of geriatric depression. Roose et al. (1987) used nortriptyline doses of 87–92 mg/day with mean serum nortriptyline levels of 92 ng/ml, and imipramine doses of 240–280 mg/day with mean serum imipramine plus desipramine levels greater than 300 ng/ml. Nortriptyline levels of 50–150 ng/ml and desipramine levels above 125 ng/ml have been found necessary for antidepressant efficacy in elderly patients in other reports (Dagon 1990; Young and Meyers 1991) and Georgotas et al. (1986) confirmed that roughly the same nortriptyline therapeutic window (50–180 ng/ml) applied to elderly patients that is usually reported in younger adults (50–150 ng/ml) (Rubin et al. 1985).

In a study of desipramine in unipolar nonpsychotic depression in patients over age 60 (Nelson et al. 1985), the minimum effective desipramine level was 115 ng/ml, the same value found in a comparison group of patients under age 60. Doses of 125–350 mg/day were necessary in this study, and geriatric patients who did not respond initially improved when the dose was raised until the blood level was in the therapeutic range. These findings suggest that although lower doses and blood levels might be used initially, the dose should be increased in nonresponding patients until the serum level is in the therapeutic range for imipramine, desipramine, nortriptyline, and possibly amitriptyline or until the patient responds. However, side effects are more likely to occur at higher doses, and adverse effects are not correlated with blood levels, especially of parent compounds.

Neuropsychiatric Side Effects of HCAs

Some side effects of HCAs are particularly problematic in the neuropsychiatric setting. Examples are summarized in Table 29–2 (Ahronheim 1992; Alexopoulos 1992; Baldessarini and Marsh 1990; Bryner and Winograd 1992; Davidson 1989; Demuth et al. 1985; Herman et al. 1990; Jick et al. 1992; Paradis et al. 1992; Rizos et al. 1988; Rockwell et al. 1988; Roose et al. 1987, 1991; Yassa et al. 1987; Young and Meyers 1991; Young et al. 1985).

Special Consideration When Using HCAs in Geriatric Neuropsychiatry

Before treating depression in elderly patients with brain disease, an attempt should be made to discontinue medications and treat illnesses that cause depression. When antidepressants are indicated, tertiary amine TCAs should be avoided. Secondary amine TCAs and newer "atypical" HCAs such as bupropion and the selective serotonin uptake inhibitors are better tolerated.

Dementia.   Patients with diffuse brain disease or with dysfunction of the right hemisphere may lose the capacity to express affect directly and may express coexisting depression as negativism, emotional lability, hostility, catatonia, or cognitive disturbance out of proportion to the actual lesion (E. D. Ross and Rush 1981). Despite some controversy (see below) about whether antidepressants can improve cognition and behavior in dementia patients, a trial of an antidepressant or ECT may be the only means of determining how much disability may be attributable to unrecognized depression in these patients. Antidepressants that should be considered under these circumstances are those that are less likely to aggravate cognitive deficits such as sertraline, fluoxetine, bupropion, and the secondary amine TCAs. Acute confusion after ECT may be greater in some dementia patients, but the underlying dementia is not exacerbated (Dubovsky, in press).

Parkinson's disease.   The anticholinergic properties of tertiary amine antidepressants such as imipramine and amitriptyline could be useful in Parkinson's disease; however, the same properties aggravate the cognitive deficits that are often present and have additive side effects with other anticholinergic drugs that parkinsonian patients may be taking. Because of its dopaminergic properties, bupropion improves parkinsonian symptoms in about one-third of patients (Cummings 1992). The monoamine oxidase inhibitor (MAOI) L-deprenyl (selegiline), which is used as a primary treatment for Parkinson's disease, is an even more appropriate choice. Stimulants also have dopaminergic properties that could benefit some parkinsonian patients. The neuroleptic attributes of amoxapine contraindicate its use in the presence of Parkinson's disease. Because of their potential to produce extrapyramidal side effects, selective serotonin uptake inhibitors probably should also be avoided in patients with Parkinson's disease. Independent of its impact on depression, ECT has been shown to improve parkinsonism, especially with the on-off phenomenon (Cummings 1992; Dubovsky, in press). Bromocriptine, an antiparkinsonian dopamine agonist, may have antidepressant properties in some patients, but this and other antiparkinsonian drugs also may cause depression.

Seizure disorders.   In sufficient doses, all antidepressants have the potential to lower the seizure threshold (Davidson 1989), an effect that only rarely causes spontaneous seizures in patients who do not have neurolog-

Table 29–2. Some neuropsychiatric and related side effects of heterocyclic antidepressants

Side Effect	Manifestations and comments	Medications
Cardiovascular	Orthostatic hypotension; may cause falls when patient goes to bathroom in middle of night.	Tricyclic antidepressants, trazodone, maprotiline; less marked with secondary amines and newer antidepressants
	Type I antiarrhythmic effect causes suppression of ventricular arrhythmias and slowing of conduction. Conduction-repolarization abnormalities with nortriptyline correlated with concentration of E-10-hydroxy-nortriptyline.	Tricyclic antidepressants: not fluoxetine, paroxetine, or bupropion
	Tachycardia not as marked in older as in younger patients.	Imipramine, amitriptyline, clomipramine, trimipramine, doxepin, and maprotiline
	Aggravation of ventricular tachyarrhythmias.	Trazodone ?other serotonergic antidepressants
Sedation	Histamine, subtype 1 (H_1), receptor blockade causes oversedation, impaired memory and cognition, worsening of organic mental syndromes, and reduced new learning.	Amitriptyline, trimipramine, doxepin, maprotiline, trazodone, and clomipramine
Psychomotor impairment	Impaired driving. Tolerance often develops after 1–2 months.	Amitriptyline, imipramine, trimipramine, doxepin, clomipramine, and trazodone
Central anticholinergic syndrome	Anxiety, agitation, confusion, restlessness, disorientation, assaultiveness, and psychosis.	Amitriptyline, imipramine, clomipramine, trimipramine, doxepin, and maprotiline
Decreased seizure threshold	Usually involves aggravation of preexisting seizure disorders. Incidence of seizures probably less than 0.4–4 per 1,000 in nonepileptic patients taking therapeutic doses. Dose-related phenomenon for all antidepressants.	Bupropion, maprotiline, amoxapine, and tertiary amine tricyclic antidepressants, but not sertraline
Extrapyramidal	Parkinsonism caused by dopamine receptor blockade by amoxapine and inhibition of dopamine release resulting from serotonergic action of selective serotonin uptake inhibitors.	Amoxapine, fluoxetine, ?other serotonin uptake inhibitors, and high doses of imipramine and amitriptyline
	Akathisia has mechanism similar to parkinsonism.	Amoxapine, fluoxetine, and ?other serotonin uptake inhibitors
	Tardive dyskinesia: orofacial dyskinesia reported in 18 patients, only 6 of whom were taking antidepressant more than 4 months, suggesting chance association except for amoxapine.	Amoxapine, imipramine, amitriptyline, nortriptyline, clomipramine, trazodone, doxepin, nomifensine, and tranylcypromine
Falls	Caused by sedation, orthostatic hypotension, and impaired balance.	Imipramine, amitriptyline, doxepin, trazodone, and clomipramine
Neuromuscular	Tremor and myoclonus.	Tricyclic antidepressants, and maprotiline
	Peripheral neuropathy.	Amitriptyline
	Proximal myopathy.	Imipramine
Sleep disorders	Vivid dreams, nightmares, and insomnia.	Desipramine, nortriptyline, protriptyline, and fluoxetine
Auditory disturbance	Tinnitus.	Most tricyclic antidepressants
Gastrointestinal	Weight gain.	Many tricyclic antidepressants
	Anorexia, nausea, and significant weight loss.	Fluoxetine
Urological	Urinary retention.	Amitriptyline, imipramine, trimipramine, doxepin, and maprotiline
	Priapism not yet reported in elderly.	Trazodone
	Sexual dysfunction may respond to yohimbine, cyproheptadine, trazodone.	Serotonin uptake inhibitors

ical predisposing factors (Jick et al. 1992). For most antidepressants, the dose at which seizures may occur are considerably higher than the usually therapeutic range, but in the cases of bupropion and maprotiline, doses that can produce seizures (greater than 450 and 225 mg/day, respectively, in younger adults) overlap therapeutic doses (Davidson 1989). Doses of these drugs at which epilepsy may be aggravated in older patients are not known, but because they may be close to the geriatric therapeutic range it is wise to avoid bupropion and maprotiline in older epileptic patients. Amoxapine, which can cause intractable seizures in elderly patients, should not be taken at all by these patients (Litovitz and Troutman 1983). Doxepin, secondary amine TCAs, and MAOIs are relatively safe in epileptic patients. In one study of younger adults (C. K. Cohen et al. 1990), sertraline at a mean dose of 117 mg/day did not lower the seizure threshold.

HCA Interactions

HCAs interact with many other medications that are prescribed in geriatric neuropsychiatry. Some important examples are listed in Table 29–3 (Bailey et al. 1992; Dagon 1990; Rizos et al. 1988; Sargenti et al. 1988; Young and Meyers 1991).

Alternatives to HCAs

When interactions, side effects, or lack of efficacy limit the usefulness of HCAs or when the patient is severely ill, ECT is an obvious consideration, even in the presence of epilepsy, dementia, or delirium (see Chapter 30). Stimulants (discussed below) are useful in treating apathetic depression associated with neurological illness. In doses of 40–90 mg/day buspirone has antidepressant properties in younger patients (Rickels et al. 1991), and augmentation of HCAs with buspirone in doses of 10–60 mg/day can be as effective as lithium augmentation with fewer side effects in older patients with brain disease.

Exposure to 2,500–10,000 lux of light for 0.5–2 hours has been found to be an effective treatment for seasonal affective disorder and some cases of nonseasonal depression. Like any antidepressant, artificial bright light can induce hypomania. The incidence of seasonal affective disorder and the effectiveness of bright light in the geriatric population has not been studied formally, but consideration of this treatment is warranted in patients with a seasonal variation of mood who cannot tolerate antidepressant side effects. Medications that sensitize the lens and retina of the eye to phototoxicity, including imipramine, fluoxetine, lith-

Table 29–3. Some potential heterocyclic antidepressant interactions

Medication	Interacting medication	Interaction
Tricyclic antidepressants (TCAs)	Anticholinergic drugs	Additive anticholinergic effects
	Tranquilizers, sedatives, and low-potency neuroleptics	Increased sedation
	Low-potency neuroleptics and antihypertensive drugs	Increased orthostatic hypotension
	Antihypertensives (clonidine, guanethidine, bethanidine, and debrisoquin)	Decreased effect of both classes
	Adding TCA to antihypertensive	Hypertensive crisis
	Type I antiarrhythmics	Additive antiarrhythmic effect, prolonged Q-T interval, widened QRS complex, and increased risk of bundle branch block
	Directly acting sympathomimetics	Potentiation of sympathomimetic
	Disulfiram	Increased activity of both classes
	Cimetidine	Increased TCA levels
Selective serotonic uptake inhibitors	Lithium, tryptophan, buspirone, and other serotonergic drugs	Headache and serotonin syndrome
	Monoamine oxidase inhibitors	Fatal serotonin syndrome
All heterocyclic antidepressants	Neuroleptics other than flupenthixol	Increased levels of both classes; clinically relevant for antidepressant
	Stimulants	Increased antidepressant levels
	Anticonvulsants	Decreased antidepressant levels
	Cholestyramine	Decreased antidepressant levels

ium, chlorpromazine, thioridazine, and propranolol, should be used with great caution, if at all, in elderly patients who are exposed to bright light or who spend much time in the sun (Roberts et al. 1992).

Monoamine Oxidase Inhibitors (MAOIs)

Currently undergoing a renaissance, MAOIs are as effective as TCAs in treating geriatric depression (Georgotas et al. 1986). In fact, because activity of the B form of MAO increases with aging and is even higher in Alzheimer patients (Alexopoulos 1992), MAOIs may be particularly appropriate choices in geriatric neuropsychiatry (Rockwell et al. 1988), especially in the presence of apathy and low motivation (Salzman 1990). Depressed patients with physical symptoms of anxiety that mimic neurological disease such as light headedness, dizziness, numbness, and paresthesias may be candidates for MAOIs, especially in the presence of rejection sensitivity, mood reactivity, and intolerance of or lack of response to HCAs (Pare 1985).

Neurological Uses of MAOIs

At doses of 5–10 mg/day, selegiline is a treatment for Parkinson's disease that does not interact with other antiparkinsonian drugs or tyramine-containing foods. Selegiline was found in several open studies and one single-blind investigation to improve anxiety, depression, and cognitive dysfunction in Alzheimer patients (Schneider and Sobin 1992). Because they suppress rapid-eye-movement (REM) sleep and have alerting properties, MAOIs can be used to treat narcolepsy.

Available Preparations

Three classes of MAOIs (Alexopoulos 1992) are now in use in the United States (Table 29–4). Tranylcypromine has amphetamine-like properties and is the most stimulating of the MAOIs. Inhibition of MAO does not persist as long after tranylcypromine is discontinued as it does after withdrawal of other MAOIs. The antidepressant dose of selegiline (20–40 mg/day) is higher than the antiparkinsonian dose. However, side effects may be less troublesome than with other MAOIs.

MAOI Metabolism and Dosing in the Elderly

MAOIs are metabolized by acetylation, which is not affected by aging; however, plasma levels in elderly pa-

tients are usually higher with a given dose, probably because of slowing of additional metabolic steps (Alexopoulos 1992). Initial doses, rate of dosage increment, and final doses therefore are lower for geriatric patients than for younger patients. However, the dose of MAOI necessary to inhibit MAO is not always lower than that in younger patients (Alexopoulos 1992), and some elderly depressed patients require the same MAOI doses as do younger patients (Young and Meyers 1991). In addition, half of the Caucasian population are "rapid acetylators," an effect that is not attenuated by age. These individuals may require higher doses than those recommended by the manufacturer, which by and large are not based on prospective dose-response studies.

Neuropsychiatric Side Effects of MAOIs

MAOIs produce more side effects in elderly patients than do HCAs (Georgotas et al. 1988). Some examples are listed in Table 29–5 (Alexopoulos 1992; Georgotas et al. 1986, 1988; Lawrence 1985; Lieberman et al. 1985; Meyler and Herxheimer 1968; Pare 1985; Sargenti et al. 1988).

Special Considerations When Using MAOIs in Geriatric Neuropsychiatry

Although seizures have occurred in nonepileptic patients after overdose of MAOIs, in therapeutic doses these drugs are safe for epileptic patients. Patients with carcinoid or pheochromocytoma should not be given MAOIs because of the risk of fatal serotonergic or hy-

Table 29–4. Monoamine oxidase inhibitors in use in the United States

Medication (by class)	Trade name	Starting dose (mg)	Daily dose[a] (mg)
Hydrazine			
Phenelzine	Nardil	7.5	15–60
Isocarboxazid	Marplan	5	10–30[b]
Nonhydrazine			
Tranylcypromine	Parnate	5	10–40
Pargyline	Eutonyl[c]	5	10–40
Phenylethylamine			
Selegiline (L-deprenyl)	Eldepryl	5	10–40[d]

[a]Higher doses may be necessary.
[b]Experience in elderly patients limited.
[c]Recently withdrawn due to poor sales.
[d]Antiparkinsonian dose = 5–10 mg.

pertensive reactions. Selegiline is an appropriate first choice for the treatment of depressed parkinsonian patients, although at higher doses (see below) it could interact with levodopa, bromocriptine, and dietary substances. Elderly patients often take over-the-counter preparations they do not consider medications and therefore do not think about when warned about potential MAOI interactions. The major risk of MAOIs in dementia patients is that they will not remember the dietary restrictions (Young and Meyers 1991). MAOIs do not aggravate cardiac conduction delays (Young and Meyers 1991).

MAOI Interactions

MAOIs have two potentially dangerous interactions. The first is the hypertensive reaction that occurs with foods that are high in tyramine content and with certain medications. Hypertensive reactions occur because MAOIs irreversibly inhibit both MAO-A, which is found in the gut and the brain, and MAO-B, which is found in the brain but not the gut. Because MAO-A metabolizes ingested tyramine (a pressor amine found in many foods) before it can be absorbed into the bloodstream, inhibition of the enzyme results in increased intestinal absorption of tyramine and an amplified pressor response that is augmented by decreased tyramine metabolism in sympathetic nerve ganglia. Hypertensive crises are no more common in elderly patients than in other patients (Georgotas et al. 1986), but they are more dangerous in patients with fragile cerebral vasculature. Because selegiline is selective for MAO-B at antiparkinsonian doses and there-

fore does not inhibit intestinal MAO, tyramine in the gastrointestinal tract is degraded normally. However, at doses above 10 mg/day selegiline loses its selectivity and inhibits MAO-A, producing tyramine reactions.

A study of traditionally proscribed foods found that the tyramine content of most of them is so low that massive amounts (e.g., 50 glasses of wine) would have to be ingested to produce a hypertensive reaction (Shulman et al. 1989). The investigators suggested that a more realistic list would include all cheese except cottage cheese and cream cheese, concentrated yeast extract, sauerkraut, broad bean pods, aged meats, salami, air-dried sausage, old chicken liver, protein extracts, spoiled protein-containing foods, pure soy products, and Chinese food. Patients should refrain from sympathomimetic drugs including most cold preparations, decongestants, and anorectics. Antihistamines, acetaminophen, Cepacol, Sucrets, plain Robitussin, and plain Alka-Seltzer are safe, but Alka-Seltzer Plus is not. Dextromethorphan, which has serotonergic properties, should be avoided because of the risk of serotonin syndrome (described below). Dark fermented tap beer, even if it is nonalcoholic should be avoided.

Experience with younger patients suggests that a 10-mg tablet of nifedipine chewed and placed under the tongue for rapid absorption can blunt the severity of hypertensive reactions (Clary and Schweitzer 1987) until the more definitive treatment of phentolamine 2–5 mg iv can be given. This approach has not been studied in the elderly. Chlorpromazine should not be used to treat hypertensive reactions because of the risk of dangerous hypotensive and anticholinergic side effects in geriatric neuropsychiatric patients.

Table 29–5. Neuropsychiatric side effects of monoamine oxidase inhibitors (MAOIs)

Side effect	Manifestations	Comments
Altered brain function	Sedation, activation, headache, paradoxical reactions, memory loss, confusion, ataxia, irritability, insomnia, mania, and psychosis	Abrupt withdrawal can cause insomnia, nightmares, mania, psychosis, and delirium.
Autonomic dysfunction	Postural hypotension, anticholinergic side effects, and sexual dysfunction	Phenelzine and isocarboxazid most anticholinergic.
Peripheral nervous system dysfunction	Peripheral neuropathy, paresthesias, gait disturbance, and falls	Caused by direct neurotoxicity or interference with B_6 metabolism. Pyridoxine replacement may be helpful.
Neuromuscular irritability	Twitching, myoclonus, muscle tension, tremor, and muscle and joint pain	May reflect mild serotonin syndrome. Nocturnal myoclonus occurs in 10%–15% of patients taking phenelzine. No tolerance.
Sexual dysfunction	Anorgasmia and impotence	Cyproheptadine occasionally helpful. Avoid yohimbine.

Because serotonin is metabolized by MAO-A, the second type of dangerous MAOI interaction is with serotonergic substances such as L-tryptophan, meperidine, dextromethorphan, and the serotonergic antidepressants imipramine, clomipramine, fluoxetine, sertraline, paroxetine, and possibly buspirone (Salzman 1992; Sargenti et al. 1988); other TCAs can be safely combined with MAOIs if the TCA is started first and low initial doses of each medication are used. Serotonin syndrome is a neurotoxic condition characterized by ataxia, hyperreflexia, myoclonus, excitation, diaphoresis, dysarthria, paresthesias, fever, confusion, delirium, seizures, coma, hypotension, and fatal cardiac arrhythmias (Lieberman et al. 1985).

MAOIs interact with a number of other kinds of compounds, some of which are listed in Table 29–6 (Lieberman et al. 1985; Meyler and Herxheimer 1968; Pare 1985; Salzman 1992; Sargenti et al. 1988).

Stimulants

Stimulants increase central release of norepinephrine, dopamine, and serotonin and may have direct serotonin agonist properties (Hoffman and Lefkowitz 1990). Stimulants (available preparations of which are listed in Table 29–7 [Alexopoulos 1992; Salzman 1992]) have been found superior to placebo in some double-blind studies of geriatric depression and depression in dementia patients, especially those who are apathetic and unmotivated (Chiarello and Cole 1987; Rockwell et al. 1988). Chiarello and Cole (1987) suggested that a preference for coffee may be an indication of a good response to a stimulant. However, stimulants cannot be considered proven treatments for depression and their long-term benefits are generally questioned.

Depression in neurologically ill patients may respond within a few weeks to stimulants, although dose-finding studies have not been conducted. Cognitive deterioration was found in one study (Holmes et al. 1989) to improve along with depression when human immunodeficiency virus (HIV) encephalopathy was treated with stimulants. Tolerance to the antidepressant effect generally has not been noted in older neuropsychiatric patients (Kaufman et al. 1984), and appetite and sleep improve when the depression remits. The medication can often be withdrawn after a few months without return of symptoms (Kaufman et al. 1984), but chronic treatment has also been successful in some instances (Chiarello and Cole 1987).

Stimulants can also be used to augment HCAs in treatment-resistant geriatric depression. One strategy for patients who cannot tolerate therapeutic doses of HCAs is to administer a lower dose of HCA and increase the blood level with a stimulant, avoiding side effects associated with products of first-pass metabolism. Intermittent treatment of bipolar depression with a stimulant can reduce the risk of antidepressant-induced hypomania or mood cycling. The major neurological uses of stimulants are in the treatment of narcolepsy and of apathy and cognitive deterioration in chronic organic mental syndromes.

Stimulant Metabolism and Dosing in Geriatric Neuropsychiatry

Until formal data have accumulated about stimulant metabolism in the elderly, low initial doses and gradual

Table 29–6. Some potential monoamine oxidase inhibitor (MAOI) interactions

Medication	Interaction
Hydrazine[a] plus nonhydrazine[b] MAOI	Fever, hypertension, convulsions, stroke, and coma
Levodopa	Hypertension; less with carbidopa
Amantadine	Hypertension
General anesthetics, sedatives, narcotics, antihistamines, neuroleptics, and antiparkinsonian drugs	Potentiation of central nervous system depression due to inhibition of hepatic metabolism
Antihypertensive drugs	Increased hypotension
Insulin	Increased hypoglycemic effect
Reserpine and tetrabenazine	Excitation
Aspartame	Headache and diaphoresis
Bupropion	Increased bupropion toxicity

[a]Phenelzine and isocarboxazid.
[b]Tranylcypromine and pargyline.

Table 29–7. Commonly used central nervous system stimulants

Medication	Trade name	Starting dose (mg)	Usual daily dose (mg)
Dextroamphetamine	Dexedrine	2.5	2.5–60
Methylphenidate	Ritalin	2.5	2.5–60
Pemoline	Cylert	37.5	37.5–112.5

increments (e.g., by 2.5 mg/day of methylphenidate every week) are recommended (Table 29–7). Doses of 5–15 mg/day are often successful in antidepressant augmentation, and 10–40 mg/day are successful as primary treatment for depression in elderly neurologically ill patients.

Neuropsychiatric Side Effects of Stimulants

Stimulant side effects are usually dose related, toxicity being rare at doses less than 15 mg/day (Hoffman and Lefkowitz 1990). Many of the adverse effects in Table 29–8 represent excessive CNS and cardiovascular stimulation (Ahronheim 1992; Hoffman and Lefkowitz 1990; Rockwell et al. 1988; Young and Meyers 1991).

Special Considerations When Using Stimulants in Geriatric Neuropsychiatry

The dopaminergic properties of stimulants could be useful for depressed parkinsonian patients, but the same effect aggravates chorea and psychosis and may lower the seizure threshold. As discussed below, a trial of stimulants in dementia patients may help identify the component that is attributable to depression.

Stimulant Interactions

Stimulants raise blood levels of TCAs, neuroleptics, and other medications that are metabolized by the P450 system.

Antimanic Drugs

The risk of mania does not increase with age (Young and Klerman 1992), but bipolar disorder does not "burn out" with age either (Shulman et al. 1992; Snowdon 1991; Young and Meyers 1991). Mania or hypomania account for 5%–10% of all mood disorders treated in elderly patients (Young and Klerman 1992), and

5%–10% of all bipolar patients become ill for the first time after age 50 (Yassa et al. 1988). Even in the geriatric population, having had previous episodes of depression without mania is no guarantee of a unipolar illness, as up to 25 years may elapse between the onset of depression and the first manic episode (Snowdon 1991).

As is true of depression, mania in the elderly is more frequently a neuropsychiatric condition than it is in younger patients because it is often an expression of neurological disease (Snowdon 1991) and because manifestations of early-onset bipolar disorder can be modified later in life by coexisting organic brain disease (Young and Klerman 1992). In various reports, 24%–36% of cases of late-onset bipolar disorder have been associated with overt neurological disease (Shulman et al. 1992; Young and Meyers 1991), which is often present before the onset of mania (Snowdon 1991). The severity of the neurological component is indicated by a retrospective study in which half of 50 elderly manic patients were dead of medical causes after 6 years of follow-up (Shulman et al. 1992).

One common neurological precipitant of mania is stroke, especially in association with right-sided lesions of the frontal cortex, basal ganglia, thalamus, or basotemporal cortex or preexisting subcortical atrophy. Other neurological causes of late-onset mania include adrenal steroids, calcium replacement, levodopa, antidepressants, bronchodilators, decongestants, vitamin B_{12} deficiency, hyperthyroidism, epilepsy, and trauma or degenerative, vascular, or neoplastic disease of the right hemisphere (Dagon 1990; Snowdon 1991; Yassa et al. 1988; Young and Klerman 1992).

The frequent association of geriatric mania with neurological disease leads to a high frequency of cognitive dysfunction (Young and Klerman 1992) and resistance to lithium (Hardy et al. 1987; Young and Klerman 1992). Treatment of neurological causes and withdrawal of medications that cause mania may lead to improvement, but additional antimanic treatments are often necessary.

Table 29–8.   Neuropsychiatric side effects of stimulants

Side effect	Manifestations
Stimulation	Agitation, restlessness, tremor, diaphoresis, hyperreflexia, confusion, cognitive deterioration, paranoia, hallucinations, suicidal and homicidal behavior, and convulsions
Cardiovascular stimulation	Tachycardia, hypertension, hypotension, headache, palpitations, arrhythmias, angina, circulatory collapse, and cerebral hemorrhage

Lithium is the first choice for the treatment and prophylaxis of mania in the elderly. Lithium augmentation can be useful for bipolar and, to a lesser extent, unipolar depression (Jefferson 1990; Roy and Pickar 1985); obsessive-compulsive disorder (Jefferson 1990; Jenike 1990); and schizophrenia (Jefferson 1990).

Neurological Uses of Lithium

Lithium has been noted in uncontrolled studies to ameliorate cluster headaches, Huntington's disease, and spasmodic torticollis. Lithium-induced leukocytosis is a treatment for leukopenia caused by chemotherapy for cancer and autoimmune disease. Reduced renal water conservation caused by lithium may counteract the syndrome of inappropriate secretion of antidiuretic hormone, which can complicate some tumors and infections of the CNS.

Metabolism and Dosing in Elderly Patients

Because of age-related reduction of renal clearance and volume of distribution, only one-half to two-thirds of the usual adult dose is necessary to achieve the same plasma level as in younger patients (Liptzin 1992; Young and Meyers 1991). Lithium half-life is usually (Ahronheim 1992; Liptzin 1992), but not always (Hardy et al. 1987), increased to about 40 hours, resulting in a longer time to reach a steady state (Liptzin 1992) with a corresponding delay in onset of therapeutic action, as well as slower elimination after discontinuation. Because of the prolonged half-life, lithium doses should not be increased more frequently than once a week (Ahronheim 1992; Liptzin 1992). The risk of neurotoxic side effects probably warrants even slower dosage adjustments in elderly neuropsychiatric patients.

Clinical lore holds that the therapeutic effect of lithium occurs at lower blood levels, as well as lower doses, in the elderly (Salzman 1990). There is, however, no empirical evidence for this assertion (Hardy et al. 1987; Young and Meyers 1991). Low starting doses (e.g., 75–150 mg/day) and maintenance doses (e.g., 600–1,200 mg/day) are appropriate (Ahronheim 1992; Liptzin 1992), but the dose should be raised if the patient does not respond and the blood level is not in the usual adult therapeutic range. Single daily doses of lithium enhance compliance, reduce adverse effects, and are safe in elderly patients (Hardy et al. 1987; Mellerup and Plenge 1990).

Neuropsychiatric Side Effects of Lithium

Lithium toxicity is common at serum levels greater than 1.5–2.0 mEq/L, but toxicity may occur at therapeutic levels, especially in elderly patients with CNS disease (Hardy 1987; Liptzin 1992). Toxicity produces a coarse tremor, ataxia, vertigo, dysarthria, disorientation, nausea, and vomiting. Severe intoxication is associated with muscle fasciculations, hyperreflexia, confusion, delirium, seizures, and coma. Irreversible memory loss, brain damage, cerebellar symptoms, and motor deficits may occur following lithium intoxication (Saxena and Maltikarjuna 1988).

Lithium side effects, which occur at therapeutic levels, are more frequent at blood levels above 0.8 mEq/L, although the prophylactic effect is more reliable at higher levels, at least in younger adults (Gelenberg et al. 1989; Vestergaard et al. 1988). Hypokalemia increases the risk of neurological side effects (Jefferson and Greist 1977). Common CNS lithium side effects are summarized in Table 29–9 (Griffin 1992; Liptzin 1992; Rizos et al. 1988; Salzman 1990; Saul 1985; Schneider and Sobin 1992; Young and Meyers 1991).

Special Considerations When Using Lithium in Geriatric Neuropsychiatry

Lithium can lower the seizure threshold and induce seizures in nonepileptic patients (Massey and Folger 1984). However, in one report (Shukla et al. 1988), therapeutic lithium levels did not increase seizure frequency or anticonvulsant requirement in a small group of epileptic bipolar patients. The use of lithium in elderly patients with seizure disorders has not been investigated formally, but anticonvulsants with antimanic properties (see below) should be considered for such patients. Because lithium occasionally causes extrapyramidal side effects, it can be problematic in parkinsonian patients. Cognitive side effects of lithium are poorly tolerated by patients with dementia. Because lithium slows the rate of depolarization of the sinus node and conduction through the atrioventricular node, electrocardiogram and cardiac function should be followed closely in elderly patients with heart disease.

Lithium Interactions

Neurotoxic interactions between lithium and neuroleptics, which consist mainly of extrapyramidal and neuromuscular syndromes or delirium (F. Miller and Menninger 1987) may represent aggravation of lithium neurotoxicity by the neuroleptic, additive neurotoxic effects, or a true interaction between the two classes of medication. Neurotoxicity is more common with higher neuroleptic doses and higher lithium levels and may be irreversible in a few cases (Cohen and Cohen 1974; Izzo and Brody 1985). A neurotoxic interaction with clozapine that included confusion, delirium, incoordination, dystonias, and myoclonus has also been reported (Blake et al. 1992). Because neuroleptics are mainly used to control agitation and psychosis until the antimanic action of lithium develops, it has been recommended that the risk of neurotoxicity could be lessened by deferring lithium therapy until the patient's behavior is under control, at which point the neuroleptic can be gradually withdrawn (Chou 1991). Other interactions of lithium with drugs used in geriatric neuropsychiatry are summarized in Table 29–10 (Abernathy 1992; Ahronheim 1992; Chou 1991; Jefferson 1990; Liptzin 1992; P. J. Perry et al. 1984; Rizos et al. 1988; Salzman 1990; Young and Meyers 1991).

Alternatives to Lithium

ECT is clearly effective for mania in elderly patients (Black et al. 1987). None of the medications that have been used in younger manic patients as alternatives or adjuncts to lithium have been studied systematically in the elderly population (Young and Meyers 1991), but some anecdotal experience has accumulated.

Carbamazepine, the best studied of the alternatives to lithium, may be particularly useful in patients with mixed, rapidly cycling, and lithium-resistant bipolar disorders, although tolerance to prophylaxis of mood disorders may develop (Post 1990). Carbamazepine is an obvious choice for bipolar patients with abnormal electroencephalography (EEG) results or epilepsy and is better tolerated than lithium in elderly patients with brain damage. However, carbamazepine can cause confusion and neurotoxicity in some of these patients, especially when combined with other antimanic drugs or neuroleptics, and older patients may be unable to tolerate the sedation it causes. Carbamazepine can also be useful for trigeminal neuralgia, but is less so for other kinds of neuropathic pain (Ahronheim 1992).

Because carbamazepine induces its own metabolism, the half-life tends to decline over a month or so from 36 to 10–20 hours (Ahronheim 1992). Some therapeutic, as well as some toxic, effects of carbamazepine can be attributed to an active epoxy metabolite (Ahronheim 1992). The initial dose of carbamazepine in elderly patients should be 50–100 mg (Ahronheim 1992; Salzman 1990). The therapeutic dose for epilepsy, and presumably for mood disorders, in older patients is thought to be 300–1,200 mg/day (Liptzin 1992; Salzman 1990); higher doses may be necessary for pain control (Ahronheim 1992). Neuropsychiatric

---

Table 29–9. Neuropsychiatric side effects of lithium

Side effect	Manifestations and comments
Neuromuscular	Tremor, ataxia, dysarthria, incoordination, myoclonus. Falls may result from ataxia and incoordination. Elderly more prone to tremor and myoclonus.
Mental	Impaired memory, concentration and consciousness, anterograde amnesia, aphasia, confusion, dazed feeling, and flat affect.
Extrapyramidal	Parkinsonism.
Degenerative	Parkinsonism and Creutzfeldt-Jakob-like syndrome.
Intracranial	Pseudotumor cerebri.
Electroencephalographic	Generalized slowing, disorganization of background rhythm, epileptiform discharges, rapid-eye-movement (REM) suppression, and seizures.
Endocrine	Hyperparathyroidism may produce mental and neuromuscular symptoms, especially depression or mania. Hypothyroidism may initiate rapid cycling or confusion.
Renal	Polyuria and polydipsia not more common in elderly. Lithium does not cause or accelerate renal failure in elderly patients. Nephrogenic diabetes insipidus may be reduced by amiloride, which reduces lithium transport into collecting duct.

side effects and interactions of lithium are noted in Tables 29–11 and 29–12 (Ahronheim 1992; Liptzin 1992; Salzman 1990).

Valproic acid appears to be a most useful agent for some bipolar patients with abnormal EEG results, rapid cycling, mixed affective states, and resistance to other medications (Chou 1991). A few reports have emerged in which valproate was effective in elderly bipolar patients (for a review, see Liptzin 1992). Starting doses of 125 mg/day and total daily doses of 125–1,800 mg/day, with blood levels of 50–150 ng/ml have been

recommended (Liptzin 1992; Salzman 1990), but these can only be considered estimates in neurologically ill geriatric patients. Some valproate side effects and interactions are noted in Tables 29–11 and 29–12.

Verapamil in doses of 240–480 mg/day has been used in elderly bipolar patients with dementia with good results and minimal side effects (Dubovsky et al. 1986). Nimodipine and other "second generation" calcium channel blocking agents that may have applications in dementia (see below) could also be useful for geriatric bipolar illness complicated by dementia or cerebrovascular disease. Side effects and interactions of calcium channel blockers are included in Tables 29–11 and 29–12.

Table 29–10. Some potential lithium interactions

Medication	Interaction
Neuroleptics, carbamazepine, clonazepam, and calcium channel blockers	Neurotoxicity and increased extrapyramidal side effects
Thiazide diuretics and angiotensin-converting enzyme (ACE) inhibitors	Increase in serum lithium level by 35%
Furosemide and amiloride	No effect on lithium clearance
Theophylline, aminophylline, and ?caffeine	Increased lithium clearance, decreased lithium half-life
Nonsteroidal antiinflammatory drugs	Increase in serum lithium level by 50%
Tetracyclines, spectinomycin, and metronidazole	Increased serum lithium concentration
Iodine	Increased risk of hypothyroidism
Beta-blockers	Increased serum lithium concentrations
Fluoxetine	Increased serum lithium concentrations

Antianxiety Drugs

Benzodiazepines and azapirones have become the primary treatments for generalized anxiety in elderly patients. Benzodiazepines are most appropriately used to treat acute anxiety or insomnia in response to a discrete stress (Salzman 1990). Because generalized anxiety disorder is chronic and recurrent, ongoing treatment is often necessary. Azapirones are better tolerated by chronically anxious patients with organic brain disease because these drugs do not impair higher cortical function, but their delayed onset of action makes them ineffective when used on an as-needed basis.

Alprazolam has been most thoroughly studied as a treatment for panic disorder, but other benzodiazepines appear to be effective if administered in equivalent doses. Clonazepam has uses in the treatment of acute mania (Chouinard and Penry 1985), although

Table 29–11. Neuropsychiatric side effects of alternatives to lithium

Alternative	Side effect	Manifestation
Carbamazepine	Neurotoxicity	Ataxia, dizziness, sedation, lethargy, dipolpia, cognitive impairment, irritability, confusion, restlessness, and seizures
	Neuroendocrine	Syndrome of inappropriate secretion of antidiuretic hormone and hypocalcemia
	Hematologic	Transient leukopenia
	Hypersensitivity	Agranulocytosis, aplastic anemia, thrombocytopenia, rash, hepatitis, and pneumonitis
Valproic acid	Neurotoxicity	Sedation, ataxia, tremor, and increased appetite
	Dermatologic	Rash and alopecia
	Gastrointestinal	Anorexia, nausea, vomiting, and hepatitis in 1/50,000 adults
Verapamil	Neurological	Sedation, dizziness, headache, and occasional extrapyramidal signs
	Cardiovascular	Flushing, hypotension, and cardiac slowing

some of its apparent antimanic effect could be secondary to sedation, which is difficult for many older neuropsychiatric patients to tolerate. Alprazolam and perhaps other benzodiazepines may have antidepressant properties in mixed anxiety-depression, but antidepressants and/or azapirones have a much wider margin of safety for this indication in neurologically ill elderly patients. Azapirones can be used to augment antidepressants in the treatment of depression and obsessive-compulsive disorder.

Neurological Uses of Anxiolytics

Clonazepam is used to treat generalized, myoclonic, and absence seizures (Chouinard and Penry 1985). Clonazepam may also be useful in pain syndromes such as trigeminal neuralgia that are associated with paroxysmal dysesthesias, burning sensations and hyperesthesias (Bouckonis and Litman 1985), and paroxysmal choreoathetosis and neuroleptic-induced akathisia (Chouinard and Penry 1985). Intravenous diazepam is a well-known treatment for status epilepticus. Intravenous benzodiazepines have been used for severe agitation in delirious patients. Buspirone is emerging as a treatment for intermittent aggressive behavior in dementia patients (these applications are described below).

Available Preparations

Benzodiazepines can be divided into short and long half-life preparations. As a general rule, the long half-life drugs are poorly tolerated by elderly neuropsychiatric patients because accumulation leads to sedation,

amnesia, psychomotor impairment, ataxia, and falls (Ray 1992). Properties of benzodiazepines used to treat anxiety are summarized in Table 29–13 (Abernathy 1992; Ahronheim 1992; Regestein 1992; Salzman 1992; Salzman et al. 1983). (Benzodiazepine hypnotics are discussed below.)

Metabolism and Dosing

Unlike antidepressants, anticonvulsants, and low-potency neuroleptics, benzodiazepines do not induce their own metabolism (Salzman 1992). Diazepam, chlordiazepoxide, clorazepate, prazepam, halazepam, and flurazepam have long elimination half-lives that are prolonged two to three times in elderly patients (Regestein 1992), resulting in a longer time to reach a steady state and drug accumulation over time (Salzman et al. 1983). Long half-life benzodiazepines also have complex hepatic oxidative metabolism that produces desmethyldiazepam, an active metabolite with a half-life in elderly patients of 80–130 hours (Salzman 1990, 1992; Salzman et al. 1983).

Hydroxylated benzodiazepines such as oxazepam, lorazepam, alprazolam, triazolam, and temazepam have intermediate and shorter half-lives and simpler metabolic pathways that are not affected as significantly by aging (Salzman 1990, 1992; Salzman et al. 1983). Such medications do not accumulate in the elderly and are quicker to reach a steady state. Despite long half-lives in elderly patients, benzodiazepines are often given in divided dose to minimize periods of intoxication caused by blood level peaks. Recommended dosage ranges for geriatric neuropsychiatry are noted in Table 29–13.

Table 29–12. Some potential interactions of alternatives to lithium

Alternative	Medication	Interaction
Carbamazepine	Lithium	Neurotoxicity
	Anticonvulsants, neuroleptics, benzodiazepines, and coumadin	Decreased blood level of the other medication caused by enzyme induction
	Fluoxetine	Increased carbamazepine levels
	Neuroleptics	Neurotoxicity
	Cimetidine, erythromycin, and isoniazid	Increased carbamazepine levels
Valproic acid	Aspirin	Increased valproate levels
	Other anticonvulsants	Increased risk of hepatotoxicity, possibly caused by toxic intermediates of valproate metabolism
	Clonazepam	Absence status epilepticus
Verapamil	Carbamazepine, lithium	Increased carbamazepine and lithium levels, neurotoxicity
	Lithium, beta-blockers	Additive cardiac slowing

Neuropsychiatric Side Effects of Benzodiazepines

The older CNS seems to be more prone to benzodiazepine toxicity, perhaps due to increased sensitivity of the benzodiazepine receptor (Salzman 1992). Patients with disease of the brain may be even more vulnerable to adverse effects of CNS depression caused by benzodiazepines such as excessive sedation, memory impairment, confusion, falls, or paradoxical reactions. As they get older, geriatric patients may develop benzodiazepine toxicity at doses that were previously well tolerated (Regestein 1992). Common benzodiazepine side effects are discussed in Table 29–14 (Ahronheim 1992; Hart et al. 1991; Ray 1992; Regestein 1992; Salzman 1991, 1992; Salzman et al. 1983; Young and Meyers 1991).

Benzodiazepine Dependence and Withdrawal

Physical dependence on benzodiazepines can occur after treatment for months with therapeutic doses, especially with shorter half-life compounds (Salzman 1991). On abrupt discontinuation, three kinds of syndromes may occur, all of which are more severe and prolonged in elderly patients with impaired central

Table 29–13. Some benzodiazepine anxiolytics

Medication	Starting dose (mg)	Therapeutic dose (mg)	Half-life (hours)	Comments
Midazolam	2.5	5–15	1–3	Used intravenously for agitation and orally for sleep. Use for anxiety in elderly patients not studied.
Lorazepam	0.5	0.5–4	12–18	Does not accumulate in elderly patients.
Alprazolam	0.25	0.25–2.0	17–24	Increased half-life in elderly patients. Has 2 active metabolites.
Oxazepam	10	10–90	10–14	Active metabolite of diazepam with no active metabolites of its own. Slow onset of action due to slow absorption.
Clonazepam	0.125	0.25–2	100	Very sedating.
Diazepam	2	2–10	75–90	Metabolized to desmethyldiazepam, an active metabolite with half life of 194 hours.
Chlordiazepoxide	5	20–40	30	Metabolized to desmethyldiazepam and desmethyl-chlordiazepoxide, both active.
Prazepam	5	10–15	See diazepam	These 3 prodrugs (precursors) are demethylated to desmethyl-diazepam, the major active metabolite.
Clorazepate	3.75	7.5–30		
Halazepam	5	10–40		

Table 29–14. Neuropsychiatric side effects of benzodiazepines

Side effect	Manifestations	Comments
Central depression	Sedation, paradoxical excitement, disinhibition, suspiciousness, agitation, aggression, wandering, ataxia, falls, and delirium	Sedation persists up to 2 weeks after discontinuation of long half-life benzodiazepines. Tolerance may develop with careful dosage increases. Benzodiazepines likely to produce falls, the most common cause of injury in the elderly population.
Cognitive dysfunction	Confusion, anterograde amnesia, dementia-like syndrome, and aggravation of dementia	Rebound insomnia more common with triazolam and other very short half-life benzodiazepines; less with alprazolam.
Psychomotor impairment	Impaired driving	Elderly neuropsychiatric patients more vulnerable to psychomotor impairment. Benzodiazepines implicated more frequently than alcohol or other medications in accidents involving elderly. Automobile accidents second most common cause of injury in the elderly.
Electroencephalographic changes	Decreased alpha, increased low-voltage fast activity, especially in frontal regions	Depressed patients with increased rapid-eye-movement (REM) density may develop nightmares or vivid dreams due to increased REM activity by benzodiazepines.

nervous systems (Busto et al. 1986; Noyes et al. 1988; Salzman 1991). Relapse (return of the original anxiety symptoms) occurs gradually over weeks to months in 60%–80% of chronically anxious patients. Rebound, an intensification of the original symptoms lasting several days, appears within hours to days in one-quarter to three-quarters of patients. Withdrawal, which appears within hours to a day or two of stopping short half-life benzodiazepines and within days to weeks of discontinuing longer half-life preparations, adds to anxiety autonomic symptoms and new CNS symptoms. Withdrawal symptoms may be even more delayed and prolonged in older patients who continue to take benzodiazepines or other CNS depressants intermittently. Withdrawal after a single dose of benzodiazepines with very short half-lives such as triazolam and midazolam may produce confusion and amnesia, especially in patients with organic brain disease (Regestein 1992; Salzman 1992).

Special Considerations When Using Benzodiazepines in Geriatric Neuropsychiatry

Benzodiazepines are obvious considerations for anxious epileptic patients, but many geriatric patients with dementia, cerebellar disease, or psychomotor impairment tolerate these drugs poorly. Benzodiazepines are often more effective and better tolerated than antiparkinsonian drugs for neuroleptic-induced akathisia.

Chronic use of benzodiazepines can aggravate cognitive deficits in dementia patients and cause dementia in neurologically intact patients. The use of these and all CNS depressants should, therefore, be reviewed before diagnosing or treating primary dementia.

Withdrawal from benzodiazepines and other CNS depressants can produce a variety of neuropsychiatric syndromes (Table 29–15) that are easily mistaken for neurological illness in elderly patients. These syndromes often appear when a new physician becomes concerned about a patient's use of tranquilizers and discontinues them when the patient runs out of medication, or when the medication is abruptly discontinued after admission to a hospital or other facility. The latter problem often develops because a patient does not consider use of the benzodiazepine important enough to report it to the physician or conceals use of the drug out of shame or fear that the physician will disapprove, as a result of which the doctor underestimates the patient's drug intake. Family members can be important sources of information about the patient's use of medications prescribed by other doctors

or obtained over the counter. Toxicology screening is usually negative during an abstinence syndrome, but may reveal other unsuspected substances.

Withdrawal from any combination of CNS depressants can be diagnosed with the barbiturate tolerance test (D. E. Smith and Wesson 1970); however, experience with this test in the elderly population has not been reported in the literature. Specific dosage guidelines have not been studied formally in geriatric patients, but one recommendation would be that if phenobarbital is used 45- to 60-mg doses should be administered on an empty stomach once signs of withdrawal appear. These doses are repeated every 2–6 hours until intoxication begins to develop. Signs of withdrawal and/or intoxication (e.g., level of consciousness, dysarthria, postural hypotension, hyper- or hyporeflexia, and nystagmus) should be recorded before and 1 hour after each dose to determine the next dose. Once definite intoxication appears or when 300–500 mg of phenobarbital have been administered in a 24-hour period, the total amount is divided into four doses given every 6 hours, and the phenobarbital is withdrawn by about 10% per day. Each specific dose is determined by the patient's overall course and response to the last dose. Phenobarbital often begins to accumulate after 4–8 days, and it may be necessary to withdraw the drug more rapidly at this point. A pentobarbital withdrawal protocol can also be used (Dubin et al. 1986), but experience with this approach in elderly patients is even more limited.

Benzodiazepine Interactions

As indicated in Table 29–16, benzodiazepines have pharmacokinetic, as well as pharmacodynamic, interactions with medications in common use in neuropsychiatry (Salzman 1992).

Table 29–15. Manifestations of central nervous system depressant withdrawal

Anxiety, panic, insomnia, agitation, restlessness, and irritability	Tinnitus and seasickness
	Amnesia
	Psychosis
Hypersensitivity to light and noise	Delirium
	Seizures
Headache, dizziness, and diaphoresis	
Myalgia, tremor, and muscle twitching	

Alternatives to Benzodiazepines

The only currently available azapirone is buspirone, which has been shown to be effective for generalized anxiety in older, as well as younger, patients (Salzman 1992). Buspirone in doses of 5–30 mg/day is preferable to benzodiazepines for chronic anxiety in elderly brain injury patients because it does not impair cognition or psychomotor function in patients with intact nervous systems (Hart et al. 1991) and because it may reduce agitation in dementia patients (see below). However, buspirone is not effective when given intermittently.

Buspirone, gepirone, and ipsapirone have been shown to have primary antidepressant properties in younger patients, but the high doses that are necessary (40–90 mg/day) are difficult for many geriatric patients to tolerate. More moderate doses (e.g., 10–40 mg/day) may augment the antidepressant or anti-obsessional effect of antidepressants, the only adverse reactions of concern being headache, nausea, dizziness, and mild serotonin syndrome with highly serotonergic antidepressants. Because buspirone inhibits presynaptic dopamine autoreceptors it may enhance dopaminergic transmission and therefore could be useful for some parkinsonian patients. The same effect could produce abnormal movements, but there is no reason why this drug should cause tardive dyskinesia as it does not block postsynaptic dopamine receptors.

TCAs, even if they are not sedating, have been found to be as effective as benzodiazepines in the treatment of generalized anxiety disorder. In many studies it is not clear whether patients might also be depressed, but the presence of depression was excluded in at least one study (Hoehn-Saric et al. 1988). Because relatively high doses of benzodiazepines may be necessary to treat panic disorder, antidepressants other than bupropion are more appropriate choices for patients with panic disorder complicated by neurological syndromes who would be expected to be sensitive to benzodiaze-

pine adverse effects and discontinuation syndromes.

Antihistamines (e.g., hydroxyzine or diphenhydramine 10–25 mg daily to qid) are frequently used as anxiolytics or sleeping pills in elderly dementia patients (Ahronheim 1992; Salzman 1992). However, the antianxiety effect is unpredictable, and tolerance to the sedative effect usually occurs rapidly. The most appropriate use of antihistamines in geriatric neuropsychiatry may be to sedate a patient for an EEG as they have minimal effects on this measure.

Antipsychotic Drugs

Antipsychotic drugs are effective for all forms of psychosis. Well-established indications include schizophrenia, bipolar disorder, and psychotic unipolar depression. In low doses, antipsychotic drugs can be helpful in psychiatric syndromes commonly encountered in geriatric neuropsychiatry such as organic hallucinosis, organic delusional syndrome, paraphrenia, and late-onset paranoia (Young and Meyers 1991). Pimozide with or without antidepressants has been found effective for monosymptomatic hypochondriacal delusions and delusions of parasitosis (Dagon 1990). The use of antipsychotics to control agitation in neurologically impaired patients is discussed below.

Neurological Uses for Antipsychotic Drugs

Antipsychotic drugs can be used to treat interictal psychoses (Dagon 1990), as can ECT (Dubovsky, in press). Low doses of most neuroleptics other than thioridazine can ameliorate nausea and vomiting caused by cancer chemotherapy, autonomic dysfunction, vestibular syndromes, and related conditions (Richelson 1985). Low doses of chlorpromazine can stop intractable hiccups, and the phenothiazine trimeprazine, which does not have antipsychotic properties, is an antipruritic agent. Haloperidol and pimozide are often used to control chorea and other involuntary movements in Huntington's disease and Tourette syndrome. (The uses of neuroleptics in delirium and dementia are discussed later in this chapter.)

Available Preparations

All currently available antipsychotic drugs except clozapine are neuroleptics (from the Greek for "to clasp the neuron") in that they control psychosis and pro-

Table 29–16.   Some benzodiazepine interactions

Medication	Interaction
Central nervous system depressants	Increased sedation, confusion, amnesia, and psychomotor impairment
Opioids	Increased respiratory depression
Cimetidine	Increased benzodiazepine levels
Anticonvulsants and adrenal steroids	Decreased benzodiazepine levels

duce neurological side effects. In neuropsychiatric practice, antipsychotic drugs do not differ in efficacy. Side effect profiles, however, differ dramatically. Some characteristics of antipsychotic drugs as used in geriatric neuropsychiatry are summarized in Table 29–17 (Ahronheim 1992; Lohr et al. 1992; Salzman 1990).

Metabolism and Dosing

As with other lipid-soluble medications in elderly patients, the volume of distribution of neuroleptics is increased and metabolism is slowed, resulting in a longer time to reach steady state and prolonged therapeutic, as well as toxic, effects (Lohr et al. 1992; Wragg and Jeste 1988). Reduced dopaminergic transmission in the elderly may contribute to the development of neurological and antipsychotic effects at lower blood levels (Lohr et al. 1992). Some low-potency neuroleptics (e.g., chlorpromazine and thioridazine) induce their own metabolism and have complex metabolic pathways with many active metabolites. Butyrophenones and thioxanthenes appear to have only inactive metabolites (Ko et al. 1985). In a few studies of Alzheimer patients, the effective plasma concentration of haloperidol to control agitation and psychosis was less than the 4–18 ng/ml range thought to represent the therapeutic range for schizophrenia, although most Alzheimer patients cannot tolerate higher levels anyway (Devanand et al. 1992).

In acutely ill younger patients, intramuscular injection of neuroleptics avoids first-pass metabolism and increases bioavailability. However, this route is usually too painful and too unpredictably absorbed in older patients with decreased muscle mass (Lohr et al. 1992; Wragg and Jeste 1988). (Intravenous use of neuroleptics is discussed below.)

Table 29–17. Antipsychotic medications

Medication (by class)	Starting dose (mg)	Usual daily dose (mg)	Comments
Phenothiazines			
Chlorpromazine	10	10–300	Many active metabolites from complex hepatic and gastrointestinal metabolism. Hypotension prohibits parenteral use in elderly patients.
Thioridazine	10	10–300	Use in elderly patients limited by anticholinergic and cardiac side effects.
Triflupromazine	10	10–75	Moderate sedation, hypotension, and extrapyramidal side effects.
Acetophenazine	10	10–100	
Mesoridazine	10	10–200	Thioridazine metabolite. May be useful in some treatment-resistant psychoses.
Perphenazine	2	4–20	Midrange in potency and side effects.
Trifluoperazine	1	2–15	More extrapyramidal side effects than perphenazine.
Fluphenazine	0.25	0.5–6	Most potent phenothiazine.
Fluphenazine decanoate and enanthate	0.25 ml	0.25–0.5 ml every 2–3 weeks	Erratic absorption due to decreased muscle mass in elderly individuals.
Thioxanthenes			
Thiothixene	1	1–15	Similar to trifluoperazine in potency and side effects.
Chlorprothixene	10	10–100	Similar to chlorpromazine in potency and side effects.
Butyrophenone			
Haloperidol	0.25	0.25–8	Intramuscular dose poorly tolerated by elderly patients.
Diphenylbutylpiperidine			
Pimozide	0.25	0.25–4	Calcium channel and dopamine, subtype 2 (D_2), receptor blocking properties. Useful for atypical psychoses, but high incidence of cardiotoxicity.
Dibenzoxazepine			
Loxapine	10	10–100	Metabolized to amoxapine. May have special applications in psychotic depression and schizophrenia with secondary depression.
Dihydroindolone			
Molindone	5	10–100	Not associated with weight gain or seizures.
Dibenzodiazepine			
Clozapine	12.5	25–450	Useful in Parkinson's disease.

Neuropsychiatric Side Effects of Antipsychotic Drugs

Antipsychotic drugs are frequently prescribed for older agitated and psychotic neuropsychiatric patients, but these patients are particularly vulnerable to neurological side effects summarized in Table 29–18 (Ahronheim 1992; Almeida 1991; Lohr et al. 1992; Satlin et al. 1992; Wragg and Jeste 1988; Yassa et al. 1991; Young and Meyers 1991). Elderly dementia patients are at increased risk of extrapyramidal side effects, possibly as a result of degenerative changes in nigrostriatal pathways, higher blood levels with a given dose, and longer duration of treatment with greater cumulative neuroleptic exposure (Young and Meyers 1991). Tremor, rigidity, and bradykinesia are more common side effects in older patients, whereas dystonia occurs less frequently than in younger patients (Young and Meyers 1991).

Tardive dyskinesia occurs in 40%–70% of patients taking neuroleptics chronically (Ereshefsky et al. 1989; Yassa et al. 1991). The risk of tardive dyskinesia in older patients is higher in women and in patients with a history of acute extrapyramidal side effects, brain damage, longer neuroleptic exposure, mood disorder, medical illness, concurrent use of antiparkinsonian drugs, and drug holidays (Almeida 1991; Lohr et al. 1992). Tardive dyskinesia in the elderly must be distinguished from loose dentures and from spontaneous dyskinesias, which occur in 5% of elderly individuals who have not been exposed to neuroleptics (Yassa et al. 1991).

Whereas tardive dyskinesia eventually resolves after discontinuation of the medication in 80% of younger adults, remission after the neuroleptic is withdrawn occurs in only one-third to one-half of geriatric patients (Almeida 1991; Yassa et al. 1991; Young and Meyers 1991). The best strategy for dealing with tardive dyskinesia in older neurologically ill patients, therefore, is to reduce the risk of its occurrence. Useful approaches to achieving this goal include using the lowest possible dose and avoiding drug holidays, antiparkinsonian drugs, and rapid dose escalations (Wragg and Jeste 1988).

Several experimental treatments for tardive dyskinesia have been introduced with variable success. Calcium channel blockers ameliorate dyskinetic movements in animals and people, but have not been studied extensively (Dubovsky 1986). Vitamin E has been thought to improve tardive dyskinesia in 21%–45% of patients in whom symptoms have been present for less than 5 years (Egan et al. 1992). However, a 6-week double-blind placebo-controlled study of 1,600 IU of vitamin E daily in 18 patients, one-third of whom were older than 53, found meaningful improvement in only a few (Egan et al. 1992). Clozapine, which is technically not a neuroleptic, reduced tardive dyskinesia by 50% or more in 43% of cases, with greatest efficacy in tardive dystonia and severe tardive dyskinesia (Lieberman et al. 1991). This effect does not appear to represent temporary masking of tardive dyskinesia with eventual exacerbation of the syndrome, as occurs with neuroleptics.

Neuroleptic malignant syndrome, which has been reported in 0.5%–1.0% of patients taking neuroleptics (Guze and Baxter 1985), has been associated most frequently with high-potency neuroleptics, but it has also been reported with low-potency neuroleptics, clozapine, metoclopramide, carbidopa-levodopa, and withdrawal of amantadine and carbidopa-levodopa (Mueller 1985; Pelonero et al. 1985). Older patients seem to be somewhat less vulnerable to neuroleptic malignant syndrome, but the risk is increased in the elderly population by brain damage, other forms of neurological disease, and debilitation (Mueller 1985). Waiting more than 2 weeks before readministering neuroleptics after an episode of neuroleptic malignant syndrome, using low doses of low-potency neuroleptics of a different class, and carefully monitoring vital signs, mental status, and extrapyramidal side effects may decrease the risk of another episode of neuroleptic malignant syndrome (Rosebush and Stewart 1989).

Although tardive dyskinesia and neuroleptic malignant syndrome can occur with clozapine, they are much less frequent than they are with neuroleptics (Kane et al. 1988). However, clozapine is difficult to administer to elderly neuropsychiatric patients for several reasons. The risk of agranulocytosis may increase with age, especially in Ashkenazi Jewish patients (Gelenberg 1992). In addition, sedation, orthostatic hypotension, hypersalivation, hyperthermia, and akathisia are common side effects (Wilson 1992). The incidence of seizures with clozapine reported by the manufacturer is 1%–2% at doses less than 300 mg/day and 4%–6% at doses of 300–600 mg/day; however, Wilson (1992) found a rate of seizures up to 8%. The manufacturer has reported 9 (incidence 1 in 3,000 patients) nonfatal cases of respiratory and/or cardiac arrest with clozapine, in some instances in patients who were also taking benzodiazepines.

Table 29–18. Neuropsychiatric side effects of antipsychotic drugs

Side effect	Manifestations	Comments
Central nervous system depression	Sedation, confusion, and memory impairment.	Tolerance may develop within 1–3 weeks if dose is increased slowly.
α-Adrenergic blockade	Orthostatic hypotension.	May produce falls, especially in patients with extrapyramidal side effects.
	Priapism.	Especially with chlorpromazine and thioridazine. Not yet reported in elderly patients.
Akathisia	May be acute or tardive. Subjective experience of restlessness may be impaired in elderly patients.	Most common neuroleptic-induced movement disorder. Treat with decreased neuroleptic dose or addition of beta-blocker or benzodiazepine.
Parkinsonism	Tremor, rigidity, bradykinesia, stiffness, shuffling gait, sialorrhea, and loss of postural reflexes.	Occurs in 75% of elderly patients. May cause falls. Try to lower dose before adding antiparkinsonian drug. Amantadine may produce less anticholinergic toxicity than other antiparkinsonians.
Dystonia	Spasm of face, neck, and extraocular muscles. Less frequent in elderly patients than in younger patients. Not dose related in elderly patients.	Treat with lower neuroleptic dose, anticholinergic drug (e.g., 0.5–1 mg benztropine), or diphenhydramine 25 mg.
Pisa syndrome	Dystonic reaction in which body is flexed to one side.	Responds to same treatment as dystonia.
Rabbit syndrome	Tardive orofacial dyskinesia with 5-Hz lip movements resembling rabbit chewing.	Responds to anticholinergic medications.
Tardive dyskinesia	Orofacial movements most common in elderly patients. Next in order of frequency are movements of feet, neck, shoulders, trunk, diaphragm, pharynx, and intercostal muscles. May be associated with cognitive impairment in elderly schizophrenic patients.	Acute extrapyramidal side effects may predict later tardive dyskinesia in geriatric patients. Tardive dyskinesia is more frequent and more persistent in elderly patients.
Catatonia	Waxy flexibility, catalepsy, negativism, mutism, staring, echolalia, and echopraxia.	Responds to withdrawal of neuroleptic and to amantadine or antiparkinsonian drugs.
Neuroleptic malignant syndrome	Extrapyramidal signs and autonomic dysfunction. Rigidity, dystonia, tremor, fever, tachycardia, unstable blood pressure, diaphoresis, increased serum creatine phosphokinase and white count, and myoglobinuria.	Has been reported in elderly as well as in younger patients.
Seizures	Spontaneous seizures or decreased seizure threshold.	Most frequent with clozapine, loxapine, and low-potency neuroleptics. Older patients more susceptible to seizures, especially with history of seizures, central nervous system disease, or recent electroconvulsive therapy.
Photosensitivity	Increased sensitivity of skin and eyes to sun. May persist for months after drug is discontinued.	May sensitize eye to toxic effects of sun or bright light.
Pigmentary retinopathy	Irreversible pigment deposition in retina.	With doses of thioridazine greater than 800 mg/day.
Syndrome of inappropriate secretion of antidiuretic hormone	Hyponatremia may produce confusion or seizures.	Water retention may be aggravated by additional direct effect of neuroleptic on kidney.
Hypothermia	Temperature dysregulation that does not progress to neuroleptic malignant syndrome.	Especially with clozapine and phenothiazines in hypothyroid patients.
Electrocardiogram	Electrocardiogram changes; sudden death rare.	Thioridazine and pimozide.

Special Considerations When Using Antipsychotic Drugs in Geriatric Neuropsychiatry

Treatment of behavioral problems associated with delirium and dementia with neuroleptics is considered in later sections of this chapter. Clozapine, loxapine, and low-potency neuroleptics should not be administered to patients with seizure disorders; haloperidol and molindone seem safest for such patients (Fenwick 1989). Because dopamine blockade by neuroleptics elevates prolactin levels, great caution is necessary using these medications with prolactin-secreting pituitary tumors and possibly breast cancer.

Agitation and psychosis in patients with Parkinson's disease may be related to dementia or to dopaminergic drugs. If changing the medication does not relieve psychosis, clozapine in doses of 6.25–275 mg/day has been found effective (Bajulaize and Addonizio 1992; Lohr et al. 1992), even if dopamine agonists are continued (Wolk and Douglas 1992). Neuroleptics are poorly tolerated by patients with Parkinson's disease, but ECT may improve the neurological illness, as well as the psychosis (Dubovsky, in press).

Antipsychotic Drug Interactions

Antipsychotic agents interact with many neurological and cardiovascular drugs. Some examples are listed in Table 29–19 (Ayd 1986; Bailey et al. 1992; Dagon 1990; Kahn et al. 1990; D. D. Miller 1991; Rizos et al. 1988; Sargenti et al. 1988; Sassim and Grohmann 1988).

Alternatives to Antipsychotic Drugs

In neurologically ill patients with catatonia, mania, depression, schizoaffective, schizophreniform, and some schizophrenic psychoses (Van Valkenberg and Clayton 1983), as well as delirium (Dubovsky, in press), ECT can be more rapidly effective and better tolerated than neuroleptics. When neuroleptics are necessary, benzodiazepines, reserpine, baclofen, or droperidol may augment the antiagitation, but not the antipsychotic, effect, reducing the amount of neuroleptic needed for behavioral control (Bodkin 1990; Richelson 1985). Benzodiazepines alone may ameliorate catatonia (Fricchione 1989).

Treatment of Insomnia in Geriatric Neuropsychiatry

Complaints of disturbed sleep are more common in elderly patients than in younger patients (Spiegel 1990). Some complaints reflect diminished efficiency and more frequent interruptions of sleep. In other cases, neurological or medical disorders disrupt sleep (Regestein 1992; Salzman 1992; Spiegel 1990). Dementia and delirium are associated with reversal or fragmentation of the sleep-wake cycle, more awakenings, and decreased total, stage 4 and REM sleep. These changes are aggravated by sleeping pills and other CNS depressants, but may be corrected by entrainment to normal light-dark cycles. Grief, depression, and anxiety are common causes of disturbed sleep in the elderly that respond to specific therapies.

Table 29–19. Some antipsychotic drug interactions

Medication	Interaction
Central nervous system depressants	Increased sedation, confusion, falls
Guanethidine	Decreased antihypertensive effect
Lithium	Increased extrapyramidal side effects
Anticholinergic antiparkinsonian drugs, cimetidine, and antacids	Decreased neuroleptic levels caused by inhibition of gastrointestinal absorption
Anticonvulsants	Decreased neuroleptic levels caused by increased metabolism
Tricyclic antidepressants	Increased levels of both; clinically significant only for tricyclic antidepressant
Levodopa	Decreased antiparkinsonian effect due to dopamine receptor blockade
Propranolol	Increased levels of both classes
Benzodiazepines	Physical collapse with clozapine
Carbamazepine	Increased risk of fatal bone marrow suppression with clozapine

Medical and neurological causes of insomnia in the elderly include chronic pain, nocturnal myoclonus, restless legs syndrome, sleep apnea, and gastroesophageal reflux. Many psychoactive substances used by geriatric patients can produce insomnia (Table 29–20).

Although geriatric patients often request a medicine for insomnia, more often than not the best approach is to stop medications the patient is already taking, especially sleeping pills. Up to one-third of elderly people and 20%–40% of patients in intermediate care facilities take benzodiazepine sleeping pills regularly. However, these drugs lose their effectiveness after 20–30 days, after which they are taken to prevent withdrawal insomnia. Sleep architecture may remain abnormal for some time after the hypnotic is withdrawn.

The initial approach to geriatric insomnia should also include discontinuing substances such as caffeine and alcohol that disrupt sleep and treating illnesses that cause insomnia. Sleep hygiene should be ensured through measures such as increasing daytime activity, avoiding naps, keeping the room at a comfortable temperature, providing a time to review the day's activities prior to getting into bed, and not spending time in bed when the patient is not asleep.

When these measures are not effective, a hypnotic medication may be appropriate. Benzodiazepine sleeping pills are best used for time-limited insomnia in reaction to identifiable stress; when these medications are to be given chronically, intermittent dosing may prolong their effectiveness. Short half-life benzodiazepines listed in Table 29–21 (Greenblatt et al. 1991; Johnson et al. 1990; Regestein 1992; Salzman 1990; Spiegel 1990) do not accumulate in the elderly, but they may produce early-morning awakening and rebound insomnia when used for more than 1–2 weeks. Longer half-life preparations are more likely to produce daytime sedation and psychomotor impairment.

Quazepam, a new hypnotic that is selective for the benzodiazepine type 1 receptor, should not produce as much daytime sedation, impairment of memory and psychomotor function (attributed in part to benzodiazepine-type 2 receptors), or withdrawal syndromes (attributed in part to peripheral type benzodiazepine receptors) as do nonselective benzodiazepines. However, quazepam is metabolized to desalkylflurazepam, a nonselective flurazepam metabolite that accumulates with chronic treatment. Zolpidem, a new benzodiazepine type 1 receptor selective agonist sleeping pill, has

Table 29–20. Substances that cause sleep disturbances in elderly individuals

Caffeine (stimulant effect lasts 12–20 hours)
Nicotine
Alcohol
Activating antidepressants
Diuretics
Antiarrhythmics
Beta-blockers
Chronic use of sleeping pills

Table 29–21. Benzodiazepine hypnotics

Medication	Dose (mg)	Half-life (hours)	Comments
Triazolam	0.125[a]	2–5	Clearance reduced in elderly. Even lowest dose in elderly patients may produce next-day anxiety, agitation, anterograde amnesia, irritability, and insomnia due to withdrawal or rebound.
Midazolam	5–15	1–3	Minimal psychomotor impairment.
Temazepam	10–30	10–20	Higher doses occasionally helpful for some treatment resistant patients. Peak plasma levels occur 1 hour after ingestion.
Flurazepam	15	100–200	Not recommended for elderly patients because of accumulation and central nervous system depression.
Quazepam	7.5–15	Not studied in elderly patients	Parent drug is selective for benzodiazepine type 1 receptor but desalkylflurazepam metabolite is nonselective and has long half-life.
Estazolam	0.5–1	Not studied in elderly patients	Similar to other high-potency benzodiazepines (e.g., triazolam).

[a]This dose effective in older, but not younger, adults.

not yet been found to have a nonselective metabolite that might complicate continued treatment.

Of the available alternatives to benzodiazepines for the treatment of insomnia in geriatric neuropsychiatry (Regestein 1992; Salzman 1990; Spiegel 1990), sedating antidepressants (e.g., 25–75 mg of trazodone or 10–25 mg of doxepin) are most reliable, even in nondepressed patients. However, these drugs may cause daytime hangover and sedation. Antihistamines (e.g., 25–50 mg of diphenhydramine) can be useful sedatives in patients with pruritus, but they may produce bothersome anticholinergic side effects and daytime sedation that increase impairment of memory and psychomotor performance in patients with brain disease. Aspirin in doses of 325–650 mg/day can have mild hypnotic properties for some patients and may counteract sleep disruption caused by adrenal steroids and bronchodilators. In contrast, over-the-counter sleeping pills, which are frequently used by elderly patients, are not particularly effective and cause daytime sedation and anticholinergic effects (Balter and Uhlenhuth 1991).

Treatment of Delirium in Elderly Patients

Agitation due to delirium in elderly patients requires urgent intervention when the patient is at risk of injury, dehydration, cardiovascular collapse, or gross noncompliance with essential medical therapy. Emergency pharmacotherapy in such situations has never been subjected to controlled studies, but clinical experience has accumulated with a number of intravenous medications, especially haloperidol, benzodiazepines, and droperidol. As discussed in Chapter 30, one to four ECT treatments can be rapidly effective in ameliorating delirium of any etiology. The barbiturate tolerance test discussed earlier should be considered before any other treatment when delirium could be the result of withdrawal from CNS depressants.

Intravenous haloperidol therapy is started with a 1- to 5-mg dose. In patients of mixed ages on a coronary care unit, Tesar et al. (1985) recommended escalating haloperidol doses rapidly to 30–75 mg administered as frequently as necessary to control agitation. In cases unresponsive to repeated intravenous doses of haloperidol, an intravenous haloperidol drip at 5–25 mg/hour may be effective (Fernandez et al. 1988). Although extrapyramidal side effects are common with intramuscular administration, they are relatively rare with the intravenous route (Fernandez et al. 1988).

In their work with delirium patients with metastatic cancer of the brain, many of whom were elderly, Adams et al. (1986) began with haloperidol 3 mg iv followed by lorazepam 0.5–1.0 mg. If the patient did not improve within 20 minutes, 5–10 mg of haloperidol was combined with or followed by 2–10 mg of lorazepam; individual doses of haloperidol did not exceed 10 mg. When pain was felt to contribute to delirium, Fernandez et al. (1988) added 0.5–4.0 mg of hydromorphone to each dose of the other intravenous medications. Patients unresponsive to other treatments have had amobarbital added to intravenous haloperidol and lorazepam, surprisingly without disinhibition or respiratory depression (Adams et al. 1986). Hypercortisolemia, hypoxemia, and hypothyroidism may contribute to resistance to intravenous haloperidol and/or lorazepam (Adams et al. 1986).

According to these investigators, one of these regimens usually ameliorates severe agitation within 90 minutes. Many patients need no further treatment, whereas some require additional intravenous or oral doses of 5–10 mg of haloperidol, possibly augmented with 0.5 mg of lorazepam (Adams 1988; Fernandez et al. 1988). The longest reported duration of intravenous therapy was 3 months, in a terminally ill patient with an intractable behavioral disorder.

In a survey of British practitioners, Pilowsky et al. (1992) found that initial intravenous doses of 10–60 mg/day of haloperidol or 10–80 mg/day of diazepam, followed by 20–40 mg of haloperidol and/or 10–40 mg of diazepam, respectively, were used most frequently for uncontrollable agitation in neurological and primary psychiatric illness. Intravenous droperidol, a butyrophenone used as an anesthetic, has also been found to be an effective antiagitation agent in delirium (Szuba et al. 1992; Pilowsky et al. 1992). Droperidol, which is associated with an 8% incidence of extrapyramidal side effects in emergency dosing, has higher potency, more rapid onset of action, and a shorter half-life than haloperidol (Szuba et al. 1992). In an average dose of 7 mg, droperidol is equally effective intramuscularly, with an equally low incidence of extrapyramidal syndromes, making it appealing in patients who are so agitated or have such fragile veins that intravenous dosing is not practical.

In intravenous doses of 5–15 mg, the tranquilizing effect of midazolam, a lipophilic high-potency 1,2-benzodiazepine, occurs quickly, while rapid elimination prevents accumulation and excessive sedation (Bond et al. 1989). Intravenous midazolam controls violent and self-destructive behavior in mentally re-tarded younger patients (Bond et al. 1989), but has not been studied in the geriatric population. Amnesia after a single intravenous dose is common, but this is not an issue for delirium patients.

Treatment of Lethal Catatonia

ECT is the treatment of choice for lethal catatonia, an unusual syndrome of catatonia, neurological signs, and fever (Mann et al. 1986). Pennati et al. (1991) reported that intravenous dantrolene was helpful for two elderly patients taking imipramine or diazepam who developed catatonia, leukocytosis, and fever. Because of the possible relationship of lethal catatonia to ex-trapyramidal syndromes, neuroleptics should not be administered.

Treatment of Problem Behaviors in Dementia Patients

Elderly patients with brain damage often develop wan-dering, agitation, shouting, unexpected violent out-bursts, and unprovoked hostility toward loved ones (C. A. Ross 1992). Most of these patients are treated by one or more psychotropic medications that are consid-ered essential by caretakers. However, reducing the use of such agents does not increase the incidence of problem behaviors (Avorn et al. 1992). It is therefore important to consider withdrawing medications that could be aggravating confusion or causing delirium, especially benzodiazepines and anticholinergic drugs (Schor et al. 1992). Even aspirin can cause delirium in susceptible patients.

Because of the risk of oversedation, confusion, falls, paradoxical excitement, and further cognitive im-pairment, benzodiazepines are poor choices for treat-ing behavioral disturbances in dementia patients (Risse and Barnes 1986). Low doses of neuroleptics, the most frequently administered drugs for all behav-ioral disturbances, are really most appropriate first choices when aggression is caused by hallucinations or paranoia (C. A. Ross 1992).

In some studies, neuroleptics have been found su-perior to placebo in controlling agitation, insomnia, irritability, and hostility in geriatric neuropsychiatry (Risse and Barnes 1986; Young and Meyers 1991), but their apparent benefit, which is only modest (Schnei-der and Sobin 1992), depends on sedative side effects and not a primary action, and they may aggravate cog-nitive and motor impairment (Ahronheim 1992; Risse and Barnes 1986; Wragg and Jeste 1988). In some stud-ies of dementia patients, only 15%–40% have demon-strated clinically meaningful improvement with neuroleptics, whereas more than 20% have exhibited increased confusion and motor symptoms (Goldstein and Birnbom 1976; G. R. Smith et al. 1974). Even re-ports of positive effects are difficult to interpret be-cause dementia patients in these reports have been diagnostically heterogeneous and the longest thera-peutic trial was 3 months (Risse and Barnes 1986).

In double-blind studies, propranolol in doses of 10-600 mg/day has been shown to be effective in reduc-ing pacing, assaultiveness, and agitation in elderly de-mentia patients (Lohr et al. 1992; Salzman 1990; Schneider and Sobin 1992). Pindolol and nadolol have also been found to reduce impulsivity and assaultive-ness in double-blind studies of dementia patients (Schneider and Sobin 1992). Improvement with beta-blockers is often delayed 4–6 weeks (Risse and Barnes 1986; Silver and Yudofsky 1985). Elderly patients who do not have high levels of vagal tone may tolerate these medications without excessive cardiac slowing, but congestive heart failure, heart block, sinus bradycar-dia, insulin-dependent diabetes mellitus, asthma, and possibly chronic obstructive pulmonary disease are contraindications (Lohr et al. 1992; Risse and Barnes 1986; Salzman 1990). High doses of beta-blockers may cause hallucinations and aggravate aggression (Schnei-der and Sobin 1992). Beta-blockers increase blood lev-els of neuroleptics and anticonvulsants.

As summarized in Table 29–22, open trials and case series of elderly dementia patients have suggested additional potential treatments for agitation and other behavioral problems (Chambers et al. 1982; Coccaro et al. 1990; Good et al. 1991; Hope et al. 1991; Lawlor et al. 1991; Lohr et al. 1992; Ratey et al. 1992; Risse and Barnes 1986; Rizos et al. 1988; Salzman 1990; Satlin et al. 1992; Schneider and Sobin 1992; Welch and Sovner 1992; Wragg and Jeste 1988). Evaluation of these treat-ments is complicated by variable duration of treatment and a lack of control subjects.

Drug Treatment of Cognitive Deterioration

The most common cause of dementia in elderly indi-viduals is Alzheimer's disease (E. Perry and Court

1992). However, at least 20% of cases of dementia have a reversible cause (Ahronheim 1992), one of the most important of which is depression. The intimate relationship between depressive "pseudodementia" (more accurately the dementia syndrome of depression) and neurological dementia makes it difficult to differentiate them from each other (Rockwell et al. 1988; Roth 1976). Up to 89% of patients with the dementia syndrome of depression eventually develop Alzheimer's or other dementias (Gottfries and Hesse 1990), a far greater number than would be expected with the passage of time alone. This observation raises the possibility that in some cases depression may enhance prodromal cognitive deficits of dementia that later evolve on their own even if they improve temporarily when the depression remits.

Even when dementia is present, depression can make a substantial contribution to cognitive decline. In addition, depression in dementia patients may be expressed as additional cognitive or behavioral decline (E. D. Ross and Rush 1981). A trial of an antidepressant may therefore be warranted in dementia patients for whom other reversible causes are not found, even if a patient does not meet formal criteria for major depressive disorder. Because sedating and anticholinergic antidepressants further impair cognitive function (Tariot 1992), antidepressants of first choice for this indication are bupropion, serotonin uptake inhibitors, or second-

Table 29–22. Medications used to treat disruptive behavior in dementia

Medication	Dose (mg/day)	Adverse effects	Special indications	Proposed Mechanisms
Neuroleptics	Haloperidol 0.25–5	Confusion, falls, extrapyramidal syndromes, and tardive dyskinesia	Agitation due to psychosis	Sedation. Antipsychotic action only in psychotic patients.
Beta-blockers	Propranolol 60–600 pindolol 40–60	Bradycardia, hypotension, psychosis, aggravation of asthma, diabetes, and heart failure	Unpredictable violent outbursts	?Decreased arousal.
Lithium	15–1,500	Cognitive deterioration and neurotoxicity	Mood disorder, episodic symptoms	Mood stabilization in patients with covert mood disorders
Carbamazepine	50–2,000	Neurotoxicity, confusion, ataxia, disorientation, and increased agitation	Abnormal electro-encephalogram (EEG) and mood disorder	Anticonvulsant, decreased affective lability.
Valproic acid	125–1800	Oversedation, confusion, and clumsiness	Abnormal EEG and mood disorder	As with carbamazepine.
Trazodone (sometimes with tryptophan)	50–500	Oversedation and confusion	Mood disorder	Not related to sedation. Serotonergic or antidepressant action may be important.
Fluoxetine, ? other serotonin uptake inhibitors	5–20	Agitation, anxiety, insomnia, akathisia, extrapyramidal syndromes, and serotonin syndrome	Mood disorder	As with trazodone.
Buspirone	10–20, sometimes up to 80	Agitation, headache, and nausea	Anxiety, depression, and unpredictable agitation	Serotonergic action or treatment of unrecognized depression
Selegiline	5–10	Oversedation and hypotension	Parkinson's disease	Serotonergic effect.
Antihistamines	25–100	Oversedation, anticholinergic, and delirium	Pruritus and allergies	Sedation and antianxiety.
Stimulants	Dextroamphetamine 10–20	Overstimulation, hypertension, psychosis	Lack of response to other treatments	?Paradoxical effect.
Dextromethorphan[a]	90–180	Sedation and serotonin syndrome	Upper respiratory infection	Serotonergic, ? N-methyl-D-aspartate (NMDA) antagonist.

[a]Reported only in younger dementia patients.

ary amine TCAs for which correlations exist between blood levels and clinical response.

Many strategies have been introduced for treating the actual cognitive decline of primary degenerative dementia. Although there is a compelling need for treatments for cognitive deterioration, most studies of these strategies leave much to be desired. Even if statistically significant improvement in various rating scales is found, the improvement may be barely noticeable to patient and family (Bracco and Amaducci 1990), or the rating scales may not reflect meaningful target symptoms (Gauthier et al. 1991; Lebowitz 1992). Conversely, medications that do not improve dementia may still be useful if they just slow deterioration. Drugs aimed at one neurotransmitter system may not be effective because multiple transmitters are affected in Alzheimer's disease (Lebowitz 1992), but if drugs with broader spectra of action are used the actual mechanism of any positive effect is obscure.

Although a few positive preliminary findings have been reported, there is no proven treatment for dementia. Even in the face of only a slight chance of benefit, however, continuing to try new treatments can be a concrete representation of ongoing hope. On the other hand, if treatments do emerge with the potential to slow the progress of severe dementia but not to restore function, ethical considerations in prolonging suffering and increasing the cost of caring for a patient who remains severely ill may be complex.

Cholinergic Therapies

In view of acetylcholine's role as a neurotransmitter of memory, and the cognitive impairment produced by drugs that interfere with central cholinergic transmission, the selective loss of cholinergic neurons in Alzheimer's disease has been felt to be etiologically important (Branconnier et al. 1992; Farlow et al. 1992; Gauthier et al. 1991). Medications that increase brain acetylcholine levels may have promise in the treatment of Lewy body dementia (E. Perry and Court 1992), but have had disappointing results in many cases of Alzheimer's disease (Bracco and Amaducci 1990; Tariot 1992). The lack of more consistently positive findings may reflect the heterogeneity of Alzheimer's disease, the involvement of other neurotransmitter systems, or perhaps such massive cholinergic neuronal destruction that the system is no longer capable of responding to exogenous manipulation (Branconnier et al. 1992).

Acetylcholine precursors have generally been found ineffective in Alzheimer's disease (Gottfries and Hesse 1990; Tariot 1992), which is not surprising in view of the loss of neurons capable of utilizing precursors. Even though cholinergic muscarinic receptors are preserved in Alzheimer's disease, trials of bethanechol and arecoline, nonselective muscarinic cholinergic agonists, have not yielded positive results (Gauthier et al. 1991). Research therefore has turned to cholinesterase inhibitors as a means of increasing cholinergic tone. Oral physostigmine in a dose of 8 mg/day for 3 weeks improved performance on a test of auditory learning, but this was not clinically meaningful (Sevash et al. 1991). Because physostigmine has a half-life of only 30 minutes, it is not a practical chronic treatment (Bracco and Amaducci 1990).

Tacrine (1,2,3,4-tetrahydro-9-acridinamine monochloride monohydrate [or THA]) is a reversible cholinesterase inhibitor with a longer duration of action. Early studies reporting positive results suggested that 40%–50% of Alzheimer's disease patients who tolerate tacrine, or 30% of all patients, had some meaningful improvement, although it was not clear whether this might last longer than 3 months (Small 1992). Three double-blind placebo-controlled studies of tacrine have appeared in recent years.

A multicenter phase 3 study supported by the company holding the patent on tacrine (trade name Cognex) enrolled 468 patients age 50 or older with probable Alzheimer's disease (Growdon 1992). After a 6-week placebo washout, patients received one of the following treatments: placebo for 6 weeks followed by tacrine 20 mg for 6 weeks; tacrine 20 mg for 12 weeks; tacrine 20 mg for 6 weeks followed by tacrine 40 mg for 6 weeks; tacrine 40 mg for 12 weeks; or tacrine 40 mg for 6 weeks followed by tacrine 80 mg for 6 weeks. The longest trial on any tacrine dose, therefore, was 12 weeks. Patients taking 80 mg of tacrine demonstrated an average increase of 3.7 points on the Alzheimer's Disease Assessment Scale (ADAS) versus an increase of 0.1 point on placebo. Assessments by physicians and caretakers of patients' cognitive and global functioning also increased on the higher tacrine dose.

Eagger et al. (1992) noted a 2-point improvement in Mini Mental State Exam (MMSE) scores that was maximal at 4 weeks and sustained over 12 weeks in patients taking tacrine 150 mg/day. Improvement was more marked when serum tacrine concentrations exceeded 8 ng/ml (Eagger and Levy 1992).

Although the clinical significance of findings of

the first two studies was not addressed, Davis et al. (1992) did consider clinical correlations of test scores. To maximize the likelihood of finding patients who would respond to tacrine, these investigators enrolled only Alzheimer's disease patients older than 50 who demonstrated improvement in ADAS scores of at least 4 points after taking 40 or 80 mg of tacrine for 6 weeks. During a subsequent 6-week double-blind phase, these patients received either placebo or the dose of tacrine that had seemed helpful during the preliminary phase. Patients taking tacrine had a smaller decrement of cognitive function than did the patients taking placebo that was statistically significant mainly for word recognition memory. The difference could have been explained by a greater decline of cognitive functioning in the placebo group caused by withdrawal from tacrine given during the initial phase. The placebo group returned to previous levels of functioning when tacrine was reinstituted. However, none of the differences between tacrine and placebo was detectable clinically.

In an editorial on recent tacrine studies, Growdon (1992) noted that tacrine probably does have a measurable effect on cognition, but it is "clinically trivial." To the degree that tacrine is helpful for some patients, long-term benefits would be expected to be limited by continued degeneration of cholinergic neurons (Ahronheim 1992). Because 10%–25% of patients taking tacrine develop reversible increases in serum transaminase levels, especially alanine aminotransferase (Farlow et al. 1992; Small 1992), the Food and Drug Administration concluded that without more convincing evidence of meaningful sustained improvement, the risk-benefit ratio of tacrine did not justify release of the drug (Food and Drug Administration 1991).

Another line of investigation that may have more promise involves the role of the intracellular calcium ion (Ca^{2+}) in neuronal degeneration (Branconnier et al. 1992; Choi 1988). All known cytotoxic processes, including ischemia, toxins, immune mechanisms, and genetically programmed cell death (apoptosis) increase free intracellular Ca^{2+} concentration ($[Ca^{2+}]_i$). Whereas the Ca^{2+} stimulates many crucial cellular actions, including learning and gene activation, excessive elevations of $[Ca^{2+}]_i$ activate enzymes such as proteases that degrade structural proteins and phospholipases, which break down the cell membrane and liberate arachidonic acid and xanthine oxidase. Arachidonic acid can be oxidized to cytotoxic free radicals and xanthine oxidase can facilitate the formation of superoxide radicals.

Elderly patients may be more vulnerable to Ca^{2+}-induced neurotoxicity because resting $[Ca^{2+}]_i$ increases with age due to prolonged calcium influx through potential dependent channels. As some people get older, $[Ca^{2+}]_i$ may gradually increase to the point at which apoptotic genes are activated, stimulating pathological processes that further promote the rise in $[Ca^{2+}]_i$ until it reaches cytotoxic levels. If progression of the increase in resting $[Ca^{2+}]_i$ with age could be delayed, $[Ca^{2+}]_i$ might not reach levels that initiate neurotoxicity during the normal lifespan.

Sustained increases of $[Ca^{2+}]_i$ can be produced by excitatory amino acids (excitotoxins) such as glutamate (Choi 1988; Garthwaite 1991; Manev et al. 1990). In moderate concentrations, excitatory amino acids facilitate learning and neuronal development; however, excessive release and decreased uptake inhibition of excitotoxins have been implicated in various forms of brain damage, including Alzheimer's disease. One study, for example, found elevated cerebrospinal fluid levels of free glutamate in 10 early Alzheimer's disease patients compared with control subjects (Pomara et al. 1992).

Through their interaction with specific receptors, the best studied of which is the N-methyl-D-aspartate (NMDA) receptor, glutamate and other excitotoxins produce sustained influx of Ca^{2+} through a receptor-operated calcium channel that persists after the excitotoxin is withdrawn. The NMDA receptor also facilitates translocation of the ubiquitous intracellular enzyme protein kinase C to the cell membrane, where it is activated by Ca^{2+}. Protein kinase C phosphorylates cytotoxic calcium-dependent proteins and enhances further Ca^{2+} influx by phosphorylating calcium channels.

One approach to reducing excitotoxicity involves the noncompetitive NMDA antagonists such as MK-801, ketamine, and dextromethorphan. These drugs bind to a phencyclidine (PCP) receptor linked to the NMDA complex to attenuate Ca^{2+} influx. In animals with ligated cerebral arteries, MK-801 improves learning and reduces neuronal death in regions such as the hippocampus and neocortex, where high concentrations of NMDA receptors are found and vulnerability to glutamate neurotoxicity seems greatest (Albers et al. 1989). Like all drugs that bind to the PCP receptor, noncompetitive NMDA antagonists could have psychotomimetic effects (Albers et al. 1989).

Another approach to reducing excitotoxicity and Ca^{2+}-stimulated neurotoxicity is to attenuate elevations of $[Ca^{2+}]_i$ by reducing calcium influx through potential dependent channels. In a 12-week preliminary analysis of a double-blind phase 3 study of Alzheimer's disease (supported by the company owning the patent to the drug), nimodipine—a lipid-soluble dihydropyridine calcium channel blocking agent—was found to slow progression of memory impairment compared with placebo (Tollefson 1990). Extension of the study over 6 months supported the preliminary findings and suggested slower deterioration in patients with more severe dementia, but it was not clear how frequently improvement on cognitive testing translates into clinically meaningful results. In addition, nimodipine currently is extremely expensive.

Vasodilators do not really increase cerebral perfusion and may even reduce circulation through the brain through a steal effect, resulting in hypoperfusion. Drugs that used to be thought of as vasodilators therefore may be more appropriately classified with the nootopics (metabolic enhancers) (Jenike et al. 1990). The best studied of the vasodilator-nootopics is Hydergine, a mixture of three hydrogenated ergot alkaloids, that was reported to be helpful in 18 studies of mild dementia (Bracco and Amaducci 1990; Gottfries and Hesse 1990; Tariot 1992); the measure most consistently improved by Hydergine in these studies was mood (Jenike et al. 1990).

A double-blind study found no difference between 3 mg and 12 mg of Hydergine over the course of a year in ratings of dementia and functioning, but because there was no placebo control it was impossible to state whether either dose was actually helpful (Jenike et al. 1990). A recent double-blind placebo-controlled study found Hydergine to be of no benefit at all to patients with moderate dementia (Thompson et al. 1990). In general, convincing evidence of the capacity of any of the vasodilator-nootopics listed in Table 29–23 to slow or reverse deterioration of Alzheimer's disease over more than a few months has not yet emerged.

Many other treatments for Alzheimer's disease and other dementias are being investigated, with varying degrees of success. Representative examples are described in Table 29–23 (Bracco and Amaducci 1990; Crapper-Mclachlan et al. 1991; Crook et al. 1991, 1992a, 1992b; Gottfries and Hesse 1990; Henderson et al. 1989; Lindvall et al. 1990; Spagnoli et al. 1991; Tariot 1992). Even though none of these treatments have been proven to be effective, trying a number of them can help to maintain hope in patients and families who view medication as a concrete representation of the physician's unwillingness to give up.

Psychiatric Side Effects of Neurological Drugs

Psychiatric syndromes commonly are caused by the many medications taken by elderly neurologically ill patients, even those that are not lipophilic. Some important reactions are noted in Table 29–24 (Kulkarni et al. 1992; Lohr et al. 1992; Medical Letter 1985). Whenever possible, the offending medicine should be withdrawn before adding psychiatric treatments. (Further discussion of these medications can be found in Chapter 27.)

Summary

Many Axis I disorders are true neuropsychiatric syndromes in the elderly in that psychiatric symptoms in this population are often produced or aggravated by neurological dysfunction. Treating such syndromes is complicated by the sensitivity of the older nervous system to the toxic, but probably not the therapeutic, effects of psychotropic medications and by interactions of psychotropic medications with the many neurological drugs taken by elderly patients. Many of the more frequently used medicines for geriatric neuropsychiatric conditions, especially the sedating and anticholinergic TCAs and neuroleptics and the long half-life benzodiazepines, are poorly tolerated. Secondary amine TCAs, new generation antidepressants, and high-potency neuroleptics are better tolerated alternatives. Short half-life benzodiazepines are appropriate choices for some acutely anxious or agitated patients, but anxiety and insomnia in patients with organic brain disease often is better managed with azapirones or antidepressants.

Severe agitation in delirium patients can be treated emergently with ECT or with intravenous haloperidol, droperidol, or benzodiazepines. Intermittent explosive outbursts and other behavioral disturbances respond to β-adrenergic blocking agents, buspirone, lithium, anticonvulsants, some antidepressants, and possibly stimulants. Neuroleptics should be avoided for this indication unless nothing else is effective. There is no proven treatment for dementia itself, and recent highly publicized trials of tacrine have yielded equivocal results. Calcium channel blockers, L-deprenyl, and possibly NMDA antagonists may have some potential.

Table 29–23.   Experimental treatments for dementia

Treatment (by class)	Comments
Vasodilators	
Hydergine	Any reproducible improvement is in mood.
Nafronyl oxalate	Improved mood, cognition, and behavior in one study. May increase oxygen consumption and adenosine phosphate (ATP) production.
Nicotinic acid	Unclear benefit.
Vitamin E	Unclear benefit.
Nootopics	
Piracetam	Inconsistent results.
Gingko biloba extract	May be useful in multi-infarct dementia. Positive preliminary results in Europe. Double-blind study now underway in United States.
NMDA Antagonists	
MK-801	Positive animal studies. Could be psychotogenic in humans.
Dextromethorphan	May improve disruptive behavior, as well as cognition.
Calcium channel blockers	
Nimodipine	Well tolerated but expensive. May slow deterioration.
Nicardipine	Not yet studied formally but could be as effective as nimodipine at somewhat lower cost.
MAO-B inhibitors	
Selegiline	May be useful in view of increased MAO-B levels in Alzheimer's disease. Mild improvement in memory after low doses administered for 6 months has been reported.
Precursors	
Phosphatidylserine	May help to maintain membrane fluidity. Improved neuropsychological test performance reported in subjects with memory loss associated with aging. Not clearly helpful in Alzheimer's disease.
Acetyl-L-carnitine	Slowed deterioration in various outcome measures over 12 months in one study.
Linopardine	Increases central nervous system release of acetylcholine, serotonin, and dopamine.
	No clear clinical benefit demonstrated yet.
Neuropeptides	
Adrenocorticotropic hormone	Benefit not demonstrated.
Vasopressin	Use based on evidence of memory deficits in vasopressin-deficient animals corrected by giving vasopressin and possible benefit to patients with central diabetes insipidus. May improve mood and attention, but not cognition, in Alzheimer's disease. Available only as a nasal snuff that is difficult for dementia patients to administer.
Thyrotropin-releasing hormone (TRH)	Unconfirmed preliminary positive results.
Vitamins	
Vitamin B_{12}	23% incidence of low B_{12} levels in Alzheimer's disease, possibly due to reduced gastrointestinal absorption.
Heavy metal chelators	
Desferrioxamine	Chelates iron and aluminum. Slowed decline over 2 years compared with lecithin and placebo in one study.
Narcotic Antagonists	
Naltrexone, naloxone	No improvement over 5 weeks in one study.
Neural transplantation	
Fetal dopaminergic neurons	Restores striatal dopamine synthesis and improves parkinsonism. Similar strategies not studied in Alzheimer's disease.

Note.   NMDA = *N*-methyl-D-aspartate; MAO-B = monoamine oxidase–B.

Table 29–24. Psychiatric side effects of neurological drugs

Syndrome	Drugs	Syndrome	Drugs
Depression	Adrenal steroids	Psychosis	Adrenal steroids
	Amantadine		Anticonvulsants
	Asparaginase		Asparaginase
	Cimetidine		Bromocriptine
	Digoxin		Cimetidine
	Indomethacin		Cisplatin
	Levodopa		Cyclophosphamide
	Methyldopa		Digoxin
	Metoclopramide		Isoniazid
	Narcotics		Levodopa
	Procainamide		Lisuride
	Propranolol		Pergolide
	Reserpine		Procainamide
	Thiazide diuretics		Propranolol
Mania	Adrenal steroids		Quinidine
	Baclofen		Ranitidine
	Bromocriptine		Sulindac
	Captopril		Tocainide
	Cimetidine	Sleep disorder and	Antidepressants
	Dextromethorphan	bad dreams	Baclofen
	Indomethacin		Bromocriptine
	Isoniazid		Cimetidine
	Levodopa		Levodopa
Confusion	Asparaginase		Lisuride
	Aspirin		Pergolide
	Cyclophosphamide		Propranolol
	Cisplatin		
	Opiates		
	Pentazocine		
	Ranitidine		
	Sulindac		
	Any medication in patients with brain damage		

References

Abernathy DR: Psychotropic drugs and the aging process: pharmacokinetics and pharmacodynamics, in Clinical Geriatric Psychiatry, 2nd Edition. Edited by Salzman C. Baltimore, MD, Williams & Wilkins, 1992, pp 61–76

Adams F: Emergency intravenous sedation of the delirious medically ill patient. J Clin Psychiatry 49 (suppl):22–26, 1988

Adams F, Fernandez F, Anderson BS: Emergency pharmacotherapy of delirium in the critically ill cancer patient. Psychosomatics 27 (suppl):33–37, 1986

Ahronheim JC: Handbook of Prescribing Medications for Geriatric Patients. Boston, MA, Little, Brown, 1992

Albers GW, Goldberg MP, Choi DW: N-methyl-D-aspartate antagonists: ready for clinical trial in brain ischemia? Ann Neurol 25:398–403, 1989

Alexopoulos GS: Treatment of depression, in Clinical Geriatric Psychiatry, 2nd Edition. Edited by Salzman C. Baltimore, MD, Williams & Wilkins, 1992, pp 137–174

Almeida JH: Neuroleptic side-effects: the "rabbit syndrome." International Journal of Geriatric Psychiatry 6:537–539, 1991

Avorn J, Soumerai SB, Everitt DE, et al: A randomized trial of a program to reduce the use of psychoactive drugs in nursing homes. N Engl J Med 327:168–173, 1992

Ayd F: Prophylactic antiparkinsonian drug therapy: pros and cons. International Drug Therapy Newsletter 21:5–6, 1986

Bailey DN, Coffee JJ, Anderson B, et al: Interaction of tricyclic antidepressants with cholestyramine in vitro. Ther Drug Monit 14:339–342, 1992

Bajulaize R, Addonizio G: Clozapine in the treatment of psychosis in an 82-year-old woman with tardive dyskinesia (letter). J Clin Psychopharmacol 12:364–365, 1992

Baldessarini RS, Marsh E: Fluoxetine and side effects. Arch Gen Psychiatry 47:191–192, 1990

Balter MB, Uhlenhuth EH: The beneficial and adverse effects of hypnotics. J Clin Psychiatry 52 (7, suppl):16–23, 1991

Black DW, Winokur G, Nasrallah A: Treatment of mania: a naturalistic study of electroconvulsive therapy vs lithium in 438 patients. J Clin Psychiatry 48:132–139, 1987

Blake LM, Marks RC, Luchins DJ: Reversible neurologic symptoms with clozapine and lithium. J Clin Psychopharmacol 12:297–299, 1992

Bodkin JA: Emerging uses for high-potency benzodiazepines in psychotic disorders. J Clin Psychiatry 51 (suppl):41–46, 1990

Bond WS, Mandos LA, Kurtz MB: Midazolam for aggressivity and violence in three mentally retarded patients. Am J Psychiatry 146:925–926, 1989

Bouckonis AJ, Litman RE: Clonazepam in the treatment of neuralgic pain syndromes. Psychosomatics 26:933–936, 1985

Bracco L, Amaducci L: Drug development for the treatment of dementia, in Clinical and Scientific Psychogeriatrics, Vol 2. The Interface of Psychiatry and Neurology. Edited by Bergener M, Finkel SI. New York, Springer, 1990, pp 260–287

Branconnier RJ, Branconnier ME, Wadshe TM, et al: Blocking the Ca^{2+} activated cytotoxic mechanisms of cholinergic neuronal death: a novel treatment strategy for Alzheimer's disease. Psychopharmacol Bull 28:175–181, 1992

Bryner C, Winograd CH: Fluoxetine in elderly patients: is there cause for concern? J Am Geriatr Soc 40:902–905, 1992

Busto V, Sellers EM, Naranjo C, et al: Withdrawal reaction after long-term therapeutic use of benzodiazepines. N Engl J Med 315:854–859, 1986

Chambers CA, Bain J, Rosebottom R, et al: Carbamazepine in senile dementia and overactivity: a placebo controlled double blind trial. IRCS Medical Science 10:505–506, 1982

Chiarello RJ, Cole JO: The use of psychostimulants in general psychiatry: a reconsideration. Arch Gen Psychiatry 44:286–295, 1987

Choi DW: Glutamate neurotoxicity and diseases of the nervous system. Neuron 1:623–634, 1988

Chou JCY: Recent advances in the treatment of acute mania. J Clin Psychopharmacol 11:3–21, 1991

Chouinard G, Penry JK: Neurologic and psychiatric aspects of clonazepam: an update. Psychosomatics 26 (suppl):1–37, 1985

Clary C, Schweitzer E: Treatment of MAOI hypertensive crisis with sublingual nifedipine. J Clin Psychiatry 48:249–250, 1987

Coccaro EF, Kramer E, Zemishlany A, et al: Pharmacologic treatment of noncognitive behavioral disturbances in elderly demented patients. Am J Psychiatry 147:1640–1645, 1990

Coffey CE, Weiner RD, Djang WT, et al: Brain anatomic effects of electroconvulsive therapy. Arch Gen Psychiatry 48:1013–1021, 1991

Coffey CE, Wilkinson WE, Weiner RD, et al: Quantitative cerebral anatomy in depression: a controlled magnetic resonance imaging study. Arch Gen Psychiatry 50:7–16, 1993

Cohen CK, Shrivastava R, Mendels J, et al: Double-blind, multicenter comparison of sertraline and amitriptyline in elderly depressed patients. J Clin Psychiatry 51 (12, suppl B):28–33, 1990

Cohen WJ, Cohen NH: Lithium carbonate, haloperidol and irreversible brain damage. JAMA 230:1283–1287, 1974

Crapper-Mclachlan DR, Dalton AJ, Krick TPA, et al: Intramuscular desferrioxamine in patients with Alzheimer's disease. Lancet 337:1304–1308, 1991

Crook TH, Tinklenberg J, Yesavage J, et al: Effects of phosphatidylserine in age-associated memory impairment. Neurology 41:644–649, 1991

Crook T, Petrie W, Wells C, et al: Effects of phosphatidylserine in Alzheimer's disease. Psychopharmacol Bull 28:61–66, 1992a

Crook T, Wilner E, Rothwell A, et al: Noradrenergic intervention in Alzheimer's disease. Psychopharmacol Bull 28:67–70, 1992b

Cummings JL: Depression and Parkinson's disease: a review. Am J Psychiatry 149:443–454, 1992

Dagon EM: Other organic mental syndromes, in Verwoerdt's Clinical Geropsychiatry, 3rd Edition. Edited by Bienenfeld D. Baltimore, MD, Williams & Wilkins, 1990, pp 85–105

Davidson J: Seizures and bupropion: a review. J Clin Psychiatry 50:256–261, 1989

Davis KL, Thal LJ, Gamzu ER, et al: A double-blind placebo-controlled multicenter study of tacrine for Alzheimer's disease. N Engl J Med 327:1953–1959, 1992

Demuth GW, Breslov RE, Drescher J: The elicitation of a movement disorder by trazodone: case report. J Clin Psychiatry 46:535–536, 1985

Devanand DP, Cooper MA, Sackeim HA, et al: Low dose oral haloperidol and blood levels in Alzheimer's disease: a preliminary study. Psychopharmacol Bull 28:169–173, 1992

Dubin WR, Weiss KJ, Dorn JM: Pharmacotherapy of psychiatric emergencies. J Clin Psychopharmacol 6:210–222, 1986

Dubovsky SL: Calcium antagonists: a new class of psychiatric drugs? Psychiatric Annals 16:724–728, 1986

Dubovsky SL, Franks RD, Allen S, et al: Calcium antagonists in mania: a double blind placebo control study of verapamil. Psychiatry Res 18:309–320, 1986

Dubovsky SL: Electroconvulsive therapy, in Comprehensive Textbook of Psychiatry, 6th Edition. Edited by Kaplan H, Sadock BJ. Baltimore, 1993 (in press)

Eagger S, Levy R: Serum levels of tacrine in relationship to clinical response in Alzheimer's disease. International Journal of Geriatric Psychiatry 7:115–119, 1992

Eagger S, Morant N, Levy R, et al: Tacrine in Alzheimer's disease: time course of changes in cognitive function and practice effects. Br J Psychiatry 160:36–40, 1992

Egan MF, Hyde TM, Albers GW, et al: Treatment of tardive dyskinesia with vitamin E. Am J Psychiatry 149:773–777, 1992

Ereshefsky L, Watanabe MD, Tran-Johnson TK: Clozapine: an atypical antipsychotic agent. Clinical Pharmacy 8:691–709, 1989

Farlow M, Gracon SI, Hershey LA, et al: A controlled trial of tacrine in Alzheimer's disease. JAMA 268:2523–2529, 1992

Fenwick P: The nature and management of aggression in epilepsy. J Neuropsychiatry Clin Neurosci 1:418–425, 1989

Fernandez F, Holmes VF, Adams F, et al: Treatment of severe refractory agitation with a haloperidol drip. J Clin Psychiatry 49:239–241, 1988

Food and Drug Administration: Tacrine as a treatment for Alzheimer's disease: an interim report from the FDA. N Engl J Med 324:349–352, 1991

Fricchione G: Catatonia: a new indication for benzodiazepines? Biol Psychiatry 26:761–765, 1989

Garthwaite J: Glutamate, nitric oxide and cell-cell signalling in the nervous system. Trends in Neurological Science 14:60–67, 1991

Gauthier S, Gauthier L, Bouchard R, et al: Treatment of Alzheimer's disease: hopes and reality. Can J Neurol Sci 18:394–397, 1991

Gelenberg AJ: Clozapine agranulocytosis update. Biological Therapies in Psychiatry 15:37–40, 1992

Gelenberg AJ, Kane JM, Keller MB, et al: Comparison of standard and low serum levels of lithium for maintenance treatment of bipolar disorder. N Engl J Med 231:1489–1493, 1989

Georgotas A, McCue RE, Hapworth W, et al: Comparative efficacy and safety of MAOIs versus TCAs in treating depression in the elderly. Biol Psychiatry 21:1155–1166, 1986

Georgotas A, McCue RE, Cooper TB, et al: How effective and safe is continuation therapy in elderly depressed patients? Arch Gen Psychiatry 45:929–932, 1988

Goldstein SE, Birnbom F: Piperacetazine versus thioridazine in the treatment of organic brain disease: a controlled double-blind study. J Am Geriatr Soc 24:355–359, 1976

Good D, Davis CM, Liem P, et al: The use of seligiline in Alzheimer's patients with behavior problems. J Clin Psychiatry 52:342–345, 1991

Goodman WK, Charney DS: Therapeutic applications and mechanisms of monoamine oxidase and heterocyclic antidepressant drugs. J Clin Psychiatry 46:6–22, 1985

Gottfries CG, Hesse C: Pharmacotherapy in psychogeriatrics: an update, in Clinical and Scientific Psychogeriatrics, Vol 2: The Interface of Psychiatry and Neurology. Edited by Bergener M, Finkel SI. New York, Springer, 1990, pp 288–313

Greenblatt DJ, Harmatz JS, Shapiro L, et al: Sensitivity to triazolam in the elderly. N Engl J Med 324:1691–1698, 1991

Griffin JP: A review of the literature on benign intracranial hypertension associated with medication. Adverse Drug React Toxicol Rev 11:41–57, 1992

Growdon JH: Treatment for Alzheimer's disease? N Engl J Med 327:1306–1308, 1992

Guze BH, Baxter LR: Neuroleptic malignant syndrome. N Engl J Med 313:163–166, 1985

Hardy BG, Shulman KI, Mackenzie SE, et al: Pharmacokinetics of lithium in the elderly. J Clin Psychopharmacol 7:153–158, 1987

Hart RP, Colenda CC, Hamer RM: Effects of buspirone and alprazolam on the cognitive performance of normal elderly subjects. Am J Psychiatry 148:73–77, 1991

Henderson VW, Roberts E, Wimer C, et al: Multicenter trial of naloxone in Alzheimer's disease. Ann Neurol 25:404–406, 1989

Herman JV, Brotman AW, Pollack MH, et al: Fluoxetine-induced sexual dysfunction. J Clin Psychiatry 51:27–29, 1990

Hoehn-Saric R, McLeod DR, Zimmerl WD: Differential effects of alprazolam and imipramine in generalized anxiety disorder. J Clin Psychiatry 49:293–301, 1988

Hoffman BB, Lefkowitz RJ: Adrenergic receptor antagonists, in Goodman and Gilman's The Pharmacological Basis of Therapeutics, 8th Edition. Edited by Gilman AG, Rall TW, Nies AS, et al. New York, Pergamon, 1990, pp 187–243

Holmes VF, Fernandez F, Levy JK: Psychostimulant response in AIDS-related complex patients. J Clin Psychiatry 50:5–8, 1989

Hoogiverf B: Amitriptyline treatment of painful diabetic neuropathy: an inadvertent single-patient clinical trial. Diabetes Care 8:526–527, 1985

Hope RA, Patel V, Series H, et al: Dexamphetamine may reduce hyperactivity in dementia: a case study using direct observation. International Journal of Geriatric Psychiatry 6:165–169, 1991

Izzo KL, Brody R: Rehabilitation in lithium toxicity. Arch Phys Med Rehabil 66:779–782, 1985

Jefferson JW: Lithium: the present and the future. J Clin Psychiatry 51 (suppl):4–8, 1990

Jefferson JW, Greist JH: Primer of Lithium Therapy. Baltimore, MD, Williams & Wilkins, 1977

Jenike MA: Approaches to patients with treatment-refractory obsessive-compulsive disorder. J Clin Psychiatry 51 (suppl):15–21, 1990

Jenike MA, Albert M, Baer L, et al: Ergot mesylates for Alzheimer's disease: a year-long double blind trial of 3 mg vs 12 mg daily. Int J Ger Psychiatry 5:375–380, 1990

Jick SS, Jick H, Knauss TA, et al: Antidepressants and convulsions. J Clin Psychopharmacol 12:241–245, 1992

Johnson LC, Chernick DA, Sateia MJ: Sleep, performance, and plasma levels in chronic insomniacs during 14-day use of flurazepam and midazolam: an introduction. J Clin Psychopharmacol 10:5S–9S, 1990

Kahn EM, Schulz C, Perel JM, et al: Change in haloperidol level due to carbamazepine: a complicatory factor in combined medication for schizophrenia. J Clin Psychopharmacol 10:54–57, 1990

Kane JM, Honigeld G, Singer J, et al: Clozapine for treatment-resistant schizophrenia. Arch Gen Psychiatry 45:789–796, 1988

Kaufman MW, Cassem N, Murray G, et al: The use of methylphenidate in depressed patients after cardiac surgery. J Clin Psychiatry 45:82–84, 1984

Ko GN, Korpi ER, Linnoila M: On the clinical relevance and methods of quantification of plasma concentrations of neuroleptics. J Clin Psychopharmacol 5:253–262, 1985

Kulkarni J, Horne M, Butler E, et al: Psychotic symptoms resulting from intraventricular infusion of dopamine in Parkinson's disease. Biol Psychiatry 31:1225–1227, 1992

Lauterbach EC, Schiveri MM: Amelioration of pseudobulbar affect by fluoxetine: possible alteration of dopamine-related pathophysiology by a selective serotonin reuptake inhibitor. J Clin Psychopharmacol 11:392–393, 1991

Lawlor BA, Sunderland T, Mellow AM, et al: A pilot placebo controlled study of chronic m-CPP administration in Alzheimer's disease. Biol Psychiatry 30:140–144, 1991

Lawrence JM: Reactions to withdrawal of antidepressants, antiparkinsonian drugs, and lithium. Psychosomatics 11:869–877, 1985

Lebowitz BD: Developments in treatment of Alzheimer's disease. Psychopharmacol Bull 28:59–60, 1992

Lieberman JA, Kane JM, Reife R: Neuromuscular effects of monoamine oxidase inhibitors. J Clin Psychopharmacol 5:217–220, 1985

Lieberman JA, Saltz BL, Johns CA, et al: The effects of clozapine on tardive dyskinesia. Br J Psychiatry 158:503–510, 1991

Lindvall O, Brundin P, Widner H, et al: Grafts of fetal dopamine neurons survive and improve motor function in Parkinson's disease. Science 247:574–577, 1990

Lipsey JR, Robinson RG, Pearlson GD, et al: Nortriptyline treatment of post-stroke depression: a double-blind study. Lancet 1:297–300, 1984

Liptzin B: Treatment of mania, in Clinical Geriatric Psychiatry, 2nd Edition. Edited by Salzman C. Baltimore, MD, Williams & Wilkins, 1992, pp 175–188

Litovitz TL, Troutman WG: Amoxapine overdose: seizures and fatalities. JAMA 250:1069–1071, 1983

Lohr JB, Jeste DV, Harris MJ, et al: Treatment of disordered behavior, in Clinical Geriatric Psychiatry, 2nd Edition. Edited by Salzman C. Baltimore, MD, Williams & Wilkins, 1992, pp 80–113

Manev H, Costa E, Wrobewski JT, et al: Abusive stimulation of excitatory amino acid receptors: a strategy to limit neurotoxicity. FASEB J 4:2789–2797, 1990

Mann SC, Caroff SN, Bleier HR: Lethal catatonia. Am J Psychiatry 143:1374–1378, 1986

Massey EW, Folger WN: Seizures activated by therapeutic levels of lithium carbonate. South Med J 77:1173–1175, 1984

Mathew NT: Prophylaxis of migraine and mixed headache: a randomized controlled study. Headache 21:105–109, 1981

Max MB, Lynch SA, Muir J, et al: Effects of desipramine, amitriptyline and fluoxetine on pain in diabetic neuropathy. N Engl J Med 326:1250–1256, 1992

McMahon FJ, DePaulo JR: Clinical features of affective disorders and bereavement. Current Opinion in Psychiatry 5:580–584, 1992

Medical Letter: Drugs that cause psychiatric symptoms. Med Lett Drugs Ther 26:75–78, 1985

Mellerup ET, Plenge P: Side effects of lithium. Biol Psychiatry 28:464–465, 1990

Meyler L, Herxheimer A: Side effects of Drugs. Baltimore, MD, Williams & Wilkins, 1968

Miller DD: Effect of phenytoin on plasma clozapine concentration in two patients. J Clin Psychiatry 52:23–25, 1991

Miller F, Menninger J: Correlation of neuroleptic dose and neurotoxicity in patients given lithium and a neuroleptic. Hosp Community Psychiatry 38:1219–1221, 1987

Mueller PS: Neuroleptic malignant syndrome. Psychosomatics 26:654–662, 1985

Nelson JC, Jatlow PI, Mazure C: Desipramine plasma levels and response in elderly melancholic patients. J Clin Psychopharmacol 5:217–220, 1985

Noyes R, Garvey MJ, Cook BL: Benzodiazepine withdrawal: a review of the evidence. J Clin Psychiatry 49:382–389, 1988

Paradis CF, Stack JA, George CJ, et al: Nortriptyline and weight change in depressed patients over 60. J Clin Psychopharmacol 12:246–250, 1992

Pare CMB: The present status of monoamine oxidase inhibitors. Br J Psychiatry 146:576–584, 1985

Pato MT, Murphy DL, DeVane CL: Sustained plasma concentrations of fluoxetine and/or norfluoxetine four and eight weeks after fluoxetine discontinuation (letter). J Clin Psychopharmacol 11:224–225, 1991

Pelonero AL, Levenson JL, Silverman JL: Neuroleptic therapy following neuroleptic malignant syndrome. Psychosomatics 26:946–947, 1985

Pennati A, Sacchetti E, Calzeroni A: Dantrolene in lethal catatonia (letter). Am J Psychiatry 148:268, 1991

Perry E, Court J: Biological correlates of dementia. Current Opinion in Psychiatry 5:554–560, 1992

Perry PJ, Calloway RA, Cook BL, et al: Theophylline-precipitated alterations of lithium clearance. Acta Psychiatr Scand 69:528–539, 1984

Pilowsky LS, Ring H, Shine PJ, et al: Rapid tranzuilisation: a survey of emergency prescribing in a general psychiatric hospital. Br J Psychiatry 160:831–835, 1992

Pollock BG, Perel JM, Altieri LP, et al: Debrisoquine hydroxylation phenotyping in geriatric psychopharmacology. Psychopharmacol Bull 28:163–167, 1992

Pomara N, Singh R, Deptula D, et al: Glutamate and other CSF amino acids in Alzheimer's disease. Am J Psychiatry 149:251–254, 1992

Post RM: Non-lithium treatment for bipolar disorder. J Clin Psychiatry 51 (suppl):9–19, 1990

Rabins PV, Pearlson E, Aylward E, et al: Cortical magnetic resonance imaging changes in elderly inpatients with a major depression. Am J Psychiatry 148:617–620, 1991

Ratey JJ, Leveroni CL, Miller AC, et al: Low-dose buspirone to treat agitation and maladaptive behavior in brain-injured patients: two case reports (letter). J Clin Psychopharmacol 12:362–364, 1992

Ray WA: Psychotropic drugs and injuries among the elderly: a review. J Clin Psychopharmacol 12:386–396, 1992

Regestein QR: Treatment of insomnia in the elderly, in Clinical Geriatric Psychopharmacology, 2nd Edition. Edited by Salzman C. Baltimore, MD, Williams & Wilkins, 1992, pp 235–253

Richelson E: Pharmacology of neuroleptics in use in the United States. J Clin Psychiatry 46:8–14, 1985

Rickels K, Amsterdam JD, Clary C, et al: Buspirone in major depression: a controlled study. J Clin Psychiatry 52:34–38, 1991

Risse SC, Barnes R: Pharmacologic treatment of agitation associated with dementia. J Am Geriatr Soc 34:368–376, 1986

Rizos AL, Sargenti CJ, Jeste DV: Psychotropic drug interactions in the patient with late-onset depression or psychosis. Psychiatr Clin North Am 11:253–275, 1988

Roberts JE, Renne CE, Dillon J, et al: Exposure to bright light and the concurrent use of photosensitizing drugs. N Engl J Med 326:1500–1501, 1992

Robinson RG, Kubos KL, Starr LP, et al: Mood disorders in stroke patients: importance of location of lesion. Brain 107:81–93, 1984

Rockwell E, Lam RW, Zisook S: Antidepressant drug studies in the elderly. Psychiatr Clin North Am 11:215–231, 1988

Roose SP, Glassman AH, Giardina EGV, et al: Tricyclic antidepressants in depressed patients with cardiac conduction disease. Arch Gen Psychiatry 44:273–275, 1987

Roose SP, Dalak GW, Glassman AH, et al: Cardiovascular effects of bupropion in depressed patients with heart disease. Am J Psychiatry 148:512–516, 1991

Rosebush P, Stewart T: Neuroleptic malignant syndrome. Am J Psychiatry 146:717–725, 1989

Rosenblatt RM, Reich J, Dehrung D: Tricyclic antidepressants in the treatment of depression and chronic pain: analysis of the supporting evidence. Anesth Analg 63:1025–1032, 1984

Ross CA: Alzheimer's disease and other neuropsychiatric disorders. Current Opinion in Psychiatry 5:561–566, 1992

Ross ED, Rush AJ: Diagnosis and neuroanatomical correlates of depression in brain damaged patients. Arch Gen Psychiatry 38:1344–1354, 1981

Roth M: The psychiatric disorders of later life. Psychiatric Annals 6:417–445, 1976

Rovner BW: Aging and the central nervous system, in Verwoerdt's Clinical Geropsychiatry, 3rd Edition. Edited by Bienenfeld D. Baltimore, MD, Williams & Wilkins, 1990, pp 17–25

Roy A, Pickar D: Lithium potentiation of imipramine in treatment-resistant depression. Br J Psychiatry 148:528–533, 1985

Rubin EH, Biggs JT, Preshorn SH: Nortriptyline pharmacokinetics and plasma levels: implications for clinical practice. J Clin Psychiatry 46:418–424, 1985

Ruegg RG, Zosook S, Swerdlow NR: Depression in the aged: an overview. Psychiatr Clin North Am 11:83–94, 1988

Salzman C: Clinical guidelines for the use of antidepressant drugs in geriatric patients. J Clin Psychiatry 46 (10, sec 2):38–44, 1985

Salzman C: Treatment of agitation, anxiety and depression in dementia. Psychopharmacol Bull 24:39–42, 1988

Salzman C: Principles of psychopharmacology, in Verwoerdt's Clinical Geropsychiatry, 3rd Edition. Edited by Bienenfeld D. Baltimore, MD, Williams and Wilkins, 1990, pp 234–249

Salzman C: The APA task force report on benzodiazepine dependence, toxicity and abuse. Am J Psychiatry 148:151–152, 1991

Salzman C: Clinical Geriatric Psychiatry, 2nd Edition. Baltimore, MD, Williams & Wilkins, 1992

Salzman C, Shader RI, Greenblatt DJ, et al: Long vs short half-life benzodiazepines in the elderly: kinetics and clinical effects of diazepam and oxazepam. Arch Gen Psychiatry 40:293–297, 1983

Sargenti CJ, Rizos AL, Jeste DV: Psychotropic drug interactions in the patient with late-onset psychosis and mood disorder, part I. Psychiatr Clin North Am 11:235–252, 1988

Sassim N, Grohmann R: Adverse drug reactions with clozapine and simultaneous application of benzodiazepines. Pharmacopsychiatry 21:306–307, 1988

Satlin A, Volicer L, Ross V, et al: Bright light treatment of behavioral and sleep disturbances in patients with Alzheimer's disease. Am J Psychiatry 149:1028–1032, 1992

Saul RF: Pseudotumor cerebri secondary to lithium carbonate. JAMA 253:2869–2871, 1985

Saxena S, Maltikarjuna P: Severe memory impairment with acute overdose lithium toxicity. Br J Psychiatry 152:853–854, 1988

Schiffer RB, Herndon RM, Rudide RA: Treatment of pathological laughing and weeping with amitriptyline. N Engl J Med 312:1480–1482, 1985

Schneider LS, Sobin PB: Non-neuroleptic treatment of behavioral symptoms and agitation in Alzheimer's disease and other dementias. Psychopharmacol Bull 28:71–79, 1992

Schor JD, Levkoff SE, Liptsitz LA, et al: risk factors for delirium in hospitalized elderly. JAMA 267:827–831, 1992

Sevash S, Guterman A, Villalon AV, et al: Improved verbal learning after outpatient oral physostigmine therapy in patients with dementia of the Alzheimer type. J Clin Psychiatry 52:300–303, 1991

Shukla S, Mukherjee S, Decina P: Lithium in the treatment of bipolar disorders associated with epilepsy: an open study. J Clin Psychopharmacol 8:201–204, 1988

Shulman KI, Walker SE, Mackenzie S, et al: Dietary restriction, tyramine, and the use of monoamine oxidase inhibitors. J Clin Psychopharmacol 9:397–402, 1989

Shulman KI, Tohen M, Satlin A, et al: Mania compared with unipolar depression in old age. Am J Psychiatry 149:341–345, 1992

Silver JM, Yudofsky S: Propranolol for aggression: literature review and clinical guidelines. International Drug Therapy Newsletter 20:9–12, 1985

Small GW: Tacrine for treating Alzheimer's disease. JAMA 268:2564–2565, 1992

Smith DE, Wesson DR: A new method for treatment of barbiturate dependence. JAMA 213:294–295, 1970

Smith GR, Taylor CW, Linkous P: Haloperidol vs thioridazine for the treatment of psychogeriatric patients: a double-blind clinical trial. Psychosomatics 15:134–137, 1974

Snowdon J: A retrospective case-note study of bipolar disorder in old age. Br J Psychiatry 158:485–490, 1991

Spagnoli A, Cucca U, Menasce G, et al: Long-term acetyl-L-carnitine treatment in Alzheimer's disease. Neurology 41:1726–1732, 1991

Spiegel R: Sleep, sleep disorders and the regulation of vigilance in physiological and pathological aging, in Clinical and Scientific Psychogeriatrics, Vol 1: The Holistic Approaches. Edited by Bergener M, Finkel SI. New York, Springer, 1990, pp 216–249

Storey P, Trumble M: Rectal doxepin and carbamazepine therapy in patients with cancer. N Engl J Med 327:1318–1319, 1992

Szuba MP, Bergmen KS, Baxter LR, et al: Safety and efficacy of high dose droperidol in agitated patients. J Clin Psychopharmacol 12:144–145, 1992

Tariot PN: Neurobiology and treatment of dementia, in Clinical Geriatric Psychiatry, 2nd Edition. Edited by Salzman C. Baltimore, MD, Williams & Wilkins, 1992, pp 277–299

Tesar GE, Murray GB, Cassem VH: Use of high-dose intravenous haloperidol in the treatment of agitated cardiac patients. J Clin Psychopharmacol 5:344–347, 1985

Thompson TL, Filley C, Mitchell D, et al: Lack of efficacy of hydergine in patients with Alzheimer's disease. N Engl J Med 323:445–448, 1990

Tollefson G: Short-term effects of the calcium channel blocker nimodipine (bay-e-9736) in the management of primary degenerative dementia. Biol Psychiatry 27:1133–1142, 1990

Van Valkenberg C, Clayton PJ: Electroconvulsive therapy and schizophrenia. Biol Psychiatry 20:699–700, 1983

Vestergaard P, Poulstrup I, Schou M, et al: Prospective studies in a lithium cohort. Acta Psychiatr Scand 78:434–441, 1988

Welch L, Sovner R: The treatment of a chronic organic mental disorder with severe mental retardation. Br J Psychiatry 161:118–120, 1992

Wilson WH: Clinical review of clozapine treatment in a state hospital. Hosp Community Psychiatry 43:700–703, 1992

Wolk SI, Douglas CJ: Clozapine treatment of psychosis in Parkinson's disease: a report of five consecutive cases. J Clin Psychiatry 53:373–376, 1992

Wragg RE, Jeste DV: Neuroleptics and alternative treatments: management of behavioral symptoms and psychosis in Alzheimer's disease and related conditions. Psychiatr Clin North Am 11:195–212, 1988

Yassa R, Camille Y, Belzile L: Tardive dyskinesia in the course of antidepressant therapy: a prevalence study and review of the literature. J Clin Psychopharmacol 7:243–246, 1987

Yassa R, Nair NPV, Iskandar H: Late-onset bipolar disorder. Psychiatr Clin North Am 11:117–129, 1988

Yassa R, Nastase C, Cvejic J, et al: The Pisa syndrome (or pleurothotonus): prevalence in a psychogeriatric population. Biol Psychiatry 29:942–945, 1991

Young RC, Klerman GL: Mania in late life: focus on age at onset. Am J Psychiatry 149:867–876, 1992

Young RC, Meyers BS: Psychopharmacology, in Comprehensive Review of Geriatric Psychiatry. Edited by Sadavoy J, Lazarus LW, Jarvik LF. Washington DC, American Psychiatric Press, 1991, pp 435–467

Young RC, Alexopoulos GS, Shamoian CA, et al: Plasma 10-hydroxynortriptyline and ECG changes in elderly depressed patients. Am J Psychiatry 142:866–868, 1985

Zis AP, Goodwin FK: Major affective disorder as a recurrent illness. Arch Gen Psychiatry 36:835–839, 1979

30

Electroconvulsive Therapy in Geriatric Neuropsychiatry

John T. Pritchett, M.D.
Charles H. Kellner, M.D.
C. Edward Coffey, M.D.

Introduction

If major depression were not a serious public health problem in the elderly population, there would be no need to discuss electroconvulsive therapy (ECT) in this book. Unfortunately, major depression is one of the most common and serious illnesses in elderly patients (see Chapter 12). In addition to death from suicide, depressive illness itself is associated with significant mortality from medical illness (Avery and Winokur 1976). ECT remains the "gold standard" treatment for serious depression and, as such, requires careful consideration as a therapeutic modality. Such consideration is particularly relevant because there is evidence that ECT is especially safe and effective in elderly patients (Consensus Conference 1985) and because of the sensitivity to the side effects of antidepressant medication experienced by the geriatric population. With the burgeoning of psychopharmacological treatments for depression over the past 30 years, many may have believed that ECT was well on its way to extinction; however, we are now no longer sanguine about the efficacy of antidepressant medications for all patients. Even with the most sophisticated psychopharmacological treatment combinations, a substantial proportion of patients remains severely ill. For these patients, it is fortunate, and sometimes even life saving, that ECT is still available.

The case for ECT is strengthened by its remarkable record of safety. ECT compares favorably with any procedure in all of medicine for its low morbidity and mortality. With recent advances in ECT treatment technique, the safety profile of the treatment continues to be refined, and ECT has enjoyed a resurgence as a much more mainstream treatment in the psychiatric armamentarium. Furthermore, it has a predictably rapid onset of effect and can be performed in both inpatient and outpatient settings.

It is widely known that ECT is most commonly used for the treatment of severe depression. In this chapter, we discuss in depth its use for this indication, but, as this is a textbook of neuropsychiatry, we also evaluate ECT as a treatment for organic affective disorders such as poststroke depression, as well as for neurological disorders such as Parkinson's disease. As the mind-body dualism separating the fields of psychiatry and neurology dissolves, investigators and clinicians will have further opportunities to explore the potent effects of ECT on brain, as well as mind, functions.

ECT in Geriatric Practice

Considerable evidence exists to demonstrate that a large proportion of patients receiving ECT are elderly. Kramer (1985) reviewed patterns of ECT use in California from 1977 to 1983 and found that the probability of receiving ECT increased with the age of the patient. Patients 65 years and older were given ECT at a rate of 3.86/10,000 population, as compared with 0.85/10,000 in those 25–44 years old. In a study of 5,729 psychiatric admissions over 3 years, Malla (1988) found that patients who received ECT in general hospitals were significantly older than those who did not receive ECT. Babigian and Guttmacher (1984) reviewed a massive amount of data from the Monroe County (New York) Psychiatric Case Register over three different 5-year epochs. They found that among first-hospitalization patients, ECT recipients were significantly more likely to be older.

Several features of the natural history of major depressive illness help to explain the frequent use of ECT in elderly patients. Post (1992) has recently reviewed data suggesting that major affective disorders increase both in severity and in cycle frequency with increasing age. In a review of the course of illness of late-onset depression, Alexopoulos (1990) cited evidence for an association between high relapse rates and later onset of illness (Zis and Goodwin 1979). Thus in the geriatric population, the frequency and severity of depressive illness, along with increased sensitivity to adverse effects of antidepressant medications, combine to make ECT an attractive and often-used treatment option (Benbow 1987, 1989; Weiner 1982).

Medical Physiology of ECT in Elderly Patients

The data on the physiology of ECT have been compiled largely from mixed-age samples of subjects, and, to our knowledge, few data focus specifically on the physiology of ECT in elderly patients. Clearly, the myriad physiological changes that accompany an ECT seizure take on particular significance in the elderly population, in whom medical illnesses involving multiple organ systems are so common. In a study of 33 elderly patients (mean age = 74 years) receiving ECT, Gaspar and Samarasinghe (1982) found a 75% incidence of major or minor medical risk factors for ECT. Of greatest importance are the physiological effects of

ECT on the brain and cardiovascular system. As described below, modifications in ECT technique may be required in patients who have cardiovascular or brain disease.

Cerebral Physiology of ECT

With ECT, an electrical stimulus is used to depolarize cerebral neurons and thereby produce a generalized cerebral seizure. The mechanism by which ECT seizures are propagated is not well understood. Bilateral ECT appears to lead to seizure generalization via direct stimulation of the diencephalon, whereas seizures induced with unilateral stimulation may begin focally in the stimulated cortex and then generalize via corticothalamic pathways (Staton 1981).

During the initial phase of the induced seizure, electroencephalographic (EEG) activity is variable, consisting of patterns of low-voltage fast activity and polyspike rhythms. These patterns correlate with tonic or irregular clonic motor movements. With seizure progression, EEG activity evolves into a pattern of hypersynchronous polyspikes and waves that characterize the clonic motor phase. These regular patterns begin to slow and eventually disintegrate as the seizure ends, sometimes terminating abruptly in a "flat" EEG (Weiner and Krystal et al. 1993). The extent to which this typical ictal EEG pattern may be altered by brain changes associated with aging has not been studied.

Transient cumulative changes also occur in the interictal EEG in response to a course of ECT. Increased predominance of delta activity on interictal EEG is seen as a function of the number of treatments given in a course of ECT and their rate of administration (Fink 1979). Asymmetric (left greater than right) decreases in average EEG frequency after a course of ECT have been correlated with increasing age of the patient (Volavka et al. 1972). The interictal EEG returns to baseline by 30 days after the ECT course in most patients (Abrams 1992). The effects of aging on the severity and persistence of these interictal EEG changes have not been extensively studied.

The ECT-induced seizure is also associated with a variety of transient and benign changes in cerebral physiology, including increases in cerebral blood flow, cerebral blood volume (resulting in a transient rise in intracranial pressure), and cerebral metabolism of oxygen and glucose (Bolwig et al. 1977; Broderson et al. 1973; Prohovnik et al. 1986). The brief rise in intracranial pressure is rarely of clinical consequence, but it is the reason for the well-known proscription against ECT in patients with space-occupying mass lesions. Postictally, cerebral blood flow and metabolism are decreased for at least several days after the seizure and then return to normal values. Transient disruptions in blood-brain barrier permeability also occur (Bolwig et al. 1977) and may account for the short-lived increase in T_1 relaxation times observed on brain magnetic resonance imaging (MRI) after ECT (Mander et al. 1987; Scott et al. 1990). The effects of age and associated brain changes on these physiological responses have not been defined.

Cardiovascular Physiology of ECT

ECT results in a marked activation of the autonomic nervous system, and the relative balance of parasympathetic and sympathetic nervous system activity determines the observed cardiovascular effects. Vagal (parasympathetic) tone is increased during and immediately after administration of the electrical stimulus, and this may be manifested by bradycardia or even a brief period of asystole. With development of the seizure, activation of the sympathetic nervous system occurs, resulting in a marked increase in heart rate, blood pressure, and cardiac workload. Peripheral stigmata of sympathetic activation may also be observed and include piloerection and gooseflesh. The tachycardia and hypertension continue through the ictus and generally end along with the seizure. Shortly after the seizure, there may be a second period of increased vagal tone that may be manifested by bradycardia and various dysrhythmias, including the appearance of ectopic beats. As the patient awakens from anesthesia, there may be an additional period of increased heart rate and blood pressure as a result of arousal and further sympathetic outflow (Welch and Drop 1989).

The cardiovascular responses during ECT combine to produce an increase in myocardial oxygen demand and a decrease in coronary artery diastolic filling time. Transient electrocardiographic (ECG) changes in the ST segment and T waves are seen in some patients during the procedure, although it is unclear whether these findings are related to myocardial ischemia. A direct effect of central nervous system stimulation on cardiac repolarization has been proposed as an alternative mechanism (Welch and Drop 1989). No corresponding rise in cardiac enzymes has been found to accompany these ECG changes (Braasch and Demaso 1980).

A recent echocardiographic study done during and after ECT treatments found transient regional wall motion abnormalities more often in patients with ST-T changes in ECG, suggesting a period of demand myocardial ischemia (Messina et al. 1992). The clinical significance of these findings remains to be evaluated in future studies.

Only a few modern studies have examined the effects of age on the cardiovascular response to ECT. With regard to vagal effects, Shettar et al. (1989) randomly assigned 19 patients (mean ±SD age = 51 ± 21 years, range = 19–84 years) to receive ECT with or without pretreatment with glycopyrrolate, the drug condition being reversed at the subsequent ECT treatment (i.e., each patient served as his or her own control). For both the placebo and glycopyrrolate conditions, there was no correlation between age and length of poststimulus asystole. With regard to sympathetic effects, two controlled studies of mixed-age samples that included elderly patients found no relationship between age and ECT-induced changes in heart rate, blood pressure, or rate-pressure product (Prudic et al. 1987; Webb et al. 1990). Another study of relatively younger patients (mean age = 43 years, range = 20–64 years) actually observed a significant inverse correlation between age and increases in blood pressure and rate-pressure product (Huang et al. 1989).

Although these results suggest that age, per se, is not associated with the extent of the cardiovascular response to ECT, these findings must be interpreted cautiously. Some of the subjects in these studies (especially those who were older) were also receiving antihypertensive drug therapy that may have attenuated their cardiovascular response to the treatments, and (as discussed below) other clinical observations suggest that at least some elderly patients with cardiovascular disease may be at risk for marked elevations in pulse and blood pressure during ECT (Bodley and Fenwick 1966; Gerring and Shields 1982; Zielinski et al. 1993).

Diagnostic Indications and Efficacy

Major Depression

The most common indication for ECT in the elderly population remains depression, both unipolar and bipolar. The typical scenario for the use of ECT in depressed elderly patients is as a second-line treatment, after patients have failed a medication trial or have

been intolerant of the side effects of medication. ECT may be used as a first-line intervention, however, in certain situations: severe suicidality, inanition and malnutrition, history of previous response to ECT, or patient preference (American Psychiatric Association 1990).

Several clinical studies of mixed-age samples with various diagnoses have found increasing age to be associated with a favorable outcome from ECT (Black et al. 1993; Carney et al. 1965; Coryell and Zimmerman 1984; Folstein et al. 1973; Gold and Chiarella 1944; Kahn et al. 1959; Mendels 1965; Roberts 1959; Strömgren 1973). A small number of studies have directly examined the effects of ECT in depressed elderly subjects, but results are somewhat difficult to compare because of differences in patient samples (e.g., size and diagnosis), ECT technique (e.g., stimulus waveform and dosage and electrode placement), and assessment methodology (Table 30–1). Nevertheless, reported response rates range from 63%–98%, clearly demonstrating that increasing age, per se, does not limit the effectiveness of ECT for depressive illness. In a recent prospective study, Wilkinson et al. (1993) stratified 78 patients receiving ECT into four age groups (18–39, 40–64, 65–74, and 75–88). Affective and cognitive measures were obtained before and after ECT. The investigators found a significant ($P < .05$) positive correlation between increasing age and good response to ECT.

A retrospective chart review of 112 consecutive geriatric hospital admissions compared outcome in depressed patients who had received ECT versus those who had received tricyclic antidepressants (nonrandom assignment) and found that ECT was associated with a better response rate (81% versus 62%) and a lower morbidity rate (0% versus 27%) (Meyers and Mei-Tal 1985–86). There are, however, no controlled, prospective, randomized studies comparing the efficacy and side effects of ECT versus drug therapy for treatment of depression in elderly patients.

Because major depression in elderly patients appears to respond well to ECT, there may be little need to correlate specific clinical features with ECT response. However, in data derived largely from mixed-age samples, a particularly good response to ECT has been associated with the presence of psychosis, catatonia, pseudodementia, pathological guilt, anhedonia, agitation, and neurovegetative signs (Greenberg and Fink 1992; Salzman 1982; Zorumski et al. 1988). A prospective study in 29 elderly patients corroborated guilt, anhedonia, and agitation as positive prognostic signs

Table 30–1. Studies of electroconvulsive therapy (ECT) as a treatment for geriatric depression

Author	Subjects	Methods	Findings
Fraser and Glass 1980	29 patients (8 men and 21 women) Age range 64–86 years "Depressive illness" by Feighner criteria	Prospective ECT two times/week; chopped sine waveform; randomized assignment to bilateral (*n* = 16) versus right uni-lateral electrode placement (*n* = 13) Blinded ratings of outcome	Both groups had significant reductions in HRSD scores at 3 weeks after the last treatment, at which point 28 (97%) of the 29 patients showed a "satisfactory" clinical outcome. No group differences in therapeutic response. Average time to reorientation after the fifth ECT was 32.8 minutes for bilateral ECT and 9.5 minutes for right unilateral ECT. WMS scores improved during ECT, and at 3 weeks post-ECT all scores were normal. No group differences.
Gaspar and Samarasinghe 1982	33 patients (9 men and 24 women) Age range 66–88 years (mean ±SD = 73.9 ± 5.7 years) Depression in 28 of 33 patients (85%); diagnostic criteria unspecified	Prospective ECT two times/week for 3–4 weeks, then one time/week. Mean number of ECT treatments = 8.7 (range 2–29), bilateral Outcome rated as good, inter-mediate, or poor	Good outcome in 26 patients (79%); intermediate outcome in 3 patients (9%); poor outcome in 4 patients (12%).
Karlinsky and Shulman 1984	33 inpatients (11 men and 22 women) Age range 62–85 years, (mean ±SD = 73.2 ± 5.0 years) DSM-III major depression, single episode *n* = 12 (36.4%); major depression, recurrent *n* = 18 (54.5%); bipolar disorder *n* = 3 (9.1%)	Retrospective ECT two or three times/week; sine wave; unilateral *n* = 23 (69.7%), bilateral *n* = 3 (9.1%), both *n* = 7 (21.2%) Nonblinded rating of outcome by author's consensus from clinical progress notes Follow-up at 3 and 6 months	Immediate "good" response *n* = 14 (42.4%), "moderate" response *n* = 12 (36.4%), "poor" response *n* = 7 (21.2%). During the 6-month follow-up, 23 patients (69.7%) remained out of hospital, and 6 patients (18.2%) received more ECT. Only one complication (pneumonia), and even this patient was able to complete the ECT course.
Burke et al. 1985	30 patients (7 men and 23 women) Age range 60–82 years (mean = 72 years) DSM-III major depression *n* = 24, bipolar disorder *n* = 5	Retrospective Average number of ECT treat-ments = 9 (range = 1–25); brief pulse; bilateral in 70% Outcome rating (4-point scale) assessed by review of medical records	92% of patients with major depression improved, and 69% showed complete symptom resolution.
Burke et al. 1987	136 patients (39 men and 97 women) Mean age of total sample = 48 years: 96 subjects less than 60 years old (mean ±SD = 39 ± 12.19 years), and 40 subjects were more than 60 years old (mean ±SD = 69 ± 6.43 years) 81% of total sample major affective disorder; diagnoses of elderly subgroup unspecified	Sine wave current; 87% bilateral, 73% unilateral; mean ±SD number of ECT treatments = 9 ± 3.6	70% of total sample had a complete resolution of affective symptoms (61% less than 60 years old and 75% more than 60 years old). Complications were found to increase with age (35% older group versus 18% younger group).

(continued)

Table 30–1.   Studies of electroconvulsive therapy (ECT) as a treatment for geriatric depression *(continued)*

Author	Subjects	Methods	Findings
Kramer 1987	50 inpatients (9 men and 41 women) Age range 61–88 years (mean = 74.1 years) DSM-III major depression $n = 49$; schizophrenia $n = 1$	Retrospective ECT three times/week; brief pulse current; bilateral electrode placement in all patients Nonblinded assessment by author's chart review	46 patients (92%) noted "much improved" after ECT. No serious medical complications.
Godber et al. 1987	163 patients (43 men and 120 women) Mean age = 86 years, all more than 65 years old Primary depression by Feighner criteria in 153 (93.8%) patients, psychotic symptoms in 80 (49%) patients	ECT two times/week for most patients, three times/week for some those slow to respond; sinusoidal waveform; right unilateral electrode placement $n = 155$ (95%) (mean number of treatments = 11.2)	83 (51%) patients "fully recovered"; 37 (23%) patients "much improved"; 34 (21%) poor response.
Magni 1988	30 patients (14 men and 16 women) Mean age = 73.9 years DSM-III major depression	Retrospective ECT two to three times/week initially, then once weekly; all bilateral; minimum 7 ECT treatments (range 7–12) Independent clinical ratings by two psychiatrists	19 patients (63%) responded to ECT.
Coffey et al. 1988	44 inpatients (18 men and 26 women) with leukoencephalopathy Age range 60–86 years, mean = 73 DSM-III diagnosis of major depression in all	Retrospective ECT three time/week; brief-pulse "moderately suprathreshold" stimulus; average number of ECT treatments = 9 (range 6–14); outcome ratings by attending physician and ward treatment team from medical records	"Excellent" response in 54%, "good" response in 44%.
Coffey et al. 1989	51 inpatients (15 men and 36 women) Age range 60–90 years, (mean 71.3 years) DSM-III major or bipolar depression ($n = 49$), organic affective disorder ($n = 2$)	Prospective ECT three times/week; brief-pulse; unilateral ($n = 38$), bilateral ($n = 3$), unilateral bilateral ($n = 10$); mean number of ECT treatments = 9 (range 5–18) Nonblinded observer and patient self-ratings	42 (82%) met criteria for full therapeutic response. No association between magnetic resonance imaging (MRI) brain white matter abnormalities and ECT response.
Mulsant et al. 1991	42 inpatients, 7 men and 35 women Age range 60–89 years, (mean ±SD 73.5 ± 7.3 years) DSM-III diagnosis of major depression.	Prospective ECT three times/week; brief-pulse current Unilateral $n = 29$ (89%); bilateral $n = 3$ (7%); switch from unilateral to bilateral $n = 10$ (24%); mean number of ECT treatments = 8.3 (range 4.13) Outcome by HRSD, BPRS, MMSE given by research nurses	28 patients (67%) had an excellent response to ECT (decrease in HRSD 50%). 38 patients had a decrease in BPRS score. No significant change in group MMSE mean scores.

(continued)

Table 30–1. Studies of electroconvulsive therapy (ECT) as a treatment for geriatric depression *(continued)*

Author	Subjects	Methods	Findings
Rubin et al. 1991	101 inpatients (19 men and 82 women) Mean ±SD age = 76.0 ± 6.4 years DSM-III unipolar depression	Retrospective 46 (46%) patients received ECT (technique not described), some in combination with antidepressant drug therapy, 65 (64%) received anti-depressant drug therapy only; nonrandomized Nonblinded retrospective ratings of outcome by "unit director"	Relative to patients treated with drug therapy, those who received ECT had significantly lower final BDI scores, a greater reduction in BDI scores, and a higher frequency of ratings of "major improvement" (42% versus 78%, respectively).
Kellner et al. 1992	15 patients (11 men and 4 women) Age range 53–87 (mean age = 69.9 years) DSM-III major depression	Prospective Blinded ratings of outcome measures including cognitive assessment and antidepressant response Bilateral electrode placement; brief pulse stimulus; randomized assignment to ECT one time/week versus 3 times/week for 3 weeks	All patients improved. HRSD scores decreased from 27 to 12 in the three-times/week group, and from 29 to 20 in one-time/week group. No difference in cognitive effects between groups.
Wilkinson et al. 1993	78 patients (23 men and 55 women) Four age groups (18–39, 40–64, 65–74, and 75–88) 43 patients more than 65 years old (mean = 68.96 years in 65–74 group and 79.50 years in 75–88 group) DSM-III major depression with melancholia or psychosis	Prospective ECT two times/week Right unilateral electrode placement $n = 5$ (6%); remainder bilateral (mean number of treatments = 7.9) Nonblinded cognitive and affective ratings Postive response to ECT defined as 50% or greater reduction in Montgomery Asberg Depression Rating Scale	Positive response to ECT in 73% of patients over age 65 and 54% of patients under age 65. Significant positive correlations between increasing age and both response to ECT, and more improvement in cognition on MMSE with ECT.

Note. Feighner criteria (see Feighner et al. 1972); HRSD = Hamilton Rating Scale for Depression (Hamilton 1960); WMS = Wechsler Memory Scale (see Wechsler 1987); DSM-III = Diagnostic and Statistical Manual of Mental Disorders, 3rd Edition (American Psychiatric Association 1980); BPRS = Brief Psychiatric Rating Scale (Overall and Gorham 1962); MMSE = Mini-Mental State Exam (Folstein et al. 1975; BDI = Beck Depression Inventory (Beck 1978).

(Fraser and Glass 1980). Multiple studies have found particularly good ECT response in patients with delusional depression, compared with a nonpsychotic group (Mulsant et al. 1991; Pande et al. 1990; Wilkinson et al. 1993), although other studies have found no difference (Rich et al. 1984a, 1986; Solan et al. 1988). The use of ECT in agitated or psychotic elderly patients may spare them exposure to neuroleptic agents. This consideration is important, given the high risk for tardive dyskinesia and drug-induced Parkinsonism in elderly patients (Jenike 1985).

Several authors have also attempted to identify predictors of nonresponse to ECT. In a retrospective study, Magni et al. (1988) compared elderly patients who responded to ECT to those who did not respond and found that physical illness during the index episode, fewer negative life events preceding the onset of the index episode, and prior depressive episodes of long duration were predictive of nonresponse to ECT. Other investigators have found that longer duration of the index episode predicts poorer outcome (Fraser and Glass 1980; Karlinsky and Shulman 1984). Previous courses of ECT and increased age at the time of first treatment with ECT have been linked with a slower response rate to ECT, without affecting eventual positive outcome (Rich et al. 1984b; Salzman 1982). These limited data should not discourage the clinician from attempting a trial of ECT in patients with any of the above predictors of nonresponse. Clinical experience suggests that many elderly patients with these putative predictors of nonresponse often improve with ECT treatment.

Efforts at using biological markers to predict ECT response in elderly patients have met with equivocal success. A variety of probes have been investigated in mixed-age patient samples including the dexamethasone suppression test (DST) and other neuroendocrine tests (Kamil and Joffe 1991; Swartz 1993), as well as polysomnographic studies (Coffey et al. 1988). However, none of these laboratory studies appear to be strong "state-specific" markers for major depressive illness, and data are conflicting on whether they can be used serially to follow the course of ECT, predict outcome, or predict early relapse. Nevertheless, a recent report by Devanand et al. (1991) suggested that consideration of complex technical factors in neuroendocrine testing may enhance the clinical utility of such assessments in ECT.

Mania

Although a vast clinical experience supports the efficacy of ECT in treating both the manic and the depressed phases of bipolar illness in elderly patients, formal data in this population are lacking. In a relatively young mixed-age population (mean age = 37 years), Small et al. (1988) randomized patients to receive either lithium or ECT for acute mania and found that those treated with ECT improved more during the first 8 weeks of the trial, with equivalent response rates thereafter. ECT appeared to be particularly effective in mixed bipolar states and agitated mania, conditions that tend to become more prevalent as the illness becomes more chronic and refractory (Calabrese et al. 1993). Many elderly patients with bipolar disorder have reached this more severe phase of the illness and thus may be expected to show a particularly good response to ECT. Anticonvulsant medications are often effective in mixed bipolar disorder (Calabrese 1993), although we are not aware of efficacy studies testing this use of anticonvulsants in elderly subjects. It is of interest that ECT also has powerful anticonvulsant properties (Sackeim et al. 1983). The question of whether bilateral ECT is more effective than nondominant unilateral ECT in the treatment of mania remains controversial (Small et al. 1991).

Schizophrenia and Other Psychotic Disorders

No controlled data exist on the use of ECT in elderly patients with schizophrenia. ECT has been used in relatively younger patients with this illness, where the presence of affective or catatonic features, or a history of response to ECT, correlates with good outcome (American Psychiatric Association 1990). ECT is not very effective for the chronic, residual phase of the illness with predominant negative features (Weiner and Coffey 1988). These "deficit" states become more common as the illness progresses (Kaplan and Sadock 1988) and thus should be highly represented in elderly schizophrenic populations, although controlled data on this issue are lacking.

ECT has also been used in elderly patients with other psychotic disorders. Botteron et al. (1991) reported three elderly patients with late-onset psychosis treated with ECT. None of the patients had major depression or dementia. Two patients with substantial structural brain changes on MRI (lateral ventricular enlargement and deep white matter hyperintensities) did not respond to ECT. A third patient with bilateral caudate hyperintensities and normal subcortical white matter did respond to ECT. As discussed below, we have noted an excellent ECT response for major depression in patients with subcortical hyperintensities on MRI, including those with psychotic symptoms and late-age onset (Coffey et al. 1989). To the best of our knowledge, there are no data on the efficacy of ECT in patients with late-onset functional psychoses, such as paraphrenia.

ECT in Elderly Patients With Concomitant Neurological Disease

A growing clinical literature suggests that ECT may be effective for affective disorders in patients with brain disease (Dubovsky 1986; Hsiao et al. 1987; Weiner and Coffey 1993; Zwil et al. 1992). In some cases, the neurobiological effects of ECT have also been used to treat the neurological disorder. Issues related to modifications in the technique of ECT in patients with cerebral disease are discussed below.

Affective disorder in dementia. Twenty percent to 30% of patients with dementia have significant concomitant depression, and 10%–15% of patients diagnosed with dementia actually have the pseudodementia of depression (Price and McAllister 1989).

Depression may be difficult to diagnose in dementia patients. Some dementia patients may be too ill to generate depressive complaints, with affective disorder manifesting itself chiefly as agitated, screaming behavior with neurovegetative signs. Personal or family history of affective disorder may be helpful in formulating a case for depression in these patients (Fogel 1988). Thorough treatment of depression in patients with dementia often does much to enhance quality of life and functional status. (The effectiveness of drug therapy for depression in patients with dementia is discussed in Chapter 29.)

Fisman (1988) recently reported the case of a man with major depression and profound pseudodementia who was diagnosed incorrectly as having Alzheimer's disease for 14 years before he received successful treatment of his affective disorder with ECT. In a literature review of 56 patients with dementia and depression treated with ECT, Price and McAllister (1989) found a 73% response rate of depression. ECT effectively treated depression in several subtypes of organic dementia including senile dementia of the Alzheimer's type, multi-infarct dementia, and normal pressure hydrocephalus, as well as the dementias of Parkinson's disease and Huntington's disease (Price and McAllister 1989). Choice of electrode placement was not specified in the majority of cases reviewed. Nearly one-third of patients with dementia also had an improvement in cognition following ECT. Delirium was a relatively infrequent complication of ECT in these patients, with an overall occurrence of 21%, clearing by the time of discharge in all but 1 patient.

Dementia does not appear to be worsened by ECT. Still, to minimize cognitive side effects from ECT, patients with dementia may require special attention to issues of concomitant medications, electrode placement, and frequency of treatments. Prospective studies are required to accurately address the question of the efficacy and side effects of ECT in depressed patients with dementia.

Parkinson's disease. As discussed in Chapter 22, depression is common in patients with Parkinson's disease, and its treatment with medication may be complicated. Serious shortcomings also limit the pharmacological treatment of the parkinsonism itself. Levodopa therapy for Parkinson's disease is often accompanied by serious side effects and does little to retard the progression of the illness. Increasing doses of the medication are required to maintain motor func-tion, but at the expense of more and more debilitating side effects such as hallucinations, dyskinesias, and the "on-off" syndrome. Neuroleptics may improve the psychoses and dyskinesia, but at the expense of increased parkinsonism. This situation has led to recent attempts at grafting fetal mesencephalic tissue into the brains of Parkinson's patients. Despite some recent encouraging results, these experiments remain fraught with difficulty at multiple levels (Fahn 1992).

In this setting, reports of the efficacy of ECT in Parkinson's disease offer hope that a safe and effective treatment may become a more routine part of the therapeutic armamentarium for this disease (Table 30–2). Case reports document that ECT is effective in treating both the motor manifestations of Parkinson's disease and the commonly associated depression (for a review, see Kellner and Bernstein 1993). Interestingly, a dissociation often exists between improvement in motor symptoms and mood, with some patients improving in one but without change in the other (for a review, see Kellner and Bernstein 1993).

A group of Swedish investigators (Andersen et al. 1987) has done the most methodologically rigorous trial of ECT in Parkinson's disease. Using a double-blind, controlled crossover design comparison of real ECT with sham ECT, 9 (82%) of 11 nondepressed elderly patients with the "on-off" syndrome experienced substantial improvement in parkinsonian symptoms with ECT, lasting from 2 to 6 weeks. Sham ECT was ineffective. Nine patients received bilateral ECT (8 responded; 1 did not respond) and 2 patients received right unilateral ECT (1 responded; 1 did not respond). A total of five to six treatments were given during the active phase of the trial. The stimulus dosing strategy was not fully detailed in the report.

In a prospective naturalistic study, Douyon et al. (1989) studied seven patients with both Parkinson's disease and major depression. Significant improvement in motor function was noted after only two bilateral treatments. Following an average of seven bilateral ECT treatments with "just above threshold" stimulus dosing, mean scores on the New York University Parkinson's Disease Rating Scale decreased from 65 to 32 (51% improvement). Patients remained well, without further ECT, for a period of 4 weeks to 6 months. Although all patients had an initial Hamilton Rating Scale for Depression score of greater than 20, follow-up ratings were done on only four patients. Depression scores decreased by a mean of 50% in these patients. In another prospective naturalistic study, Zervas and

Table 30–2. Electroconvulsive therapy (ECT) for the treatment of Parkinson's disease

Study	*N* patients	Diagnosis	ECT course	Treatment response
Fromm 1959	8	Parkinson's disease	5–6 bilateral ECT treatments	Improvement: 5 patients Mild improvement: 2 patients No improvement: 1 patient
Lebensohn et al. 1975	2	Parkinson's disease and depression (1 patient) Parkinson's disease and bipolar, depressed (1 patient)	4–6 ECT treatments (electrode placement unknown)	Improvement in Parkinson's symptoms: 2 patients Improvement in depressive symptoms: 2 patients
Brown 1973	7	Parkinson's disease Major depression	Average of 8 ECT treatments (electrode placement unknown)	No improvement in Parkinson's symptoms No improvement in depression
Lipper and Bermanzohn 1975	1	Parkinson's disease Psychotic depression	7 ECT treatments (electrode placement unknown)	Marked improvement in depression Improvement in Parkinson's symptoms
Dysken et al. 1976	1	Parkinson's disease Depression	12 bilateral ECT treatments	Improvement in Parkinson's symptoms Improvement in depressive symptoms
Asnis 1977	1	Parkinson's disease Psychotic depression	6 bilateral ECT treatments	Improvement in Parkinson's symptoms Improvement in depressive symptoms
Yudofsky 1979	1	Parkinson's disease Psychotic depression	10 ECT treatments (electrode placement unknown)	Improvement in Parkinson's symptoms Improvement in depressive symptoms
Balldin et al. 1980	5	Parkinson's disease (5 patients) Parkinson's disease and depression (3 patients)	4–8 bilateral ECT treatments	Improvement in Parkinson's symptoms: all 5 patients Improvement in depressive symptoms: all 3 patients
Balldin et al. 1981	9	Parkinson's disease	3–8 bilateral ECT treatments	Marked improvement: 5 patients Slight improvement: 2 patients No improvement: 2 patients
Ward et al. 1980	5	Parkinson's disease	6 bilateral ECT treatments	No improvement: 5 patients
Holcomb et al. 1983	1	Parkinson's disease Depression	14 ECT treatments (electrode placement unknown)	Improvement in Parkinson's symptoms Improvement in depressed mood
Levy et al. 1983	1	Parkinson's disease Major depression	10 ECT treatments (electrode placement unknown)	Improvement in Parkinson's symptoms Resolution of depressive symptoms
Young et al. 1985	1	Parkinson's disease Major depression Dementia	7 right unilateral ECT treatments	Improvement in Parkinson's symptoms No improvement in depressed mood or cognitive function
Jaeckle and Dilsaver 1986	1	Parkinson's disease Bipolar, depressed	9 bilateral ECT treatments	Improvement in Parkinson's symptoms Improvement in depressed mood
Andersen et al. 1987	11	Parkinson's disease	Sham control Bilateral (9 patients) Right unilateral (2 patients)	Improvement: 9 out of 11 patients
Burke et al. 1988	3	Parkinson's disease Depression	5–8 right unilateral ECT treatments	Improvement in Parkinson's symptoms: 2 patients No improvement in Parkinson's symptoms: 1 patient Improvement in depressed mood: 3 patients

(continued)

Table 30–2. Electroconvulsive therapy (ECT) for the treatment of Parkinson's disease *(continued)*

Study	N patients	Diagnosis	ECT course	Treatment response
Atre-Vaidya and Jampala 1988	1	Parkinson's disease Mania	12 bilateral ECT treatments	Improvement in Parkinson's symptoms Resolution of manic symptoms
Roth et al. 1988	1	Parkinson's disease Bipolar, manic	10 right unilateral ECT treatments	Improvement in Parkinson's symptoms Resolution of manic symptoms
Birkett 1988	5	Parkinson's disease Major depression	Right unilateral ECT (number unknown)	Improvement in Parkinson's symptoms; 4 patients No improvement in Parkinson's symptoms: 1 patient Improvement in depressive symptoms: 4 patients No improvement in depressive symptoms: 1 patient
Douyon et al. 1989	7	Parkinson's disease Major depression	Average of 7 bilateral ECT treatments	Improvement in depressed mood: 7 patients Improvement in Parkinson's symptoms: 7 patients
Lauterbach and Moore 1990	1	Parkinson's disease Major depression	9 ECT treatments (electrode placement unknown)	Improvement in Parkinson's symptoms Improvement in depression
Zervas and Fink 1991	4	Parkinson's disease	8–12 ECT treatments Bilateral: 3 patients Right unilateral: 1 patient	Improvement in Parkinson's symptoms: all 4 patients
Friedman and Gordon 1992	5	Parkinson's disease Major depression	7–12 ECT treatments Bilateral: 1 patient Right unilateral: 3 patients Electrode placement unknown: 1 patient	Improvement in depressed mood: 4 patients Improvement in Parkinson's symptoms: 3 patients
Holzer et al. 1992	1	Parkinson's disease Major depression	8 right unilateral ECT treatments	Improvement in Parkinson's symptoms Improvement in depressed mood
Oh et al. 1992	11	Parkinson's disease Major depression: 10 patients Mania: 1 patient	3–9 ECT treatments Bilateral: 1 patient Right unilateral: 9 patients Switch from unilateral to bilateral: 1 patient	Minor improvement in Parkinson's symptoms: 2 patients Improvement in psychiatric symptoms: 6 patients Post-ECT delirium: 7 patients

Fink (1991) described the successful ECT treatment of four nondepressed elderly patients with severe refractory Parkinson's disease. Three of the four patients received bilateral ECT. Stimulus dosing strategies were not specified. Improvement in parkinsonism rating scores of 20%–40% was observed. Two patients were successfully treated with ongoing maintenance ECT, but once it was discontinued, both patients relapsed within 4 to 6 weeks. Finally, ECT has also been found to be effective for neuroleptic-induced parkinsonism (Hermesh et al. 1992).

Rasmussen and Abrams (1991) have suggested

that the primary indication for ECT in Parkinson's disease be refractoriness to, or intolerance of, antiparkinsonian medication in patients with severe disability from the disease. They have recommended that ECT for Parkinson's disease be initiated with right unilateral placement at substantially suprathreshold electrical dosage, with a switch to bilateral ECT if no response is seen after three right unilateral treatments. It should be noted, however, that some patients with Parkinson's disease may be at increased risk for developing delirium during ECT (Figiel et al. 1991), a complication that could be worsened by use of bilateral electrode placement. For patients who have clearly benefited from ECT, Rasmussen and Abrams (1991) recommended a maintenance ECT regimen titrated to the longest intertreatment interval that will maintain improvement.

The mechanism by which ECT benefits Parkinson's patients is unclear. Studies by Rudorfer et al. (1988) have shown significant increases in cerebrospinal fluid homovanillic acid, the primary metabolite of dopamine in the central nervous system, following a course of ECT. In addition to these presumed presynaptic effects, Fochtmann (1988) has found increased dopamine, subtype 1 (D_1), receptor binding in the substantia nigra of rats given electrically induced seizures. She has hypothesized that these changes may be associated with other changes in the dopamine system, including upregulation of postsynaptic dopamine, subtype 2 (D_2), receptors in the striatum. Another potential dopamine-enhancing mechanism may be the temporary disruption of the blood-brain barrier seen with ECT (Bolwig et al. 1977), allowing an increase in brain concentrations of levodopa. Whatever the mechanism by which dopamine potentiation may occur, levodopa dosage may need to be decreased during a course of ECT to avoid dyskinesia and delirium, presumably related to dopamine overactivity.

Poststroke depression.   As discussed in Chapter 23, about one-third of patients will develop significant depression in the 2 years following a stroke (Robinson and Price 1982). In a placebo-controlled trial, Lipsey et al. (1984) found a statistically significant improvement in poststroke depression treated with nortriptyline. Other uncontrolled studies have found a 47%–52% response rate to psychostimulants in this population (Finklestein et al. 1987; Lingam et al. 1988). However, patients with stroke are often quite ill and medically debilitated, leading to intolerance of pharmacotherapy. In the study by Lipsey et al. (1984), 35% of patients assigned to receive nortriptyline dropped out because of medication intolerance.

Clinical reports suggest ECT may also be effective for the treatment of poststroke depression. In a retrospective chart review of 14 patients with poststroke depression (mean age = 66 years) treated with ECT at the Massachusetts General Hospital, Murray et al. (1986) found that 86% had marked improvement in depression after ECT. Apparently, no patient exhibited any worsening of neurological deficit, and although formal measures of cognitive status were not reported, 5 of the

6 patients with "cognitive impairment" pre-ECT showed lessening of this deficit after ECT.

Currier et al. (1992) published retrospective data on 20 geriatric patients with poststroke depression treated with ECT at the same hospital, using predominantly nondominant unilateral electrode placement. A "marked or moderate response" to ECT was observed in 95% of patients. No patient experienced any exacerbation of preexisting neurological deficits, but 3 patients exhibited "minor encephalopathic complications" (prolonged postictal confusion and amnesia) and 2 patients developed "severe interictal delirium requiring neuroleptics." Of note, 7 (37%) patients relapsed within a mean of 4 months of discontinuing ECT, despite ongoing maintenance drug therapy.

Elderly psychiatric patients with no clinical history of stroke often have subcortical white matter hyperintensities on MRI, which are believed to be evidence of ischemic cerebrovascular disease. Coffey et al. (1989) found a high rate (82%) of response to ECT in depressed patients with these MRI findings, many of whom had been refractory to antidepressant drug therapy. In addition, the majority of the patients tolerated the course of ECT without major systemic or cognitive side effects. In summary, ECT may be effective for poststroke depression, but controlled prospective data are needed to confirm this clinical impression and to identify patients potentially at risk for the adverse cognitive effects of the treatment.

Other neuropsychiatric illnesses.   A variety of other organic mental syndromes in elderly patients may improve with ECT, including catatonia and delirium from many different causes (Hsiao et al. 1987; Weiner and Coffey 1993). Indeed, the antidelirium effect of ECT may occur even in the absence of improvement in the conditions that originally caused the delirium. Of course, a careful neuropsychiatric evaluation is required in such instances so as to clarify the etiology, including those conditions that might increase the risk of ECT (see below).

Issues of ECT Treatment Technique Relevant to Elderly Patients

Pre-ECT Evaluation

When a patient is referred for ECT, a focused evaluation of indications and risk factors for the treatment should ensue. The patient's current mental status, neuropsychiatric history (including all recent somatic therapies and any history of ECT), and family psychiatric history should be reviewed. Evaluation of medical risk factors for the treatment should focus on the central nervous system, the heart, the musculoskeletal system, and the upper gastrointestinal tract. Any history of head trauma or surgery, seizures, focal or general neurological complaints, angina, congestive heart failure, bony fractures, osteoporosis, spinal disease or trauma, or esophageal reflux should be elicited. Personal or family history of problems with anesthesia should be determined. Handedness should be assessed because of its relevance to nondominant unilateral electrode placement. Because the hand used for writing is often a fallible measure, patients should be asked which hand they use to throw a ball, cut with a knife, and so on (American Psychiatric Association 1990). A minority of left-handed patients and patients with mixed dominance may have language localized to the right hemisphere. For this reason, if significant confusion is observed in a left-handed patient after the first right unilateral ECT, consideration should be given to the use of bilateral or left unilateral electrode placement at the next session. The time required for the patient to become fully oriented after the treatment can be measured for each electrode placement, and the treatment series can then be continued using the laterality associated with less confusion.

A careful documentation of baseline affective and cognitive status is essential in elderly patients before ECT. In our clinical experience, the Hamilton or Montgomery Asberg Depression Rating Scales and the Mini-Mental State Exam are often helpful standardized instruments that may be followed at intervals throughout the ECT course.

A physical examination, basic laboratory tests (serum electrolytes and blood count), and an ECG should be obtained before ECT. Special care should be given to the neurological examination, including the funduscopic examination to rule out papilledema. Further studies, such as spine X-rays, EEG, brain computed tomography (CT) or MRI, and cardiac functional evaluations should be ordered as clinically indicated. Our clinical practice involves the routine use of brain CT or MRI and EEG in elderly patients. The elderly have an increased incidence of clinically significant incidental brain findings (e.g., aneurysm, subdural hematoma, undiagnosed primary or metastatic brain tumor, and evidence of increased intracranial

pressure), and neuroimaging may have predictive value as a tool to detect increased risk for some ECT side effects (discussed below). The EEG can be helpful in making the differential diagnosis between pseudodementia and dementia in some cases (Leuchter 1991). A baseline EEG to determine background frequency may also be helpful for use as a comparison in cases of prolonged encephalopathy after ECT.

For patients with serious cardiovascular disease, consultation with a cardiologist is often indicated. Once the decision to proceed with ECT has been made, the cardiologist should be asked how best to maximize the patient's cardiovascular function in preparation for, and during, the ECT.

A careful evaluation of the patient's medication is required for optimal ECT. Traditionally, all psychotropics are stopped before ECT, although neuroleptics may be used if necessary. Lithium taken in proximity to ECT has been linked to an increased incidence of delirium and seizures (Weiner et al. 1980). These effects may be related to an increase in brain lithium concentration, due to transient opening of the blood-brain barrier with ECT. Most patients should not receive lithium for several days before or after ECT (Kellner et al. 1991a).

Antidepressants are usually stopped to avoid cumulative cardiac and central nervous system side effects (Kellner et al. 1991a). Studies in the early 1960s found no added benefit with tricyclic antidepressant and ECT combination therapy (Seager and Bird 1962). In a retrospective chart review of 84 geriatric depressed patients, however, Nelson and Benjamin (1989) found improved outcome with tricyclic antidepressant and ECT combination therapy, measured by the need for fewer treatments. No increase in side effects occurred in the combination group. The study is severely limited by its retrospective design and the fact that the ECT-only group presumably contained more medically ill patients, in whom antidepressant drug therapy may have been stopped for fear of complication (Nelson and Benjamin 1989).

Benzodiazepines may impair the intensity of the therapeutic seizure, thereby decreasing treatment response (Pettinati et al. 1986). The use of these agents in elderly patients may also theoretically increase their susceptibility to cognitive side effects from ECT. Benzodiazepine use should be minimized or stopped before ECT.

In patients with epilepsy, the anticonvulsant effect of ECT itself may allow for a temporary decrease in anticonvulsant dosage. There are few reported data about the effects of carbamazepine and valproate on the efficacy of ECT.

Several other specific pharmacological issues require attention. Theophylline levels should be monitored closely, as high blood levels during ECT have been associated with status epilepticus (Abrams 1992). Echothiophate, an organophosphate glaucoma medication that irreversibly inhibits cholinesterase and pseudocholinesterase, may cause prolonged apnea with succinylcholine and should be avoided (Zorumski et al. 1988). Patients should receive any required cardiac, antireflux, or other medications with a sip of water the morning of their ECT.

A final and critically important component of the pre-ECT evaluation is the informed consent procedure. According to the 1990 American Psychiatric Association Task Force report on the practice of ECT, adequately informed consent should involve "1) the provision of adequate information, 2) a patient who is capable of understanding and acting intelligently upon such information, and 3) the opportunity to provide consent in the absence of coercion" (American Psychiatric Association 1990, p. 64). Compared with younger patients, those over 65 appear to be less aware that they can refuse ECT (Malcolm 1989). With the increased prevalence of cognitive impairment in elderly patients, competency to consent becomes a major issue, and the education of both the patient and family becomes essential. This is also a time in the patient's life cycle when children are becoming increasingly responsible for their parents, and this may need to be included in the consent process. Incompetent patients may require the judicial appointment of a legal guardian for consent. (For a pertinent sample of an informed consent document, see American Psychiatric Association 1990.)

ECT Technique

ECT is commonly given in the United States as a series of single treatments on alternate mornings. For the geriatric age group, it is typically performed in an inpatient setting. Patients have been previously screened for coexisting medical conditions, indications for treatment, and competency to consent. The treatment team consists of a psychiatrist, an anesthesiologist, and specially trained nursing personnel. ECT is typically given in either a special treatment suite or the recovery area of an operating room suite. Patients should

have nothing to eat or drink for at least 8 hours before treatment. The short-acting barbiturate methohexital is given in a dose of approximately 1 mg/kg body weight iv, followed by the depolarizing neuromuscular blocker succinylcholine given in a dose of 0.75–1.5 mg/kg body weight iv. Adequacy of neuromuscular blockade is monitored by the use of a peripheral nerve stimulator or by clinical assessment of relaxation, including loss of reflexes and tone.

Throughout the procedure, the patient is ventilated with 100% oxygen and monitored using a pulse oximeter. Heart rate and blood pressure are also closely monitored. After the insertion of a specially designed rubber bite block into the mouth, a predetermined electrical stimulus is delivered across electrodes placed on the patient's properly prepared scalp. Typically, a generalized seizure ensues, lasting from 30 to 90 seconds. The seizure is monitored by observation of brain ictal activity on EEG and by the motor manifestations of the seizure, using a blood pressure cuff inflated above systolic pressure on the right ankle to prevent access of the succinylcholine to that extremity. Ventilatory support is continued until the patient emerges from the anesthesia, and further recovery is provided in an environment with as little stimulation as possible. The entire procedure takes about 20 minutes, and patients are often able to have breakfast within an hour of the time of treatment.

A typical course of ECT consists of 6–12 treatments, although occasional patients may require fewer or more treatments to achieve full response. The treatment schedule is often modified in elderly patients because of their sensitivity to cognitive side effects, with treatments given once or twice, rather than three times, per week (American Psychiatric Association 1990). ECT is stopped when the patient is felt to have achieved maximal clinical improvement or when further improvement is not noted between treatments. Special attention is then given to maintenance treatment with either medication or ECT (see below).

Anesthesia Considerations

Anesthesia decisions during ECT are influenced by the physiology of the elderly patient. Because methohexital is an anticonvulsant and because the seizure threshold is often increased in elderly patients, the lowest effective anesthetic dose is desirable. Because methohexital dosing is based on lean body mass, the required methohexital dosage in many elderly patients may be less than 1 mg/kg total body weight (Fragen and Avram 1990).

The use of succinylcholine may also require special consideration in the elderly patient. Succinylcholine stimulates muscarinic cholinergic receptors in the sinus node and may cause bradycardia, especially if serial doses are required. This effect may be pronounced in patients receiving beta-blockers and those with evidence of preexisting conduction delay on ECG, conditions frequently found in elderly patients. Pretreatment with anticholinergics, such as atropine, may block this bradycardiac effect. Patients with extensive burns or trauma may have an exaggerated extracellular release of potassium in response to succinylcholine (Miller and Savarese 1990). The alternative use of a nondepolarizing muscle relaxant should be considered in these patients. Myalgia following ECT may be due to either the fasciculation caused by succinylcholine or the excessive motor movement during the seizure. Fasciculation may be blocked for subsequent ECT treatments by a small pretreatment dose of d-tubocurare (e.g., 3 mg).

Intragastric pressure also increases with succinylcholine, related to abdominal skeletal muscle fasciculation; however, the risk of gastric reflux and aspiration is reduced by an increase in esophageal pressure above the lower esophageal sphincter (Miller and Savarese 1990). Certain groups of elderly patients (e.g., those with hiatal hernia, gastroparesis, or morbid obesity) are at risk for significant gastroesophageal reflux during the procedure, with subsequent risk for aspiration pneumonitis (Zibrak et al. 1988). Smokers are particularly prone to morbidity from aspiration (Lichtor 1990). In these patients, additional strategies beyond nothing-by-mouth (NPO) status may be used to decrease gastric volume and acidity during ECT. Premedication with histamine, subtype 2 (H2), receptor antagonists or sodium citrate decreases gastric acidity, and metoclopramide increases lower esophageal sphincter tone and promotes gastric emptying (Lichtor 1990).

Stimulus Dosing

Seizure threshold (the amount of electricity required to elicit a seizure) increases with age (Sackeim et al. 1991). This effect is believed to be the result of a decrease in the excitability of the brain, but may also be partially due to increases in skull thickness (electrical resistance) with aging. Older patients thus require higher ECT stimulus intensities (dosage) than do younger patients, but the optimal stimulus dosage for ECT has yet to be defined. Recent data in mixed-age samples suggest that barely suprathreshold stimulus intensities may be ineffective (especially for unilateral nondominant ECT) (Sackeim et al. 1993), whereas excessive stimulus dosing has been linked to more cerebral toxicity (Weiner et al. 1986). Given these data, our clinical practice is to use stimulus dosing in unilateral ECT that is 1.5–2.5 times the patient's seizure threshold. This method requires a predetermination of the patient's seizure threshold, which may be done routinely at the first ECT session by fixed incremental increases in stimulus intensity over successive stimulations until a seizure results (Sackeim et al. 1987). For bilateral ECT, we use a stimulus dose that is 1.5 times the seizure threshold, as the efficacy of this modality appears to be less sensitive to dosing effects than that of unilateral ECT.

Seizure threshold increases during ECT (the well-known anticonvulsant effect), necessitating increases in stimulus dosage during the course of therapy (Coffey et al. 1990; Sackeim 1991; Sackeim et al. 1991). This effect does not appear to be more pronounced in elderly patients, but because this population has a higher initial seizure threshold some older patients may eventually require stimulus intensities during their course of treatment that exceed the maximal settings of the ECT device. In such instances, we have found caffeine to be an effective and well-tolerated strategy for augmenting ECT seizures in elderly patients (Coffey et al. 1987, 1990; Lurie and Coffey 1990). The effects of cerebral disease and age-related changes in brain structure on ECT seizure threshold have not been described but are currently under study in our laboratory.

Electrode Placement

The choice of unilateral or bilateral ECT in the elderly patient is often a complex one. Studies in mixed-age samples suggest that right unilateral ECT has fewer cognitive side effects (Weiner et al. 1986). Most research has also found unilateral and bilateral ECT to be equivalent in efficacy (American Psychiatric Association 1990); however, those studies that do find differences between the two methods consistently favor bilateral ECT (for a review, see Abrams 1992).

Few studies have addressed the issue of electrode placement specifically in elderly patients. In a meta-analysis of the literature, Pettinati et al. (1986) found a trend for improved efficacy in elderly patients with bilateral treatment. In the only reported randomized study, 29 elderly depressed patients were assigned either to unilateral or bilateral ECT two times a week (Fraser and Glass 1980). Stimulus dosing strategies were unclear. No group differences were observed in therapeutic response or memory performance after ECT, but those subjects randomized to bilateral electrode placement required more time to recover orientation after the fifth ECT treatment (Table 30–1). Whether the effects of cerebral disease or age-related structural brain changes modify the therapeutic or adverse effects of unilateral versus bilateral ECT in elderly patients has not been studied.

Thus limited data exist to guide the choice of ECT electrode placement in elderly patients with neuropsychiatric illness. Our approach is to begin with right unilateral ECT in the elderly, switching to bilateral ECT if minimal or no response is seen by the fifth or sixth treatment. Because bilateral ECT may have a more rapid onset of action, it may be considered the treatment of choice in urgently ill patients. If intolerable cognitive side effects develop with bilateral ECT, patients may be switched to unilateral ECT once their affective disorder has begun to respond.

Maintenance ECT

Major depression is increasingly recognized as a chronic, relapsing condition. Some studies have found 6-month relapse rates as high as 50% for patients initially responsive to antidepressant medications who are then given no form of maintenance therapy (Prien and Kupfer 1986). Similarly high rates of relapse have been noted following ECT response if no form of maintenance therapy is given (Jarvie 1954). Frank et al. (1990) found that relapse rates following response to pharmacotherapy can be substantially reduced by continuation of full dosage of antidepressant medication.

ECT is one of the few treatments in modern medicine that is commonly stopped as soon as it has proven effective. Usual clinical practice involves placing patients on maintenance pharmacotherapy after successful ECT. Because these are often patients who had initially failed to respond to medication therapy, it is not surprising that Sackeim et al. (1990) found a 50% relapse rate at 1 year for patients placed on medication after response to ECT. There was a particular pro-

pensity to relapse within the first 4 months after successful ECT.

An evolving literature in mixed-age samples indicates that maintenance ECT is safe and effective in the prevention of depressive relapse, with several promising retrospective reports in elderly patients (for a review, see Monroe 1991). Thienhaus et al. (1990) described six elderly patients with major mood disorder treated with maintenance ECT for a period of 1–6 years. While receiving maintenance ECT, patients had a significant decline in average annual inpatient hospital days, compared with a similar period prior to the use of maintenance ECT.

Dubin et al. (1992) reported the successful use of maintenance ECT for an average of 22 months in a group of eight patients over age 75. The single patient in the case series who required rehospitalization had been removed from maintenance ECT by her attending psychiatrist and placed on fluoxetine prior to her relapse. There were no significant adverse events associated with maintenance ECT in this case series.

Loo et al. (1991) described the use of maintenance ECT in seven elderly patients over an average of 3 years. Mean time in the hospital during this 3-year period decreased to 3 weeks, compared with 27 weeks for the 3 years prior to the start of maintenance ECT. Patients had 1.4 recurrences of illness during the maintenance ECT period, compared with 4.7 recurrences over the 3 years preceding maintenance ECT.

In one of the few prospective studies to date, we (Clarke et al. 1989) evaluated 27 patients free of psychotropic medications (mean age = 65; range = 26–90) assigned to a maintenance ECT protocol after initial ECT response. Only 8% of patients who completed the maintenance ECT protocol required rehospitalization, whereas 47% of those who dropped out of the protocol relapsed (a statistically significant difference).

Studies comparing maintenance ECT with maintenance pharmacotherapy following ECT response are lacking in the literature. As of this writing, a multisite study comparing nortriptyline, nortriptyline plus lithium, and placebo after successful ECT has been initiated with funding from the National Institute of Mental Health. Further prospective studies comparing maintenance ECT with medication are also required.

Maintenance ECT typically involves single treatments given initially at weekly intervals and then titrated to every 4–8 weeks, as the patient's depressive symptoms allow. The increased interval between maintenance treatments results in less cognitive side effects than a course of ECT, leading to the suggestion that bilateral treatment may be the modality of choice for maintenance ECT (Kellner 1991c). Several factors determine whether the treatments are best done on an outpatient basis. Patients must be reliably NPO for 6–8 hours before treatment, except for taking any required premedications with only a sip of water. Patients must also have an adequate support system to assure observation and care for several hours after treatment. If these factors are problematic as an outpatient, or if the patient has complex medical or recovery needs, an overnight stay in the hospital may be required.

Adverse Effects of ECT and Their Management

The safety of ECT compares favorably with any treatment requiring general anesthesia. The mortality is variously reported as approximating one death per 10,000 treatments (the same as general anesthesia for minor surgery) (American Psychiatric Association 1990), or as low as 0.2 deaths per 10,000 treatments (Kramer 1985). Kroessler and Fogel (1993) compared the mortality on long-term follow-up of 65 depressed patients age 80 or older who had been treated with ECT with that of patients treated with other modalities. These investigators found a 2-year survival of 54% in the group treated with ECT, versus 90% in the group treated with medications. This group difference was found to be related to more severe depression and physical illness in the patients who had received ECT. The course of ECT itself was remarkably well-tolerated by these elderly patients, with a median interval of 20 months between receiving ECT and time of death. The authors called for further attention to medical comorbidity as a prognostic factor in future outcome studies of geriatric depression.

Cardiovascular Side Effects

A proportion of elderly patients referred for ECT will have serious preexisting cardiovascular disease. Common cardiac conditions such as hypertension, angina, previous myocardial infarction, atrial and ventricular arrhythmia, aneurysm, and conduction system disease all require evaluation and optimized treatment before ECT to minimize the chance of adverse effects from the hemodynamic events that occur during ECT.

Studies have compared the cardiovascular complication rate of ECT in older and younger patients,

finding an increase in transient and treatable complications in the elderly. In a nonblinded, retrospective chart review of 293 patients, Alexopoulos et al. (1984) found cardiovascular complications in 9% of the older-than-65 group, compared with 1% in the less-than-65 group. Cardiac ischemia, arrhythmia, hypertension, and congestive heart failure were the most common complications, although the vast majority were not clearly temporally related to ECT and did not prevent the successful completion of treatment.

Burke et al. (1987) conducted a similar retrospective chart review of 136 subjects, 30% of whom were over age 60. Sine wave bilateral ECT was used in 85% of cases. They found a cardiorespiratory complication rate of 15% in patients over age 60, compared with 3% in those under 60. Complications were correlated with the number of cardiovascular medications the patient was receiving, with more medication presumably marking those with more cardiovascular illness. These complications did not affect treatment response.

The effect of increasing age on complications during ECT has been further documented in a retrospective chart review of 81 elderly patients by Cattan et al. (1990). Most patients received bilateral ECT, with a switch to right unilateral placement ($n = 21$) if required by cognitive side effects. They found a 36% cardiovascular complication rate in patients over age 80, compared with 12% in younger geriatric patients. As would be expected, patients in the over-80 group had significantly more medical diagnoses and were receiving more cardiovascular medication than those in the younger group.

Recently, Zielinski et al. (1993) studied the rate of cardiac complications in a group of 40 depressed patients (mean age = 68.9, range = 54–84 years) with serious preexisting cardiac disease (left ventricular impairment, conduction delay, and ventricular arrhythmias) compared with a group of 40 depressed patients without cardiac disease (mean age = 68.3 years, range = 55–83). Not surprisingly, the group with preexisting cardiac disease had more complications. However, most of the complications were transient (e.g., brief arrhythmias or increases in ectopy), and 38 of the 40 cardiac patients were able to complete their course of ECT. Interestingly, this group of depressed patients with cardiac disease had even more difficulty with adverse cardiac effects from prior trials of tricyclic antidepressants; fully 11 out of 21 had been forced to stop tricyclic treatment because of cardiovascular complications. Further prospective studies, carefully controlled for severity of cardiovascular and other medical disease, are needed to evaluate the effects of age on cardiovascular complications with ECT.

Increasingly sophisticated medical management during ECT should decrease the cardiovascular risk of treatment for elderly patients (Weiner and Coffey 1993). The primary areas of concern are bradycardia, tachycardia, hypertension, and ventricular arrhythmia. Anticholinergic premedications (atropine and glycopyrrolate) may be used to prevent vagally induced bradycardia, but in elderly patients their use may be complicated by confusion, tachycardia, constipation, and urinary retention. As such, we reserve the use of anticholinergic premedication for patients who develop unusually prolonged or severe bradyarrhythmias. The method of serial stimulations to determine a patient's seizure threshold (described earlier) may involve administration of subconvulsive stimuli, with a vagal surge unaccompanied by the sympathetic outflow associated with a seizure. The use of this method, as well as the presence of conduction delay on the ECG, may also indicate the need for pretreatment with anticholinergic medications.

Hypertension and tachycardia during ECT in elderly patients may be attenuated by short-acting intravenous adrenergic blockers such as labetalol or esmolol (Howie et al. 1990; Stoudemire et al. 1990). It should be kept in mind that beta-blockers have anticonvulsant effects and their use during ECT may theoretically limit the intensity of the ECT seizure and, in turn, its therapeutic potency. Kalayam and Alexopoulos (1989) have described the safe use of sublingual nifedipine before administration of anesthesia in an elderly patient with a severe hypertensive response to ECT. Hydralazine (an α-adrenergic antagonist), as well as nitroglycerine (sublingual, transdermal, or intravenous), may also be used when clinically indicated. Trimethaphan produces transient sympathetic and parasympathetic ganglionic blockade and is considered the cardiovascular agent of choice at some institutions (Maneksha 1991). Although the hemodynamic responses to ECT are robust, they are well-tolerated by most patients, including the elderly (Webb et al. 1990). In addition, indiscriminate use of antihypertensive medication may lead to clinically significant hypotension in elderly patients. As such, we do not routinely attempt to blunt the cardiovascular response to ECT in elderly patients unless such changes are extreme or are clearly associated with evidence of cardiovascular compromise. Finally, patients receiving adrenergic

blockers should probably receive anticholinergic premedication to prevent a disproportionate decrease of sympathetic tone below parasympathetic tone, with resultant bradycardia (Abrams 1992).

Significant posttreatment ventricular ectopy (multifocal premature ventricular contractions [PVCs] or several consecutive PVCs) may be treated with lidocaine (1–1.5 mg/kg body weight). Because of its anticonvulsant properties, lidocaine should be given after termination of seizure (Drop and Welch 1989). Stoudemire et al. (1990) found that ventricular ectopy could be reduced with pretreatment with labetalol.

Cerebral Side Effects

There is no evidence that ECT causes structural brain damage (Weiner 1984). Carefully controlled prospective brain imaging studies in humans reveal no changes in brain structure for up to 6 months after a course of ECT (Coffey 1993; Coffey et al. 1991). Neuropathological studies in animals, including cell counts in regions thought to be at highest risk, fail to find evidence of brain damage when the seizures are induced under conditions that approximate standard clinical practice (i.e., when the seizures are spaced, relatively brief, and modified by oxygenation and muscle relaxation). Furthermore, studies of the pathophysiology of seizure-induced structural brain damage in animals indicate that the conditions necessary for injury do not apply to the modern practice of ECT (Weiner 1984).

The incidence of cerebrovascular complications with ECT is exceedingly rare. ECT has been given successfully to a patient with cerebral aneurysms, with close management of blood pressure elevation (Drop and Welch 1989). A recent report of intracerebral hemorrhage in a normotensive patient during ECT was probably related to cerebral amyloid angiopathy (Weisberg et al. 1991). We know of no other report of intracerebral hemorrhage with ECT, nor of any documented case of ischemic stroke during the treatment.

The interval required between an acute cerebral infarction and the initiation of safe ECT is unclear. Alexopoulos et al. (1984) reported the uneventful delivery of ECT 4 days after a cerebral infarct (whether it was hemorrhagic or ischemic was not specified), and Murray et al. (1986) reported successful ECT 1 month after ischemic stroke. Patients with a recent cerebral infarction may have more friable vasculature with a propensity to rebleed. These patients require time for cerebral vessels to heal before ECT, with careful management of blood pressure during the procedure. Titratable antihypertensive agents with short half-lives (e.g., esmolol or nitrates) are helpful in this situation. Care must be taken to avoid hypotension in all elderly patients with cerebrovascular disease.

Other intracranial processes are risk factors for ECT. As described above, intracranial mass lesions and increased intracranial pressure are among the most serious risk factors for ECT. In a retrospective literature review, Maltbie et al. (1980) examined 28 cases of patients (mean age = 47; range = 20–80) with brain tumor treated with ECT. Only 34% of patients improved, and 74% showed neurological deterioration, with 29% dead of neurological complications within a month of ECT. This study was flawed by a form of recall bias, with cases involving dramatic outcomes more likely to be reported. As well, a previously undiagnosed brain tumor would be more likely diagnosed during a treatment course involving complications than during an uneventful ECT course. Abrams (1992) reviewed reports of several cases of safe delivery of ECT to patients with brain tumors, mostly meningiomas, and ascribed the lessened risk to small, slow-growing tumors that have no associated increased intracranial pressure. There is no report of safe ECT prospectively given to a patient with documented increased intracranial pressure (Abrams 1992). Subdural hematomas may require evacuation before ECT (Abrams 1992).

Side Effects in Other Organ Systems

Other organ systems that may be impaired in the elderly patient need to be considered before ECT, including the lungs, bones, eyes, and teeth. Pulmonary status should be optimized before ECT. Patients with severe chronic obstructive pulmonary disease (COPD) and carbon dioxide retention may require special ventilatory strategies during the treatment (Abrams 1992). Pneumonia secondary to aspiration of gastric contents may occur rarely during ECT (Alexopoulos et al. 1989; Karlinsky and Shulman 1984). If possible, ECT treatment should be withheld until resolution of the pneumonia.

Patients with osteoporosis, spinal disc disease, or spondylosis may require increased muscular relaxation during ECT. Such patients may require succinylcholine doses of at least 1.0–1.5 mg/kg body weight, and they require careful attention to clinical evidence of adequate relaxation (e.g., loss of reflexes, tone, and disap-

pearance of fasciculation) prior to delivery of the stimulus. Kellner et al. (1991b) reported the safe treatment of a patient with osteoporosis and cervical spondylosis with multiple subluxations of the cervical spine using succinylcholine doses of 1.3 mg/kg body weight.

Because ECT produces a transient increase in intraocular pressure, patients with chronic open-angle glaucoma should receive their eye drops before ECT. As noted earlier, echothiophate, an irreversible cholinesterase inhibitor, should be stopped several days before ECT. Patients with acute closed-angle glaucoma or retinal detachment should be stabilized before ECT and followed closely by an ophthalmologist during an ECT course.

Dentition that is loose, decayed, or asymmetric may increase the risk of dental injury during ECT. A major proportion of malpractice litigation with ECT surrounds dental issues (Slawson 1985). Scrupulous attention should be paid to the insertion of a specially designed, firm, rubber bite block before delivery of the ECT stimulus. The tongue, cheeks, and lips must be kept clear of the clenching teeth. The bite block should be used even with edentulous patients. Occasionally, upper or lower dentures may be kept in place during the treatment to facilitate airway management. In patients with only a few remaining, and possibly loose, teeth, dental consultation or alternative bite block strategies (with the aim of shifting bite pressure to the molars) may be helpful (Welch 1993).

Cognitive Side Effects

The cognitive side effects of ECT include acute postictal confusion, interictal delirium, and amnesia. The severity of these adverse effects is increased with bilateral electrode placement, sine waveform, higher stimulus dose relative to seizure threshold, and more frequent treatments. Conversely, cognitive side effects are reduced with right unilateral electrode placement, brief-pulse waveform, lower stimulus dose relative to seizure threshold, and longer intervals between treatments (American Psychiatric Association 1990). Although it has been suggested that elderly patients may be at greater risk for these cognitive side effects than are younger patients, the controlled data on this issue are limited.

Acute postictal disorientation. Studies in mixed-age samples of adults have reported that increasing age is associated with longer or more severe disorientation immediately after ECT (Burke et al. 1987; Calev et al. 1991; Daniel et al. 1987; Sackeim et al. 1987). Of studies that have focused on the elderly subjects, Fraser and Glass (1978) measured time to recovery of full orientation in nine depressed elderly patients who received ECT in courses that alternated electrode placement (i.e., unilateral at one treatment, followed by bilateral at the next treatment, and so on). When comparing these reorientation times to those found in the extant literature for younger patients, they observed that recovery in elderly patients took five times as long for unilateral treatment and nine times as long for bilateral treatment. Recovery time after bilateral ECT increased cumulatively over the course of ECT, and with closer spacing of treatments. No such relationship was found for unilateral ECT. In a subsequent study of 29 depressed elderly patients randomly assigned to courses of either unilateral ($n = 13$) or bilateral ($n = 16$) sine wave ECT, Fraser and Glass (1980) found significantly longer reorientation times after the fifth ECT for patients receiving bilateral treatments (32.8 minutes) than for those receiving unilateral treatments (9.5 minutes) (Table 30–1). In contrast to the bilateral group, patients receiving unilateral ECT showed a significant shortening in recovery time from the first to the last treatment.

Interictal delirium.   In a small proportion of patients, ECT will be associated with more prolonged disorientation and even frank delirium. Most studies evaluating interictal delirium in elderly patients have used disorientation as a measure, rather than the full DSM-III-R (American Psychiatric Association 1987) criteria for delirium. In a retrospective study of 136 patients receiving mainly bilateral, sine-wave ECT, Burke et al. (1987) found disorientation (confusion severe enough to alter treatment plan) in 18% of patients older than 60 versus in 13% of younger patients. This incidence increased to 25% for patients over age 75. The retrospective study of Alexopoulos et al. (1984), using mostly bilateral (waveform not specified) ECT, also found a somewhat greater incidence of confusion (disorientation to time, place, and person) in elderly patients (12.6%) than in younger patients (9.6%). Cattan et al. (1990), using primarily bilateral or combination bilateral-unilateral sine-wave ECT, found no significant difference in the frequency of severe disorientation (defined functionally by interference in ward activities) between elderly patients 65 to 80 years old (45%, $n = 42$) and those over 80 (59%, $n = 39$.). In the Al-

exopoulos et al. (1984) study, the elderly patients with a history of underlying organic brain disease were found to have higher levels of severe post-ECT confusion than were the younger patients, suggesting that baseline cerebral impairment may increase the risk of adverse cognitive effects of ECT.

Several studies have implicated subcortical structural disease in the development of interictal delirium with ECT. We have found subcortical gray and white matter lesions to be more extensive in elderly patients who developed a prolonged interictal delirium during a course of ECT. Most of these patients were able to continue ECT, with no decline in expected treatment response. All patients were free of delirium 1 week post-ECT (Coffey et al. 1989; Figiel et al. 1990). The specificity of subcortical disease in producing delirium after ECT is further suggested by Martin et al. (1992), who found that poststroke patients with lesions of the caudate nucleus had a 92% incidence of delirium during ECT. Patients with a previous stroke in other brain regions had the same incidence of delirium as did a group of elderly depressed control (no stroke) subjects receiving ECT (Martin et al. 1992). In a prospective study of seven consecutive patients with Parkinson's disease, Figiel et al. (1991) found a 100% incidence of interictal delirium during a course of ECT. The deliria took 7–21 days to clear, longer than is typical, but 86% of patients recovered from depression. Whether the delirium was due to subcortical disease versus increased intracerebral concentration of levodopa (due to transient breakdown of the blood-brain barrier with ECT) is unknown.

In summary, transient periods of acute post-ECT disorientation are common in patients undergoing ECT. Although the duration and severity of these episodes may increase with age, the majority of elderly patients appear to recover their orientation within 60–120 minutes of the treatment. In the small percentage of elderly patients who develop more prolonged confusion or frank delirium, underlying cerebral impairment may be contributory, especially dysfunction of the basal ganglia. Clearly, more research is needed in a larger number of elderly patients to characterize post-ECT confusion and to identify its risk factors, including the effects of preexisting cerebral impairment.

Amnesia.   A course of ECT is associated with transient disturbances in memory, including both retrograde and anterograde amnesia. Retrograde amnesia (forgetting of material known before the ECT) may extend back to several months prior to the treatment and is more pronounced with bilateral electrode placement, sine waveform, grossly suprathreshold stimulus intensity, and increased treatment frequency (Abrams 1992). These same factors also increase anterograde amnesia (forgetting of material learned after the start of ECT). These side effects subside within weeks of completing ECT, but some patients may have permanent loss of specific memories for some events that occurred before, during, or shortly after the treatment course. Although some patients may report persistent memory difficulties, objective testing has demonstrated that ECT does not produce persistent impairment in the ability to remember past information or acquire new information (American Psychiatric Association 1990).

Given the large body of data on the amnestic effects of ECT, it is surprising that relatively little controlled research has examined the contribution of age as a risk factor (Abrams 1992; Calev et al. 1993; Fink 1979). Some (Fromholt et al. 1973; Hesche et al. 1978), but not all (d'Elia and Raotma 1977; Strömgren et al. 1976), early studies found that ECT-induced amnesia is worse in older patients. Zervas et al. (1993) recently examined age effects on memory in the context of a study comparing two-times-a-week versus three-times-a-week bilateral ECT using contemporary techniques (pulse waveform given at "moderately suprathreshold" stimulus intensity). The sample consisted of 42 inpatients with a mean ±SD age of 53.5 ± 16.1 years; no patient was older than 65 years however. Significant correlations were found between age and decrements in retrograde memory at 1–3 days after the end of ECT, but not at 1 month or 6 months posttreatment. Age was also correlated with decrements in verbal anterograde memory acutely at 1-month post-ECT (but not at 6-months post-ECT) and with changes in figural anterograde memory acutely and at 6-months post-ECT.

In the study by Fraser and Glass (1980) (also see Table 30–1), all elderly patients showed impairment of memory function before ECT, but during treatment memory improved and was normal in all patients at 3 weeks after completion of the ECT course. No group differences were found on the basis of electrode placement. Memory performance has also been reported to improve in elderly patients with the pseudodementia of depression who are treated successfully with ECT (Reynolds et al. 1987).

In summary, there are relatively few controlled data to support the "clinical wisdom" that elderly pa-

tients are at greater risk for the amnestic side effects of ECT. More work is needed in a larger number of elderly patients (especially in the "old old") to characterize the extent and severity of ECT-induced amnesia and to identify relevant risk factors, including the effects of preexisting cerebral impairment. At this time, prudent recommendations for lessening ECT amnesia in the elderly include the use of unilateral electrode placement and brief pulse stimuli, avoiding maximally suprathreshold stimulus dosage, and lessening the frequency of treatments (e.g., giving ECT on Monday and Friday instead of Monday, Wednesday, and Friday).

Psychosocial Issues

In addition to its myriad biological effects, ECT involves important intrapsychic and interpersonal effects. A powerful treatment, during which the patient is put to sleep and has an electrical stimulus delivered to the head, may arouse predictable fears and fantasies in the patient. Issues of trust and autonomy over one's body while in a vulnerable position may predominate, especially in patients with a previous history of trauma. Patient education, in particular educational videotapes, may be quite effective and reassuring for these fears. Patients who are vulnerable to idealized fantasies of a nurturant, all-caring, supportive other may overvalue the ECT procedure and practitioner. Conversely, these patients may excessively devalue the treatment when their distorted expectations are not realized. Such patients may be at increased risk for a bad psychological outcome from the treatment. Overidealization of the treatment should be challenged by the ECT practitioner, firmly grounding the informed consent process in factual information.

Patient attitude surveys find that those undergoing ECT typically find the experience no more upsetting than a trip to the dentist (Fox 1993; Hughes et al. 1981; Malcolm 1989). In the only study that has systematically examined the effects of age on patients' perception and knowledge of ECT, Malcolm (1989) found that patients over age 65 had less knowledge of the procedure before treatment, and were also less fearful of it. In addition, fewer elderly patients viewed the treatment as frightening after completing a course of ECT.

Medicolegal issues surrounding the use of ECT in elderly patients include the informed consent process (discussed above), do-not-resuscitate (DNR) orders, and consideration of driving after ECT. A patient with

DNR status may still experience improved quality of life with aggressive treatment of his or her affective disorder and may still be considered for ECT (Sullivan et al. 1992). Strategies for the management of major complications that could occur during ECT should be discussed with the patient and the family prior to treatment. Patients should not drive until that point after a course of ECT when cognitive side effects have significantly resolved. This issue may be an especially sensitive one for elderly patients who value driving as a way of maintaining their mobility and functional independence.

Conclusions

Fifty-five years after its introduction, ECT remains a cornerstone of the treatment of severe affective disorder and selected other neuropsychiatric illnesses in elderly patients. Recent modifications in ECT technique have reduced the risk of severe side effects in this population. There is, however, a paucity of controlled data comparing the efficacy and safety of ECT versus pharmacotherapy in the elderly population. ECT also appears to be an effective treatment in patients with preexisting brain disease and in some cases may even benefit the underlying neurological disorder. Further study is needed to determine the impact of age-related changes in brain structure and/or function and of preexisting cerebral disease on the beneficial and adverse effects of ECT in geriatric patients.

References

Abrams R: Electroconvulsive Therapy, second edition. New York, Oxford University Press, 1992

Alexopoulos GS: Clinical and biological findings in late-onset depression, in American Psychiatric Press Review of Psychiatry, Vol 9. Edited by Tasman A, Goldfinger SM, Kaufman CA. Washington, DC, American Psychiatric Press, 1990, pp 249–262

Alexopoulos GS, Shamoian CJ, Lucas J, et al: Medical problems of geriatric psychiatric patients and younger controls during electroconvulsive therapy. J Am Geriatr Soc 32:651–654, 1984

Alexopoulos GS, Young RG, Abrams RC: ECT in the high-risk geriatric patient. Convulsive Therapy 5:75–87, 1989

American Psychiatric Assocation: Diagnostic and Statistical Manual of Mental Disorders, 3rd Edition. Washington, DC, American Psychiatric Association, 1980

American Psychiatric Assocation: Diagnostic and Statistical Manual of Mental Disorders, 3rd Edition, Revised. Washington, DC, American Psychiatric Association, 1987

American Psychiatric Association: The Practice of Electroconvulsive Therapy: Recommendations for Treatment, Training and Privileging. Washington, DC, American Psychiatric Association, 1990

Andersen K, Balldin J, Gottfries CG, et al: A double-blind evaluation of electroconvulsive therapy in Parkinson's disease with "on-off" phenomena. Acta Neurol Scand 76:191–199, 1987

Asnis G: Parkinson's disease, depression, and ECT: a review and case study. Am J Psychiatry 134:191–195, 1977

Atre-Vaidya N, Jampala V: Electroconvulsive therapy in parkinsonism with affective disorder. Br J Psychiatry 152:55–58, 1988

Avery E, Winokur G: Mortality in depressed patients treated with electroconvulsive therapy and antidepressants. Arch Gen Psychiatry 33:1029–1037, 1976

Babigian HM, Guttmacher LB: Epidemiologic considerations in electroconvulsive therapy. Arch Gen Psychiatry 41:246–253, 1984

Balldin J, Eden S, Granerus A-K, et al: Electroconvulsive therapy in Parkinson's syndrome with "on-off" phenomenon. Journal of Neural Transmission 47:11–21, 1980

Balldin J, Granerus A-K, Lindstedt G, et al: Predictors for improvement after electroconvulsive therapy in parkinsonian patients with "on-off" symptoms. Journal of Neural Transmission 52:199–211, 1981

Beck AT: Depression Inventory. Philadelphia, PA, Philadelphia Center for Cognitive Therapy, 1978

Benbow SM: The use of electroconvulsive therapy in old age psychiatry. International Journal of Geriatric Psychiatry 2:25–30, 1987

Benbow SM: The role of electroconvulsive therapy in the treatment of depressive illness in old age. Br J Psychiatry 155:147–152, 1989

Birkett DP: ECT in parkinsonism with affective disorder (letter). Br J Psychiatry 152:712–713, 1988

Black DW, Winokur G, Nasrallah A: A multivariate analysis of the experience of 423 depressed inpatients treated with electroconvulsive therapy. Convulsive Therapy 9:112–120, 1993

Bodley PO, Fenwick PBC: The effects of electroconvulsive therapy on patients with essential hypertension. Br J Psychiatry 112:1241–1249, 1966

Bolwig T, Hertz M, Paulson O, et al: The permeability of the blood-brain barrier during electrically induced seizures in man. J Clin Invest 7:87–93, 1977

Botteron K, Figiel GS, Zorumski CF: Electroconvulsive therapy in patients with late-onset psychoses and structural brain changes. J Geriatr Psychiatry Neurol 4:44–47, 1991

Braasch ER, Demaso DR: Effect of electroconvulsive therapy on serum isoenzymes. Am J Psychiatry 137:625–626, 1980

Brodersen P, Paulson OB, Bolwig TG, et al: Cerebral hyperemia in electrically induced epileptic seizures. Arch Neurol 28:334–338, 1973

Brown G: Parkinsonism, depression and ECT (letter). Am J Psychiatry 132:1084, 1973

Burke WJ, Rutherford JL, Zorumski CF, et al: Electroconvulsive therapy and the elderly. Compr Psychiatry 26:480–486, 1985

Burke WJ, Rubin EH, Zorumski CF, et al: The safety of ECT in geriatric psychiatry. J Am Geriatr Soc 35:516–521, 1987

Burke W, Peterson J, Rubin E: Electroconvulsive therapy in the treatment of combined depression and Parkinson's disease. Psychosomatics 29:341–346, 1988

Calabrese JR, Woyshville MJ, Kimmel SE, et al: Mixed states and bipolar rapid cycling and their treatment with divalproex sodium. Psychiatric Annals 23(2):70–78, 1993

Calev A, Cohen R, Tubi N, et al: Disorientation and bilateral moderately suprathreshold titrated ECT. Convulsive Therapy 7:99–110, 1991

Calev A, Pass HL, Shapira B, et al: ECT and memory, in The Clinical Science of ECT. Edited by Coffey CE. Washington, American Psychiatric Press, 1993, pp 125–142

Carney MWP, Roth M, Garside RF: The diagnosis of depressive syndromes and the prediction of ECT response. Br J Psychiatry 111:659–674, 1965

Cattan RA, Barry PP, Mead G, et al: Electroconvulsive Therapy in Octogenarians. J Am Geriatr Soc 38:753–758, 1990

Clarke TB, Coffey CE, Hoffman GW, et al: Continuation therapy for depression using outpatient electroconvulsive therapy. Convulsive Therapy 5:330–337, 1989

Coffey CE: Structural brain imaging and electroconvulsive therapy, in Clinical Science of ECT. Edited by Coffey CE. Washington, DC, American Psychiatric Press, 1993, pp 73–92

Coffey CE, Weiner RD, Hinkle PE, et al: Augmentation of ECT seizures with caffeine. Biol Psychiatry 22:637–649, 1987

Coffey CE, Figiel GS, Djang WT, et al: Leukoencephalopathy in Elderly Depressed Patients Referred for ECT. Biological Psych 24:143–161, 1988

Coffey CE, Figiel GS, Djang WT, et al: White matter hyperintensity on magnetic resonance imaging: clinical and neuroanatomic correlates in the depressed elderly. J Neuropsychiatry Clin Sci 1:135–144, 1989

Coffey CE, Figiel GS, Weiner RD, et al: Caffeine augmentation of ECT. Am J Psychiatry 147:579–585, 1990

Coffey CE, Weiner RD, Djang WT, et al: Brain anatomic effects of ECT: a prospective magnetic resonance imaging study. Arch Gen Psychiatry 48:1013–1021, 1991

Consensus Conference: Electroconvulsive therapy. JAMA 254:2103–2108, 1985

Coryell W, Zimmerman M: Outcome following ECT for primary unipolar depression: a test of newly proposed response predictors. Am J Psychiatry 141:862–867, 1984

Currier MB, Murray GB, Welch CC: Electroconvulsive therapy for post-stroke depressed geriatric patients. J Neuropsychiatry Clin Neurosci 4:140–144, 1992

Daniel WF, Crovitz HF, Weiner RD: Neuropsychological aspects of disorientation. Cortex 23:169–187, 1987

d'Elia G, Raotma H: Memory impairment after convulsive therapy: influence of age and number of treatments. Archives of Psychiatry and Neurological Sciences 223:219–226, 1977

Devanand DP, Sackeim HA, Lo ES, et al: Serial dexamethasone suppression tests and plasma dexamethasone levels. Arch Gen Psychiatry 48:525–533, 1991

Douyon R, Serby M, Klutchko B, et al: ECT and Parkinson's disease revisited: a "naturalistic" study. Am J Psychiatry 146:1451–1455, 1989

Drop LJ, Welch CA: Anesthesia for electroconvulsive therapy in patients with major cardiovascular risk factors. Convulsive Therapy 5:88–101, 1989

Dubin WR, Jaffe R, Roemer R, et al: The efficacy and safety of maintenance ECT in geriatric patients. J Am Geriatr Soc 40:706–709, 1992

Dubovsky SL: Using electroconvulsive therapy for patients with neurological disease. Hosp Community Psychiatry 37:819–825, 1986

Dysken M, Evans H, Chan C, et al: Improvement of depression and parkinsonism during ECT: a case study. Neuropsychobiology 2:81–86, 1976

Fahn S: Fetal-tissue transplants in Parkinson's disease. N Engl J Med 327:1589–1590, 1992

Feighner JP, Robins E, Guze SB, et al: Diagnostic criteria for use in psychiatric research. Arch Gen Psychiatry 26:57–63, 1972

Figiel GS, Coffey CE, Djang WT, et al: Brain magnetic resonance imaging findings in ECT-induced delirium. J Neuropsychiatry Clin Neurosci 2:53–58, 1990

Figiel GS, Hassen MA, Zorumski C, et al: ECT-induced delirium in depressed patients with Parkinson's disease. Journal of Neuropsychiatry 3:405–411, 1991

Fink M: Convulsive Therapy: Theory and Practice. New York, Raven, 1979

Finklestein SD, Weintraub RJ, Karmooz N, et al: Antidepressant drug treatment for post-stroke depression: a retrospective study. Arch Phys Med Rehabil 68:772–778, 1987

Fisman M: Intractable depression and pseudodementia: a report of two cases. Can J Psychiatry 33:628–630, 1988

Fochtmann L: A mechanism for the efficacy of ECT in Parkinson's disease. Convulsive Therapy 4:321–327, 1988

Fogel BS: Electroconvulsive therapy in the elderly: a clinical research agenda. International Journal of Geriatric Psychiatry 3:181–190, 1988

Folstein M, Folstein S, McHugh PR: Clinical predictors of improvement after electroconvulsive therapy of patients with schizophrenic, neurotic reactions and affective disorders. Biol Psychiatry 7:142–152, 1973

Folstein MF, Folstein SE, McHugh PR: Mini-Mental State: a practical method for grading the cognitive state of patients for the clinician. J Psychiatr Res 12:189–198, 1975

Fox HA: Patients' fear and objection to electroconvulsive therapy. Hosp Community Psychiatry 44:357–360, 1993

Fragen RJ, Avram MJ: Barbiturates, in Anesthesia, 3rd Edition, Vol 1. Edited by Miller RD. New York, Churchill Livingstone, 1990, pp 225–242

Frank E, Kupfer DJ, Perel JM, et al: Three-year outcomes for maintenance therapies in recurrent depression. Arch Gen Psychiatry 47:1093–1099, 1990

Fraser RM, Glass IB: Recovery from ECT in elderly patients. Br J Psychiatry 133:524–528, 1978

Fraser RM, Glass IB: Unilateral and bilateral ECT in elderly patients: a comparative study. Acta Psychiatr Scand 62:13–31, 1980

Friedman J, Gordon N: Electroconvulsive Therapy in Parkinson's disease: a report on five cases. Convulsive Therapy 8:204–210, 1992

Fromholt P, Christensen AL, Strumgren LS: The effects of unilateral and bilateral electroconvulsive therapy on memory. Acta Psychiatr Scand 49:466–478, 1973

Fromm GH: Observation on the effects of electroshock treatment in patients with parkinsonism. Bulletin of Tulane University 18:71–73, 1959

Gaspar D, Samarasinghe LA: ECT in psychogeriatric practice: a study of risk factors, indications and outcome. Compr Psychiatry 23:170–175, 1982

Gerring JP, Shields HM: The identification and management of patients with high risk for cardiac arrhythmias during modified ECT. J Clin Psychiatry 43:140–143, 1982

Godber C, Rosenvinge H, Wilkinson D, et al: Depression in old age: prognosis after ECT. International Journal of Geriatric Psychiatry 2:19–24, 1987

Gold L, Chiarella CJ: The prognostic value of clinical findings in cases treated with electric shock. J Nerv Ment Dis 100:577–583, 1944

Greenberg L, Fink M: The use of electroconvulsive therapy in geriatric patients. Clin Geriatr Med 8:349–354, 1992

Hamilton M: A rating scale for depression. J Neurol Neurosurg Psychiatry 23:56–62, 1960

Hermesh H, Aizenberg D, Friedberg G, et al: Electroconvulsive therapy for persistent neuroleptic-induced akathisia and parkinsonism: a case report. Biol Psychiatry 31:407–411, 1992

Hesche J, Roder E, Theilgaard A: Unilateral and bilateral ECT: a psychiatric and psychological study of therapeutic effect and side-effects. Acta Psychiatr Scand Suppl 275:1–180, 1978

Holcomb H, Sternberg D, Heninger G: Effects of electroconvulsive therapy on mood, parkinsonism and tardive dyskinesia in a depressed patient: ECT and dopamine systems. Biol Psychiatry 18:865–873, 1983

Holzer JC, Giakas WJ, Mazure CM, et al: Dysarthria during ECT given for Parkinson's disease and depression. Convulsive Therapy 8:201–203, 1992

Howie MB, Black HA, Zvar AD, et al: Osmolal reduces autonomic hypersensitivity and length of seizures induced by electroconvulsive therapy. Anesth Analg 71:384–388, 1990

Hsiao JK, Messenheimer JA, Evans DL: ECT and neurological disorders. Convulsive Therapy 3:121–136, 1987

Huang KC, Lucas LF, Tsueda K, et al: Age-related changes in cardiovascular function associated with electroconvulsive therapy. Convulsive Therapy 5:17–25, 1989

Hughes J, Barraclough BM, Reeve W: Are patients shocked by ECT? J R Soc Med 74:283–285, 1981

Jaeckle R, Dilsaver S: Covariation of depressive symptoms, parkinsonism, and post-dexamethasone plasma cortisol levels in a bipolar patient: simultaneous response to ECT and lithium carbonate. Acta Psychiatr Scand 74:68–72, 1986

Jarvie H: Prognosis of depression treated by electric convulsive therapy. BMJ 1:132–134, 1954

Jenike MA: Handbook of Geriatric Psychopharmacology. Littleton, MA, PSG Publishing, 1985

Kahn RL, Pollack M, Fink M: Sociopsychologic aspects of psychiatric treatment in a voluntary mental hospital: duration of hospitalization, discharge ratings and diagnosis. Arch Gen Psychiatry 1:565–574, 1959

Kalayam B, Alexopoulos GS: Nifedipene in the treatment of blood pressure rise after ECT. Convulsive Therapy 5:110–113, 1989

Kamil R, Joffe RT: Neuroendocrine testing in electroconvulsive therapy (in Electroconvulsive Therapy. Edited by Kellner CH). Psychiatr Clin North Am 14(4):961–970, 1991

Kaplan HI, Sadock BJ: Schizophrenia in Synopsis of Psychiatry, 5th Edition. Baltimore, MD, Williams & Wilkins, 1988, pp 253–269

Karlinsky H, Shulman KI: The clinical use of electroconvulsive therapy in old age. J Am Geriatr Soc 32(3):183–186, 1984

Kellner CH, Bernstein HJ: ECT as a treatment for neurologic illness, in Clinical Science of Electroconvulsive Therapy. Edited by Coffey CE. Washington, DC, American Psychiatric Press, 1993, pp 183–210

Kellner CH, Nixon DW, Bernstein HJ: ECT-drug interactions: a review. Psychopharmacol Bull 27:595–609, 1991a

Kellner CH, Tolhurst JE, Burns CM: ECT in the presence of severe cervical spine disease. Convulsive Therapy 7:52–55, 1991b

Kellner CH, Burns CM, Bernstein HJ, et al: Electrode placement in maintenance electroconvulsive therapy 7:61–62, 1991c

Kellner CH, Monroe RR, Pritchett J, et al: Weekly ECT in geriatric depression. Convulsive Therapy 8(4):245–252, 1992

Kramer BA: Use of ECT in California, 1977–1983. Am J Psychiatry 142:1190–1192, 1985

Kramer BA: Electroconvulsive therapy use in geriatric depression. J Nerv Mental Dis 175:233–235, 1987

Kroessler D, Fogel B: Electroconvulsive therapy for major depression in the oldest old. American Journal of Geriatric Psychiatry 1(1):30–37, 1993

Lauterbach E, Moore N: Parkinsonism-dystonia syndrome and ECT. Am J Psychiatry 147:1249–1250, 1990

Lebensohn Z, Jenkins R: Improvement of parkinsonism in depressed patients treated with ECT. Am J Psychiatry 132:283–285, 1975

Leuchter A: Electroencephalography, in Comprehensive Review of Geriatric Psychiatry. Edited by Sadavoy J, Lazarus LW, Jarvik LF. Washington, DC, American Psychiatric Press, 1991, pp 273–283

Levy L, Savit J, Hodes M: Parkinsonism: improvement by electroconvulsive therapy. Arch Phys Med Rehabil 64:432–433, 1983

Lichtor JL: Psychological preparation and preoperative medication in anesthesia, 3rd Edition, Vol 1. Edited by Miller RD. New York, Churchill Livingstone, 1990, pp 895–928

Lingam VR, Lazarus LW, Groves L, et al: Methylphenidate in treating post-stroke depression. J Clin Psychiatry 49:151–153, 1988

Lipper S, Bermanzohn P: Electroconvulsive therapy in patients with parkinsonism (letter). Am J Psychiatry 132:457, 1975

Lipsey JR, Robinson RG, Pearlson GD: Nortriptyline treatment of post-stroke depression: a double-blind study. Lancet 1:297–300, 1984

Loo H, Galinowski A, De Carvalho W, et al: Use of maintenance ECT for elderly depressed patients (letter). Am J Psychiatry 148:810, 1991

Lurie SN, Coffey CE: Caffeine-modified ECT in depressed patients with medical illness. J Clin Psychiatry 51:154–157, 1990

Magni G, Fisman M, Helmes E: Clinical correlates of ECT-resistant depression in the elderly. J Clin Psychiatry 49:405–407, 1988

Malcolm K: Patients' perceptions and knowledge of electroconvulsive therapy. Psychiatric Bulletin 13:161–165, 1989

Malla AK: Characteristics of patients who receive electroconvulsive therapy. Can J Psychiatry 33:696–701, 1988

Maltbie AA, Wingfield MS, Volow MR, et al: Electroconvulsive therapy in the presence of brain tumor. J Nerv Ment Dis 168:400–405, 1980

Mander AJ, Whitfield A, Keen DM, et al: Cerebral and brain stem changes after ECT revealed by nuclear magnetic resonance imaging. Br J Psychiatry 151:69–71, 1987

Maneksha FR: Hypertension and tachycardia during electroconvulsive therapy: to treat or not to treat? Convulsive Therapy 7:28–35, 1991

Martin M, Figiel G, Mattingly G, et al: ECT-induced interictal delirium in patients with a history of CVA. J Geriatr Psychiatry Neurol 5:149–155, 1992

Mendels J: Electroconvulsive therapy and depression, I: the prognostic significance of clinical factors. Br J Psychiatry 111:675–681, 1965

Messina AG, Paranicas M, Katz B, et al: Effect of electroconvulsive therapy on the electrocardiogram and echocardiogram. Anesth Analg 75:511–514, 1992

Meyers BS, Mei-Tal V: Empirical study on an inpatient psychogeriatric unit: biological treatment in patients with depressive illness. Int J Psychiatry Med 15:111–124, 1985–86

Miller RD, Savarese JJ: Pharmacology of muscle relaxants and their antagonists, in Anesthesia, 3rd Edition. New York, Churchill Livingstone, 1990, pp 389–435

Monroe RR: Maintenance electroconvulsive therapy. Psychiatr Clin North Am 14:947–960, 1991

Mulsant BH, Rosen J, Thornton JE, et al: A prospective naturalistic study of electroconvulsive therapy in late-life depression. J Geriatr Psychiatry Neurol 4:3–13, 1991

Murray GB, Shea V, Conn DK: Electroconvulsive therapy for post-stroke depression. J Clin Psychiatry 47(5):258–260, 1986

Nelson JP, Benjamin L: Efficacy and safety of combined ECT and tricyclic antidepressant drugs in the treatment of depressed geriatric patients. Convulsive Therapy 5:321–329, 1989

Oh JJ, Rummans TA, O'Conner MK, et al: Cognitive impairment after ECT in patients with Parkinson's disease and psychiatric illness (letter). Am J Psychiatry 149:271, 1992

Overall JE, Gorham DR: The Brief Psychiatric Rating Scale. Psychol Rep 10:799–812, 1962

Pande AC, Grunhaus LJ, Haskett, et al: Electroconvulsive therapy in delusional and non-delusional depressive disorder. J Affect Disord 19(3):215–219, 1990

Pettinati HM, Mathisen KS, Rosenberg J, et al: Meta-analytical approach to reconciling discrepancies in efficacy between bilateral and unilateral electroconvulsive therapy. Convulsive Therapy 2:7–17, 1986

Post RM: Transduction of psychosocial stress into the neurobiology of recurrent affective disorder. Am J Psychiatry 149:999–1010, 1992

Price TRP, McAllister TW: Safety and efficacy of ECT in depressed patients with dementia: a review of clinical experience. Convulsive Therapy 5:61–74, 1989

Prien R, Kupfer D: Continuation drug therapy for major depressive episodes: how long should it be maintained? Am J Psychiatry 143:18–23, 1986

Prohovnik I, Sackeim HA, Decina P, et al: Acute reductions of regional cerebral blood flow following electroconvulsive therapy (in Electroconvulsive Therapy: Clinical and Basic Research Issues. Edited by Malitz S, Sackeim HA). Ann N Y Acad Sci 462:249–262, 1986

Prudic J, Sackeim HA, Decina P, et al: Acute effects of ECT on cardiovascular functioning: relations to patient and treatment variables. Acta Psychiatr Scand 75:344–351, 1987

Rasmussen K, Abrams R: Treatment of Parkinson's disease with electroconvulsive therapy. Psychiatr Clin North Am 14:925–933, 1991

Reynolds CF, Perel JM, Kupfer DJ, et al: Open-trial response to antidepressant treatment in elderly patients with mixed depression and cognitive impairment. Psychiatry Res 21:111–122, 1987

Rich CL, Spiker DG, Jewell SW, et al: DSM-III, RDC, and ECT: depressive subtypes and immediate response. J Clin Psychiatry 45:14–18, 1984a

Rich CL, Spiker DG, Jewell SW, et al: The efficiency of ECT, I: response rate in depressive episodes. Psychiatry Res 11:167–176, 1984b

Rich CL, Spiker DG, Jewell SW, et al: ECT response in psychotic versus nonpsychotic unipolar depressives. J Clin Psychiatry 47:123–125, 1986

Roberts JM: Prognostic factors in the electroshock treatment of depressive states, I: clinical features from history and examination. Journal of Mental Science 105:693–702, 1959

Robinson RG, Price TR: Post-stroke depressive disorders: a follow-up study of 103 patients. Stroke 13:635–641, 1982

Roth S, Mukherjee J, Sackeim H: Electroconvulsive therapy in a patient with mania, parkinsonism and tardive dyskinesia. Convulsive Therapy 4:92–97, 1988

Rubin EH, Kinsoherf DA, Wehrman SA: Response to treatment of depression in the old and very old. J Ger Psychiatry Neurol 4:65–70, 1991

Rudorfer M, Risby E, Hsaio J, et al: ECT alters human mono-amines in a different manner from that of antidepressant drugs. Psychopharmacol Bull 24:396–399, 1988

Sackeim HA: Are ECT devices underpowered? Convulsive Therapy 7:233–236, 1991

Sackeim HA, Decina P, Prohovnik I, et al: Anticonvulsant and antidepressant properties of electroconvulsive therapy: a proposed mechanism of action. Biol Psychiatry 18:1301–1310, 1983

Sackeim HA, Decina P, Kanzler M, et al: Effects of electrode placement on the efficacy of titrated, low-dose ECT. Am J Psychiatry 144:1449–1455, 1987

Sackeim HA, Prudic J, Devanand DP, et al: The impact of medication resistance and continuation pharmacother-apy on relapse following response to electroconvulsive therapy in major depression. J Clin Psychopharmacol 10:96–104, 1990

Sackeim HA, Devanand DP, Prudic J: Stimulus intensity, sei-zure threshold, and seizure duration: impact on the effi-cacy and safety of electroconvulsive therapy. Psychiatr Clin North Am 14:803–843, 1991

Sackeim HA, Prudic J, Devanand DP, et al: Effects of stimulus intensity and electrode placement on the efficacy and cognitive effects of electroconvulsive therapy. N Engl J Med 328:839–846, 1993

Salzman C: Electroconvulsive therapy in the elderly patient. Psychiatr Clin North Am 5:191–197, 1982

Scott AI, Douglas RH, Whitfield A, et al: Time course of ce-rebral magnetic resonance changes after electroconvul-sive therapy. Br J Psychiatry 156:551–553, 1990

Seager CP, Bird RL: Imipramine with electrical treatment in depression: a controlled trial. Journal of Mental Science 108:704–707, 1962

Shettar MS, Grunhaus L, Pande AC, et al: Protective effects of intramuscular glycopyrrolate on cardiac conduction during ECT. Convulsive Therapy 5:349–352, 1989

Slawson P: Psychiatric malpractice: the electroconvulsive therapy experience. Convulsive Therapy 1:195–203, 1985

Small JG, Klapper MH, Kellams JJ, et al: ECT compared with lithium in the management of manic states. Arch Gen Psy-chiatry 45:727–732, 1988

Small JG, Milstein V, Small IF: Electroconvulsive therapy for mania. Psychiatr Clin North Am 14:887–903, 1991

Solan WJ, Khan A, Avery DH, et al: Psychotic and non-psychotic depression: comparison of response to ECT. J Clin Psychiatry 49:97–99, 1988

Staton RD: Electroencephalographic recording during bitemporal and unilateral non-dominant hemisphere (Lancaster position) electroconvulsive therapy. J Clin Psy-chiatry 42:264–269, 1981

Stoudemire A, Knos G, Gladson M, et al: Labetalol in the control of cardiovascular responses to electroconvulsive therapy in high-risk depressed medical patients. J Clin Psychiatry 51(12):508–512, 1990

Strömgren LS: Unilateral versus bilateral electroconvulsive therapy. Acta Psychiatr Scand Suppl 240:5–65, 1973

Strömgren LS, Christensen AL, Fromholt P: The effects of unilateral brief-interval ECT on memory. Acta Psychiatr Scand 54:336–346, 1976

Sullivan MO, Ward NG, Laxton A: The woman who wanted electroconvulsive therapy and do-not-resuscitate status. Gen Hosp Psychiatry 14:204–209, 1992

Swartz CM: Clinical and laboratory predictors of ECT re-sponse, in Clinical Science of Electroconvulsive Therapy. Edited by Coffey CE. Washington, DC, American Psychi-atric Press, 1993, pp 53–71

Thienhaus OJ, Margletta S, Bennett JA: A study of the clinical efficacy of maintenance ECT. J Clin Psychiatry 51(4):141–144, 1990

Volavka J, Feldstein S, Abrams R, et al: EEG and clinical change after bilateral and unilateral electroconvulsive therapy. Electroencephalogr Clin Neurophysiol 32:631–639, 1972

Ward C, Stern GM, Pratt R, et al: Electroconvulsive therapy in parkinsonian patients with the "on-off" syndrome. Journal of Neural Transmission 49:133–135, 1980

Webb MC, Coffey CE, Saunders WR, et al: Cardiovascular re-sponse to unilateral electroconvulsive therapy. Biol Psy-chiatry 28:758–766, 1990

Wechsler D: Wechsler Memory Scale—Revised. San Antonio, TX, Psychological Corporation, 1987

Weiner RD: The role of electroconvulsive therapy in the treatment of depression in the elderly. J Am Geriatr Soc 30:710–712, 1982

Weiner RD: Does ECT cause brain damage? Behavioral and Brain Sciences 7:1–53, 1984

Weiner RD, Coffey CE: Indications for use of electroconvul-sive therapy, in American Psychiatric Press Review of Psy-chiatry, Vol 7. Edited by Frances AJ, Hales RE. American Psychiatric Press, 1988, pp 458–481

Weiner RD, Coffey CE: Electroconvulsive therapy in the med-ical and neurological patient, in Psychiatric Care of the Medical Patient. Edited by Stoudemire A, Fogel B. New York, Oxford University Press, 1993, pp 207–224

Weiner RD, Krystal AD: EEG monitoring of ECT seizures, in Clinical Science of Electroconvulsive Therapy. Edited by Coffey CE. Washington, DC, American Psychiatric Press, 1993, pp 93–109

Weiner RD, Whanger AD, Erwin CW, et al: Prolonged confu-sional state and EEG seizure activity following concurrent ECT and lithium use. Am J Psychiatry 137:1452–1453, 1980

Weiner RD, Rogers HJ, Davidson JRT, et al: Effects of stimu-lus parameters on cognitive side effects. Ann N Y Acad Sci 462:315–325, 1986

Weisberg LA, Elliott D, Mielke D: Intracerebral hemorrhage following electroconvulsive therapy. Neurology 41:1849, 1991

Welch CA: ECT in medically ill patients, in Clinical Science of Electroconvulsive Therapy. Edited by Coffey CE. Wash-ington, DC, American Psychiatric Press, 1993, pp 167–182

Welch CA, Drop LJ: Cardiovascular effects of ECT. Convul-sive Therapy 5:35–43, 1989

Wilkinson AM, Anderson DN, Peters S: Age and the effects of ECT. International Journal of Geriatric Psychiatry 8:401–406, 1993

Young R, Alexopoulos G, Shamoian A: Dissociation of motor response from mood and cognition in a parkinsonian pa-tient treated with ECT. Biol Psychiatry 20:566–569, 1985

Yudofsky SC: Parkinson's disease, depression and electroconvulsive therapy: a clinical and neurobiologic synthesis. Compr Psychiatry 20:579–581, 1979

Zervas I, Fink M: ECT for refractory Parkinson's disease. Convulsive Therapy 7:222–223, 1991

Zervas IM, Calev A, Jandorf L, et al: Age-dependent effects of electroconvulsive therapy on memory. Convulsive Therapy 9:39–42, 1993

Zibrak JD, Jensen WA, Bloomingdale K: Aspiration pneumonitis following electroconvulsive therapy in patients with gastroparesis. Biol Psychiatry 24:812–814, 1988

Zielinski, RJ, Roose SP, Devanand DP, et al: Cardiovascular complications of ECT in depressed patients with cardiac disease. Am J Psychiatry 150:904–909, 1993

Zis AP, Goodwin FK: Major affective disorder as a recurrent illness: a critical review. Arch Gen Psychiatry 36:835–839, 1979

Zorumski CF, Rubin EH, Burke WJ: Electroconvulsive therapy for the elderly. Hosp Community Psychiatry 39:643–647, 1988

Zwil A, McAllister TW, Price TRP: Safety and efficacy of ECT in depressed patients with organic brain disease: review of a clinical experience. Convulsive Therapy 8:103–109, 1992

31

Psychosocial Therapies

Linda Teri, Ph.D.
Susan M. McCurry, Ph.D.

Introduction

Historically, it was believed that older adults were not good candidates for nonpharmacological, psychotherapeutic interventions (Freud 1924). However, in the past several decades, increasing numbers of researchers have studied the psychosocial issues confronting aging adults, and their response to individual and group therapies (for a discussion of this trend, see Teri and Logsdon 1992). Recent reviews have summarized the empirical literature on the application of psychosocial therapies with depressed older adults (Niederehe 1994; Teri et al. 1994). Reviews are also available relating to specific psychotherapeutic interventions with elderly patients, including behavioral assessment and treatment of anxiety (Hersen and van Hasselt 1992), reduction of insomnia (Engle-Friedman and Bootzin 1991), behavioral management of dementia (Fisher and Carstensen 1990a), use of reminiscence therapy (Thornton and Brotchie 1987), and group interventions for family caregivers (Toseland and Rossiter 1989). In this chapter, we summarize the main psychotherapeutic techniques currently in use with elderly patients that have been tested experimentally and review the empirical literature in which these techniques have been applied to specific elder populations. Further, we describe some special considerations underlying assessment and treatment of older adults. Finally, we identify future directions for clinical practice and research with aging populations.

Common Psychotherapeutic Interventions

A number of recent reference texts have summarized the physical, developmental, environmental, cognitive, social, and psychological factors that impact and guide psychotherapeutic interventions with older adults (e.g., Birren and Schaie 1990; Birren et al. 1992). The vast majority of controlled, experimental outcome studies that exist on psychotherapy with older adults fall into the broad categories of psychoeducational or cognitive-behavior therapy (CBT). Psychoeducational therapies emphasize the didactic presentation of psychological theories and techniques and the practice of these techniques in everyday situations. In contrast, CBT refers to an approach that combines the conceptual and applied work of various cognitive and behavioral-social learning theorists such

as Beck (see Beck et al. 1979) and Lewinsohn (see Lewinsohn et al. 1984). In CBT interventions, it is generally assumed that psychiatric disturbances are learned and maintained through a combination of cognitive distortions and behavioral or environmental events. Therefore, treatment seeks to change the cognitive and behavioral context in which the disturbance is occurring.

Although CBT conceptually includes psychoeducational strategies, it goes beyond them to provide systematic skill training in cognitive and behavioral techniques. For example, CBT can involve using specific techniques such as providing new information, teaching problem-solving strategies, correcting skills deficits, modifying ineffective communication patterns, and changing the physical environment in which problems arise. Homework assignments to supplement in-session interventions are frequently given. Although specific treatment protocols vary, all CBT approaches tend to be active and focused on solving specific, current, day-to-day problems, rather than seeking global personality change. It should be noted that in practice, the terms *psychoeducational* and *cognitive-behavioral* are often used interchangeably to refer to similar intervention strategies.

There have also been a few controlled studies that compared the use of psychodynamic or insight-oriented approaches with either CBT or pharmacotherapy in depressed elderly subjects. The dynamic approaches used in these studies differ from CBT interventions in their emphasis on the importance of the therapeutic alliance and in their interest in historical causes of current client behavior. Typically, patients are not taught new specific skills in therapy, nor is homework outside of session considered an essential aspect of treatment. Rather, greater import is assigned to patients' ongoing emotional experience. Therapeutic techniques such as reflection or interpretation of patient resistance are often used, and the therapist tends to be less directive than in CBT. Brief dynamic or insight-oriented approaches do, however, also focus on specific problem resolution within a limited number of therapy sessions (Bellak and Small 1965). One form of psychodynamic therapy that has been used in empirical treatment outcome studies with depressed elderly patients, interpersonal psychotherapy (IPT) (Klerman et al. 1984), is particularly interesting because it offers a research-oriented operationalization of psychodynamic treatment, which historically has not been empirically based.

There is also a small empirical literature on the effectiveness of reminiscence and/or life review therapy for elderly patients. Reminiscence is defined as "the act or process of recalling the past . . . a narration of past experiences" (American Heritage Dictionary 1985). In reminiscence therapy, elderly patients are encouraged to remember the past and to share their memories, either with a therapist or with peers, as a way of increasing self-esteem and social intimacy. It is often highly directive and structured, with the therapist picking each session's reminiscence topic. In life review therapy, past experiences are not only recalled, but an effort is made to reexperience old conflicts and rework them into a therapeutic resolution. In other words, life review is one form of reminiscence, designed to produce a better understanding and acceptance of past events (Butler 1963). In the clinical intervention literature, however, *reminiscence* and *life review* are often loosely used as interchangeable terms for any individual or group narrative therapy that encourages patients to remember and describe the past.

Finally, the experimental literature includes a number of isolated studies in which "supportive" interventions of various types have been compared to one another or to no-treatment controls. Specifics regarding these various interventions are discussed throughout the chapter. However, it is worthwhile to note that many of these nonspecific interventions use techniques that are drawn from CBT, insight-oriented, or reminiscence approaches; for example, patients may be taught specific behavior skills, relaxation techniques, or problem-solving strategies.

Psychotherapy for Depression in Elderly Patients

Much of the psychotherapeutic research that has been conducted with elderly patients has focused on the treatment of depression. Depression is thought to affect approximately 15% of the community-dwelling people over age 65, and up to 25% of nursing home residents (National Institutes of Health 1991) (see also Chapter 12, this volume). Depression symptoms are also prevalent among elderly medical patients or dementia patients and their caregivers (Gallagher et al. 1989; Kim and Hershey 1988; Teri and Wagner 1992). Nevertheless, epidemiological studies indicate that older adults are underserved by mental health providers. It has been estimated that only 10% of the elderly

population in need of psychiatric treatment receives this care (National Institutes of Health 1991). Because recurrence of depressive episodes is common throughout the life span, and suicide rates for elderly adults are greater than for younger adults, this lack of psychosocial treatment in geriatric patients is a cause of concern. Fortunately, the empirical literature on depression treatment with elderly patients has yielded generally encouraging results.

CBT and Psychodynamic Psychotherapy

Cognitive-behavioral approaches have been used in the treatment of depression in elderly patients. For example, CBT has been reported with geriatric outpatients and inpatients, medically healthy and ill older adults, and in both group and individual intervention settings. Some of the research describing the efficacy of CBT is in the form of case reports, clinical writings, and controlled clinical trials (e.g., Baum and Gallagher 1987; Griffin and Waller 1985; Steuer and Hammen 1983; Teri and Gallagher-Thompson 1991; Teri and Uomoto 1991; Waller and Griffin 1984; Yost et al. 1986). There is also a small, but growing, experimental literature that suggests CBT may be an effective treatment for depression in elderly patients.

Much of the empirical data published thus far on the efficacy of CBT with geriatric subjects has come from Thompson, Gallagher-Thompson, and their colleagues (Table 31–1). Several of these studies compared cognitive and behavioral approaches with a brief psychodynamic or insight-oriented approach. For example, Gallagher and Thompson (Gallagher and Thompson 1982, 1983; L. W. Thompson and Gallagher 1985) examined the comparative effectiveness of short-term individual cognitive, behavior, and brief insight-relational therapy in a sample of 30 elderly outpatient volunteers diagnosed as having a major depressive disorder (MDD). A substantial decrease in depression symptoms was obtained for subjects in all three groups by the end of treatment, and this decrease was maintained at 1 year. However, maintenance of treatment gains was not comparable across the three conditions: depressive symptoms increased for subjects in the brief relational-insight therapy group, beginning as early as 6 weeks posttreatment with no such relapse evident for subjects in the cognitive or behavioral conditions.

Subsequent studies (L. W. Thompson and Gallagher 1984) repeated the comparison of cognitive, be-

Table 31–1.   Empirical studies of cognitive-behavioral or psychodynamic therapy

Study	Sample population	Sample age (years)	Treatment	Treatment duration
Zarit et al. 1981	47 volunteer women	Mean = 64	Memory training group Personal growth group	7 sessions in 4 weeks
Gallagher and Thompson 1982, 1983; L. W. Thompson and Gallagher 1985[a]	30 outpatients with major depressive disorder (MDD)[b]	Mean = 66–69 (range = 59–80)	Individual cognitive therapy (CT) Individual behavior therapy (BT) Individual insight-oriented therapy	16 sessions in 12 weeks
Jarvik et al. 1982	32 MDD outpatients (drug trial) 26 MDD outpatients (group therapy)	Range = 55–81	Imipramine Doxepin Placebo	36 weeks
Steuer et al. 1984	33 outpatient volunteers with MDD	Median = 66 (range = 55–78)	Group cognitive-behavior therapy (CBT) Group psychodynamic therapy	46 sessions in 9 months
L. W. Thompson et al. 1983	56 volunteer attendees	Mean = 68 (range = 60–82)	Coping with depression group course: Professional instructors Nonprofessional instructors	6 weeks
Fry 1984	28 outpatients	Mean = 65 (range = 67–80)	CBT group CBT group after wait-list control	12 sessions in 4 weeks
L. W. Thompson and Gallagher 1984	37 outpatients with MDD	Mean = 67	Individual CT Individual BT Individual dynamic Wait-list control	16–20 sessions in 3–4 months
Sloane et al. 1985; Schneider et al. 1986[a]	55 outpatients with MDD	Mean = 64 (all subjects older than 60)	Individual interpersonal psychotherapy Nortriptyline Pill placebo	16 weeks
L. W. Thompson and Gallagher 1986; L. W. Thompson et al. 1987, 1988; Gaston et al. 1988, 1989; Marmar et al. 1989; Gallagher-Thompson et al. 1990[a]	91 outpatients with MDD	Mean = 67	Individual CT Individual BT Individual psychodynamic Wait-list control	16–20 sessions in 3–4 months
Beutler et al. 1987	56 outpatients with MDD	Mean = 70–71 for all groups (all subjects older than 65)	Alprazolam Placebo (medication) CBT group and alprazolam CBT group and placebo	20 sessions
Scogin et al. 1987	29 mildly depressed volunteers	Mean = 68–72	Individual cognitive bibliotherapy Individual delayed (cognitive) bibliotherapy Attention-control reading	Self-paced
Scogin et al. 1989, 1990	67 community residents	Mean = 68	Individual cognitive bibliotherapy Individual behavioral bibliotherapy Wait-list control	4 weeks
L. W. Thompson et al. 1991	67 older adult outpatient volunteers	?	Desipramine Individual CBT Medication and CBT combined	? sessions in 3–4 months

[a]Studies cited together reported on subsamples of the larger randomized clinical trial.
[b]Studies that identified subjects as diagnosed with MDD are specified; other studies may or may not have included subjects with MDD diagnosis.

havior, and brief dynamic therapies with elderly adults with MDD. Once again, significant decreases were demonstrated in depression, with no significant between-group differences. When these approaches were compared to a 6-week delayed-treatment control condition (Gallagher-Thompson et al. 1990; L. W. Thompson and Gallagher 1986; L. W. Thompson et al. 1987), equivalent treatment gains were once again evidenced across modalities at the end of therapy. Other authors have reported similar results. For example, Fry (1984) found group-format CBT to be effective in reducing depression in geriatric subjects in both immediate and delayed treatment conditions, although in his study (compared with the previous studies) patients were experiencing a wider (including milder) range of depressive symptoms before treatment. CBT strategies have also been shown to be effective in treating depression in elderly patients whether such techniques are taught by professional or peer instructors (L. W. Thompson et al. 1983) and through self-paced or time-limited bibliotherapy (Scogin et al. 1987, 1989, 1990).

CBT has also been compared to pharmacotherapy for treating depression in the elderly population. Jarvik, Steuer, and their colleagues (Jarvik et al. 1982; Steuer et al. 1984) conducted two concurrent studies with geriatric outpatients who met DSM-III criteria (American Psychiatric Association 1980) for major depression. In one study (Jarvik et al. 1982), they compared the response of patients who received either imipramine, doxepin, or a placebo drug. In the other study (Steuer et al. 1984), patients were assigned to either a CBT or a psychodynamic group therapy condition. Results indicated that all medication and therapy conditions were better than a placebo in reducing depression, and no significant differences between active conditions (imipramine versus doxepin; CBT versus dynamic therapy) were observed. Medication therapy initially (at 26 weeks) was associated with a higher full remission rate than was psychotherapy (45% versus 12%, respectively) (Jarvik et al. 1982). However, patients in the medication group also had a higher treatment dropout rate and greater number of subjects who showed no improvement by the end of treatment (36 weeks) than did the psychotherapy group. Furthermore, by the end of treatment, 40% of all patients who completed psychotherapy had achieved a full remission in depression, eliminating the early advantage found in medication recipients. Slightly better results for the CBT than the psychodynamic groups were observed, but because subjects were enrolled in an open-

trial fashion (nonrandomized), these conclusions are difficult to interpret (Steuer et al. 1984).

Beutler et al. (1987) compared the relative and combined effectiveness of alprazolam and group cognitive therapy in geriatric patients with major depression. Patients were randomly assigned to a 20-week, therapy-plus-medication (alprazolam or placebo) or medication-only condition. Subjects in all conditions showed reductions in depression symptoms (as rated by interviewers using the Hamilton Depression Rating Scale [HDRS; Hamilton 1967]) after 1 month of treatment, and gains were maintained through follow-up sampling (3 months posttreatment). However, patient self-reports of depression (using the Beck Depression Inventory [BDI; Beck 1967]) and sleep disturbance showed continued improvement after 1 month and at follow-up only for subjects who were in the group therapy condition. A significantly larger number of patients who received cognitive therapy were asymptomatic by the end of follow-up than were those who received medication without psychotherapy. No significant differences were reported for subjects receiving therapy with or without active medication.

More recently, Gallagher and Thompson have conducted randomized controlled clinical trials comparing the efficacy of CBT in treating depressed elderly patients with the use of desipramine, either singly or in combination with CBT (L. W. Thompson et al. 1991). Patients in the combined treatment group had significantly greater reductions in depression than did those in the desipramine-only group, but not those in the CBT-only group. No significant differences in depression measures were observed in subjects who received either desipramine or CBT alone.

IPT has been shown to have effectiveness equivalent to that of nortriptyline at 6 and 16 weeks in the acute treatment of geriatric patients with major depression and to be associated with lower dropout rates (Schneider et al. 1986; Sloane et al. 1985). In an ongoing study, Reynolds, Frank, and their colleagues (see Niederehe 1994) are comparing recurrent elderly depressive patients randomized to maintenance treatment with IPT, nortriptyline, or a combination of both. Data from these types of well-controlled comparison studies will be instrumental in furthering our understanding of the efficacy of psychotherapy with depressed elderly patients.

A variety of factors have been identified that may influence treatment effects observed in depression studies using CBT and dynamic interventions with elderly patients. These factors include endogeneity of depression (Gallagher and Thompson 1983), the presence of a personality disorder (L. W. Thompson et al. 1988), severity of the depression at the onset of treatment (Beckham 1989), patient expectancies for change (Gaston et al. 1989), and the patient's role in the development of the therapeutic alliance (Gaston et al. 1988; Marmar et al. 1989). It has also been suggested that therapist misconceptions about elderly patients' limited capacity for behavior change may lead clinicians to underutilize psychotherapy and underestimate its potential effectiveness with older patients (Fry 1986; Lazarus and Weinberg 1982). However, no empirical studies have been conducted to examine the relationship between therapist factors and treatment outcome in the elderly population.

In summary, there is a small, but significant, empirical literature showing the effectiveness of CBT and psychodynamic therapies in treating depression in physically healthy, elderly patients (the few studies with physically frail or otherwise impaired, depressed individuals are reviewed below). There is evidence that symptom improvements obtained with psychotherapy are equal to those found with pharmacotherapy and that psychotherapy may be associated with lower dropout rates than pharmacological interventions alone. A wide variety of CBT formats, including individual and group interventions, bibliotherapy, and variants of CBT (cognitive only, behavioral only, and CBT), have all produced reductions in depression. In many studies, treatment gains have been maintained up to 1 year follow-up. The psychotherapy literature has primarily focused on community-residing volunteers diagnosed as having MDD; however, some studies have shown psychotherapy to be effective with milder depressive symptoms as well. There have not yet been any empirical studies comparing CBT or psychodynamic treatments with depressed older adults in psychiatric inpatient settings. However, the research methodologies and standardized assessment instruments that have been used in outpatient studies with CBT and psychodynamic interventions should be applicable to future research with depressed geriatric inpatients as well.

Reminiscence and Life Review Therapies

Empirical trials have been conducted using reminiscence and life review to reduce depression and anxiety (measured by a variety of self-report measures) and to increase feelings of self-esteem and life satisfaction in

older elderly patients (Table 31–2). Although results have generally been promising, findings have been inconsistent. For example, Fielden (1990) observed that life satisfaction and socialization increased more among reminiscence group participants than among participants of a "here-and-now," current events group conducted at a sheltered housing complex. In contrast, Lappe (1987) and Rattenbury and Stones (1989) found that both reminiscence and current events discussion groups were effective in improving elderly patients' ratings of psychological well-being. In yet another set of studies, reminiscence activities produced no significant effects on measures of depression, anxiety, or self-esteem (Hedgepeth and Hale 1983; Perrotta and Meacham 1981).

A number of variables may contribute to the differential impact of reminiscence on psychological well-being, including the frequency and duration of the intervention (Baines et al. 1987; Lappe 1987), patient age (Youssef 1990), whether or not the reminiscence is conducted in long-term care or community settings (Fielden 1990; Lieberman and Falk 1971; Molinari and Reichlin 1985), what measures of change are used to assess treatment outcome (Berghorn and Schafer 1987), and whether environmental stimuli (e.g., music) are used to enhance the reminiscence process (Bennett and Maas 1988). The amount of structure provided to the reminiscence activity may also affect treatment outcome. For example, it has been suggested that systematic life review techniques are clinically more powerful than simple recollections of the past. Fry (1983) found that "structured" reminiscence was more successful than "unstructured" reminiscence in lowering depression posttests and significantly raised reports of self-confidence and adequacy. Haight (1988) compared structured life review reminiscing with nonstructured "friendly home visits," and found life review participants reported increased amounts of life satisfaction and increased psychological well-being. Structured life review strategies have been found to be as effective as systematic relaxation training (Ingersoll and Silverman 1978) and CBT (Harp Scates et al. 1986) in reducing anxiety and improving life satisfaction or self-esteem.

It has also been suggested that the impact of reminiscence techniques may differ when they are used in an individual or group therapy format. For example, some authors have noted that studies using individual reminiscence have produced positive outcomes less consistently than have group interventions (Watt and

Wong 1991). However, other authors have reported improvements in mood following individual reminiscence procedures (Fallot 1980; Fry 1983) and have even suggested that individual interventions may be the treatment of choice for life review with geriatric subjects (Haight 1988). There is also some concern that the terms *reminiscence* and *life review* actually describe multiple, distinct psychological processes and that these processes may significantly alter the effectiveness of reminiscence as a therapeutic technique (Watt and Wong 1991). Indeed, the conceptual differences between simple reminiscence and active life review have been considered by several authors (see Merriam 1980; Molinari and Reichlin 1985; Watt and Wong 1991). However, to date there has been no empirical attempt to define operationally the processes of reminiscence and life review or to test their differential impact with selected clinical populations.

In summary, although the numbers of empirical studies using reminiscence and life review with geriatric outpatients are limited, there is evidence that both can help reduce negative mood and improve life-

Table 31–2. Empirical studies of reminiscence therapy with older adults

Study	Sample population	Sample age (years)	Treatment	Treatment duration
Ingersoll and Silverman 1978	17 community elders	Mean = 70	Behavioral group Reminiscence/life review group	8 sessions
Fallot 1980	36 female out-patients	Mean = 66 (range = 46–85)	Individual reminiscence Individual nonreminiscence	2 sessions
Perrota and Meacham 1981	21 community elders	Mean = 75–80	Individual reminiscence Individual current life events No-treatment control	5 sessions
Fry 1983	162 depressed outpatients	Median = 68 (range = 65–82)	Individual structured reminiscence Individual unstructured reminiscence Attention-only control	5 sessions
Hedgepeth and Hale 1983	60 female outpatients	Mean = 76 (range = 60–98)	Individual reminiscence (past successes) Individual reminiscence (present positive events) No-reminiscence control	1 session
Harp Scates et al. 1986	50 outpatients	Mean = 75 (all subjects older than 65)	CBT group Reminiscence group Activity condition	6 sessions in 3 weeks
Lappe 1987	83 NH residents	Mean = 83	Reminiscence group Current events group	10 weeks (half met two times/week; other half met one time/week)
Bennett and Maas 1988	26 NH female patients	Mean = 82	Music-based life review group Verbal life review group	6 sessions
Haight 1988	60 homebound elderly	Mean = 73–79 (all subjects older than 50)	Individual life review sessions Control ("individual friendly visits") No-treatment control	6 sessions
Rattenbury and Stones 1989	24 NH residents for all groups	Mean = 83–87	Reminiscence group Current topics group No-treatment control	8 sessions
Fielden 1990	31 sheltered housing residents	Mean = 74–75	Reminiscence group "Here-and-now" group	9 sessions
Youssef 1990	66 female NH residents (65–74 years)	All subjects older than 65	Reminiscence group Reminiscence group (75+ years) No-treatment control	6 sessions in 5 weeks

Note. NH = nursing home or long-term residential setting.

satisfaction and self-esteem. However, nonsignificant findings have been reported in several studies, which has led to speculation about factors that increase the efficacy of reminiscence strategies. Studies have shown that structured life review strategies may be more effective than simple narrative reminiscence. There is also evidence that life review conducted in individual or group format may produce differential treatment effects; however, no well-designed comparison studies to confirm either of these hypotheses have been conducted. There has been no attempt to identify which clinical groups are more likely to benefit from reminiscence or which are at risk to develop iatrogenic effects. In contrast to the CBT and psychodynamic treatments described above, none of the reminiscence studies reviewed here were conducted with patients diagnosed as having major depression.

Other Therapy Interventions

The remaining empirical studies conducted on psychotherapy with elderly patients used a variety of intervention techniques to modify depression, anxiety, and other symptoms of emotional distress (see Table 31–3). As noted earlier, these techniques are commonly drawn from the CBT, dynamic and insight-oriented, or reminiscence therapies. For example, several studies have used meditation-relaxation and cognitive change techniques. DeBerry (1982) found that relaxation-meditation training was effective in reducing self-reports of anxiety but not depression in a group of depressed elderly women. Similar results were found using meditation in a later study in which the investigators compared relaxation techniques with cognitive restructuring (DeBerry et al. 1989); however,

Table 31–3. Empirical studies (miscellaneous) with older adults

Study	Sample population	Sample age (years)	Treatment	Treatment duration
Nevruz and Hrushka 1969	36 psychiatric inpatients	Mean = 70	Structured therapy group Unstructured therapy group	24 sessions in 12 weeks
Mulligan and Bennett 1977	23 isolated outpatients	Mean = 77 (all subjects older than 67)	Social visits (individuals at home) Control visits (2 visits only)	1 hour every 2 weeks for 6 months
DeBerry 1982	36 depressed women	Mean = 63–79	Group relaxation-meditation Group relaxation-meditation with follow-up tapes Pseudo-relaxation control group	10 weeks (plus 10 weeks of daily practice for group relaxation-meditation with follow-up tapes
Lieberman and Bliwise 1985	108 outpatients	Range = 60–83	Professional-led support group Peer-led support group	36 sessions in 9 months
Franzke 1987	84 community-dwelling subjects	All subjects older than 65	Assertiveness training groups No-treatment control	6 sessions
Ong et al. 1987	20 discharged inpatients (most in day hospital program)	Mean = 74	Support group (psychodynamic and problem-solving) No-added-treatment control	Weekly sessions for 9 months
Alexander et al. 1989	73 NH patients and NH residents	Mean = 81	Individual transcendental meditation Individual mindfulness training Individual mental relaxation Wait-list control	4 sessions in 12 weeks
DeBerry et al. 1989	32 outpatients	Mean = 69 (range = 65–75)	Relaxation-meditation group Cognitive restructuring group Pseudo-treatment control (pseudo-relaxation)	20 sessions in 10 weeks
Reich and Zautra 1989	25 bereaved, 25 disabled, and 58 (matched) control subjects	Mean = 71	Perceived control intervention Placebo contact No-contact control	4 sessions in 10 weeks

Note. NH = nursing home or long-term residential setting.

cognitive interventions alone produced no significant changes in either depression or trait anxiety. Interestingly, Alexander et al. (1989) found that both meditation and "mindfulness" training resulted in improvements in cognitive functioning, blood pressure readings, and 3-year survival rates, despite the fact that no changes in anxiety or depression were associated with either intervention.

Some studies have focused on providing depressed elderly patients with skills training. Participation in assertiveness training has been shown to successfully improve effectiveness in interpersonal situations and ratings of self-acceptance (Franzke 1987). Reich and Zautra (1989) found that four sessions of individual therapy, designed to enhance perceived control, significantly increased participation in positive activities and decreased psychological distress in bereaved and disabled elderly subjects. However, these improvements were not maintained after the treatment was discontinued.

Other studies have examined the impact of therapy on subjects' long-term functioning. For example, isolated community-dwelling elderly people who received regular "social visits" in their home for 6 months were more likely to be living independently in the community at 6-month follow-up than were control subjects (Mulligan and Bennett 1977). Geriatric psychiatric patients who participated in weekly psychodynamic problem-solving groups for 9 months had a lower rehospitalization rate, despite the fact that no changes in depression symptoms were observed for participants (Ong et al. 1987). Therapy has even been shown to influence geriatric psychiatric patients' willingness to leave state hospital wards and try community placement options (Nevruz and Hrushka 1969).

In summary, a variety of nonspecific psychosocial interventions have been used with geriatric subjects. Although a few studies have included psychiatric inpatients, the majority have been conducted with outpatient volunteers. These studies have shown that different combinations of relaxation, cognitive restructuring, emotional support, and skills training can improve self-ratings of depression, anxiety, and self-acceptance. There is also evidence that psychosocial interventions lead to improvements in long-term survival rates and reduced rehospitalization for chronically ill psychiatric patients. However, long-term maintenance of improvements in mood or generalization of newly learned skills has not been consistently reported after therapy discontinuation.

Psychotherapy for Depression in Elderly Patients With Dementia

CBT and Psychodynamic Psychotherapy

There is a growing literature describing the management of behavior problems in dementia (for a review, see Fisher and Carstensen 1990a). Until recently, however, relatively little attention has been given to the treatment of depression in dementia patients, despite its prevalence and impact on functional status (Teri and Wagner 1992).

The use of CBT to treat depression in dementia patients has also been described. Although data are currently unavailable, Gallagher-Thompson and colleagues have reported good success using cognitive techniques with mildly impaired patients (Teri and Gallagher-Thompson 1991). Teri and colleagues (Teri and Uomoto 1991; Teri et al. 1991) have also developed an ongoing treatment study with Alzheimer's disease patients diagnosed as having major or minor depression and their caregivers at the University of Washington Medical Center. This study integrates knowledge gained from decades of clinical writings geared to help caregivers cope with the problems of patients with dementia (Zarit 1989) and empirical work showing that behavioral interventions are effective in treating depression in younger and older patients without dementia (Gallagher and Thompson 1982; Lewinsohn et al. 1984).

From this perspective, depression is viewed as a series of behaviors that are learned and maintained through positive and negative reinforcement contingencies (Lewinsohn et al. 1980). Consequently, the central aim of treatment is to reduce or eliminate depression behaviors by altering the contingencies that maintain them, as well as by introducing new contingencies to stimulate and maintain nondepressive behaviors. In the University of Washington study, treatment consists of eight 60-minute sessions, once per week, with patients and caregivers participating in varying degrees. The goals of treatment are to teach caregivers behavioral strategies for improving patient depression by 1) increasing pleasant events and decreasing unpleasant events and 2) using behavioral problem-solving strategies to alter the contingencies that relate to depression and associated behavior problems. Caregiver-patient pairs are randomly assigned in a double-blind controlled clinical trial to either behavioral or wait-list control conditions.

Data obtained thus far indicate significant reductions in depression on standardized measures (such as the HDRS and the Cornell Depression in Dementia Scale [Alexopoulos et al. 1988]) for patients in the behavior therapy conditions, but not for those in the wait-list condition. Seventy-three percent of patients in behavior therapy improved over the course of treatment, whereas only 5% improved on the wait list. In addition, caregivers of patients who were in the behavior therapy condition showed significant reductions in depression, but those on the wait list did not. This latter finding was unexpected, as patient depression alone was the treatment target. Increased skill in patient management, the availability of regular therapeutic support, and the reduced depression in the family member with dementia most likely explain these added benefits. Thus behavioral treatment of patients with dementia may have the additional advantage of improving the caregiver's affect and the quality of his or her caregiving, both of which are important areas often not assessed in typical outcome studies (Teri et al. 1992).

Reminiscence and Life Review Therapies

Both reminiscence and life review techniques have also been used with confused, depressed elderly patients in long-term care settings (Baines et al. 1987; Goldwasser et al. 1987; Orten et al. 1989). In these studies, reminiscence storytelling was conducted in a group format (Table 31–4). Specific topics or themes were suggested by staff, sometimes with the assistance of personal artifacts, newspapers, music, or other memorabilia used to stimulate residents' memories. Results of all three studies found that simple reminiscing led to reductions in depression and improvements in social functioning for the confused participants. However, changes were not maintained over time for all treatment groups. It was suggested that the inexperience of group facilitators and heterogeneity in level of patient impairment may have negatively impacted long-term treatment effects (Goldwasser et al. 1987; Orten et al. 1989). Interestingly, Baines et al. (1987) found that reminiscence groups did improve long-term interactions between nursing home staff and patients; they suggested this might be a result of increased staff understanding of patient needs and their caretaking role.

In summary, CBT has been reported effective in reducing major and minor depression in outpatients diagnosed as having progressive dementing illnesses such as Alzheimer's disease. There is also evidence that treatment for depression in patients with Alzheimer's disease can improve caregivers' mood, even when treatment does not specifically focus on the caregiver. Although the empirical literature on use of CBT with dementia patients and their caregivers is still in its infancy, such positive early results warrant further investigation. In long-term residential settings, reminiscence techniques have been used to improve mood and social functioning with severely impaired dementia patients. However, changes associated with use of

Table 31–4.   Empirical studies with cognitively disabled depressed elderly patients

Study	Sample population	Sample age	Treatment	Treatment duration
Baines et al. 1987	30 NH residents	Mean = 82 (range = 72–90)	Reality orientation-reminiscence group Reminiscence-reality orientation group No-treatment control	40 sessions/16 weeks (1, 2 crossover at 8 weeks)
Goldwasser et al. 1987	27 NH patients with dementia	Mean = 82 (range = 70–97)	Reminiscence group Supportive (attention/placebo) group No-treatment control	10 sessions in 5 weeks
Orten et al. 1989	56 inpatients with dementia	Mean = 83 (range = 58–101)	Reminiscence group No-treatment control	16 sessions
Teri et al. 1991	60 Alzheimer's disease patients w/ major or minor depression and caregiver	Mean = 75 (range = 53–93)	Individual BT Individual problem solving Wait-list control	9 sessions

Note. NH = nursing home or long-term residential setting.

reminiscence are not well sustained once treatment is discontinued, at least for the more cognitively impaired residents.

Psychotherapy With Medically Ill Elderly Patients

Elderly patients represent a disproportionally high percentage of the medical illnesses, disabilities, and utilization of health care services in the United States (Keuthen and Wisocki 1991). Because they also represent one of the fastest growing segments of American society, there is concern that the demand for geriatric medical services will eventually exceed available resources. In response, an increasing number of practitioners have begun exploring the supplemental role of psychosocial interventions in geriatric health care. For

example, a number of studies have shown that the use of mental health services leads to a reduction in medical care, particularly in-hospital stays for people over age 55 (Mumford et al. 1984). Use of behavioral interventions has been shown to improve elderly patients' compliance with difficult medical procedures and their participation in wellness programs and exercise regimens (Gutman et al. 1977; Kirschenbaum et al. 1987; Matteson 1989). Recent books have described the application and efficacy of psychological interventions with chronic pain and medical rehabilitation in elderly patients (Hartke 1991; Saxon 1991).

The few controlled experimental studies using psychosocial interventions with medically ill geriatric patients have focused on patients' abilities to cope with chronic or life-threatening illness (Table 31–5). Most of these studies have used a combination of supportive,

Table 31–5. Empirical studies in health care settings with older adults

Study	Sample population	Sample age (years)	Treatment	Treatment duration
Godbole and Verinis 1974	61 rehabilitation inpatients with physical disabilities	Mean = 69 (range = 38–82)	Individual confrontational therapy Individual supportive therapy No-treatment control	6–12 sessions in 2–4 weeks
Ibrahim et al. 1974	118 cardiac patients	Range = 35–65 (67% of subjects older than 50)	Supportive group therapy No-treatment control	50 weeks
Gruen 1975	70 hospitalized cardiac patients	Range = 40–69	Individual supportive counseling No-treatment control	5–6 days/week until discharge (mean = 3 weeks)
Kaplan and Kozin 1981	28 female rheumatoid arthritis patients	Mean = 46–51 (range = 23–63)	Education and supportive counseling group Education only group	1 education and 12 counseling sessions
Spiegel et al. 1981	58 female breast cancer patients	Mean = 54–55	Support group No-treatment control group	Support group met weekly for 1 year
Evans et al. 1982	84 isolated visually impaired volunteers	Mean = 61–62 (range = 53–78 years)	Group problem solving by telephone No-treatment control group	8 sessions
Oldenberg et al. 1985	46 cardiac patients	Mean = 56 (range = 29–69)	Individual education/relaxation/ counseling Individual education/relaxation Standard care control	10 sessions (counseling) education and relaxation instructions on audiotape
Shearn and Fireman 1985	105 rheumatoid arthritis patients	Mean = 55–58	Stress management group Support group No-treatment control	10 sessions
Keefe et al. 1990	99 osteoarthritis patients	Mean = 64	Pain coping skills (cognitive-behavior therapy) group Arthritis education group Standard care control	10 sessions
Greer et al. 1992	156 cancer patients	Mean = 51–52 (range =18–74)	Individual CBT group No-treatment control	0–13 sessions over 4 months (median = 5 sessions)

educational, and problem-solving strategies. In one of the earliest studies, Godbole and Verinis (1974) studied 51 elderly patients with a mixture of physical disabilities, including cardiovascular and respiratory disease. Subjects were randomly assigned to a "confrontational," support, or no-treatment control condition. Patients in both active conditions showed significant improvements on measures of depression, anxiety, hopelessness, and somatic complaints compared with control subjects. In a later intervention, Evans et al. (1982) provided problem-solving group therapy by telephone to legally blind elderly patients. Participants showed increases in activity levels and decreases in self-reports of loneliness although no changes in actual social involvement were observed.

Studies have also examined the use of psychotherapy with cancer patients. Spiegel et al. (1981) found that metastatic breast cancer patients who attended a year-long, nondirective support group reported significantly less anxiety, fatigue, and confusion, as well as improved coping strategies, compared with control subjects. Greer et al. (1992) studied newly diagnosed cancer patients who participated in individual CBT sessions to learn a combination of relaxation techniques, cognitive coping strategies, and communication skills for improving interpersonal relationships. Participants reported significantly less anxiety, helplessness, fatalism, and depression, and significantly greater positive adjustment toward their disease than did no-treatment controls. Statistical improvements were maintained at 4-month follow-up.

Cardiovascular disease (including stroke and heart disease) represents another important medical problem in geriatric patients that may be amenable to psychotherapeutic intervention (Cohen-Cole 1989; Lipsey and Parikh 1989). A number of authors have suggested that group psychotherapy with stroke patients can improve social and psychological functioning (e.g., Butcher et al. 1984; Imes 1984). Research has also described the utility of various depression treatment measures for assessing poststroke depression in geriatric patients (Agrell and Dehlin 1989). Surprisingly, there have been no empirical studies demonstrating the efficacy of psychotherapy with this population. Data are available, however, on the use of psychosocial interventions with heart disease patients.

Ibrahim et al. (1974) compared cardiac patients assigned to a weekly supportive therapy group with control subjects. Therapy participants had slightly better survival rates and showed a smaller rise in social alienation than did control subjects during the study period, although no significant differences on psychological, physical, or social measures were obtained. In contrast, Gruen (1975) found that patients who were seen almost daily for supportive counseling and education while in intensive care after a heart attack scored lower on measures of anxiety and depression during hospitalization than did control subjects. Differences in anxiety between groups were maintained at 4-month follow-up, and treatment group subjects also tended to be less restricted in activity at follow-up than were the no-treatment control subjects. Oldenburg et al. (1985) found that patients receiving either brief individual counseling (6 to 10 sessions) and education or education alone after hospitalization for a heart attack reported better psychological and life-style functioning at 3-, 6-, and 12-month follow-up than did those in a routine care comparison group.

Finally, there is a growing literature examining the impact of psychosocial treatments on disability, pain, and depression in adults with rheumatoid or osteoarthritis (Mullen et al. 1987). Keefe et al. (1990) found that patients with osteoarthritic knee pain who received a combination of training in pain coping skills and arthritis education reported significantly lower amounts of pain and psychological disability (anxiety and depression) than did patients who either received only arthritis education or standard medical care. However, earlier intervention studies with rheumatoid arthritis patients yielded less promising results. For example, Kaplan and Kozin (1981) found no differences between rheumatoid patients who only received information about their disease and patients who received information and participated in 12 nondirective group counseling sessions. Shearn and Fireman (1985) also found no significant differences in measures of depression, life satisfaction, or functional disability between rheumatoid arthritis patients and control subjects who participated in either stress management or mutual support groups for 10 weeks. Thus interventions designed to treat psychological disability and pain behaviors in medical patients may be differentially effective with select populations. Other factors that have been suggested as having possibly confounding effects on treatment outcome in medically ill elderly patients include patients' ages and whether or not the spouse is involved in treatment (Keefe et al. 1990).

In summary, although the number of available controlled studies is still small and contains mixed results, there is evidence that psychosocial interventions are a valuable supplement to some of the medical conditions that impact older adults. Most studies have sampled medical outpatients, and all have used some form of psychoeducational, problem-solving, or supportive intervention strategy. Significant improvements in depression, anxiety, hopelessness, and coping have been reported with cancer, heart disease, and arthritis patients. Slight improvements in survival rate and lower risks for rehospitalization have also been described. However, data are difficult to compare across studies because duration and type of treatment are highly variable and individualized to medical diagnosis and disease severity.

Psychotherapy With Geriatric Caregivers

The American Association of Retired Persons (1986) has estimated that more than 5 million community-dwelling elderly people in this country require some form of assistance to maintain independent living. The vast majority of this assistance comes from family members, usually spouses or grown children (who are often themselves elderly or beyond middle age). Caregiving is often a difficult task associated with increased levels of depression, anxiety, insomnia, marital conflict, alcohol and medication use, and medical illness (Cantor 1983; Clipp and George 1990; Coppel et al. 1985; Farkas 1980; Gaynor 1989; Pruchno and Potashnik 1989; Rabins et al. 1982). Recent reviews by Toseland and Rossiter (1989) and Zarit and Teri (1991) have summarized the research on various psychoeducational, psychotherapeutic, and self-help interventions that have been used with caregivers. These authors have noted the lack of methodological rigor that characterizes most of these studies and the relatively modest treatment effects that have been reported. However, they also point out the difficulty in expecting short-term supportive or educational interventions to have substantial impact, given the complexity and duration of the caregiving role.

A number of empirical studies have been conducted with heterogeneous groups of caregivers and patient types. Greene and Monahan (1987, 1989) recruited community-dwelling caregivers whose levels of stress placed their elderly patient at risk for being institutionalized. The majority of patients were living with their care providers (77%) and had at least one major medical illness (89%); fewer than one-fifth (14%) were diagnosed as having Alzheimer's disease. Significant reductions in caregiver anxiety, depression, and burden levels were observed following 8 weeks of group counseling, which contained supportive, educational, and relaxation components. However, improvements were not maintained at 4-month follow-up, and no caregiver or patient characteristics were associated with any outcome. Lovett and Gallagher (1988) studied 107 family caregivers whose patients had a mixture of moderate to severe memory impairment (40% of patients) and a variety of medical conditions and disabilities. Caregivers who attended 10 weeks of either a behaviorally based group focusing on increasing pleasant events or a cognitive, problem-solving group experienced decreases in depression and increases in morale that were not observed in wait-list control subjects. Perceived self-efficacy had a greater relationship to improvement on outcome measures than did the abundance of pleasant social events in the caregiver's life.

A few studies have attempted to control for heterogeneity of care providers by focusing on caregivers of patients with specific disabling conditions rather than on caregivers in general (Table 31–6). For example, Evans et al. (1988) found that caregivers of stroke patients who either 1) participated in educational classes on the physical and psychosocial consequences of stroke or 2) participated in education plus seven additional CBT counseling sessions scored significantly higher at 6-month and 1-year follow-ups on measures of family functioning, communication, and problem solving than did caregivers who did not receive these services. Families receiving counseling had significantly higher levels of patient adjustment than those receiving education alone or no education or counseling services. This is particularly important given that 1) anxiety and depression are common following strokes (Gass and Lawhorn 1991); 2) left untreated, depressive symptoms may not spontaneously resolve over time (Egelko et al. 1989); and 3) level of depression and stroke recovery are strongly related to the quality of patients' family relationships and response to stroke-related disability (Evans et al. 1987; S. C. Thompson et al. 1989).

Other studies have focused on caregivers of patients with Alzheimer's disease or other progressive dementias. Haley et al. (1987) recruited community-dwelling caregivers who saw the dementia patient at least once a week. They found no improvements in caregivers' self-reports of psychological or social functioning after participation in 10 weeks of either support-only or support-with-skills-training groups.

Mohide et al. (1990) compared live-in caregivers who received a combination of education, respite, and group support with caregivers who had standard contact with standard community home nursing services. Although neither group showed improvements in depression or anxiety after 6 months, caregivers who received the combination treatment did report more increases in perceived quality of life and satisfaction

with nursing services and their caregiving role than did the conventional care recipients. Chiverton and Caine (1989) provided a brief (3-session) educational intervention designed to inform caregiving spouses about Alzheimer's disease and to teach a range of communication and behavioral strategies for improving patient care. Participants scored higher on posttreatment measures of competence (including emotional coping) and knowledge than did control subjects; however, no

Table 31–6. Empirical treatment studies with caregivers of patients with dementia or physically frail elderly adults

Study	Sample population	Sample age (years)	Treatment	Treatment duration
Greene and Monahan 1987, 1989	289 caregivers of dementia patients and medically ill patients (34 groups)	Mean = 58	Group support, education, and group relaxation training No-treatment control (self-selected nonparticipants)	8 sessions
Haley et al. 1987	54 family caregivers of dementia patients	Mean = 78	Support group Support and stress management group Wait-list control	10 sessions in 4 months (7 weekly, 2 every other week, 1 after month delay)
Scharlach 1987	37 daughters (of 24 elderly mothers)	Mean = 50 (daughters) (range = 38–62)	Cognitive-behavior therapy (CBT) group Supportive/educational group Wait-list control	2 sessions
Zarit et al. 1987	119 family caregivers of elderly dementia patients	Mean = 62	Support group Individual and family counseling Wait-list control	8 sessions
Evans et al. 1988	188 caregivers of stroke patients	Mean = 61–63	Education group Education and CBT (education group and individual CBT) Standard care control	2 sessions education; 7 sessions CBT
Lovett and Gallagher 1988	107 caregivers of frail elders	Mean = 59	Behavioral group Problem-solving group Wait-list control	10 sessions
Chiverton and Caine 1989	40 spouses of dementia patients	Mean = 71 (range = 58–87)	Education group No-treatment control	3 sessions in 4 weeks
Toseland et al. 1989	56 daughters/daughters-in-law caretakers of frail elderly patients	Mean = 50–55 (range = 35–66)	Professionally led support and education group Peer-led support group Respite-only control	8 sessions
Mohide et al. 1990	60 caregivers of dementia patients	Mean = 66–69	Caregiver support program (home visits, respite care, and support group) Conventional care control (home nursing)	6 months
Toseland et al. 1990	154 daughters/daughters-in-law caretakers	Mean = 50–52	Individual supportive therapy Support group Respite-only control	8 sessions
Toseland and Smith 1990	87 daughters/daughters-in-law caretakers	Mean = 50	Individual "action-oriented" therapy with professional counselor Individual "action-oriented" therapy with peer counselor No-treatment control	8 sessions

follow-up data to assess maintenance of treatment effects were obtained.

Zarit et al. (1987) reported reductions in family caregivers' burden level and psychiatric symptoms following an 8-week education and problem-solving support group or 8 weeks of individual and family counseling. Furthermore, reductions were maintained at 1-year follow-up. However, the observed treatment effects were no greater than the changes observed in wait-list control subjects at posttest.

Toseland and colleagues limited their caretaking sample to adult daughters and daughters-in-law who were caring for parents with two or more chronic disabilities. In a series of articles, they compared the effectiveness of peer-led versus professionally led "action-oriented" support groups for caregivers (Toseland et al. 1989), peer-led versus professionally led individual counseling (Toseland and Smith 1990), and group versus individual (regardless of peer or professional leadership status) treatment effects (Toseland et al. 1990). Significant improvements on measures of well-being and social support and decreases in psychiatric symptoms occurred as a result of both the peer-led and the professionally led interventions, regardless of whether caregivers were seen in an individual or group context. However, greater reductions in psychiatric symptoms tended to be associated with individual and professional-led treatment, whereas greater increases in social support were found in the group and peer-led interventions.

All of these studies focused on caregivers of frail, medically disabled, or cognitively impaired elderly individuals. There is also a small literature investigating the utility of psychosocial interventions with family and friends of older adults before they assume the caregiving role. Scharlach (1987) examined whether the relationship between adult daughters and their elderly widowed mothers could be improved while the mothers were still functioning independently. Daughters were assigned to either a cognitive-behavioral condition, which focused on reducing unrealistic feelings of responsibility, or a supportive-educational condition, in which daughters were encouraged to become more aware of their mothers' needs. Daughters who attended the cognitive-behavioral seminars had greater reductions in feelings of burden than did control subjects or participants in the supportive-educational seminar. Further, cognitive-behavioral subjects reported subjectively greater improvements in their relationships with their mothers, and the mothers reported significantly less loneliness, after the intervention than did participants in the other two conditions. Although this is only a single study, it raises the interesting possibility that psychosocial interventions may serve a preventative function with individuals who are likely to become future caregivers.

In summary, the empirical literature on psychosocial interventions with caregivers is small and has produced inconsistent findings. There is evidence that brief individual or group treatment, with either professional therapists or caregiver peers, can lead to reductions in self-reports of caregiver distress. With caregivers of stroke patients, treatment also appears to improve family relationships, as well as caretaker problem-solving and communication skills. Unfortunately, many caregiver studies have not collected follow-up data, and, when available, improvements in psychological functioning at posttreatment have been inconsistently maintained over time.

Psychotherapy With Elderly Patients in Long-Term Care Settings

A move into a long-term care setting can be difficult, or even traumatic, for many older adults. Consequently, there is growing interest in the use of psychosocial interventions to help ease some of the acute adjustment problems associated with long-term residential care. Recent reviews have identified the interventions most commonly used with nursing home residents (Burckhardt 1987; Gugel 1989; Karuza and Katz 1991), and the importance of proper instrument selection to measure treatment outcome in long-term care settings (Mosher-Ashley 1987; Rabins et al. 1987). Common interventions include reality orientation, validation therapy, supportive interventions, and a variety of behavior modification techniques (including interpersonal skill training and activity enhancement). These interventions emphasize cognitive training, sensory stimulation, and physical rehabilitation, rather than improvements in social functioning. Staff training programs also exist. The majority of these programs have also been geared toward teaching staff to manage specific problem patient behaviors (e.g., Burgio and Burgio 1986; Fisher and Carstensen 1990b; Maletta 1992; Sperbeck and Whitbourne 1981), although there are also some that have examined the impact of counseling on patients' initial and long-term adjustment to nursing home life (Table 31–7).

Dye and Erber (1981) described a program in which newly admitted residents participated in support groups (with or without family members) to discuss the events that led to their move, any problems encountered during the admission process, and problem-solving strategies for coping with institutional life. Patients who participated in the resident-only group had lower levels of anxiety and higher internal locus of control scores than did either control subjects or patients who were in family groups. However, at 6-month follow-up, the resident-only group was significantly more agitated and had lower health self-rating scores than did members of the family and control groups.

Other studies examining residents' long-term adjustment to institutionalization have found similar problems in generalization and maintenance. Lindell (1978) reported positive changes in self-concept in long-term residential center and nursing home patients who participated in nondirective support groups; however, changes were only maintained in those subjects who continued to meet with their group regularly after the formal research study ended. Hussian and Lawrence (1981) found that depressed nursing home patients initially showed improvements in mood as a result of systematic increases in daily activity or training in problem-solving skills. However, after 2 weeks, only those subjects who both increased their daily activity and learned new problem-solving strate-

Table 31–7. Empirical studies in long-term care with elderly patients

Study	Sample population	Sample age (years)	Treatment	Treatment duration
Power and McCarron 1975	30 NH patients	Mean = 84 (range = 70–98)	Individual interactive contact (including physical touching and socialization) No-treatment control	15 weeks
Langer and Rodin 1976	91 NH patients	Range = 65–90	Responsibility/choice condition Comparison condition	Single group intervention
Schulz 1976	42 NH patients	Mean = 82 (range = 67–96)	Scheduled visits; subjects choose appointment time Scheduled visits; subjects do not choose appointment time Nonscheduled random visits No-visit comparison	2 months
Berger and Rose 1977	25 NH patients	Mean = 77 (range = 48–97)	Individual interpersonal skill training Individual discussion control Assessment-only control	3 sessions
Lindell 1978	39 NH patients	Mean = 81–82 (all subjects older than 65)	Group supportive therapy No-treatment control	Therapy: 16 sessions in 8 weeks; control: 3 sessions in 8 weeks
Langer et al. 1979	54 NH patients	Mean = 79–80	Individual high reciprocal self-disclosure Individual low reciprocal self-disclosure No-interview control Pretest-only control	4 sessions over 6 weeks
Dye and Erber 1981	52 recently admitted NH patients	Mean = 80	Resident-only group Resident-family group No-treatment control	7 sessions
Hussian and Lawrence 1981	36 depressed NH patients	Mean = 74 (all subjects older than 60)	Social reinforcement for activity Problem solving (individual) Wait-list control Social reinforcement plus problem solving Problem solving plus social reinforcement Information control	10 sessions in 2 weeks
Moran and Gatz 1987	59 NH residents	Mean = 76	Task-oriented group Insight-oriented group Wait-list control	12 sessions

Note. NH = nursing home or long-term residential setting.

gies continued to show improved mood. At 3-month follow-up, no gains were maintained. Thus although support at the time of transition into a nursing home appears to enhance patients' immediate functioning, it may not be sustained unless other factors are developed to maintain it.

Interpersonal factors have been shown to be particularly influential in patients' psychosocial functioning in long-term care settings. For example, Power and McCarron (1975) found that increasing the depressed geriatric patients' physical contact with staff, their verbal conversation, and their social interaction with peers led to reductions in self-reported and observed depression in the patients. Other studies have suggested that sustained, successful coping in long-term care settings is affected by residents' perception of their autonomy and situational control (Langer and Rodin 1976; Schulz 1976) and that social interaction may be associated with improvements in immediate memory, alertness, and self-initiation (Langer et al. 1979).

Moran and Gatz (1987) found that nursing home residents who participated in an interpersonal task group (which developed a welcoming project for incoming residents) showed significant improvements in feelings of self-control and increases in scores of life satisfaction. Berger and Rose (1977) found that interpersonal skills could be effectively taught to nursing home residents, although in their study skills did not generalize to novel, unpracticed situations. Thus although increases in quantity and quality of interpersonal contacts may enhance patients' adjustment and successful functioning in long-term care facilities, it may be necessary for staff to provide ongoing opportunities and assistance if these improvements are to maintained.

In summary, there have been relatively few empirical studies on the use of psychotherapeutic interventions with residents of long-term care settings. There is a large nursing home literature that describes the impact of cognitive training, sensory stimulation, and management of specific behavior problems (such as incontinence). However, because these studies do not have improved mood or social functioning as their targets of intervention, they have not been reviewed in this chapter. The few studies that have examined the impact of psychotherapy on psychological functioning in residential settings suggest that treatment can improve patient self-concept, reduce depression, and enhance social interaction. It appears, however, that

changes are not well maintained without ongoing therapeutic support.

Summary and Future Research Directions

Several conclusions can be drawn from the literature thus far on the efficacy of psychosocial interventions with older adults. First, a variety of interventions have been studied with physically healthy, community-dwelling older adults. Cognitive-behavioral strategies have generated the most empirical research, although psychodynamic, reminiscence, and various supportive techniques have also been studied with this population. Each has been found to be effective in decreasing depression, and a few studies have shown this treatment effectiveness to be equal or superior to pharmacotherapeutic interventions. There is some evidence that improvements resulting from CBT are better maintained at follow-up than those from the other treatment forms, but there are too few long-term outcome comparison studies to evaluate how robust these findings are.

Although research is less plentiful, there is also empirical evidence for the efficacy of CBT and its variants with medically ill patients and patients with dementia, elderly caregivers, and residents of long-term care institutions. A few studies have also found that psychodynamic therapy, reminiscence and life review activities, and supportive interventions can reduce negative mood and improve life satisfaction and self-esteem in disabled or institutionalized older adults and their caregivers. In some cases, long-term improvements (e.g., in reduced rehospitalization or nursing home placement) were reported even in the absence of reductions in acute depression ratings.

A variety of factors have been identified that may contribute to differential treatment effects across studies. These include patient variables, such as the presence of premorbid personality disorders, severity of symptoms at the onset of treatment, cognitive capacity, and patient feelings of control or expectancies for change. Specific treatment variables have also been implicated in differential outcomes. For example, structured life review strategies may be more effective than simple reminiscence, participation of family members may enhance treatment impact, and treatment with professional therapists may produce greater reductions in psychiatric symptoms than peer-led interventions. In therapy with patients in long-term settings, and in outpatient therapy with caregivers, successful maintenance of therapeutic gains appears contingent on ongoing, or at least periodic, therapy contact. Both group and individual therapy formats have been successful with older patients.

Much additional research is needed to examine the efficacy of psychosocial interventions with elderly patients. Unfortunately, many psychosocial interventions currently in use with older adults are based on uncontrolled case studies and anecdotal reports. The controlled studies that have been conducted represent a mixture of cognitive-behavioral, psychodynamic, relaxation, supportive counseling, and educational techniques. There are, as yet, no data to indicate which components of particular interventions are efficacious in improving psychological, physical, or social functioning of subjects. Oftentimes, treatment protocols are poorly described, making replication or comparison across studies difficult. Thus more rigorous treatment definition is needed. There is little empirical research on the impact of therapist or environmental variables (including institutional or familial factors) on therapy outcome. The cultural, environmental, familial, and health factors that are likely to impact treatment efficacy must be systematically investigated. The intervention literature has tended to focus primarily on the management of pathological cognitive or emotional disorders. The challenges of normal aging deserve attention as well.

Additional research is needed to identify how long interventions should be continued to maximize treatment impact and to establish strategies for generalization and maintenance once the intervention ends. In the studies reported here, therapy duration ranged from a single or few sessions to months or years; in some cases, even subjects within a given study are exposed to different numbers of sessions over variable lengths of time. Clarifying the significance of this variable may be particularly important for older adults with chronic physical or social circumstances that have precipitated psychosocial intervention. Because therapy outcome is dependent on how psychosocial functioning is defined and measured, research is also needed to identify assessment instruments that are carefully validated, sensitive to expected changes, and appropriate for use with various elderly populations and in specialized contexts.

Given the number of older adults who are medically ill and living in long-term care settings, it is surprising that there are so few controlled studies

examining the psychosocial impact of physical disability and institutionalization in geriatric patients. Future research with such patients may benefit from using single-case design strategies. Although such strategies necessarily use small numbers of individuals, they can provide good information with little disruption to medical or residential facilities. Validity of results could be maximized by applying such designs to multiple settings and using a broad range of reliable assessment instruments. Such designs may also offer an opportunity for the conjoint impact of pharmacological and psychosocial interventions on functioning to be evaluated with a range of elderly populations.

In summary, despite the need for additional research, the limited data available on psychosocial interventions with older adults are surprisingly consistent and encouraging. A variety of behavioral and supportive interventions have produced improvements in psychological functioning in physically healthy, depressed older subjects, as well as in institutionalized or medically ill geriatric patients and their caregivers. Treatment gains from psychological interventions are often comparable to their medical counterparts. Research now needs to focus on improving gains and clarifying which strategies are maximally effective for which patient groups.

References

Agrell B, Dehlin O: Comparison of six depression rating scales in geriatric stroke patients. Stroke 20:1190–1194, 1989

Alexander CN, Langer EJ, Newman RI, et al: Transcendental meditation, mindfulness, and longevity: an experimental study with the elderly. J Pers Soc Psychol 57:950–964, 1989

Alexopoulos GS, Abrams RC, Young RC, et al: Cornell Scale for depression in dementia. Biol Psychiatry 23:271–284, 1988

American Association of Retired Persons: A Profile of Older Persons: 1986. Washington, DC, American Association of Retired Persons, 1986

American Heritage Dictionary, Second College Edition. Boston, MA, Houghton Mifflin, 1985

American Psychiatric Association: Diagnostic and Statistical Manual for Mental Disorders, 3rd Edition. Washington, DC, American Psychiatric Association, 1980

Baines S, Saxby P, Ehlert K: Reality orientation and reminiscence therapy. Br J Psychiatry 151:222–231, 1987

Baum D, Gallagher D: Case studies of psychotherapy with dying persons. Clinical Gerontologist 7:41–50, 1987

Beck AT: Depression, Experimental, and Theoretical Aspects. New York, University of Pennsylvania Press, 1967

Beck AT, Rush AJ, Shaw BF, et al: Cognitive Therapy for Depression. New York, Guilford, 1979

Beckham EE: Improvement after evaluation in psychotherapy of depression: evidence of a placebo effect? J Clin Psychol 45:945–950, 1989

Bellak L, Small L: Emergency Psychotherapy and Brief Psychotherapy. New York, Grune & Stratton, 1965

Bennett SL, Maas F: The effect of music-based life review on the life satisfaction and ego integrity of elderly people. British Journal of Occupational Therapy 51:433–436, 1988

Berger RM, Rose, SD: Interpersonal skill training with institutionalized elderly patients. J Gerontol 32:346–353, 1977

Berghorn FJ, Schafer DE: Reminiscence intervention in nursing homes: what and who changes? Int J Aging Hum Dev 24:113–125, 1987

Beutler LE, Scogin F, Kirkish P, et al: Group cognitive therapy and alprazolam in the treatment of depression in older adults. J Consult Clin Psychol 55:550–556, 1987

Birren JE, Schaie KW (eds): Handbook of the Psychology of Aging, 3rd Edition. San Diego, CA, Academic Press, 1990

Birren JE, Sloane RB, Cohen GD (eds): Handbook of Mental Health and Aging, 2nd Edition. San Diego, CA, Academic Press, 1992

Burckhardt CS: The effect of therapy on the mental health of the elderly. Res Nurs Health 10:277–285, 1987

Burgio KL, Burgio LD: Behavior therapies for urinary incontinence in the elderly. Clin Geriatr Med 2:809–827, 1986

Butcher J, Smith E, Gillespie C: Short-term group therapy for stroke patients in a rehabilitation centre. Br J Med Psychol 57:283–290, 1984

Butler RN: The life review: an interpretation of reminiscence in the aged. Psychiatry 26:65–76, 1963

Cantor M: Strain among caregivers: a study of experience in the U.S. Gerontologist 23:597–604, 1983

Chiverton P, Caine ED: Education to assist spouses in coping with Alzheimer's disease: a controlled trial. J Am Geriatr Soc 37:593–598, 1989

Clipp EC, George LK: Psychotropic drug use among caregivers of patients with dementia. J Am Geriatr Soc 38:227–235, 1990

Cohen-Cole SA: Depression and heart disease, in Aging and Clinical Practice: Depression and Coexisting Disease. Edited by Robinson RG, Rabins PV. New York, Igaku-Shoin, 1989, pp 27–39

Coppel DB, Burton C, Becker J, et al: Relationships of cognitions associated with coping reactions to depression in spousal caregivers of Alzheimer's disease patients. Cognitive Therapy and Research 9:253–266, 1985

DeBerry S: The effects of meditation-relaxation on anxiety and depression in a geriatric population. Psychotherapy: Theory, Research and Practice 19:512–521, 1982

DeBerry S, Davis S, Reinhard KE: A comparison of meditation-relaxation and cognitive/behavioral techniques for reducing anxiety and depression in a geriatric population. Journal of Geriatric Psychiatry 22:231–247, 1989

Dye CJ, Erber JT: Two group procedures for the treatment of nursing home patients. Gerontologist 21:539–544, 1981

Egelko S, Simon D, Riley E, et al: First year after stroke: tracking cognitive and affective deficits. Arch Phys Med Rehabil 70:297–302, 1989

Engle-Friedman M, Bootzin RR: Insomnia as a problem for the elderly, in Handbook of Clinical Behavior Therapy with the Elderly Client. Edited by Wisocki PA. New York, Plenum, 1991, pp 273–298

Evans RL, Werkhoven W, Fox HR: Treatment of social isolation and loneliness in a sample of visually impaired elderly persons. Psychol Rep 51:103–108, 1982

Evans RL, Bishop DS, Matlock A, et al: Prestroke family interaction as a predictor of stroke outcome. Arch Phys Med Rehabil 68:508–512, 1987

Evans RL, Matlock, A, Bishop DS, et al: Family intervention after stroke: Does counseling or education help? Stroke 19:1243–1249, 1988

Fallot RD: The impact on mood of verbal reminiscing in later adulthood. Int J Aging Hum Dev 10:1979–1980, 1980

Farkas S: Impact of chronic illness on the patient's spouse. Health Soc Work 5:39–46, 1980

Fielden MA: Reminiscence as a therapeutic intervention with sheltered housing residents: a comparative study. British Journal of Social Work 20:21–44, 1990

Fisher JE, Carstensen LL: Behavior management of the dementias. Clinical Psychology Review 10:611–629, 1990a

Fisher JE, Carstensen LL: Generalized effects of skills training among older adults. Clinical Gerontologist 9:91–107, 1990b

Franzke AW: The effects of assertiveness training on older adults. Gerontologist 27:13–16, 1987

Freud S: On psychotherapy, in Collected Papers, Vol 1. London, Hogarth Press, 1924, pp 249–263

Fry PS: Structured and unstructured reminiscence training and depression among the elderly. Clinical Gerontologist 1:15–37, 1983

Fry PS: Cognitive training and cognitive-behavioral variables in the treatment of depression in the elderly. Clinical Gerontologist 3:25–45, 1984

Fry PS: Depression, Stress, and Adaptations in the Elderly: Psychological Assessment and Intervention. Rockville, MD, Aspen, 1986

Gallagher DE, Thompson LW: Treatment of major depressive disorder in older adult outpatients with brief psychotherapies. Psychotherapy: Theory, Research and Practice 19:482–490, 1982

Gallagher DE, Thompson LW: Effectiveness of psychotherapy for both endogenous and nonendogenous depression in older adult outpatients. J Gerontol 38:707–712, 1983

Gallagher D, Rose J, Rivera P, et al: Prevalence of depression in family caregivers. Gerontologist 29:449–456, 1989

Gallagher-Thompson D, Hanley-Peterson P, Thompson LW: Maintenance of gains versus relapse following brief psychotherapy for depression. J Consult Clin Psychol 58:371–374, 1990

Gass CS, Lawhorn L: Psychological adjustment following stroke: an MMPI study. Psychological Assessment 3:628–633, 1991

Gaston L, Marmar CR, Thompson LW, et al: Relation of patient pretreatment characteristics to the therapeutic alliance in diverse psychotherapies. J Consult Clin Psychol 56:483–489, 1988

Gaston L, Marmar CR, Gallagher D, et al: Impact of confirming patient expectations of change processes in behavioral, cognitive, and brief dynamic psychotherapy. Psychotherapy 26:296–302, 1989

Gaynor S: When the caregiver becomes the patient. Geriatric Nursing 10:121–123, 1989

Godbole A, Verinis JS: Brief psychotherapy in the treatment of emotional disorders in physically ill geriatric patients. Gerontologist 14:143–148, 1974

Goldwasser AN, Auerbach SM, Harkins SW: Cognitive, affective, and behavioral effects of reminiscence group therapy on demented elderly. Int J Aging Hum Dev 25:209–222, 1987

Greene VL, Monahan DJ: The effect of a professionally guided caregiver support and education group on institutionalization of care receivers. Gerontologist 27:716–721, 1987

Greene VL, Monahan DJ: The effect of a support and education program on stress and burden among family caregivers to frail elderly persons. Gerontologist 29:472–477, 1989

Greer S, Moorey S, Baruch JD, et al: Adjuvant psychological therapy for patients with cancer: a prospective randomised trial. BMJ 304:675–680, 1992

Griffin M, Waller MV: Group therapy for the elderly: one approach to coping. Clinical Social Work Journal 13:261–271, 1985

Gruen W: Effects of brief psychotherapy during the hospitalization period on the recovery process in heart attacks. J Consult Clin Psychol 43:223–232, 1975

Gugel R: Psychosocial interventions in the nursing home, in Principles and Practice of Nursing Home Care. Edited by Katz PR, Calkins E. New York, Springer, 1989, pp 212–224

Gutman GM, Herbert CP, Brown SR: Feldenkrais versus conventional exercises for the elderly. J Gerontol 32:562–572, 1977

Haight BK: The therapeutic role of a structured life review process in homebound elderly subjects. J Gerontol 43:P40–P44, 1988

Haley WE, Brown SL, Levine EG: Experimental evaluation of the effectiveness of group intervention for dementia caregivers. Gerontologist 27:376–382, 1987

Hamilton M: Development of a rating scale for primary depressive illness. British Journal of Social and Clinical Psychology 6:278–296, 1967

Harp Scates SK, Randolph DE, Gutsch KU, et al: Effects of cognitive-behavioral, reminiscence, and activity treatments on life satisfaction and anxiety in the elderly. Int J Aging Hum Dev 22:141–146, 1986

Hartke RJ: Psychological Aspects of Geriatric Rehabilitation. Gaithersburg, MD, Aspen, Inc, 1991

Hedgepeth BE, Hale WD: Effect of a positive reminiscing intervention on affect, expectancy, and performance. Psychol Rep 53:867–870, 1983

Hersen M, van Hasselt VB: Behavioral assessment and treatment of anxiety in the elderly. Clinical Psychology Reviews 12:619–640, 1992

Hussian RA, Lawrence PS: Social reinforcement of activity and problem-solving training in the treatment of depressed institutionalized elderly patients. Cognitive Therapy Research 5:57–69, 1981

Ibrahim MA, Feldman JG, Sultz HA, et al: Management after myocardial infarction: a controlled trial of the effect of group psychotherapy. Int J Psychiatry Med 5:253–268, 1974

Imes C: Interventions with stroke patients: EMG biofeedback, group activities, cognitive retraining. Cogntive Rehabilitation 2:4–17, 1984

Ingersoll B, Silverman A: Comparative group psychotherapy for the aged. Gerontologist 18:201–206, 1978

Jarvik LF, Mintz JM, Steuer J, et al: Treating geriatric depression: a 26-week interim analysis. J Am Geriatr Soc 30:713–717, 1982

Kaplan S, Kozin F: A controlled study of group counseling in rheumatoid arthritis. J Rheumatol 8:91–99, 1981

Karuza J, Katz PR: Psychosocial interventions in long-term care: a critical overview, in Advances in Longterm Care, Vol 1. Edited by Katz PR, Kane RL, Mezey MD. New York, Springer, 1991, pp 1–27

Keefe FJ, Caldwell DS, Williams DA, et al: Pain coping skills training in the management of osteoarthritic knee pain: a comparative study. Behavior Therapy 21:49–62, 1990

Keuthen N, Wisocki PA: Behavioral medicine for the health concerns of the elderly, in Handbook of Clinical Behavior Therapy With the Elderly Client. Edited by Wisocki PA. New York, Plenum, 1991, pp 363–381

Kim KY, Hershey LA: Diagnosis and treatment of depression in the elderly. Int J Psychiatry Med 18:211–221, 1988

Kirschenbaum DS, Sherman J, Penrod JD: Promoting self-directed hemodialysis: measurement and cognitive-behavioral intervention. Health Psychol 6:373–385, 1987

Klerman GL, Weissman MM, Rounsaville BJ, et al: Interpersonal Psychotherapy of Depression. New York, Basic Books, 1984

Langer EJ, Rodin J: The effects of choice and enhanced personal responsibility for the aged: a field experiment in an institutional setting. J Pers Soc Psychol 34:191–198, 1976

Langer EJ, Rodin J, Beck P, et al: Environmental determinants of memory improvement in late adulthood. J Pers Soc Psychol 37:2003–2013, 1979

Lappe JM: Reminiscing: the life review therapy. Journal of Gerontological Nursing 13:12–16, 1987

Lazarus LW, Weinberg J: Psychosocial intervention with the aged. Psychiatr Clin North Am 5:215–227, 1982

Lewinsohn PM, Sullivan JM, Grosscup SJ: Changing reinforcing events: an approach to the treatment of depression. Psychotherapy: Theory, Research and Practice 17:322–334, 1980

Lewinsohn PM, Antonuccio DO, Steinmetz JL, et al: The Coping With Depression Course. Eugene, OR, Castalia, 1984

Lieberman MA, Bliwise NG: Comparisons among peer and professionally directed groups for the elderly: implications for the development of self-help groups. International Journal of Group Psychotherapy 35:155–175, 1985

Lieberman MA, Falk JM: The remembered past as a source of data for research on the life cycle. Human Development 14:132–141, 1971

Lindell AR: Group therapy for the institutionalized aged. Issues in Mental Health Nursing 1:77–86, 1978

Lipsey JR, Parikh RM: Depression and stroke, in Aging and Clinical Practice: Depression and Coexisting Disease. Edited by Robinson RG, Rabins PV. New York, Igaku-Shoin, 1989, pp 186–201

Lovett S, Gallagher D: Psychoeducational interventions for family caregivers: preliminary efficacy data. Behavior Therapy 19:321–330, 1988

Maletta GJ: Treatment of behavioral symptomatology of Alzheimer's disease, with emphasis on aggression: current clinical approaches. Int Psychogeriatr 4:117–130, 1992

Marmar CR, Gaston L, Gallagher D, et al: Alliance and outcome in late-life depression. J Nerv Ment Dis 177:464–472, 1989

Matteson MA: Effects of a cognitive behavioral approach and positive reinforcement on exercise for older adults. Educational Gerontology 15:497–513, 1989

Merriam S: The concept and function of reminiscence: a review of the research. Gerontologist 20:604–609, 1980

Mohide EA, Pringle DM, Streiner DL, et al: A randomized trial of family caregiver support in the home management of dementia. J Am Geriatr Soc 38:446–454, 1990

Molinari V, Reichlin RE: Life review reminiscence in the elderly: a review of the literature. Int J Aging Hum Dev 20:81–92, 1985

Moran JA, Gatz M: Group therapies for nursing home adults: an evaluation of two treatment approaches. Gerontologist 27:588–591, 1987

Mosher-Ashley PM: Procedural and methodological parameters in behavioral-gerontological research: a review. Int J Aging Hum Dev 24:189–229, 1987

Mullen PD, Laville EA, Biddle AK, et al: Efficacy of psychoeducational interventions on pain, depression, and disability in people with arthritis: a meta-analysis. J Rheumatol 14:33–39, 1987

Mulligan MA, Bennett R: Assessment of mental health and social problems during multiple friendly visits: the development and evaluation of a friendly visiting program for the isolated elderly. Int J Aging Hum Dev 8:43–65, 1977

Mumford E, Schlesinger HJ, Glass GV, et al: A new look at evidence about reduced cost of medical utilization following mental health treatment. Am J Psychiatry 141:1145–1158, 1984

National Institutes of Health: Diagnosis and Treatment of Depression in Late Life (Consensus Development Conference Statement, vol 9, no 3). November 4–6, 1991

Nevruz N, Hrushka M: The influence of unstructured and structured group psychotherapy with geriatric patients on their decision to leave the hospital. Int J Group Psychotherapy 19:72–78, 1969

Niederehe G: Psychosocial therapies with depressed older adults, in Diagnosis and Treatment of Depression in Late Life. Edited by Schneider LS, Reynolds CF, Lebowitz BD, et al. Washington, DC, American Psychiatric Press, 1994, pp 293–315

Oldenburg B, Perkins RJ, Andrews G: Controlled trial of psychological intervention in myocardial infarction. J Consult Clin Psychol 53:852–859, 1985

Ong YL, Martineau F, Lloyd C, et al: A support group for the depressed elderly. International Journal of Geriatric Psychiatry 2:119–123, 1987

Orten JD, Allen M, Cook J: Reminiscence groups with confused nursing center residents: an experimental study. Soc Work Health Care 14:73–86, 1989

Perrotta P, Meacham JA: Can a reminiscing intervention alter depression and self-esteem? Int J Aging Hum Dev 14:23–30, 1981

Power CA, McCarron LT: Treatment of depression in persons residing in homes for the aged. Gerontologist 27:132–135, 1975

Pruchno R, Potashnik S: Caregiving spouses: physical and mental health in perspective. J Am Geriatr Soc 37:697–705, 1989

Rabins PV, Mace NL, Lucas MJ: The impact of dementia on the family. JAMA 248:333–335, 1982

Rabins PV, Rovner BW, Larson DB, et al: The use of mental health measures in nursing home research. J Am Geriatr Soc 35:431–434, 1987

Rattenbury C, Stones MJ: A controlled evaluation of reminiscence and current topics discussion groups in a nursing home context. Gerontologist 29:768–771, 1989

Reich JW, Zautra AJ: A perceived control intervention for at-risk older adults. Psychol Aging 4:415–424, 1989

Saxon SV: Pain Management Techniques for Older Adults. Springfield, IL, Charles C Thomas, 1991

Scharlach AE: Relieving feelings of strain among women with elderly mothers. Psychol Aging 2:9–13, 1987

Schneider LS, Sloane RB, Staples FR, et al: Pretreatment orthostatic hypotension as a predictor of response to nortriptyline in geriatric depression. J Clin Psychopharmacol 6:172–176, 1986

Schulz R: Effects of control and predictability on the physical and psychological well-being of the institutionalized aged. J Pers Soc Psychol 33:563–573, 1976

Scogin F, Hamblin D, Beutler LE: Bibliotherapy for depressed older adults: a self-help alternative. Gerontologist 27:383–387, 1987

Scogin F, Jamison C, Gochneaur K: Comparative efficacy of cognitive and behavioral bibliotherapy for mildly and moderately depressed older adults. J Consult Clin Psychol 57:403–407, 1989

Scogin F, Jamison C, Davis N: Two-year follow-up of bibliotherapy for depression in older adults. J Consult Clin Psychol 58:665–667, 1990

Shearn MA, Fireman BH: Stress management and mutual support groups in rheumatoid arthritis. Am J Med 78:771–775, 1985

Sloane RB, Staples FR, Schneider LS: Interpersonal therapy versus nortriptyline for depression in the elderly, in Clinical and Pharmacological Studies in Psychiatric Disorders. Edited by Burrows GD, Norman TR, Dennerstein L. London, John Libby, 1985, pp 344–346

Sperbeck DJ, Whitbourne SK: Dependency in the institutional setting: a behavioral training program for geriatric staff. Gerontologist 21:268–275, 1981

Spiegel D, Bloom JR, Yalom I: Group support for patients with metastatic cancer. Arch Gen Psychiatry 38:527–533, 1981

Steuer JL, Hammen CL: Cognitive-behavioral group therapy for the depressed elderly: issues and adaptations. Cognitive Therapy and Research 7:285–296, 1983

Steuer JL, Mintz J, Hammen CL, et al: Cognitive-behavioral and psychodynamic group psychotherapy in treatment of geriatric depression. J Consult Clin Psychol 52:180–189, 1984

Teri L, Gallagher-Thompson D: Cognitive-behavioral interventions for treatment of depression in Alzheimer's patients. Gerontologist 31:413–416, 1991

Teri L, Logsdon RG: The future of psychotherapy with older adults. Psychother 29:81–87, 1992

Teri L, Uomoto J: Reducing excess disability in dementia patients: training caregivers to manage patient depression. Clinical Gerontologist 10:49–63, 1991

Teri L, Wagner AW: Alzheimer's disease and depression. J Consult Clin Psychol 60:379–391, 1992

Teri L, Logsdon R, Wagner A, et al: The caregiver role in behavioral treatment of depression in dementia patients, in New Directions in Alzheimer's Disease and Family Stress. Edited by Light E, Lebowtiz B, Niederehe G. New York, Springer, 1991 pp 7–13

Teri L, Rabins P, Whitehouse P, et al: Management of behavior disturbance in Alzheimer's disease: current knowledge and future directions. Alzheimer Dis Assoc Disord 6:77–88, 1992

Teri L, Curtis J, Gallagher-Thompson D, et al: Cognitive-behavior therapy with depressed older adults, in Diagnosis and Treatment of Depression in Late Life. Edited by Schneider LS, Reynolds CF, Lebowitz BD, et al. Washington, DC, American Psychiatric Press, 1994, pp 279–291

Thompson LW, Gallagher D: Efficacy of psychotherapy in the treatment of late-life depression. Advances in Behavior Research and Therapy 6:127–139, 1984

Thompson LW, Gallagher D: Depression and its treatment in the elderly. Aging 348:14–18, 1985

Thompson LW, Gallagher D: Psychotherapy for late-life depression. Generations 10:38–41, 1986

Thompson LW, Gallagher D, Nies G, et al: Evaluation of the effectiveness of professionals and nonprofessionals as instructors of "Coping with Depression" classes for elders. Gerontologist 23:390–396, 1983

Thompson LW, Gallagher D, Breckenridge JS: Comparative effectiveness of psychotherapies for depressed elders. J Consult Clin Psychol 55:385–390, 1987

Thompson LW, Gallagher D, Czirr R: Personality disorder and outcome in the treatment of late life depression. J Geriatr Psychiatry 21:133–146, 1988

Thompson LW, Gallagher-Thompson D, Hanser S, et al: Treatment of late-life depression with cognitive/behavioral therapy or desipramine. Poster presented at the annual meeting of the American Psychological Association, San Francisco, CA, August 1991

Thompson SC, Sobolew-Shubin A, Graham MA, et al: Psychosocial adjustment following a stroke. Soc Sci Med 28:239–247, 1989

Thornton S, Brotchie J: Reminiscence: a critical review of the empirical literature. Br J Clin Psychol 26:93–111, 1987

Toseland RW, Rossiter CM: Group interventions to support family caregivers: a review and analysis. Gerontologist 29:438–448, 1989

Toseland RW, Smith GC: Effectiveness of individual counseling by professional and peer helpers for family caregivers of the elderly. Psychol Aging 5:256–263, 1990

Toseland RW, Rossiter CM, Labrecque MS: The effectiveness of peer-led and professionally led groups to support family caregivers. Gerontologist 29:465–471, 1989

Toseland RW, Rossiter CM, Peak T, et al: Comparative effectiveness of individual and group interventions to support family caregivers. Soc Work 35:209–217, 1990

Waller M, Griffin M: Group therapy for depressed elders. Geriatric Nursing 5:309–311, 1984

Watt LM, Wong PT: A taxonomy of reminiscence and therapeutic implications. Journal of Gerontological Social Work 16:37–57, 1991

Yost E, Beutler L, Corbishley MA, et al: Group Cognitive Therapy: A Treatment Approach for Depressed Older Adults. New York, Pergamon, 1986

Youssef FA: The impact of group reminiscence counseling on a depressed elderly population. Nurse Pract 15:32,35–38, 1990

Zarit SH: Issues and directions in family intervention research, in Alzheimer's Disease Treatment and Family Stress: Directions for Research. Edited by Light E, Lebowitz BD. Rockville, MD, National Institute of Mental Health, 1989, pp 458–486

Zarit SH, Teri L: Interventions and services for family caregivers. Annual Review of Gerontology and Geriatrics 11:241–265, 1991

Zarit SH, Cole KD, Guider RL: Memory training strategies and subjective complaints of memory in the aged. Gerontologist 21:158–164, 1981

Zarit SH, Anthony CR, Boutselis M: Interventions with caregivers of dementia patients: comparison of two approaches. Psychol Aging 2:225–232, 1987

32

Neuropsychiatry in Nursing Homes

Barry W. Rovner, M.D.
Ira R. Katz, M.D.

Introduction

Existing research demonstrates that nursing homes are the modern mental institutions for elderly people in the United States. Unfortunately, training of nursing home staff and physicians, processes of care, and the recognition and treatment of mental disorders lag behind the current state of scientific knowledge in psychiatry (Rovner and Katz 1992). Consequently, the nursing home represents one of the greatest current challenges in clinical neuroscience. Although it is important to recognize the promise of basic and clinical research for developing treatments that may prevent or cure Alzheimer's disease, it is also necessary to apply scientific knowledge about the relationships between brain disease and behavior to develop strategies for caring for patients with dementia on a day-to-day basis.

Although the prevalence of nursing home residency for those over 65 is about 5%, 20%–50% of people over 65 will live in nursing homes at some point before death (German et al. 1992).

The cost of their care is enormous:

> In 1989 the total cost of nursing home care was $47.9 billion, or 8% of all health care expenditures. This was a 12% increase from the year before, and exceeded the 9% average increase observed for the 1980s overall. The bulk (64%) of nursing home expenditures are financed by public programs, either directly through Medicaid (43%) or Medicare (about 3%), or indirectly from transfer payments (i.e., the Medicaid mandated contributions from the resident's social security income; 18%). Given the projected considerable increase in the number and proportion of older Americans, the use of and expense associated with nursing homes has become an issue of considerable national concern. (Wolinsky et al. 1992, p. 173)

How much of a concern is evident in a recent study of projected nursing home costs. Kemper et al. (1991) estimated that it will cost $60 billion to pay for future nursing home care for Americans who turned 65 in 1990. This projection is based on data that indicate that 43% of this cohort will enter a nursing home during their lives and will spend an average of 2.8 years there. Other research has shown that the growth rate for nursing home beds during the past decade has not kept pace with the increase in the population of older people. Harrington et al. (1992) found wide variations across states in this ratio, with the most severe under-

supply in the northeast, resulting in a serious problem of access. Citing the work of Nyman regarding nursing homes in Wisconsin, they noted, "an increase in the number of elderly in an area, while holding beds constant, is positively associated with the number of private nursing home patients and negatively associated with the number of Medicaid patients" (Harrington et al., p. 179). They concluded that this represents a crowding-out effect that is consistent with excess demand and nursing homes' preference for private patients. As the bed supply continues to decline relative to the elderly population, issues of access and quality become even more important to study.

Recognizing that the dementia syndrome, so prevalent in this population, is the syndromatic expression of a brain disease and not the consequence of normal aging has been a major conceptual advance only relatively recently accepted by the nursing home industry and the governmental agencies that regulate them. Gradually, making the diagnosis of dementia in nursing homes has become an acceptable, indeed a required, practice (e.g., PASARR [preadmission screening and annual resident review] regulations of the 1987 Nursing Home Reform Act). However, recognizing dementia syndromes as brain diseases has led to a denial, of sorts, of the noncognitive behavioral aspects of these disorders such as depression, delusions, hallucinations, and states of agitation. Although supervision and provision of assistance in activities of daily living are essential components of care for dementia patients in the nursing home, these noncognitive psychiatric symptoms frequently accompany the dementia syndrome and determine both the patients' needs for care and the quality of care they receive.

History

The modern nursing home can trace its origins to the almshouses and mental institutions of the 19th century, which, transformed incrementally by public policies, have come to resemble hospital facilities. As such, these once derided places have gained respectability through their identification with the more credible medical institution. Along with that credibility has come the expectation that patients would be cared for with the expertise, knowledge, and technology characteristic of the best hospitals. The policies, procedures, and staffing patterns of most nursing homes are, in fact, based on this model:

Indeed, nursing homes appear, at first glance, like a patient-care floor in a general hospital. As in a hospital, the center of activity, and often the physical center of the floor, is a nursing home station. A high-fronted desk, wide enough to permit 2 or 3 people to sit at it, looks out onto the corridor. Behind it and to the sides are books and manuals, miscellaneous supplies, racks filled with patients' charts, lockable medicine cabinet, and perhaps doors to a supply room and a staff bathroom or lounge. Not infrequently, diplomas or state licenses hang on the wall behind the nursing station, along with other official-looking documents, all neatly framed. (Vladeck 1980; p. 7)

As in hospitals, most patients in nursing homes have medical disorders such as high blood pressure, strokes, heart disease, arthritis, and diabetes (Johnson and Grant 1985; p. 38). They are cared for by nurses and seen by physicians, and they receive medications. The patients are expected more or less to lie in bed passively and receive the ministrations of the nursing staff.

The reality of the nursing home, however, is not reflected by the sterility of the medical model. Patients have moved from sickbeds to gerichairs, and the nursing home now echoes the bedlam of the psychiatric hospital in the era before the development of specific treatments:

The characteristic picture is that of a dozen residents arrayed in front of a television or sitting in a hall, each staring ahead. If anyone is talking, it is mostly to herself. (Vladeck 1980; p. 26)

Epidemiology

The change in the kinds of patients cared for in nursing homes over the past 20 years is related to the aging of the population and the increasing prevalence of dementing conditions. Patients with these conditions, unlike their primarily medically ill counterparts, are in need of medical attention as a result of their mental, rather than their physical, symptoms.

These changes are evident in successive nursing home surveys. The 1977 National Nursing Home Survey indicated that approximately 57% of patients had "chronic brain syndrome" or "senility." By 1985, 63% were so diagnosed. However, these surveys have relied on nonclinician reviews of nursing records and interviews with nursing staff rather than on psychiatrists' di-

rect examination of patients. Cross-sectional studies such as these cannot reveal whether psychiatric or behavior disorders are the cause or consequence of institutionalization. Furthermore, none has used current diagnostic terms such as those specified in DSM-III-R (American Psychiatric Association 1987). Thus, until recently, no studies were carried out on the prevalence of mental disorders among new admissions to nursing homes in which psychiatrists examined large, systematically ascertained samples and made diagnoses according to modern diagnostic criteria. In 1987 to 1989, as part of a National Institute of Aging Study, we (Rovner et al. 1990a) evaluated 454 new admissions to eight Baltimore area proprietary nursing homes. The overall objective of our study was to analyze mental morbidity among nursing home residents, establish its magnitude and type, and assess its influence on quality of life.

The following list shows the prevalence of psychiatric disorders divided into 4 mutually exclusive diagnostic groups based on the presence and type of psychopathology:

1. *Dementia complicated:* Patients with dementing disorders complicated by the co-occurrence of depression, delusions, or delirium ($n = 123$, 27.1% of the entire sample; 40.2% of all dementia patients)
2. *Dementia only:* Patients with dementing disorders without delusions, depression, or delirium ($n = 183$, 40.3%)
3. *Other psychiatric disorders:* non-dementia patients with affective disorders or schizophrenia ($n = 58$, 12.8%)
4. *No psychiatric disorder:* those without any disorder ($n = 90$, 19.8%)

Overall, 364 new admissions (80.2%) had a psychiatric disorder according to the examining research psychiatrists. The most common diagnosis was dementia ($n = 306$, 67.4%). The most frequent etiology of dementia was primary degenerative dementia of the Alzheimer's type ($n = 172$, 37.9% of the entire sample) followed by multi-infarct dementia ($n = 81$, 17.8% of the entire sample). Other dementia syndromes included the dementia syndrome of depression, Parkinson's disease, and brain tumor. Of the patients without dementia ($n = 148$, 32.6%), 58 (12.8% of the entire sample) had a psychiatric disorder such as affective disorder ($n = 47$, 10.4%) or schizophrenia ($n = 11$, 2.4%).

In spite of these epidemiological and clinical realities, nursing homes continue to model themselves after general rather than neuropsychiatric hospitals. The medical staffs consist primarily of internists, family practitioners, or general practitioners, and the nursing staff consists primarily of individuals trained in medical-surgical nursing. Because neither the training of the nursing nor medical staffs, or their approaches to care, have changed in accord with the changes in the population, the original conceptualization of nursing homes as diminutive hospitals is no longer applicable. Furthermore, the fact that the majority of nursing home patients have conditions known to be associated with states of psychopathology including delirium, depression, delusions, and hallucinations and behavior disorders such as agitation, combativeness, and wandering has added an unanticipated sense of acuity and disturbance to the environment. Overwhelmed, nursing home staff have turned to restraints and psychotropic medications to manage these psychiatric syndromes and behavior disorders, often in an indiscriminate and uninformed way. Ironically, nursing homes have returned to their origins as mental institutions in that most patients have mental disorders without cures, have disruptive behaviors that are difficult to manage, and are frequently physically and chemically restrained.

Use of Medications in Nursing Homes

There are data from controlled clinical trials in the nursing home and in other settings that demonstrate that antipsychotic medications can be modestly effective in the short-term treatment of agitation and related behavior disturbances in patients with dementia (Schneider et al. 1990). However, recognition of the frequent misuse of psychotropic drugs and their adverse consequences (e.g., hip fractures [Ray et al. 1987b] and cognitive impairment [Rovner et al. 1988]) has led to federal legislation restricting the use of neuroleptics and sedative-hypnotics (Omnibus Budget Reconciliation Act [OBRA] 1987). Before this legislation, our Baltimore nursing home study found that 34% of dementia patients without delusions or hallucinations received neuroleptics, as did 21.4% of residents without dementia and 6.7% of patients with no psychiatric diagnosis at all.

Prescribing a neuroleptic now requires documentation of a specific psychiatric diagnosis and behavioral indications. Garrard et al. (1991) estimated that had these regulations been in effect from 1976 to 1985,

50% of neuroleptic use in almost 9,000 nursing home residents would have been out of compliance. Ray et al. (1987a) conducted a controlled trial of the efficacy of an education visit in reducing inappropriate antipsychotic prescribing for nursing home patients and found that, although well received, the visit did not change prescribing practices. More recently, however, studies have demonstrated the feasibility of reducing the use of these medications without apparent adverse clinical consequences (Avorn et al. 1992).

We (Rovner et al. 1992) found a 36% reduction in prescriptions for neuroleptics from the 3 months before OBRA went into effect until 3 months afterward with no increase in prescriptions for sedative-hypnotics. The same trends were sustained 1 year later. Although quality assurance data for the prevalence of medical events such as bed sores, weight loss, falls with fractures, adverse incidents, urinary tract infections, and deaths revealed small but significant changes, the data were difficult to interpret because comparable data from previous years were unavailable. However, our study provided a limited glimpse into the impact of these regulations and their potential effects.

Many nursing home studies have also demonstrated the inadequate treatment of depression in nursing homes. Heston et al. (1992) found that of 868 persons with depression only 10% were treated with antidepressants. More received neuroleptics and benzodiazepines, but most received no treatment at all.

We (Katz et al. 1990; Rovner et al. 1991) have demonstrated the high prevalence of depression in nursing homes and have also documented low rates of recognition and treatment. In a series of studies from the Philadelphia Geriatric Center, we found in 1989 that the prevalence of major depression was 20% and that depression was associated with medical disorders that complicated diagnosis and treatment (Parmelee et al. 1989). In 1991, we showed that pain was associated with depression, particularly when a physical problem also contributed as a potential source of pain (Parmelee et al. 1991). We hypothesized that either pain causes depression and/or that depression intensifies pain. In 1992, we showed an increased mortality rate with major depression that appeared to be attributable to its correlation with ill health (Parmelee et al. 1992a). In contrast, studying a different sample of patients and using different methods to control for medical illness, we found that depression was an independent risk factor for mortality over and above severity of medical illness (Rovner et al. 1991). Depression increased the risk of death for depressed patients by 59%. In 1992, we (Parmelee et al. 1992b) found a 6.6% incidence of major depression over 1 year and showed that 40% of patients who were depressed on initial evaluation showed no remission after 1 year.

Given the high prevalence of depression and its serious adverse consequences, our 1990 study evaluating the efficacy of nortriptyline in the treatment of major depression for elderly patients residing in residential care settings stands as a landmark study demonstrating both the promise and difficulties of treating depression in nursing homes (Katz et al. 1990). Sixty percent of treated patients were shown to have improved substantially. However, many patients refused or were uncooperative with the study or had unstable medical conditions that prevented treatment. Our study also indicated, therefore, the need for new clinical trials, possibly testing electroconvulsive therapy (ECT) and medications with fewer anticholinergic and cardiovascular side effects to advance the care of patients with depression in nursing homes.

Recognizing the limitations of current neuropsychiatric treatment in nursing homes, the American Association for Geriatric Psychiatry, the American Geriatrics Society, and the American Psychiatric Association published a position statement on psychotherapeutic medications in nursing homes (1992). The tenets of the statement are

1. Optimizing the use of psychotherapeutic medications will require additional support for both clinical training and research.
2. Appropriate use of psychotherapeutic medications for the treatment of patients with diagnosed psychiatric disorders is an important component of the medical and mental health care of nursing home residents.
3. The basic principles underlying the treatment of psychiatric disorders and behavioral problems in nursing homes are identical to those for the treatment of geriatric patients in other settings.
4. Nursing home residents with Alzheimer's disease and other dementias should be evaluated to determine whether they are experiencing affective, psychotic, and behavioral systems; when such symptoms are present they should be treated.
5. Psychiatric disorders such as depression are common in nursing home residents and require treatment. These disorders frequently coexist with, as well as complicate, the disabling chronic medical

and neurological disorders that make long-term care necessary.

Sakauye and Camp (1992) described a consultation-liaison psychiatry program in a teaching nursing home to meet these objectives by implementing five guiding principles: 1) making the patient human to the staff, 2) assuming no behavior is random, 3) looking for depression or psychosis as a source of problems, 4) reducing medications and medication doses, and 5) creating a more homelike environment.

Inappropriate medication use in nursing home residents is not limited to psychotropic drugs. Beers et al. (1991) reviewed the literature indicating inappropriate use of antihypertensives, nonsteroidal anti-inflammatory agents, oral hypoglycemics, analgesics, and a variety of other commonly prescribed medications. They proposed explicit criteria defining the inappropriate use of these medications and also suggested that these criteria may be useful for quality assurance review and clinical practice guidelines.

Special Care Units

Special dementia care units in nursing homes have evolved as potentially innovative approaches to care. The underlying theory of treatment generally is based on the identification and treatment of excess disability and compensation for lost abilities through environmental and social support, as well as on systematic evaluations of residents for potentially reversible medical and neuropsychiatric disorders. These units are generally costly to develop, as they require modification of existing designs or creation of new ones, as well as recruitment and training of personnel at higher staff-patient ratios. They often charge higher daily rates, and therefore the care that they provide may be out of reach for most nursing home patients with dementia.

The Office of Technology Assessment (1992) recently completed a report of dementia care units in nursing homes and estimated that 10% of nursing homes have such units. Ohta and Ohta (1988) were among the first, however, to note the variability among dementia units and the heterogeneity of the patients who reside in them. Perhaps for these reasons, it has been difficult to assess the effectiveness of such units. Gold et al. (1991) found that such units appeared to be associated with care of a higher quality than that on traditional units, but that the quality of special care units was by no means uniform. Holmes et al. (1990) compared the characteristics of dementia patients residing on these units with their counterparts on other units within the same facilities and found that the two groups differed in levels of cognitive impairment, behavior, functioning, and physical status. Perhaps most revealing, they found that, despite a higher prevalence of behavioral disorders among special care patients, their staff did not view the disturbances as more severe and suggested that the specialized staff were able to adjust to these behaviors. Sloane et al. (1991) conducted a case control study of 625 patients with dementia on 31 specialized dementia units and 32 traditional units in five states. They found that specialized care units can reduce the use of physical restraints, but perhaps not that of psychotropic drugs, and that different variables determine the use of physical restraints and psychotropic medications in the two types of units.

Several recent studies have been conducted to evaluate the outcome of treatment on special care units. Benson et al. (1987) reported increased levels of mental, emotional, and self-care functioning for patients admitted to a specialized unit. We (Rovner et al. 1990b) compared the outcomes of dementia patients residing on this specialized unit with other patients from the same facility over a 1-year period and found that the functional capacity of those on this unit remained stable, whereas that of the others declined.

Principles of Care

In practice, the perceptions of nursing staff are critical components determining whether a behavior disorder is present or not. Different observers may have differing views about whether a particular behavior is an expected and accepted occurrence or a disturbance that offends or threatens caretakers and the homeostasis of the environment. In this light, the definition of a behavior disorder includes elements of the inherent dispositions of the patient, the observer, and their interaction within the environment. This point underscores the importance of education of people who provide care in the nursing home environment.

Perhaps it is not unreasonable to consider nursing homes as places beset with an epidemic of dementia. This line of reasoning is useful because it leads to two relevant concepts of public health care, namely the contribution of the environment to provoking and sustaining aspects of disease and the development of preventive procedures and practices. To understand the contribution of the environment, we must understand the nature of the underlying disease. Dementia patients have experienced a loss in their capacity to know and reason about the world, which is reflected in impairments in several discrete cognitive areas including memory, language, and visuospatial perception. Once the disease state is recognized as the cause of dementia, its impact in the nursing home can be illuminated by identifying its particular impairments and the disabilities and handicaps that emerge from them.

Impairment refers to the symptoms or clinical manifestation of the brain damage. For example, *memory impairment* ("amnesia") refers to the loss of ability to learn, store, or retrieve new information. *Disability* refers to the loss in functional ability consequent to the impairment. Thus, patients with amnesia are unable to recall recent events. *Handicap* refers to the social disadvantage that results from the disability. In this example, patients with amnesia are excluded from nursing home activities because of their forgetfulness. Making these distinctions enables physicians and nursing home personnel to comprehend the variety of symptoms and behaviors of dementia patients and their consequences as they occur in the nursing home.

The underlying brain disease exists independent of the environment, but how the disease manifests itself (i.e., whether a behavior disorder emerges or not as a symptom of disease) reflects the interaction of a number of processes. A clarifying distinction in this regard is the recognition of *predisposing features* and *precipitating factors*. Dementia patients are predisposed to behavior disturbances on the basis of 1) specific syndromes marked by depression, delusions, and hallucinations; 2) delirium secondary to metabolic disturbances, infections, medications; and 3) poor impulse control, impaired judgment, and dysregulation of mood secondary to the brain damage. Precipitating factors may be environmental events such as recent nursing home placement, change of rooms, changes in caregivers, uninformed approaches to care, or exposure to threatening activities or circumstances that overwhelm cognitive capacities.

This reasoning leads to parallel but distinctive treatment interventions. From the neuropsychiatric perspective, recognizing that a patient's behavior is the reflection of brain disease, rather than of a willful or manipulative nature, and that depression, delirium, delusions, and hallucinations may represent biological aberrations and symptoms of the underlying disease directs treatment toward the somatic therapies found to be beneficial in other neuropsychiatric patients with these symptoms.

Although neurological influences are important in the genesis of behavior disorders, psychosocial influences are important as well. Patients are exposed to environments and persons that they may not fully comprehend or recognize, predisposing them to a sense of uncertainty, frustration, and lack of direction. Because of these predispositions, the provocations or precipitating factors in the environment may lead to behavior disturbance. It is thus important to understand the behavior in its social context so that interventions can be designed within that context to prevent the emergence of behavior disorders.

Importance of Activity Programs

Though there is no direct evidence that lack of activities in nursing homes is directly detrimental to health, it very well may be so. Spector and Takada (1991) found that residents with moderate levels of activity participation were less likely to decline or die than residents with lower levels of participation. Deprivation may also aggravate the underlying conditions: "the essence of aggravated aging is that environmental factors increase the morbidity of a group whose morbidity is expected to be high so that the effect of the environmental factors is overlooked" (Evans 1984, p. 353).

Appreciation of these observations shifted nursing home regulatory emphasis from the physical qualities of nursing homes to the outcome of care they provide. Nursing homes were directed to develop ways to facilitate the highest practical level of functioning for patients. These interventions, aimed at an entire population, may improve the care of a substantial proportion of nursing home patients by reducing unnecessary physical and chemical restraints. However, broad interventions such as these are not particularly sensitive to the continuing individual needs of many patients. In fact, despite the beneficent intentions of OBRA 1987, the proposed rules continue to fall short of improving the psychosocial rehabilitation of patients.

Psychosocial Rehabilitation in Nursing Homes

The concept of psychosocial rehabilitation, particularly as a form of psychiatric treatment, began with the

observations of Pinel, who, in the late 18th century, was appointed the director of the mental institutions of Paris, the Bicêtre and the Salpêtrière. Pinel recognized the overuse of restraints and prohibited their use and replaced them with clinical programs providing social activity, physical activity, and physical comfort. These innovations were designed to achieve the highest level of psychosocial functioning for patients. In this sense, they anticipated the modern definition of psychosocial rehabilitation, which attempts to "enable an individual who suffers from long-term mental illness to develop to the fullest extent of his or her capacities" (Bachrach 1992, p 1456).

In 1856, Connolly wrote,

The old system placed all violent or troublesome patients in the position of dangerous animals. The new system regards them as afflicted persons whose brain and nerves are diseased and who are to be restored to health, comfort, and reason. (p. 53)

Quoting Pinel, he wrote,

We seek a mild air for the consumptive, and place the asthmatic in an atmosphere which does not irritate him, and keep a patient with heart disease on level ground; and on the same prophylactic and curative principles, we must remove from an insane person every influence that could further excite his brain . . . for these reasons, a residence in a well-ordered asylum deserves to be ranked among the most efficacious parts of direct treatment. (p. 73)

Given that the prevalence of dementia and behavior disorders is high in nursing homes and that there is yet no primary treatment for the brain disease itself, treatment should focus on prevention of behavior disorders. In this case, preventive treatment begins by emphasizing the importance of environmental factors. Dementia patients are unable to adapt easily to their environment because their neuropsychiatric illness produces loss of intellectual functioning and decreased adaptability. Thus the environment must be arranged to meet the needs of the patient. In the absence of a properly arranged "fit" between environment and patient needs, behavior disorders are inevitable.

What then is the current environment of nursing homes that may contribute to behavior disorders? As suggested earlier, nursing home approaches to care have been based on a medical model that no longer fulfills the needs of the patients. Neither the training of the staff nor the approaches of care facilitate recognition of the environment's influence on disease. As Pinel suggested, the environment must be shaped around the patient to facilitate recovery or, at the very least, to prevent further decline.

Behavior disorders, whatever their pathogenic mechanisms, usually lead to restrictive forms of management such as restraints and neuroleptics, which may further contribute to decrements in function and independence. However, if one pathogenic mechanism leading to behavior disorders includes the relative deprivation of the environment, then its modification holds promise as a means of primary prevention. Goldstein (1952), studying the behavioral changes of patients with brain damage, noted two important aspects of their behavior. First, he observed that patients with brain damage may appear emotionally dull but that there is no diminution of their emotions. The extent to which they are so perceived, however, results in disturbances of mood being minimized or ignored. Second, patients with brain damage, despite their perceived or apparent constrictions of mood, thought, and behavior, are, in fact, capable of cheerful activity and constructive behavior when appropriate stimuli and occasion are properly supplied by those around them.

The extent to which patients with dementia are believed not to experience emotion nor to enjoy meaningful activity has led to some unfortunate consequences in nursing homes, not the least of which are that treatable depression is unrecognized and that rehabilitative efforts are neglected. Thus the potentially provocative circumstances of the environment, combined with the impaired judgment, impulse control, and frustration tolerance of the patient with brain damage, dispose the situation to behavior disturbances. Goldstein (1952) called the disturbances "disordered or catastrophic conditions" (in contrast to the ordered conditions of patients experiencing success). He described the catastrophic reaction as follows:

> A patient may look animated, calm, in a good mood, well-poised, collected, and cooperative when he is confronted with tasks he can fulfill; the same patient may appear dazed, become agitated, change color, start to fumble, become unfriendly, evasive, and even aggressive when he is not able to fulfill the task. His overt behavior appears very much the same as a person in the state of anxiety. (p. 255)

Goldstein (1952) stressed the importance of experiences of success or "self-realization" for dementia patients to sustain the "ordered condition" and avoid the disordered or catastrophic one. Goldstein defined "anxiety" as a catastrophic condition in which self-realization is not possible—a condition that may be produced by a variety of events, all of which have in common the following:

> There is a discrepancy between the individual's capacities and the demands made on him, and this discrepancy makes self-realization impossible. This may be due to external or internal conditions, physical or psychological. (p. 257)

Goldstein (1952) further suggested that the patient can be maintained in an ordered condition through protective mechanisms that guarantee success and avoid situations of task failure:

> [The patients] like to be in a familiar room in which everything is organized in a definitive way . . . the patients themselves cannot voluntarily arrange things in a definite way [and must rely on others to maintain] those arrangements which they can handle. This allows for some ordered form of behavior and for some kind of self-realization. Only as long as the environment is so organized by the people around him, and that no tasks arise that he cannot fulfill . . . can catastrophic reactions be avoided. (p. 259)

Activity programs in nursing homes designed to accord with the patients' level of cognitive impairment represent interventions that may improve patients' sense of self, minimize anxiety, and protect them from catastrophic conditions. As Goldstein (1952) noted, such activities enable patients. . .

> To keep themselves busy with things that they are able to do as a protection against things that they cannot cope with. The activities which engross them need not be of great value in themselves. Their usefulness consists apparently in the fact that they protect the patient. (p. 258)

Even though the cognitive and behavioral impairments of dementia patients persist, and quite likely worsen after a time, these patients may show a decrease in behavior disorders and catastrophic reactions because routine and nonthreatening circumstances become predictable aspects of their day-to-day lives.

Legal Issues in Nursing Homes

The recently enacted Patient Self-Determination Act (PSDA) requires federally funded nursing facilities to inform patients of their rights under state law: 1) to make decisions to accept or refuse medical or surgical treatment and 2) to formulate advanced directives. Advanced directives allow currently competent patients to record the nature and kind of medical procedures they desire should they become incompetent in the future. These directives decrease the probability that a guardianship hearing will be necessary. Most states allow two types of advanced directives, the living will and the durable power of attorney.

As previously discussed, the prevalence of dementing conditions and other psychiatric disorders in nursing homes is high. This situation suggests that many nursing home patients may not be competent at the time of admission to execute properly advanced directives or to give consent to medical procedures. Thus, although the PSDA may improve autonomy in decision making for nursing home residents, a large proportion may not understand this right. We (Janofosky and Rovner 1993) recently investigated the current prevalence of advanced directives among nursing home patients ($n = 186$). Of 29 residents assessed to be competent, 14 (48%) had a durable power of attorney or a living will. One person (3.5%) had a guardian. The remaining 14 patients (48.5%) had no advanced directive. One hundred fifty-seven patients were assessed as not competent, and 61 (39%) of them had a durable power of attorney or a living will, 44 (28%) had a guardian, and the remaining 52 (33%) had no form of advanced directive.

The primary finding of this study was that substantial numbers of nursing home residents lacked either a guardian or an advanced directive. This finding is particularly troubling for competent patients who are at high risk of becoming incompetent as time passes. These data stress the importance of identifying, as early as possible, competent patients at high risk of becoming incapable of making their own health care decisions in the future. These patients need to be thoroughly informed about their right to formulate an advanced directive. Although the PSDA requires patients to be informed of their right to formulate advanced directives on admission to a nursing home, for those already incompetent it is too late. Patients who become incompetent before executing an advanced directive

lose the ability to inform their physicians and the world in general about their preference if or when they are unable to speak knowingly for themselves.

Conclusions

Although many of these clinical observations and recommendations may seem obvious, and even though they have constituted essential elements of care in other medical and neuropsychiatric settings, they are new to the care of patients in nursing homes. One need only recall that recognizing the high prevalence of dementia and the excessive use of restraints and psychotropic medications are recent advances, when we look forward to what remains to be accomplished in the care of nursing home patients. The lack of knowledge, lack of interest, and lack of resources on these matters have all contributed to what had been the "acceptable" standard of care of "warehousing" in nursing homes. As a result, few administrators or physicians in nursing homes have emphasized the need for psychosocial rehabilitation for dementia patients or organized a system of care to provide it.

Compounded by the lack of public awareness and the reluctance of federal agencies to provide reimbursement for it, psychosocial rehabilitation programs, despite OBRA language that supports them, are far from being regular and essential aspects of nursing home care. These efforts should be "intertwined" with and become "innate" elements of reasonable and expected care. To prevent behavior disorders and decline secondary to inactivity, these programs should enable patients to achieve their highest level of functioning and well-being. As Bachrach (1992) noted,

> [Although] the gains that some can make are so small as to seem out of proportion to the effort it takes on the part of patient and personnel to produce them . . . they are so important that the institution must give each long-term patient encouragement and help to achieve his maximum of restoration. (p. 172)

We are stressing the importance of psychosocial rehabilitation and, even more basically, humanistic treatment of nursing home residents with dementia or other neuropsychiatric disorders. All too often, such appeals set off empty debates about the relative importance of high technology versus highly personal approaches to care. This debate would be pointless here. There is a need for vigorous approaches to neuropsychiatric diagnosis for all patients with dementia and behavioral disturbances to identify those with hallucinations, delusions, depression, and delirium. There is also a need for assessment of deficits (e.g., amnesia, aphasia, apraxia, and agnosia) and ensuring that all aspects of nursing home care are carried out with the knowledge of these deficits. Here there must be interactions between clinical neuroscience and front line staff. If environmental interventions are to prevent or treat behavior disturbances they must be more than well-intentioned humanistic endeavors, they must be inferred from what is known of the nature of the cognitive deficits in dementia, both in general and in the individual patient.

To provide this level of care, a complete revision of the nursing home industry will be required to meet acceptable standards of neuropsychiatric care for patients in nursing homes. Zimmer et al. (1993) discussed the disparity between the ideals and the realities of nursing home medical directorship and indicated that, to fill the role adequately, greater financial commitment by facilities and reimbursement systems will be necessary. In the absence of such leadership, it will be difficult to implement other promising and innovative efforts, such as enriched educational and practice programs for nursing staff, the use of geriatric nurse practitioners, and collaborative relationships with psychiatrists. Future efforts and directions to improve nursing home care might profitably follow the successful approaches already used in modern psychiatric, neuropsychiatric, and rehabilitation hospitals.

Summary

In this chapter, we reviewed the high prevalence of neuropsychiatric conditions and behavior disturbances in nursing homes. We discussed how nursing homes, as they currently exist, are based on a medical model that may not be appropriate for the problems of their patients and are staffed by personnel who direct their care toward the treatment of medical conditions, but not neuropsychiatric ones. This situation may lead to inappropriate use of physical and chemical restraints, the inability to reduce behavior disorders, and failure to improve the psychosocial functioning of patients. Improving the care of patients with neuropsychiatric disorders in nursing homes requires appreciation of the brain damaged state and how environmental circumstances contribute to both the genesis of problems and the potential for maximizing patients' cognitive, emotional, and physical functioning.

References

American Association for Geriatric Psychiatry, the American Geriatrics Society, and the American Psychiatric Association: Position statement: psychotherapeutic medications in the nursing home. J Am Geriatr Soc 40:946–949, 1992

American Psychiatric Association: Diagnostic and Statistical Manual of Mental Disorders, 3rd Edition, Revised. American Psychiatric Association, 1987

Avorn J, Soumerai SB, Everitt DE, et al: A randomized trial of a program to reduce the use of psychoactive drugs in nursing homes. N Engl J Med 327:168–173, 1992

Bachrach LL: Psychosocial rehabilitation and psychiatry in the care of long-term patients. Am J Psychiatry 149:1455–1463, 1992

Beers MH, Ouslander JG, Rollinghter I, et al: Explicit criteria for determining inappropriate medication use in nursing homes. Arch Intern Med 151:1825–1837, 1991

Benson DM, Cameron D, Humbach E, et al: Establishment and impact of a dementia unit within the nursing home. J Am Geriatr Soc 35:319–323, 1987

Connolly J: Treatment of the Insane Without Restraints. London, Smith, Elder, 1856

Evans JG: Prevention of age-associated loss of autonomy: epidemiological approaches. Journal of Chronic Disease 37:353–363, 1984

Garrard J, Makriss L, Dunham T, et al: Evaluation of neuroleptic drug use by nursing home elderly under proposed Medicare and Medicaid regulations. JAMA 265: 463–467, 1991

German PS, Rovner BW, Burton LC, et al: The role of mental morbidity in the nursing home experience. Gerontologist 32:152–158, 1992

Gold D, Sloane P, Mathew L, et al: Special care units: a typology of care settings for memory-impaired older adults. Gerontologist 31:467–475, 1991

Goldstein K: The effect of brain damage on the personality. Psychiatry 15:245–260, 1952

Harrington C, Preston S, Grant L, et al: Revised trends in states' nursing home capacity. Health Affairs 11:170–180, 1992

Heston LL, Garrard J, Makris L, et al: Inadequate treatment of depressed nursing home elderly. J Am Geriatr Soc 40:1117–1122, 1992

Holmes D, Teresi J, Weiner A, et al: Impact associates with special care units in long-term care facilities. Gerontologist 30:178–181, 1990

Janofsky JS, Rovner BW: Prevalence of advanced directives and guardianship in nursing home patients. J Geriatr Psychiatry Neurol 6:214–216, 1993

Johnson CL, Grant LA: The Nursing Home in American Society. Baltimore, MD, Johns Hopkins University Press, 1985

Katz IR, Simpson GM, Curlik SM, et al: Pharmacologic treatment of major depression for elderly patients in residential care settings. J Clin Psychiatry 51 (suppl):41–48, 1990

Kemper P, Spillman BC, Murtaugh CM: A lifetime perspective on proposals for financing nursing home care. Inquiry 28:333–344, 1991

Office of Technology Assessment: Special Care Units for Persons With Dementia. Washington, DC, Congress of the United States Office of Technology Assessment, 1992

Ohta RJ, Ohta BM: Special units for Alzheimer's disease patients: a critical look. Gerontologist 28:803–808, 1988

Parmelee P, Katz IR, Lawton MP: Depression among institutionalized aged: assessment and prevalence estimation. J Gerontol 44:M22–M29, 1989

Parmelee P, Katz IR, Lawton MP: The relation of pain to depression among institutionalized aged. J Gerontol 1:P15–P21, 1991

Parmelee P, Katz IR, Lawton MP: Depression and mortality among institutionalized aged. J Gerontol 47:P3–P10, 1992a

Parmelee P, Katz IR, Lawton MP: Incidence of depression and long-term care settings. J Gerontol 47:M189–M196, 1992b

Ray WA, Blazer DD, Schaffner W, et al: Reducing antipsychotic drug prescribing for nursing home patients: a controlled study of the effect of an educational visit. Am J Pub Health 77:1448–1450, 1987a

Ray WA, Griffin MR, Schaffner W, et al: Psychotropic drug use and the risk of hip fracture. N Engl J Med 316:363–369, 1987b

Rovner BW, Katz IR: Psychiatric disorders in the nursing home: a selective review of studies related to clinical care. International Journal of Geriatric Psychiatry 7:75–82, 1992

Rovner BW, David A, Lucas-Blaustein MJ, et al: Self care capacity and anticholinergic drug levels in nursing homes. Am J Psychiatry 145:107–109, 1988

Rovner BW, German PS, Broadhead J, et al: The prevalence and management of dementia and other psychiatric disorders in nursing homes. Int Psychogeriatr 2:13–24, 1990a

Rovner BW, Lucas-Blaustein J, Folstein MF, et al: Stability over one year in patients admitted to a nursing home dementia unit. International Journal of Geriatric Psychiatry 5:77–82, 1990b

Rovner BW, German PS, Brandt LJ, et al: Depression and mortality in nursing homes. JAMA 265:993–996, 1991

Rovner BW, Edelman BA, Cox MP, et al: The impact of antipsychotic drug regulations (OBRA 1987) on psychotropic prescribing practices in nursing homes. Am J Psychiatry 149:1390–1392, 1992

Sakauye KM, Camp CJ: Introducing psychiatric care into nursing homes. Gerontologist 32:849–852, 1992

Schneider L, Pollock VE, Liness SA: A meta-analysis of controlled trials of neuroleptic treatment in dementia. J Am Geriatr Soc 38:553–563, 1990

Sloane PJ, Matthew LJ, Scarborough M, et al: Physical and pharmacologic restraint of nursing home patients with dementia: impact of specialized units. JAMA 265:1278–1282, 1991

Spector WD, Takada HA: Characteristics of nursing homes that affect resident outcomes. Journal of Aging and Health 3:427–454, 1991

Vladeck BC: Unloving Care: The Nursing Home Tragedy. New York, Basic Books, 1980

Wolinsky FD, Callahan CM, Fitzgerald JF, et al: The risk of nursing home placement and subsequent death among older adults. Journal of Gerontology 47:S173–S182, 1992

Zimmer JG, Watson NM, Levenson SA: Nursing home medical directors: ideals and realities. J Am Geriatr Soc 41:127–130, 1993

Index

Page numbers printed in **boldface** type refer to tables or figures

A68 epitopes, **41**, 46
Abbreviated Injury Scale, 481
Abstinence from benzodiazepines, 311
Accident death rates, 21, **22**
Acetazolamide, **572**
Acetophenazine, 613–614, **614**
Acetylcholine
    age-related changes, 54, **54**
    behavioral alterations associated
        with, 90, **90**
    disorders associated with, 91
    indications for, 622
    origins and destinations, 90, **90**
Acquired immunodeficiency syndrome
    AIDS dementia complex, 379, 380
    etiology, 313, 536
    MRI findings, 538, **538**
    neurological complications of, 537–538
ACTH. See Adrenocorticotropic
        hormone
Activities of daily living
    assessments of, 28
    percentage of elderly with difficulties
        in, 28, **28**, **29**
    percentage of elderly with
        independence in, 29, **29**
    poststroke depression effects on,
        460–461, **462**
Activity assessment, 102–103
Activity programs, 689, 690
Acute confusional state. See also
        Delirium
    drug-induced, 556–558
Acute disseminated encephalomyelitis,
        530
Acyclovir, **570**
Adapin. See Doxepin
Addiction. See also Dependence;
        Withdrawal
    to heroin, 313
    to illicit drugs, 313–314
    with limbic system dysfunction, **82**,
        82–83
    to narcotics, 313, 343
    to prescription analgesic drugs, 313
Adenoma pathology, 524
Adjustment disorder, 245, 443
Adrenal medullary tissue grafting, 437
Adrenal steroids
    drug interactions, **613**
    side effects, 561, **562**, **626**
α-Adrenergic blockade, drug-related,
        615, **616**
α-Adrenergic blockers, drug
        interactions, 554, **555**
Adrenergic system
    challenge studies, 580–581, **581**

pharmacological probes of, 580–582
Adrenocorticotropic hormone, side
        effects, **572**
Adrenoleukodystrophy, 532–533
Affect
    aspects of, 103
    assessment of, 103
    definition, 244
    flattened, 103
Affective blunting, 103
Affective disorders
    in Alzheimer's disease, 246
    definition, 244
    ECT treatment, 640–641
    late-life–onset schizophrenia
        comparison, 273–274
    neurobiology of aging with, 62
    organic, 255
    in Parkinson's disease, 441
    prevalence rates, 26, **26**
Affective dysprosody, 83–84, **84**
Age-associated memory impairment
    alternative approaches, 149
    background, 146–147
    biological bases, 154
    clinical assessment, 122
    constructs, 147–155
    definition, 147–148, 153, 154
    diagnostic criteria, 148, 151–152, 153
    as diagnostic entity, 153–154
    future research strategies, 154–155
    NIMH psychometric criteria, 147
Age-consistent memory impairment,
        147, 153
Age-related memory decline
    alternative approaches, 149
    biological bases, 154
    constructs, 147–155
    definition, 148
Aggression, 90, **90**
Aging. See also Successful aging
    of autonomic nervous system, 58
    of brain, 7, 36–38, 41–51, 51–53
    of brain structure, 164–173
    cellular, 43–44
    demographics of, 8
    EEG abnormalities, 216–217
    epidemiology of, 18–33
    genomic alterations, 46–47
    molecular neuropathology of, 44–46,
        46–48
    neurobiology of, 35–69
    neurophysiological alterations,
        216–240
    normal, 131
    pathological, 50–51, 328
    PET studies, 203–206, **204**

premature, 304
    sexual, 59–60
    sleep in, 328
    systemic effects, 63
    theories of, 36, 47
    worldwide, 20, **20**
Agitation
    definition, 102
    drug-induced, **568–574**
    drug treatment, 624
Agnosia
    clinical assessment of, 121
    environmental, **80**, 83–84, **84**
Agoraphobia
    alcohol problems, 288
    prevalence, **281**, 281
    treatment, 290
AIDS. See Acquired immunodeficiency
        syndrome
Akathisia
    acute, 417
    drug-related, **284**, 285, 562, **563**, 615,
        616
    haloperidol side effect, 362
    tardive, 417
Albuterol, **572**
Alcohol
    drug interactions, 554, **555**
    early- vs. late-onset problems, 302
    intoxication in elderly, 305
    neurotoxicity, 304–305
    pathophysiological effects, 300
    protective value against heart disease,
        302–303
    side effects, **571**
    therapeutic use and health
        maintenance value, 302
    withdrawal, **284**, 285, 305–306, 558
    withdrawal delirium, 357
Alcohol abuse, 300. See also Alcoholism
    comorbidity with anxiety disorders,
        288
    incidence rates, 26
    management of, 309
    neuropsychiatric aspects, 302–303
    prevalence rates, 26, **26**
    reactive, 302
Alcohol-associated disorders
    dementia, 382
    insomnia, 307
    mood disorders, 307–308
    movement disorder, 308
    organic mental disorders
        epidemiology, 302
        management, 308–309
        neuropsychiatric aspects, 302–309
        subacute, 305–306

Alcohol use disorders
　clinical features, 303
　complications, 303
　course, 303–304
　epidemiology, 302
　neuropsychiatric aspects, 302–309
　psychiatric comorbidity in, 308
　screening and diagnosis, 303
Alcoholic cognitive deterioration,
　reversible, 306
Alcoholic dementia, 306–307, **307**
Alcoholism
　in anxiety, 288
　brain structure abnormalities, 9, 11
　chronic, 304, 305
　depressive symptoms, 307–308
　laboratory abnormalities, **303**, 303
　memory impairment of, 382
　mood symptoms, 252
　neuropsychology, 304
　prevalence of, 302
Alertness assessment, 113
Alexithymia, 83–84, **84**
Allocortex
　hippocampal, 74, **75**
　neuronal alterations in aging, 45, **49**
Alprazolam
　dependence, 309
　depression treatment, 665
　indications for, 609–610
　metabolism and dosing, 610, **611**
　pharmacokinetics of, **289**, 290
Alternating patterns/programs
　assessment, 118, **118**
Alzheimer's Association, 394–395
Alzheimer's disease
　affective syndromes, 246
　alcoholic dementia and, 306–307
　brain atrophy with, 42, **43**, **44**, **45**
　cholinergic challenge studies, 580
　cholinergic deficiency, 91
　classification, 390
　clinical features, **398**
　cognitive features, 391
　comorbidity, 27
　constructional disturbance, **136**, 137
　depressive symptoms, 247, 670–671
　diagnosis, 394
　differential diagnosis, 392
　in Down's syndrome, 46
　environmental risks, 391
　epidemiology, 390–391
　familial, 46
　frontal lobe dementia
　　differentiation, **398**
　hearing loss with, 61
　incidence rates, 26
　Lewy body variant of, 439
　MAO alterations, 57
　mood symptoms, 246–248
　mortality data, 22
　myoclonus in, 427
　neurochemistry of, 393
　neuroimaging studies, **392**, 392–393
　neuropathology, **38–39**, 40, 41, **41**,
　　46, 55, 57–58, 393–394

neuropsychiatric features, 391–392,
　394
neuropsychological profile, **139**,
　139–140
NINCDS criteria for, 51
olfactory deficits, 60
pathological overlap with aging,
　50–51
PET studies, 209
prevalence, 8
psychotherapy for patient caregivers,
　673–675, **674**
with psychotic symptoms, **264**, 265
rating scales, 108
risk factors, 390
serotonergic challenge studies, 583
sleep disturbances, 326, 328
thyrotropin-releasing hormone
　stimulation test in, 587
treatment, 394–395, 622–624
visual impairment, 61
white matter alterations, 51
Amantadine
　depression treatment, 443–444
　dopaminergic challenge studies, **585**,
　　585–586
　drug interactions, **605**, 605
　fatigue treatment, 530
　Parkinson's disease treatment, 437
　side effects, 558, **568**, **626**
Ambitendency, 103
Ambulation changes, 560
Amiloride, 608, **609**
γ-Aminobutyric acid. *See* GABA
Aminophylline, 608, **609**
Amitriptyline
　available preparations, 599, **599**
　contraindications, 248
　depression treatment, 255, 498
　drug metabolism and dosing, **445**,
　　600
　emotional lability treatment, 530
　neurological uses, 598–599
　pharmacological properties, **446**
　seizure threshold effect, **518**, 518
　side effects, 343, 446, 600, **601**
Amnesia. *See also* Memory impairment
　of Alzheimer's disease, 391
　clinical assessment, 122
　in ECT, 652–653
　with limbic system dysfunction, **82**
　nonverbal, **80**
　pharmacological challenge studies,
　　578
　posttraumatic, 482
　with thalamic nuclei dysfunction, 86
　verbal, **80**
Amoxapine
　available preparations, 599, **599**
　oral dose, **445**
　pharmacological properties, **446**
　seizure threshold effect, **518**, 518
　side effects, 446, 600, **601**
Amphetamines
　challenge studies, **578**, 581, **581**
　side effects, 561, **562**, **571**, **572**

Amphotericin B, **570**
Amusia, **80**
Amygdala-hippocampal complex
　atrophy, **169**, 169–170
Amyloid deposits, **41**, 46, 51, 394
Amyotrophic lateral sclerosis, 395, 400
Amytal interview, 102
Anafranil. *See* Clomipramine
Analgesics
　abuse, 313
　neuropsychiatric side effects, **568**
　pain treatment, 342
Anarithmetia, **80**
Androgens, effects on sexual function,
　561, **562**
Anergic-abulic states, 498
Anesthesia
　delirium with, 558
　ECT considerations, 646–647
　local blocks, 345
Aneurysms, 459–460
Angiotensin-converting enzyme
　inhibitors, 608, **609**
Animal models
　of delirium, 358
　neurobiology of aging, 62–63
　of traumatic brain injury, 491
Animal Naming Test, 138, 139
Anomia, 396, 441
Anosodiaphoria, 107
Anosognosia, 107
　definition, 467
　poststroke, 467–469, **473**
　　clinical correlates, 467–469
　　mechanism, 469
　　prevalence, 467–469
Anosognosia Questionnaire, 467, **468**
Anoxia
　brain injury with, 40
　effects in elderly, 531–532
　myoclonus after, 426
Antacids, **617**
Antiarrhythmics
　drug interactions, **602**
　side effects, 559, 561, **568**
Anticholinergics
　depression treatment, 443–444
　drug interactions, **602**, **617**
　Parkinson's disease treatment, 437
　side effects, 556–557, 558, 561, **562**,
　　569
Anticholinesterase, **572**
Anticoagulants, 554, **555**
Anticonvulsants
　advances, 12
　drug interactions, 518, **519**, **602**, **613**,
　　617
　pain treatment, 344
　side effects, 558, **569**, **626**
Antidepressants. *See also specific agents by
　name*; Tricyclic antidepressants
　anxiety relief, 290–291
　behavior treatment, **384**, 384
　depression treatment, 313, 465
　dosages, **445**
　drug interactions, 554, **555**

guidelines for use, **446**, 447
heterocyclic, 598–603
indications for, 598
mood changes with, 252
pain treatment, 343–344
panic disorder treatment, 313
pharmacodynamics, **553**
pharmacokinetics, 256
pharmacology, 255, **446**
seizure threshold effect, **518**, 518
side effects, 446, 465, 557, **569**, **626**
sleep disturbances treatment, 329
Antidiarrheals, **570**
Antiepileptic drugs, 512, 517, **517**
Antihistamines
    anxiety relief, 291, 613
    behavior treatment, 620, **621**
    drug interactions, **605**, 605
    side effects, **570**
Antihypertensives, 252, 557, 561, **562**,
    568, **602**, **605**, 605
Antimalarials, **570**
Antimanic drugs, 606–607
Antimicrobials, **570**
Antineoplastics, **571**
Antiparkinsonian drugs, 558, 559, **568**,
    605, 605
Antiphospholipid antibody syndrome,
    542
Antipsychotics
    alternatives, 617
    available preparations, 613–614, **614**
    behavior treatment, **384**, 384
    drug interactions, 617, **617**
    indications for, 613
    metabolism and dosing, 614
    neurological uses, 613
    pain treatment, 344
    seizure threshold effect, **518**, 518
    side effects, 344, 615, **616**
    special considerations in geriatric
        neuropsychiatry, 617
Antisocial personality, **26**
Antispasmodics, **569**
Anxiety
    about crime, 283
    in Alzheimer's disease, 246
    after concussion, 285
    definition, 280, 690
    differential diagnosis, 286–287, **287**
    drug-induced, 285, 451, 558, **568–574**
    evaluation of, 286
    generalized
        in Parkinson's disease, **442**, 448
        treatments, **292**
    laboratory investigations, 286
    with limbic system dysfunction, 82, **82**
    with medical illness, 10, **284**, 284–286
    morbid, 280
    neurobiology of, 283–284
    with neurotransmitter disturbances,
        90, **90**
    with pain, 338
    with Parkinson's disease, 248, 285
    pharmacological challenge studies,
        578

poststroke, 250, 285, 465–466, 472, **473**
    clinical correlates, 465–466
    frequency, 465
    mechanism, 465–466
    phenomenology, 465
    rating scales, 108, 286
    symptoms, 280, **280**
    after traumatic brain injury, 493
    treatment of, 289–292, 609–613
Anxiety disorders
    in alcoholics, 308
    brain structure and, **6**, 7, 9
    with chronic pain, 338–339
    complications of, 287–289
    DSM-IV classification, 280, **280**
    epidemiological studies, 280–281
    future research directions, 292–293
    medical illness and, 10
    neuropsychiatric aspects, 280–296
    in Parkinson's disease, 448
    phenomenology, 281–283
    prevalence, **26**, 281, **281**
    treatments, 291–292, **292**
Anxiolytics
    available preparations, 610, **611**
    indications for, 609–610
    metabolism and dosing, 610
    neurological uses, 610
    pain treatment, 344
Apathy, poststroke, 466–467, 472, **473**
    clinical correlates, 466
    clinical-pathological correlates,
        466–467
    mechanism of, 466–467
    prevalence, 466
Apathy Scale, **466**, 466
Aphasia, **80**, 122–123
Aphasia Screening Test, 138
Aphasia syndromes, 123, **123**
Apomorphine challenge studies, **585**,
    585–586
Appearance assessment, 101–102
Apperception, self-disturbances of, 106
Apraxia, 79, **80**, 120–121
Aprindine, **572**
Aprosodia, **80**
Arecoline challenge studies, **578**, 579,
    579
Arousal. *See also* Sleep
    assessment of, 113, 114
    basal forebrain regulation, 356
    brain stem regulation, 357
    central systems, 356
    hypothalamic-cortical regulation,
        356–357
    reduced, 121
    reticular activating system, 356
Arsenic, **572**
Arteriosclerosis, 44, **46–48**, 51–52, 52
Arteriosclerotic dementia, 371
Arteriosclerotic encephalopathy,
    subcortical, 374, 530–531
Arteriovenous malformations, brain
    changes with, 459–460
Arteritis, temporal, 540–541
Arthritis, prevalence rates, 27, **27**

Asendin. *See* Amoxapine
Asparaginase, **571**, **626**
Aspartame, **572**, **605**, 605
Aspirin, **626**
Association nuclei, 85–86, **87**
Asterixis, **409**
Astrocytes
    age-related alterations, 43, **46**, 49
    normal, 37, **37**
Astrocytomas, 524, 526
Atenolol, 360–361, **361**
Atherosclerosis
    age-related, 52, 63
    death rates, 21, **22**
    definition, 52
Atherosclerotic thrombosis, brain
    changes with, 459
Athetosis, 419
Atrophy
    brain, 41, **41–44**, 43
        generalized, **166**, 167, **168**
        imaging studies, **186–189**
        regional, 167–170, **169**
    cortical, **41**, 42
        age-related ratings, 166, **166**, **168**
        with chronic alcoholism, 305
    focal lobar, 395, **399**, 399–400
    multiple system, 424
Atropine, **569**, 570
Attention
    clinical assessment, **113**, 113–114
    neuropsychological assessment of,
        134–136, **135**
    neurotransmitter disturbances, 90, **90**
    pharmacological challenge studies,
        578
Attention disorders, clinical assessment,
    121–122
Auditory Consonant Trigrams, imaging
    correlation studies, **192–194**
Auditory evoked potentials, 220, 221
Auditory functions, age-related
    alterations, 60, 61
Autism, neurobiology of aging and, 62
Autonomic nervous system
    aging of, 58
    drug-induced dysfunction, **604**
Aventyl. *See* Nortriptyline
Avoidance patterns, with panic
    disorder, 282, **282**
Azathioprine, **571**
6-Azauridine, **571**
AZT. *See* Zidovudine

Back pain, anxiety with, 338
Baclofen
    GABA-ergic challenge studies,
        583–584, **584**
    side effects, **572**, **626**
    tardive dyskinesia treatment, 419
Bacterial infections
    in dementia, 379
    neuropsychiatric aspects, 539
Bacterial meningitis
    cerebrospinal fluid profile, **535**
    features, 539

Balance impairments, drug-related, 310
Balint's syndrome, 229–230
Barbiturates
    seizure threshold effect, **518**, 518
    side effects, 252, **569**, **571**
Basal forebrain, cholinergic
        projections, 356
Basal ganglia
    functional overview, 406–408, **407**
    tumor manifestations, 527
Basal ganglia-thalamocortical motor
        circuits, 406–408, **407**
Bear-Fedio Inventory, 515–516
Beck Anxiety Inventory, 286
BEHAVE-AD, 108
Behavior
    assessment of, 119
    neurobiological basis of, 72–96
    pharmacological challenge studies,
        578
    phenomenology of, 101
    violent, 83–84, **84**
Behavior therapy
    benefits of, 671
    for dementia, 670
    for pain relief, 345–346
Behavioral changes. *See also*
        Catastrophic reaction
    from chronic complex partial
        seizures, 107
    with dementia, 384, **384**, **385**
    drug treatment, 620, **621**
    with frontal-subcortical circuit
        disorders, 88–89, **89**
    and geriatric neuropsychiatry, 9–11,
        10
    ictally related, **512**, 512–513
    neurological diseases among elderly
        with, 8
    with neurotransmitter disturbances,
        90, **90**
    rating scales, 108
    after traumatic brain injury, 492
Behavioral disorders
    in epilepsy, **510**, 510, 516
        etiology and pathology, 516–517
        ictally related, **512**, 512–513
        neuropsychological, 512
        psychosocial, 511–512
    management of, 690
    neurochemical, 89–93
    prevention of, 689
    with thalamic nuclei dysfunction,
        86
    in traumatic brain injury, 494
Behavioral Inhibition System, 284
Behavioral neuroanatomy, Yakovlev
        model, 72–74, **73**
Behavioral neurology, geriatric
        neuropsychiatry comparison, 5–6
Behcet's syndrome, neuropsychiatric
        aspects, 542–543
Benton Facial Recognition Test, 174,
        192–194
Benton Visual Retention Test, **135**, 137
Benzene, **573**

Benzodiazepines. *See also specific drugs by
        name*
    abuse pattern, 309
    alternatives, 613
    antagonist challenge studies, **578**,
        583–584, **584**
    anxiety treatment, 289–290
    available preparations, 610, **611**
    challenge studies, **578**, 583–584, **584**
    dependence, 611–612
        epidemiology, 309–310
        neuropsychiatric aspects, 309–313
        symptoms, 309
        treatment, 312–313
    discontinuance phenomena, 309,
        310–312
    drug distribution changes with aging,
        10
    drug interactions, 612, **613**, **617**
    drug metabolism and dosing, 610
    hypnotics, **618**, 618
    long-term, 290, **290**, 312
    neurological uses, 610
    pain treatment, 344
    pharmacokinetics, **289**, 290
    psychiatric effects, 559–560, 611, **611**
    seizure threshold effect, **518**, 518
    sexual effects, 561, **562**
    side effects, 310, 344, 558, **569**, **571**
    sleep disturbances treatment, 329
    sleep disturbances with, 560–561
    special considerations in geriatric
        neuropsychiatry, 612
    withdrawal, 611–612
        effects, 558, 612, **612**
        outcome, 311–312
        signs and symptoms, 310–311
Benztropine, 437, **569**
Bereavement, sleep effects, 328
Beta-blockers
    for anxiety, 291
    behavior treatment, 620, **621**
    drug interactions, 608, **609**
    sleep disturbances with, 561
Beta power, age-related changes, 221
Bethanidine, **568**, **602**
Bibliotherapy, for depression, 666
Binswanger's disease, 51, **52**, 374,
        530–531
Biofeedback, 345
Biperidine, **568**
Bipolar disorder, DSM-III-R
        classification, 245
Black elderly. *See also* Elderly
    life expectancy, 20–21, **21**
    median income, 19–20
    mortality rates, 21
    population changes, 19, **19**
Black-white mortality crossover, 21
Bleomycin, **571**
Block Design Test, 136, 138, 174
Blood-brain barrier, age-related
        changes of, 53
Blood tests, **303**, 303
Blunting, affective, 103
Body size, effects on brain imaging, 161

Bon bon sign, 417
Borderzone infarction dementia, **373**,
        374
Boston Diagnostic Aphasia
        Examination, **135**, 138, 139
Boston Naming Test, 139, 141
Botulinum toxin, 419, 424
Bradyphrenia, 102, 442
Brain. *See also* Cerebral hemispheres
    abscess, **535**, 539
    aging, 7, 41, **41**
        anatomic imaging, 159–194
        cellular, **41**, 43–44, **46**
        genomic, 46–47
        molecular, 44–46, **46–48**
        neuronal, 38–40, **41**
        normal vs. abnormal, 36–38, **37**
        structural, 41–51
        transmitter systems, 53–58, **54**
    atrophy of, 41, **41**, **42**
        age-related, 42–43, **43–46**, 166,
            167–170, **168**, **186–189**
        with Alzheimer's disease, 42, **43–45**
        definition, 42
        drug-related, 310
        generalized, 167
        in multiple sclerosis, 529–530
        PET findings, **204**, 205
        regional, 167–170, **169**
    behavioral regions, 72
    ECT effects, 635, 650–651
    iron, 172–173
    late-life–onset schizophrenia
            changes, 267–271, **268**
    neuroimaging
        functional, 195–213
        methodological issues, 160–164
        parameters, 170–173
        quantitative, 164
        after traumatic brain injury,
            496–497
    qualitative measures, 164
    quantitative measures, 164
    RNA content, 49
    structural changes
        age-related, 41–51, 164–173,
            174–175
        with late-life–onset schizophrenia,
            267–269, **268**
    tissue imaging characteristics,
            171–172
    tumors
        anxiety with, 285
        EEG abnormalities, 524–525
        MRI abnormalities, 525, **525**
Brain diseases. *See also specific diseases
        and disorders by name*
    cost of, 9
    manifestations, 8, 41, **41**
    prevalence rates, 7
Brain dysfunction
    drug-induced, **604**
    neuropsychiatric syndromes
            associated with, 83–84, **84**
Brain injury. *See also* Traumatic brain
        injury

anoxic, 40
definition, 480
in old old, 488
primary, 483
secondary, 483–484
traumatic, 481–507
Brain reserve capacity, 500
Brain stem
aging, 40, **41**
neuronal groups, 357
tumor manifestations, 527
Brain stem auditory evoked potentials, 224
Bridling, 417
Brief Psychiatric Rating Scale, 108
Broca's area asymmetries, 78
Brodmann's areas, 74
Bromide, **573**
Bromocriptine
depression treatment, 443–444
dopaminergic challenge studies, **585**, 585–586
Parkinson's disease treatment, 437, 443–444
side effects, 558, **568**, **626**
Bronchitis, prevalence rates, **27**
Bronchodilators, sympathomimetic, 554, **555**
Brown-Peterson Interference Test, **192–194**
Bupropion
available preparations, 599, **599**
behavior treatment, **384**, 384
depression treatment, 249
drug interactions, **605**, 605
oral dose, **445**
pharmacological properties, **446**
seizure threshold effect, **518**, 518
sexual effects, 561, **562**
side effects, 447, **569**, 600, **601**
Buspirone
antidepressant properties, 613
for anxiety, 290
behavior treatment, **384**, 385, 620, **621**
for benzodiazepine withdrawal, 312
drug interactions, **602**
effects on sexual function, 561, **562**
neurological uses, 610
tardive dyskinesia treatment, 419
Butorphanol, **342**, 342–343
Butyrophenones, **569**, 613–614, **614**

Caffeine
anxiety-like symptoms with, 284, **284**
challenge studies, **578**
drug interactions, 608, **609**
and panic attacks, 283, 284
side effects, **571**, **572**
CAGE test, 303
Calcification
intracranial, 170–171
physiological, 171
Calcium
intracellular, 623–624
neuropsychiatric side effects, **573**

Calcium channel blockers
drug interactions, 608, **609**
experimental, 624, **625**
tardive dyskinesia treatment, 419
Calculation assessment, **113**, 116–117
California Verbal Learning Test, **135**, 137
CAMCOG, imaging correlation studies, **192–194**
Cancellation tests, visual, **135**, 135
Cancers
death rates, 21, **22**
incidence rates, 24
leading sites, 21, 24
psychotherapy for, 672
Cannabinols, **571**
Capgras syndrome, **105**, 105
Captopril
anticholinergic effects, 360–361, **361**
drug interactions, 554, **555**
side effects, 568, **626**
Carbamazepine
behavior treatment, **384**, 385, 620, **621**
for benzodiazepine withdrawal, 312
depression treatment, 498
drug interactions, 518, **519**, 554, **555**, 608, **609**, 617
mania treatment, 12, 608–609
seizure treatment, 517, **517**
side effects, **569**, 608–609, **609**
β-Carboline, GABA-ergic challenge studies, 583–584, **584**
Carbon dioxide
challenge studies, **578**
and panic attacks, 283
Carbon disulfide, **573**
Carbon monoxide, neuropsychiatric effects, 88–89, **89**, **573**
Carcinomatosis, meningeal, 380
Cardiac glycosides, neuropsychiatric side effects, **568**
Cardiovascular disease
with anxiety, 284, **284**
mood symptoms, 251–252
panic disorder with, 289
psychotherapy for, 672
Cardiovascular drugs
psychotic and affective symptoms, 558–559
side effects, 557
sleep disturbances with, 561
Cardiovascular system
age-related alterations, 63, **63**
ECT effects, 635–636, 649–650
Caregivers, psychotherapy for
empirical studies, 673–675, **674**
Cataracts, prevalence rates, **27**
Catastrophic reaction
in Alzheimer's disease, 247
definition, 469, 690
with lateralized brain dysfunction, 83–84, **84**
in stroke, 469–470, 472, **473**
Catastrophic Reaction Scale, 469, **469**

Catatonia
akinetic, 121
components of, 102–103
drug-related, 615, **616**
treatment, 620
Catecholamines, mechanism of action, 336
Category Test, **135**, 136
Caudate disorders, behavioral abnormalities associated with, 88–89, **89**
Center for Epidemiological Studies Depression Scale, 154–155
Central nervous system
age-related alterations, 58
alcohol sensitivity, 304
drug-related depression, 615, **616**
drug vulnerability, 551–552
infections, 533, **534**, 543
inflammatory disorders, 540–543, **541**
neuroendocrine probes, 586–587
peptide probes, 587–588
pharmacological probes, 579–586
radiation effects, 532
tumors, 524–527, 543
vasculitis, isolated, 541–542
Central nervous system depressants, drug interactions, **617**
Central nervous system stimulants, side effects, **572**
Cephalosporins, **570**
Cerebellar disease, tremor in, 410
Cerebellar outflow tremor, **409**, 410
Cerebellum
aging, 40, **41**
drug-induced ataxia, 562, **563**
Cerebral blood flow. *See also* Regional cerebral blood flow
MRI of, 173
PET of, 195–213
Cerebral embolism, 459
Cerebral glucose metabolism. *See also* Regional cerebral metabolic rate for glucose
age-related decrease, **205**, 205–206
PET studies, 197–198, **199**, 202–203, **203**
Cerebral hemispheres
age-related atrophy, **169**, 169–170
asymmetries
anatomic, 78–79
cognitive, 79–80, **80**
clinical deficits resulting from lesions, 79–80, **80**
dominance, 78–80
laterality, 78–80
specialization, 78–80
white matter
age-related alterations, 51–53
connections, 76–78, **78**
Cerebral metabolic rate for glucose. *See* Global gray cerebral metabolic rate for glucose; Regional cerebral metabolic rate for glucose
Cerebral metabolic rate for oxygen, PET studies, 199–202, **200–201**

Cerebral tumors, intellectual impairment pattern with, 380
Cerebrospinal fluid spaces, aging studies, **183–185**
Cerebrotendinous xanthomatosis, 533
Cerebrovascular diseases
    classification, 458–459
    death rates, 21, **22**
    diagnostic criteria, **372**
    with late-life–onset psychosis, **264**, 265
    neuropsychiatric aspects, 457–475
    prevalence rates, **27**
Chemotherapy
    and anxiety, 287
    neurological complications of, 532
Chemotherapy-related leukoencephalopathy, 532
Chest pain, anxiety with, 338–339
Chloral hydrate, **569, 571**
Chlorazepate, **569**
Chlordiazepoxide
    available preparations, 610, **611**
    metabolism and dosing, 610, **611**
    pharmacokinetics of, **289**, 290
    side effects, 290, **290**
Chlormethiazole, **553**
m-Chlorophenylpiperazine challenge studies, **582**, 582–583
Chlorpheniramine, **570**
Chlorpromazine
    available preparations, 613–614, **614**
    contraindications, 604
    drug interactions, 554, **555**
    seizure threshold effect, **518**, 518
Chlorpropamide, 554, **555**
Chlorprothixene, 613–614, **614**
Cholecystokinin challenge studies, **578**
Cholestyramine
    drug interactions, **602**
    effects on sexual function, 561, **562**
Choline
    challenge studies, 579, **579**
    neuropsychiatric effects, **573**
Cholinergic deficit, **41**
Cholinergic systems
    age-related alterations, 53–55, **54**
    challenge studies, 579, **579**
    magnocellular, 54
    pathways, 90–91, **91**, 356
    pharmacological probes of, 579–580
    in sleep, 329
Cholinergic therapies, indications for, 622–624
Choreas
    causes, 411, **411**
    definition, 411
    drug-induced, 562, **563**
    neuropsychiatric aspects, 411–419
    neurotransmitter disturbances, 90, **90**
    senile, 413, 415–416
    vascular, 416
Chronic conditions, prevalence of, 26–27, **27**
Chronic interictal schizophrenic disorder, **514**, 514–515
Chronic obstructive pulmonary disease

death rates, 21, **22**
panic disorder with, 286
Chronically mentally ill patients, neurobiology of aging in, 62
Cimetidine
    anticholinergic effects, 360–361, **361**
    drug interactions, 554, **555**, **602**, **613**, **617**
    side effects, **570**, 626
Ciprofloxacin, **570**
Circadian timekeeping, conceptual model, 324–325, **325**
Cisplatin, **626**
Clinical assessment
    introduction, 100
    of memory, 155–156
    purpose of, 100
Clinical history, 112–113
Clinical interview
    goal, 131
    style, 100–101
Clinical training, 6
Clomethiazole, **569**
Clomiphene citrate, **572**
Clomipramine
    for anxiety, 290–291
    available preparations, 599, **599**
    efficacy, 290
    seizure threshold effect, **518**, 518
    side effects, 600, **601**
Clonazepam
    behavior treatment, **384**, 385
    drug interactions, 518, **519**, 608, **609**
    indications for, 609
    metabolism and dosing, 610, **611**
    neurological uses, 610
    pharmacokinetics of, **289**, 290
    seizures treatment, 517, **517**
    side effects, **569**
Clonidine
    adrenergic challenge studies, 581, **581**
    for benzodiazepine withdrawal, 312
    drug interactions, 554, **555**, **602**
    effects on sexual function, 561, **562**
    neuropsychiatric side effects, **568**
    tardive dyskinesia treatment, 419
Clonus, **409**
Clorazepate
    available preparations, 610, **611**
    metabolism and dosing, 610, **611**
    pharmacokinetics of, **289**, 290
    side effects, 290, **290**
Clotrimazole, **570**
Clozapine
    available preparations, 613–614, **614**
    delusions treatment, 450
    drug interactions, **617**
    seizure threshold effect, **518**, 518
    side effects, **569**, 615
    tardive dyskinesia treatment, 419
Cobalamin (vitamin B$_{12}$), experimental therapy with, 624, **625**
Cobalamin (vitamin B$_{12}$) deficiency
    dementia caused by, 381
    mood symptoms, 252

Cocaine
    abuse, 313
    side effects, 561, **562, 572, 573**
Codeine
    anticholinergic effects, 360–361, **361**
    for pain treatment, **342**, 342–343
Coexisting dementia and depression, 255
Cognition, definition, 391
Cognitive-affective disorder, 255
Cognitive-behavior therapy
    for anxiety, 291–292
    for cancer, 672
    for depression, 663–666
    for depression in dementia, 669–670, 671
    efficacy, 677–678
    empirical studies, **664**
    future research directions, 677–678
    for pain, 345
    pharmacotherapy comparison, 665
    principles, 662
Cognitive dysfunction
    depression-related, 141
    in multiple sclerosis, **528**, 528–529
    after traumatic brain injury, 492
Cognitive function
    clinical assessment of, 120–121
    ECT effects, 651–653
    of hemispheres, 79–80, **80**
    neuropsychological tests of, 134–139, **135**
    pharmacological challenge studies, **578**
Cognitive impairment
    after alcohol withdrawal, 305–306
    depression-induced, 255, 461, **463**
    drug-induced, 310, 556–558, 608, **609**
    drug treatment, 620–622
    incidence rates, 26
    from lesions, 79–80, **80**
    not amounting to dementia, 150
    in Parkinson's disease, 441
    prevalence rates, 26, **26**
    psychotherapy for patient caregivers, 673–675, **674**
    rating scales, 108
    reversible alcoholic, 306
Cognitive impairment syndromes, assessment of, 121–124
Cognitive reserve capacity, 500
Cognitive restructuring techniques, 291
Coherence
    FASCICLE-PA measure, 228–229, **231**
    qEEG measure, 227–230, **231, 232**, 233–234
    VISUAL measure, 228–229, **232**
Collagen-vascular diseases
    mood changes with, 252
    neuropsychiatric aspects, 542–543
Commonwealth-Harvard study on delirium, 355
Comorbidity, 27
Complex partial seizures, 510, **511**
Compliance, 551
Comprehension assessment, 115

Computed tomography
  advances in, 11
  of aging brain, 159–194
    brain tissue characteristics, 171–172
    intracranial calcification, 170–171
    neuropsychological correlations, 174
    plane of imaging, 163
    studies, **179–182, 183–185, 186–189**
  in Alzheimer's disease, **392**, 392
  with brain tumors, 525
  with depression-induced cognitive impairment, 255
  in frontal lobe dementia, **392**
  in Huntington's disease, 412–413, **413**
  with mood disorders, 253–254
  neuropsychological correlations studies, **192–194**
  in Parkinson's disease, 441
  sensitivity and specificity, 246
  after traumatic brain injury, 496–497
  X-ray, 162
Concentration assessment, 113–114, 122
Concordance, 227, **229**
Concussion, 285, 482
Confusion. *See also* Delirium
  drug-related, 450, 556–558, **604**, 608, **609, 613, 617, 626**
  with neurotransmitter disturbances, 90, **90**
  in Parkinson's disease, **442**
Confusion Assessment Method, 353
Consciousness
  clouding, 363
  level of, 113
Consortium to Establish a Registry of Alzheimer's Disease, word list learning test, 155
Constructional disturbance, **80**
Content (term), 101
Continuous performance, 114
Continuous Performance Test, 135
Contraceptives. *See* Oral contraceptives
Contrecoup injuries, 483
Controlled Oral Word Association Test, 138
Conversion hysteria, 83–84, **84**
Copulatory dyskinesia, 417
Cordance mapping, 227, **228, 229**, 234
  in depression, 227, **230**
Cornell Scale for Depression in Dementia, 247
Coronary artery disease, alcohol-protective hypothesis, 303
Coronary heart disease, incidence rates, 24
Corpora amylacea, 44
Cortex. *See also* Neocortex
  age-related alterations, 40, **40, 41**, 41, **49**
  anterior cingulate, **88**, 88
  atrophy of, **41**, 42
    age-related ratings, 166, **166, 168**
    with chronic alcoholism, 305
  cerebral
    deafferentation, **226**, 226–227, **228**

  subcortical connections, 85–89
  dorsolateral prefrontal circuits, **87**, 87–88, **88**
  frontal subcortical circuits, 86–89, **87, 88**
    behavioral abnormalities associated with, 88–89, **89**
    neurobehavioral syndromes associated with, 87–88
  heteromodal association, 75, **77**
  histological organization, 74, **74**
  mesial temporal, **38–39**, 40, **40**, 51
  motor circuit, 86–87
  multimodal association, **75**
  oculomotor circuit, 87
  orbitofrontal, **88**, 88
  paralimbic, 74, **75**, 81
  primary auditory, 74
  primary motor, 74, **75, 76**
  primary sensory, **75, 76**
  primary somatosensory, 74
  primary visual, 74
  role in regulation of sleep and arousal, 356–357
  temporal asymmetries, 78–79, **79**
  thalamic relationships, 85–86, **86**
  unimodal association areas, 75, **75, 76**
Cortical dementia, 440, **440**
Corticosteroids, side effects, 559, **571, 572**
Corticotropin-releasing factor, age-related alterations, 57
Corticotropin-releasing hormone stimulation test, 586–587
Costs
  of brain disorders, 9
  of nursing homes, 684
Cotard's syndrome, **105**, 105
Coumarins, **553**
CPSs. *See* Complex partial seizures
Cranial dystonia, 422
Creutzfeldt-Jakob disease
  cerebrospinal fluid profile, 534, **535**
  clinical course, 534
  in dementia, 379
  diagnosis of, 383
  incidence of, 534
  myoclonus in, 426–427
  neuropathology, 534
Crime, anxiety about, 283
CT. *See* Computed tomography
Cushing's syndrome, anxiety-like symptoms, **284**, 285
Cyanocobalamin deficiency, dementia caused by, 381
Cyclobenzaprine, **573**
Cyclophosphamide, **626**
Cycloserine, **570**
Cyclosporin A, **573**
Cyclothymia, DSM-III-R classification, 245
Cylert. *See* Pemoline
Cyproheptadine, **573**
Cytoskeleton, age-related alterations, 45–46

Danazol, **572**
Dapsone, **570**
de Clerambault syndrome, **105**, 105
Deafferentation
  cortical, **226**, 226–227, **228**
  qEEG diagnosis of, 230–232
Death, leading causes in elderly, 21, **22**
Debrisiquin, **602**
Decision making rights, of elderly, 12–13
Decongestants, mood changes with, 252
Deformity or orthopedic impairment, prevalence rates, **27**
Delayed Recall Index, 153, 155
Delirious mania, 255
Delirium
  activated patients, 354, **355**, 363
  agitated, 467
  animal models, 358
  classification of states, 265
  dementia and, 360
  depressive, 513, 515
  diagnosis of, 224, 352–355
  diagnostic criteria, **450**
  differentiating subtypes, 355
  drug-induced, 360–361, 450, 556–558, **568–574**
  DSM-IV criteria, **352**, 352
  EEG findings, 218, 357–358
  epidemiology, 355–356
  etiology, 354–355, 358, **359**
  hyperalert/hyperactive patients, 354
  hypoalert/hypoactive patients, 354
  interictal, 652
  mood changes with, 252
  neurobiology of, 356–357
  neuropsychiatric aspects, 351–365
  neurotransmitter disturbances, 90, **90**
  in Parkinson's disease, **442**
  pathophysiology, 357–358
  phenomenology, 354
  qEEG diagnosis and assessment, 224
  risk factors, 358–360, **359**
  sedative-hypnotic withdrawal, 357
  somnolent patients, 354, **355**, 363
  symptoms of, 356
  terminology, 352–355
  treatment of, 361–363, **362**, 619–620
Delusions
  assessment of, 104–105
  brain structure and, 9
  common themes, 105, **105**
  definition, 105
  drug-related, 449–450
  management of, 449–450
  mood-congruent, 244
  with neurotransmitter disturbances, 90, **90**
  in Parkinson's disease, **442**
  in stroke, 467
Dementia. *See also* Frontal lobe dementias; Multi-infarct dementia; Vascular dementia
  in adrenoleukodystrophy, 533
  alcoholic, 306–308, **307**, 382
  anxiety-like symptoms, 285

Dementia *(continued)*
    arteriosclerotic, 371
    behavior disturbances, 8
        drug treatment, **384**, 384, **385**, 620,
            621
        ECT treatment, 640–641
        precipitating features, 688
        predisposing features, 688
    brain structure and, 9
    clinical features, 440, **440**
    definition, 377, 438–439
    and delirium, 360
    depression and, 247
    diagnostic criteria, **372**, **438**, 438
    differential diagnosis, 621
    as disease, 684
    EEG findings, 217, **219**, **222**, **229**, 383
    epidemiology of, 24–26
    HIV-1–associated, 538
    in Huntington's disease, 414–415
    hydrocephalic, 376–377
    hypoperfusion of watershed
        (borderzone infarction), **373**,
        374
    incidence rates, 25–26
    infectious disorders in, 379–380
    laboratory studies, 383, **383**
    lacking distinctive histologic features,
        395, 399, **399**
    mixed, 371
    neoplasia-associated, 380–381
    neuroimaging studies, 383, **383**
    neuropsychiatric symptoms, 370
    neuropsychological profiles, **139**,
        139–140
    neurotransmitter disturbances, 55,
        90, **90**
    nondegenerative causes, 370, **371**,
        384–385
    in nursing homes, 685
    nutritional causes, 370, **371**, 381–382
    paraneoplastic, 381
    in Parkinson's disease, 437–442
    population-based studies, 25–26
    posttraumatic, 370, **371**, 382
    prevalence of, 8, 24–25, 685
    prevention of, 689
    psychotherapy for patient caregivers,
        673–675, **674**
    qEEG diagnosis, 221–224
    questionable, 150
    in schizophrenia, 379
    seizures in, 512
    senile, 437, 552
    sleep disturbances, 328
    small-vessel disease, **373**, 374
    standard evaluation, 382–383, **383**
    strategic single-infarct, **373**, 373–374
    subcortical, **139**, 140, 374, 439, 440,
        440
    survival rates, 22
    systemic diseases that lead to, 392
    treatment of
        considerations for, 383–384
        electroconvulsive therapy, 448
        experimental, 624, **625**

    in nursing homes, 689–690
    pharmacotherapy, 600, 620–622,
        624
    true, 377
Dementia care units, 687–688
Dementia-like syndrome, **568–574**
Dementia of the Alzheimer type. *See
    also* Alzheimer's disease
    disconnection in, 229–230
    qEEG diagnosis, 221–224, 227–230,
        228, **231**, **232**
    sleep disturbances, 326
Dementia syndrome of depression
    classification, 370, **371**
    definition, 255, 377
    diagnosis, 378
    neuroimaging findings, 378
    neuropsychological profile, **139**, 141,
        377–379
    prognosis, 378
Demographics
    of aging, 8
    of traumatic brain injury, 489, **489**
Demyelination
    causes, 527, **528**, 543
    disorders, 527–533
Denial of Illness Scale, 467, **468**
Dependence. *See also* Addiction
    benzodiazepine, 309–313
    nicotine, 314–315
        in alcoholics, 308
Depersonalization, 106
Depigmentation, **56–57**
Deprenyl
    anxiety relief, 451
    for depression, 443–444
    side effects, 447
L-Deprenyl. *See* Selegiline
Depressants, withdrawal effects, 612,
    612
Depression. *See also* Dementia
    syndrome of depression; Major
    depression
    adjustment disorder with, 245
    in alcoholics, 307–308
    in Alzheimer's disease, 246, 247–248,
        251, 391
    biological markers, 253
    brain structure abnormalities, 9, 11
    with cardiovascular disease, 251–252
    with chronic pain, 337–338
    cognitive dysfunction with, 141, 255
    comorbidity, 27
    cordance mapping, 227, **230**
    CT abnormalities, 253–254
    and dementia, 247
    differential diagnosis, 286–287, **287**
    dopamine association, 91
    drug-related, 252, 450, 558–560,
        568–574, **626**
    EEG abnormalities, 217–218
    in epilepsy, 515
    frontal-subcortical circuit disorders,
        88–89, **89**
    full, 445, **445**
    incidence rates, 26

    late-onset
        brain changes, **268**
        PET changes, 270
    life events effects on, 326–327
    limbic system dysfunction, **82**
    masked, 338
    medical illness and, 10
    minor, 245, 250
    MRI abnormalities, **230**, 254
    with multi-infarct dementia, 251
    in multiple sclerosis, **528**, 529
    neurobiology of aging with, 62
    neurotransmitter deficits, 90, **90**, 338
    in nursing homes, 686–687
    organic mental disorder with, 141
    in Parkinson's disease, 248–249, 285,
        443–448, 598
        clinical features, 443
        electroconvulsive therapy for,
            447–448
        general considerations, 443
        model for, 249
        pathophysiology, 443
        pharmacotherapy for, 443–447
        prevalence, **442**
        subtypes, 445, **445**
        treatment, 249
    partial, 445, **445**
    PET studies, 209, **210**
    pharmacological challenge studies,
        578
    poststroke, 6, **6**, 460–465, 472, **473**,
        598
        clinical correlates, 460–461, **462**,
            463
        clinical-pathological correlates,
            462–465, **464**
        diagnosis of, 250
        ECT treatment, 644
        features, 250
        frequency, 460
        mechanism, 462–465, **464**
        phenomenology, 460, **461**
        prevalence rates, 249–250
        treatment, 251, 465, **465**
    psychosocial effects, 326
    rating scales, 108
    as series of behaviors, 669
    sleep effects, 324, 328
    symptoms, 244–245, **245**
    with thyroid disturbance, 252
    after traumatic brain injury, 252, 493
        diagnostic process and tools, 496
        pharmacotherapy, 498
    treatment of, 255–256, 530
        bibliotherapy, 666
        electroconvulsive therapy, 634
        in nursing homes, 686–687
        psychotherapy, 663–669
        stimulants, 605
    with vitamin deficiencies, 252
    white matter alterations, 51
Depressive delirium, 513, 515
Depressive pseudodementia, 209
Depressive stupor, 255
Depth perception, reduced, **80**

Derailment, 104
Derealization, 106
Descriptive phenomenology, definition, 101
Descriptive psychopathology, definition, 101
Desensitization therapy, for anxiety, 292
Design fluency, **80**, 119
Desipramine
    adrenergic challenge studies, 581, **581**
    available preparations, 599, **599**
    behavior treatment in dementia, **384**, 384
    for depression in Parkinson's disease, 249
    drug interactions, 554, **555**
    drug metabolism and dosing, **445**, 600
    pharmacological properties, **446**
    seizure threshold effect, **518**, 518
    side effects, 446
Deslanoside, **553**
Desyrel. See Trazodone
Dexamethasone, nonsuppression theories, 586–587
Dexamethasone suppression test, 249, 586–587
Dexedrine. See Dextroamphetamine
Dextroamphetamine
    available preparations, **605**
    seizure threshold effect, **518**, 518
Dextromethorphan
    behavior treatment, 620, **621**
    psychiatric side effects of, **626**
Diabetes mellitus
    anxiety-like symptoms, **284**, 285
    death rates, 21, **22**
    prevalence rates, **27**
Diazepam
    antidepressant benefits, 255
    available preparations, 610, **611**
    dependence, 309
    metabolism and dosing, 610, **611**
    neurological uses, 610
    pharmacodynamics, **553**
    pharmacokinetics, **289**, 290
    side effects, 290, **290**
    tardive dyskinesia treatment, 419
Diazepam-binding inhibitor, 358
Dibenzodiazepine, 613–614, **614**
Dibenzoxazepine, 613–614, **614**
Dichloralphenazone, **553**
Dicyclomine, **569**
Diet
    and anxiety, 284, **284**
    and dementia, 370, **371**, 381–382
Diethyl-m-toluamide, **573**
Diethylpropion, **572**
Differential diagnosis, neuropsychological testing in, 139–141
Diffuse Lewy body disease, 439
Digit Span Test, 113–114, **135**, 135, **192–194**, 354
Digit Symbol Test, 174, **192–194**
Digitalis, 559

Digoxin
    drug interactions, 554, **555**
    side effects, 360–361, **361**, 557, 559, **626**
Dihydroergotamine, 376
Dihydroindolone, 613–614, **614**
Diltiazem
    anticholinergic effects, 360–361, **361**
    drug interactions, 554, **555**
    neuropsychiatric side effects, **573**
    pharmacodynamics, **553**
Diogenes syndrome, 303
Diphenhydramine
    for anxiety, 291
    pharmacodynamics, **553**
    side effects, **570**
Diphenoxylate, **570**, 573
Diphenylbutylpiperidine, **614**
Dipyridamole, 360–361, **361**
Disability, definition of, 688
Disconnection, in dementia of the Alzheimer type, 229–230
Disconnection syndromes
    qEEG diagnosis of, 227–230, **231**, **232**
    related fiber tracts, 77–78, **78**
Discontinuance phenomena, 309, 310–312
Discordance, 227
Disopyramide, **568**
Disorientation
    acute postictal, 651–652
    right-left, 121
Dissociation, in epilepsy, 516
Disulfiram
    drug interactions, 554, **555**, **602**
    effects on sexual function, 561, **562**
    neuropsychiatric side effects, **573**
Diuretics. See also Thiazide diuretics
    effects on sexual function, 561, **562**
DNA, age-related alterations, 50
DNA markers, for Huntington's disease, 413
Do-not-resuscitate (DNR) status, 653–654
Dopamine
    age-related changes, 54, **54**, 57
    behavioral alterations associated with, 90, **90**
    disorders associated with, 91
    mechanism of action, 336
    origins and destinations, 90, **90**
    tardive dyskinesia treatment with antagonists, 419
Dopamine β-hydroxylase levels, 55
Dopaminergic systems
    age-related alterations, **54**, 56–57, **56–57**
    challenge studies, 584–586, **585**
    pathways, 91, **91**
Dorsolateral frontal convexity syndrome, **124**, 124
Down's syndrome, 46, 390
Doxepin
    antidepressant benefits, 255
    available preparations, 599, **599**
    behavior treatment, **384**, 384

oral dose, **445**
pharmacological properties, **446**
seizure threshold effect, **518**, 518
side effects, 600, **601**
Dressing apraxia, 121
Dressing disturbance, **80**
Drive assessment, **118**, 118
Driving, as ethical issue, 12
Drug abuse. See also Substance abuse
    in alcoholics, 308
    underrecognition of, 556
Drug holidays, 418
Drugs. See also Pharmacotherapy; specific drugs by name, by class
    absorption, 552, **554**
    adverse effects, **284**, 285, 551–552
    anticholinergic effects, 360, **361**
    associated with neuropsychiatric syndromes, 556–562
    CNS vulnerability to, 551–552
    disposition factors in elderly, **554**
    distribution, 553, **554**
    drug interactions, 255–256, 554, **555**
    elimination half-life, 597
    excretion, 553–554, **554**
    and geriatric neuropsychiatry, 9–11, **10**
    metabolism, 10–11, 553–554, **554**, 597
    mood changes with, 252
    in nursing homes, 686–687
    over-the-counter, 550, 556
    pharmacodynamics, **553**
        CNS vulnerability, 551–552
        definition, 596
    pharmacokinetics, 336, 552–554, 596
    polypharmacy effects, 554, **555**
    prescription
        effects on sexual function, 561, **562**
        factors to consider with elderly patients, 563
        frequency of use, 550
        most frequently prescribed, **550**, 550
        in nursing homes, 686–687
        that produce anxiety, 285
    side effects, 255–256, 426, 624, **626**
    steady state concentration, 597
    that produce tremor, 410
    toxicity, 360–361, 382
    use
        effects on brain imaging, 162
        by elderly, 10
        frequency of, 550
    volume of distribution, 596
DST. See Dexamethasone suppression test
Dyazide, 360–361, **361**
Dynamic psychotherapy, for anxiety disorders, 291
Dyscalculia, assessment of, 117
Dyskinesia
    copulatory, 417
    drug-induced, 562, **563**
    spontaneous orofacial, 415
    tardive, 416–419
Dyslexia, neurobiology of aging with, 62

Dysmegaiopsia, 106
Dysphonia, spasmodic, 422
Dysprosody
    affective, 83–84, **84**
    motor, 103
Dysthymia
    diagnostic criteria, **444, 460**
    DSM-III-R classification, 245
    with pain, 338
Dystonia
    axial, 423
    classification, 421
    cranial, 422
    disorders that simulate, **421**
    drug-related, 423, 562, **563**, 615, **616**
    etiology, 421, **421**
    focal, 421–422
    generalized, 421
    idiopathic, 421–422, **421**, 423
    multifocal, 421
    neuropsychiatric aspects, 419–424
    oromandibular, 413, **414**, 422
    psychogenic, 424
    secondary, **421**, 423–424
    segmental, 421
    task-specific, 422
    transient, 423
    treatment, 424
Dystonic tremor, 419
Dystrophic neurites, 46, **49**, 50

Early-onset schizophrenia, brain
        changes, **268**
Eating disorders, in Alzheimer's
        disease, 391
Echo de pensees, 106
Echopraxia, 103
Edentulous orodyskinesia, 415
Education
    agenda for, 13
    effects on brain imaging, 161–162
    of elderly women, 30
Elation
    in Alzheimer's disease, 246
    with neurotransmitter disturbances,
        90, **90**
Elavil. *See* Amitriptyline
Eldepryl. *See* Selegiline
Elderly
    ADL and IADL independence, 29, **29**
    ADL and IADL limitations, 28, **28**, **29**
    decisionmaking rights of, 12–13
    definition, 18, 550
    functional limitations of, 27–28
    health diversity of, 29–30
    institutionalization of, 28–29
    leading causes of death in, 21, **22**
    life expectancy of, 20–21, **21**
    living arrangements, 19
    marital status, 19
    median income, 19–20
    mortality rates, 21–23, **22**, **23**
    neurological diseases with behavioral
        manifestations among, 8
    neuropsychiatric aspects of
        neurological disease in, 367–574

neuropsychiatric aspects of
        psychiatric disorders in, 241–365
neuropsychiatric assessment of,
        97–109
    population, 8, 20, **20**
    psychiatric illness in, 8–9
    racial composition of, 19, **19**
    sex ratio, 19, **20**
Elderly early-onset schizophrenia
    classification, 264, **264**
    definition, 264
    symptoms, 263, **264**
Elderly men
    alcohol abuse incidence, 26
    life expectancy, 20–21, **21**
    living arrangements, 19
    marital status, 19
    median income, 19–20
    mental disorders prevalence, 26, **26**
    mortality rates, 21
    in nursing homes, 29, **29**
    risk of heart disease in, 24
    sexual decline, 59
    suicide rates, 26
Elderly women
    ADL and IADL limitations, 28
    alcohol abuse incidence, 26
    education of, 30
    heart disease risk, 24
    life expectancy, 20–21, **21**
    living arrangements, 19
    marital status, 19
    median income, 19–20
    mental disorders prevalence, 26, **26**
    mortality rates, 21
    in nursing homes, 29, **29**
Electroconvulsive therapy (ECT)
    adverse effects of, 649–653
        amnestic, 653
        cardiovascular, 649–650
        cerebral, 650–651
        cognitive, 651–653
    anesthesia considerations, 646–647
    cardiovascular physiology, 635–636
    cerebral physiology, 635
    with concomitant neurological
        disease, 640–644
    for depression, 249, 251, 256,
        447–448
    efficacy, 636–644
    in geriatric practice, 634
    indications for, 634, 636–644
    informed consent procedure, 646
    issues relevant to elderly patients,
        644–649
    maintenance, 648–649
    malpractice litigation, 651
    for mania, 256, 608
    medical physiology in elderly,
        634–636
    medicolegal issues, 653–654
    pharmacological issues, 645–646
    pre-ECT evaluation, 644–646
    principles, 633–659
    psychiatric uses, 447
    psychosocial issues, 653–654

risk factors, 651
    studies, **637–639**
    technique, 646, 647–648
Electroencephalography
    advantages of, 216
    with brain tumors, 524–525
    conventional, 216–218
    with delirium, 353, 357–358
    with dementia, 383
    desynchronized, 220
    history of, 216
    limitations of, 216
    neurophysiology of abnormalities,
        226–227
    rate of use, 218
    synchronized, 220
Embolism, cerebral, 459
Emotion, hemisphericity of, 83–84
Emotional incontinence, 245, 470
Emotional lability
    in Alzheimer's disease, 246
    description, 245–246
    in multiple sclerosis, **528**, 529
    in stroke, 470–471, **473**
    treatment, 530
Emotional state assessment, 103–104
Enalapril, **553**
Encephalitis
    herpes simplex, 536
    paraneoplastic limbic, 527
Encephalomalacia, subcortical, 51
Encephalomyelitis, acute disseminated,
        530
Encephalopathy
    dementing metabolic and toxic, 370,
        371, 381–382
    hepatic, 224
    subcortical arteriosclerotic, 374,
        530–531
Endep. *See* Amitriptyline
Endocrine agents, side effects, **572**
Endocrine disorders
    anxiety-like symptoms, **284**, 285
    mood changes, 252
Endocrine system, responses to
        dexamethasone suppression test,
        586–587
Enkephalin, 93
Environmental agnosia, **80**, 83–84, **84**
Ephedrine, **572**
Epidemiologic Catchment Area
        Program, 26, **26**, 280–281, 324
Epidemiology. *See also specific measures by
        name*
    of aging, 18–33
    of chronic conditions, 26–27
    of neuropsychiatric disorders, 24–26
    risk measures, 23–24
Epidural abscess, neuropsychiatric
        aspects, 539
Epilepsia partialis continua, **409**
Epilepsy
    behavioral disorders in, **510**, 510, 516
        etiology, 516–517
        pathology, 516–517
    clinical aspects, 510–511

definitions, 510
demography, 510
depression in, 515
interictal psychopathology, 513–517
interictal psychosis, 513–515
mood changes with, 252
neuropsychiatric aspects, 509–521
personality characteristics, 515–516
posttraumatic, 484
progressive myoclonic, 424
psychiatric disturbances in, 516–517, **517**
schizophreniform psychosis in, 513–515
suicide in, 515
treatment, 517–519
Epileptic discharges, periodic lateralizing, 512–513
Epileptic myoclonus, 424
Epileptic seizures. *See also* Seizures
classification, 510–511, **511**
differential diagnosis, 511
Epinephrine, **572**
Episodic dyscontrol, in epilepsy, 516
Erotomania, **105**, 105
Estazolam, **618**, 618
Estrogens, effects on sexual function, 561, **562**
Etat lacunaire (lacunar state), 374
Ethanol. *See also* Alcohol
side effects, **569**
Ethchlorvynol, seizure threshold effect, **518**, 518
Ethical issues, 12–13
Ethionamide, **570**
Ethosuximide
drug interactions, 518, **519**
seizures treatment, 517, **517**
side effects, **569**
Euphoria
with lateralized brain dysfunction, 83–84, **84**
in multiple sclerosis, **528**, 529
Euthanasia, 12
Eutonyl. *See* Pargyline
Evoked potentials
age-related changes, 220–221
auditory, 220, 221
clinical usefulness, 233, 234
diagnosis of deafferentation with, 230–232
diagnosis of delirium with, 224
diagnosis of dementia with, 223
endogenous or cognitive, 220
P300 latency measures, 223–224
somatosensory, 220, 221, 224, 230
stimulus bound or exogenous, 220
visual, 220, 221, 224
Executive Interview, 108
Executive skills
categories of, **118**, 118
clinical assessment, **113**, 117–120
impairments
in frontal lobe dementia, 396
in multiple sclerosis, 529
in Parkinson's disease, 441

neuropsychological assessment, **135**, 136–137
Exposure, for management of phobias, 291
Extended Scale for Dementia, imaging correlation studies, **192–194**

Facial discrimination, impaired, **80**
Facial Recognition Test, **135**, 138
Fahr's disease, behavioral abnormalities associated with, 88–89, **89**
Falls, drug-related, 310, **617**
Family considerations, after traumatic brain injury, 499–500
Family history, and late-onset schizophrenia, 265–266, **266**
Famous Events Test, 137
Famous Faces Test, 137
FASCICLE-PA measure, 228–229, **231**
Fatigue
in multiple sclerosis, **528**, 529
treatment, 530
FDG. *See* Fluorodeoxyglucose
Fear. *See also* Paranoia
of victimization, 283
Fenfluramine
effects on sexual function, 561, **562**
serotonergic challenge studies, **582**, 582–583
side effects, **572**
Fetal tissue transplantation
intrastriatal grafting, 437
Parkinson's disease treatment, 249
Fibroblast growth factor, 59
Fight or flight response, 283, 581
Finger Oscillation Test, **135**, 138
Fixed test batteries, 132–134
Flavoxate, **571**
Fluorodeoxyglucose, cerebral metabolism, 197–198, **199**
Fluoxetine
available preparations, 599, **599**
behavior treatment, **384**, 385, 620, **621**
drug interactions, 608, **609**
efficacy, 291
emotional lability treatment, 530
neurological uses, 599
oral dose, **445**
pain treatment, 344
pharmacological properties, **446**
seizure threshold effect, **518**, 518
side effects, 446–447, 561, **562**, **569**
Fluphenazine
for anxiety, 291
available preparations, 613–614, **614**
seizure threshold effect, **518**, 518
Flurazepam, 290, **290**, **618**, 618
Flutamide, **573**
Fly-catcher's tongue, 417
Focal lobar atrophy, 395, **399**, 399–400
Folic acid deficiency
dementia caused by, 381–382
mood symptoms, 252
Forebrain, basal cholinergic projections, 356

Forgetfulness. *See also* Amnesia; Memory impairment
age-inappropriate, 150–151
benign senescent, 146, 148, 154
late-life, 147, 153–154
senescent, 149, 150
Form (term), 101
Formication, 107
Foster homes, alcohol-free, 309
Fourier transformation, 219
Framingham Heart Study, 24
Fregoli syndrome, 105, **105**
Fries, James, theories of aging, 36
Frontal lobe atrophy, age-related, **169**, 169–170
Frontal lobe dementias
classification, 390
clinical features, 395–397, 397–401, **398**
differential diagnosis, **398**
epidemiology, 395
neuroimaging studies, **392**
neuropathological findings, 397
neuropsychological profile, **139**, 140
non-Alzheimer type, 395, 399, **399**
nosology, 395
pathological features, 397–401
primary, **399**
secondary, **399**, 400–401
Frontal lobe disorders
clinical assessment, 123–124
neuropsychiatric symptoms, **124**, 124
Frontal lobe dysfunction
pseudo-depressed personality disorders of, 395
pseudo-psychopathic personality disorders of, 395
Frontal lobe tumors, neuropsychiatric manifestations, 526
Frontal-subcortical circuit disorders, behavioral changes, 88–89, **89**
Functional assessment, 125
Functional impairment, threshold for, 500
Fungal infections, neuropsychiatric aspects, 539
Fungal meningitis, cerebrospinal fluid profile, **535**
Furosemide
anticholinergic effects, 360–361, **361**
drug interactions, 554, **555**, 608, **609**
pharmacodynamics, **553**

GABA, mechanism of action, 336
GABAergic systems
age-related alterations, 58
challenge studies, 583–584, **584**
pathways, 90, **90**, 92
Gait disorders, drug-induced, 560
Galveston Orientation and Amnesia Test, 482
Gate theory, of pain medication, 335
Gedankenlautwerden, 106
Gender factors
brain imaging, 161
late-onset schizophrenia, 266, **266**

Gender factors *(continued)*
PET studies, **204**, 205
psychiatric disorders, 9
General anesthetics, drug interactions, **605**, 605
General Memory Index, 153
Generalized anxiety
in Parkinson's disease, **442**, 448
treatments, **292**
Generalized tonic-clonic seizures, classification, 510, **511**
Genomic function, age-related alterations, 46–50
Gepirone, 613
Geriatric Depression Scale, 108
Geriatric neuropsychiatry
behavioral neurology comparison, 5–6
clinical training, 6
convergent results, **6**, 6–7
definition, 4
as discipline, 4–6, **5**
education agenda, 13
emergence and growth of, 7
ethical issues, 12–13
introduction, 4–15
medical illness and, 9–11, **10**
medications and, 9–11, **10**
neuroimaging advances, 11–12
neuropsychiatry comparison, 4–5
patient care agenda, 13
PET in, 208–209
psychiatry comparison, 5
research agenda, 13
treatment advances, 12
Geriatric neuropsychology, methodological issues, 130–131
Gerstmann-Straüssler-Scheinker syndrome, 533–534
Gerstmann's syndrome, 526
Geste antagoniste, 422
Gilles de la Tourette syndrome, 428, 449
Glasgow Coma Scale, 113, **481**, 481
Glasgow Outcome Scale, 482
Gliosis, progressive subcortical
classification, **399**
clinical and pathological features, 399
definition, 395
Global Deterioration Scale, 125
Global gray cerebral metabolic rate for glucose, age-related decrease, **205**, 205–206
Globus pallidus disorders, behavioral abnormalities associated with, 88–89, **89**
Glucose
cerebral metabolism. *See also* Regional cerebral metabolic rate for glucose
age-related decrease, **205**, 205–206
PET studies of, 197–198, **199**, 202–203, **203**
challenge studies, **578**
Glutamate
origins and destinations, 90, **90**
projection system, 92–93

Glutamate receptors, age-related alterations, 58
L-Glutamine, **573**
Glutethimide, seizure threshold effect, **518**, 518
Glycine, 93
Gompertz Law, 36
Grand mal seizures, 510
Grandeur, delusions of, **105**, 105
Granulomatous angiitis, 541–542
Granulovacular degenerations, 44, **46–48**
Graying of the population, **18**, 18–20
Griseofulvin, **570**
Grooved Pegboard Test, **135**, 138
Group therapy
benefits of, 669
for caregivers, 675
for depression, 665, 666
for nursing home residents, 677
for stroke, 672
Growth factors, 59
Growth hormone, 60
GTCSs. *See* Generalized tonic-clonic seizures
Guanethidine
drug interactions, 554, **555**, **602**, **617**
side effects, 252, **568**
Guilt, delusions of, 105

Halazepam
available preparations, 610, **611**
metabolism and dosing, 610, **611**
pharmacokinetics of, **289**, 290
Hallucinations
auditory, 106
autoscopic, 106
drug-related, 449
elementary, 106
extracampine, 106
functional, 106
in Parkinson's disease, **442**
release, 467
secondary, 467
in stroke, 467, 472
tactile, 107
visual, 106
drug-induced, **568–574**
Hallucinogens, side effects, **571**
Hallucinosis
peduncular, 467
poststroke, 472
secondary, 467
Haloperidol
anxiety relief, 291
available preparations, 613–614, **614**
behavior treatment, **384**, 384, 620, **621**
delirium management, 362–363
delusions treatment, 450
drug interactions, 554, **555**
intravenous, 619
seizure threshold effect, **518**, 518
Halothane, **573**
Halstead-Reitan Neuropsychological Battery, 131–133, **133**, 138

Hamilton Anxiety Rating Scale, 286
Hamilton Rating Scale for Depression, 108, 247, 645
Hand sequences, 118
Handedness, effects on brain imaging, 161
Handicap, definition of, 688
Hasegawa Dementia Scale, imaging correlation studies, **192–194**
Head injury. *See also* Traumatic brain injury
anxiety with, 285
definition, 480
mood symptoms, 252
Hearing loss
age-related, 60, 61
prevalence rates, 27, **27**
Heart disease
death rates, 21, **22**
incidence rates, 24
protective value of alcohol against, 302–303
Heavy metals
experimental chelators, 624, **625**
neuropsychiatric side effects, **573**
Hebrew Rehabilitation Center for the Aged, 355
Hemiballismus, 416
Hemidystonia, 421
Hemifacial spasm, 427
Hemiparesis
left-sided, **80**
right-sided, **80**
Hemisensory loss
left, **80**
right, **80**
Hemorrhage, intracranial, 459
Heparin, **553**
Hepatic encephalopathy, qEEG diagnosis and assessment, 224
Heroin addiction, 313
Herpes simplex encephalitis
cerebrospinal fluid profile, **535**
neuropsychiatric aspects, 536
Herpes simplex infection, in dementia, 379
Heterocyclic antidepressants
alternatives, 602–603
available preparations, 599, **599**
drug interactions, 602, **602**
indications for, 598
metabolism and dosing, 599–600
neurological uses, 598–599
side effects, 600, **601**
special considerations in geriatric neuropsychiatry, 600–602
Hip fractures, drug-related, 310
Hippocampal allocortex, 74, **75**
Hippocampus
age-related alterations
cellular, **38–39**, 38–40, **40**
neuronal, **38–39**, 38–40, **40**, 40, **41**, 43
neuronal pathways, **38–39**, 38–40
normal, 38, **38–39**
Hirano bodies, 44, 45, **46–48**

Hispanic elderly. *See also* Elderly
  median income, 20
  population changes, 19, **19**
Histamine₁ blockers, side effects, **570**
Histamine₂ blockers, side effects, 557,
  559, **570–571**
Histaminergic system, 90, **90**, 93
Homonymous hemianopia
  left, **80**
  right, **80**
Hopkins Verbal Learning Test, **135**, 137
Hormonal agents, effects on sexual
  function, 561, **562**
Hospitalized patients, psychiatric illness
  and, 10
Human immunodeficiency virus–type
  1–associated minor
  cognitive/motor disorder, 538
Human immunodeficiency virus–type 1
  dementia complex, cerebrospinal
  fluid profile, **535**
Human immunodeficiency virus–type 1
  (HIV-1) infection
  in dementia, 379
  diagnosis of, 538
  neuropsychiatric manifestations,
    536–538
  neurospychiatric manifestations, **537**
  signs and symptoms, 537
Huntington's disease
  anxiety with, 285
  behavioral abnormalities, 88–89, **89**
  course, 412
  dementia of, 414–415
  diagnosis, 412–413, **413**
  differential diagnosis, 413, **414**
  DNA markers, 413
  genetics of, 412
  late-onset, 412
  mood disorder, 251
  movement disorders, 411–412
  neurochemistry, 413–415
  neuropathology, 449
  neuropsychological features, 140, 412
  pathology, 413–415
  PET abnormalities, 413, 415
  psychiatric features, 412
  treatment, 415
Hydergine, 376, 624
Hydralazine, **568**
Hydrocephalic dementia
  diagnosis, 377
  evaluation of, 377
  neuropsychiatric aspects, 376–377
  treatment, 377
Hydrocephalus
  classification, 370, **371**
  normal-pressure, 41, **42**, 376–377
  obstructive, 524
Hydrochlorothiazide, 360–361, **361**
Hydromorphone, **342**, 342–343
Hydroxyzine
  anxiety relief, 291
  seizure threshold effect, **518**, 518
Hyoscyamine, **569**, **571**
Hyperactivity, definition, 102

Hyperfrontality index, 202
Hyperintensity
  periventricular, 374, **375**
  subcortical, **190–191**
  white matter, 374, **375**
Hyperkinetic movement disorders
  characteristics, 406
  neuropsychiatric aspects, 405–431
  treatment, 429
Hyperorality, in frontal lobe dementia,
  396
Hyperparathyroidism, anxiety-like
  symptoms, **284**, 285
Hyperpituitarism, anxiety-like
  symptoms, **284**, 285
Hypersexuality
  in frontal lobe dementia, 396
  with limbic system dysfunction, **82**
  in multiple sclerosis, **528**, 529
Hypertension
  age-related, 63
  animal models, 62
  during ECT, 650
  essential, 58
  prevalence rates, **27**
Hyperthyroidism
  anxiety-like symptoms, **284**, 285
  anxious or agitated, 285
  apathetic, 285
  mood changes, 252
Hypnotherapy, 345
  for pain relief, 345
Hypnotics. *See also* Sedative-hypnotics
  benzodiazepine, **618**, 618
Hypochondriacal delusions, **105**
Hypoglycemia, anxiety-like symptoms,
  284, 285
Hypoglycemics, 554, **555**
Hypokinetic movement disorders,
  characteristics, 406
Hypoparathyroidism, anxiety-like
  symptoms, **284**, 285
Hypoperfusion of watershed dementia,
  neuropsychiatric aspects, **373**, 374
Hypopituitarism, anxiety-like
  symptoms, **284**, 285
Hyposexuality
  in epilepsy, 516–517
  with limbic system dysfunction, **82**
Hypotension
  orthostatic, 58
  postural, 58
Hypothalamic-pituitary-adrenal axis,
  age-related alterations, 60
Hypothalamic-pituitary axis, age-related
  alterations, 59–60
Hypothalamic tumors, neuropsychiatric
  manifestations, 527
Hypothalamus
  age-related alterations, 59–60
  role in regulation of sleep and
    arousal, 356–357
Hypothermia, drug-related, 615, **616**
Hypothyroidism, mood symptoms, 252
Hypoxia, effects in elderly, 531–532
Hysteria, conversion, 83–84, **84**

Ibuprofen
  anticholinergic effects, 360–361, **361**
  neuropsychiatric side effects, **568**
Ictally related behavioral alterations, in
  seizures, **512**, 512–513
Idazoxan challenge studies, 581, **581**
Idea, overvalued, 105
Ideomotor apraxia, 121
Illicit drug abuse
  in alcoholics, 308
  neuropsychiatric aspects, 313–314
Imaging. *See also* Neuroimaging; *specific
  modalities by name*
  of aging brain, 159–194
  analysis methods, 163–164
  of brain iron, 172–173
  general considerations, 163–164
  head movement artifacts, 163
  measures, 164
  methodological issues, 160–164
  modalities for, 162–163
  parameters, 170–173
  phantom calibration, 163
  study design, 160–161
  subject selection, 161–162
  techniques, 162–163
  after traumatic brain injury, 496–497
Imipramine
  available preparations, 599, **599**
  contraindications, 248
  depression treatment, 249
  drug metabolism and dosing, **445**,
    599–600
  efficacy, 290
  pharmacological properties, **446**
  seizure threshold effect, **518**, 518
  side effects, 600, **601**
Imitation behavior, assessment of, 119
Immediate Recall test, 155
Immune system, age-related alterations,
  61–62
Impairment, definition of, 688
Incidence, definition, 23
Income, of elderly, 19
Indifference, 83–84, **84**
Indole hallucinogens, **571**
Indomethacin, 252, **568**, **626**
Infarction, behavioral abnormalities
  associated with, 88–89, **89**
Infectious disorders
  cerebrospinal fluid profiles, 534,
    535
  of CNS, 533–540, 543
  in dementia, 370, 371, 379–380
  mood changes with, 252
  myoclonus secondary to, 426
Inflammatory disorders, of CNS,
  540–543
Influenza, death rates, 21, **22**
Informed consent, 646
Injury Severity Scale, 481
Insight
  assessment of, 107
  definition, 107
Insight-oriented approaches,
  intervention strategies, 662

Insomnia
   alcohol-associated, 307
   with anxiety, 288–289
   drug-related, **604**
   treatment, 329, 617–619
Institutionalization, of elderly, 28–29
Instrumental activities of daily living,
      28, 29
Insulin
   anticholinergic effects, 360–361, **361**
   drug interactions, 554, **555**, **605**, 605
Insulin-like growth factor, 59
Intellectual impairment, poststroke
      depression effects on, 460
Intellectual processes, assessment of,
      136
Intelligence
   crystallized, 196
   fluid, 196
   neuropsychological assessment of,
      135
Interferon, **571**
Interleukin-1, 61
Interleukin-2, 61
International Classification of Diseases,
      22
Interpersonal psychotherapy
   for depression, 665
   intervention strategy, 662
Intoxication, alcohol, 305
Intracranial calcification, 170–171
Intracranial hemorrhage, brain
      changes, 459
Intracranial tumors
   clinical features, 380
   diagnosis, 381
   pathology, 524
Iodine, 608, **609**
Iproniazid, **570**
Ipsapirone, 613
Iron, brain imaging of, 172–173
Ischemia Scale, 371, 392
Ischemic heart disease, prevalence
      rates, **27**
Isocarboxazid
   available preparations, 603, **603**
   drug interactions, **605**, 605
   neuropsychiatric side effects, **604**
Isoetharine, **572**
Isoniazid, **570**, **626**
Isoproterenol, **553**, **572**
Isosafrole, **573**
Isosorbide dinitrate, 360–361, **361**

Janimine. *See* Imipramine
Jealousy, delusions of, **105**, 105
Judgment, assessment of, 107
Judgment of Line Orientation test, **135**,
      138

Ketamine, **571**
Kety-Schmidt technique, of functional
      neuroimaging, 196–197
Kidney function
   age-related alterations, 63, **63**
   drug distribution and, 11

Klüver-Bucy syndrome, 396, **398**
Kuru, 534

La belle indifference, 107
Lactate
   challenge studies, **578**
   and panic attacks, 283
Lacunae, brain changes, 459
Lacunar state (etat lacunaire), 374
Lafora's disease, 424
Language
   clinical assessment, 104, **113**,
      115–116
   as lateralized function, 79
   neuropsychological assessment, **135**,
      138
Language decline
   in Alzheimer's disease, 391
   in frontal lobe dementia, 396
   in Parkinson's disease, 440–441
Lanoxin, 360–361, **361**
Late-life forgetfulness
   definition, 147, 153, 154
   as diagnostic entity, 153–154
Late-life–onset psychoses
   brain changes, 267–271, **268**
   classification, **264**, 264–265
   course and prognosis, 272
   definition, 262, 264–265
   diagnosis, 264–265
   ECT treatment, 640
   epidemiology, 263
   historical background, 262–263
   investigational scheme, 265, **266**
   multi-infarct disease relationship,
      272–273
   neuropsychiatric aspects, 261–277
   neuropsychological testing, 271
   PET abnormalities, 269–270, **270**
   prevalence, 263
   SPECT abnormalities, 269
   treatment and treatment response,
      271–272
Late-life–onset schizophrenia
   affective disorder comparison,
      273–274
   brain changes, 267–271, **268**, 274
   classification, 264, **264**
   clinical picture, 263–264
   definition, 262, 264
   epidemiology, 263
   neuropathology, 270–271
   phenomenology, 263–264
   prevalence, 263
   risk factors, 265–267, **266**, 274
   symptoms, 263, **264**
Late-onset mania. *See also* Mania
   biological markers, 253
   epidemiology, 252–253
   treatment, 256
Late paraphrenia. *See also*
      Late-life–onset schizophrenia
   classification, 264, **264**
   clinical phenomenology, 263–264
   definition, 262–263, 264
   PET abnormalities, 269–270, **270**

Lateral prefrontal syndrome,
      behavioral abnormalities
      associated with, 88–89, **89**
Lateralizing epileptic discharges,
      periodic, 512–513
Learning assessment, 115–116
Lecithin challenge studies, **578**, 579,
      579
Legal issues, in nursing homes, 691
Lethal catatonia, treatment, 620
Leukoaraiosis, 51, **52**, 374
Leukodystrophy, metachromatic, 532
Leukoencephalopathy
   postradiation and
      chemotherapy-related, 532
   progressive multifocal, 538
Levodopa
   challenge studies, **585**, 585–586
   depression treatment, 443–444
   drug interactions, **605**, 605, **617**
   Parkinson's disease treatment, 436
   pharmacodynamics, **553**
   side effects, 252, 436, 450–451, 561,
      562, **568**, **626**
Levorphanol, **342**, 342–343
Lewy bodies, 44, **46–48**, 50, 439
Leyton Obsessional Inventory, 449
Lidocaine, **568**
Life events, effects on sleep, 326–327
Life expectancy, 20–21, **21**
Life review therapy
   for anxiety, 666–668
   for depression, 666–668
   for depression in dementia, 670–671
   efficacy, 663, 667–668
Limbic encephalitis, paraneoplastic, 527
Limbic striatum, 88
Limbic system
   asymmetries, 83
   cortical components, 80–81, **81**
   neuropsychiatric disorders associated
      with, 81–82, **82**
   nuclei function and anatomic
      relationships, 85–86, **87**
Lipofuscin, in brain, 44, **46–48**
Lisuride, **568**, **626**
Lithium
   alternatives, 608–609, **609**
   antidepressant benefits, 255
   behavior treatment, 620, **621**
   drug distribution changes with aging,
      10
   drug interactions, 554, **555**, **602**,
      607–608, **609**, **617**
   drug metabolism and dosing, 607
   efficacy, 256
   indications for, 607
   neurological uses, 607
   neurotoxicity, 608, **609**
   seizure threshold effect, **518**, 518
   side effects, 447, 561, **562**, **569**, 607,
      608
   special considerations in geriatric
      neuropsychiatry, 607
   toxicity, 607
Liver disease, alcohol-related, 303

Liver function, drug distribution and, 10–11
Living arrangements, of elderly, 19
Local anesthetic blocks, 345
Logical Memory Test, 152, 155
Long-term care, psychotherapy for elderly patients in, 675–677
empirical studies, 675–677, **676**
Loperamide, **570**
Lorazepam
available preparations, 610, **611**
dependence, 309
metabolism and dosing, 610, **611**
pharmacokinetics of, **289**, 290
Loxapine
available preparations, 613–614, **614**
seizure threshold effect, **518**, 518
Ludiomil. *See* Maprotiline
Luria-Nebraska Neuropsychological Battery, 132, **133**, 133–134
Lyme disease
cerebrospinal fluid profile, **535**
neurological manifestations, 540

Macroadenomas, 526
Magnetic resonance angiography, with brain tumors, 525
Magnetic resonance imaging
advances in, 11
of aging brain, 159–194
neuropsychological correlations, 174
studies, **179–182**, **183–185**, **186–189**, **190–191**, **192–194**
in AIDS, 538, **538**
in Alzheimer's disease, **392**, 393
analysis methods, 164
of brain iron, 172–173
brain tissue characteristics, 172
with brain tumors, 525, **525**
of cerebral blood flow, 173
in depression, **230**
in frontal lobe dementia, **392**
intracranial calcification, 170–171
with late-life–onset psychosis, 268
with mood disorders, 254
with multiple sclerosis, 530, **531**
with Parkinson's disease, 441–442
phantom calibration, 163
sensitivity and specificity, 246
technique, 162–163
after traumatic brain injury, 496–497
with vascular dementia, 374, **375**
Magnetic resonance spectroscopy
age-related findings, 173
in Alzheimer's disease, **392**, 393
in frontal lobe dementia, **392**
Magnocellular neurons, 54
Major depression
diagnostic criteria, **444**, **460**
DSM-III-R classification, 245
ECT treatment, 636–640, **637–639**
epidemiology, 252
incidence rates, 26
with lateralized brain dysfunction, 83–84, **84**
poststroke, 460, **461**

after stroke, 250
symptoms, **245**
Malpractice litigation, 651
Manganese
side effects, **573**
toxicity, 88–89, **89**
Mania
in Alzheimer's disease, 246–247
delirious, 255
drug-related, 252, 450–451, 558–560, **568–574**, **604**, **626**
drug treatment, 606–607, 608–609
ECT treatment, 640
electroconvulsive therapy, 447
with frontal-subcortical circuit disorders, 88–89, **89**
after head trauma, 252
late-onset
biological markers, 253
epidemiology, 252–253
treatment, 256
with lateralized brain dysfunction, 83–84, **84**
with limbic system dysfunction, **82**
with multi-infarct dementia, 251
in multiple sclerosis, **528**, 529
neurological causes, 606
new-onset, 252–253
in Parkinson's disease, 249, **442**, 448
poststroke, 250, **473**
clinical correlates, 471–472
mechanism, 472
prevalence, 471–472
with thalamic nuclei dysfunction, 86
after traumatic brain injury, 493
Mannerisms, definition, 102
MAO. *See* Monoamine oxidase
Maprotiline
available preparations, 599, **599**
drug interactions, 554, **555**
oral dose, **445**
pain treatment, 344
seizure threshold effect, **518**, 518
side effects, **569**, 600, **601**
Marchiafava-Bignami disease, 531
Marijuana use, 313
Marital status, of elderly, 19
Marplan. *See* Isocarboxazid
Masked depression, 338
Mattis Dementia Rating Scale, 125, **192–194**
McGill Pain Questionnaire, 341
Mebeverine, **573**
Mecamylamine challenge studies, 579, **579**
Meclizine, **573**
Medial frontal syndrome
behavioral abnormalities associated with, 88–89, **89**
neuropsychiatric symptoms, **124**, 124
Median income, of elderly, 19
Medical illnesses
with anxiety, **284**, 284–286
with anxiety disorders, 287–288
and geriatric neuropsychiatry, 9–11, **10**

prevalence in elderly, 10
psychiatric illness and, 10
psychotherapy for, 671–673
risk of, 23–24
sleep effects, 326
Medical therapy
CNS effects of, 551–552
concomitant physical illness, 554, **554**
environmental factors, 554–556
neuropsychiatric aspects, 549–566
special considerations for geriatric patients, 550–556
Medications. *See* Drugs; Pharmacotherapy; *specific medications by name, by class*
Meditation training, 668–669
Mefloquine, **570**
Meige's syndrome, 415
Melancholia, 245
Memory
clinical assessment, **113**, 114–115, 155–156
ECT effects, 653
neuropsychological assessment, **135**, 137–138
pharmacological challenge studies, **578**
primary (short-term or immediate), 146
secondary (long-term or recent), 146
tertiary (remote), 146
Memory decline, age-related, 148
alternative approaches, 149
biological bases, 154
constructs, 147–155
Memory disorders
clinical assessment, 122
with depression-induced cognitive impairment, 255
Memory impairment. *See also* Amnesia
age-associated, 145–157
alternative approaches, 149
biological bases, 154
clinical assessment, 122
constructs of, 147–155
age-consistent, 147
definition of, 688
drug-related, **604**
in multiple sclerosis, 529
neurotransmitter disturbances, 90, **90**
in Parkinson's disease, 440
Memory tests
differential sensitivity of, 152–153
objective, 155
Meningeal carcinomatosis, 380
Meningiomas, 524, 526
Meningitis
bacterial, **535**, 539
fungal, **535**
Meningoencephalitis
aseptic, **535**
neuropsychiatric aspects, 536
Menopause, 59
Mental disorders
epidemiology of, 26
prevalence rates, 26, **26**

Mental retardation
    mood changes with, 252
    neurobiology of aging with, 62
Mental status examination
    clinical, 113–121
    clinical history, 112–113
    cognitive, 121–124
    cognitive domains, 113, **113**
    components of, 101, **102**
    functional, 125
    goals of, 112
    introduction, 112
    rating scales, 124–125
    technique, 113
Mentally ill patients, neurobiology of
        aging in, 62
Mepacrine, **573**
Meperidine, **342**, 342–343
Meprobamate
    seizure threshold effect, **518**, 518
    side effects, **569**, **571**
Mercury, **573**
Mesoridazine, 613–614, **614**
Metabolic deficiencies, mood
        symptoms, 252
Metabolic disturbances, myoclonus
        secondary to, 426
Metabolic encephalopathies,
        dementing, 381–382
    classification, 370, **371**
Metachromatic leukodystrophy, 532
Methadone, **342**, 342–343
Methaqualone, **518**, 518
Methoserpidine, **573**
3-Methoxy-4-hydroxylphenylglycol
        levels, 55
N-Methyl-D-aspartate antagonists,
        experimental, 624, **625**
1-Methyl-4-phenyl-1,2,3,6-
        tetrahydropyridine, 434
Methyldopa
    drug interactions, 554, **555**
    side effects, **568**, **626**
α-Methyldopa
    anticholinergic effects, 360–361, **361**
    effects on sexual function, 561, **562**
Methylphenidate
    antidepressant benefits, 255
    available preparations, **605**
    depression treatment, 498
    dopaminergic challenge studies, **585**,
        585–586
    pharmacokinetics of, 256
    poststroke mood disorders
        treatment, 251
    seizure threshold effect, **518**, 518
    side effects, **572**
Methylxanthines, 561
Methysergide, **573**
Metoclopramide
    drug interactions, 554, **555**
    side effects, **573**, **626**
Metoprolol, 360–361, **361**
Metrizamide, **573**
Metronidazole
    drug interactions, 608, **609**

side effects, **570**
Michigan Alcoholism Screening Test,
        303
Microadenomas, pituitary, 526
Midazolam, **618**, 618
    available preparations, 610, **611**
    intravenous, 619–620
    metabolism and dosing, 610, **611**
Milkmaid grip, 411
Mindfulness training, 669
Mini-Mental State Exam
    CT correlations, 174
    delirium subscales, 352–353, **354**
    description, 107–108, 124–125, 153,
        155, 352, 392, 645
    imaging correlation studies, **192–194**
    sample page, **353**
Minnesota Heart Survey, 24
Minnesota Multiphasic Personality
        Inventory, 337
Minor depression
    definition, 250
    postroke, 250
    symptoms, 245
Mithramycin, **571**
Mitmachen, 103
Mobility disorders, drug-induced, 560
Molindone
    available preparations, 613–614, **614**
    delusions treatment, 450
    seizure threshold effect, **518**, 518
    side effects, **570**
Monoamine oxidase, age-related
        alterations, 57
Monoamine oxidase inhibitors
    available preparations, 603, **603**
    drug interactions, **602**, 604–605, **605**
    experimental, 624, **625**
    indications for, 603
    metabolism and dosing, 603
    neurological uses, 603
    pain treatment, 343–344
    seizure threshold effect, **518**, 518
    side effects, 561, **562**, **569**, **571**, 603,
        604
    special considerations in geriatric
        neuropsychiatry, 603–604
Montgomery Asberg Depression Rating
        Scales, 645
Mood
    assessment of, 103, 341
    definition, 244
    delusional, 105
    after stroke, 250
    after traumatic brain injury, 492
Mood disorders
    alcohol-associated, 307–308
    with chronic pain, 337–338
    classification, 246
    definition, 244
    differential diagnosis, 246
    idiopathic
        biological markers, 253
        epidemiology, 252–253
        neuroimaging, 253–255
        neuropsychiatric aspects, 252–256

with lateralized brain dysfunction,
        83–84, **84**
    with limbic system dysfunction, 81–82
    neuropsychiatric aspects, 243–259
    in Parkinson's disease, 441
    syndromic, 244–246
    treatment, 246, 255–256
Mood symptoms
    mood syndromes comparison,
        244–246
    neuropsychiatric disorders with,
        246–252
Mood syndromes
    diagnosis of, 244–245
    DSM-III-R classification, 245
    DSM-IV classification, 244–245
    mood symptoms comparison,
        244–246
    neuropathology, 256
    prevalence, 256
    signs and symptoms, 256
    treatment, 256
Morphine, **342**, 342–343, **553**
Mortality
    black-white crossover, 21
    cause-specific, 21–22
    with panic disorder, 289
    rates, 21–23, **22**, **23**
Motor activity
    assessment of, 102–103
    decreased, 102
Motor dysprosody, 103
Motor nuclei, function and anatomic
        relationships, 85–86, **87**
Motor processes
    clinical evaluation of, 138–139
    neuropsychological assessment of, **135**
Movement disorders
    alcohol-associated, 308
    drug-induced, 561–562, **563**
    in Huntington's disease, 411–412
    hyperkinetic, 405–431
    hypokinetic, 406
    rhythmical, **409**
MPTP. See 1-Methyl-4-phenyl-1,2,3,6-
        tetrahydropyridine
MRI. See Magnetic resonance imaging
MRS. See Magnetic resonance
        spectroscopy
Multi-infarct dementia. See also Vascular
        dementia
    classic, 265
    definition, 371
    multi-infarct disease comparison, 272
    neuropsychiatric aspects, **373**, 373
    qEEG diagnosis, 222, 227–230,
        230–232, **231**, **232**
Multi-infarct disease
    classification, **264**, 265
    definition, 265
    late-life–onset psychosis relationship,
        272–273
    multi-infarct dementia comparison,
        272
Multidisciplinary clinics, for pain relief,
        346

Multifocal leukoencephalopathy, progressive, 538
Multilingual Aphasia Examination, **135**
Multiple sclerosis
    anxiety with, 285
    clinical features, 528
    diagnosis of, 530
    epidemiology, 527–528
    mood changes with, 252
    MRI findings, 530, **531**
    neurological signs and symptoms, 528
    neuropsychiatric features, **528**, 528–530, 543
        treatment, 530
    pathophysiology, 530
    treatment, 530
Multiple system atrophy, 424
Multiple system degenerations, differential diagnosis, 436
Mutism, akinetic, 121
Myasthenia gravis, anxiety with, 285
Myocardial infarction
    anxiety levels, 287
    risk rates, 24
Myoclonic epilepsy, progressive, 424
Myoclonus
    causes, 424, **425**
    definition, 424
    drug-induced, 562, **563**
    EEG abnormalities, 424
    epileptic, 424
    essential, 425–426
    idiopathic, 425–427
    neuropsychiatric aspects, 424–427
    nocturnal, 425
    palatal, 427
    physiological, 425
    postanoxic, 426
    related to dementing and neurodegenerative diseases, 426–427
    rhythmical, **409**
    secondary, 426–427
    segmental, 427
    spinal, 427

Nadolol, 620
Nalidixic acid, **570**
Naloxone challenge studies, **578**
Naming assessment, 115–116
Naproxen, **568**
Narcotics
    addiction, 313, 343
    drug interactions, **605**, 605
    effects on sexual function, 561, **562**
    experimental antagonists, 624, **625**
    pain treatment, **342**, 342–343
    side effects, 343, **568**, **626**
    withdrawal effects of, 558
Nardil. See Phenelzine
National Health Interview Survey, 26–27
National Institute for Neurological and Communicative Disorders and Stroke, criteria for Alzheimer's disease, 51

National Institute of Mental Health, criteria for AAMI, 147
    applicability of, 151–152
National Institute of Mental Health Self-Rating Scale, 582
National Institute of Neurological and Communicative Disorders and Stroke-Alzheimer's Disease and Related Disorders Association, 392
National Institutes of Health Consensus Development Conference on Sleep Disorders in late life, 324
Necrosis, death rates, 21, **22**
Negativism, 103
Neglect
    left-sided, **80**
    right-sided, **80**
    unilateral, 122
Neocortex
    age-related alterations, 43, 45, **46**, **49**
    functional organization, 74–76, **75**
    hemispheric specialization, laterality, and dominance, 78–80
    histological organization, 74, **74**
    white matter connections, 76–78
Neoplastic disorders
    CNS, 524–527, 543
    dementing, 380–381
        classification, 370, **371**
    demography, 524
    laboratory evaluations, 524–525
    neuropsychiatric manifestations, 526–527
    pathology, 524
    physiology, 524
    treatment and prognosis, 525–526
Nephritis/necrosis, death rates, 21, **22**
Nerve growth factor, 58–59
Nervous system
    age-related changes, 596
    median zone, 72, **73**, 84–85, **93**, 93
    paramedian-limbic zone, 72–73, **73**, 80–84, **93**, 93
    supralimbic-neocortical zone, 73, **73**, 74–80, **93**, 93
    Yakovlev model, 72–74, **73**
Neural transplantation, experimental, 624, **625**
Neurites
    dystrophic, 46, **49**, 50
    noradrenergic, 55
Neuroacanthocytosis, behavioral abnormalities associated with, 88–89, **89**
Neuroanatomy, behavioral, 72–74
Neurobehavioral Cognitive Status Examination, 108, 125
Neurobehavioral Rating Scale, 108, 125, 482
Neurobehavioral syndromes, frontal lobe, 87–88
Neurobiology
    of aging, 35–69, 62–63
    of anxiety, 283–284
    of behavior, 72–96
    of delirium, 356–357

Neuroborreliosis
    cerebrospinal fluid profile, **535**
    neurological manifestations, 540
Neurochemistry, and behavior, 89–93
Neurocircuitry, in sleep, 328–329
Neuroendocrine probes, 586–587, 588
Neurofibrillary tangles, **41**, 45–46, **49**, **50**, 50–51
    in Alzheimer's disease, 394
Neuroimaging. See also specific modalities by name
    advances in, 11–12
    functional, 195–213
    of idiopathic mood disorders, 253–254
    Kety-Schmidt technique, 196–197
    methodological issues, 160–164
    parameters, 170–173
    quantitative, 164
    schizophrenia findings, 273
    after traumatic brain injury, 496–497
    Xenon-133 technique, 196–197
Neuroleptic malignant syndrome, 362–363, 615, **616**
Neuroleptics. See also specific agents by name
    advances in, 12
    anxiety relief, 291
    behavior treatment, 620, **621**
    contraindications, 624
    delirium management, 362
    drug interactions, **602**, **605**, 605, 608, **609**
    late-onset psychosis treatment, **271**, 271–272
    neuropsychiatric side effects of, 615
    in nursing homes, 686–687
    side effects, 285, 362–363, 410, 558, 561, **562**, **569–570**
Neurological diseases. See also specific diseases and disorders by name
    with anxiety symptoms, **284**, 285
    with behavioral manifestations, 8
    in HIV-1 infection, **537**, 537–538
    neuropsychiatric aspects, 367–574
Neuromelanin, in brain, 44, **46–48**
Neurons
    age-related alterations, **37**, 37–40, **41**, 43, **46**
    magnocellular, 54
    normal, 37, **37**
Neuropathy, peripheral, 285
Neuropeptides
    age-related alterations, 57
    CNS probes, 587–588
    experimental, 624, **625**
Neuropil, 37
Neuropsychiatric assessment
    of activity, 102–103
    of appearance, 101–102
    clinical, 100
    of elderly patients, 97–109
    of emotional state, 103–104
    of insight and judgment, 107
    interview style, 100–101
    of perceptual disturbances, 106–107

Neuropsychiatric assessment *(continued)*
    of personality, 107
    rating scales, 107–108
    of speech and language, 104
    terminology, 101
    of thought content, 104–106
Neuropsychiatric disorders. *See also*
        specific diseases and disorders by name
    drug-induced, 556–562, **568–574**
    ECT treatment, 644
    epidemiology of, 24–26
    frontal-subcortical circuit, 88–89, **89**
    lateralized, 83–84, **84**
    with limbic system dysfunction,
        81–83, **82**
    with mood symptoms, 243–259,
        246–252
    sleep effects, 326
    in stroke, 460–473
Neuropsychiatry
    definition, 4, 5
    geriatric neuropsychiatry
        comparison, 4–5
    in nursing homes, 683–693
Neuropsychological assessment
    cognitive functioning tests, 134–139,
        135
    fixed test battery approaches,
        132–134
    flexible approach, 134
    goals, 130
    introduction, 130
    methodological issues, 130–131
    process, 131–132
Neuropsychological impairment
    with frontal-subcortical circuit
        disorders, 88–89, **89**
    after traumatic brain injury, 492
Neuropsychological tests
    administration of, 132
    in differential diagnosis, 139–141
    ecological validity of, 141–142
    with geriatric norms, 131
    imaging correlation studies, **192–194**
    of late-life–onset psychosis, 271
    selection of, 132
Neuropsychology, of alcoholism, 304
Neuropsychopharmacology, geriatric,
    595–631
Neurosis, nocturnal, 283
Neurosyphilis, cerebrospinal fluid
    profile, **535**
Neurotoxicity
    alcohol, 304–305
    lithium, 608, **609**
Neurotransmitters
    age-related alterations, 551–552
    behavioral alterations, 90, **90**
    mechanism of action, 335–336
    origins and destinations, 90, **90**
    in sleep, 328–329
    types of, 89–90
Neurotrophic factor, brain-derived, 58
Neurotrophins, 58
Nicotine
    challenge studies, **578**, 579, **579**

dependence
    in alcoholics, 308
    complications and comorbidities,
        314–315
    epidemiology, 314
    replacement systems, 315
    transdermal patch, 315
Nicotine-dependence disorder, 314
Nicotine polacrilex gum, 315
Nifedipine
    anticholinergic effects, 360–361, **361**
    drug interactions, 554, **555**
    neuropsychiatric side effects, **568**, 604
Nihilism, delusions of, **105**, 105
Nitrazepam, **553**
Nitrofurantoin, **570**
Nitroglycerin
    anticholinergic effects, 360–361, **361**
    drug interactions, 554, **555**
Nitrous oxide, **571**
Nocturnal neurosis, 283
Nomifensine, 600, **601**
Noncompliance, 551
Nonsteroidal anti-inflammatory drugs
    drug interactions, 554, **555**, 608, **609**
    side effects, 557, 559, **568**
Nootopics, 624, **625**
Noradrenaline
    age-related changes, 54, **54**, 55
    behavioral alterations, 90, **90**
    origins and destinations, 90, **90**
Noradrenergic systems
    age-related alterations, **54**, 55, **56–57**
    neurites, 55
    pathways, 91–92, **92**
Norepinephrine, mechanism of action,
    336
Norethisterone, **572**
Normal-pressure hydrocephalus, 41, **42**,
    376–377
Normalization, forced (or
    paradoxical), 513
Norpramin. *See* Desipramine
Nortriptyline
    available preparations, 599, **599**
    behavior treatment, **384**, 384
    depression treatment, 249, 255, 465,
        465
    metabolism and dosing, 599–600
    oral dose, **445**
    pharmacokinetics of, 256
    pharmacological properties, **446**
    poststroke mood disorders
        treatment, 251
    seizure threshold effect, **518**, 518
    side effects, 343, 446, 600, **601**
NSAIDs. *See* Nonsteroidal
    anti-inflammatory drugs
Nursing Home Reform Act, 684
Nursing home residents
    group therapy for, benefits of, 677
    psychotherapy for, 675–677, **676**
Nursing homes
    activity programs, 689, 690
    consultation-liaison psychiatry
        program, 687

costs, 684
    epidemiology of, 685–686
    history of, 684–685
    legal issues in, 691
    medications in, 686–687
    neuropsychiatry in, 683–693
    percentage of elderly in, 28–29, **29**
    prevalence of psychiatric disorders,
        685
    principles of care, 688–689
    psychosocial rehabilitation in,
        689–690
    special care units, 687–688
Nutritional deficiency, dementing, 370,
    371, 381–382
Nyquist frequency, 219

Obesity, SNS alterations with, 58
Obsessive-compulsive disorder
    brain structure, **6**, 6–7, 11
    with frontal-subcortical circuit
        disorders, 88–89, **89**
    hemispheric relationships, 83–84, **84**
    with limbic system dysfunction, 82, **82**
    neuropathology of, 448–449
    neurotransmitter disturbances, 90, **90**
    in Parkinson's disease, 448–449
    prevalence, **281**, 281
    treatment, 291, **292**
Occipital lobe tumors, neuropsychiatric
    manifestations, 526–527
Occupational palsies, 422
Office of Technology Assessment, report
    of dementia care units, 687–688
Olfactory senses, age-related
    alterations, 60
Oligodendrogliomas, 524, 526
Ondansetron challenge studies, **582**,
    582–583
Opioids
    abuse, 313
    drug interactions, **613**
    pain treatment, 335, **342**, 342–343
    side effects, **571**, **626**
Oral benzodiazepines, seizure
    threshold effect, **518**, 518
Oral contraceptives, side effects, **572**
Orbitofrontal syndrome
    behavioral abnormalities, 88–89, **89**
    neuropsychiatric symptoms, **124**, 124
Organic affective disorder, 255
Organic mental disorders
    alcohol-associated, 302–309, **304**
        epidemiology, 302
        management, 308–309
        subacute, 305–306
    atypical, 305–306
    depression-induced, 141
    with pain, 340
Organophosphates, neuropsychiatric
    side effects, **573**
Orodyskinesia, edentulous, 415
Orofacial dyskinesia, spontaneous, 415
Oromandibular dystonia, 413, **414**, 422
Orthopedic impairment, prevalence
    rates, **27**

Orthostatic tests, adrenergic challenge
    studies, 581, **581**
Orthostatic tremor, 410
Osteoarthritis, psychosocial therapy for,
    672
Over-the-counter drugs
    frequency of use, 550
    side effects of, 556
Overvalued idea, 105
Oxandrolone, **573**
Oxazepam
    available preparations, 610, **611**
    metabolism and dosing, 610, **611**
    pharmacokinetics of, **289**, 290
Oxotremorine challenge studies, **578**
Oxprenolol, 291
Oxybutynin, **571**
Oxygen-15 water, PET with, 207–208, **208**
Oxygen consumption, PET studies of
    rCBF and, 199–202, **200–201**
Oxymetholone, **573**
Oxyprenolol, **568**

Pain
    acute, 340
    anatomy and pathophysiology, 334–336
    ascending pathways, **334**, 334–335
    assessment of, 340–341
    chronic
        behavioral reinforcers, 345–346
        as emotion, 337
    chronic degenerative, 336
    descending pathways, 335
    endogenous control system, 335
    gate theory, 335
    neuropsychiatric aspects, 333–350
    neurotransmitter deficits, 338
    nonorganic, 337, 339
    organic, 337, 339
    perception of, 336–337
    pharmacotherapy for, 341–342
    postoperative, 341
    prevalence of, 336–337
    psychiatric disorders with, 337–340
    psychosocial factors, 337
    socioeconomic factors, 339
    somatoform disorders, 339
    treatment, 341–346
        multidisciplinary, 346
        organic modalities, 345
        psychotherapeutic, 345–346
Pain-prone patients, 337
Palsy
    occupational, 422
    progressive supranuclear
        behavioral abnormalities, 88–89, **89**
        transmitter systems alterations, 55
    pseudobulbar, 103
    supranuclear gaze, 87
Pamelor. *See* Nortriptyline
Pancuronium, **553**
Panic disorders
    with acute pain, 339
    alcohol abuse with, 288
    avoidance patterns, 282, **282**
    with chest pain, 339

with COPD, 286
incidence rates, 26
mortality due to cardiovascular
    disease with, 289
neuroanatomical hypothesis, 284
neurobiology of, 283
prevalence, **281**, 281
treatment, 290, **292**
Paraneoplastic syndromes, 527
Paranoia
    brain changes, 268–269
    classification, 265
Paranoid delusions, 105
Paranoid psychoses, without
        hallucinations
    classification, **264**, 264–265
    definition, 264–265
Paraphilias
    with limbic system dysfunction, **82**
    with neurotransmitter disturbances,
        90, **90**
Paraphrenia
    historical background, 262–263
    late, 262–264, **264**
        brain changes, 268–269
Parasympathetic nervous system
    aging of, 58
    drug-induced dysfunction, **604**
Pargyline
    available preparations, 603, **603**
    drug interactions, **605**, 605
Parietal lobe tumors, neuropsychiatric
        manifestations, 526
Parinaud's syndrome, 527
Parkinsonism
    alcohol-associated, 308
    classification, **435**
    clinical features, 434
    differential diagnosis, **435**, 435–436
    dopamine association, 91
    drug-related, 562, **563**, 615, **616**
    neuropsychiatric aspects, 433–456
    neurotransmitter disturbances, 55,
        90, **90**
    toxins that cause, 434
    treatment of, 437
        electroconvulsive therapy, 447–448
Parkinson's disease
    affect, 441
    age of onset, 435
    anxiety in, 285, 448
    behavioral abnormalities, 88–89, **89**
    bradyphrenia in, 442
    cognitive impairment, 441
    comorbidity, 27
    CT abnormalities, 441
    dementia and, 8
    depression in, 285, 443–448, 598
        subtypes, 445, **445**
    depressive disorders and, 8
    differential diagnosis, **435**, 435–436
    dopamine association, 91
    dopaminergic challenge studies,
        585–586
    drug-related conditions in, 449–450
    epidemiology, 434–435

language deficits, 440–441
management of, 451
mania in, 448
memory deficits, 440
mood symptoms, 248–249
MRI abnormalities, 441–442
neuronal alterations with, 58
neuropsychiatric aspects, 433–456
neuropsychological profile, 140
obsessive-compulsive disorder in,
    448–449
on-off episodes, 248
PET findings, 255, 442
prevalence, 8, **434**, 434
psychiatric manifestations, 442–451
psychosis in, 449
risk factors, 434–435
sleep disturbances, 328
treatment of, 436–437
    antidepressants, 600
    electroconvulsive therapy,
        641–644, **642–643**
    pharmacotherapy, 617
tremor in, **409**
visuospatial impairments, 441
Parkinson's disease dementia
    clinical features, 439–441
    neuroimaging, 441–442
    neuropsychiatric aspects, 437–442
    overview, 437–438
    pathology, 439
    prevalence, 438
    treatment, 442
Parlodel. *See* Bromocriptine
Parnate. *See* Tranylcypromine
Paroxetine, 599, **599**
Partial seizures
    chronic complex, 107
    classification, 510, **511**
Pathological Laughter and Crying
    Scale, 470, **471**, **477–478**
Patient care agenda, 13
Patient history, clinical, 112–113
Patient interviews, 100–101, 131
Patient Self-Determination Act, 691
Paxil. *See* Paroxetine
Peduncular hallucinosis, 467
Pemoline
    available preparations, **605**
    fatigue treatment, 530
    side effects, **572**
Penicillins, side effects, **570**
Pentazocine
    pain treatment, **342**, 342–343
    pharmacodynamics, **553**
    side effects, **573**, **626**
Pentoxifylline, 376
Peptide probes, 587–588
Peptidergic systems, age-related
    alterations, **54**, 57
Perceptual disturbances, assessment of,
    106–107
Pergolide
    anxiety relief, 451
    Parkinson's disease treatment, 437
    side effects, 450–451, **568**, **626**

Periodic lateralizing epileptic
    discharges, 512–513
Peripheral neuropathy, anxiety with,
    285
Periventricular hyperintensity, 374, **375**
    age-related, **166**, 170, **171**
Permax. *See* Pergolide
Perphenazine
    available preparations, 613–614, **614**
    delusions treatment, 450
Persecution, delusions of, 105, **105**
Personal relevance disorders, 83–84, **84**
Personality
    assessment of, 107
    epileptic characteristics, 515–516
    premorbid, **266**, 266–267
    schizoid, 265
Personality changes
    with limbic system dysfunction, 82,
        82
    in multiple sclerosis, **528**, 529
    after traumatic brain injury, 493
Personality disorders
    in alcoholics, 308
    clusters of, 107
    organic, 107
    pseudo-depressed, 395
    pseudo-psychopathic, 395
Pertofrane. *See* Desipramine
PET. *See* Positron-emission tomography
Pharmacodynamics
    age-related changes, **553**
    CNS vulnerability, 551–552
    definition, 596
Pharmacokinetics
    age-related changes, 336, 552–554
    definition, 596
    disposition factors in elderly, **554**
    drug absorption, 552, **554**
    drug distribution, 553, **554**
    drug excretion, 553–554, **554**
    drug metabolism, 10–11, 553–554,
        554, 597
    elimination half-life, 597
    steady state concentration, 597
    volume of distribution, 596
Pharmacological challenges
    adrenergic studies, 580–582, **581**
    basic concepts, 579–580
    choice of dependent variables,
        579–580
    cholinergic studies, **579**, 579–580
    dopaminergic studies, 584–586, **585**
    drug specificity, 579
    GABA-ergic studies, 583–584, **584**
    serotonergic studies, 582–583, **583**
    underlying age and medical
        condition of subject, 580
Pharmacological probes, **578**, 578,
    579–586, 588
Pharmacotherapy. *See also* Drugs; *specific
    drugs by name*
    for AD-associated psychiatric
        symptoms, 394
    for behavioral changes in dementia,
        384, 384, **385**

cognitive-behavior therapy
    comparison, 665
    for delirium management, 362, **362**
    for depression in Alzheimer's
        disease, 248
    for depression in Parkinson's disease,
        443–447
    for Huntington's disease, 415
    for multiple sclerosis
        neuropsychiatric manifestations,
        530
    for neurobehavioral sequelae of
        traumatic brain injury, 497–498
    for pain treatment, 341–342
Phenacemide, **569**
Phenacetin, **568**
Phencyclidine
    challenge studies, **578**
    side effects, **571**
Phendimetrazine, 561, **562**
Phenelzine
    available preparations, 603, **603**
    drug interactions, **605**, 605
    efficacy, 290
    side effects, 446, **604**
Phenindione, **573**
Phenmetrazine, **572**
Phenobarbital
    for benzodiazepine withdrawal, 312
    drug interactions, 518, **519**
    seizures treatment, 517, **517**
Phenomenology, descriptive, 101
Phenothiazines
    available preparations, 613–614, **614**
    drug interactions, 554, **555**
    side effects, **569**
Phenylephrine, **572**
Phenylpropanolamine, **572**
Phenytoin
    drug interactions, 518, **519**, 554, **555**
    pain treatment, 344
    seizures treatment, 517, **517**
    side effects, **569**
Phobias
    alcohol abuse with, 288
    prevalence, **281**, 281
    treatments, **292**
Phobic disorder, in Parkinson's disease,
    448
Phonagnosia, **80**, 83–84, **84**
Phosphorous, neuropsychiatric side
    effects, **573**
Photosensitivity, drug-related, 615, **616**
Physical examination, of psychiatry, 101
Physostigmine challenge studies, **578**,
    579, **579**
Pick's disease
    classification, **399**
    clinical and pathological features,
        397–399
    EEG abnormalities, **229**
    neuropsychological profile, 140
    SPECT diagnosis, **229**
    type II, 399
Pigmentary retinopathy, drug-related,
    615, **616**

Pimozide
    available preparations, 613–614, **614**
    seizure threshold effect, **518**, 518
Pindolol, behavior treatment, 620, **621**
Pineal tumors, neuropsychiatric
    manifestations, 527
Piperazines, seizure threshold effect,
    518, 518
Piribedil, **568**
Pisa syndrome, drug-related, 615, **616**
Pituitary tumors
    neuropsychiatric manifestations, 527
    pathology, 524
    treatment, 526
Pizotifen, **574**
Planning ability assessment, 119
Platelet-derived growth factor, 59
Plicamycin, **571**
Pneumonia/influenza, death rates, 21,
    22
Podophyllin, **570**
Polyarteritis nodosa, neurological
    manifestations, 541
Polycythemia rubra vera, chorea in, 416
Polypharmacy, neuropsychiatric effects
    in elderly, 554, **555**
Population, graying of the, **18**, 18–20
Poriomania, 513
Porteus Maze Test, **135**, 137
Positron-emission tomography
    advances in, 11
    of aging, 199–208
        factors influencing, 203–206, **204**
    in Alzheimer's disease, 209, **392**, 393
    basic principles, 197–199, **198**
    with brain tumors, 525
    of cerebral glucose metabolism,
        197–198, **199**
    in Creutzfeldt-Jakob disease, 534, **535**
    in dementia, 209, **210**, **228**
    with depression in Parkinson's
        disease, 249
    experimental approaches, 206–208
    in frontal lobe dementia, **392**, 396
    in geriatric neuropsychiatry, 208–209
    in Huntington's disease, 413
    in late-life–onset schizophrenia,
        269–270, **270**
    in mood disorders, 254–255
    with oxygen-15 water, 207–208, **208**
    in Parkinson's disease, 442
    partial volume effect, **204**, 205
    of rCBF, 198–199, 199–202, **200–201**
    of rCMRglc, 202–203, **203**
    of rCMRO$_2$, 199–202, **200–201**
    specificity and sensitivity, 393
    after stroke, 250–251
    after traumatic brain injury, 497
    in vascular dementia, 375, **376**
Postanoxic states, 531–532
Postconcussion syndrome, 285, 482
Posterior fossa tumors,
    neuropsychiatric manifestations,
    527
Posthypoxic states, 531–532
Postradiation leukoencephalopathy, 532

Posttraumatic amnesia state, 482
Posttraumatic Neurobehavioral
     Screening Inventory, 495, **495**,
     506–507
Posttraumatic stress disorder
     prevalence, 281
     treatments, **292**
Potassium, drug interactions, 554, **555**
Poverty, delusions of, **105**, 105
Praxis, 79, **113**
Prazepam
     available preparations, 610, **611**
     metabolism and dosing, 610, **611**
     pharmacokinetics of, **289**, 290
Prazosin, **568**
Prednisolone, 360–361, **361**
Prefrontal cortical disorders, behavioral
     abnormalities, 88–89, **89**
Premature aging
     with chronic alcoholism, 304
     definition, 304
Premorbid personality, and late-onset
     schizophrenia, **266**, 266–267
Prescription drugs
     effects on sexual function, 561, **562**
     factors to consider with elderly
          patients, 563
     frequency of use, 550
     most frequently prescribed, **550**, 550
     in nursing homes, 686–687
     that produce anxiety, 285
President's Test, imaging correlation
     studies, **192–194**
Prevalence, definition, 23–24
Primidone
     drug interactions, 518, **519**
     seizures treatment, 517, **517**
Prion infections, 533–534
Problem behaviors, drug treatment,
     620, **621**
Procainamide, **568**, **626**
Procaine, **570**, **574**
Procarbazine, **574**
Procyclidine, **568**, **574**
Programming assessment, **118**, 118
Progressive multifocal
     leukoencephalopathy
     cerebrospinal fluid profile, **535**, 538
     neurological manifestations, 538
Progressive myoclonic epilepsy, 424
Progressive subcortical gliosis
     classification, **399**
     clinical and pathological features, 399
     definition, 395
Progressive supranuclear palsy
     behavioral abnormalities, 88–89, **89**
     transmitter systems alterations, 55
Propafenone, **574**
Propantheline, **569**
Propranolol
     anticholinergic effects, 360–361, **361**
     anxiety relief, 291
     behavior treatment, **384**, 385, 620,
          621
     for benzodiazepine withdrawal, 312
     drug interactions, **617**

pharmacodynamics, **553**
     side effects, 561, **562**, **568**, **571**, **626**
     tardive dyskinesia treatment, 419
Prosopagnosia, **80**, 83–84, **84**
Protein synthesis, age-related
     alterations, 49–50
Protriptyline
     available preparations, 599, **599**
     oral dose, **445**
     seizure threshold effect, **518**, 518
     side effects, 600, **601**
Prozac. *See* Fluoxetine
Pseudo-depressed personality disorders
     of frontal lobe dysfunction, 395
Pseudo-psychopathic personality
     disorders of frontal lobe
     dysfunction, 395
Pseudobulbar affect, 470
Pseudobulbar palsy, 103
Pseudodementia, 141, 209, 255, 377
Pseudoephedrine, **572**
Psuedohallucinations, 106
Psychiatric assessment, terminology,
     101
Psychiatric disorders. *See also specific*
     disorders by name
     neuropsychiatric aspects, 241–365
     in nursing homes, 685
     with pain, 337–340
     in Parkinson's disease, **442**, 442–451
     in traumatic brain injury, 495–497
Psychiatric history, 341
     effects on brain imaging, 162
Psychiatric illnesses. *See also specific*
     disorders by name
     in elderly population, 8–9
     gender differences, 9
     in hospitalized patients, 10
     and medical illnesses, 10
Psychiatry
     geriatric neuropsychiatry
          comparison, 5
     physical examination of, 101
Psychodynamic therapy
     for anxiety disorders, 291
     for depression, 663–666
     for depression in dementia, 669–670
     empirical studies, **664**
     intervention strategies, 662
Psychoeducation
     intervention strategies, 662
     after traumatic brain injury, 499
Psychological conflicts, and pain, 339
Psychomotor impairment
     in Alzheimer's disease, 391
     description, 102
     drug-related, 310, **613**
Psychomotor speed, clinical evaluation
     of, 138–139
Psychopathology
     descriptive, 101
     rating scales, 108
Psychopharmacology. *See also specific*
     drugs and classes of drugs by name
     age-related changes relevant to, 596
     principles, 596–598

Psychoses
     acute atypical, 467
     acute organic, 467
     brain changes, 267–271, **268**
     diagnosis of, 354
     drug-induced, 449–450, 558–560,
          568–574, **604**, **626**
     electroconvulsive therapy for, 447,
          640
     interictal, 513–515
     late-onset, 262–277
          ECT treatment, 640
          neuroleptic treatment, **271**,
               271–272
     with limbic system dysfunction, 81, **82**
     in multiple sclerosis, **528**, 529
     with neurotransmitter disturbances,
          90, **90**
     in Parkinson's disease, **442**, 449
     pharmacological challenge studies,
          578
     poststroke, 467, **473**
          clinical-pathological correlates, 467
          mechanism, 467
          prevalence, 467
     schizophrenic, 513–515, 516
     secondary, 467
     with seizures, 513
     senile, 262, 437
     symptoms of first rank, 105–106
     temporal lobe abnormalities, 6, **6**
     without defined neuropathology,
          264, 265
Psychosocial illness, sleep effects, 326
Psychosocial rehabilitation
     importance of, 691–692
     in nursing homes, 689–690
Psychosocial therapy
     benefits, 672–673
     for delirium management, 362, **362**
     future research directions, 677–678
     principles, 661–682
     for rheumatoid or osteoarthritis, 672
Psychostimulants, 561
Psychotherapy. *See also specific*
     interventions by name
     for anxiety disorders, 291–292, **292**
     benefits of, 669
     for cancer patients, 672
     for cardiovascular disease, 672
     for caregivers, 673–675, **674**
     common interventions, 662–663
     for depression, 663–669
     for depression in dementia, 669–671
     empirical studies, **668**
     impact on long-term functioning, 669
     interpersonal, 662, 665
     interventions, 668–669
     for long-term care patients, 675–677,
          676
     for medically ill patients, 671–673,
          671
     for multiple sclerosis, 530
     for pain treatment, 345–346
     after traumatic brain injury,
          498–499

Psychotic affective patients, classification, **264**, 265
Psychotropics
distribution of, 597
drug interactions, 518, **519**
effects on sexual function, 561, **562**
excretion, 597–598
metabolism of, 597
psychiatric effects of, 559–560
seizure threshold effect, **518**, 518
PTSD. *See* Posttraumatic stress disorder
Pulmonary disorders, with anxiety, **284**, 285–286
Pulmonary function, age-related alterations, 63, **63**
Purdue Pegboard Test, **135**, 138
Purkinje cells, 37, **37**

Quantitative electroencephalography (qEEG)
advantages, 233–234
age-related changes, 220–221, **222**
alternative methods, 225
coherence, 227–230, **231**, **232**
FASCICLE-PA measure, 228–229, **231**
VISUAL measure, 228–229, **232**
concordance maps, 227
cordance mapping, 227, **228**, **229**
diagnosis of delirium with, 224
diagnosis of dementia with, **219**, 221–224, **222**
discordance maps, 227
future, 232–233
limitations of, 224–226
new methods for interpreting, 226–233
sensitivity, 225
technique, 218–220
Quazepam, **618**, 618–619
Quinidine, **568**, **626**

Rabbit syndrome, 410, 615, **616**
Radiation-related leukoencephalopathy, 532
Radiation therapy, delayed effects of, 532
Rancho Los Amigos Scale, 482
Ranitidine
anticholinergic effects, 360–361, **361**
side effects, **571**, **626**
Rapid-eye-movement (REM) sleep, 324
Rating scales. *See also specific tests by name*
for anxiety, 286
cognitive, 124–125
neuropsychiatric, 107–108
neuropsychological, 131–132, 139–142
rCBF. *See* Regional cerebral blood flow
rCMRglc. *See* Regional cerebral metabolic rate for glucose
Reading comprehension assessment, 115
Recall assessment, 115
Regional cerebral blood flow
PET studies, 198–199, 199–202, **200–201**
experimental approaches, 206–208

reduced
age-related, 206–207
with chronic alcoholism, 305
Regional cerebral metabolic rate for glucose
PET studies, 202–203, **203**
experimental approaches, 206–208
factors influencing, 203–206, **205**
reduced levels
age-related, 206–207, **207**
with dementia, 209
with depression, 209
Regional cerebral metabolic rate for oxygen, PET studies, 199–202, **200–201**
Rehabilitation
psychosocial, 691–692
after traumatic brain injury, 499–500
Reitan-Indiana Aphasia Screening Test, **135**
Relaxation training
for anxiety relief, 291, 292
for pain relief, 345
Release hallucinations, 467
REM sleep, 324
Reminiscence, definition, 663
Reminiscence therapy
for anxiety, 666–668
for depression, 666–668
for depression in dementia, 670–671, **670**
efficacy, 663, 667–668
empirical studies, **667**
individual vs. group, 666–667
Remote memory
assessment of, 115
evaluation of, 137–138
Renal function
age-related alterations, 63, **63**
drug distribution and, 11
Repetition assessment, 115
Research agenda, 13
Reserpine
drug interactions, **605**, 605
effects on sexual function, 561, **562**
side effects, **568**, **571**, **626**
Residential center patients, psychotherapy for, 675–677
empirical studies, 675–677, **676**
Response control assessment, **118**, 118–119, **119**, **120**, **121**
Rest tremor, 408, **409**
Restless legs syndrome, 425
Reticular activating system, thalamocortical components, 85, **85**
Reverse digit span, 114
Reverse sequences, 114
Reversible alcoholic cognitive deterioration, 306
Rey Auditory-Verbal Learning Test, **135**, 137, 152
Rey-Osterrieth Complex Figure Test, **135**, **136**, 136–138
Rheumatoid arthritis, psychosocial therapy for, 672

Rhythm
impaired, **80**
tapping, 118
Rhythmical movement disorders, **409**
Right-left disorientation, clinical assessment of, 121
Ritalin. *See* Methylphenidate
Rivermead Behavioral Memory Test, 155
RNA
age-related alterations, 50
brain content, 49
RO 15-1788 challenge studies, **578**, 583–584, **584**
Rochester, Minnesota studies, 24, 25–26

Salbutamol, **574**
Salicylates
drug interactions, 554, **555**
neuropsychiatric side effects, **568**
Salicylic acid, anticholinergic effects, 360–361, **361**
Schaffer collaterals, 38, **38–39**
Schedules for Clinical Assessment in Neuropsychiatry, bottom up approach, 496
Schizoid personality, classification, 265
Schizophrenia. *See also* Late-life–onset schizophrenia
in alcoholics, 308
brain changes, **268**
clinical phenomenology, 263–264
CT abnormalities, **268**
dementia in, 379
ECT treatment, 640
EP abnormalities, 231–232
hemispheric relationships, 83–84, **84**
MRI abnormalities, **268**, 268, **269**, 273
neurobiology of aging with, 62
old vs. young patients, 263–264, **264**
pathoplastic age-associated features, 264
PET abnormalities, **268**, 269–270, **270**
prevalence rates, **26**
rCBF abnormalities, **268**
SPECT abnormalities, **268**, 269, 273
symptoms, 263, **264**
of first rank, 105–106
temporal lobe abnormalities, 6, **6**
Schizophrenic psychosis
in epilepsy, 513–515
etiology and pathology, 516
Scopolamine
challenge studies, **578**, **579**, 579–580
side effects, **569**
Sedative-hypnotics
effects on sexual function, 561, **562**
side effects, **569**
withdrawal, **284**, 285
delirium, 357
effects, 558
Sedatives, drug interactions, **602**, **605**, 605
Seizure disorders
antidepressant treatment, 600–602
EEG abnormalities, 218

Seizure threshold
    drug effects, **518**, 518
    during ECT, 647
Seizures
    AED control, 512
    classification, 510–511, **511**
    in dementing disorders, 512
    differential diagnosis, 511
    drug-related, 608, **609**, 615, **616**
    ECT-induced, 635
    generalized, 510
    grand mal, 510
    neuropsychological impact, 512
    nonepileptic, 511
    partial
        chronic complex, 107
        classification, 510, **511**
    psychosocial impact, 511–512
    psychotic symptoms and frequency
        correspondence, **514**, 514
Seleginine
    available preparations, 603, **603**
    behavior treatment, 620, **621**
    drug interactions, 604–605
    neurological uses, 603
    Parkinson's disease treatment, 12,
        249, 436–437
    special considerations in geriatric
        neuropsychiatry, 604
Self, disturbances of apperception, 106
Semantic anomia, 396
Senescent forgetfulness
    age-inappropriate, 150
    defined, 149
Senile chorea, 413, 415–416
Senile dementia
    of the Alzheimer type, 552
    in Parkinson's disease, 437
Senile plaques, **41**, **49**, **50**, 50–51, 55
Senile psychoses, 262, 437
Senile squalor, 303
Senile tremor, 409
Senses, age-related alterations, 60–61
Sensory deficits
    age-related, 60–61
    and late-onset schizophrenia, 266, **266**
Sensory nuclei, function and anatomic
    relationships, 85–86, **87**
Septicemia, death rates, 21, **22**
Serial 7s, 114
Serotonergic drugs, drug interactions,
    602
Serotonergic systems
    age-related alterations, **54**, 55, **56–57**
    challenge studies, 582–583, **583**
    origins and destinations, 90, **90**
    pathways, 92, **93**
    pharmacological probes, 582–583
    in sleep, 329
Serotonin
    age-related changes, 54, **54**, 55
    behavioral alterations, 90, **90**
Serotonin reuptake inhibitors, 290, 291
Serotonin syndrome, 605
Serotonin uptake inhibitors, 600, **601**,
    602

Sertraline
    available preparations, 599, **599**
    efficacy, 291
    oral dose, **445**
    pain treatment, 344
    side effects, **569**
Severe medical disease, risk of, 23–24
Sex. *See* Gender factors
Sex ratio, of elderly population, 19, **20**
Sexual dysfunction
    in Alzheimer's disease, 391
    drug-related, 451, 561, **562**, **604**
    with limbic system dysfunction, 82, **82**
    in multiple sclerosis, **528**, 529
Sexual function
    age-related changes, 59, 561
    and late-onset schizophrenia, 266, **266**
Short Portable Mental Status
    Questionnaire, 125
Shy-Drager syndrome, 424, 427
Sick role, 345
Sight. *See also* Visual impairments
    age-related alterations, 60, 61
Signal transduction, age-related
    alterations, 58
Simple partial seizures, 510, **511**
Sinemet CR, 436
Sinequan. *See* Doxepin
Single photon emission computed
    tomography
    advances in, 11
    in Alzheimer's disease, **392**, 393
    with amyotrophic lateral sclerosis,
        400, 400
    with brain tumors, 525
    in frontal lobe dementia, **392**, 396,
        397, **398**
    with late-life–onset psychosis, 269
    with mood disorders, 254–255
    specificity and sensitivity, 393
    after traumatic brain injury, 497
    with vascular dementia, 375
Skills training, 669
Sleep. *See also* Arousal
    age-dependent changes, 327
    neurocircuitry and neurotransmitters
        in, 328–329
    non-REM, 324
    in pathological aging, 328
    REM, 324
    spousal bereavement impact, 328
    in successful aging, 320, 327–328
    terminology, 324
    in usual aging, 328
Sleep disorders
    in Alzheimer's disease, 391
    biopsychosocial model, 323–331
    drug-induced, 560–561
    in late life, 323–331
Sleep disturbances
    alcohol-associated, 307
    with anxiety, 288–289
    conceptual model, 324–325, **325**
    drug-related, 451, **626**
    life events affects, 326–327
    medical burden affects, 325–326

    neuropsychiatric burden affects, 326
    prevalence, 324
    psychosocial burden affects, 325–326
    substances that cause, **618**, 618
    treatment of, 329, 344, 384
Sleep efficiency, definition, 324
Sleeping pills, **618**, 618
Small-vessel disease dementia, **373**, 374
Smell, age-related alterations, 60
Smoking. *See also* Nicotine
    cessation, 315
    complications and comorbidities,
        314–315
    depression symptoms, 314–315
    prevalence, 314, 315
Social drinkers, cognitive functioning, 304
Social phobia
    alcohol problems, 288
    treatments, **292**
Social support, importance of, 325–326
Social visits, benefits of, 669
Socioeconomic status, effects on brain
    imaging, 161–162
Somatic delusions, **105**
Somatoform pain disorders, 339
Somatosensory evoked potentials, 220,
    221, 224, 230
Spasm, hemifacial, 427
Spasmodic dysphonia, 422
Spasmodic torticollis, 422
Spasticity, treatment, 530
Special care units, 687–688
Special senses, age-related alterations,
    60–61
SPECT. *See* Single photon emission
    computed tomography
Spectinomycin, 608, **609**
Spectral analysis, 219, **219**
Speech
    assessment of, 104, 115
    clinical evaluation of, 138
    empty, 123
Spirochete infections, 539–540
Spontaneous orofacial dyskinesia, 415
Spontaneous speech, assessment of, 115
Spousal bereavement, sleep effects, 328
SPSs. *See* Simple partial seizures
Startle syndromes, 426
State-Trait Anxiety Inventory, 286
State-Trait Personality Inventory, 338
Stereotypes, definition, 102
Steroids
    drug interactions, **613**
    side effects, 252, 559, 561, **562**, **571**,
        572, **626**
Stimulants
    analgesia, 335
    available preparations, **605**
    behavior treatment, 620, **621**
    drug interactions, **602**, 606
    indications for, 605
    metabolism and dosing, 605–606
    neuropsychiatric side effects of, 606,
        606
    special considerations in geriatric
        neuropsychiatry, 606

Stimulation-produced analgesia, 335
Stimulus boundedness, **120**, 120, **121**
Strength of Grip Test, **135**
Streptomycin, **570**
Stress, sleep disturbances with, 326
Stress buffering, 326–327, 328
Stroke
    anosognosia in, 467–469, **473**
    anxiety in, 465–466, 472, **473**
    apathy in, 466–467, 472, **473**
    behavioral alterations, 8
    catastrophic reactions, 469–470,
        472–473, **473**
    comorbidity, 27
    depression in, 6, **6**, 460–465, 472,
        473, 598, 644
    emotional lability in, 470–471, **473**,
        473
    group psychotherapy for, 672
    incidence rates, 24, **25**
    mania in, 471–472, **473**, 473
    mood complications, 249–251
    neuropsychiatric syndromes in,
        472–473, **473**
    prevalence, 8, 27, **27**
    prevention, 12
    psychosis in, 467, **473**
    risk factors, 249
    vascular dementia and, 8
Stroop Test, **135**, 135–136, **192–194**
Stupor, depressive, 255
Subacute combined degeneration, 531
Subcortical arteriosclerotic
        encephalopathy, 374, 530–531
Subcortical brain, age-related
        alterations, 40, **41**, 43
Subcortical dementias
    clinical features, 374, 439, 440, **440**
    neuropsychological profile, **139**, 140
    pathology, 439
Subcortical encephalomalacia, 51
Subcortical gliosis, progressive
        classification, **399**
    clinical and pathological features,
        399
    definition, 395
Subcortical hyperintensity
    age-related, 166, **166**, 170, **171**, **172**,
        173, **190–191**
    neuropsychological correlations
        studies, **192–194**
Subcortical lesions, anxiety with, 285
Subdural hematomas
    diagnosis of, 382
    posttraumatic, 484, **485**
Substance abuse. *See also* Alcohol abuse
    assessment principles, 300–302
    with chronic pain, 339–340
    concepts, **298**, 299
    DSM-IV criteria, **299**
    highlights, 315
    ICD-10 criteria, **299**
    management principles, 300–302
    neuropsychiatric aspects, 297–321
    risk factors, 299–300, **300**
    terminology, **298**, 299

treatment, 315
    underrecognition of, 556
Substance P, 93
Substance use disorders
    assessment, 300–301
    risk factors, 299–300, **300**
Successful aging, 131, 320, 327–328
Succinylcholine, 646–647
Sudden death, risk rates, 24
Suicide
    alcohol problems, 303
    assessment of potential for, 103–104
    depression and, 9
    in epilepsy, 515
    rates in elderly, 26
    risk factors, 341
Sulfamethoxazole, 554, **555**, **570**
Sulfonamides, **570**
Sulfonylureas, 554, **555**
Sulindac, **626**
Superman hallucinations, 106
Supplement on Aging, 27, 28
Support groups, for multiple sclerosis,
        530
Supranuclear gaze palsy, 87
Supranuclear palsy, progressive
    behavioral abnormalities, 88–89, **89**
    transmitter systems alterations, 55
Surmontil. *See* Trimipramine
Surveillance and Epidemiology End
        Results program, 24
Survivor effect, definition, 161
Sydenham's chorea
    behavioral abnormalities, 88–89, **89**
    neuropathology of, 449
Sylvian fissure asymmetries, 78
Symmetrel. *See* Amantadine
Sympathetic nervous system, aging of,
        58
Sympathomimetics
    bronchodilators, 554, **555**
    drug interactions, **602**
    effects on sexual function, 561, **562**
    side effects, **572**
Symptom Checklist-90 revised, 286
Symptoms of first rank, assessment of,
        105–106
Syncope, differential diagnosis, 511
Syndrome of inappropriate antidiuretic
        hormone secretion, drug-related,
        608, **609**, 615, **616**
Synthesis assessment, **118**, 118, 119
Syphilis, 539–540
Systemic diseases, 370, **371**, 381, 392.
        *See also specific diseases and disorders
        by name*
Systemic lupus erythematosus
    antiphospholipid antibody syndrome
        in, 542
    CNS manifestations, 543
    neuropsychiatric manifestations, 542
    pathological features, 542

Tachycardia, during ECT, 650
Tacrine, 12, 622–623
Tardive akathisia, 417

Tardive dyskinesia
    classical, 417
    definition, 416
    differential diagnosis, 413, **414**,
        417–418, **418**
    dopamine receptor supersensitivity
        hypothesis of, 416, 417, 418
    drug-related, 615, **616**
    epidemiology, 418
    management of, **420**
    neuropsychiatric aspects, 416–419
    pathophysiology, 418
    prevention, 418–419
    signs and symptoms, 417
    subtypes, 416–417, **417**
    treatment, 419, 615
Tau epitope, 46, **49**
Temazepam, **553**, **618**, 618
Temporal arteritis, 540–541, 543
Temporal lobes
    age-related atrophy, **169**, 169–170
    tumors, 526
TENS. *See* Transcutaneous electrical
        nerve stimulation
Tetrabenazine, **574**, **605**, 605
Tetracyclines, **570**, 608, **609**
Thalamic disorders, behavioral
        abnormalities, 86, 88–89, **89**
Thalamotomy, Parkinson's disease
        treatment, 437
Thalamus
    cortical relationships, 85–86, **86**
    nuclei function and anatomic
        relationships, 86, **87**
    role in sleep and arousal, 356
    tumors, 527
Thallium, **574**
Theophyllines
    anticholinergic effects, 360–361, **361**
    drug interactions, 554, **555**, 608, **609**
    neuropsychiatric side effects, **574**
Thiazide diuretics
    drug interactions, 554, **555**, 608, **609**
    psychiatric side effects of, **626**
Thiocarbanilide, **570**
Thioridazine
    available preparations, 613–614, **614**
    behavior treatment, **384**, 384
    delusions treatment, 450
    drug interactions, 554, **555**
    seizure threshold effect, **518**, 518
Thiothixene
    available preparations, 613–614, **614**
    behavior treatment, **384**, 384
    seizure threshold effect, **518**, 518
    side effects, **569**
Thioxanthenes, 613–614, **614**
Thought content assessment, 104–106
Thought insertion, 106
Thrombosis, atherosclerotic, 459
Thyroid disturbances, mood changes,
        252
Thyroid function, abnormalities of, 60
Thyroid hormones, side effects, **572**
Thyrotropin releasing hormone, age-
        related alterations of secretion, 60

Thyrotropin-releasing hormone stimulation test, 587
Thyroxine, 561, **562**
Ticlopidine, 12
Tics
 causes, 428, **428**
 drug-induced, 562, **563**
 neuropsychiatric aspects, 427–428
 with neurotransmitter disturbances, 90, **90**
Timolol, 360–361, **361**
Tinkertoy Test, **135**, 136, 137
Tip-of-the-tongue phenomenon, 441
Titubation, 410
Tobacco dependence
 in alcoholics, 308
 complications and comorbidities, 314–315
 epidemiology, 314
Tocainide, **626**
Tofranil. See Imipramine
Token Test, 468
Tolbutamide, **553**
Tolerance, definition, **299**
Touch, age-related alterations, 60
Tourette's syndrome, 428, 449
Tower of London Test, **135**, 137
Toxic disorders, dementing, 382
 classification, 370, **371**
Toxic encephalopathies, dementing, 381–382
 classification, 370, **371**
Toxic states, classification, 265
Toxicity. See also Neurotoxicity
 drug, 360–361, 382
 lithium, 607
 manganese, 88–89, **89**
Toxins that cause parkinsonism, 434
Trail Making Test, **135**, 174
Training, clinical, 6
Tranquilizers, **602**. See also Sedatives; specific drugs by name
Transcutaneous electrical nerve stimulation, 335, 341, 345
Transdermal nicotine patch, 315
Transient ischemic attacks, 459
Transmitter systems, age-related alterations, 53–58, **54**
Tranylcypromine
 available preparations, 603, **603**
 drug interactions, **605**, 605
 side effects, 600, **601**
Trauma, dementia after, 382
Trauma Coma Data Bank, 489
Traumatic brain injury
 affective symptoms after, 492
 behavioral disorders in, 494
 causes, 485–486, **487**
 classification, 480–483
  by mechanism or cause of injury, 480–481
  by severity of injury, 481–482
  by stages of recovery and outcome, 482–483
 demographics of, 489, **489**
 epidemiology, 485–485

future directions, 500
incidence rates, 485, **486**
methodological issues, 480
mortality rates, **490**, 491, **492**
neurobehavioral sequelae, 493–494, 500–501
 diagnosis, 495–497
 diagnostic process and tools, 496
 early considerations, 497
 imaging, 496–497
 management, 495, 497–500
 pharmacological strategies, 497–498
 psychotherapeutic strategies, 498–499
 rehabilitation and family considerations, 499–500
 treatment principles, 500–501
neuropsychiatric aspects, 481–507
outcome, 486–495
 age differences, 488–491, **490**, **491**, 494–495, **495**
 behavioral, 491–494
 global, 487–491
 initial, 487
 longer-term, 487–488
 neurobehavioral, 491–495
 predictors, 495
pathophysiology and sequelae of, 483–485
scales, 481
special consideration for geriatric populations, 484–485
terminology, 480
Trazodone
 antidepressant benefits, 255
 available preparations, 599, **599**
 behavior treatment, 620, **621**
 behavior treatment in dementia, **384**, 384
 effects on sexual function, 561, **562**
 oral dose, **445**
 pain treatment, 344
 pharmacological properties, **446**
 poststroke depression treatment, 251, 465
 seizure threshold effect, **518**, 518
 side effects, 446, 447, **569**, 600, **601**
Tremor
 cerebellar, **409**, 410
 cerebellar outflow, **409**, 410
 classification, **409**
 definition, 408
 differential diagnosis, **409**
 drug-induced, 562, **563**, **604**, 608, **609**
 dystonic, 419
 essential, **409**, 409–410
 familial, 409
 kinetic, 408, **409**
 midbrain or rubral, **409**, 410
 neuropsychiatric aspects, 408–410
 orthostatic, **409**, 410
 in Parkinson's disease, **409**
 physiological, 408–409
  drug-induced, 562, **563**
 postural, 408, **409**
 primary writing, **409**, 410

psychogenic, **409**
 rabbit syndrome, 410
 rest, 408, **409**
 senile, 409
Trental. See Pentoxifylline
Triamcinolone, **572**
Triazolam, **618**, 618
Tricyclic antidepressants. See also specific drugs by name
 as anxiolytics, 613
 challenge studies, **578**
 dosages, **445**
 drug interactions, 554, **555**, **602**, 605, **617**
 effects on sexual function, 561, **562**
 pain treatment, 343–344
 posttraumatic depression treatment, 498
 side effects, 343, **569**, **571**, 600, **601**
Trifluoperazine
 available preparations, 613–614, **614**
 behavior treatment in dementia, **384**, 384
Triflupromazine, 613–614, **614**
Trihexyphenidyl
 dopaminergic challenge studies, **585**, 585–586
 neuropsychiatric side effects, **568**
 Parkinson's disease treatment, 437
Trimethoprim, 554, **555**, **571**
Trimipramine
 available preparations, 599, **599**
 oral dose, **445**
 seizure threshold effect, **518**, 518
 side effects, 600, **601**
Trophic factors, age-related alterations, 58–59
Tryptophan
 drug interactions, **602**
 neuropsychiatric side effects, **574**
 serotonergic challenge studies, **582**, 582–583
Tryptophan hydroxylase levels, 55
Tumors. See also Neoplastic disorders
 brain
  anxiety with, 285
  EEG abnormalities, 524–525
 cerebral, 380
 cognitive impairment from, 79–80, **80**
 deep midline, 527
 frontal lobe, 526
 intracranial, 380, 381
 mood changes with, 252
 myoclonus secondary to, 426
 occipital lobe, 526–527
 parietal lobe, 526
 posterior fossa, 527
 subcortical, 285
 temporal lobe, 526
Twilight states, 513
Tyrosine hydroxylase levels, 55

UBOs. See Unidentified bright objects
Unidentified bright objects, 268, **269**, 273
Use it or lose it theory of aging, 36

Valproic acid
 behavior treatment, 620, **621**
 drug interactions, 518, **519**, 554, **555**
 mania treatment, 12, 609
 pain treatment, 344
 seizures treatment, 517, **517**
 side effects, **569**, 609, **609**
 tardive dyskinesia treatment, 419
Vascular chorea, 416
Vascular dementia. *See also* Multi-infarct
  dementia
 classification, 370, **371**, **372**
 clinical features, 371, **372**
 diagnostic criteria, **372**
 epidemiology, 371
 evaluation of, 374–375
 incidence rates, 26
 mood symptoms, 251
 neuroimaging findings, 374, **375**
 neuropsychiatric aspects, 370–376
 neuropsychological profile, **139**, 140
 stroke and, 8
 subtypes, **373**, 373–374
 treatment, 375–376
Vasculitis
 isolated CNS, 541–542
 neuropsychiatric aspects, 540–542
Vasoactive intestinal peptide, 93
Vasodilators
 classification, 624
 experimental, 624, **625**
Ventricular-brain ratio
 in depression, 253–254
 effects of aging on, 165
Ventricular size, effects of aging on,
  164–167, **165**, **166**
 imaging studies, **179–182**
Ventriculomegaly, **41**, 42, **42**
Verapamil
 drug interactions, 554, **555**
 mania treatment, 609
 pharmacodynamics, **553**
 side effects, 609, **609**
Veratrum, **574**
Verbal fluency
 assessment, 119
 definition, 529
 in multiple sclerosis, 529
 reduced, **80**
Victimization fear, 283
Vincristine, **571**
Violent behavior, hemispheric
  relationships, 83–84, **84**

Viral infections, 536–538
Viral meningoencephalitides, 536
Visual evoked potentials, 220, 221, 224
Visual Form Discrimination Test, **135**,
  138
Visual hallucinations, drug-related, 449,
  568–574
Visual impairments
 age-related, 60–61
 prevalence rates, 27, **27**
Visual Memory Span test, 135
Visual memory tests, **135**, 135, 137
Visual Reproduction Test, 137, 152,
  153, 174
Visuomotor processes, assessment, **113**,
  116, 116, **117**, **135**, 138
Visuospatial impairments
 in Alzheimer's disease, 391
 characteristic features, 116, **117**
 in Parkinson's disease, 441
Visuospatial processes, assessment, **113**,
  116, 116, **117**, **135**, 138
Vitamin B$_{12}$, experimental therapy
  with, 624, **625**
Vitamin B$_{12}$ deficiency
 dementia caused by, 381
 mood symptoms, 252
Vitamin deficiencies, mood symptoms,
  252
Vitamin E, tardive dyskinesia treatment,
  419
Vivactil. *See* Protriptyline

Wada test, 83–84
Warfarin
 anticholinergic effects, 360–361, **361**
 pharmacodynamics, **553**
Wearing it out theory of aging, 36
Wechsler Adult Intelligence
  Scale-Revised, 131, **135**, 136, 147,
  151
Wechsler Memory Scale, 137
Wechsler Memory Scale-Revised
 description, **135**, 135, 137, 155
 imaging correlation studies, **192–194**
 normative data, 131, 146
 sensitivity, 153
Wellbutrin. *See* Bupropion
Wepman Auditory Discrimination Test,
  135
Wernicke-Korsakoff syndrome, 306
Wernicke's area asymmetries, 78, **79**
White elderly. *See also* Elderly

life expectancy, 20–21, **21**
 median income, 20
 mortality rates, 21
 suicide rates, 26
White matter
 age-related alterations, 51–53
 association fibers, 76–78, **77**, **78**
 commissural fibers, **77**, 77–78, **78**
 connections, 76–78
 disconnection syndromes
  qEEG diagnosis of, 227–230
  related fiber tracts, 77–78, **78**
 hyperintensities, 374, **375**
 projection fibers, 76, **78**
Wilson's disease
 anxiety with, 285
 behavioral abnormalities, 88–89, **89**
Wisconsin Card Sorting Test, **135**, 136,
  192–194, 396
Withdrawal
 alcohol, 305–306
 benzodiazepine, 311–312
 definition, **299**
Withdrawal delirium, alcohol or
  sedative-hypnotic, 357
Women. *See also* Elderly women;
  Gender factors
 postmenopausal changes, 561
Word list learning test, 155
Word salad, 104
World population, elderly, 20, **20**
Writer's cramp, 422
Writing tremor, primary, **409**, 410

X-ray CT, technique, 162
Xanthomatosis, cerebrotendinous, 533
Xenon-133 technique, of functional
  neuroimaging, 196–197

Yakovlev model, of nervous system,
  72–74, **73**
Yohimbine
 challenge studies, **578**, 581, **581**
 neuropsychiatric side effects, **574**
 and panic attacks, 283
Young early-onset schizophrenia,
  symptoms, 263, **264**

Zidovudine, **574**
ZK 93426 challenge studies, **578**,
  583–584, **584**
Zoloft. *See* Sertraline